CORE CURRICULUM FOR

# NEONATAL INTENSIVE CARE NURSING

FIFTH EDITION

EDITED BY

M. TERESE VERKLAN, PhD, CCNS, RNC, FAAN

Professor/Neonatal Clinical Nurse Specialist
Graduate School of Basic Sciences
School of Nursing
The University of Texas Medical Branch
Galveston, Texas

MARLENE WALDEN, PhD, RN, NNP-BC, CCNS

Nurse Scientist, Advanced Practice Providers Administrative Services
Texas Children's Hospital;
Assistant Professor
Pediatrics-Newborn Section
Baylor College of Medicine
Houston, Texas

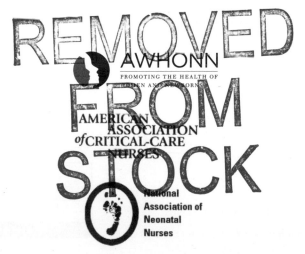


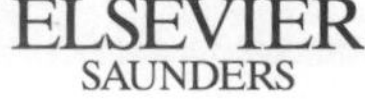
ELSEVIER
SAUNDERS

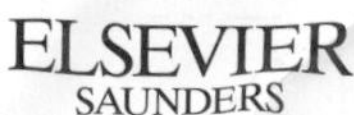

3251 Riverport Lane
St. Louis, Missouri 63043

CORE CURRICULUM FOR NEONATAL INTENSIVE CARE NURSING ISBN: 978-0-323-22590-8



**Library of Congress Cataloging-in-Publication Data**

Core curriculum for neonatal intensive care nursing / edited by M. Terese Verklan, Marlene Walden. – Fifth edition.
p.; cm.
Neonatal intensive care nursing
Includes bibliographical references and index.
ISBN 978-0-323-22590-8 (pbk.: alk. paper)
I. Verklan, M. Terese, editor of compilation. II. Walden, Marlene, 1956- editor of compilation. III. Association of Women's Health, Obstetric, and Neonatal Nurses, issuing body. IV. American Association of Critical-Care Nurses, issuing body. V. National Association of Neonatal Nurses, issuing body. VI. Title: Neonatal intensive care nursing.
[DNLM: 1. Neonatal Nursing–methods–Outlines. 2. Intensive Care, Neonatal–methods–Outlines. WY 18.2]
RJ253.5
618.92'01–dc23

2013045759

*Content Manager:* Laurie K. Gower
*Senior Content Development Specialist:* Heather Bays
*Publishing Services Manager:* Deborah L. Vogel
*Project Manager:* Brandilyn Flagg
*Designer:* Teresa McBryan

Printed in the United States of America

Last digit is the print number: 9 8 7 6 5 4 3 2 1

# Foreword

Continuing the unique partnership that began in 1996, the Association of Women's Health, Obstetric and Neonatal Nurses; the National Association of Neonatal Nurses; and the American Association of Critical-Care Nurses have collaborated once again on this fifth edition of the *Core Curriculum for Neonatal Intensive Care Nursing*.

These three major nursing specialty organizations have produced a landmark document already recognized for its far-reaching influence on neonatal intensive care nursing. The editors collaborated with each other to ensure a high-quality product, and dozens of contributors and reviewers supported the effort with the gift of expert knowledge.

We applaud Terese Verklan and Marlene Walden and the many collaborators who responded to their editorial leadership. We recognize and appreciate their commitment to ensuring through this valuable reference that critically ill infants and their families receive safe and optimal care, benefitting from the latest knowledge and best practices in the field.

**Karen Harris, MSN, RN, WHNP-BC**
President, Association of Women's Health,
Obstetric and Neonatal Nurses

**Cheryl A. Carlson, PhD, APRN, NNP-BC**
President, National Association of Neonatal Nurses

**Vicki Good, RN, MSN, CENP**
President, American Association of Critical-Care Nurses

*To Mom, Cindy, Paul, and Theresa George—thank you*
*for showing me I have no boundaries. And in loving memory of my father.*
**MTV**

*In loving memory of my mother, Wanda, and my twin sister, Sharlene,*
*who taught me so much about love and caring for others.*
*Also to my professional colleagues who teach me so much;*
*but most important, to the babies and families who have taught me*
*the art of neonatal nursing.*
**MW**

# Contributors

**Debra Armentrout, RN, MSN, NNP-BC, PhD**
Associate Professor
Track Administrator
NNP Program
School of Nursing
University of Texas Medical Branch
Galveston, Texas

**Teresa Bailey, RN, MSN, NNP-BC**
Neonatal Nurse Practitioner
Seton Family of Hospitals
Pediatrix Medical Group
Austin, Texas

**Kathleen Benjamin, RN, MSN, NNP-BC**
Neonatal Nurse Practitioner
Children's Hospital of Colorado
Aurora, Colorado

**S. Louise Bowen, NNP-BC, MSN, DNP(c)**
Instructor
College of Nursing
South University
Tampa, Florida

**Holly A. Boyd, RN, MSN, NNP-BC**
Neonatal Nurse Practitioner
Neonatal Nurse Practitioner Service
Texas Children's Hospital
Houston, Texas

**Marina Boykova, MSc**
Doctoral Student
College of Nursing
University of Oklahoma
Oklahoma City, Oklahoma

**Wanda T. Bradshaw, RN, MSN, NNP-BC, PNP**
Assistant Professor
School of Nursing
Duke University
Durham, North Carolina

**M. Colleen Brand, PhD, RN, NNP-BC**
Neonatal Nurse Practitioner
Neonatal Nurse Practitioner Service
Texas Children's Hospital
Houston, Texas

**Leigh Ann Cates, MSN, APRN, NNP-BC, RRT-NPS, CHSE**
Neonatal Nurse Practitioner
Newborn Service
Texas Children's Hospital
Houston, Texas;
Assistant Professor
School of Nursing
NNP Program
University of Texas Medical Branch
Galveston, Texas

**William Diehl-Jones, BSc, BScN, MSc, PhD**
Adjunct Professor
Faculty of Nursing
University of Manitoba
Winnipeg, Manitoba, Canada

**Georgia R. Ditzenberger, PhD, NNP-BC**
Assistant Professor
Division of Neonatology
Department of Pediatrics
UW-Madison School of Medicine and Public Health;
Adjunct Faculty
School of Nursing
UW-Madison
Director UWMF NICU Neonatal Advanced Practice Provider Team;
Manager
Neonatal Simulation
Madison, Wisconsin

**Christine D. Domonoske, PharmD**
Neonatal Clinical Specialist
Pharmacy
Children's Memorial Hermann Hospital
Houston, Texas

**Ann Donze, RN, MSN, NNP-BC**
Neonatal Nurse Practitioner
Newborn Intensive Care Unit
St. Louis Children's Hospital
St. Louis, Missouri

**Linda Lane Ehret, MSN, APRN, NNP-BC**
Neonatal Nurse Practitioner
Pediatrix Medical Group
Denver, Colorado

**Debbie Fraser, MN, RNC-NIC**
Associate Professor
Athabasca University;
Advanced Practice Nurse
Department Faculty of Health Disciplines/NICU
St. Boniface General Hospital
Winnipeg, Manitoba, Canada

**Susan Arana Furdon, MS, RN, NNP-BC**
Neonatal Clinical Nurse Specialist/Nurse Practitioner
Department of Nursing
The Children's Hospital at Albany Medical Center
Albany, New York

**Martha Goodwin, RNC, NNP**
Nurse Practitioner
Children's Mercy
Kansas City, Missouri

**Brenda Hueske Halbardier, PhD(c), NNP**
Assistant Professor
Department of Pediatrics
Division of Neonatal-Perinatal Medicine
University of Texas–Houston Medical School
Houston, Texas

**Pat Hummel, PhD, APRN, NNP-BC, PCPNP-BC**
Neonatal Nurse Practitioner
Neonatal Intensive Care Unit;
PCPNP, Coordinator, Neonatal Developmental Follow-up Program
Loyola University Medical Center
Maywood, Illinois

**Helen M. Hurst, DNP, RNC-OB, APRN-CNM**
Graduate Coordinator and Assistant Professor
Nursing
University of Louisiana at Lafayette
Lafayette, Louisiana

**Carole Kenner, PhD, RN, FAAN**
Executive Director
Council of International Neonatal Nurses
Boston, Massachusetts

**Barbara Elizabeth Pappas, MSN, ARNP, NNP-BC**
Neonatal Nurse Practitioner
Blank Children's Hospital
Des Moines, Iowa

**Deanna Lynn Robey, RNC, BSN, CLNC**
Neonatal Clinical Nurse
Blank Children's Hospital
Des Moines, Iowa

**Sharyl L. Sadowski, MSN, APN, NNP-BC**
Clinical Faculty–Pediatric Nursing
Marcella Niehoff School of Nursing
Loyola University
Maywood, Illinois

**Julieanne Schiefelbein, DNP, MA (Ed), NNP-BC, CPNP, NPY-BC**
Neonatal Nurse Practitioner
NICU
Intermountain Health Care;
Director
Neonatal Nurse Practitioner Program
College of Nursing
University of Utah
Salt Lake City, Utah

**Jan Sherman, PhD, RN, NNP-BC**
Adjunct Associate Professor
Colleges of Nursing
University of Missouri
St. Louis, Missouri and Columbia, Missouri;
Department of Child Health
School of Medicine
University of Missouri
Columbia, Missouri

**Bonita Shviraga, PhD, RN, CNM**
Aurora Nurse-Midwives Manager
The Medical Center of Aurora
Aurora, Colorado

**Joan Renaud Smith, PhD, RN, NNP-BC**
Neonatal Nurse Practitioner
Newborn Intensive Care Unit
St. Louis Children's Hospital
St. Louis, Missouri

**Carol Turnage Spruill, RN, MSN, CNS, CPHQ, NTMNC**
Clinical Nurse Specialist
Clinical Effectiveness and Safety
Children's Memorial Hermann Hospital
Houston, Texas

**Leann Sterk, RN, MSN, CNP, CNS**
Neonatal Nurse Practitioner
NICU
Rapid City Regional Hospital
Rapid City, South Dakota

**Laura Stokowski, RN, MS**
Staff Nurse
Inova Fairfax Hospital
Fairfax, Virginia

**Tanya Sudia-Robinson, PhD, RN**
Professor
Georgia Baptist College of Nursing
Mercer University
Atlanta, Georgia

**Diane M. Szlachetka, APRN, NNP-BC**
Neonatal Nurse Practitioner
Division of Newborn Medicine
Baystate Medical Center
Springfield, Massachusetts

**Karen A. Thomas, PhD**
Professor
Family and Child Nursing
University of Washington
Seattle, Washington

**Carol Ingals Tyner, RN, MSN, NNP-BC**
Neonatal Nurse Practitioner
Neonatal Nurse Practitioner Service
Texas Children's Hospital
Houston, Texas

**M. Terese Verklan, PhD, CCNS, RNC, FAAN**
Professor/Neonatal Clinical Nurse Specialist
Graduate School of Basic Sciences
School of Nursing
The University of Texas Medical Branch
Galveston, Texas

**Marlene Walden, PhD, RN, NNP-BC, CCNS**
Nurse Scientist, Advanced Practice Providers Administrative Services
Texas Children's Hospital;
Assistant Professor
Pediatrics-Newborn Section
Baylor College of Medicine
Houston, Texas

**Diana J. Wilson, RN, MSN, NNP-BC**
Neonatal Nurse Practitioner
Neonatal Nurse Practitioner Service
Texas Children's Hospital;
Instructor
Pediatrics-Newborn Section
Baylor College of Medicine
Houston, Texas

**Catherine L. Witt, MS, NNP-BC**
Coordinator
NNP Program
Loretto Heights School of Nursing
Regis University
Denver, Colorado

# Reviewers

**Sandra Sundquist Beauman, MSN, RNC-NIC**
Clinical Research Coordinator
Department of Pediatrics
University of New Mexico Health Sciences Center
Albuquerque, New Mexico

**Melissa Renee Beck, RN, MSN, NNP-BC**
Neonatal Nurse Practitioner
Pitt County Memorial Hospital
Greenville, North Carolina

**Bobby B. Bellflower, DNSc, NNP-BC**
Neonatal Nurse Practitioner
LeBonheur Children's Hospital;
Assistant Professor/Option Coordinator NNP Program
Memphis, Tennessee

**Wanda Todd Bradshaw, RN, MSN, NNP-BC, PNP, CCR**
Assistant Professor
School of Nursing
Duke University
Durham, North Carolina

**Denise Casey, RN, MS, CPNP, CCRN**
Clinical Nurse Specialist
Children's Hospital Boston
Boston, Massachusetts

**Denise M. Cole, MS, RNC-NIC**
Coordinator
Oklahoma Perinatal Care Project
Obstetrics and Gynecology
The University of Oklahoma Health Sciences Center
Oklahoma City, Oklahoma

**Elizabeth Drake, RN, MN, CNNP, CNS**
NICU Clinical Nurse Specialist
CHOC Children's at Mission Hospital
Mission Viejo, California

**Janet E. Fogg, PhD, RNC-NIC, CNE**
Assistant Professor of Nursing
Professor-in-Charge
Professional Graduate Programs
Hershey Campus Coordinator
Pennsylvania State University
University Park, Pennsylvania

**Dodi Gauthier, MEd, RNC-OB, CEFM**
Perinatal Educator and Direct Care Nurse
Birth Center/Antepartum Units
Santa Barbara Cottage Hospital
Santa Barbara, California

**Michelle LaBrecque, RN, MSN, CCRN**
Clinical Nurse Specialist
Neonatal ICU
Children's Hospital Boston
Boston, Massachusetts

**Carie Linder, MSN, RNC-NIC, ARNP-BS**
Neonatal Nurse Practitioner
Wesley Medical Center
Wichita, Kansas;
Integris Baptist Medical Center
Oklahoma City, Oklahoma

**Arlene Lovejoy, MS, RNP, CNS, RNC-NIC, C-NPT, RRT**
Clinical Nurse Specialist and Pediatric Nurse Practitioner
Los Angeles County + University of Southern California Medical Center
Los Angeles, California

**Andrea C. Morris, MSN, RNC-NIC, CCRN**
Neonatal Clinical Nurse Specialist
Neonatal Intensive Care
Citrus Valley Medical Center–QVC
West Covina, California

**Mindy Morris, MS, RNC, CNS, NNP-BC**
Neonatal Nurse Practitioner
Children's Hospital of Orange County
Orange, California

**Caitlin O'Brien, BSN, RN, CCRN**
Clinical Educator
Neonatal Intensive Care Unit
Children's Hospital Boston
Boston, Massachusetts

**Melissa Otoya, BSN, MSN-CNL, RNC**
Neonatal Nurse Practitioner
Children's Hospital of Orange County
Orange, California

**Julieanne H. Schiefelbein, DNP, MA (Ed), NNP-BC, CPNP, NPY-BC**
Assistant Professor (Clinical)
College of Nursing
University of Utah;
Neonatal Nurse Practitioner
Intermountain Healthcare
Salt Lake City, Utah

**Elizabeth L. Sharpe, MSN, ARNP, NNP-BC**
Neonatal Nurse Practitioner
Pediatrix Medical Group
West Palm Beach, Florida

**Pamela Scott Spivey, MSN, APRN, CCNS**
Neonatal Clinical Nurse Specialist
Newborn Center
Texas Children's Hospital
Houston, Texas

**Robin L. Watson, MN, RN, CNS, CCRN**
Quality & Safety Integration Officer
Harbor-UCLA Medical Center
Torrance, California

# Preface

The provision of intensive care to the high-risk neonate challenges every neonatal care provider. Research and refinements in technology have made "high-tech" modalities such as ECMO, nitric oxide, and hypothermia available to many more hospitals. The art and science of neonatal nursing is never stochastic. We learn from scientists, researchers, multidisciplinary colleagues, and of course, our infants and their families. At a minimum, we are expected to enhance our application of clinical knowledge by utilizing an evidence-based approach to improve patient outcomes. The role of the nurse is frequently to bring together all of the pieces of the puzzle to ensure comprehensive, clinically excellent, and compassionate care to sick newborns and their families.

The fifth edition of *Core Curriculum for Neonatal Intensive Care Nursing* is intended as a clinical resource. It is divided into sections and designed in an outline format so that it may be used as an easy reference. The first section, *Antepartum, Intrapartum, and Transition to Extrauterine Life*, addresses clinical issues related to factors that affect the fetus and the neonate's ability to successfully adapt to postnatal life. Information is also presented as to how we can assist in the recognition of the high-risk fetus/neonate and plan interventions that support the physiologic demands of the neonate during transition. *Cornerstones of Clinical Practice* presents concepts common to the delivery of quality care to all high-risk newborns and families. A new chapter has been added that addresses the late preterm infant specifically since recent research has indicated this group of neonates has a high risk of morbidity and mortality when they are treated the same way as a healthy term neonate. The third section, *Pathophysiology: Management and Treatment of Common Disorders*, provides a systems approach to the assessment and management of the disease processes high-risk neonates commonly present with. The last section, *Professional Practice*, focuses on the caregiver to strengthen competency with respect to research use, in addition to providing an overview of universal ethical and legal issues that may be encountered in the practice of neonatal nursing.

This text is the collaborative effort of the three major nursing specialty associations: the Association of Women's Health, Obstetric and Neonatal Nurses (AWHONN); the American Association of Critical-Care Nurses (AACN); and the National Association of Neonatal Nurses (NANN). The book brings together experts in the care of the high-risk neonate, all having the common goal of providing a comprehensive resource for the management and care of sick newborns. We are honored to be the editors of such an outstanding collaborative effort.

**M. Terese Verklan**

**Marlene Walden**

# Contents

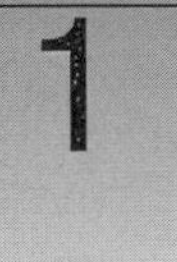

CHAPTER 1

# Uncomplicated Antepartum, Intrapartum, and Postpartum Care

BONITA SHVIRAGA

**OBJECTIVES**

1. Identify normal physiologic changes of each system in pregnancy.
2. Describe parameters to assess gestational age and establish pregnancy dating.
3. Discuss genetic screening options for pregnancy.
4. Identify medications that may cause congenital malformations.
5. Outline components of prenatal care, including history, physical, laboratory, and diagnostic testing.
6. Explain tests of fetal lung maturity.
7. Identify six methods of antepartum fetal surveillance.
8. Discuss the normal stages of labor and delivery.
9. Describe low-risk labor management, including fetal monitoring guidelines.
10. Discuss normal immediate postpartum recovery and related postpartum nursing assessments and management.

Antepartum, intrapartum, and postpartum care are not usually included within the practice parameters of the neonatal nurse. Yet an understanding of the normal processes of pregnancy, birth, and postpartum recovery provides a framework for beginning to understand factors that affect the developing fetus and the high-risk neonate. This chapter discusses uncomplicated antepartum, intrapartum, and postpartum nursing care. In addition, an overview of the normal physiologic changes that can be expected in a healthy mother is included.

## TERMINOLOGY

A. **Calculation of gestation:** 280 days, 40 postmenstrual weeks, or 10 lunar months counted from the first day of the last menstrual period. (Actual duration of gestation from conception to estimated date of delivery is 38 weeks, assuming a 28-day cycle.)
B. **Trimesters:** division of gestation into three segments of approximately equal duration.
   1. First trimester: 0 to 12 weeks.
   2. Second trimester: 13 to 27 weeks.
   3. Third trimester: 28 to 40 weeks.
C. **Preterm, late preterm, term, and post-term pregnancy:** *preterm*, less than 37 completed weeks; *late preterm*, $34^{0/7}$ to $36^{6/7}$ weeks; *term*, 37 to 42 weeks; and *post-term*, greater than 42 weeks.

## NORMAL MATERNAL PHYSIOLOGIC CHANGES BY SYSTEMS

A. **Alimentary tract and perinatal nutrition (Blackburn, 2013).**
   1. During pregnancy there is an increased caloric need of 300 kcal/day to support the growing fetus and increased maternal metabolic rate, resulting in a caloric requirement of 2500 kcal/day during pregnancy (Pillitteri, 2010). Pregnant teenagers need an additional 100 to

200 kcal/day. Total recommended weight gain for women with normal body mass index (BMI) is 25 to 35 pounds, and for underweight women a gain of up to 40 pounds may be recommended (American College of Obstetricians and Gynecologists [ACOG], 2013b). Limiting weight gain to 11 to 20 pounds is recommended for obese women (ACOG, 2013b).

2. An inadequate intake of folic acid has been associated with neural tube defects (NTDs) (London et al., 2011). It is likely that the functional mechanism for folate's effect on NTDs is its epigenetic role in DNA methylation and histones (Ross and Desai, 2012). Routine supplementation of folic acid 0.4 to 0.8 mg is recommended for women of childbearing age or planning a pregnancy to assist in the prevention of NTDs (U.S. Preventive Services Task Force, 2009). Women with a previously affected child should take folic acid 4 mg daily for 4 weeks prior to conception and throughout the first 3 months of gestation (Gregory et al., 2012).
3. Approximately 50% of pregnancies are affected by morning sickness during the first trimester, which is associated with increased levels of human chorionic gonadotropin (hCG) and progesterone (Pillitteri, 2010).
4. The stomach loses tone and has decreased motility and delayed emptying time because of the effects of progesterone.
5. Relaxation of the pyloric sphincter and upward displacement of the diaphragm in combination with increased intra-abdominal pressure from the enlarging uterus can result in gastroesophageal reflux and heartburn.
6. The small bowel has reduced motility and hypertrophy of the duodenal villi to increase absorption of nutrients. Constipation is a problem because of mechanical obstruction from the uterus, reduced motility, and increased water absorption.
7. The gallbladder has decreased muscle tone and motility after 14 weeks as a result of the effects of progesterone. High levels of estrogen may decrease water absorption by the gallbladder's mucosa, leading to dilute bile with resulting inability to sequester cholesterol. This increase in cholesterol may lead to gallstone formation during the second and third trimesters of pregnancy. Decreased gallbladder tone may also lead to increased retention of bile salts, resulting in pruritus and cholestasis gravidarum. Cholestasis gravidarum has been associated with increased risk of stillbirth and preterm deliveries (Kroumpouzos, 2007).
8. The liver is displaced upward by the enlarging uterus. Estrogen may cause altered production of plasma proteins, bilirubin, serum enzymes, and serum lipids. Alterations in laboratory values such as reduced serum albumin, elevated alkaline phosphatase, and elevated serum cholesterol may mimic liver disease. Serum levels of bilirubin, aspartate aminotransferase (AST), and alanine aminotransferase (ALT) are unchanged in normal pregnancy and may be used as an indicator of hepatic compromise during pregnancy. During labor, alkaline phosphatase levels may increase further, and AST, ALT, and lactate dehydrogenase levels may increase as a result of stress of labor.

**B. Respiratory system (Blackburn, 2013).**

1. The increased vascularity and vascular congestion of the upper respiratory tract resulting from increased levels of estrogen causes hypersecretion of mucus from the nasopharynx, resulting in nasal stuffiness, sinus congestion, and epistaxis (nosebleed) during pregnancy (Lowdermilk et al., 2012).
2. Maternal oxygen requirements increase during pregnancy as a result of increased maternal metabolic rate, fetal oxygen requirements, and increased tissue mass (Lowdermilk et al., 2012).
3. The chest wall profile changes. Increased levels of estrogen and relaxin cause relaxation of intercostal ligaments with resulting increased chest expansion and chest circumference and an increase in the subcostal margin angle (Cunningham et al., 2010). The diaphragm is elevated by 4 cm in the third trimester (Lowdermilk et al., 2012).
4. Respiratory changes during pregnancy include a 30% to 40% increase in tidal volume, a 20% to 30% decrease in expiratory reserve volume, a 20% decrease in residual volume, and a 20% decrease in functional residual capacity (Pillitteri, 2010). Forced expiratory volume does not change in pregnancy and is a reliable indicator of asthma status in pregnant women. Progesterone, estradiol, and prostaglandins increase the sensitivity of the respiratory center to carbon dioxide (Lowdermilk et al., 2012). Maternal $Paco_2$ levels decrease to 32 mm Hg and

oxygen levels rise to 106 mm Hg early in pregnancy to allow fetal–placental exchange (Pillitteri, 2010). As a result of these cumulative respiratory changes, pregnant women may experience physiologic dyspnea. To prevent the maternal acidosis due to the carbon dioxide levels from the fetus, mild hyperventilation occurs. This hyperventilation may increase to cause respiratory alkalosis. According to Cunningham et al. (2010), progesterone lowers the threshold and increases chemosensitivity to carbon dioxide; in response to the respiratory alkalosis, plasma bicarbonate levels decrease from 26 to 22 mmol/L, creating a slight increase in blood pH that shifts the oxygen dissociation curve to the left. Although pulmonary function is not impaired, respiratory diseases may be more serious during pregnancy (Cunningham et al., 2010).

**C. Skin (Blackburn, 2013).**

1. Because of elevated levels of estrogen, spider angiomas are frequently seen on the neck, face, throat, and arms. Palmar erythema is common in two thirds of white women and one third of African American women (Cunningham et al., 2010).
2. Striae gravidarum occur in women with a genetic predisposition to stretching of the skin or connective tissue. Stretching due to the increased activity of adrenocorticosteroids, estrogens, and relaxin may cause separation and rupture of areas of connective tissue of the skin, leading to pink or red streaks on the abdomen, thighs, and breasts (Lowdermilk et al., 2012; Pillitteri, 2010). After pregnancy, striae do not completely resolve; however, they turn a silvery-white color (Pillitteri, 2010).
3. Increased pigmentation is due to increased levels of estrogen, progesterone, and melanocyte-stimulating hormone. This is most marked on the nipples, areolas, perineum, and midline of the lower portion of the abdomen (commonly called the linea nigra).
4. Sun-sensitive hyperpigmentation of the face, called chloasma or melasma and also referred to as the "mask of pregnancy," results in a dark, blotchy appearance of the face, forehead, and upper lip and occurs in 45% to 70% of women. There is a genetic predisposition to melasma.
5. During gestation a greater percentage of the hair remains in the anagen (growth) phase, which decreases normal hair loss. Hair loss commonly occurs between 2 and 4 months after delivery and is due to an increase in the telogen (resting) phase of hair growth. The hair returns to a normal growth phase within 1 to 5 months (Kroumpouzos, 2012).
6. Changes in secretory glands occur during pregnancy. Sebaceous gland activity changes are variable, with resulting changes in acne unpredictable (Kroumpouzos, 2012). Eccrine sweat gland activity increases as a result of increased thyroid activity, body weight, and metabolic activity and may result in miliaria and dyshidrotic eczema.
7. Changes in the nails are uncommon but may occur beginning in the first trimester. These changes include brittleness, distal separation of the nail bed, subungual hyperkeratosis, whitish discoloration (leukonychia), and transverse grooving (Kroumpouzos, 2012). The cause is unknown.

**D. Urinary system (Blackburn, 2013).**

1. Structural renal changes begin during the first trimester and are a result of estrogen, progesterone, and prostaglandin $E_2$ secretion; pressure from the enlarging uterus; and increase in blood volume (Lowdermilk et al., 2012). The kidneys enlarge, the ureters dilate, hyperplasia of the smooth muscle walls of the ureters occurs, and the ureters elongate (Lowdermilk et al., 2012). Hydronephrosis occurs in 80% of pregnant women. Bladder capacity also increases to 1000 mL (Pillitteri, 2010). The consequences of these changes include the following:
   a. An increase in asymptomatic bacteriuria that may lead to cystitis and pyelonephritis.
   b. Difficulty in diagnosing obstruction on x-ray examination and interference with studies of glomerular filtration, renal blood flow, and tubular function. Accuracy of 24-hour urine collection results may also be affected.
   c. Vesicoureteral reflux, which may occur especially during the third trimester, as a result of decreased bladder tone.
2. Urodynamic and hemodynamic changes also occur in the renal system during pregnancy.
   a. Mean 24-hour urine output increases from 1475 to 1919 mL, and the mean number of daily voids increases as well.

b. The renal plasma flow increases by 75%, with a 25% decrease in the third trimester (Gordon, 2012). The increased renal plasma flow is accompanied by an increase in glomerular filtration rate of 50%, which leads to an increase in creatinine clearance and a decrease in nitrogen levels, as reflected by decreased blood urea nitrogen (BUN) and serum creatinine levels (Pillitteri, 2010).
c. An increased filtration of sodium is balanced by an increased reabsorption of sodium by the renal tubules.
d. The lower renal threshold for glucose excretion negates using urine glucose measurements in the management of diabetes mellitus.
e. Proteinuria of trace to 1+ may occur as a result of an increased load of amino acids. Although this level of proteinuria may not indicate pathology, the pregnant woman with proteinuria and hypertension should be evaluated for preeclampsia (Lowdermilk et al., 2012).

**E. Cardiovascular system (Blackburn, 2013; Cunningham et al., 2010).**

1. There is an increase in maternal blood volume by 1500 mL or 30% to 50% from the end of the first trimester, peaking at 28 to 32 weeks (Lowdermilk et al., 2012). If plasma volume increases faster than red blood cell (RBC) production, a hemodilutional pseudoanemia may result (Pillitteri, 2010).
2. There is an increase in maternal heart rate, which increases by 10 to 20 beats above the nonpregnant state by the third trimester. Stroke volume increases during the first and second trimesters and then decreases during the third trimester. Pregnancies with multiples have a greater increase in maternal cardiac output.
3. Because the heart is displaced leftward and upward by the enlarging uterus, the cardiac silhouette increases on x-ray films.
4. Altered cardiac sounds in pregnancy include splitting of the first heart sound, an audible $S_3$ heart sound, systolic flow murmurs (90% of pregnant women), and transient diastolic murmurs (20% of pregnant women).
5. Blood pressure remains at the prepregnancy level in the first trimester and drops during the second trimester at approximately 24 weeks of gestation by 5 to 10 mm Hg systolic and 10 to 15 mm Hg diastolic. It returns to normal prepregnancy levels at the end of pregnancy.
6. Between 20 and 24 weeks of gestation, pressure on and resulting obstruction of the inferior vena cava may occur in the supine position. The resulting 25% fall in cardiac output is called supine hypotension. Positioning the mother in a lateral position or with lateral displacement of the uterus with placement of a wedge under her hip assists in the prevention of supine hypotension.
7. Blood stagnates in the lower extremities because of compression of the pelvic veins and the inferior vena cava, contributing to dependent edema, varicosities of the legs and vulva, and hemorrhoid formation.

**F. Breasts (Blackburn, 2013).**

1. Early changes in the breasts (beginning by 4 weeks of gestation) include tingling, heaviness, tenderness, and enlargement in response to increased levels of estrogen (Lowdermilk et al., 2012). These symptoms usually subside at the end of the first trimester.
2. The areolas enlarge and darken. Sebaceous glands on the areolae increase activity in preparation for lactation and therefore become more prominent (Kroumpouzos, 2012).
3. Estrogen, progesterone, human placental lactogen (hPL), hCG, prolactin, and luteal and placental hormones cause hyperplasia of the breast tissue and development of lactiferous ducts and lobular alveolar tissue during the second and third trimesters (Lowdermilk et al., 2012; Pillitteri, 2010). Physical examination may reveal palpable milk ducts and excretion of colostrum from the nipples.
4. Colostrum, which is a high-protein precursor of breast milk, may be expressed as early as the fourth month of pregnancy (Pillitteri, 2010).
5. The breast is capable of lactogenesis after 16 weeks. Compared to milk produced after a term delivery, the milk produced after delivery of a preterm infant (i.e., <34 weeks) has higher protein content; higher antiinfective properties, including secretory immunoglobulin A and lactoferrin; and higher oligosaccharides, fat, sodium, chloride, and iron.

G. **Skeletal changes (Gordon, 2012).**
  1. Compensating for the anteriorly positioned growing uterus, the lower portion of the back curves. This lordosis shifts the center of gravity backward over the lower extremities and causes low back pain, a common complaint in pregnancy.
  2. Sacroiliac and pubic symphysis joints loosen during pregnancy because of the hormone relaxin.
  3. Alteration in the center of gravity, loosening of the joints, and an unsteady gait increase the risk of falls in pregnancy.
  4. Numbness, tingling, weakness, and aching in the upper extremities are a result of marked lordosis. Symptoms are the result of anterior flexion of the neck in the cervicodorsal region, producing traction on the brachial plexus and ulnar and median nerves (Lowdermilk et al., 2012).
  5. Although serum calcium levels decrease during pregnancy, serum ionized calcium levels are unchanged. The National Institutes of Health (2013) recommends 1300 mg of calcium for women 14 to 18 years of age and 1000 mg of calcium for women 19 to 50 years of age during pregnancy and lactation.
  6. Bone turnover is low in the first trimester and then increases in the third trimester when peak fetal calcium transfer occurs; however, osteoporosis is not associated with pregnancy bone turnover.

H. **Hematologic changes (Blackburn, 2013; Gordon, 2012).**
  1. Plasma volume is increased 15% by the end of the first trimester, undergoes a rapid expansion during the second trimester, peaks at 32 to 34 weeks, and then plateaus near term. Plasma volume at or near term is 40% to 45% (~1500 mL) above prepregnant levels (Cunningham et al., 2010).
  2. The white blood cell (WBC) count rises progressively during pregnancy and labor. Prepregnancy levels range from 5000 to 12,000 cells/microliter (mcL) and increases up to 25,000 cells/mcL in labor and the early postpartum period.
  3. The RBC count rises up to 33% during the first trimester, with an average increase of 30% to 35% throughout pregnancy. The increase in plasma volume changes the ratio of RBCs to plasma, causing a drop in hematocrit. This "physiologic anemia of pregnancy" reaches the lowest levels at 30 to 34 weeks; then as the hematocrit begins to rise, a closer to normal ratio of RBCs to plasma results in a higher hematocrit near term.
  4. Iron requirements are increased by 800 mg in pregnancy, with total fetal requirements of 350 to 400 mg of iron (Pillitteri, 2010). Fetal iron requirements are greatest during the third trimester. Serum ferritin levels fall until 30 to 32 weeks, with the greatest decrease between 12 and 25 weeks.
  5. Pregnancy has been called a "hypercoagulable state." The platelet count decreases slightly, but remains within the normal range. Fibrinogen is increased by 50% to 80%, and factors VII through X increase (Pillitteri, 2010). Bleeding and clotting times remain normal. The incidence of thromboembolism increases five- to six-fold and is greatest during the postpartum period (Pettker and Lockwood, 2012).
  6. Pregnancy is known to result in altered immunologic function so that the "foreign fetus" is accommodated. Therefore, a decrease in cellular immunity may account for improvement of certain autoimmune diseases in pregnancy and an increased susceptibility to infection. The humoral immune system characterized by antibody-mediated immunity remains intact.

I. **Endocrine and metabolic changes (Blackburn, 2013).**
  1. **Thyroid:** The thyroid enlarges during pregnancy; however, there is little transplacental transfer of the hormones triiodothyronine ($T_3$) and thyroxine ($T_4$). Thyroid-binding globulin (TBG) increases during the first trimester owing to the effects estrogen has on the liver. TBG plateaus by 20 weeks and results in increases in total $T_4$ and total $T_3$ levels (Mestman, 2012). hCG has thyrotropic activity and can activate thyroid-stimulating hormone (TSH) receptors and also increase secretion of $T_4$ (Blackburn, 2013). Serum portions of $T_3$ and $T_4$ are normal unless a maternal iodine deficiency is present or there are abnormalities of the thyroid gland (Mestman, 2012). Increased hCG levels are associated with decreased TSH levels in early pregnancy. There is a transient decrease in TSH during the first trimester, with a return to normal levels by the second trimester. Fetal thyroid function appears to be independent of maternal thyroid function.

2. **Carbohydrate metabolism (Cunningham et al., 2010):**
   a. Characterized by mild fasting hypoglycemia, postprandial hyperglycemia, and hyperinsulinemia.
   b. The basal metabolic rate is increased by 25%.
   c. Peripheral resistance to insulin is referred to as the "diabetogenic effect of pregnancy." Its purpose is to ensure a sustained postprandial supply of glucose for the fetus. By term there is a 50% to 70% reduction in the action of insulin. The hormones responsible for this effect are hPL, progesterone, and estrogen. hPL may increase lipolysis, leading to increased free fatty acids, which increases tissue resistance to insulin.
   d. Glucose is actively transported to the fetus; however, insulin and glycogen do not cross the placenta. During pregnancy, hyperglycemic states rapidly change to fasting states, resulting in hypoglycemia. In this fasting state, there is an increase in levels of fatty acids, triglycerides, and cholesterol. This switch in fuels from glucose to lipids is referred to as accelerated starvation, and ketonuria rapidly occurs.

## ANTEPARTUM CARE

**A. Initial antepartum visit.**

1. A thorough obstetric history is obtained:
   a. Gravidity (G), indicating the number of pregnancies, and parity (P), indicating the number of births. The obstetric history is often written as "G_P_ _ _ _". Four-number parity is often used, which includes the number of elective and spontaneous abortions and the number of living children.
      (1) *G* indicates the number of times the woman has been pregnant, including this pregnancy.
      (2) *P* represents the number of term deliveries, number of preterm deliveries, total number of abortions (elective and spontaneous before 20 weeks, including ectopic pregnancies), and number of living children.
      (3) For example, G5P1121 indicates this is a woman's fifth pregnancy; she has had one term delivery, one preterm delivery, two abortions, and has one living child.
   b. Information regarding course of pregnancy and delivery: Weeks of completed gestation for each pregnancy, weight of newborn at birth, any maternal or neonatal complications, duration of labor in hours, type of delivery (vaginal, forceps, vacuum, or operative), reason for any cesarean delivery as well as any information known about uterine scar and postoperative course.
   c. Medical history and review of systems, including infections (hepatitis, human immunodeficiency virus [HIV], herpes simplex virus [HSV], rubella, varicella, sexually transmitted infections, and tuberculosis), psychosocial assessment, substance use, and family history.
   d. Genetic history: ethnicity; maternal age (>35 years); paternal age (>50 years); family history of genetic disorders, such as Down syndrome, fragile X syndrome; NTD; mental retardation; and cystic fibrosis. Ethnic predispositions to certain genetic disorders are:
      (1) African Americans: sickle cell anemia.
      (2) Ashkenazi Jews: Tay–Sachs disease, Canavan disease, familial dysautonomia.
      (3) Cajuns: Tay–Sachs disease.
      (4) French Canadians: Tay–Sachs disease.
      (5) Mediterranean descent: β-thalassemia and sickle cell disease.
      (6) Southeast Asians: α-thalassemia.
   e. History of pregnancy loss or neonatal death (Blackburn, 2013).
   f. Exposure to teratogens (Blackburn, 2013).
   g. History of current pregnancy.
   h. Review of systems.
2. Perform a complete physical examination, including a complete pelvic examination.
3. Initial laboratory work (Table 1-1), including genetic screening blood work such as screens for ethnically linked disorders.

■ TABLE 1-1
■ ■ **Routine Initial Prenatal Screening Tests***

| Test | Reason for Screening Test |
|---|---|
| Blood type, Rh status, antibody screen | Identifies fetuses at risk of isoimmune disease |
| Hemoglobin or hematocrit | Baseline laboratory studies: rule out anemia |
| Hemoglobin electrophoresis in patients with African/African American ethnicity | Screen at-risk populations to determine carrier status and determine indication to screen partner. Also, women with sickle cell trait have higher risk of bacteriuria in pregnancy. |
| Cystic fibrosis carrier testing | Cystic fibrosis testing is recommended for all couples planning a pregnancy, particularly for those ethnic groups at highest risk (e.g., whites and Ashkenazi Jews) to determine carrier status and determine if partner screening is indicated |
| Rubella antibody screen | Identifies women susceptible to acquiring rubella during pregnancy; susceptible women should be immunized *after* delivery |
| Hepatitis B surface antigen | Identifies women whose offspring can be treated at birth to prevent hepatitis B infection |
| Hepatitis C antibody | Screen at-risk women |
| Serologic test for syphilis (VDRL or RPR) | Treatment reduces fetal/neonatal morbidity; mandated by law in most states |
| Human immunodeficiency virus I and II | Identifies women for treatment and perinatal therapy to decrease transmission to the fetus |
| Urinalysis | |
| Glucose, ketones, protein | Screen for diabetes, pregnancy-induced hypertension, and renal disease |
| RBCs, WBCs, bacteria | Possible urinary tract infection |
| Diabetes screen (new patient if high risk, and 24 to 28 weeks) | Fasting and glucose tolerance tests to rule out gestational diabetes |
| Papanicolaou smear | Identifies cervicitis and precancerous and cancerous lesions |
| *Neisseria gonorrhoeae* and *Chlamydia*[†] cultures | Identify treatable sexually transmitted diseases, most of which can cause fetal or neonatal morbidity |
| Quad screen (maternal serum for AFP, human chorionic gonadotropin, estriol) | Tests done at 15 to 20 weeks at mother's discretion after counseling; AFP screens for neural tube defects, Down syndrome; combination of three tests very sensitive in identifying Down syndrome |

Adapted from Clinic Protocol for Department of Obstetrics and Gynecology, University of Colorado Health Sciences Center; O'Neill, P., Davies, J., LeBel, A., and Hobbins, J.: Maternal factors affecting the newborn. In P.J. Thureen, J. Deacon, J.A. Hernandez, and D.M. Hall (Eds.): *Assessment and care of the well newborn* (2nd ed.). St. Louis, 2005, Elsevier Saunders.

*AFP*, α-Fetoprotein; *RBCs*, red blood cells; *RPR*, rapid plasma reagin; *VDRL*, Venereal Disease Research Laboratory; *WBCs*, white blood cells.

*Laboratory tests may vary from one center to another. Ultrasonography is considered by some to be a screening tool for congenital anomalies.

[†]Some centers also screen for *Mycoplasma hominis* and group B streptococcus colonization.

## Assessment of Gestational Age

A. **Last menstrual period (LMP):** Estimating gestational age by counting from the LMP is a reliable method.
   1. A menstrual history should include frequency and duration of menstrual periods, heaviness of menstrual flow, menarche, and hormonal contraceptive use.
   2. The estimated date of delivery (EDD) or due date may be determined by Nägele's rule:

$$\text{EDD} = \text{First day of LMP} - 3 \text{ months} + 7 \text{ days} + 1 \text{ year}$$

B. **Pelvic examination and fundal height.**
   1. Determination of the size of the uterus during an early examination (before 12 to 14 weeks) is relatively accurate if the mother is of normal height and not grossly obese.
   2. Fundal height measurements (in centimeters) are made from 20 weeks on to assess growth and approximate gestational age ± 2 cm. The uterus is generally at the umbilicus at 20 weeks.
   3. In mothers who have significantly increased BMIs, ultrasound is indicated to monitor fetal growth.

C. **Quickening is the first feeling of fetal movement.**
   1. Primigravida: has quickening by 18 to 20 weeks.
   2. Multigravida: has quickening by 16 to 18 weeks.

D. **Fetal heart tones:** Can be detected by an electronic Doppler device as early as 9 weeks and commonly by 12 weeks, and may be auscultated with a fetoscope by 19 to 20 weeks. Today the fetoscope is rarely used in developed countries, but may still be used in the developing world.

E. **Ultrasonography (Platt, 2005).**
   1. Crown–rump measurement during the first trimester (6 to 12 weeks) most accurately reflects gestational age ±4.7 days with 95% accuracy (Richards, 2012). Gestational sac measurements prior to 6 weeks of gestation are not as accurate and should be followed up with subsequent ultrasound when the fetus is visible.
   2. Fetal heart motion and fetal pole can be detected by real-time ultrasonography as early as 6 weeks of gestation by vaginal ultrasonography (Richards, 2012).
   3. Biparietal diameter (BPD) is the most frequently used method of establishing gestational age; it is most accurate between 12 and 20 weeks. The BPD has an accuracy of ±7 days between 14 and 21 weeks with a 95% confidence interval (Richards, 2012).
   4. Abdominal circumference can be used to assess gestational age and intrauterine growth restriction. Use of abdominal circumference to assess gestational age is best done before 14 weeks.
   5. Fetal femur length may also be used to determine gestational age in the second trimester and is accurate ±7 days.
   6. Reliability of ultrasound dating after 26 weeks is low and reliability of single parameters is poor. Beyond 30 weeks of gestation, accuracy of ultrasound measurements is ±2 to 3 weeks (Richards, 2012). Assessment of multiple parameters along with serial ultrasounds may be done to determine gestational age.

## Genetic Screening

A. **All patients who present for care at less than 20 weeks should be offered noninvasive and invasive genetic screening regardless of age (ACOG, 2011b).**

B. **Noninvasive screening for chromosomal abnormalities (ACOG, 2011b).**
   1. First-trimester integrated screening at 10 to 14 weeks includes ultrasound measurement of fetal nuchal translucency and/or biochemical markers. Biochemical markers include α-fetoprotein (AFP), β-hCG, unconjugated estriol, inhibin A, and pregnancy-associated plasma protein A (PAPP-A).
   2. Serum integrated biochemical marker screening in first and second trimesters where nuchal translucency measurement is not an option. Single report in second trimester.
   3. Nuchal translucency is a more reliable screen for multiples because interpretation of biochemical markers is difficult in multiple gestations (Simpson et al., 2012).
   4. All patients should be offered screening for cystic fibrosis, and if carrier status is detected then the partner should be screened and, if indicated, counseled (ACOG, 2011c).
   5. Second-trimester ultrasound at 18 to 20 weeks for review of systems.
   6. Second-trimester biochemical marker screening at 15 to 20 weeks: screens for open NTDs, Down syndrome, trisomy 13, and trisomy 18. For other potential genetic problems, screens with up to four markers—AFP, estriol, hCG, and inhibin A—with increased detection of chromosomal abnormalities with additional markers.

C. **Invasive screening.**
   1. Chorionic villus sampling (CVS) at 9 to 11 weeks: transabdominal or transvaginal aspiration of trophoblastic tissue with a catheter under ultrasound guidance (Simpson et al., 2012). Risk of pregnancy loss is similar to amniocentesis. If CVS is performed for an increased risk of NTD, cystic hygroma, or other suspected anomaly, then the risk is increased (Simpson et al., 2012).
   2. Amniocentesis at 18 to 20 weeks: aspiration of approximately 20 mL of amniotic fluid with a spinal needle inserted through the maternal abdomen into the uterine cavity under ultrasound guidance. Direct chromosomal analysis of fluid and AFP measurement are performed. Risk of procedural pregnancy loss: 1 in 400 (Simpson et al., 2012).

## Antepartum Visits

A. **Frequency:** Obstetric visits are recommended every 4 weeks until 28 weeks, then every 2 to 3 weeks until 36 weeks, and then weekly; however, the number of visits can be decreased dependent on risk (Gregory et al., 2012).
B. **Routine assessments:** Weight, blood pressure, fundal height, fetal presentation, fetal heart tones, fetal movement, abnormal bleeding or discharge, signs of preterm labor, signs of preeclampsia, psychosocial state.
C. **Laboratory and diagnostic assessments.**
   1. 24- to 28-week visit:
      a. A 50-g oral glucose challenge test for gestational diabetes is performed. A level greater than 135 mg/dL is abnormal. A 3-hour oral glucose tolerance test is performed on all patients with an abnormal oral glucose challenge test screen result. The diagnosis of gestational diabetes is made if two values are elevated (plasma values: fasting, 92-126 mg/dL; at 1 hour, 180 mg/dL; and at 2 hours, 153 mg/dL (Blackburn, 2013).
      b. Obtain repeat hemoglobin and hematocrit determinations to recheck for anemia. Repeat at 36 weeks if anemia is detected.
   2. 28-week visit: obtain a repeat antibody titer for Rh-negative mothers; administer Rh immunoglobulin, 300 mg, if no anti-D antibody has been detected.
   3. Ultrasonography may be indicated to evaluate fetal growth, amniotic fluid volume, Doppler flow, or placental assessment.
   4. 36-week visit: repeat HIV, syphilis, gonorrhea, and chlamydia cultures if indicated.
   5. 35- to 37-week visit: obtain a vaginal/rectal group B streptococcus (GBS) culture. If the woman is penicillin allergic, then sensitivities for erythromycin and clindamycin should be obtained if the culture is GBS positive (Centers for Disease Control and Prevention [CDC], 2010). The culture result is reliable for 5 weeks (CDC, 2010).

## Antepartum Fetal Surveillance

A. **Fetal movement counts or fetal kick counts.**
   1. Fetal movement periods last approximately 40 minutes, and quiet periods last approximately 20 minutes (Greenberg et al., 2012).
   2. Decrease in fetal movements precedes fetal death; therefore, fetal movement counts are a cost-effective method to monitor fetal well-being (Greenberg et al., 2012).
   3. The American College of Obstetricians and Gynecologists (2013a) describes two methods for fetal movement counting. A woman may be instructed to count fetal movements over a 2-hour period up to 10 movements. If the infant moves less than 10 times in 2 hours, there is cause for concern and further testing, such as NST, is indicated. Alternatively, a woman may be asked to count fetal movements for 1 hour three times per week. If counts equal or exceed her baseline counts, it is reassuring; if the count is less than baseline, then further testing is indicated.
B. **Nonstress test (NST).** This is the most widely used screening method for fetal well-being. It is indicated for patients at risk of placental insufficiency and may be started as early as 30 to 32 weeks of gestation.
   1. Some indications for NST include post-term pregnancy, diabetes mellitus, hypertension, previous stillbirths, intrauterine growth restriction, decreased fetal movements, and Rh disease (ACOG, 2013a).
   2. Testing is repeated once or twice weekly. A *reactive* NST result is two fetal heart rate (FHR) accelerations, defined as a 15-beat rise from baseline that lasts for at least 15 seconds with return to baseline during a 20-minute period. A *nonreactive* test result is no FHR accelerations after 40 minutes (Greenberg et al., 2012; Nageotte, 2010).
   3. A reactive test result is reassuring, and with a false-negative rate of 0.3% (Nageotte, 2010). A nonreactive result is an indication for further testing.
C. **Contraction stress test (CST).**
   1. The CST evaluates the reserve function of the placenta. Indications for use are the same as for use of the NST. The CST is most often used after a nonreactive NST result (Greenberg et al., 2012).

2. Done by evaluating fetal heart tracing during three spontaneous or induced 40- to 60-second or longer moderate contractions in a 10-minute period (Nageotte, 2010). Contractions can be induced through nipple stimulation (endogenous oxytocin) or intravenous oxytocin challenge test (exogenous).
3. The CST simulates a labor pattern and allows the fetus to be stressed as in normal labor. The CST evaluates for FHR decelerations in relation to the onset of uterine contractions.
   a. A positive CST result is defined as late decelerations of the FHR that are present with the majority of contractions in a 10-minute window. Delivery should be considered with a positive CST result.
   b. Findings may also be considered suspicious or equivocal, unsatisfactory, or as showing tachysystole. These cases require retesting in the next 24 hours for adequate interpretation of fetal well-being (Greenberg et al., 2012).
   c. The false-negative rate (stillbirth within 1 week of negative antepartum test) is 0.04%; however, 30% of positive CSTs do not require intrapartum interventions (Nageotte, 2010).

D. **Biophysical profile (Greenberg et al., 2012).**
1. The biophysical profile uses real-time ultrasonography to evaluate five parameters, each receiving either 0 or 2 points; the maximum score is 10 points, with management based on the assigned score. The five parameters are: NST, fetal breathing, gross body/limb movements, fetal tone, and amniotic fluid.
2. Modified biophysical profile: NST/amniotic fluid index (AFI).
   a. NST is an indicator of present fetal condition.
   b. AFI is a marker of longer-term fetal status.

E. **Amniotic fluid assessment.**
1. Decreased amniotic fluid volume (oligohydramnios) is associated with uteroplacental insufficiency. It may also be indicative of fetal genitourinary or lung anomalies. There is an increased incidence of perinatal morbidity and mortality with oligohydramnios (Moore, 2010).
2. Polyhydramnios may be associated with chromosomal disorders, anatomic anomalies such as tracheoesophageal fistula, maternal diabetes, preterm delivery, and perinatal mortality (Gilbert, 2012).
3. Measurement of amniotic fluid:
   a. Single deep vertical pocket measurement of 2 cm is considered adequate (Greenberg et al., 2012).
   b. The four-quadrant measure is the AFI, and it varies by gestational age. AFI of less than 5 at term is used as cutoff for oligohydramnios (Moore, 2010).

## Laboratory Assessments for Documenting Fetal Lung Maturity (Locatelli, 2010)

A. Lecithin/sphingomyelin (L/S) ratio ≥2.0 indicates fetal lung maturity and occurs when fetal lung surfactant is present in amniotic fluid (at approximately 35 weeks). Positive predictive value is 98%.

B. Phosphatidylglycerol (PG), a minor component of surfactant, is also present in amniotic fluid at approximately 35 weeks and increases rapidly at 37 weeks. PG is reported as present or absent with a positive predictive value of 95% to 100%. Measurement of PG is a more reliable test of lung maturity in mothers with diabetes than is measurement of the L/S ratio.

C. Fetal lung maturity assay measures surfactant/albumin ratio in amniotic fluid. It is less expensive, is easier to perform, and has fewer false-negative results than the L/S ratio or PG measurement. Positive predictive value is 96% to 100%. Values greater than 55 are considered mature, and values of 35 to 55 are considered borderline.

D. Lamellar body counts are produced by type II pneumocytes and are a direct measurement of a storage form of surfactant (Greenberg et al., 2012). Test is inexpensive and may be performed in 15 minutes with less than 1 mL of amniotic fluid. Values of 30,000 to 40,000/mcL indicate pulmonary maturity. Results have a 97% to 98% negative predictive value. Meconium has a minimal effect on values, increasing count by approximately 5000/mcL, and bloody fluid may slightly increase the count.

## Maternal Infections

**A. TORCH infections (Table 1-2).**
1. Acronym rarely used as diagnostic grouping but frequently used clinically to refer to five infectious diseases: *t*oxoplasmosis, *o*thers (e.g., parvovirus, congenital syphilis), *r*ubella, *c*ytomegalovirus infection, and *h*erpes simplex. They all cross the placenta and may adversely affect the fetus.

**B. Sexually transmitted infections (Table 1-3).**

**C. Other communicable diseases (Table 1-4).**

**D. Chorioamnionitis (Thureen et al., 2005).**
1. An infection of the chorion, amnion, and amniotic fluid that may cause perinatal morbidity and mortality; usually associated with prolonged labor and ruptured membranes, but can also be found in women with intact membranes.
2. Usually an ascending infection, commonly caused by *Escherichia coli*, group B streptococcus (GBS), anaerobic streptococci, and bacteroids.

**E. Infection with GBS.**
1. Approximately 10% to 30% of women are colonized with GBS (Dinsmoor, 2010). Colonization can be transient, chronic, or intermittent.
2. GBS may cause severe invasive disease in neonates. The majority of neonatal GBS infections occur during the first week of life and present as sepsis or pneumonia (CDC, 2010). There has been a 70% decline in neonatal GBS infection since intrapartum prophylaxis was instituted in the 1990s, and further reduction was noted with the implementation of universal screening in 2002 (CDC, 2010). The infection rate is 5.1 in 1000 infants born to colonized mothers without risk factors and increases to 41 in 1000 infants if there is premature labor and delivery, prolonged rupture of membranes, or intrapartum fever (Dinsmoor, 2010).
3. All women should be screened at 35 to 37 weeks of gestation for rectal–genital group B streptococcus. Cultures done ≤5 weeks prior to delivery have a 95% to 98% negative predictive value; after 5 weeks the negative predictive value declines (CDC, 2010). Any woman with positive culture results should be given antibiotic prophylaxis during labor according to CDC guidelines (2010).

# NORMAL LABOR AND BIRTH

**A. Stages and phases of labor:** There are three stages of labor.
1. First stage: onset of contractions to complete dilatation; has three phases.
   a. Latent phase: onset of labor to time when the slope of cervical dilatation changes.
   b. Active phase: approximately 4 cm to complete cervical dilatation. Maximum slope is from 5 to 9 cm and is time when labor progresses rapidly.
   c. Transition: portion of active phase from 8 to 10 cm with intense contraction and beginning of descent.
2. Second stage: complete dilatation to delivery of infant. Maximum fetal descent coincides with transition and second stage.
3. Third stage: time from delivery of infant to delivery of placenta.

## Intrapartum Labor Management

**A. Admission.**
1. History, review of prenatal records, contractions, membrane status, bleeding, fetal movement, and nutritional status.
2. Physical examination: vital signs, fetal heart tones, contraction pattern, abdominal examination (Leopold's maneuvers, estimated fetal weight, scars), extremities, vaginal examination (dilatation, effacement, station), pelvis, examination if history warrants to assess for ruptured membranes (Amnisure©, Nitrazine, ferning, pooling, Valsalva maneuver). Nitrazine, pooling, and ferning are nonspecific tests for detection of ruptured membranes. Amnisure© (PAMG-1) is an immunoassay test that is more specific and sensitive for ruptured membranes.

TABLE 1-2
**TORCH Infections**

| Infection/ Incubation | Transmission | Detection | Maternal Effects | Neonatal Effects | Incidence and Prevention |
|---|---|---|---|---|---|
| Cytomegalovirus<br>Incubation: unknown | Intimate contact with infected secretions (breast milk, cervical mucus, semen, saliva, and urine)<br>Transplacentally<br>Organ transplantation | IgM titer | Clinically "silent"; only 1% to 5% acquire symptoms: low-grade fever, malaise, arthralgia, hepatomegaly | Infection is most likely to occur with maternal primary infection; 90% of infected infants are free of symptoms at birth, but 5% to 15% of these may have long-term sequelae, 5% with severe involvement at birth: IUGR, microcephaly, periventricular calcification, deafness, blindness, chorioretinitis, mental retardation, hepatosplenomegaly | Primarily occurs in 1% to 2% of pregnant women; 90% of adult population in United States are seropositive. Rigorous personal hygiene throughout pregnancy to prevent infection if not infected |
| Herpes simplex virus<br>Incubation: 2 to 10 days | Intimate mucocutaneous exposure<br>Passage through an infected birth canal<br>Ascending infection, especially with rupture of membranes<br>Transplacentally (rare) if initial infection occurs during pregnancy | Suspect with vesicles on cervix, vagina, or external genital area; painful lesions<br>Presumptive diagnosis by fluorescent antibody or Papanicolaou smear on vesicular fluid<br>Confirm diagnosis by vesicle culture | Painful genital lesions<br>Primary infection commonly associated with fever, malaise, myalgias<br>Numbness, tingling, burning, itching, and pain with lesions<br>Lymphadenopathy<br>Urinary retention | Rare transplacental transmissions have resulted in miscarriages<br>Mortality rate of 5% to 60% if neonatal exposure is with active primary infection<br>Neurologic or ophthalmic sequelae<br>Disseminated infection in 70% of cases, with jaundice, respiratory distress, and CNS involvement | Estimated 300,000 new cases per year<br>1:3000 to 20,000 live births with perinatal transmission<br>Up to 80% of women delivering infected infants have no history of genital herpes; cesarean delivery if known active infection<br>Avoid genital contact when male has penile lesions; use condoms |

| | | | | | |
|---|---|---|---|---|---|
| Rubella<br>Incubation: 14 to 21 days | Nasopharyngeal secretions<br>Transplacentally | Serologic antibody titer testing (IgG-specific rubella antibody)<br>Virus isolation from throat | Pink maculopapular rash on face, neck, arms, and legs lasting 3 days<br>Lymph node enlargement, fever, malaise, headache<br>History of exposure 3 weeks earlier | Fetal infection rate greatest before 11 weeks and after 35 weeks, but severe sequelae occur with first-trimester infection; includes deafness (60% to 70%), eye defects (10% to 30%), CNS anomalies (10% to 25%), congenital heart disease (10% to 20%) | Since introduction of vaccine in late 1960s, rubella is rare<br>Occurs more commonly in springtime<br>Vaccine is contraindicated during pregnancy; vaccinate susceptible women postpartum |
| Toxoplasmosis (protozoa, *Toxoplasma gondii*)<br>Incubation: 2 to 3 weeks | Eating raw meat containing *T. gondii*<br>Ingesting *T. gondii* cysts secreted in feces of infected cats<br>Transplacentally<br>Impossible to transmit to others because the infecting organisms are tissue bound and are not secreted | Serologic antibody testing<br>ELISA | 90% of infected women have no symptoms<br>Posterior cervical lymphadenopathy<br>Malaise<br>Premature labor and delivery | Severity varies with gestational age (usually, earlier infection results in more severe effects)<br>Neurologic, ophthalmologic, and co-sequelae are variable<br>IUGR<br>Hydrocephalus<br>Microcephaly | Incidence varies throughout the world (1 to 4 infants per 1000 live births)<br>20% to 30% of U.S. women have been exposed<br>Incidence of congenital toxoplasmosis infection in the United States is 1:1000 to 8000<br>Reduce contact with cats during pregnancy |

From Thureen, P.J., Davies, J.K., Lebel, A., and Hobbins, J.C.: Maternal factors affecting the newborn. In P.J. Thureen, J. Deacon, J.A. Hernandez, and D.M. Hall (Eds.): *Assessment and care of the well newborn* (2nd ed.). St. Louis, 2005, Elsevier Saunders.

*CNS*, Central nervous system; *ELISA*, enzyme-linked immunosorbent assay; *IgG*, immunoglobulin G; *IgM*, immunoglobulin M; *IUGR*, intrauterine growth restriction; *TORCH*, *t*oxoplasmosis, *o*ther infections (e.g., congenital syphilis), *r*ubella, *c*ytomegalovirus infection, and *h*erpes simplex.

■ TABLE 1-3
■ ■ **Sexually Transmitted Infections**

| Infection/Agent/ Incubation | Detection | Maternal Effects | Neonatal Effects | Incidence |
|---|---|---|---|---|
| Acquired immunodeficiency syndrome<br>Human immunodeficiency virus<br>Incubation: variable, months to years | ELISA for screening<br>Western blot or indirect immunofluorescence assay<br>p24 antigen for acute infection before seroconversion | | 30% chance of transmission from infected mother<br>Syndrome develops in up to 65% of infected infants within a few months after birth | 1991: estimated 200,000 cases in the United States; 0.15% of all women who delivered were infected |
| Chlamydiosis<br>Bacterium: *Chlamydia trachomatis*<br>Incubation: variable but more than 1 week | Culture of endocervical and urethral specimens<br>ELISA or fluorescent antibody | Most cases asymptomatic<br>Mucopurulent cervicitis on swab specimen is less sensitive and specific<br>Occasionally premature rupture of membranes, preterm labor, IUGR, infertility, chorioamnionitis | 30% to 40% of exposed infants have conjunctivitis<br>Frequently associated with other sexually transmitted infections | Most common sexually transmitted infection<br>3% to 18% have pneumonia<br>Estimated 4 million cases occur annually in the United States, with prevalence rates in female patients of 8% to 20%<br>70% of infections may be asymptomatic |
| Gonorrhea<br>Bacteria: *Neisseria gonorrhoeae*, gram-negative diplococcus<br>Incubation: 10 days | Endocervical, oral, or rectal cultures<br>Genital or blood cultures<br>Gram stain of lesions | 60% to 80% of those infected are free of symptoms<br>Occasionally pelvic peritonitis, premature rupture of membranes, postpartum endometritis, chorioamnionitis, increased infertility, ectopic pregnancy | Purulent conjunctivitis<br>Sepsis or meningitis | More than 1 million cases are reported in the United States each year<br>Incidence in pregnancy ranges from 1% to 10%, depending on the population |

| | | | | |
|---|---|---|---|---|
| Human papillomavirus<br>Incubation: unknown (3 months to years) | Single or multiple irregular painless papules in the genital or perianal area<br>Colposcopy used as adjunct in equivocal situations<br>Cervical cytologic testing | Significant number of lesions enlarge during pregnancy<br>Usually multicentric in pregnancy<br>Viral lesions probably more frequent in pregnant women because of increased hormone levels<br>Increasing incidence noted in STI clinics and private offices<br>Peak occurrence at ages 15 to 35<br>Associated with other STIs | Potential transmission of laryngeal papillomas<br>Very rare ($<$1:1000 to 1500 pregnancies in which mothers have genital condyloma) | Estimated 40 to 60 million people infected worldwide |
| Syphilis<br>Spirochete: *Treponema pallidum*<br>Incubation: 3 weeks on average | VDRL test<br>Rapid plasma reagin test<br>Fluorescent treponemal antibody absorption test | Primary chancre: painless ulcerative lesion<br>Secondary syphilis: fever and malaise, red macules on palms or soles of feet<br>Generalized lymphadenopathy<br>Early latent (positive serologic finding $<$1 year's duration) syphilis<br>Latent (cardiovascular) syphilis<br>Neurosyphilis | Vary depending on gestation<br>Stillbirth<br>IUGR<br>Nonimmune hydrops<br>Premature labor | 100,000 cases are reported in the United States each year; 80% of these women are of reproductive age<br>3850 cases of congenital syphilis in 1992<br>70% to 100% fetal transmission rate in primary maternal disease |
| Trichomoniasis<br>Protozoa: *Trichomonas vaginalis*<br>Incubation: 4 to 20 days | "Wet prep" saline examination<br>Papanicolaou smear<br>Dysuria<br>Urinalysis | Malodorous, discolored vaginal discharge | Infant contact through infected vagina<br>Usually asymptomatic | Not reported to CDC but estimated in as many as 20% of pregnancies<br>Estimates of 10% to 15% of all cases of vaginitis |

From Thureen, P.J., Davies, J.K., Lebel, A., and Hobbins, J.C.: Maternal factors affecting the newborn. In P.J. Thureen, J. Deacon, J.A. Hernandez, and D.M. Hall (Eds.): *Assessment and care of the well newborn* (2nd ed.). St. Louis, 2005, Elsevier Saunders.

*CDC*, Centers for Disease Control and Prevention; *ELISA*, enzyme-linked immunosorbent assay; *IUGR*, intrauterine growth retardation; *STI*, sexually transmitted infection; *VDRL*, Venereal Disease Research Laboratory.

TABLE 1-4
**Other Communicable Diseases**

| Infection/ Agent/ Incubation | Mode of Transmission | Maternal Effects | Neonatal Effects | Incidence and Prevention |
|---|---|---|---|---|
| Influenza virus<br>Incubation: 24 to 72 hours | Respiratory secretions | Usually brief but incapacitating disease<br>Death occurs from secondary bacterial pneumonia | Any risk of malformation has been confined to first trimester<br>Most studies fail to support teratogenicity | Killed virus vaccine<br>Vaccine during pregnancy is indicated if mother is at medical risk because of other diseases |
| Mumps<br>Paramyxovirus<br>Incubation: 16 to 18 days | Respiratory secretions | Spontaneous abortion rate is increased twofold | Teratogenicity is unknown | Avoid pregnancy for 3 months after vaccination |
| Parvovirus B19 (fifth disease)<br>DNA virus<br>Incubation: 4 to 14 days | Respiratory secretions | Erythema<br>Elevated temperature<br>Arthralgia | Spontaneous abortions | Risk for women with primary infection during the first 20 weeks of pregnancy is 15% to 17%<br>200,000 to 300,000 cases in the United States each year |
| Hepatitis B | Sexually<br>Perinatally<br>Transplacentally<br>Blood, stool, and saliva transmission | Fever, jaundice, malaise, hepatosplenomegaly<br>Premature labor | Increased stillbirth rate<br>Infected infants usually symptom-free at birth | One third of infants born to HBsAg-positive mothers will have HBsAg/HBeAg positivity and anti-HBe negativity |
| Varicella (chickenpox)<br>Varicella-zoster virus<br>Incubation: 11 to 21 days | Probably by aerosolized respiratory droplets<br>Portal of entry is the respiratory tract<br>Transplacentally | Severe in adults<br>Risk of premature labor as a result of high temperature<br>Risk of varicella pneumonia appears to be increased during pregnancy | 2% of infants with maternal infection in the first trimester have cutaneous scarring, eye abnormalities, and retardation<br>At risk if maternal rash onset 5 days before to 2 days after delivery; severe disseminated neonatal disease may develop, and one third die | 90% of women are immune<br>In the United States, occurs in less than 0.1% of pregnancies |

From Thureen, P.J., Davies, J.K., Lebel, A., and Hobbins, J.C.: Maternal factors affecting the newborn. In P.J. Thureen, J. Deacon, J.A. Hernandez, and D.M. Hall (Eds.): *Assessment and care of the well newborn* (2nd ed.). St. Louis, 2005, Elsevier Saunders.

*DNA*, Deoxyribonucleic acid; *HBe*, hepatitis B "e"; *HBeAg*, hepatitis B "e" antigen; *HBsAg*, hepatitis B surface antigen.

B. **Management of low-risk patient (Macones et al., 2008).** The patient should be identified as being low or high risk on the basis of available data. ACOG (2013a) recommends that low-risk patients have auscultation of FHR every 30 minutes in the first stage and every 15 minutes in the second stage, and high-risk patients every 15 minutes in the first stage and every 5 minutes in the second stage.
 1. A Category II or Category III FHR detected by auscultation is indication for electronic fetal monitoring: bradycardia, tachycardia, or FHR decelerations.
 2. Electronic fetal monitoring—Eunice Shriver Kennedy National Institute of Child Health and Human Development terminology is currently recommended. FHR patterns are described according to their baseline, variability, accelerations, and decelerations.
  a. FHR baseline evaluated over a 10-minute segment (Macones et al., 2008).
   (1) Normal baseline is 110 to 160 beats per minute (bpm). It is determined by approximating the FHR to increments of 5 bpm. There must be at least 2 minutes of identifiable baseline.
   (2) Bradycardia is less than 110 bpm for 10 minutes or greater.
   (3) Tachycardia is greater than 160 bpm for 10 minutes or greater.
  b. FHR baseline variability is fluctuations in FHR over a 10-minute window that are determined by the peak to trough in bpm. Variability is classified as:
   (1) Absent variability: amplitude range undetectable.
   (2) Minimal variability: amplitude greater than undetectable but less than 5 bpm.
   (3) Moderate variability: amplitude 6 to 25 bpm.
   (4) Marked variability: greater than 25 bpm.
  c. Accelerations are an abrupt increase in FHR to the peak in less than 30 seconds by at least 15 beats and lasting at least 15 seconds. A prolonged acceleration is $\geq$2 minutes but less than 10 minutes. In fetuses less than 32 weeks, an FHR acceleration is $\geq$10 beats lasting $\geq$10 seconds.
  d. Decelerations are decreases in FHR and are classified in relationship to their occurrence relative to the contractions as well as based on various characteristics of the deceleration. They are classified as early, late, or variable. Recurrent decelerations occur $\geq$50% of the time in a 20-minute window, and intermittent decelerations occur less than 50% of the time in a 20-minute window.
  e. Sinusoidal FHR patterns are undulating sine wave patterns with a cycle of 3 to 5/minute that persists for $\geq$20 minutes.
  f. FHR patterns are classified by category:
   (1) Category I: Normal FHR reflecting normal acid–base balance and can be followed in routine manner, without intervention.
   (2) Category II: Indeterminate FHR not predictive of abnormal fetal acid–base balance. These tracings require continued surveillance and reevaluation.
   (3) Category III: Abnormal FHR tracing predictive of abnormal fetal acid–base balance. Requires prompt evaluation and possible intervention to resolve the abnormal pattern or delivery.
  g. Uterine activity may be measured by external palpation, external tocodynamometer, or intrauterine pressure catheter to assess frequency, duration, and intensity of contractions. Uterine activity is classified as follows:
   (1) Normal: $\leq$5 contractions in 10 minutes averaged over 30 minutes.
   (2) Tachysystole: greater than 5 contractions in 10 minutes averaged over 30 minutes.

C. **Second-stage management.**
 1. Fetal descent/pushing.
  a. ACOG (2011a) recommends adherence to a 2-hour time limit for primipara and 1 hour for multipara (3 hours for primipara and 2 hours for multipara with epidurals). Research has shown no significant relationship between second-stage duration and perinatal mortality, 5-minute Apgar scores less than 7, neonatal seizures, or admission to a neonatal intensive care unit (Varney et al., 2004). Current recommendations state that critical factor is time of duration of active pushing rather than overall duration (Roberts and Hanson, 2007); therefore, passive descent and evaluation of fetal descent relative to time spent actively pushing is advised.

**D. Third stage—time from the birth of the baby to the delivery of the placenta.**

1. Normal duration from 0 to 30 minutes.

## PUERPERIUM: "FOURTH TRIMESTER"

The period from delivery through the sixth week is known as the "fourth trimester." Under the Newborns' and Mothers' Health Protection Act of 1996, minimum federal standards mandate health plans to provide coverage for 48 hours after a normal vaginal birth and 96 hours after a cesarean birth unless the attending health care provider and mother agree on early discharge (Crum, 2006b).

**A. Uterine involution.**

1. Involution begins immediately after delivery. The fundus is generally firm at the level of the umbilicus and generally decreases by one finger breadth daily. It is not palpable abdominally by 2 weeks.

**B. Breasts/breastfeeding.**

1. During the first 2 to 3 postpartum days, high-protein colostrum secretion provides the infant with nutrition. It also has high concentrations of immunoglobulin A, lactoferrin, and oligosaccharide to protect the infant against infection (Blackburn, 2013).
2. On the second or third postpartum day, milk secretion begins and breast engorgement may occur. Engorgement generally resolves spontaneously within 24 to 36 hours. In nonbreastfeeding mothers, lactation ceases within 1 week.
3. Mature milk is established by the end of the first or second week. Milk production is based on supply–demand, and suckling provides a sensory nerve stimulus to secrete prolactin and oxytocin to increase milk production (Blackburn, 2013).
4. Establishment of breastfeeding is facilitated by early initiation of breastfeeding, rooming-in, breastfeeding on demand, not using pacifiers, and not providing formula supplementation unless medically indicated. Postpartum breastfeeding support contributes to successful initiation and continuation of breastfeeding.

**C. Immunizations.**

1. Rubella vaccination should be administered in the immediate postpartum period to all women who are not immune (Crum, 2006a). $Rh_o$(D) immune globulin (RhoGAM) suppresses the immune response; therefore, if the woman needs $Rh_o$(D) immune globulin and a rubella vaccine, the rubella vaccine can be delayed until the postpartum week 6 visit or, if given with $Rh_o$(D) immune globulin, she should be retested for rubella immunity 3 months after administration (Crum, 2006b).
2. $Rh_o$(D) immune globulin (300 mcg given intramuscularly) is administered prophylactically to Rh-negative women antepartally at 28 weeks and within 72 hours of bleeding, injury, trauma, and amniocentesis. After delivery, it is administered to Rh-negative women with an Rh-positive fetus to prevent sensitization from fetal–maternal transfusion of Rh-positive fetal erythrocytes (Crum, 2006b).
3. Tdap (tetanus, diphtheria, and acellular pertussis): It is recommended that all pregnant women receive Tdap at 27 to 36 weeks of gestation. Women who have not previously received a dose of Tdap, including breastfeeding women, should receive Tdap immediately postpartum (CDC, 2012).

**D. Emotional changes.**

1. Postpartum blues may occur from birth to 14 days postpartum. Mild, transient symptoms of emotional lability may be caused by hormonal changes, sleep deprivation, role adjustment, and physiologic changes. Symptoms may be more intense if there are neonatal problems.
2. Postpartum depression may occur from birth throughout 6 months postpartum, and evaluation includes diagnostic criteria for depression. There are various screening tools such as the Beck or Edinburgh Postpartum Depression scales. A rare severe form of postpartum depression is postpartum psychosis, which may encompass suicidal thoughts or delusional behaviors.
3. Postpartum thyroiditis may cause symptoms of fatigue and depression. Women with postpartum depression should be evaluated for thyroiditis.

## REFERENCES


American College of Obstetricians and Gynecologists: Intrapartum fetal heart rate monitoring: Nomenclature, interpretation, and general management principles. *Practice Bulletin No. 106*. Washington, DC, 1999 reaffirmed 2013a, American College of Obstetricians and Gynecologists.

American College of Obstetricians and Gynecologists: Weight gain during pregnancy. *Committee Opinion No. 548*. Washington, DC, 2013b, American College of Obstetricians and Gynecologists.

American College of Obstetricians and Gynecologists: Dystocia and augmentation of labor. *Practice Bulletin No. 49*. Washington, DC, 2003 reaffirmed 2011a, American College of Obstetricians and Gynecologists.

American College of Obstetricians and Gynecologists: Screening for fetal chromosomal abnormalities. *Practice Bulletin No. 77*. Washington, DC, 2011b, American College of Obstetricians and Gynecologists.

American College of Obstetricians and Gynecologists: Update on carrier screening for cystic fibrosis. *Committee Opinion No. 486*. Washington, DC, 2011c, American College of Obstetricians and Gynecologists.

Blackburn, S.T.: *Maternal, fetal, and neonatal physiology: A clinical perspective* (4th ed.). St. Louis, 2013, Elsevier Saunders.

Centers for Disease Control and Prevention: Tdap for pregnant women: Information for providers. 2012. Retrieved from http://www.cdc.gov/vaccines/vpd-vac/pertussis/tdap-pregnancy-hcp.htm.

Centers for Disease Control and Prevention: 2010 Guidelines for the Prevention of perinatal group B streptococcal disease. Revised guidelines from CDC 2010. *MMWR Recommendations and Reports*, 59 (RR-10):1–36, 2010. Retrieved November 19, 2010, from http://www.cdc.gov/groupbstrep/guidelines/guidelines.html.

Crum, K.: Maternal physiologic changes. In D.L. Lowdermilk, and S.E. Perry (Eds.): *Maternity nursing* (7th ed.). St. Louis, 2006a, Elsevier Mosby, pp. 454–465.

Crum, K.: Nursing care during the fourth trimester. In D.L. Lowdermilk and S.E. Perry (Eds.): *Maternity nursing* (7th ed.). St. Louis, 2006b, Elsevier Mosby, pp. 466–495.

Cunningham, F.G., Leveno, K.J., Bloom, S.L., et al.: *Williams' obstetrics:* (23rd ed.). New York, 2010, McGraw-Hill.

Dinsmoor, M.: Group B streptococcus. In J.R. Queenan, J.C. Hobbins, and C.Y. Spong (Eds.): *Protocols for high-risk pregnancies* (5th ed.). Hoboken, NJ, 2010, Wiley-Blackwell, pp. 334–339.

Gilbert, W.: Amniotic fluid disorders. In S.G. Gabbe, J.R. Niebyl, and J.L. Simpson (Eds.): *Obstetrics: Normal and problem pregnancies* (6th ed.). Philadelphia, 2012, Elsevier Saunders, pp. 759–768.

Gordon, M.: Maternal physiology. In S.G. Gabbe, J.R. Niebyl, and J.L. Simpson (Eds.): *Obstetrics: Normal and problem pregnancies* (6th ed.). Philadelphia, 2012, Elsevier Saunders, pp. 42–65.

Greenberg, M.B., Druzin, M.L., Smith, J., et al.: Antepartum fetal evaluation. In S.G. Gabbe, J.R. Niebyl, and J.L. Simpson (Eds.): *Obstetrics: Normal and problem pregnancies* (6th ed.). Philadelphia, 2012, Elsevier Saunders, pp. 237–263.

Gregory, K.D., Niebyl, J., and Johnson, T.: Preconception and prenatal care: Part of the continuum. In S.G. Gabbe, J.R. Niebyl, and J.L. Simpson (Eds.): *Obstetrics: Normal and problem pregnancies* (6th ed.). Philadelphia, 2012, Elsevier Saunders, pp. 102–124.

Kroumpouzos, G.: Dermatologic disorders of pregnancy. In S.G. Gabbe, J.R. Niebyl, and J.L. Simpson (Eds.): *Obstetrics: Normal and problem pregnancies* (6th ed.). Philadelphia, 2012, Elsevier Saunders, pp. 1084–1097.

Kroumpouzos, G.: Intrahepatic cholestasis of pregnancy. In S.G. Gabbe, J.R. Niebyl, and J.L. Simpson (Eds.): *Obstetrics: Normal and problem pregnancies* (5th ed.). Philadelphia, 2007, Churchill Livingstone, pp. 1112–1113.

Locatelli, A.: Indices of maturity. In J.T. Queenan, J.C. Hobbins, and C.Y. Spong (Eds.): *Protocols for high-risk pregnancies* (5th ed.). Hoboken, NJ, 2010, Wiley-Blackwell, pp. 99–106.

London, M.L., Ladewig, P.A., Ball, J.W., et al.: *Maternal & child nursing care*. New York, 2011, Pearson.

Lowdermilk, D.L., Perry, S.E., Cashion, M.C., et al.: *Maternity nursing*. (10th ed.). St. Louis, 2012, Elsevier Mosby.

Macones, G.A., Hankins, G., Spong, C.Y., et al.: The 2008 National Institute of Child Health and Human Development workshop on electronic fetal monitoring: Update on definitions, interpretation, and research guidelines. *JOGNN*, 37:510–515, 2008.

Mestman, J.H.: Thyroid and parathyroid diseases in pregnancy. In S.G. Gabbe, J.R. Niebyl, and J.L. Simpson (Eds.): *Obstetrics: Normal and problem pregnancies* (6th ed.). Philadelphia, 2012, Elsevier Saunders, pp. 922–952.

Moore, T.: Oligohydramnios. In J.R. Queenan, J.C. Hobbins, and C.Y. Spong (Eds.): *Protocols for high-risk pregnancies* (5th ed.). Hoboken, NJ, 2010, Wiley-Blackwell, pp. 399–413.

Nageotte, M.P.: Antepartum testing. In J.T. Queenan, J.C. Hobbins, and C.Y. Spong (Eds.): *Protocols for high-risk pregnancies* (5th ed.). Hoboken, NJ, 2010, Wiley-Blackwell, pp. 92–98.

National Institutes of Health: Dietary supplement fact sheet: calcium. 2013. Retrieved from http://ods.od.nih.gov/factsheets/Calcium-HealthProfessional/.

Pettker, C. and Lockwood, C.J.: Thromboembolic disorders. In S.G. Gabbe, J.R. Niebyl, and J.L. Simpson (Eds.): *Obstetrics: Normal and problem pregnancies* (6th ed.). Philadelphia, 2012, Elsevier Saunders, pp. 980–983.

Pillitteri, A.: *Maternal and child health nursing: Care of the childbearing and childrearing family* (6th ed.). Philadelphia, 2010, Lippincott Williams & Wilkins.

Platt, L.: Routine and prenatal screening. In J.R. Queenan, J.C. Hobbins, and C.Y. Spong (Eds.): *Protocols for high-risk pregnancies* (5th ed.). Hoboken, NJ, 2005, Wiley-Blackwell, pp. 43–52.

Richards, D.S.: Obstetrical ultrasound: Imaging, dating, and growth. In S.G. Gabbe, J.R. Niebyl, and J.L. Simpson (Eds.): *Obstetrics: Normal and problem pregnancies* (6th ed.). Philadelphia, 2012, Elsevier Saunders, pp. 166–192.

Roberts, J. and Hanson, L.: Best practices in second stage labor care: Maternal bearing down and positioning. *Journal of Midwifery and Women's Health*, 52:238–245, 2007.

Ross, M.G., and Desai, M.: Developmental origins of adult health and disease. In S.G. Gabbe, J.R. Niebyl, and J.L. Simpson (Eds.): *Obstetrics: Normal and problem pregnancies* (6th ed.). Philadelphia, 2012, Elsevier Saunders, pp. 83–98.

Simpson, J.L., Richards, D.S., Otaño, L., et al.: Prenatal genetic diagnosis. In S.G. Gabbe, J.R. Niebyl, and J.L. Simpson (Eds.): *Obstetrics: Normal and problem pregnancies* (6th ed.). Philadelphia, 2012, Elsevier Saunders, pp. 211–236.

Thureen, P., Davies, J., LeBel, A., et al.: Maternal factors affecting the newborn. In P.J. Thureen, J. Deacon, J. Hernandez, and D. Hall (Eds.): *Assessment and care of the well newborn* (2nd ed.). St. Louis, 2005, W.B. Saunders, pp. 3–26.

U.S. Preventive Services Task Force: Folic acid for the prevention of neural tube defects: U.S. Preventive Services Task Force recommendation statement. *Annals of Internal Medicine*, 150(9):626–631, 2009.

Varney, H., Kriebs, J., and Gegor, C.: *Varney's midwifery* (4th ed.). Boston, 2004, Jones & Bartlett.

CHAPTER

# 2 Antepartum–Intrapartum Complications

HELEN M. HURST

**OBJECTIVES**

1. List maternal risk factors that may exist before pregnancy.
2. Discuss the effects of hypertension and diabetes on the maternal–placental–fetal complex.
3. Categorize intrapartum conditions that may result in complications for the newborn infant.
4. Assess the fetus/neonate for effects of tocolytic drugs.
5. Describe the effect on the fetus/neonate of select intrapartum crises: placental abruption, placenta previa, cord prolapse, and shoulder dystocia.
6. List neonatal complications associated with breech delivery.
7. Examine the effect of obstetric analgesia/anesthesia and cesarean birth on the newborn infant.

An understanding of maternal complications enhances the ability of the nurse to anticipate and recognize neonatal complications and intervene appropriately. The purpose of this chapter is to provide a comprehensive review of possible neonatal complications resulting from maternal risk factors. These risk factors may exist before the pregnancy or develop during the antepartum and intrapartum periods (Table 2-1).

## ANATOMY AND PHYSIOLOGY

A. **The fetus.** The fetus is a part of the maternal–placental–fetal complex.
B. **Conditions and substances that affect the pregnant woman.** These have the potential to affect placental functions of respiration, nutrition, excretion, and hormone production. Decreased placental function can in turn adversely affect the fetus.
C. **The placenta.** The placenta is the connection between the maternal and embryonic circulatory systems, facilitating metabolic and nutrient exchange. Functions of the placenta include fetal nutrition, respiration, and excretion. Placental development begins at implantation and the placenta becomes a discrete organ by 14 weeks of gestation (London et al., 2011).
D. **Placental transport mechanisms.** These mechanisms, including passive and facilitated diffusion, are affected by a number of factors (Baschat, 2011; Burton et al., 2012; Ross et al., 2012).
   1. Placental area.
      a. To supply the increased growth needs of the fetus, the placenta normally increases in size as the pregnancy advances.
      b. A placenta that is not keeping pace with fetal growth or that has decreased functional area as a result of infarct or separation does not allow optimal transport of materials between the fetus and the mother.
      c. The outcome of decreased functional placental area can include a decrease in fetal growth, fetal or neonatal distress, and even fetal or neonatal death.
   2. Concentration gradient.
      a. Passive and facilitated diffusion of unbound substances dissolved in maternal and fetal plasma occurs in the direction of lesser concentration.

■ TABLE 2-1
■ ■ **Prenatal High-Risk Factors**

| Factor | Maternal Implications | Fetal/Neonatal Implications |
|---|---|---|
| **SOCIAL-PERSONAL** | | |
| Low income level and/or low educational level | Insufficient or later antenatal care<br>↑ Risk preterm birth<br>Poor nutrition<br>↑ Risk preeclampsia | Low birth weight<br>Prematurity<br>Intrauterine growth restriction (IUGR)/ small for gestational age (SGA) |
| Poor diet | ↑ Inadequate nutrition/Inadequate weight gain<br>↑ Risk of preterm labor/birth<br>↑ Risk anemia<br>↑ Risk preeclampsia | Fetal malnutrition<br>Prematurity<br>IUGR/SGA |
| Living at high altitude | ↑ Hemoglobin | Prematurity<br>IUGR<br>↑ Hemoglobin (polycythemia) |
| Multiparity greater than 3 | ↑ Risk antepartum/postpartum hemorrhage | Anemia<br>Fetal death |
| Weight less than 45.5 kg (100 lb) | Poor nutrition<br>Cephalopelvic disproportion<br>Prolonged labor | IUGR<br>Hypoxia associated with difficult labor and birth |
| Weight more than 91 kg (200 lb) | ↑ Risk hypertension<br>↑ Risk cephalopelvic disproportion<br>↑ Risk diabetes | ↓ Fetal nutrition/perfusion<br>↑ Risk macrosomia |
| Age less than 16 years | Poor nutrition<br>Insufficient/late antenatal care<br>↑ Risk preeclampsia<br>↑ Risk cephalopelvic disproportion | Low birth weight<br>↑ Fetal demise |
| Age greater than 35 years | ↑ Risk preeclampsia<br>↑ Risk cesarean birth<br>Psychosocial issues | ↑ Risk congenital anomalies<br>↑ Chromosomal abnormalities |
| Smoking 1 pack per day/more | ↑ Risk hypertension<br>↑ Risk cancer | ↓ Placental perfusion<br>↓ $O_2$ and nutrients available<br>Low birth weight<br>IUGR<br>Preterm birth |
| Use of addicting drugs | ↑ Risk poor nutrition<br>↑ Risk infection with intravenous (IV) drugs<br>↑ Risk HIV, hepatitis C<br>↑ Risk abruptio placentae | ↑ Risk congenital anomalies<br>↑ Risk low birth weight<br>Neonatal withdrawal<br>Lower serum bilirubin |
| Excessive alcohol consumption | ↑ Risk poor nutrition<br>Possible hepatic effects with long-term consumption | ↑ Risk fetal alcohol syndrome (FAS) |
| **PREEXISTING MEDICAL DISORDERS** | | |
| Diabetes mellitus | ↑ Risk preeclampsia, hypertension<br>Episodes of hypoglycemia and hyperglycemia<br>↑ Risk cesarean birth | Low birth weight<br>Macrosomia<br>Neonatal hypoglycemia<br>↑ Risk congenital anomalies<br>↑ Risk respiratory distress syndrome |
| Cardiac disease | Cardiac decompensation<br>Further strain on mother's body<br>↑ Maternal death rate | ↑ Risk fetal death<br>↑ Perinatal mortality |

■ TABLE 2-1
■ ■ **Prenatal High-Risk Factors—cont'd**

| Factor | Maternal Implications | Fetal/Neonatal Implications |
|---|---|---|
| Anemia: Less than 11 g/dL hemoglobin, less than 32% hematocrit | Iron-deficiency anemia<br>Low energy level<br>Decreased oxygen-carrying capacity | Fetal death<br>Prematurity<br>Low birth weight |
| Hypertension | ↑ Vasospasm<br>↑ Risk of central nervous system (CNS) irritability<br>↑ Risk seizures<br>↑ Risk cerebrovascular accident (CVA)<br>↑ Risk renal damage | ↓ Placental perfusion<br>→ Low birth weight<br>Preterm birth |
| Thyroid disorder | ↑ Infertility | ↑ Spontaneous abortion |
| Hypothyroidism | ↓ Basal metabolic rate (BMR), goiter, myxedema | ↑ Risk congenital goiter |
| Hyperthyroidism | ↑ Risk miscarriage<br>↑ Preterm labor/birth<br>↑ Risk postpartum hemorrhage<br>↑ Risk preeclampsia<br>Danger of thyroid storm | ↑ IUGR/SGA<br>↑ Anemia<br>↑ Risk stillbirth<br>Mental retardation → cretinism<br>↑ Incidence congenital anomalies<br>↑ IUGR/SGA<br>↑ Risk neonatal hyperthyroidism |
| Renal disease (moderate to severe) | ↑ Risk renal failure | ↑ Risk IUGR/SGA<br>↑ Risk preterm birth |
| Diethylstilbestrol (DES) exposure | ↑ Infertility, spontaneous abortion<br>↑ Cervical incompetence<br>↑ Risk breech presentation | ↑ Risk preterm birth |
| **OBSTETRIC CONSIDERATIONS** | | |
| PREVIOUS PREGNANCY | | |
| Stillborn | ↑ Emotional/psychologic distress | ↑ Risk IUGR/SGA<br>↑ Risk preterm birth |
| Habitual abortion | ↑ Emotional/psychologic distress | ↑ Risk abortion |
| Cesarean birth | ↑ Possibility repeat cesarean birth<br>↑ Risk of uterine rupture | ↑ Risk preterm birth<br>↑ Risk respiratory distress |
| Rh or blood group sensitization | | Hydrops fetalis<br>Icterus gravis<br>Neonatal anemia<br>Kernicterus<br>Hypoglycemia |
| CURRENT PREGNANCY | | |
| Large for gestational age (LGA) | ↑ Risk cesarean birth<br>↑ Risk gestational diabetes<br>↑ Risk instrument assisted birth<br>↑ Risk preeclampsia<br>↑ Risk extensive lacerations<br>↑ Risk primary pulmonary hypertension (PPH)<br>↑ Risk shoulder dystocia | ↑ Risk birth injury<br>Hypoglycemia<br>Macrosomia<br>Hyperbilirubinemia<br>↑ Risk birth injury |
| Rubella (first trimester) | | Congenital heart disease<br>Cataracts<br>Nerve deafness<br>Bone lesions<br>Prolonged virus shedding |
| Rubella (second trimester) | | Hepatitis<br>Thrombocytopenia |

*Continued*

■ TABLE 2-1
■ ■ **Prenatal High-Risk Factors—cont'd**

| Factor | Maternal Implications | Fetal/Neonatal Implications |
|---|---|---|
| Cytomegalovirus | | IUGR<br>Encephalopathy |
| Herpesvirus type 2 | Severe discomfort<br>Concern about possibility of cesarean birth, fetal infection | Neonatal herpesvirus type 2<br>Hepatitis with jaundice<br>Neurologic abnormalities |
| Syphilis | ↑ Incidence abortion | ↑ Fetal demise<br>Congenital syphilis |
| Urinary tract infection | ↑ Risk preterm labor<br>Uterine irritability | ↑ Risk preterm birth |
| Abruptio placentae and placenta previa | ↑ Risk hemorrhage<br>Bed rest<br>Extended hospitalization<br>Pulmonary embolus | Fetal/neonatal anemia<br>Intrauterine hemorrhage<br>↑ Fetal demise |
| Preeclampsia/eclampsia | *See* Hypertension | ↓ Placental perfusion<br>→ Low birth weight |
| Multiple gestation | ↑ Risk postpartum hemorrhage<br>↑ Risk gestational diabetes<br>↑ Risk preeclampsia<br>↑ Risk placenta previa | ↑ Risk preterm birth<br>↑ Risk stillbirth<br>↑ Risk fetal demise<br>↑ Risk IUGR/SGA<br>↑ Risk malpresentation |
| Elevated hematocrit (greater than 41%) | Increased viscosity of blood | Fetal death rate 5 times normal rate |
| Spontaneous premature rupture of membranes | ↑ Uterine infection | Preterm birth<br>Fetal demise<br>Fetal/neonatal sepsis |

From Davidson, M.R., London, M.L., and Ladewig, P.A.: *Olds' Maternal-newborn nursing & women's health across the lifespan* (9th ed.). Boston, 2012, Pearson Prentice Hall, pp. 321-322.

**b.** The greater the concentration gradient, the faster will be the rate of diffusion.

**c.** Concentration gradients are maintained when dissolved substances are removed from the plasma by metabolism, cellular uptake, or excretion. For example, the excretion of $CO_2$ from the maternal lungs maintains the concentration gradient for $CO_2$, permitting fetal plasma $CO_2$ to cross from fetal plasma to maternal plasma. Inefficient maternal excretion of $CO_2$ may lead to maternal respiratory acidosis and fetal acidosis.

**3.** Diffusing distance.

**a.** The greater the distance between maternal and fetal blood in the placenta, the slower will be the diffusion rate of substances.

**b.** Any edema that develops in the placental villi increases the distance between the fetal capillaries within the villi and the maternal arterial blood in the intervillous spaces, thus slowing the diffusion rate of substances between the maternal and fetal circulations.

**c.** Edema of villi may occur in:

(1) Maternal diabetes.
(2) Transplacental infections.
(3) Erythroblastosis fetalis.
(4) Twin-to-twin transfusion syndrome (donor twin).
(5) Fetal congestive heart failure.

**d.** Thinning of the placental membrane in the second half of pregnancy decreases diffusing distance, thus increasing the functional efficiency of the placenta. However, this change also facilitates the passage of drugs in pregnancy and the intrapartum period.

**4.** Uteroplacental blood flow.

**a.** At term, uterine blood flow is 750 mL/min or more, representing 10% to 15% of the maternal cardiac output.

b. Decreased blood flow to the uterus or within the intervillous spaces will decrease the transport of substances to and from the fetus.
c. Causes of decreased uteroplacental blood flow include:
(1) Maternal vasoconstriction in hypertension, cocaine abuse, diabetic vasculopathy, and smoking.
(2) Maternal vasodilatation caused by vasodilators, antihypertensives, and regional anesthetics with sympathetic blockade actions.
(3) Decreased maternal cardiac output in supine hypotension.
(4) Decreased maternal blood flow in intervillous spaces resulting from edema of the placental villi.
(5) Tachysystole (>5 contractions in 10 minutes, averaged over 30 minutes) (American College of Obstetricians and Gynecologists [ACOG], 2010).
(6) Increased uterine resting tone.
(7) Severe maternal physical stress.
(8) Degenerative placental changes near term.

5. Fetal factors.
a. Fetal tachycardia, often seen with fetal hypoxia, is analogous to an adult's "blowing off $CO_2$"; the increased heart rate increases the delivery of $CO_2$ to the placenta for diffusion to the maternal circulation. Fetal tachycardia represents a chronic decrease in oxygen.
b. Conversely, fetal bradycardia resulting from hypoxia or anoxia leads to an increased $CO_2$ level. Fetal bradycardia, in the absence of congenital heart disease, represents an acute decrease in oxygen.
c. Umbilical cord compression leads to $CO_2$ accumulation and acidosis.
d. Fetal pH during labor is usually 0.1 to 0.15 unit less than the maternal pH; this difference increases the transport of acidophilic substances from the mother to the fetus and reduces albumin binding of drugs, resulting in a more free drug in the fetal bloodstream.

## CONDITIONS RELATED TO THE ANTEPARTUM PERIOD

### Preeclampsia and Eclampsia (Sibai, 2012; Dekker, 2011)

Hypertensive disorders in pregnancy, including gestational hypertension, preeclampsia and eclampsia, chronic hypertension, and chronic hypertension with superimposed preeclampsia, are a major cause of maternal–fetal morbidity and death in the United States. The main pathophysiologic events in preeclampsia are vasospasm, hematologic changes, and endothelial damage, leading to tissue hypoxia and multiple organ involvement.

A. **Incidence:** The incidence of hypertensive disorders is 5% to 10% of all pregnancies, with the incidence of preeclampsia at 5% to 8% of all pregnancies.

B. **Etiology/predisposing factors (Sibai, 2012; Dekker, 2011).**
1. The exact cause of preeclampsia and eclampsia has not been determined, although current theories involve an immunologic basis, genetic conflict, endothelial cell activation, abnormal trophoblast invasion, alterations in coagulation, damage to vascular endothelium, maternal predisposition, and cardiovascular maladaptation.
2. Preeclampsia and eclampsia are associated with nulliparity, extremes of maternal age (teenagers and age >40 years), family history of preeclampsia, preeclampsia in a previous pregnancy, obesity, maternal low birth weight, chronic inflammatory conditions (lupus, rheumatologic disease), a history of gestational diabetes or type 1 diabetes mellitus, chronic hypertensive or renal disease, thrombophilias (factor V Leiden mutation, antiphospholipid syndrome), multifetal gestation, or large fetus. Other predisposing factors include poor outcomes in a previous pregnancy such as placental abruption, fetal death, and intrauterine growth restriction (IUGR) in previous pregnancies.

C. **Clinical presentation.**
1. A blood pressure (BP) of 140/90 mm Hg or above after 20 weeks of gestation. Severe preeclampsia is characterized by a BP of 160/110 mm Hg or above. BP measurements must be on at least two occasions, 6 hours apart with the patient on bed rest.

2. Proteinuria (≥300 mg/dL in a 24-hour urine collection) due to decreased renal perfusion resulting in the development of glomerular capillary endotheliosis.
3. Edema is no longer considered to be a relevant factor in the diagnosis of preeclampsia, as one third of preeclamptic patients may not exhibit edema. However, if a pregnant woman demonstrates a rapid increase in generalized edema, she should be screened for preeclampsia (Dekker, 2011).
4. Other signs and symptoms: headache, hyperreflexia with clonus, visual and retinal changes, irritability, nausea and vomiting, epigastric pain, dyspnea, and oliguria.

**D. Potential complications.**

1. Maternal.
   a. Eclampsia (grand mal seizure).
   b. Cardiopulmonary failure and pulmonary edema.
   c. Hepatic failure, hemorrhage or rupture.
   d. Cerebrovascular accident.
   e. Renal cortical necrosis.
   f. Disseminated intravascular coagulation.
   g. HELLP syndrome (i.e., *h*emolysis, *e*levated *l*iver function test results, and *l*ow *p*latelet count).
   h. Retinal detachment.
   i. Stroke or death (rare).
   j. Long-term cardiovascular morbidity.
2. Placental/fetal.
   a. Premature placental aging, placental infarction, and decrease in amniotic fluid.
   b. Abruptio placentae in 1% to 4% of cases, depending upon the severity of the disease (Dekker, 2011).
   c. Fetal growth restriction (10% to 25%).
   d. Fetal hypoxia and neurologic injury (<1%).
   e. Prematurity (15% to 67%).

**E. Assessment and management (Dekker, 2011; Sibai, 2012).**

1. Severe preeclampsia.
   a. Primary goals of management include prevention of seizures (via limitation of stimuli and drug therapy), prevention of complications (via frequent systems assessments and laboratory studies), and birth of a live infant. Due to the increased risk of maternal morbidity and mortality, and the inherent risks to the fetus, there is a general consensus to deliver the baby if severe preeclampsia presents after 34 weeks of gestation.
   b. Seizure precautions.
   c. Placental–fetal function tests: continuous electronic fetal monitoring; fetal movement; ultrasonography to determine fetal age and detect IUGR; serial nonstress tests, biophysical profile, and/or umbilical artery Doppler studies; and amniocentesis to determine fetal lung maturity.
   d. Medications.
      (1) Use of intravenous (IV) magnesium sulfate as a central nervous system (CNS) depressant to prevent seizures. A transient decrease in BP often occurs. Observe fetal heart rate for decreased variability, and anticipate hypotonus in the newborn. Therapy is continued for at least 24 hours postpartum.
      (2) Use of antihypertensives is indicated when systolic BPs are greater than 160 mm Hg or diastolic BPs are greater than 110 mm Hg:
         (a) Labetalol hydrochloride. Decreases peripheral vascular resistance and, therefore, increases uteroplacental perfusion. Observe the fetal heart rate for transient bradycardia. Contraindicated in patients with bradycardia, moderate to severe asthma, and congestive heart failure.
         (b) Hydralazine (Apresoline). Should no longer be considered a first-line drug. Although effective in lowering BP, this drug has many side effects and alternative medications are preferred. Observe fetal heart rate for signs of hypoxia (tachycardia, bradycardia, or late decelerations), which can occur with a sudden decrease in maternal BP.

(3) Use of corticosteroids to increase fetal lung maturity when birth can be delayed for 24 to 48 hours and the woman is at less than 34 weeks of gestation. Infants born to mothers who are treated with antenatal steroid therapy are at decreased risk for respiratory distress syndrome, cerebrovascular hemorrhage, and death.

**e.** Delivery.

(1) The decision for delivery is based on gestational age and condition of the fetus, cervical Bishop score, presence of labor, and the presence or absence of fetal growth restriction or oligohydramnios.

(2) Severe preeclampsia is not an indication for cesarean section, and the vaginal route is preferred.

**2.** Eclampsia (Dekker, 2011; Sibai, 2012).

**a.** Immediate notification of physician or midwife.

**b.** Control of current seizure and prevention of recurrent seizures with administration of IV magnesium sulfate.

**c.** Control of severe hypertension with an antihypertensive (labetalol) to maintain the systolic BP between 140 and 160 mm Hg and the diastolic BP between 90 and 105 mm Hg.

**d.** Safety measures for woman during and after seizures to prevent injury.

**e.** Support of respirations with airway, oxygen, and suctioning, and the correction of hypoxemia and/or acidemia.

**f.** Observe fetal heart rate for transient bradycardia, rebound tachycardia, decreased variability, and late decelerations.

**g.** Continuous maternal assessment, including assessment for uterine contractions and signs of placental abruption.

**h.** Laboratory work: complete blood count (CBC), clot observation, serum creatinine, liver function tests, fibrinogen, arterial blood gases, and electrolytes.

**i.** Initiate the process of delivery according to the status of the maternal–placental–fetal complex. The mother must be stabilized before a cesarean section is performed.

**j.** Maternal emotional support.

**3.** Assessment of newborn infant for the following:

**a.** IUGR.

**b.** Preterm gestational age.

**c.** Hypoxia and acidosis.

**d.** Possible adverse drug effects on neonate:

(1) When maternal administration of high doses of magnesium sulfate occurs near the time of birth, the newborn must be observed for 24 to 48 hours for signs of magnesium toxicity (respiratory depression and neuromuscular depression, as evidenced by weakness, lethargy, hypotonia, flaccidity, and poor suck) (Davidson et al., 2012).

(2) Hypotension, bradycardia, hypoglycemia, respiratory depression, and transient tachypnea, with maternal administration of labetalol.

## Diabetes Mellitus (ACOG, 2011; Landon et al., 2012)

Women with insulin-dependent diabetes who become pregnant, and pregnant women in whom gestational diabetes mellitus (GDM) or type 1 diabetes develops, are at risk during the antepartum period due to altered carbohydrate metabolism. Therefore, the fetus/neonate is also at risk. Optimal control of maternal blood glucose concentration and anticipatory management of the newborn infant are important elements of perinatal care.

**A. Incidence:** 3% to 5% of all pregnancies are complicated by diabetes mellitus and 7% by GDM.

**B. Etiology and predisposing factors in gestational diabetes.**

**1.** In the second half of pregnancy, the secretion of human placental lactogen and lactogen increases cellular resistance to insulin. Additionally, cortisol and glycogen levels increase. The pancreas of the woman who is predisposed to diabetes cannot meet the increased demand for insulin, which leads to hyperglycemia.

**2.** Risk factors for GDM include maternal obesity, previous history of gestational diabetes, a family history of diabetes, age greater than 25 years, member of an ethnic group at risk for diabetes (Native North American, Hispanic, African American, Pacific Islanders, and

South or East Asian Americans), and prior obstetric history (infant weighing >4500 g, congenital anomaly, stillbirth, hydramnios).

C. **Clinical presentation and screening for gestational diabetes.**
   1. The American College of Obstetricians and Gynecologists recommends that all pregnant women be screened for gestational diabetes either by patient history, clinical risk factors, or a 50-g 1-hour glucose challenge test at 24 to 28 weeks of gestation.
   2. Women at high risk for GDM (severe obesity, strong family history of type 2 diabetes mellitus, previous history of gestational diabetes, impaired glucose metabolism, or glycosuria) should be screened at the first prenatal visit, because GDM may be asymptomatic or evidenced only by subtle changes. Screening should be repeated at 24 to 28 weeks of gestation, or when hyperglycemia is evident.
   3. Women with average risk for GDM should be screened with a 1-hour glucose challenge test at 24 to 28 weeks of gestation, with further testing if values are abnormal.
   4. Women who are low risk for GDM (ethnic group with a low prevalence of GDM, no known primary relative with diabetes mellitus, age <25 years, normal weight prior to pregnancy, no history of poor obstetric outcomes, no history of abnormal glucose metabolism) may not require glucose screening.

D. **Potential complications.**
   1. Maternal.
      a. Hypoglycemic reactions in the first trimester.
      b. Ketoacidosis in the second and third trimesters.
      c. Progression of vasculopathy, nephropathy, and retinopathy with preexisting diabetes.
      d. Hydramnios.
      e. Gestational hypertension and preeclampsia.
      f. Anemia.
      g. Infections such as monilial vaginitis and urinary tract infections.
      h. Increased rates of episiotomy, perineal tears, and cesarean section (Perry et al., 2010).
   2. Fetal/neonatal: Outcomes can be improved via careful attention to prepregnancy and pregnancy glycemic control.
      a. Macrosomia (weight >4000 g) with possible traumatic vaginal birth, such as with shoulder dystocia, and subsequent birth trauma. IUGR when the mother has vascular disease (Davidson et al., 2012).
      b. Fetal death.
      c. Respiratory distress syndrome.
      d. Hypoglycemia, hypocalcemia, and hypomagnesemia.
      e. Polycythemia, hyperviscosity, and hyperbilirubinemia.
      f. Cardiomyopathy with congestive heart failure.
      g. Congenital anomalies as a consequence of poorly controlled preexisting diabetes may include anencephaly, open spina bifida, holoprosencephaly, ventricular septal defects, transposition of the great vessels, sacral agenesis, or caudal dysplasia. Currently, 30% to 50% of perinatal mortality results from congenital anomalies in pregnancies in which the mother has type 1 or type 2 diabetes.

E. **Assessment and management.**
   1. In preexisting diabetes:
      a. Preconception counseling is recommended, with optimal control of blood glucose levels. Insulin is considered the therapy of choice, but oral hypoglycemics are now offered as a suitable alternative for women who cannot, or who prefer not to, take insulin. Both glyburide and metformin are being utilized in the pregnant woman; glyburide is considered superior to metformin as it does not cross the placenta and there is a decreased incidence of neonatal hypoglycemia. Although metformin crosses the placenta, there is no evidence that it is teratogenic, but women may also need insulin supplementation. The woman should begin taking 0.4 mg of folic acid daily, and continue through the first trimester, to reduce the risk for neural tube defects.
      b. Glycosylated hemoglobin tests may be performed before conception and during the pregnancy to assess glucose control during the previous 1 to 2 months, with an acceptable hemoglobin $A_{1c}$ goal of 5% to 6%.

c. Home blood glucose monitoring, diet, exercise, and either insulin pump therapy or several daily injections of insulin are prescribed to maintain euglycemia (60 to 120 mg/dL). Optimal control is associated with a decreased risk of macrosomia, respiratory distress syndrome, congenital anomalies, and perinatal death, as well as maternal urinary tract infection and preterm labor.
d. Women are evaluated early in pregnancy for evidence of diabetic retinopathy and nephropathy.
e. In the first trimester, screening for nuchal translucency, free β-human chorionic gonadotropin (β-hCG) and pregnancy-associated plasma protein A (PAPP-A) should be offered (Fraser and Farrell, 2011).
f. At 16 weeks of gestation, the woman should be offered maternal serum α-fetoprotein (MSAFP) testing, accompanied by a comprehensive ultrasound at 18 to 21 weeks to assess for the presence of neural tube defects or other anomalies. An alternative choice of testing may be the triple screen (MSAFP, maternal serum unconjugated estriol, and β-hCG) or the quad test, which includes inhibin A in addition to the three elements of the triple screen (Fraser and Farrell, 2011). Ultrasounds for fetal growth should be performed monthly between 28 and 36 weeks of gestation. Fetal and Doppler umbilical artery velocimetry is also recommended.
g. Weekly prenatal visits are made after 28 weeks, with fetal assessment by means of nonstress tests, biophysical profiles, and daily fetal movement counting.
h. Timing and mode of delivery are based upon the clinical picture of both the woman and the fetus, and some evidence suggests delivery at 38 weeks of gestation. Birth should take place in a facility with a neonatal intensive care unit (NICU).
i. Insulin may be given intravenously during labor to maintain blood glucose between 70 and 90 mg/dL. Glucose levels are monitored hourly to ensure optimum titration of insulin in order to decrease the risk of neonatal rebound hypoglycemia.
j. Before any decision is made about induction of labor, amniocentesis is performed to determine the lecithin/sphingomyelin ratio and the presence of phosphatidylglycerol. Delivery is accomplished before term if maternal or fetal complications develop.

2. In gestational diabetes:
   a. A 2000- to 2500-calorie American Diabetes Association diet comprising 50% to 60% complex carbohydrates is recommended;
   b. Self-monitoring of blood glucose is encouraged, with fasting and 2-hour postprandial glucose levels checked regularly; and
   c. Nonstress testing begins at 28 to 32 weeks of gestation.
3. In the neonate:
   a. Assess for gestational age and size (large for gestational age or IUGR).
   b. Assess for:
      (1) Respiratory distress;
      (2) Hypoglycemia, hypocalcemia, and hypomagnesemia;
      (3) Polycythemia and hyperviscosity;
      (4) Complications resulting from decreased blood flow, erythrocyte hemolysis, and thrombosis;
      (5) Congenital malformations; and
      (6) Birth injuries: fractured clavicles, intracranial bleeding, facial nerve paralysis, brachial palsy, and skull fractures.

## CONDITIONS RELATED TO THE INTRAPARTUM PERIOD

### Preterm Labor (Svigos et al., 2011; Simhan et al., 2012)

Preterm labor is labor occurring at greater than 20 and before 37 completed weeks of gestation. Preterm labor is defined as the presence of uterine contractions and documented cervical change. Threatened preterm labor is defined as the presence of uterine contractions without cervical change. The prognosis for the fetus improves with each week of pregnancy gained.

A. **Incidence:** In 2012, 11.7% of live births in the United States were preterm, and complications from prematurity are the leading cause of perinatal death (March of Dimes, 2012b).

**B. Etiology/predisposing factors.**

1. The exact cause of preterm labor is unknown, although chorioamnionitis and other infections such as periodontitis and bacterial vaginosis have been implicated.
2. A number of maternal factors have been associated with an increased incidence of preterm labor: maternal age (<15 or >35 years), socioeconomic effects (lower socioeconomic status or educational level, African American race, poor nutrition, inadequate prenatal care), medical/obstetric history (use of assisted reproductive technologies, anemia, preexisting or gestational hypertension or diabetes, previous preterm birth, prior stillbirth, grand multiparity, one or more midtrimester pregnancy losses, pregnancy termination, short interpregnancy interval, uterine anomalies and cervical insufficiency, systemic and genitourinary tract infections, hydramnios, immunologic factors, placental abruption, and placenta previa), and lifestyle factors (use of alcohol, cigarettes, and illicit drugs such as cocaine, and domestic violence or other stressors) (Perry et al., 2010).
3. Fetal factors contributing to the development of preterm labor may include fetal congenital anomalies and complications from multifetal gestation (Perry et al., 2010).
4. Risk scoring systems, designed to screen women during pregnancy, have a predictive value of only 17% to 34%. Many women who give birth before term do not have any known risk factors.

**C. Clinical presentation.**

1. Painless or painful persistent uterine contractions.
2. Low, dull, intermittent, or constant backache.
3. Intermittent or constant menstrual-like cramping.
4. Pelvic pressure.
5. Abdominal cramps, which may be accompanied by diarrhea.
6. Increased vaginal discharge, which may be mucoid, watery, or slightly bloody.
7. Spontaneous premature rupture of membranes.
8. A generalized feeling that something is wrong.
9. Progressive cervical effacement and dilatation.
   a. Cervix >3 cm dilatation/≥80% effaced: Preterm labor diagnosis is confirmed.
   b. Cervix 2 to 3 cm dilatation/<80% effaced: Preterm labor likely but not established.
   c. Cervix <2 cm dilatation/<80% effaced: Diagnosis uncertain.

**D. Potential complications.**

1. Maternal.
   a. Side effects from tocolytic agents.
   b. Emotional stress and financial issues.
   c. Complications from the mode of delivery, especially when a cesarean section is performed at less than 30 to 32 weeks of gestation as the lower uterine segment is poorly developed; there is a greater chance of infection, hemorrhage, and subsequent poor uterine function.
2. Fetal/neonatal.
   a. Preterm birth with an increase in neonatal morbidity and death.
   b. Risks associated with prematurity, such as respiratory distress syndrome, necrotizing enterocolitis, intracranial hemorrhage, seizures, septicemia, and sequelae of IUGR.
   c. Side effects from pharmacotherapeutics (tocolytic agents, antibiotics, corticosteroids).

**E. Assessment and management.**

1. Assessment of risk should be performed at the first and subsequent prenatal visits for preterm labor risk factors.
2. Patient education should be provided to all pregnant women, including the symptoms of preterm labor and the actions to take if they occur (lie down on the left side and drink several glasses of fluid; report to the physician or midwife if contractions are still occurring after 1 hour).
3. Helping high-risk women modify their risk factors and take measures to prevent preterm labor (e.g., stop smoking, improve nutrition and hydration, treat infections, decrease work hours and stress, increase rest, and avoid nipple preparation or sexual activity that may initiate signs of preterm labor).

4. Although regular cervical examinations and ultrasonographic evaluation of the cervix are being performed by some providers, these methods have not been validated as predictors of preterm birth.
5. The use of the fetal fibronectin test, performed on vaginal secretions in symptomatic women, may help prevent a false-positive diagnosis of preterm labor and prevent unnecessary and potentially harmful pharmacologic treatment.
6. ACOG and the Society for Maternal Fetal Medicine recommend that women with a singleton pregnancy, who have had a previous episode of a singleton spontaneous preterm labor or birth, or premature rupture of membranes, should receive progesterone supplementation (17α-hydroxyprogesterone caproate) (ACOG, 2008). Studies indicate a 40% decrease in the preterm birth rate of women who had a previous preterm birth, when given 17α-hydroxyprogesterone caproate.
7. Although episodes of suspected preterm labor are widely treated with bed rest, hydration, and pelvic rest, there is little evidence that these interventions are effective (Davidson et al., 2012). Antenatal corticosteroid therapy is recommended for women at risk for preterm birth who are between 24 and 34 weeks of gestation, to reduce the incidence of neonatal morbidity and death from respiratory distress syndrome and intraventricular hemorrhage.
8. When appropriate and not contraindicated, tocolytics should be used to allow enough time for antenatal corticosteroid therapy to benefit the fetus and/or for transfer of the mother to a hospital with a level III nursery.
   a. Nifedipine (Procardia), a calcium channel blocker given orally, is the primary choice for tocolysis because of its ease of administration and few maternal–fetal side effects. It is contraindicated in cardiac disease, hypertension, and intrauterine infection, and should not be administered concurrently with magnesium sulfate and β-mimetics.
   b. Magnesium sulfate, given intravenously before 32 weeks of gestation, appears to have a neuroprotective effect and may decrease the incidence of cerebral palsy. It is recommended that its use be limited to between 24 and 32 weeks of gestation. Data do not support the use of this drug as a tocolytic, and research has not demonstrated that its use prolongs pregnancy. When maternal administration of high doses of magnesium sulfate occurs near the time of birth, the neonate should be monitored for respiratory depression, and neuromuscular depression, as evidenced by weakness, lethargy, hypotonia, flaccidity, and poor suck.
   c. Prostaglandins (indomethacin) mediate contractions and are effective as tocolytics. Indomethacin is given prior to 32 weeks, orally, and use is restricted to 2 to 3 days. Maternal side effects include nausea, vomiting and dyspepsia. Contraindications to its use include fetal renal anomalies, oligohydramnios, IUGR, chorioamnionitis, ductal-dependent cardiac defects, and twin-to-twin transfusion syndrome. Fetal side effects include oligohydramnios, constriction of the ductus arteriosus, and neonatal pulmonary hypertension.
   d. Terbutaline (Brethine), a β-mimetic, has commonly been used as a tocolytic, but due to potential side effects its use should be limited to a single 0.25-mg dose subcutaneously. This may be used while a therapy with a slower onset of action is being started, or to stop contractions during the initial evaluation of the patient to assist in the diagnosis of preterm labor. Data indicate that there are few side effects for a single dose.
9. Antibiotic therapy should be instituted to prevent neonatal group B streptococcal infection, or to treat specific conditions such as urinary tract infections.
10. If the measures noted above are not successful, and the cervix continues to efface and dilate, the following measures are important:
    a. To allow the amniotic fluid to cushion the fetal skull, no rupture of the membranes is performed until close to delivery.
    b. The head is delivered in a slow, controlled fashion.
    c. Cesarean delivery is often suggested for the preterm fetus with a breech presentation because of the risk of cord prolapse and the potential risk of difficult birth of the head. There is no justification for elective cesarean delivery of all preterm infants.

## Abruptio Placentae

In abruptio placentae, the placenta separates suddenly, prematurely, and in varying degrees from the uterine wall during pregnancy or labor. It is a common cause of bleeding in the second half of pregnancy.

A. **Incidence:** Placental abruption occurs in 1 in 100 pregnancies (March of Dimes, 2013). One third of all bleeding in pregnancy results from placental abruption (Francois and Foley, 2012).
B. **Etiology/predisposing factors.**
   1. Although the cause of placental abruption has not been definitively established, there is a high correlation with hypertensive disorders during pregnancy, history of previous abruption, cocaine use, trauma, and placental abnormalities (circumvallate). Additional risk factors include uterine fibroids or malformations, rapid uterine decompression associated with polyhydramnios and multifetal pregnancy, increased parity, chorioamnionitis and intrauterine infections, inherited or acquired thrombophilias, preterm premature rupture of membranes, and maternal cigarette smoking (Francois and Foley, 2012).
C. **Clinical presentation (Francois and Foley, 2012; Murray and McKinney, 2010).**
   1. Maternal signs and symptoms.
      a. Dark or bright red vaginal bleeding, ranging from spotting to frank hemorrhage. In 20% to 30% of patients with abruption, there is no visible evidence of bleeding (Navti and Konje, 2011).
      b. Abdominal or lower back pain.
      c. Persistent cramping or sharp, continuous abdominal pain.
      d. Board-like and tender abdomen.
      e. Uterine irritability.
      f. Elevated uterine resting tone.
      g. Tachysystole.
      h. Enlargement of the uterus as blood accumulates, with increasing abdominal girth.
      i. Signs of hypovolemic shock as bleeding increases.
   2. Evidence of fetal compromise.
      a. Loss of fetal heart tones or movement.
      b. Tachycardia.
      c. Late or variable decelerations.
      d. Decreased fetal heart rate variability.
D. **Potential complications.**
   1. Maternal (Francois and Foley, 2012; Navti and Konje, 2011).
      a. Anemia.
      b. Hypovolemic shock.
      c. Couvelaire uterus (blood forced between the muscle fibers of the uterus).
      d. Disseminated intravascular coagulation.
      e. Postpartum hemorrhage.
      f. Fetomaternal hemorrhage.
      g. End-organ damage.
      h. Death.
   2. Fetal/neonatal.
      a. Anemia.
      b. Preterm birth and sequelae associated with prematurity.
      c. Hypoxemia.
      d. Hypovolemia.
      e. Greater risk for long-term neurobehavioral problems.
      f. Risk for sudden infant death syndrome and ventricular leukomalacia.
      g. IUGR.
      h. Perinatal death (10-fold increase).
E. **Assessment and management.**
   1. Any episode of bleeding during pregnancy in an Rh-negative woman requires a Kleihauer--Betke test and the administration of Rh immunoglobulin (Murray and McKinney, 2011).

2. Management decisions are based on the severity of the abruption, complications, gestational age, and maternal–fetal status.
3. Ongoing assessment of:
   a. Amount and nature of bleeding.
   b. Pain.
   c. Maternal vital signs.
   d. Fetal condition.
   e. Uterine contractions and tone.
4. Management if fetus is stable and maternal hematologic status can be maintained:
   a. Ultrasonography to locate placenta and determine degree of placental separation and location of hematoma.
   b. Bed rest in left lateral position, close assessment of abdomen for rigidity and pain, and close assessment of vaginal bleeding.
   c. Monitoring of maternal vital signs and continuous monitoring of fetal heart for tachycardia, late decelerations, and decreasing baseline variability.
   d. Insertion of large-gauge IV catheters (16- to 18-gauge) for possible administration of fluids and blood products.
   e. CBC, coagulation studies, and type and cross-match for blood.
   f. Possible collection of urine for drug screening if abuse is suspected.
   g. Possible induction of labor and/or vaginal birth.
   h. Notify the NICU and the neonatologist/pediatrician.
   i. Emotional support of woman and family.
5. Preparation for cesarean birth if evidence of fetal compromise or severe hemorrhage occurs:
   a. Inform and support parents and ensure that surgical consent is obtained.
   b. Notification of anesthesia department and NICU.
   c. Laboratory tests as above.
   d. Preparation of the abdomen for surgery (clipping of hair around incision site) and insertion of an indwelling urinary catheter.

## Placenta Previa

Placenta previa is a placenta that is implanted in the lower part of the uterus near the cervix (marginal) or in varying degrees (partial or total) over the cervix. Cervical dilatation at or near term is accompanied by bleeding from the placenta. Placenta previa is a common cause of bleeding in the second half of pregnancy, when the lower uterine segment stretches and thins.

A. **Incidence:** The incidence is 1 in 200 births in the United States (March of Dimes, 2012a).

B. **Etiology/predisposing factors (Francois and Foley, 2012).**
   1. The precise cause of placenta previa is unknown, but it occurs most frequently in multiparous and older women.
   2. Other associated and predisposing factors include previous placenta previa, increasing parity or maternal age, prior cesarean birth, living in higher altitudes, cigarette smoking, maternal race (Asian women have the highest incidence), multifetal gestation, and prior curettage.

C. **Clinical presentation (Navti and Konje, 2011).**
   1. Bright red, painless vaginal bleeding. Although the first bleeding episode may be slight in amount, more blood is usually lost in subsequent episodes.
   2. Uterine contractions occur in 10% to 20% of cases, but otherwise the uterus is usually soft and nontender.
   3. If an ultrasound is performed at less than 20 weeks of gestation, a low-lying placenta may be noted. However, at this gestational age, the lower uterine segment is not yet fully developed and this is not diagnostic of a placenta previa.
   4. Failure of presenting part of fetus to become engaged. Fetus may lie transversely or be in a breech position.

D. **Potential complications.**
   1. Maternal.
      a. Anemia.
      b. Hypovolemic shock.

c. Endometritis.
d. Decreased contractile strength of the lower uterine segment, which can lead to postpartum hemorrhage and need for hysterectomy.
e. Abnormal placental implantation (placenta accreta, percreta, and increta).
f. Air embolism.

2. Fetal/neonatal.
a. Perinatal mortality.
b. Fetal anemia.
c. Malpresentation.
d. IUGR.
e. Prematurity and subsequent sequelae.

E. **Assessment and management.**
1. Treatment and delivery decisions are based on amount of bleeding, gestational age, cervical status, grade of previa, and condition and presentation of fetus (Navti and Konje, 2011). Any episode of bleeding during pregnancy in an Rh-negative woman requires a Kleihauer–Betke test and the administration of Rh immunoglobulin to Rh-negative, unsensitized women.
2. Marginal or partial placenta previa with minimal bleeding is managed conservatively:
a. Serial ultrasounds to confirm diagnosis, rule out IUGR, and monitor fetal growth.
b. No vaginal examinations.
c. Activity restrictions at home or in the hospital determined by clinical presentation.
d. Nutritional supplements and dietary management to prevent anemia.
e. Antenatal corticosteroid therapy may be considered.
f. Avoidance of intercourse and orgasm, which can cause uterine contractions.
g. Time of delivery is based on the clinical picture but generally recommended at 37 weeks when fetal lung maturity is documented.
h. Vaginal birth can be planned if the placenta is greater than 2 to 3 cm from the cervical os (Francois and Foley, 2012).
3. Partial or total placenta previa with greater amounts of bleeding is handled as noted above, except that vaginal birth may not be possible. In addition:
a. Frequent assessment of vaginal bleeding, with pad counts and/or weighing of pads.
b. Frequent assessment of maternal vital signs and fetal heart tones, and palpation of abdomen.
c. Laboratory work: CBC, type and cross-match for possible blood transfusion.
d. With significant bleeding, placement of IV lines with 16- to 18-gauge catheters for blood administration.
e. Cesarean section is the preferred mode of delivery for a partial or complete placenta previa. Timing is dependent on the clinical picture.

## Umbilical Cord Prolapse

Umbilical cord prolapse is an event that is life threatening to the fetus and requires immediate and effective management by the nurse. It occurs when the cord falls below the presenting part or is compressed between the presenting part and the pelvis or cervix.

A. **Incidence:** Varies from 1 in 265 to 426 births, with an incidence in vertex presentations of 3% and in breech presentations of 3.7% (Davidson et al., 2012; Steer and Danielian, 2011).

B. **Etiology/predisposing factors.**
1. The fetal presenting part does not fill the pelvic inlet well, and the cord slips past it, often when the membranes rupture.
2. Predisposing factors include fetal malpresentations such as breech and transverse lie, obstetric manipulations (e.g., amniotomy and forceps), abnormally long cord, preterm labor, low birth weight fetus, multiple gestation, polyhydramnios, lack of engagement before the onset of labor, multiparity, and abnormal placentation (Davidson et al., 2012; Steer and Danielian, 2011).

C. **Clinical presentation.**
1. Cord is protruding from vagina or is palpable on vaginal examination.
2. In an occult prolapse, cord is not visible or palpable but is located between the presenting part and the pelvis or cervix.

3. More commonly occurs with a high station of presenting part, and membranes are often ruptured.
4. Fetal heart rate changes observed may include an abrupt occurrence of persistent, severe variable decelerations or bradycardia.

**D. Potential complications.**

1. Maternal.
   a. Trauma to the birth canal from rapid forceps delivery.
   b. If general anesthesia is used for surgery, may result in uterine atony with subsequent postpartum bleeding.
   c. Blood loss from cesarean birth.
   d. Emotional distress.
2. Fetal/neonatal.
   a. Fetal/neonatal complications are directly related to compression of the umbilical cord, and perinatal mortality increases as increased time elapses between cord prolapse and birth.
   b. Fetal anoxia leading to long-range neurologic complications.
   c. Fetal death.

**E. Assessment and management.**

1. Assessments on admission to labor and delivery.
   a. Presenting part and its station.
   b. Dilation of cervix.
   c. Status of membranes.
   d. Estimation of fetal weight and fetal heart rate.
2. Assessment for presence of polyhydramnios or lack of engagement of presenting part. Ambulation during labor and artificial rupture of membranes may be contraindicated if either of the above is present.
3. Assessment after artificial or spontaneous rupture of membranes.
   a. Monitor fetal heart rate for changes as indicated above.
   b. Perform vaginal examination to detect prolapse if indicated.
4. If prolapse has occurred (Steer and Danielian, 2011):
   a. Keep the examining hand in vagina to push the presenting part away from the cord and to relieve cord compression until birth of fetus. The obstetrician or midwife may also attempt to replace the prolapsed cord into the uterus.
   b. Monitor fetal heart rate continuously and palpate cord lightly for continued pulsation. Administration of oxygen, insertion of IV lines if not already present, and notification of the anesthesia and neonatology departments.
   c. An alternative measure is to insert an indwelling catheter to fill the mother's bladder with sterile saline solution in order to elevate the fetal presenting part so that it is off the cord.
   d. Help woman into knee–chest or steep Trendelenburg's position, with hips elevated and head down (Davidson et al., 2012).
   e. If the cervix is fully dilated and the fetal station is below the ischial spines, vaginal birth may be expedited. However, emergency cesarean delivery may be preferable, especially if the cervix is not fully dilated and the fetus exhibits signs of potential compromise.

## Shoulder Dystocia

Shoulder dystocia is an acute emergency in which the physician or midwife is unable to deliver the shoulders of the infant by the usual maneuvers (downward traction) after birth of the head.

**A. Incidence:** Incidence is 0.2% to 3% of all births. As this is a major obstetric emergency that must be acted upon quickly and occurs infrequently, multidisciplinary simulation drills should be instituted in the facility (Gherman, 2011).

**B. Etiology/predisposing factors.**

1. The fetal shoulders are too broad to be delivered between the symphysis pubis and the sacrum.
2. Factors associated with shoulder dystocia include maternal obesity, macrosomia, a history of previous shoulder dystocia, prolonged second stage of labor, diabetes mellitus or impaired glucose metabolism, previous birth of a macrosomic infant, and instrumented midpelvic

delivery. However, up to 50% of cases occur with fetuses less than 4000 g (Gherman, 2011; Lanni and Seeds, 2012).

C. **Clinical presentation.**
  1. Prolonged transitional phase of labor (8 to 10 cm).
  2. Prolonged second stage of labor (>2 hours).
  3. After birth of the head, it recoils against the perineum and restitution does not occur ("turtling"). The usual traction from below is not successful in delivering the neonate.

D. **Complications.**
  1. Maternal.
    a. Third- or fourth-degree lacerations.
    b. Postpartum hemorrhage.
    c. Vaginal and cervical lacerations.
    d. Ruptured uterus.
    e. Bladder atony.
  2. Fetal/neonatal.
    a. Birth injuries such as brachial palsy, Erb's palsy, facial nerve palsy, or fractured clavicle or humerus.
    b. Hypoxia.
    c. Permanent brain injury.
    d. Intrapartum or neonatal death.

E. **Assessment and management (Gherman, 2011; Lanni and Seeds, 2012).**
  1. If risks factors are present and/or the provider anticipates a possible shoulder dystocia, the neonatal team should be present for delivery.
  2. Anticipate shoulder dystocia if descent of the head is slow and estimated weight is large. Make sure the woman's bladder is empty before birth occurs.
  3. If shoulder dystocia occurs, the physician or midwife will:
    a. Use the McRoberts maneuver (maternal hip flexion; an exaggerated lithotomy position).
    b. Apply suprapubic pressure to attempt to release the anterior shoulder; the pressure may be directly downward or lateral.
    c. Turn the woman onto her side or pull the hips off the bed to free the sacrum.
    d. Turn the woman on "all fours" facing downward to widen the pelvic outlet if this can be easily accomplished (Gaskin's maneuver).
    e. Manually rotate the shoulders from the anteroposterior to the oblique diameter.
    f. Use the Woods' corkscrew maneuver, in which both hands are inserted internally to rotate the posterior shoulder to the anterior position for delivery under the pubic bone, with the maneuver repeated for the other side.
    g. Deliver the posterior arm.
    h. The expulsive efforts of the mother, as opposed to traction by the provider, are of the utmost importance.

## Breech Presentation

A. **Incidence:** Incidence is dependent on gestational age, and is 14% at 29 to 32 weeks, 2.2% to 3.7% at term, and overall 3% to 4% of all labors (Penn, 2011).

B. **Etiology/predisposing factors.**
  1. Maternal.
    a. Polyhydramnios or oligohydramnios.
    b. Uterine abnormalities (e.g., bicornuate uterus).
    c. Contracted pelvis.
    d. Use of anticonvulsant medications or alcohol abuse.
  2. Placental/fetal.
    a. Placenta previa or cornual placenta.
    b. Multifetal gestation.
    c. IUGR or fetal anomalies, especially those related to CNS problems.
    d. Short cord.
    e. Preterm fetus.

C. **Clinical presentation.**
   1. Woman feels fetus kicking in the lower abdomen.
   2. Fetal heart sounds are heard loudest above the umbilicus.
   3. Use of Leopold's maneuvers indicates head is in the fundal area and the breech is in the pelvis.
   4. On vaginal examination, it is found that the presenting part is soft, no fontanelles are felt, and the genitalia may be identified.

D. **Assessment and management.**
   1. Postural exercise, in which the woman assumes either the knee–chest or an elevated-hip posture several times a day to help the fetus turn from breech to cephalic presentation, has been suggested, but is not supported in the literature (Penn, 2011).
   2. The physician may attempt external cephalic version (after 36 weeks in nulliparas; after 37 weeks in parous women) with or without the use of a uterine relaxant and if the fetus remains in a cephalic presentation, vaginal birth. However, in many cases the fetus reverts to breech (Penn, 2011).
   3. Assessments on admission to labor and delivery:
      a. Perform Leopold's maneuvers and vaginal examination to determine presentation.
      b. Report clinical findings immediately to the physician or midwife.
   4. Ultrasonography may be ordered to confirm breech presentation, determine degree of flexion of fetal head, evaluate size of fetal head, estimate fetal weight, diagnose fetal anomalies, and locate placenta.
   5. ACOG recommends that the mode of delivery be based on the experience level of the provider, and the majority will choose elective cesarean delivery. If the provider is experienced in breech delivery, he or she may plan a delivery as long as specific guidelines are followed and the woman is provided with informed consent regarding maternal and neonatal risks (ACOG, 2012).
   6. Assessment of the neonate who was in the breech presentation may reveal:
      a. Edema of the external genitalia.
      b. A continuation of the frank breech position for a period of time after the birth.

E. **Complications.**
   1. Fetal/neonatal complications resulting from vaginal birth (Davidson et al., 2012; Penn, 2011).
      a. Prolapsed cord.
      b. Asphyxia from slow birth of fetal head or from compression of umbilical cord between pelvis and head during birth.
      c. Aspiration of amniotic fluid with potential for meconium aspiration syndrome.
      d. Genital damage in the male infant.
      e. CNS injuries such as intracranial hemorrhage, brachial plexus injury, and severed spinal cord, especially if fetal head is hyperextended.
      f. Damage to the nose and pharynx.

## OBSTETRIC ANALGESIA AND ANESTHESIA

There is no method of pharmacologic pain relief that is completely safe for all laboring women. In addition, side effects or adverse reactions in the woman affect the fetus to some degree. For this reason, nonpharmacologic methods of pain management (e.g., labor support, freedom of movement, hypnosis, acupressure and acupuncture, application of heat or cold, listening to music, breathing techniques, massage, hydrotherapy, and transcutaneous electrical nerve stimulation) can be important and useful for the laboring woman (Tsen, 2011).

### Obstetric Analgesia

Obstetric analgesia is given by either the intramuscular or the IV route and in as small a dose as possible. Any use of analgesia in the laboring woman should take into account the potential effects on the mother/fetus, effects on contractions and the progress of labor, and the medical condition of the mother (Davidson et al., 2012). Narcotic analgesics such as butorphanol tartrate (Stadol) and nalbuphine hydrochloride (Nubain) are commonly used for pain relief.

**A. Potential side effects or complications (Davidson et al., 2012).**
1. Maternal.
    a. Respiratory depression.
    b. Nausea and vomiting.
    c. Hypotension.
    d. Drowsiness and dizziness.
    e. Clammy skin and sweating.
2. Fetal/neonatal.
    a. Decreased variability of the fetal heart rate, sinusoidal pattern (Stadol).
    b. Neonatal respiratory depression.

**B. Assessment and management.**
1. Avoid administration of analgesics close to birth if possible.
2. Administer IV analgesics slowly; give during a uterine contraction to minimize amount of drug the fetus receives.
3. Observe the woman for side effects and monitor the fetal heart rate with the electronic fetal monitor or via intermittent auscultation.
4. With maternal hypotension, turn the woman onto her left side, increase IV infusion of fluids, and closely monitor the fetal heart rate and maternal BP.
5. Have naloxone (Narcan), oxygen, and ventilatory equipment available to manage potential newborn respiratory depression.
6. Document use of analgesic and transmit this information to the nursery nurse.
7. Observe the neonate for side effects of maternal analgesia.

## Obstetric Anesthesia

Several types of anesthesia are used with women in labor and delivery. General anesthesia is used primarily for emergency cesarean and complicated vaginal births when it is not possible to have immediate and effective regional anesthesia. Regional anesthesia includes continuous lumbar epidural, spinal, and pudendal block. Local anesthesia involves perineal infiltration prior to episiotomy, birth, and/or perineal repair.

**A. Potential complications with general anesthesia.**
1. Maternal (Davidson et al., 2012).
    a. Vomiting and aspiration of gastric contents, with acid pneumonitis (Mendelson's syndrome) as a consequence.
    b. Respiratory depression.
    c. Hypotension or hypertension.
    d. Tachycardia.
    e. Laryngospasm.
    f. Uterine atony.
2. Fetal/neonatal.
    a. Neonatal respiratory depression and hypotonicity.
    b. Fetal depression in proportion to the amount of anesthesia.

**B. Assessment and management with general anesthesia.**
1. The woman must have nothing by mouth while in labor if there is a strong possibility that she will receive general anesthesia.
2. Note the time of her last meal.
3. Physician may order 30 mL of clear antacid to be administered before general anesthesia to increase the pH of the stomach contents in case of aspiration.
4. Endotracheal tube and cricoid pressure are techniques used by the anesthesiologist to prevent aspiration.
5. Place a wedge under the right hip to cause displacement of the uterus from the aorta and vena cava and to prevent supine hypotensive syndrome during surgery.
6. Monitor the woman's cardiorespiratory status during and after surgery, and uterine bleeding postoperatively.
7. Monitor the newborn infant after surgery for complications.

**C. Potential complications with regional anesthetics.**

**1.** Maternal (Davidson et al., 2012; Tsen, 2011).

**a.** With spinal and epidural anesthesia:

(1) Hypotension due to sympathetic blockade.

(2) Allergic reaction to the injected anesthetic.

(3) Toxic reaction to overdose or intravascular injection, with seizure activity.

(4) Respiratory paralysis from inadvertent high spinal anesthesia.

(5) Postdural puncture headache.

(6) Failure of anesthetic to be effective.

(7) Urinary retention during labor and in the postpartum period.

(8) Formation of a hematoma that compresses the spinal cord, with potential for permanent damage.

(9) Paralysis (rare).

**b.** With epidural anesthesia:

(1) Catheter migration.

(2) Bladder distention.

(3) Prolonged second stage and subsequent increase in instrumented vaginal delivery (forceps and vacuum-assisted).

(4) Increase in the use of oxytocin (Hawkins and Bucklin, 2012).

(5) Back pain and postdural puncture headache.

(6) "Epidural shakes" and "epidural fever" (involuntary shivering that leads to an elevated temperature). Fever may also be caused by a decrease in hyperventilation and dissipation of heat (Murray and McKinney, 2011).

**c.** With pudendal block (Hawkins and Bucklin, 2012; Murray and McKinney, 2011):

(1) Sciatic nerve trauma.

(2) Perforated rectum.

(3) Anesthetic toxicity.

(4) Broad-ligament hematoma.

**2.** Fetal/neonatal.

**a.** Toxic reaction from overdose or intravascular injection.

**b.** Fetal compromise with prolonged maternal hypotension, as evidenced by late decelerations, bradycardia, and either increased or decreased variability.

**D. Assessment and management with regional anesthetics.**

**1.** Note history of allergies to local anesthetics.

**2.** Prehydrate with 500 to 1000 mL IV fluid before spinal or epidural anesthesia to minimize hypotensive effects from sympathetic blockade.

**3.** Position and reassure woman during administration of anesthetic. To prevent supine hypotension, a small roll may be placed under the right hip.

**4.** Monitor the woman's BP after administration of spinal or epidural anesthetic; monitor fetal heart rate after any type of regional anesthesia.

**5.** Monitor bladder distention and catheterize if necessary.

**6.** Complications and their management.

**a.** Hypotension.

(1) Signs and symptoms.

(a) Decreased baseline BP.

(b) Dizziness or affected vision.

(c) Nausea and vomiting.

(2) Management.

(a) Increase IV fluids.

(b) Displace uterus from aorta and vena cava.

(c) Administer oxygen and IV ephedrine as ordered.

(d) Monitor the fetal heart rate for evidence of compromise, and the fetus/newborn for side effects of ephedrine (tachycardia, jitteriness, and increased muscular activity).

**b.** High spinal.

(1) Signs and symptoms.

(a) Breast numbness, indicating a rising level of anesthesia.

(b) Sensation of inability to breathe.
(c) Respiratory arrest.
(2) Management.
(a) Notify anesthesia immediately.
(b) Maintain airway and ventilation.
(c) Observe fetal heart rate for signs of compromise.

**c.** Toxic reaction.
(1) Signs and symptoms.
(a) Metallic taste.
(b) Ringing in ears.
(c) Slurring of speech.
(d) Numbness of tongue and mouth.
(e) Seizures.
(f) Cardiovascular and respiratory depression.
(2) Management.
(a) Cardiorespiratory support.
(b) Drugs to control seizures.
(c) Monitor the newborn infant for seizures, bradycardia, apnea, and hypotonia.

**d.** Allergic reaction.
(1) Signs and symptoms.
(a) Bronchospasm.
(b) Laryngeal edema.
(c) Urticaria.
(2) Management: use of IV antihistamine such as diphenhydramine (Benadryl).

## Cesarean Delivery

**A. Incidence:** The cesarean birth rate in the United States was 32.8% in 2010. The primary cesarean section rate was 23.6% and the vaginal birth after cesarean section (VBAC) rate was 9.2% (Martin et al., 2012). Possible reasons for the increasing cesarean rate include an increase in women who have had a previous cesarean section, the use of continuous electronic fetal monitoring, increased number of labor inductions with failure of induction, decline in vaginal breech birth and VBACs, decreased operative vaginal deliveries, repeat cesareans, increased multifetal pregnancies, changes in obstetric training, medical–legal issues, parental–societal expectations of the outcome of the pregnancy, and some evidence that women may be requesting elective cesarean (Berghella and Landon, 2012; Dickinson, 2011).

**B. Indications.**

**1.** Maternal.
**a.** Previous cesarean delivery.
**b.** Cephalopelvic disproportion.
**c.** Dystocia (inadequate progress in labor).
**d.** Maternal medical conditions.

**2.** Placental.
**a.** Abruptio placentae.
**b.** Placenta previa.
**c.** Placental insufficiency.

**3.** Fetal.
**a.** Suspected fetal compromise.
**b.** Breech or other malpresentation.
**c.** Multifetal gestation.
**d.** Congenital anomalies such as myelomeningocele and anterior abdominal wall defects.

**C. Potential complications.**

**1.** Maternal.
**a.** Infection.
**b.** Anemia.
**c.** Hemorrhage.

d. Morbidity and death from anesthesia.
e. Inadvertent operative injuries.
f. Pulmonary embolus and atelectasis.
g. Thrombophlebitis.

2. Fetal/neonatal.
   a. Asphyxia.
   b. Iatrogenic preterm birth.
   c. Respiratory distress syndrome caused by retained fluid in the lungs.
   d. Persistent pulmonary hypertension (Murray and McKinney, 2011).
   e. Anemia from blood loss caused by incision of placenta and lack of full placental transfusion.

**D. Assessment and management.**

1. Perform usual interventions to prepare the woman for operative delivery.
2. Notify neonatology and pediatrician.
3. Give an antacid if ordered.
4. Remove fetal scalp electrode before surgery if present.
5. Place wedge under woman's right hip to displace the uterus to the left to avoid supine hypotension and fetal hypoxia.
6. Follow Neonatal Resuscitation Program protocols for neonatal care following birth.

## REFERENCES


American College of Obstetricians and Gynecologists: Mode of singleton term breech delivery: *ACOG Committee Opinion No. 340.* Washington, DC, November 2012, American College of Obstetricians and Gynecologists.

American College of Obstetricians and Gynecologists: Screening and diagnosis of gestational diabetes: ACOG Practice Bulletin No. 504. Washington, DC, September 2011, American College of Obstetricians and Gynecologists.

American College of Obstetricians and Gynecologists: Management of intrapartum fetal heart rate tracings: *ACOG Practice Bulletin No. 116.* Washington, DC, November 2010, American College of Obstetricians and Gynecologists.

American College of Obstetricians and Gynecologists: Use of progesterone to reduce preterm birth: ACOG Committee Opinion No. 419. Washington, DC, November 2008, American College of Obstetricians and Gynecologists.

Baschat, A.A.: Fetal growth disorders. In D. James, P. Steer, C. Weiner, and B. Gonik (Eds.): *High risk pregnancy: Management options* (4th ed.). St. Louis, 2011, Elsevier Saunders, pp. 173–196.

Berghella, V., and Landon, M.B.: Cesarean delivery. In S.G. Gabbe, J.R. Niebyl, and J.L. Simpson (Eds.): *Obstetrics: Normal and problem pregnancies* (6th ed.). Philadelphia, 2012, Elsevier Saunders, pp. 445–478.

Burton, G.J., Sibley, C.P., and Jauniaux, E.R.M.: Placental anatomy and physiology. In S.G. Gabbe, J.R. Niebyl, and J.L. Simpson (Eds.): *Obstetrics: Normal and problem pregnancies* (6th ed.). Philadelphia, 2012, Elsevier Saunders, pp. 3–22.

Davidson, M.R., London, M.L., and Ladewig, P.A.: *Olds' maternal-newborn nursing & women's health across the lifespan* (9th ed.). Upper Saddle River, NJ, 2012, Pearson Education.

Dekker, G.: Hypertension. In D. James, P. Steer, C. Weiner, and B. Gonik (Eds.): *High risk pregnancy: Management options* (4th ed.). St. Louis, 2011, Elsevier Saunders, pp. 599–626.

Dickinson, J.E.: Cesarean section. In D. James, P. Steer, C. Weiner, and B. Gonik (Eds.): *High risk pregnancy: Management options* (4th ed.). St. Louis, 2011, Elsevier Saunders, pp. 1269–1280.

Francois, K.E., and Foley, M.R.: Antepartum and postpartum hemorrhage. In S.G. Gabbe, J.R. Niebyl, and J.L. Simpson (Eds.): *Obstetrics: Normal and problem pregnancies* (6th ed.). Philadelphia, 2012, Elsevier Saunders, pp. 415–444.

Fraser, R., and Farrell, T.: Diabetes. In D. James, P. Steer, C. Weiner, and B. Gonik (Eds.): *High risk pregnancy: Management options* (4th ed.). St. Louis, 2011, Elsevier Saunders, pp. 795–811.

Gherman, R.B.: Shoulder dystocia. In D. James, P. Steer, C. Weiner, and B. Gonik (Eds.): *High risk pregnancy: Management options* (4th ed.). St. Louis, 2011, Elsevier Saunders, pp. 1185–1190.

Hawkins, J.L., and Bucklin, B.A.: Obstetrical anesthesia. In S.G. Gabbe, J.R. Niebyl, and J.L. Simpson (Eds.): *Obstetrics: Normal and problem pregnancies* (6th ed.). Philadelphia, 2012, Elsevier Saunders, pp. 362–387.

Landon, M.B., Catalano, P.M., and Gabbe, S.G.: Diabetes mellitus complicating pregnancy. In S.G. Gabbe, J.R. Niebyl, and J.L. Simpson (Eds.): *Obstetrics: Normal and problem pregnancies* (6th ed.). Philadelphia, 2012, Elsevier Saunders, pp. 887–921.

Lanni, S.M., and Seeds, J.W.: Malpresentations and shoulder dystocia. In S.G. Gabbe, J.R. Niebyl, and J.L. Simpson (Eds.): *Obstetrics: Normal and problem pregnancies* (6th ed.). Philadelphia, 2012, Elsevier Saunders, pp. 388–414.

London, M.L., Ladewig, P.A., Ball, J.W., Bindler, R.C., and Cowen, K.J.: *Maternal and child nursing care* (3rd ed.). Upper Saddle River, NJ, 2011, Pearson Education.

March of Dimes: *Pregnancy complications: placental abruption.* 2013. Retrieved April 10, 2013, from http://www.marchofdimes.com/pregnancy/complications_abruption.html.

March of Dimes: *Pregnancy complications: placenta previa.* 2012a. Retrieved April 10, 2013, from http://www.marchofdimes.com/pregnancy/complications_previa.html.

March of Dimes: *2012 premature birth report card.* 2012b. Retrieved April 11, 2013, from http://www.marchofdimes.com/mission/prematurity_reportcard.html.

Martin, J.A., Hamilton, B.E., Ventura, S.J., et al.: Births: Final data for 2010. *National Vital Statistics Reports*, 61 (1), 2012.

Murray, S.S., and McKinney, E.S.: *Foundations of maternal-newborn nursing:* (4th ed.). St. Louis, 2011, Elsevier Saunders.

Navti, O.B., and Konje, J.C.: Bleeding in late pregnancy. In D. James, P. Steer, C. Weiner, and B. Gonik (Eds.): *High risk pregnancy: Management options* (4th ed.). St. Louis, 2011, Elsevier Saunders, pp. 1037–1051.

Penn, Z.: Breech presentation. In D. James, P. Steer, C. Weiner, and B. Gonik (Eds.): *High risk pregnancy: Management options* (4th ed.). St. Louis, 2011, Elsevier Saunders, pp. 1101–1121.

Perry, S.E., Hockenberry, M.J., Lowdermilk, D.L., and Wilson, D.: *Maternal child nursing care* (4th ed.). St. Louis, 2010, Elsevier Mosby.

Ross, M.G., Ervin, M.G., and Novak, D.: Placental and fetal physiology. In S.G. Gabbe, J.R. Niebyl, and J.L. Simpson (Eds.): *Obstetrics: Normal and problem pregnancies* (6th ed.). Philadelphia, 2012, Elsevier Saunders, pp. 23–41.

Sibai, B.M.: Hypertension. In S.G. Gabbe, J.R. Niebyl, and J.L. Simpson (Eds.): *Obstetrics: Normal and problem pregnancies* (6th ed.). Philadelphia, 2012, Elsevier Saunders, pp. 779–824.

Simhan, H.N., Iams, J.D., and Romero, R.: Preterm birth. In S.G. Gabbe, J.R. Niebyl, and J.L. Simpson (Eds.): *Obstetrics: Normal and problem pregnancies* (6th ed.). Philadelphia, 2012, Elsevier Saunders, pp. 627–658.

Steer, P.J., and Danielian, P.: Fetal distress in labor. In D. James, P. Steer, C. Weiner, and B. Gonik (Eds.): *High risk pregnancy: Management options* (4th ed.). St. Louis, 2011, Elsevier Saunders, pp. 1191–1210.

Svigos, J.M., Dodd, J.M., and Robinson, J.S.: Threatened and actual preterm labor including mode of delivery. In D. James, P. Steer, C. Weiner, and B. Gonik (Eds.): *High risk pregnancy: Management options* (4th ed.). St. Louis, 2011, Elsevier Saunders, pp. 1075–1090.

Tsen, L.R.: Neuraxial analgesia and anesthesia in obstetrics. In D. James, P. Steer, C. Weiner, and B. Gonik (Eds.): *High risk pregnancy: Management options* (4th ed.). St. Louis, 2011, Elsevier Saunders, pp. 1211–1229.

CHAPTER

# 3 Perinatal Substance Abuse

JAN SHERMAN

**OBJECTIVES**

1. Discuss the direct and indirect effects of drugs of abuse on the fetus.
2. Describe the maternal conditions that are contraindications for breastfeeding.
3. Describe the maternal and neonatal characteristics associated with drug use in pregnancy.
4. Describe the physical characteristics of an infant with a neonatal narcotic abstinence syndrome.
5. List four nonpharmacologic nursing interventions appropriate for managing withdrawal.
6. Discuss the pharmacologic management of neonatal abstinence syndrome.

## OVERVIEW

Substance abuse has been an issue for society since ancient times. Over the past several decades, attention has been directed toward the use of legal and illegal substances by pregnant women. Almost all drugs are known to cross the placenta and have effects on the fetus.

The effects on the human fetus of prenatal smoking, alcohol use, and opiate use have been identified and studied over the past decades (Behnke and Smith, 2013; Hudak and Tan, 2012). Of more recent concern is the abuse of prescription drugs. In 2010, over 1.9 million people in the United States were addicted to prescription opioid pain relievers (National Institute of Drug Abuse [NIDA], 2012).

The mean hospital cost for a neonatal abstinence syndrome (NAS) admission in 2009 was $53,400. The need to decrease resource utilization and the costs of treatment as well as improve psychosocial and developmental outcomes in infants exposed to substances in utero is paramount. Methods must be developed to decrease the risk of adverse neonatal outcomes such as low birth weight (<2500 g) and mortality (Patrick et al., 2012).

Future work on NAS should involve novel approaches designed to minimize and manage opiate exposure before pregnancy, such as opioid vaccines and pharmacogenomics (McLemore et al., 2013). Treatment of mothers during pregnancy must be evidence based. Multiple individual, family, and environmental factors such as nutritional status, extent of prenatal care, neglect or abuse, and socioeconomic conditions must also be addressed (NIDA, 2011a).

A. **Prevalence (Substance Abuse and Mental Health Services Administration [SAMHSA], 2013; Patrick et al., 2012).**
   1. Exposure to substances of abuse can affect individuals across the life span, starting in utero. Each year, an estimated 400,000 to 440,000 infants (10% to 11% of all births) are affected by prenatal alcohol or illicit drug exposure.
   2. Between 2000 and 2009, the rate of newborns diagnosed with NAS increased from 1.20 to 3.39 per 1000 births.
   3. Compared with all other hospital births, newborns with NAS were significantly more likely to have respiratory diagnoses, low birth weight, feeding difficulties, and seizures.
   4. Newborns with NAS were more likely to be covered by Medicaid and reside in zip codes within the lowest income quartile.
   5. Prenatal exposure to alcohol, tobacco, and illicit drugs has the potential to cause a wide spectrum of physical, emotional, and developmental problems for these infants. The harm caused to the child can be significant and long-lasting, especially if the exposure is not detected and the effects are not treated as soon as possible.

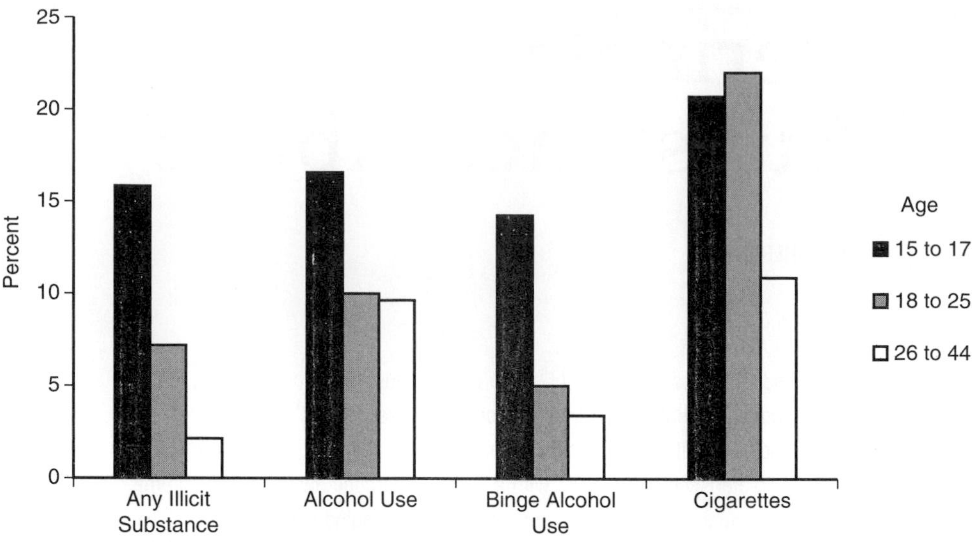


FIGURE 3-1 ■ Current substance use among pregnant women, 2008-2009 combined. (From National Institute of Drug Abuse: *Topics in brief: Prenatal exposure to drugs of abuse.* 2011. Retrieved from http://www.drugabuse.gov/publications/topics-in-brief/prenatal-exposure-to-drugs-abuse.)

6. While most pregnant women do not abuse illicit drugs, combined 2008 and 2009 data from the National Survey on Drug Use and Health found that, among pregnant women ages 15 to 44 years, the youngest ones generally reported the greatest substance use, as shown in Figure 3-1 (NIDA, 2011a).
7. Addiction to opioids (e.g., heroin, morphine, prescription pain relievers) is a serious global problem that affects the health, social, and economic welfare of all societies. An estimated 12 to 21 million people worldwide abuse opioids (NIDA, 2011b).

B. **Prescription drug abuse.**
1. Prescription drug abuse is the intentional use of a medication without a prescription, in a way other than as prescribed, or for the experience or feeling it causes. Prescription drug abuse remains a significant problem in the United States.
2. The increased use of prescription opiates in pregnant women to treat acute or chronic pain has been noted (Hudak and Tan, 2012).
3. In a recent report, chronic use of narcotic prescriptions (use for $\geq$1 intrapartum month) among pregnant women cared for at a single clinic increased five-fold from 1998 to 2008, and 5.6% of infants delivered to these women manifested signs of neonatal withdrawal (Kellogg et al., 2011).
4. Of great concern is that, in women between 15 and 17 years of age, the rate of prescription drug abuse is 23% in pregnant versus 13% in nonpregnant women (Johnston et al., 2008).

C. **Alcohol (National Institute on Alcohol Abuse and Alcoholism [NIAAA], 2010; SAMSHA, 2012; SAMHSA, 2012).**
1. Alcohol continues to be one of the most widely abused substances during pregnancy, and its effects on fetal development and infant outcomes have been well studied. Data from prenatal clinics and postnatal studies suggest that 20% to 30% of women do drink at some time during pregnancy.
2. Alcohol can disrupt fetal development at any stage during a pregnancy. Research shows that binge drinking, which means consuming four or more drinks per occasion, and regular heavy drinking put a fetus at the greatest risk for severe problems.
3. Based on data averaged over 2009 and 2010, of pregnant women ages 15 to 44 years, an estimated 10.8% reported current alcohol use, 3.7% reported binge drinking, and 1% reported heavy drinking.
4. These rates were significantly lower than the rates for nonpregnant women in the same age group (54.7%, 24.6%, and 5.4%, respectively). Binge drinking during the first trimester of pregnancy was reported by 10.1% of pregnant women ages 15 to 44 years.

D. **Tobacco (SAMHSA, 2012).**
   1. The 2-year moving average rates from 2002-2003 to 2009-2010 indicate that current cigarette use among women ages 15 to 44 years decreased from 30.7% to 26.7% for those who were not pregnant and from 18% to 16.3% for those who were pregnant.
   2. However, among those ages 15 to 17 years, the rate of cigarette smoking was higher for pregnant women than nonpregnant women, 22.7% vs. 13.4%.

## PRECONCEPTION COUNSELING AND INTERVENTIONS (AMERICAN ACADEMY OF PEDIATRICS [AAP] AND THE AMERICAN COLLEGE OF OBSTETRICIANS AND GYNECOLOGISTS [ACOG], 2012)

A. **The core topics in preconception care that should be addressed include alcohol use, tobacco use, and illicit drug use.** Behavioral counseling can be particularly effective during the preconception period and antenatal period.
B. **Preconception women who smoke cigarettes or use any other form of tobacco product should be identified and encouraged and supported in an effort to quit.** Importantly, tobacco cessation at any point during pregnancy yields substantial health benefits for the expectant mother and newborn.
C. **Smoking during pregnancy and sudden infant death syndrome (SIDS) have a strong association.** Children born to mothers who smoke during pregnancy are at increased risk of asthma, infantile colic, and childhood obesity. Cessation of smoking is recommended before pregnancy.
D. **Other important behavioral issues to address prenatally include alcohol use and misuse and the abuse of prescription and nonprescription recreational drugs.** All women should be asked about the quantity and frequency of their alcohol use. Women who are trying to become pregnant should be counseled to completely refrain from all alcohol use.
E. **Referral relationships with appropriate resources should be established and used as needed to assist women with these issues.** Women who are counseled concerning their alcohol or drug use should be followed up to assess adherence to recommendations. Table 3-1 details the major drugs of abuse (Hudak and Tan, 2012).

## TREATMENT APPROACHES FOR PREGNANT WOMEN (AAP AND ACOG, 2012)

A. **Medications.**
   1. Research shows that some medications that are effective in drug-abusing populations can also be beneficial for pregnant women and their babies. Methadone maintenance in opioid-dependent pregnant women has been used for the past 35 years, and is associated with improved birth weight and improvements in multiple areas (Kraft and van den Anker, 2012).
   2. Methadone maintenance combined with prenatal care and a comprehensive drug treatment program can improve many of the detrimental maternal and neonatal outcomes associated with untreated heroin abuse (Kraft and van den Anker, 2012).
   3. Another medication for treating opioid dependence, buprenorphine, has recently been shown to produce fewer neonatal abstinence symptoms in babies than methadone, resulting in shorter infant hospital stays (Kraft and van den Anker, 2012).
B. **Behavioral treatments.**
   1. Research has shown the value of evidence-based treatments in changing drug abuse and addiction behaviors in pregnant women. One example is contingency management, where participants are given incentives, such as small cash amounts, privileges, or prizes, for maintaining abstinence.
   2. Compared to a standard treatment condition, motivational incentive approaches appear to increase treatment retention and prolong abstinence in pregnant women with cocaine, opiate, and nicotine dependence. In general, it is important to closely monitor women who are trying to quit drug use during pregnancy and to adjust treatment as needed.

■ TABLE 3-1
■ ■ **Major Drugs of Abuse**

| Opioids | CNS Stimulants | CNS Depressants | Hallucinogens |
|---|---|---|---|
| Agonists | Amphetamines | Alcohol | Indolealkylamines (LSD, psilocin, psilocybin, DMT, DET) |
| Morphine | Dextroamphetamine (Dexedrine) | Barbiturates | Phenylethylamines (mescaline, peyote) |
| Codeine | Methamphetamine | Benzodiazepines | Phenylisopropylamines (MDA, MMDA, MDMA, MDEA) |
| Methadone | Amphetamine sulfate | Other sedative-hypnotics | Inhalants |
| Meperidine (Demerol) | Amphetamine congeners | Methaqualone (Quaalude) | Solvents and aerosols (glues, gasoline, paint thinner, cleaning solutions, nail polish remover, Freon) |
| Oxycodone (Percodan, OxyIR, Percolone, Roxicodone, Percocet, OxyContin) | Benzphetamine (Didrex) | Glutethimide (Doriden) | Nitrites |
| | Diethylpropion (Tenuate) | Chloral hydrate | Nitrous oxide |
| | Fenfluramine | Cannabinoids | |
| Propoxyphene (Darvon) | Phendimetrazine (Adipost, Bontril, Prelu-2) | Marijuana | |
| Hydromorphone (Dilaudid) | Phentermine (Adipex-P, Zantryl) | Hashish | |
| Hydrocodone (Lortab, Vicodin) | Cocaine | | |
| Fentanyl (Sublimaze) | Methylphenidate (Ritalin, Concerta) | | |
| Tramadol (Ultram, Ultracet) | Pemoline (Cylert) | | |
| Heroin | Phenylpropanolamine | | |
| Antagonists | Phencyclidines | | |
| Naloxone (Narcan) | Nicotine | | |
| Naltrexone (ReVia) | | | |
| Mixed Agonist-Antagonists | | | |
| Pentazocine (Talwin) | | | |
| Buprenorphine (Buprenex) | | | |

Adapted from Hudak, M.L., Tan, R.C., Committee on Drugs, and Committee on Fetus and Newborn, American Academy of Pediatrics: Neonatal drug withdrawal. *Pediatrics*, 129(2):e540-e560, 2012. Epub January 30, 2012. Retrieved from http://pediatrics.aappublications.org/content/129/2/e540.

*DET*, Diethyltryptamine; *DMT*, dimethyltryptamine; *LSD*, lysergic acid diethylamide; *MDA*, methylenedioxyamphetamine; *MDEA*, 3,4-methylenedioxyethamphetamine; *MDMA*, 3,4-methylenedioxymethamphetamine (ecstasy); *MMDA*, 3-methoxy-4,5-methylenedioxyamphetamine.

C. **Comorbidity associated with mental disorders.**
   1. Research suggests that pregnant women with mood or anxiety disorders are more likely to have a substance use disorder as well, and vice versa.
   2. More treatment research on co-occurring psychiatric and substance use problems in pregnant women, including an examination of mood-focused smoking cessation interventions, is needed.

## MECHANISMS OF ACTION OF DRUGS ON THE FETUS (BEHNKE AND SMITH, 2013)

Drugs can affect the fetus in multiple ways, through either direct or indirect effects.

A. **Direct effects.**
   1. Early in gestation, drugs can have significant teratogenic effects. During the fetal period, after major structural development is complete, drugs have more subtle effects, including abnormal growth and/or maturation, alterations in neurotransmitters and their receptors, and alterations in brain organization. These are considered to be the direct effects of drugs.

B. **Indirect effects.**
   1. Drugs that exert a pharmacologic effect on the mother can indirectly affect the fetus. Indirect effects of drugs of abuse on the fetus include altered delivery of nutrition to the fetus, because of either placental insufficiency or altered maternal health behaviors attributable to the mother's addiction.
   2. Maternal factors such as decreased access to/compliance with health care, increased exposure to violence, and increased risk of mental illness and infection may place the fetus at risk.

C. **Ethanol.**
   1. Ethanol easily crosses the placenta into the fetus, with a significant concentration of the drug identified in the amniotic fluid as well as in maternal and fetal blood.
   2. Ethanol has direct teratogenic effects during the embryonic and fetal stage of development as well as altered neurotransmitter levels in the brain, altered brain morphology, altered neuronal development, and hypoxia.

D. **Tobacco.**
   1. Nicotine is only one of more than 4000 compounds to which the fetus is exposed through maternal smoking. Of these, approximately 30 compounds have been associated with adverse health outcomes.
   2. Although the exact mechanisms by which nicotine produces adverse fetal effects are unknown, it is likely that hypoxia, undernourishment of the fetus, and direct vasoconstrictor effects on the placental and umbilical vessels all play a role.

E. **Marijuana.**
   1. Unlike other drugs, the placenta appears to limit fetal exposure to marijuana. The adverse effects of marijuana on the fetus are thought to be attributable to complex pharmacologic actions on developing systems, altered uterine blood flow, and altered maternal health behaviors.
   2. Marijuana can remain in the body for up to 30 days, thus prolonging fetal exposure. Smoking marijuana produces as much as 5 times the amount of carbon monoxide, which may alter fetal oxygenation, as does cigarette smoking.

F. **Opiates.**
   1. Opiates rapidly cross the placenta, with drug equilibration between the mother and the fetus. Opiates have been shown to decrease brain growth and cell development in animals.

G. **Cocaine.**
   1. Cocaine easily crosses both the placenta and the blood–brain barrier and can have significant teratogenic effects on the developing fetus.
   2. It appears that the development of areas of the brain that regulate attention and executive functioning are particularly vulnerable to cocaine. Functions such as arousal, attention, and memory may be adversely affected by prenatal cocaine exposure.

H. **Methamphetamine.**
   1. Methamphetamine readily passes through the placenta and the blood–brain barrier and stimulates the central nervous system (CNS). It is possible that the mechanism of action of methamphetamine is an interaction with and alteration of neurotransmitter systems as well as alterations in brain morphogenesis.

## IDENTIFICATION OF PRENATAL EXPOSURE

A. **Characteristics associated with drug use (AAP and ACOG, 2012).**
   1. Before the onset of withdrawal signs, the presence of maternal or infant characteristics known to be associated with drug use in pregnancy can be considered indications to screen for intrauterine drug exposure, by using meconium or urine samples.
   2. Maternal characteristics.

a. Maternal characteristics that suggest a need for screening include no prenatal care, previous unexplained fetal demise, precipitous labor, abruptio placentae, hypertensive episodes, severe mood swings, cerebrovascular accidents, myocardial infarction, and repeated spontaneous abortions.
b. Women who use illicit substances are at risk of human immunodeficiency virus (HIV) infection, acquired immunodeficiency syndrome (AIDS), herpesvirus infection, hepatitis, and syphilis, each of which can have significant adverse effects on the fetus and newborn.

3. Infant characteristics.
a. Infant characteristics that may be associated with maternal drug use include prematurity; unexplained intrauterine growth restriction; neurobehavioral abnormalities; urogenital anomalies; and atypical vascular incidents, such as cerebrovascular accidents, myocardial infarction, and necrotizing enterocolitis in otherwise healthy full-term infants.

**B. Identification of drug users (Behnke and Smith, 2013; Hudak and Tan, 2012).**

1. Two basic methods are used to identify drug users: self-report or biological specimens. Although no single approach can accurately determine the presence or amount of drug used during pregnancy, it is more likely that fetal exposure will be identified if a biological specimen is collected at the time of a structured interview (Eyler et al., 2005).
2. Self-reported history.
a. Self-reported history is an inexpensive and practical method for identifying prenatal drug exposure. This is the only method available in which information can be obtained regarding the timing of the drug use during pregnancy and the amount used.
b. However, self-report suffers from problems with the veracity of the informant and recall accuracy (AAP and ACOG, 2012).
3. Biological specimens.
a. Several biological specimens can be used to screen for drug exposure. Each specimen has its own individual variations with regard to the window of detection and the specific drug metabolites.
b. The three most commonly used specimens to establish drug exposure during the prenatal and perinatal period are urine, meconium, and hair; however, none is accepted as a "gold standard." Other specimens such as umbilical cord, cord blood, human milk, and amniotic fluid may also be tested.
c. Breast milk.
(1) A minimum of 10 mL of breast milk is required for testing (United States Drug Testing Laboratories, Inc. [USDTL], 2012b). Collection instructions can be found at http://www.usdtl.com/lactostat.html.
d. Urine.
(1) Urine has been the most frequently tested biological specimen because of its ease of collection. Urine testing identifies only recent drug use, because threshold levels of drug metabolites generally can be detected in urine only for several days. False-negative urine test results may occur in the presence of significant intrauterine drug exposure.
(2) Marijuana metabolites can be excreted for as long as 10 days in the urine of regular users and up to 30 days in chronic, heavy users. Urine is a good medium as well for the detection of nicotine, opiate, cocaine, and amphetamine exposure.
e. Meconium.
(1) Meconium is easy to collect and is a more accurate indication of exposure over a longer gestational period than urine analysis. While meconium screening may also yield false-negative test results, the likelihood is lower than with urine screening.
(2) It is hypothesized that drugs accumulate in meconium throughout pregnancy, and this is thought to reflect exposure during the second and third trimesters of pregnancy when meconium forms. Meconium has been used for the detection of nicotine, alcohol, marijuana, opiate, cocaine, and amphetamine exposure.
(3) Because meconium is heterogeneous and drugs do not appear to diffuse throughout the entire meconium mass, the pooling of multiple meconium stools is highly encouraged until the milk stool appears. For maximum sensitivity, 2 to 3 g (1 teaspoon) of meconium are necessary for testing (USDTL, 2012c). Collection instructions can be found at http://www.usdtl.com/mecstat.html.

f. Hair.
   (1) Hair is easy to collect, although some parents may decline this sampling method.
   (2) Drugs become trapped within the hair and can reflect drug use over a long period of time. Hair is useful for the detection of nicotine, opiate, cocaine, and amphetamine exposure.

g. Umbilical cord.
   (1) Umbilical cord tissue appears to be as reliable as meconium testing, with the additional benefit of availability of the tissue at the time of birth. Umbilical cord tissue performs as well as meconium in assessing fetal drug exposure to amphetamines, opiates, cocaine, cannabinoids, alcohol, and bath salts.
   (2) The cord may have a more rapid return of information to the clinician since meconium may not be passed for several days (Montgomery et al., 2006; USDTL, 2012a).
   (3) A 6-inch segment of the umbilical cord is required for testing (USDTL, 2012a). Collection instructions can be found at http://www.usdtl.com/cordstat.html.

4. Additional screenings.
   a. Additional assessment of infants of drug-abusing mothers should include possible screening for hepatitis B, hepatitis C, HIV, and other sexually transmitted infections (AAP and ACOG, 2012).

**C. Legal implications of drug screening.**

1. The legal implications of testing and the need for consent from the mother may vary among the states; therefore, health care providers should be aware of local laws and legislative changes that may influence regional practice (AAP and ACOG, 2012).
2. Each hospital should consider adopting a policy for maternal and newborn screening to avoid discriminatory practices and to comply with local laws (AAP and ACOG, 2012; Hudak and Tan, 2012).

## MEDICAL ISSUES IN THE FETAL AND NEWBORN PERIOD

**A. Fetal growth (Behnke and Smith, 2013).**

1. Fetal tobacco exposure has been a known risk factor for low birth weight and intrauterine growth restriction for more than 50 years. Decreasing birth weight has been shown to be related to the number of cigarettes smoked. However, by 24 months of age, most studies no longer demonstrate an effect of fetal tobacco exposure on growth parameters.
2. There is a vast literature on the teratogenic effects of prenatal alcohol exposure after the first description of fetal alcohol syndrome (FAS) in 1973. Growth restriction is a hallmark of FAS. More information is available from the American Academy of Pediatrics (www.aap.org) and on the National Institute on Alcohol Abuse and Alcoholism website (NIAAA, 2013).
3. Marijuana has not been associated with fetal growth restriction, particularly after controlling for other prenatal drug exposures.
4. Studies have reported lower birth weight in opiate-exposed newborn infants born at $\geq$33 weeks of gestation, independent of use of other drugs, prenatal care, or other medical risk factors.
5. Pregnant women who abuse methamphetamine are at increased risk of preterm birth, placental abruption, fetal distress, and intrauterine growth restriction at rates similar to those for pregnant women who use cocaine (Hudak and Tan, 2012).

**B. Neurobehavioral abnormalities (Behnke and Smith, 2013).**

1. Prenatal nicotine exposure may produce impaired orientation and autonomic regulation, as well as abnormalities of muscle tone.
2. Prenatal alcohol exposure may cause poor habituation and low levels of arousal along with motor abnormalities.
3. Prenatal marijuana exposure is associated with increased startles and tremors in the newborn.
4. Abnormal neurobehavior in opiate-exposed newborn infants is related to neonatal abstinence.
5. Prenatal cocaine exposure may cause irritability and lability of state, decreased behavioral and autonomic regulation, and poor alertness and orientation.

6. Prenatal methamphetamine exposure has been documented to cause abnormal neurobehavioral patterns in exposed newborn infants consisting of poor movement quality, decreased arousal, and increased stress. There are reports of long-term adverse neurotoxic effects of in-utero methamphetamine exposure on behavior, cognitive skills, and physical dexterity (Hudak and Tan, 2012).

## NEONATAL DRUG WITHDRAWAL AND ACUTE TOXICITY

A. **For all drug classes except opioids, the symptoms of NAS are usually self-limited and do not require pharmacologic treatment (Patrick et al., 2012).**
B. **Neonatal withdrawal most commonly results from intrauterine opioid exposure.** Signs and symptoms of withdrawal *worsen* as drug levels decrease. In addition to prenatal exposure, hospitalized infants who are treated with opioids or benzodiazepines to provide analgesia or sedation may be at risk of manifesting signs of withdrawal (AAP and ACOG, 2012; Behnke and Smith, 2013; Hudak and Tan, 2012).
C. **Other drugs cause signs in infants because of acute toxicity.** Signs and symptoms of acute toxicity *abate* with drug elimination (AAP and ACOG, 2012).

## NEONATAL NARCOTIC ABSTINENCE SYNDROME

A. **An opiate withdrawal syndrome was first described by Finnegan and colleagues (Finnegan et al., 1975a, 1975b).**
B. **Neonatal withdrawal most commonly results from intrauterine opioid exposure.** Infants with NAS often require prolonged hospitalization and treatment with medication (Hudak and Tan, 2012).
C. **The constellation of clinical findings associated with opioid withdrawal has been termed neonatal narcotic abstinence syndrome.** This syndrome includes a combination of physiologic and neurobehavioral signs such as sweating, irritability, increased muscle tone and activity, feeding problems, diarrhea, and seizures (Behnke and Smith, 2013; Hudak and Tan, 2012).
D. **Withdrawal signs will develop in 55% to 94% of infants exposed to opioids in utero.** Neonatal withdrawal signs also have been described in infants exposed antenatally to benzodiazepines, barbiturates, and alcohol (Behnke and Smith, 2013).
E. **Because fetal drug exposure often is unrecognized in the immediate newborn period, affected infants may be discharged to homes where they are at increased risk of a variety of medical and social problems, including abuse and neglect (AAP and ACOG, 2012; Hudak and Tan, 2012).**
F. **The specific effect of drug exposure on the fetus and newborn varies widely with the substance ingested, the amount received, and individual susceptibility.**

## COCAINE AND OTHER STIMULANTS (HUDAK AND TAN, 2012)

A. **An abstinence syndrome after intrauterine exposure to CNS stimulants such as cocaine and amphetamine has not been clearly defined.**
B. **Neurobehavioral abnormalities may occur in neonates with intrauterine cocaine exposure, most frequently on the second or third postnatal days.**
C. **These abnormalities may include irritability, hyperactivity, tremors, high-pitched cry, and excessive sucking.** Because cocaine or its metabolites may be detected in neonatal urine for as long as 7 days after delivery, observed abnormalities in exposed infants may reflect drug effect rather than withdrawal.

## OPIOIDS (HUDAK AND TAN, 2012)

A. **Opioids are a class of natural, endogenous, and synthetic compounds.** Morphine is one of many natural opioids. Codeine, heroin (diacetylmorphine), hydromorphone (Dilaudid), fentanyl (Sublimaze), and methadone are examples of synthetic opioids.

B. **Maintenance programs with methadone can sustain opioid concentrations in the mother and fetus to minimize opioid craving and prevent fetal stress.** Disadvantages of methadone include the extremely unlikely achievement of successful detoxification after delivery and a more severe and prolonged course of NAS.

C. **The synthetic opioid buprenorphine is approved for the treatment of opioid dependence.** Buprenorphine, either alone (Subutex) or in combination with naloxone (Suboxone), has been used both as a first-line treatment of heroin addiction and as a replacement drug for methadone.

D. **Buprenorphine has some advantages over methadone as a treatment of opioid addiction in pregnant women.** Infants born to mothers treated with buprenorphine had shorter hospital stays (10 vs. 17.5 days), had shorter treatment durations for NAS (4.1 vs. 9.9 days), and required a lower cumulative dose of morphine (1.1 vs. 10.4 mg) compared with infants born to mothers on methadone maintenance (Jones et al., 2010b).

## CLINICAL PRESENTATION OF OPIOID WITHDRAWAL (HUDAK AND TAN, 2012)

A. **Opioid receptors are concentrated in the CNS and the gastrointestinal tract.** As such, the predominant signs and symptoms of opioid withdrawal reflect CNS irritability, autonomic overreactivity, and gastrointestinal tract dysfunction.

B. **Onset of signs attributable to neonatal withdrawal from heroin often begins within 24 hours of birth, whereas withdrawal from methadone usually commences around 24 to 72 hours of age.** Infants exposed to buprenorphine may have an onset of withdrawal that peaks at 40 hours, and signs are most severe at 70 hours of age.

C. **Withdrawal from ethanol begins early during the first 3 to 12 hours after delivery.**

D. **Barbiturate withdrawal has a median onset of 4 to 7 days, but a wide range of 1 to 14 days.** Other sedative-hypnotics have exhibited even later onset, including as late as day 12 for diazepam and day 21 for chlordiazepoxide.

E. **Clinical features of NAS fall into two major categories: neurologic excitability (e.g., high-pitched cry, tremors, increased wakefulness) and gastrointestinal dysfunction (e.g., vomiting, fever, sweating) (see Fig. 3-1).**

## PRETERM INFANTS AND DRUG WITHDRAWAL (HUDAK AND TAN, 2012)

A. **Preterm infants have been described as being at lower risk of drug withdrawal with less severe courses.**

B. **The apparent decreased severity of signs in preterm infants may relate to developmental immaturity of the CNS, differences in total drug exposure, or lower fat depots of drug.**

C. **The clinical evaluation of the severity of abstinence may be more difficult in preterm infants because scoring tools to describe withdrawal were largely developed in term or late preterm infants.**

## ASSESSMENT OF WITHDRAWAL

A. **Several tools are available for quantifying the severity of withdrawal symptoms.**

B. **Each nursery should adopt a protocol for the evaluation and management of neonatal withdrawal, and staff should be trained in the correct use of an abstinence assessment tool.**

C. **The Finnegan instrument was created to assess severity of disease in those with known opioid exposure.** On day 2 of life, a score of 7 corresponds with the 95th percentile for nonexposed infants, meaning any score of 8 or greater is highly suggestive of in-utero opioid exposure even in infants of those women denying opioid use during pregnancy (Finnegan et al., 1975a, 1975b; Kraft and van den Anker, 2012).

D. **The modified Finnegan's Neonatal Abstinence Scoring System is the predominant tool used in the United States (Fig. 3-2).** This instrument assigns a cumulative score based on the interval observation of 21 items relating to signs of neonatal withdrawal.

**NEONATAL ABSTINENCE SCORING SYSTEM**

| System | Signs and Symptoms | Score | AM | | | | | PM | | | | | Comments |
|---|---|---|---|---|---|---|---|---|---|---|---|---|---|
| Central Nervous System Disturbances | Excessive high-pitched (or other) cry<br>Continuous high-pitched (or other) cry | 2<br>3 | | | | | | | | | | | Daily weight: |
| | Sleeps <1 hour after feeding<br>Sleeps <2 hours after feeding<br>Sleeps <3 hours after feeding | 3<br>2<br>1 | | | | | | | | | | | |
| | Hyperactive Moro reflex<br>Markedly hyperactive Moro reflex | 2<br>3 | | | | | | | | | | | |
| | Mild tremors disturbed<br>Moderate-severe tremors disturbed | 1<br>2 | | | | | | | | | | | |
| | Mild tremors undisturbed<br>Moderate-severe tremors undisturbed | 3<br>4 | | | | | | | | | | | |
| | Increased muscle tone | 2 | | | | | | | | | | | |
| | Excoriation (specific area) | 1 | | | | | | | | | | | |
| | Myoclonic jerks | 3 | | | | | | | | | | | |
| | Generalized convulsions | 5 | | | | | | | | | | | |
| Metabolic/Vasomotor/Respiratory Disturbances | Sweating | 1 | | | | | | | | | | | |
| | Fever <101° (99°–100.8° F/37.2°–38.2° C)<br>Fever >101° (38.4° C and higher) | 1<br>2 | | | | | | | | | | | |
| | Frequent yawning (>3 or 4 times/interval) | 1 | | | | | | | | | | | |
| | Mottling | 1 | | | | | | | | | | | |
| | Nasal stuffiness | 1 | | | | | | | | | | | |
| | Sneezing (>3 or 4 times/interval) | 1 | | | | | | | | | | | |
| | Nasal flaring | 2 | | | | | | | | | | | |
| | Respiratory rate >60/min<br>Respiratory rate >60/min with retractions | 1<br>2 | | | | | | | | | | | |
| Gastrointestinal Disturbances | Excessive sucking | 1 | | | | | | | | | | | |
| | Poor feeding | 2 | | | | | | | | | | | |
| | Regurgitation<br>Projectile vomiting | 2<br>3 | | | | | | | | | | | |
| | Loose stools<br>Watery stools | 2<br>3 | | | | | | | | | | | |
| | Total Score | | | | | | | | | | | | |
| | Initials of Scorer | | | | | | | | | | | | |

FIGURE 3-2 ■ Modified Finnegan's Neonatal Abstinence Scoring System. (Developed by L. Finnegan.)

## NONPHARMACOLOGIC TREATMENT

A. **Initial treatment of infants who develop early signs of withdrawal is directed at (Hudak and Tan, 2012):**
   1. Minimizing environmental stimuli (both light and sound) by placing the infant in a dark, quiet environment.
   2. Avoiding autostimulation by careful swaddling.
   3. Responding early to an infant's signals by adopting appropriate infant positioning and comforting techniques (swaying, rocking).

4. Providing frequent small volumes of hypercaloric formula or human milk to minimize hunger and allow for adequate growth (Kraft and van den Anker, 2012).
5. Caloric needs may be as high as 150 to 250 kcal/kg/day because of increased energy expenditure and loss of calories from regurgitation, vomiting, and/or loose stools.
6. The infant needs to be carefully observed to recognize fever, dehydration, or weight loss promptly.
7. The goals of therapy are to ensure that the infant achieves adequate sleep and nutrition to establish a consistent pattern of weight gain and begins to integrate into a social environment (Kraft and van den Anker, 2012).
8. Additional supportive care in the form of intravenous fluids, replacement electrolytes, and gavage feedings may be necessary to stabilize the infant's condition in the acute phase and obviate the need for pharmacologic intervention.

## PHARMACOLOGIC TREATMENT (KRAFT AND VAN DEN ANKER, 2012)

A. **Drug therapy is indicated to relieve moderate to severe signs of NAS and to prevent complications such as fever, weight loss, and seizures if an infant does not respond to a committed program of nonpharmacologic support.**

B. **Unnecessary pharmacologic treatment will prolong drug exposure and the duration of hospitalization, to the possible detriment of maternal–infant bonding.** The only clearly defined benefit of pharmacologic treatment is the short-term amelioration of clinical signs.

C. **An opioid (morphine or methadone) is the drug of first choice and the ideal treatment for opioid withdrawal symptoms associated with in-utero exposure to opiates.**

D. **Phenobarbital (identified as phenobarbitone in the British nomenclature) is often used as a rescue therapy when the maximum dose of opioid replacement therapy is reached without adequate resolution of symptoms (Hudak and Tan, 2012).**

E. **Diluted, deodorized tincture of opium has a morphine concentration of 0.4 mg/mL and an ethanol concentration of 0.19%.** This agent has been largely replaced by an ethanol-free morphine solution of 0.4 mg/mL concentration.

F. **Methadone is a long-acting opioid commonly used for abstinence treatment.** The longer half-life of methadone provides less of a flux between peak and trough levels, while also providing ease of administration at less frequent intervals.

G. **Buprenorphine is a long-acting opioid receptor agonist.** In a recent clinical trial, treatment with buprenorphine revealed a mean length of treatment of 23 days, compared with a mean length of 34 days using standard-of-care oral morphine. Adjunctive therapy with phenobarbital may be required. Buprenorphine is absorbed rapidly by the sublingual route with no evidence of aspiration in neonates.

H. **Paregoric is no longer used, because it contains variable concentrations of other opioids, as well as toxic ingredients such as camphor, anise oil, alcohol, and benzoic acid (Hudak and Tan, 2012).**

I. **Diazepam is not recommended because of a documented lack of efficacy compared with other agents and because of its adverse effects on infant suck and swallow reflexes.**

J. **Ideal treatment uses protocol-driven drug titration to control symptoms.** Regardless of the manner of dose titration, infants who do not have control of symptoms despite high doses of the initial therapy are treated with a secondary drug. After stabilization, symptom scores are used to gradually wean the controlling drug or drugs (Hudak and Tan, 2012).

## ACQUIRED OPIOID AND BENZODIAZEPINE DEPENDENCY

A. **One of the primary components in caring for critically ill children is to provide adequate and safe analgesia and sedation by using both pharmacologic and nonpharmacologic measures.**

B. **Pharmacologic treatment typically includes medications in the opioid and benzodiazepine drug classes.** If these drugs cannot safely be discontinued within a few days, physical dependence can develop and manifest with signs of withdrawal. Various weaning and treatment protocols are noted in Hudak and Tan (2012).

## SELECTIVE SEROTONIN REUPTAKE INHIBITORS (HUDAK AND TAN, 2012)

A. **Selective serotonin reuptake inhibitors (SSRIs) are a class of antidepressant medications that became available for widespread clinical use in 1988.** SSRIs are now the most frequently used drugs to treat depression both in the general population and in pregnant women.

B. **Reports have linked third-trimester use of SSRIs in pregnant women to a constellation of neonatal signs that include continuous crying, irritability, jitteriness, and/or restlessness; shivering; fever; tremors; hypertonia or rigidity; tachypnea or respiratory distress; feeding difficulty; sleep disturbance; hypoglycemia; and seizures.**

C. **The onset of these signs ranged from several hours to several days after birth and they usually resolved within 1 to 2 weeks.**

D. **A mother on treatment with an SSRI who desires to nurse her infant should be counseled about the benefits of breastfeeding as well as the potential risk that her infant may continue to be exposed to a measureable level of the SSRI with unknown long-term effects.**

## LONG-TERM EFFECTS RELATED TO PRENATAL DRUG EXPOSURE (BEHNKE AND SMITH, 2013)

A. **Tobacco.**
   1. A number of studies have identified effects of prenatal tobacco exposure on long-term behavioral outcomes extending from early childhood into adulthood. Impulsivity and attention problems have been identified in children prenatally exposed to nicotine (Hudak and Tan, 2012).
   2. In addition, prenatal tobacco exposure has been associated with hyperactivity and negative and externalizing behaviors in children. Studies of both young and older children prenatally exposed to nicotine have revealed abnormalities in learning and memory and slightly lower IQ scores.
   3. Poorer performance on arithmetic and spelling tasks has also been noted.

B. **Marijuana.**
   1. Prenatal marijuana exposure has been associated with academic underachievement, particularly in the areas of reading and spelling.

C. **Opiates.**
   1. Hyperactivity and short attention span have been noted in toddlers prenatally exposed to opiates. Older exposed children have demonstrated memory and perceptual problems.

D. **Cocaine.**
   1. Prenatal cocaine exposure has not predicted overall development, IQ, or school readiness.
   2. Deficits in attention processing and an increase in symptoms of attention-deficit/hyperactivity disorder and oppositional defiant disorder have been self-reported by the exposed children.
   3. Subtle language delays have been associated with prenatal cocaine exposure. Table 3-2 shows the summary of effects of prenatal drug exposure.

## BREASTFEEDING AND SUBSTANCE ABUSE (AAP, 2012)

A. **Caregivers are faced with weighing the risks of exposing an infant to drugs during breastfeeding against the many known benefits of breastfeeding.** Maternal substance abuse is not a categorical contraindication to breastfeeding.

B. **Adequately nourished narcotic-dependent mothers can be encouraged to breastfeed if they are enrolled in a supervised methadone maintenance program and have negative screening for HIV and illicit drugs.**

C. **Street drugs such as phencyclidine (PCP), cocaine, and cannabis can be detected in human milk, and their use by breastfeeding mothers is of concern, particularly with regard to the infant's long-term neurobehavioral development; thus they are contraindicated.**

D. **Alcohol may blunt the prolactin response to suckling and negatively affects infant motor development.**

■ TABLE 3-2
■ ■ **Summary of Effects of Prenatal Drug Exposure**

| | Nicotine | Alcohol | Marijuana | Opiates | Cocaine | Methamphetamine |
|---|---|---|---|---|---|---|
| **SHORT-TERM EFFECTS/BIRTH OUTCOME** | | | | | | |
| Fetal growth | Effect | Strong effect | No effect | Effect | Effect | Effect |
| Anomalies | No consensus on effect | Strong effect | No effect | No effect | No effect | No effect |
| Withdrawal | No effect | No effect | No effect | Strong effect | No effect | * |
| Neurobehavior | Effect | Effect | Effect | Effect | Effect | Effect |
| **LONG-TERM EFFECTS** | | | | | | |
| Growth | No consensus on effect | Strong effect | No effect | No effect | No consensus on effect | * |
| Behavior | Effect | Strong effect | Effect | Effect | Effect | * |
| Cognition | Effect | Strong effect | Effect | No consensus on effect | Effect | * |
| Language | Effect | Effect | No effect | * | Effect | * |
| Achievement | Effect | Strong effect | Effect | * | No consensus on effect | * |

From Behnke, M., Smith, V.C., Committee on Substance Abuse, and Committee on Fetus and Newborn, American Academy of Pediatrics: Prenatal substance abuse: Short- and long-term effects on the exposed fetus. *Pediatrics*, 131(3):e1009-1024, 2013. Epub February 25, 2013. Retrieved from http://pediatrics.aappublications.org/content/131/3/e1009.
*Limited or no data available.

E. **Maternal smoking is not an absolute contraindication to breastfeeding but should be strongly discouraged because it is associated with an increased incidence in infant respiratory allergy and SIDS.**
F. **Smoking should not occur in the presence of the infant so as to minimize the negative effect of secondary passive smoke inhalation.** Smoking is also a risk factor for low milk supply and poor weight gain.
G. **Methadone is not a contraindication to breastfeeding and is included in the AAP "approved" category for breastfeeding women.** Supervised methadone use is considered to be compatible with breastfeeding and has a potential benefit in reducing the symptoms associated with NAS.
H. **Mothers who are positive for HIV types 1 and 2 or untreated brucellosis should not breastfeed or provide expressed milk to their infants.** Breastfeeding should not occur if the mother has active (infectious) untreated tuberculosis or has active herpes simplex lesions on her breast.

## DISCHARGE AND FOLLOW-UP CARE (HUDAK AND TAN, 2012)

A. **Documentation of in-utero illicit substance exposure and alcohol use by the mother should preclude early discharge after birth.** Appropriate planning for discharge and subsequent follow-up care requires social work assessment and may include referral for child protective services if there is a concern about the future well-being of the infant.
B. **Long-term effects on learning and school performance, behavioral problems, and emotional instability of infants exposed to illicit drugs, alcohol, and tobacco in utero remain major concerns.**
C. **Drug exposure during development may have long-lasting effects on behavioral and cognitive outcomes.** These effects also may result from environmental factors that place drug-exposed infants at high risk of physical, sexual, and emotional abuse, neglect, and developmental delay.

## RESUMPTION OF SUBSTANCE USE AMONG RECENT MOTHERS

A. **When compared with women in the third trimester of pregnancy, nonpregnant women with children under 3 months old in the household had much higher rates of past-month alcohol use (6.2% vs. 31.9%), binge alcohol use (1% vs. 10%), cigarette use (13.9% vs. 20.4%), and marijuana use (1.4% vs. 3.8%).**

B. **These data provide indirect evidence of dramatic increases in the prevalence of substance use among mothers with babies under 3 months old based on cross-sectional reports from pregnant, parenting, and nonpregnant women.** This increase implies a resumption of substance use following childbirth (SAMHSA, 2009).

C. **Multidisciplinary long-term follow-up should include medical, developmental, and social support.** In general, a coordinated multidisciplinary approach without criminal sanctions has the best chance of helping infants and families (SAMHSA, 2009).

## FUTURE THERAPIES

A. **There is clearly an unmet medical need to develop improved pharmacologic treatment for infants with NAS.** Future research needs to determine not only the most accurate screening methods but also the most effective prevention and treatment interventions to reduce the incidence and prevalence of opioid dependence among women.

B. **Future directions may include the examination of the existing scales, particularly those based on the Finnegan scale, to discern whether it is possible to simplify the scales to include those elements most closely correlated with clinical outcomes in the management of infants with known opioid exposure (Kraft and van den Anker, 2012).**

C. **A 3-point scale consisting of hyperactive Moro reflex, mild tremors when undisturbed, and increased muscle tone has been described as discriminative between opioid-exposed and non–opioid-exposed infants, but this scale has not yet been validated in a large sample (Jones et al., 2010a).**

D. **A vaccine that blocks a wide range of opioids of abuse may have distinct advantages in battling the widespread availability of illicit and prescription opioids of abuse.** Vaccines against drugs of abuse such as heroin, cocaine, nicotine and methamphetamine are currently being studied (McLemore et al., 2013).

   1. The optimum strategy would be for a drug-dependent woman to develop immunity prior to pregnancy with periodic booster injections to maintain high antibody titers against the targeted opioid during pregnancy. While opioid vaccines will probably not replace existing agonist substitution therapy, they could serve as useful adjuncts (McLemore et al., 2013).

E. **Pharmacogenomics is the field of study encompassing the genetic basis underlying individual drug response variability.** Pharmacogenomics examines multiple genes suspected of affecting individual pharmacodynamic (drug action) and pharmacokinetic (body's response) parameters, and seeks to correlate a specific drug response with specific genetic variations. The exploration of maternal–fetal/neonatal pharmacogenomics as a new NAS treatment strategy shows promise (McLemore et al., 2013).

## REFERENCES

American Academy of Pediatrics, Policy statement: Breastfeeding and the use of human milk. *Pediatrics*, 129(3):e827–e841, 2012. Retrieved from http://pediatrics.aappublications.org/content/129/3/e827.full.

American Academy of Pediatrics and American College of Obstetricians and Gynecologists, *Guidelines for perinatal care* (7th ed.). Elk Grove Village. IL, and Washington, DC, 2012, American Academy of Pediatrics and American College of Obstetricians and Gynecologists.

Behnke, M., and Smith, V.C., Committee on Substance Abuse, and Committee on Fetus and Newborn, American Academy of Pediatrics: Prenatal substance abuse: Short- and long-term effects on the exposed fetus. *Pediatrics*, 131(3):e1009–e1024, 2013. Epub February 25, 2013. Retrieved from http://pediatrics.aappublications.org/content/131/3/e1009.

Eyler, F.D., Behnke, M., Wobie, K., et al.: Relative ability of biologic specimens and interviews to detect prenatal cocaine use. *Neurotoxicology and Teratology*, 27 (4):677–687, 2005.

Finnegan, L.P. (1990). Neonatal abstinence. In: Nelson NM, ed. *Current Therapy in Neonatal-Perinatal Medicine*. 2nd ed. Toronto, Ontario: BC Decker Inc; 1990.

Finnegan, L.P., Connaughton, J.F., Kron, R.E., and Emich, J.P., Neonatal abstinence syndrome: Assessment and management. *Addictive Diseases*, 2(1-2):141–158, 1975a.

Finnegan, L.P., Kron, R.E., Connaughton, J.F., and Emich, J.P., Assessment and treatment of abstinence in the infant of the drug-dependent mother. *International Journal of Clinical Pharmacology and Biopharmacy*, 12(1-2):19–32, 1975b.

Hudak, M.L., and Tan, R.C., Committee on Drugs, and Committee on Fetus and Newborn, American Academy of Pediatrics. Neonatal drug withdrawal. *Pediatrics*, 129(2):e540–e560, 2012. Epub January 30, 2012. Retrieved from http://pediatrics.aappublications.org/content/129/2/e540.

Johnston, L.D., O'Malley, P.M., Bachman, J.G., and Schulenberg, E., *Monitoring the future national results on adolescent drug use: Overview of key findings, 2007* (NIH Publication No. 08-6418). Bethesda, MD, 2008, National Institute of Drug Abuse.

Jones, H.E., Harrow, C., and O'Grady, K.E., Neonatal abstinence scores in opioid exposed and non-exposed neonates: A blinded comparison. *Journal of Opioid Management*, 6(6):409–413, 2010a.

Jones, H.E., Kaltenbach, K., and Heil, S.H., Neonatal abstinence syndrome after methadone or buprenorphine exposure. *New England Journal of Medicine*, 363(24):2320–2331, 2010b.

Kellogg, A., Rose, C.H., Harms, R.H., and Watson, W.J., Current trends in narcotic use in pregnancy and neonatal outcomes. *American Journal of Obstetrics and Gynecology*, 204:259.e1–259.e4, 2011.

Kraft, W.K., and van den Anker, J.N., Pharmacologic management of the opioid neonatal abstinence syndrome. *Pediatric Clinics of North America*, 59 (5):1147–1165, 2012Epub August 30, 2012.

McLemore, G.L., Lewis, T., Jones, C.H., and Gauda, E.B., Novel pharmacotherapeutic strategies for treatment of opioid-induced neonatal abstinence syndrome. *Seminars in Fetal and Neonatal Medicine*, 18(1):35–41, 2013. Epub October 9, 2012.

Montgomery, D., Plate, C., Alder, S.C., et al.: Testing for fetal exposure to illicit drugs using umbilical cord tissue vs meconium. *Journal of Perinatology*, 26(1):11–14, 2006.

National Institute of Drug Abuse, Topics in brief: *Medication-assisted treatment for opioid addiction*. 2012: Retrieved from http://www.drugabuse.gov/publications/topics-in-brief/medication-assisted-treatment-opioid-addiction.

National Institute of Drug Abuse, *Topics in brief: Prenatal exposure to drugs of abuse*. 2011a: Retrieved from http://www.drugabuse.gov/publications/topics-in-brief/prenatal-exposure-to-drugs-abuse.

National Institute of Drug Abuse, *Topics in brief: Prescription drug abuse*. 2011b: Retrieved from http://www.drugabuse.gov/publications/topics-in-brief/prescription-drug-abuse.

National Institute on Alcohol Abuse and Alcoholism, *Drinking and your pregnancy*. 2013: Retrieved from http://pubs.niaaa.nih.gov/publications/DrinkingPregnancy_HTML/pregnancy.htm.

National Institute on Alcohol Abuse and Alcoholism, *Fetal alcohol exposure*. 2010: Retrieved from http://www.niaaa.nih.gov/alcohol-health/fetal-alcohol-exposure.

Patrick, S.W., Schumacher, R.E., Benneyworth, B.D., et al.: Neonatal abstinence syndrome and associated health care expenditures: United States, 2000-2009. *JAMA*, 307(18):1934–1940, 2012. Epub April 30, 2012.

Substance Abuse and Mental Health Services Administration, *Substance-exposed infants*. 2013: Retrieved from http://www.ncsacw.samhsa.gov/resources/substance-exposed-infants.aspx.

Substance Abuse and Mental Health Services Administration, *Results from the 2010 National Survey on Drug Use and Health. Summary of national findings*. 2012. Retrieved from http://www.samhsa.gov/data/NSDUH/2k10 NSDUH/2k10Results.htm#3.1.3.

Substance Abuse and Mental Health Services Administration, Office of Applied Studies, *The NSDUH Report: Substance use among women during pregnancy and following childbirth*. May 21, 2009. Retrieved from. http://www.oas.samhsa.gov/2k9/135/PregWoSubUse.htm.

United States Drug Testing Laboratories, Inc., *CordStat*. 2012a. Retrieved from http://www.usdtl.com/cordstat.html.

United States Drug Testing Laboratories, Inc., *LactoStat*. 2012b. Retrieved from http://www.usdtl.com/lactostat.html.

United States Drug Testing Laboratories, Inc., *MecStat*. 2012c. Retrieved from http://www.usdtl.com/mecstat.html.

CHAPTER

# 4 Adaptation to Extrauterine Life

M. TERESE VERKLAN

**OBJECTIVES**

1. Identify primary features of fetal circulation.
2. Identify physiologic changes that occur during transition to extrauterine life.
3. Identify routine care considerations for a newborn infant during the transition period.
4. Identify signs and symptoms of common problems in the transition period.
5. Define the methods and intervention times for parental teaching.

The transition period is considered to be the first 6 to 10 hours of life, but more than a period of time, it is a process of physiologic change in the newborn infant that begins in utero as the child prepares for the transition from intrauterine placental support to extrauterine self- maintenance. The fetus prepares for transition during the course of gestation in such ways as storing glycogen, producing catecholamines, and depositing brown fat. The neonate's ability to accomplish the transition to extrauterine life will depend on gestational age and the quality of placental support during gestation as well as any physical defects or anomalies that may affect major organ systems.

## ANATOMY AND PHYSIOLOGY

### Characteristics of Placental–Fetal Circulation

A. **Placenta.**
   1. Blood oxygenation and elimination of waste products of metabolism. Transfer of $O_2$ and $CO_2$ across the placenta is by simple diffusion.
   2. High rate of metabolism. The placenta uses one third of all the oxygen and glucose supplied to it by the maternal circulation for its own metabolic needs.
   3. Low-resistance circuit. The placenta receives approximately 50% of fetal cardiac output.
   4. Characteristics of uterine venous blood as it enters the intervillous space: $P_{CO_2}$ of 38 mm Hg, $P_{O_2}$ of 40 to 50 mm Hg, and pH of 7.36.

B. **Fetal shunts/blood flow (Fig. 4-1) (Moore et al., 2013).**
   1. Umbilical vein ($P_{O_2}$ 32 to 35 mm Hg). It carries oxygenated blood from the placenta to the fetus.
   2. Ductus venosus. Forty percent to 60% of the umbilical venous blood bypasses the liver through the ductus venosus to the inferior vena cava (IVC). It is a low-resistance channel that allows a significant portion of relatively well-oxygenated blood to enter the heart directly; the other half passes through the liver and enters the IVC via the hepatic veins. This mixing of blood slightly lowers the $P_{O_2}$.
   3. IVC blood and the blood from the coronary sinuses ($P_{O_2}$ = 25 to 28 mm Hg). This blood is largely deflected across the right atrium, through the foramen ovale, and into the left atrium. In contrast, most of the blood from the superior vena cava (SVC), also returning to the right atrium, is deflected to the right ventricle (see item 6, below). The crista dividens (lower edge of the septum secundum) separates the flow of blood from the IVC into two streams, with 50% to 60% of the blood from the IVC being diverted across the foramen ovale into the left atrium (Blackburn, 2013) and the remainder of blood from the IVC remaining in the right atrium and mixing with poorly oxygenated blood from the SVC and coronary sinus.

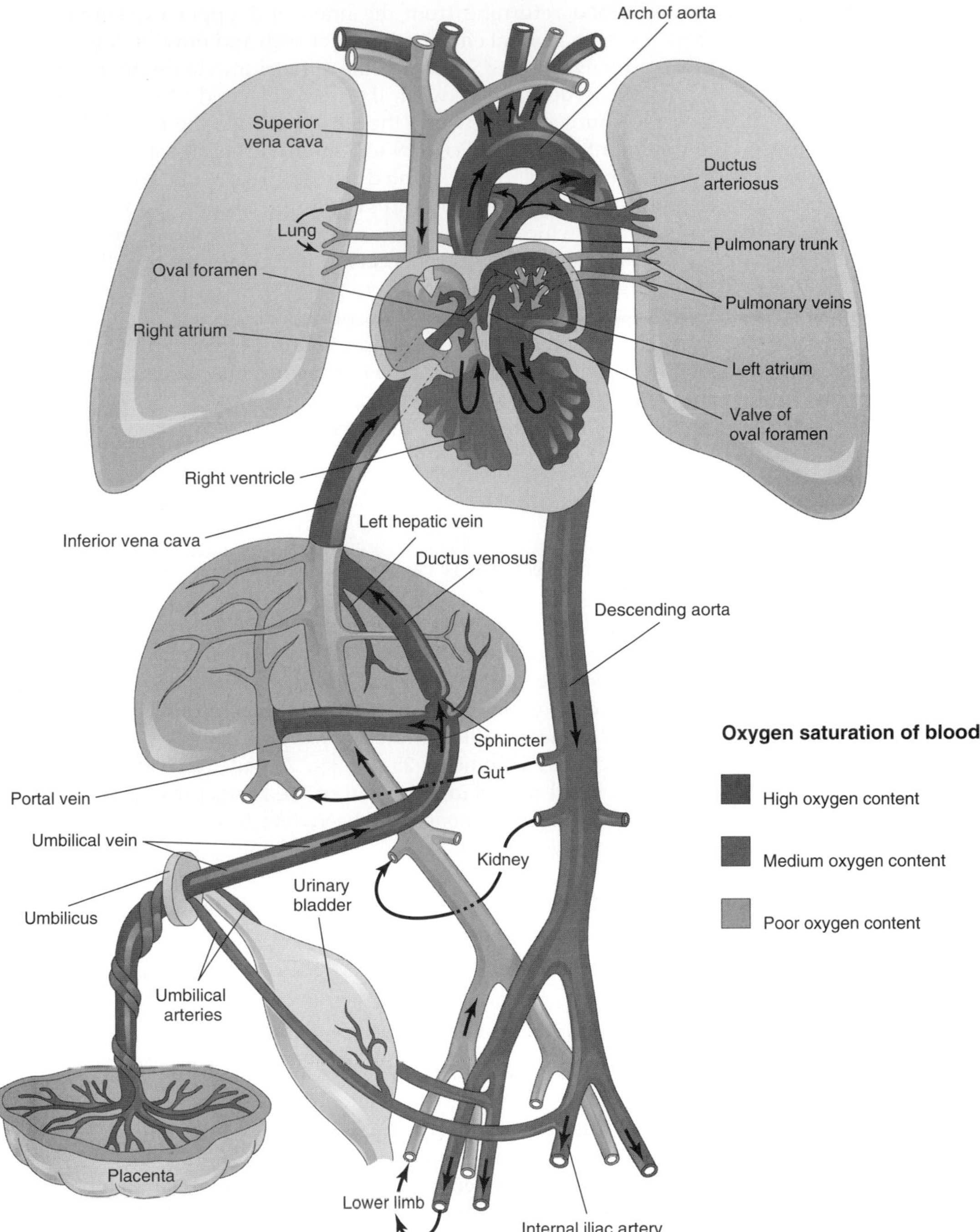


FIGURE 4-1 ■ Simplified scheme of fetal circulation. *Shaded areas* indicate oxygen saturation of the blood; *arrows* show course of fetal circulation. Organs are not drawn to scale. (From Moore, K.L., Persaud, T.V.N., and Torchia, M.G.: *The developing human: Clinically oriented embryology* [9th ed.]. Philadelphia, 2013, Elsevier Saunders.)

4. Left atrium. Blood is received from the right atrium via the foramen ovale and mixes with a small amount of blood returning from the lungs via the pulmonary veins.
5. Left ventricular blood ($Po_2 = 25$ to 28 mm Hg). Virtually all this blood is from the IVC by way of the right atrium–foramen ovale–left atrium pathway. Left ventricular blood is pumped out through the aorta to the brain from the upper part of the aortic arch. Approximately 90% of the blood from the ascending aorta feeds the coronary, carotid, and subclavian arteries and thus the brain and upper extremities.

6. The SVC. Unoxygenated blood returning from the brain and upper extremities is received by the SVC. Ninety-seven percent enters the right atrium and flows to the right ventricle through the tricuspid valve; only 3% flows to the left atrium via the foramen ovale.
7. Right atrium. Some mixing occurs here between the unoxygenated SVC blood and the oxygenated IVC blood not shunted directly into the left atrium via the foramen ovale.
8. Right ventricle. The dominant ventricle ($Po_2$=19 to 22 mm Hg) ejects about 66% of the total cardiac output. Most of the blood is shunted across the ductus arteriosus, away from the lungs, and into the descending aorta to supply the kidneys and intestines. It then divides into two arteries, which subsequently return back to the placenta.
9. Ductus arteriosus. Equal in size to the aorta, it connects the pulmonary artery to the descending aorta. The blood flows right to left (pulmonary artery to aorta) across the ductus arteriosus because of high pulmonary vascular resistance and low placental resistance. Patency is maintained by the low oxygen tension in utero and by the vasodilating effect of prostaglandin $E_2$.
10. Low pulmonary blood flow (only 10% to 12% of the right ventricular output). This results from high pulmonary vascular resistance (Blackburn, 2013).
11. Descending aorta. It supplies the kidneys and intestines, divides into two arteries, and returns blood to the placenta for oxygenation.

## Fetal Lung Characteristics

A. **Decreased blood flow.** In part, the decrease is caused by compression of the pulmonary capillaries by the fetal lung fluid.
B. **Pulmonary arteries.** The small pulmonary arteries of the fetus have a thick, muscular medial layer; they are very reactive and are actively constricted by the low $Po_2$ normally present during fetal life. Pulmonary vascular resistance increases throughout fetal life.
C. **Lung fluid secretion.** Fetal lungs actively secrete fluid; secretion of fluid is decreased near term. At term, the lungs contain 30 mL of plasma ultrafiltrate per kilogram of body weight. This is comparable to a postnatal thoracic gas volume of 25 mL/kg. An adequate fluid volume is necessary for lung development. Fluid moves into and out of the lungs through the trachea.
D. **Fetal breathing.** In-utero fetal breathing movements have been detected as early as 11 weeks of gestation. They contribute to lung development.
E. **Surfactant.** Surfactant is secreted into the amniotic fluid by the fetal lung before 20 weeks of gestation. The absolute quantity of surfactant increases throughout gestation in both the lung and amniotic fluid and can support extrauterine respiration at approximately 34 weeks of gestation.

## Fetal Metabolism and Hematology

A. **Glucose.** Fetal blood glucose concentrations are 70% to 80% of maternal blood glucose concentrations. Glucose is exchanged via the placenta by facilitated diffusion.
B. **Glycogen.** Large glycogen stores (2 to 10 times that of an adult) provide large energy reserves to sustain the newborn infant through the transition period.
C. **Hemoglobin.** Fetal hemoglobin has an increased affinity for oxygen. Fetal hemoglobin is progressively replaced by adult hemoglobin from weeks 32 to 36 of gestation and is approximately 80% of the total hemoglobin at term.

## Labor

A. **Placenta.** Maternal placental perfusion ceases with uterine contractions.
B. **Stress hormones.** High concentrations of stress hormones (predominantly norepinephrine) are released as a direct effect of the resultant hypoxia on the adrenal medulla.

## Cardiopulmonary Adaptation at Birth

A. **Cardiovascular adaptation (Fig. 4-2) (Hillman et al., 2012; Moore et al., 2013).**
   1. Umbilical cord is clamped.
      a. Placenta is separated from the circulation, and the umbilical arteries and veins constrict.

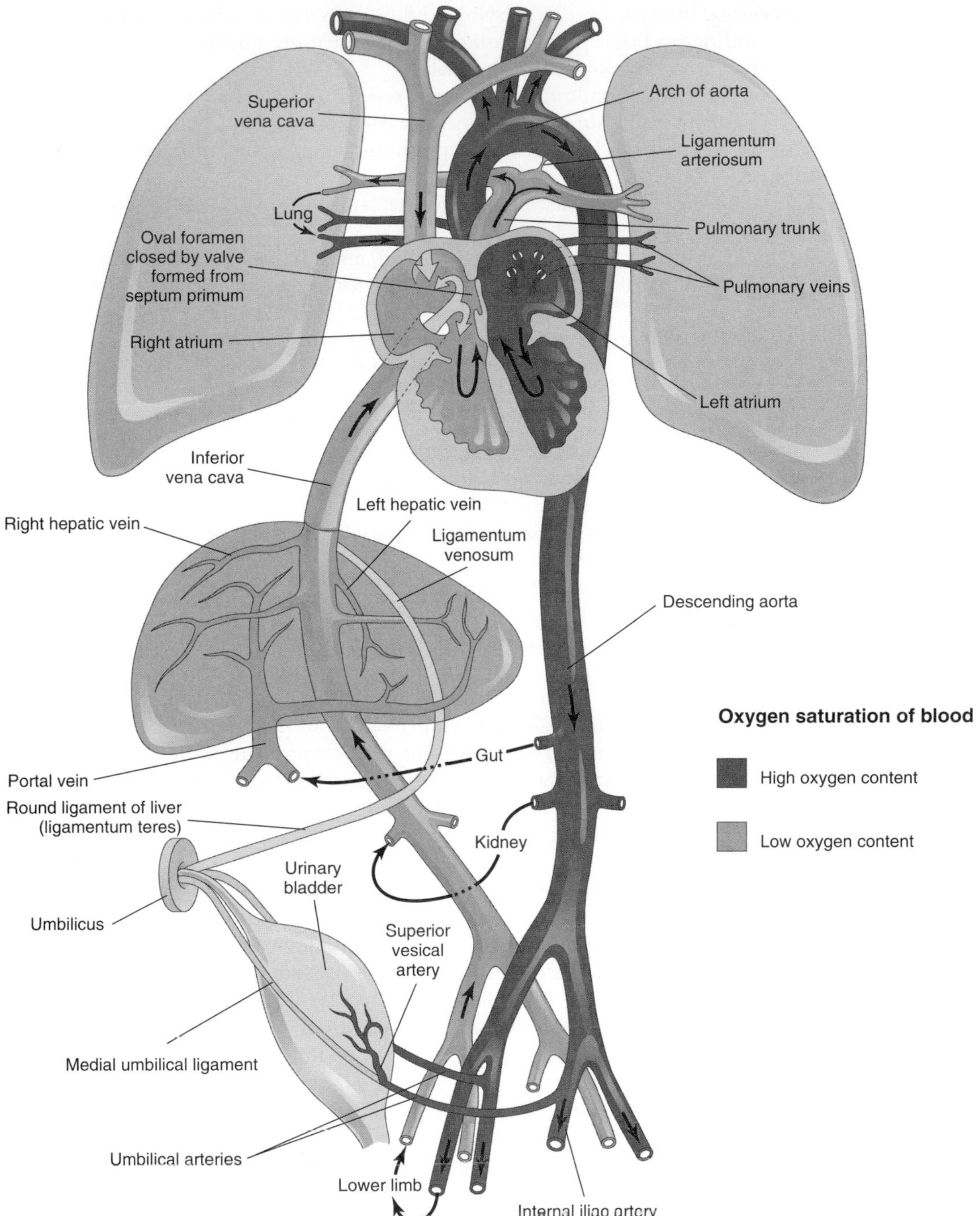


FIGURE 4-2 ■ Simplified representation of circulation after birth. Adult derivatives of fetal vessels and structures that become nonfunctional at birth are also shown. *Arrows* indicate course of neonatal circulation. Organs are not drawn to scale. (From Moore, K.L., Persaud, T.V.N., and Torchia, M.G.: *The developing human: Clinically oriented embryology* [9th ed.]. Philadelphia, 2013, Elsevier Saunders.)

b. As the low-resistance placental circuit is removed, there is a resultant increase in systemic blood pressure; the systemic vascular resistance then exceeds the pulmonary vascular resistance.

2. The three major fetal shunts (ductus venosus, foramen ovale, and ductus arteriosus) functionally close during transition (Leone and Finer, 2013).
   a. Ductus arteriosus. The lungs now provide more efficient oxygenation of the blood, and the arterial oxygen tension rises. This rise in $P_{O_2}$ is a potent stimulus to constriction of the

ductus arteriosus. Increased pulmonary blood flow increases the metabolism of circulating prostaglandins, and the loss of prostaglandins contributed by the placenta enhances the constrictive effects of oxygen on the ductus.

b. Foramen ovale. The fall in pulmonary vascular resistance results in a drop in right ventricular and right atrial pressure, and the increased systemic vascular resistance results in an increase in left atrial and left ventricular pressures, causing the foramen ovale to close against the atrial septum.
   (1) The foramen ovale becomes sealed by the deposit of fibrin and cell products during the first month of life.
   (2) Until the foramen ovale is anatomically sealed, anything that produces a significant increase in right atrial pressure can reopen the foramen ovale and allow a right-to-left shunt.

c. Ductus venosus. Absent umbilical venous return leads to closure of the ductus venosus. It functionally closes within 2 to 3 days and becomes the ligamentum venosum.

3. Postnatal circulation (see Fig. 4-2) (Hillman et al., 2012; Moore et al., 2013).
   a. Systemic venous blood enters the right atrium from the SVC and the IVC.
   b. Poorly oxygenated blood enters the right ventricle and passes through the pulmonary artery into the pulmonary circulation for oxygenation.
   c. The oxygenated blood returns to the left atrium through the pulmonary veins.
   d. This blood passes through the left ventricle and into the aorta to supply the systemic circulation with oxygenated blood.

**B. Pulmonary adaptation (Blackburn, 2013; Hillman et al., 2012).**

1. The lungs as the organ of gas exchange. Intermittent breathing begins in utero long before delivery and, after birth, is a continuation of movements and reflexes that have been well established.
2. Stimuli for initiating respiration. The mild hypercapnia, hypoxia, and acidosis that result from normal labor are due partially to the intermittent cessation of maternal–placental perfusion with contractions. The decreased pH stimulates the respiratory center directly; the low $Po_2$ and high $Pco_2$ stimulate the respiratory center by means of central and peripheral chemoreceptors (Gauda and Martin, 2013). Other stimuli include cold, light, noise, and touch.
3. Entry of air into lungs with the first breath.
   a. Aeration of the lungs drives fluid into the interstitium; it is then absorbed through the lymphatic and pulmonary circulation. The rate at which this process occurs is variable, and fine crackling rales may be audible throughout the lungs until this process is completed.
   b. The pulmonary vessels respond to the increase in $Po_2$ with vasodilation. Pulmonary vascular resistance progressively decreases until adult levels are reached by 6 to 8 weeks of age (Blackburn, 2013).
4. Inspiration of air and expansion of lungs. After the thoracic squeeze (during labor and vaginal delivery, this empties the lungs of approximately one third of the fetal lung fluid), the subsequent recoil of the chest wall causes inspiration of air and expansion of the lungs. Negative intrathoracic pressures generated with the first breath may be as high as 20 to 70 cm $H_2O$ because of the mechanical advantage created by the high resting level of the diaphragm in the nonaerated lung (Niermeyer and Clarke, 2011). Subsequent breaths in the normal newborn infant require 15 to 20 cm $H_2O$ pressure.
5. Respiratory augmentation. Head's paradoxic reflex is a vagally mediated hyperinflation triggered by distention of stretch receptors in the large airways.
6. Work of inspiration. This is predominately related to overcoming the surface tension of the walls of the terminal lung units at the gas–tissue interface. On expiration, the ability to retain air depends on surfactant (Hillman et al., 2012).
   a. Surfactant is a complete lipoprotein produced by type II alveolar pneumocytes; surfactant release increases in response to increased catecholamine levels at birth.
   b. Surfactant has the ability to lower the surface tension at an air–liquid interface.
   c. As the surfactant lowers the surface tension in the alveolus at end-expiration, it stabilizes the alveoli and prevents collapse.
7. There is an increase in the functional residual capacity with each breath. Less inspiratory pressure is thus required for subsequent breaths.

8. Lung compliance. Improves in the hours after delivery as a result of circulating catecholamines. The increased levels of catecholamines (especially of epinephrine) also clear the lungs by decreasing the secretion of the lungs' fluids and increasing their absorption through the lymphatic system.

## ROUTINE CARE CONSIDERATIONS DURING TRANSITION (GARDNER AND HERNANDEZ, 2011; ALDEN, 2012A; ALDEN 2012B; TAYLOR, WRIGHT, AND WOODRUM, 2013)

A. **Assessment/observation.** Within 2 hours of birth, the neonate's health status should be evaluated and the neonate assessed for risks that may complicate transition to extrauterine life (American Academy of Pediatrics [AAP] and American College of Obstetricians and Gynecologists [ACOG], 2012).
   1. Body measurements. Head circumference, length, and weight are recorded.
   2. Vital sign assessment. Vital signs recorded on admission will include heart rate, respiratory rate, and axillary temperature. Universal blood pressure screening in the well newborn infant is not warranted (AAP, 1993).
   3. Gestational age assessment. Weight, head circumference, and length are graphed against the assessed gestational age and medical record (refer to Chapter 7).
   4. Clinical changes. During the first hours of life, vital signs stabilize and the newborn proceeds through sleep–wake cycles associated with readiness-to-feed behaviors (Verklan, 2002). The time sequence of changes is altered in infants with low Apgar scores, immaturity, maternal medications, and intrinsic disease (refer to Chapter 5).
   5. Head-to-toe physical examination (refer to Chapter 7). The following findings seen during transition are within normal limits as the infant progresses through the physiologic changes described under cardiopulmonary adaptation, above.
      a. Skin.
         (1) Acrocyanosis. Vasoconstricted peripheral vessels result in a mottled appearance; peripheral pulses are decreased initially. (These findings are sequelae of catecholamine release, mild acidosis, and cold stress.)
         (2) Petechiae of the face and facial bruising. A vertex presentation, a rapid second stage of labor, or a tight nuchal cord may result in these skin changes. (With severe facial bruising, central color may be assessed by looking at the mucous membranes in the mouth.)
      b. Head.
         (1) The neonate's head is large relative to the body. During a vaginal delivery, considerable molding of the skull bones may take place to facilitate passage through the birth canal. Molding resolves during the first hours and days.
         (2) Caput succedaneum (edema of the presenting part of the scalp, caused by pressure that restricts the return of venous and lymph flow during vaginal delivery) may be present.
      c. Respirations/breath sounds.
         (1) Initially, coarse rales and moist tubular breath sounds. These breath sounds may continue until clearing of lung fluid is complete.
         (2) Prolonged expiratory phase.
         (3) Respiratory rate of 30 to 60 breaths per minute.
         (4) Grunting and retracting (intercostal and substernal). These findings may be present during the first hours of life as lung fluid is cleared.
      d. Heart sounds.
         (1) Second heart sound may be loud during the first 2 hours; splitting of the second heart sound is usually detectable at 2 to 4 hours of age and increases during the next 12 hours (pulmonic ahead of aortic component).
         (2) Soft grade 2/6 systolic murmur may be present; represents a left-to-right shunt across the ductus arteriosus before its closure.

e. Heart.
   (1) Normal heart rate 120 to 160 beats per minute (bpm); increased initially, with a mean peak of 180 bpm, and then decreased or irregular.
   (2) Consistently high or low heart rate suggests a pathologic condition.

f. Intestines.
   (1) Blood flow is reduced initially.
   (2) As the bowel begins to fill with air, normal motility and bowel sounds are present within 15 minutes.
   (3) The normal term neonate passes meconium within the first 24 hours after birth. If a term neonate has not passed meconium by 48 hours after birth, the lower gastrointestinal (GI) tract may be obstructed.

g. Urinary function.
   (1) Urine is normally passed within the first 24 hours after birth.
   (2) Failure to void within the first 24 hours may indicate genitourinary obstruction or abnormality.

h. Extremities. Findings may include deformities resulting from the intrauterine position.

B. **Thermoregulation considerations in the nursery (Brown and Landers, 2011).** The admission assessment and observation should be done in a controlled environment, such as a radiant warmer or incubator, that both provides warmth and prevents heat loss so that the infant maintains a normal temperature without increasing oxygen consumption, using glucose stores, or exceeding brown fat stores in the process of nonshivering thermogenesis (mediated by norepinephrine released by cold stress). Normal axillary ranges are 36.5° to 37.5° C (97.7° to 99.5° F) for the term neonate and 36.3° to 36.9° C (97.3° to 98.6° F) for the preterm neonate. Hypothermia and hyperthermia occur when the infant's attempts to maintain a normal temperature fail, which has serious metabolic consequences for the newborn infant (refer to Chapter 6).

1. Monitor temperature. Check axillary temperature every 30 minutes to 1 hour during transition while the infant is under a radiant warmer. Avoid hyperthermia (skin temperature greater than 37° C or axillary temperature greater than 37.5° C). NOTE: Monitoring the axillary temperature allows time for successful intervention before a fall in core temperature indicates failure of the body's heat-regulation mechanism.
2. First bath. Delay bath until body temperature has stabilized and is within normal limits. Check temperature 30 minutes after the bath and 1 hour after transfer to open crib.
3. Temperature. Check temperature at least every 4 hours until the infant's condition is stable, and then every 8 hours until discharge. Temperatures may need to be monitored every 30 minutes until stable.
4. Environmental temperature (incubator or warmer). Record environmental temperature with temperature checks of the infant to monitor his or her environmental requirements. NOTE: These requirements can be checked against the normal ranges of neutral thermal environmental temperature needs as a tool in evaluating an infant's condition.

C. **Transition nursery medications (AAP and ACOG, 2012; Taylor et al., 2013).**

1. Eye care. Administered to both eyes before 1 hour of age in all neonates, regardless of type of delivery.
   a. Recommendation. Apply a 1- to 2-cm ribbon of sterile ophthalmic ointment containing 0.5% erythromycin, or 1% tetracycline, or an ophthalmic solution of 2.5% povidone-iodine for prophylaxis of ophthalmia neonatorum due to *Neisseria gonorrhoeae*. Prophylaxis for *Chlamydia trachomatis* requires erythromycin or tetracycline.
   b. Procedure. Instill medication into conjunctival sac within 1 hour of birth; however, this may be delayed until after the first breastfeeding. The medication should not be flushed from the eye after application. A new tube is used for each infant.
2. Vitamin $K_1$ (phytonadione). Administer vitamin K within 1 hour of birth.
   a. Recommendation. Every neonate should receive a single parenteral 0.5- to 1-mg dose of natural vitamin K (phytonadione). Administer 0.5 mg if the infant weighs less than 1.5 kg and 1 mg if the infant weighs more than 1.5 kg.
   b. Risk of deficiency. Maternal dietary inadequacy of vitamin K, hepatic immaturity, reduced liver stores, and absence of intestinal flora predispose the child to deficiency

of vitamin K; gut bacteria are a substantial source. Vitamin K is needed to promote the hepatic biosynthesis of vitamin K–dependent clotting factors, including prothrombin (factor II), proconvertin (factor VII), plasma thromboplastin component (factor IX), and Stuart factor (factor X). Deficiency results in hemorrhagic disease of the newborn (HDN).

(1) Classic HDN. The disease occurs at 1 to 7 days of life. The infant is healthy at birth but develops cutaneous or GI bleeding. Other sites of bleeding include nasal bleeding or bleeding after circumcision. Classic HDN can be prevented with vitamin K prophylaxis.

(2) Early HDN. Maternal exposure to drugs, including warfarin, anticonvulsants, and antituberculosis drugs, may affect coagulation. Severe or life-threatening hemorrhage may occur during delivery or in the first day of life. Intracranial hemorrhage is a common complication. Early HDN is the only type that cannot be prevented by vitamin K prophylaxis.

(3) Late HDN. The late form of HDN may occur between 1 and 3 months of life. Acute intracranial hemorrhage is the most common initial finding and is often fatal or neurologically devastating. Other findings include GI or mucous membrane bleeding. Late HDN can be prevented by vitamin K prophylaxis.

**3.** Hepatitis vaccine and hepatitis B immunoglobulin (HBIG).

**a.** Rate of hepatitis B virus (HBV) infection. If the mother is hepatitis B surface antigen (HBsAg) and hepatitis B "e" antigen (HBeAg) positive, the baby has a 90% risk of HBV infection in the first 12 months if treatment is not received. There is a 20% risk of HBV infection if the mother is positive for HBsAg only (Venkatesh et al., 2011).

**b.** Chronicity. In the absence of treatment, the neonate will likely become a carrier, and eventually develop primary hepatocellular carcinoma (Venkatesh et al., 2011).

**c.** Maternal HBsAg-positive treatment recommendations:

(1) Child is bathed as soon as temperature is stable.

(2) Hepatitis B vaccine (Engerix-B, 10 mcg, or Recombivax-HB, 5 mcg) and HBIG, 0.5 mL intramuscularly (prepared from plasma to contain a high titer of antibody against HBsAg) should be administered before 12 hours of age; may be given concurrently at different sites; 85% to 95% effective in preventing both HBV infection and the chronic carrier state.

(3) Remaining doses of hepatitis B vaccine are given at 1 and 6 months of age.

**d.** Maternal HBsAg-negative treatment recommendations:

(1) Hepatitis B vaccine should be administered to all infants, including those born to HBsAg-negative mothers.

(2) Hepatitis B vaccine (Engerix-B, 10 mcg, or Recombivax-HB, 5 mcg) is administered prior to discharge from the hospital. The second dose is administered at 1 to 2 months of age and the third dose at 6 to 18 months of age.

**e.** Unknown maternal HBsAg status at delivery. Follow schedule for maternal HBsAg-positive status. Additional HBIG administration will depend on the results of maternal serologic screening done within 12 hours after delivery.

**f.** Premature infants with birth weight less than 2 kg born to HBsAg-negative mothers should receive the vaccine just before hospital discharge if the infant weighs more than 2 kg, or the dose is delayed until 2 months of age when other routine immunizations are given. All premature infants born to HBsAg-positive mothers should receive immunoprophylaxis (HBIG) and vaccine beginning as soon as possible after birth, followed by appropriate postvaccination testing (Venkatesh et al., 2011).

**D. Glucose needs/first feeding (Anderson et al., 2011; Blackburn, 2013; McGowan et al., 2011).**

**1.** The stress of delivery causes increased conversion of fats and glycogen to glucose for the increased energy needs of temperature maintenance, skeletal muscles, and breathing and crying. Breakdown products of this conversion are glucose, free fatty acids, and glycerol.

**2.** Hepatic glycogen is mobilized immediately after birth in response to the increased catecholamines to provide a continuing source of glucose to the brain in the absence of placental supply; in a healthy term infant, up to 90% of the hepatic glycogen stores may be consumed by 3 hours of life.

3. Blood glucose concentration at birth is about 85% of the maternal level. The last maternal meal, the duration of labor, the mode of delivery, the type and amount of intravenous (IV) fluids administered to the mother, and medications given to the mother all influence the actual concentration of glucose. The glucose level then falls for 1 to 2 hours, followed by an increase and stabilization at mean levels of approximately 70 mg/dL by the age of 3 hours in healthy, nonstressed infants (Jain et al., 2013).
4. A screening blood glucose test (on capillary whole blood) should be performed in infants with risk factors at 30 minutes to 1 hour of age. A glucose level less than 40 mg/dL at any time in any newborn infant is an indication for evaluation and treatment. The goal is to maintain the glucose value at greater than 40 mg/dL in the first day and greater than 40 to 50 mg/dL thereafter. NOTE: The whole-blood glucose level on the screening test is usually 10% to 15% lower than the corresponding serum or plasma level because the erythrocytes will continue to metabolize the glucose in the sample. Risk factors include the following:
   a. Asphyxia, cold stress, increased work of breathing, and sepsis, which lead to an increased metabolic response and increased use of glucose.
   b. Reduced stores of glucose in premature and small-for-gestational-age infants.
   c. Hyperinsulinemia in infants of mothers with diabetes or gestational diabetes and in large-for-gestational-age infants, resulting in rapid removal of glucose from the circulation.
   d. Any symptoms of a low blood glucose level. An infant may have jitteriness, irritability, seizures, hypothermia, temperature instability, lethargy, poor feeding, emesis, apnea, pallor, cyanosis, and weak or high-pitched cry (see also Common Problems and Clinical Presentation, item F: Metabolic Problems). NOTE: Capillary samples from an unwarmed heel may lead to a falsely low glucose value because of stasis of blood and ongoing transfer of glucose to the cells.
5. Early, frequent feedings should be given on demand; frequency is not to exceed 4 hours between feedings (maximum of 3 hours between feedings for infants weighing <2.5 kg). Allow the infant to begin feeding when he or she is demanding nutrition and when evaluation findings are within normal limits; nursing or formula feeding can be used (type of formula is by family's or physician's choice).
   a. Evaluation before feeding.
      (1) Physical examination. Bowel tones are normal, and abdomen is soft and nontender. Sucking reflex is normal, with no excessive mucus. Passage of an orogastric tube is indicated before feeding if questions exist regarding esophageal patency. Anus and nares are patent. The respiratory rate is less than 60 breaths per minute and the pattern of breathing is normal.
      (2) Contraindications to nippling the feeding or to breastfeeding (consider gavage feeding for these infants).
         (a) Choanal atresia.
         (b) Respiratory rate greater than 60 breaths per minute without other signs of respiratory distress.
         (c) Weak suck.
         (d) Absent coordination of suck and swallow.
      (3) Contraindications to any enteral feedings.
         (a) Cyanosis.
         (b) Severe birth asphyxia.
         (c) Shock.
         (d) Increased work of breathing and oxygen requirement.
         (e) Suspicion of GI obstruction.
   b. Sterile-water "test" feeding. It is difficult to evaluate an infant's ability to suck and swallow with sterile water because most infants do not like the taste and on occasion will refuse to suck or swallow; therefore, it is advisable to forgo "sips of water" in favor of a thorough evaluation before feeding.
   c. Dextrose 5%. Use of dextrose 5% is not indicated as a "test" feeding because studies show that it is more irritating to the lungs after aspiration than is formula. Moreover, it is not indicated after a feeding.

d. Guidelines for feeding in transition nursery for transient asymptomatic hypoglycemia:
   (1) May breastfeed or be offered formula (by nipple or gavage) if there are no contraindications to enteral feedings (see Contraindications, item a (3), above), and the infant is active and vigorous.
   (2) Check glucose level 1 hour after feeding is given.
e. Indications for IV glucose infusion (see Initial Stabilization of the Sick Newborn Infant):
   (1) Hypoglycemia is persistent and symptomatic.
   (2) Enteral feedings are contraindicated.
   (3) Oral feedings do not maintain normal glucose levels.
   (4) Initial glucose screening level is less than 40 mg/dL.

E. **Ongoing teaching during transition.**
   1. Discuss with family the infant's ability to see and hear, with a preference for black–white contrast initially, and the sound of a higher-pitched voice.
   2. Demonstrate or point out infant's response to stimuli (tactile, visual, auditory): self-consolability, body movements, gaze, head turning.
   3. Discuss physical findings.
      a. Transient: head molding, acrocyanosis, birth trauma, positional deformities.
      b. Permanent: congenital anomalies, birthmarks.
   4. A stable infant may stay with the family from birth through recovery to postpartum period with appropriate observation and teaching provided by all staff members in contact with the family unit.

F. **If newborn transitioned in a nursery, he or she may be transferred when the following are stable.**
   1. Temperature, heart rate, respiratory rate.
   2. Glucose level.
   3. Normal physical assessment findings, or abnormal findings that do not require continuous observation or immediate intervention or treatment.

## RECOGNITION OF THE SICK NEWBORN INFANT

### Review of Perinatal History (Rezaee et al., 2013)

A. **Ultrasonographic–biophysical profile:** estimated date of confinement, evidence of congenital anomalies, twins, breech, preterm, and intrauterine growth restriction.

B. **Medications or history of substance abuse:** alcohol, nicotine, cocaine, opiates, marijuana, amphetamines, tocolytics, anticonvulsants, anticoagulants, and analgesics/anesthetics.

C. **Maternal illnesses:** pregnancy-induced hypertension, diabetes, intrapartum fever/infection (e.g., with group B streptococcus, genital herpes simplex virus, human immunodeficiency virus, and varicella), HBsAg positive, thyroid disease, inherited disorders, and cardiac disease.

D. **Perinatal fetal distress, delivery complications:** abnormal fetal heart rate pattern, meconium staining of the amniotic fluid, rapid delivery, difficult delivery, rupture of membranes more than 18 hours before delivery.

E. **Cesarean delivery and indications:** breech presentation, fetal distress, placenta previa, abruptio placentae, cephalopelvic disproportion, failure to progress in labor.

### Physical Assessment

A. **Skin.**
   1. Cyanotic.
   2. Pale.
   3. Mottled.
   4. Cool to touch.
   5. Poor perfusion.

B. **Respiratory system.**
   1. Poor color.
   2. Tachypnea.
   3. Decreased air entry.

4. Increased work of breathing: grunting, flaring, and retracting.
5. Apnea.
6. Unequal breath sounds.
7. Oxygen requirement.

C. **Cardiovascular system.**
1. Abnormal heart sounds such as murmur.
2. Weak, absent, or unequal pulses.
3. Hepatosplenomegaly.

D. **Central nervous system.**
1. Hypertonic or hypotonic.
2. Jitteriness, tremors.
3. Lethargy.
4. Bulging fontanelle (record baseline head circumference).
5. Seizures.
6. Irritability, high-pitched cry.

E. **Morphologic features.**
1. Congenital anomalies (e.g., abdominal wall defects, imperforate anus).
2. Severe birth trauma.
3. Absent or decreased limb movement.
4. Asymmetry.

F. **GI tract.**
1. Abdominal distention (measure baseline abdominal girth).
2. Increased gastric contents on aspiration.
3. Inability to pass an orogastric tube.
4. Excessive mucus.
5. Emesis soon after birth or after first feeding.

## Diagnostic Tools (Bradshaw and Tanaka, 2011)

A. **Pulse oximetry (peripheral monitoring of oxygen saturation).**
1. Oxygen saturation ($Sa_{O_2}$) of blood is that percentage of the total hemoglobin concentration that is chemically combined with oxygen.
2. A baseline $Pa_{O_2}$ value should be obtained to confirm the infant's oxygen level.

B. **Transcutaneous oxygen tension.**
1. Measures the oxygen that has diffused from the skin capillaries through the dermis to the surface of the skin.
2. Site must have adequate perfusion as the sensor heats the skin to dilate the local blood vessels and promote diffusion of oxygen to the skin surface.
3. Sensor needs to be regularly calibrated.

C. **Arterial blood gas determinations.** If oxygen requirement persists, pulse oximetry saturations in room air are decreased and cyanosis is present.

D. **Chest x-ray examination.** Anteroposterior and lateral views are needed if respiratory distress is present or cardiac disease is suspected.

E. **Transillumination.** Use a high-intensity light placed over the side of the chest in question if pneumothorax or pneumomediastinum is suspected.

F. **Whole-blood glucose screening test or serum glucose determination if indicated by history or assessment results:** see Routine Care Considerations During Transition, item D: Glucose Needs/First Feeding.

G. **Hematocrit determination.**
1. History of blood loss.
2. Plethoric or pale infant.
3. Twins (to rule out twin-to-twin transfusion).
4. Heel-stick (capillary) samples tend to have higher results by approximately 10%.
5. Hematocrit variations. Highest hematocrit is at 2 to 4 hours of age and then progressively falls as a result of the beginning of red blood cell breakdown and the cessation of erythropoiesis in response to a comparatively oxygen-enriched environment.

H. **Complete blood cell count with differential examination of the white blood cells.**
   1. As part of a sepsis diagnostic evaluation.
   2. To screen for normal and abnormal hematologic indices.
I. **Blood culture as part of a diagnostic evaluation for sepsis.**
J. **Urine sample collection.**
   1. Urinalysis.
   2. Screening test for drugs of abuse.
K. **Lumbar puncture:** Performed at the discretion of the physician/advanced practice nurse as part of a diagnostic evaluation for sepsis.
L. **Ultrasonography, computed tomography, and magnetic resonance imaging.**
   1. Cranial evaluation for abnormal central nervous system (CNS) findings.
   2. Abdominal examination if history of two-vessel cord to rule out renal anomalies.
M. **Echocardiography and electrocardiography:** As part of a diagnostic study for a congenital cardiac defect.
N. **Passage of orogastric tube.**
   1. To check patency of esophagus in infants with excessive pooling of mucus in the oropharynx.
   2. To decompress a distended abdomen.
   3. To measure and assess gastric contents (>25 mL and/or significant bile in the stomach indicates obstruction).

## Common Problems and Clinical Presentation

A. **Birth trauma (refer to Chapter 2).**
B. **Perinatal hypoxia–ischemia (Blackburn, 2013; Scher, 2013; Volpe, 2008).**
   1. Birth asphyxia is defined as interference with gas exchange resulting in compromised oxygen delivery, accumulation of $CO_2$, and a switch to anaerobic metabolism.
   2. Fetal distress is indicated by an abnormal fetal heart rate pattern, meconium staining of the amniotic fluid, scalp pH less than 7.20, and Apgar scores less than 5 at 1 minute of age and less than 7 at 5 minutes of age.
   3. Pathophysiologic sequelae include:
      a. Decreasing $Po_2$. The tissue hypoxia that ensues leads to anaerobic metabolism with release of lactic acid into the circulation.
      b. Respiratory acidosis from elevated levels of carbon dioxide.
      c. Metabolic acidosis.
         (1) Results in high pulmonary vascular resistance.
         (2) Leads to decreased surfactant release.
      d. Hypoxic–ischemic damage to less vital organs such as kidney and gut after redistribution of blood to vital organs.
      e. The myocardium depends on its stored reserves of glycogen for energy as its supply of oxygen falls. Eventually this reserve is consumed and the myocardium is simultaneously exposed to progressively lower $Po_2$ and pH levels. The combined effects lead to reduced myocardial function with decreased blood flow to vital organs.
   4. All newborn infants have some degree of respiratory acidosis and hypoxia during labor and vaginal delivery; a healthy term infant has increased tolerance and reserves. The asphyxiated newborn infant has more prolonged hypoxia and respiratory acidosis and may have additional metabolic acidosis, hypothermia, and hypoglycemia.
   5. Clinical findings.
      a. Mild to moderate perinatal hypoxia–ischemia.
         (1) Extended awake, alert state (45 minutes to 1 hour).
         (2) Dilated pupils.
         (3) Normal muscle tone.
         (4) Active suck.
         (5) Regular or slightly increased respiratory rate.
         (6) Normal or slightly increased heart rate.

b. Moderate to severe perinatal hypoxia–ischemia.
   (1) Hypothermia.
   (2) Hypoglycemia.
   (3) Pupils constricted.
   (4) Respiratory distress manifested by grunting, flaring, retracting, tachypnea, and oxygen requirement.
   (5) Seizures (subtle and multifocal clonic; 12 to 24 hours of age).
   (6) Acute tubular necrosis following reduced blood flow to the kidneys.
   (7) Hypotonia initially, lethargy.
   (8) Bradycardia.

c. Severe perinatal hypoxia–ischemia requires constant monitoring in a level III/IV (intensive care) nursery.
   (1) Pale skin, poor perfusion, hypotension.
   (2) Cerebral edema.
   (3) Seizures.
   (4) Apnea.
   (5) Intracranial hemorrhage.

**C. Pulmonary problems (Gardner et al., 2011; Martin and Crowley, 2013).**

1. Air leak: 2% to 10% of healthy term neonates develop spontaneous air leak, as do 16% to 36% of neonates who require ventilatory support, including continuous positive airway pressure.
   a. Tachypnea, unequal breath sounds, shift of heart tones, and distant heart tones.
   b. Transillumination of chest is positive for free air.
2. Retained lung fluid, respiratory distress syndrome (because of prematurity or birth asphyxia), and pneumonia.
   a. Decreased air entry with respiratory distress syndrome and pneumonia.
   b. Increased work of breathing: grunting, flaring, and retracting.
   c. Tachypnea, apnea.
   d. Decreased saturations ($Sa_{O_2}$), cyanosis, continued oxygen requirement.
3. Aspiration syndromes (meconium, blood).
   a. Coarse rales.
   b. Tachypnea.
   c. Barrel chest.
4. Upper airway obstruction (e.g., choanal atresia or micrognathia).
5. Extrapulmonary (e.g., phrenic nerve injury with resultant diaphragmatic paralysis or eventration of the diaphragm).

**D. Cardiovascular problems (Phelps et al., 2013; Scholz and Reinking, 2013).**

1. Congenital heart disease.
   a. Acyanotic lesions.
      (1) Patent ductus arteriosus with a left-to-right shunt.
      (2) Ventricular septal defect.
      (3) Atrial septal defect.
      (4) Endocardial cushion defect or atrioventricular canal defects.
   b. Obstructive lesions.
      (1) Aortic stenosis.
      (2) Coarctation of the aorta.
      (3) Pulmonary valve stenosis or atresia.
      (4) Hypoplastic left heart syndrome.
   c. Admixture of lesions.
      (1) Normal or increased pulmonary blood flow.
         (a) Complete transposition of the great vessels.
         (b) Truncus arteriosus.
         (c) Anomalous venous connections of the pulmonary veins.
      (2) Decreased pulmonary blood flow.
         (a) Tetralogy of Fallot.
         (b) Tricuspid valve atresia.

2. Persistent fetal shunts.
   a. Patent ductus arteriosus with right-to-left shunt.
   b. Persistent pulmonary hypertension.
3. Clinical findings.
   a. Cyanosis with or without increased work of breathing, decreased oxygen saturations. NOTE: Absence of any signs of abnormal respiratory function in the presence of cyanosis suggests congenital heart disease.
   b. Unequal or absent pulses, bounding pulses, decreased blood pressure in the lower extremities, and decreased perfusion.
   c. Increased precordial activity, shift of point of maximal impulse of heart tones to right, murmur.
   d. Congestive heart failure, indicated by tachypnea, moist breath sounds, tachycardia, peripheral edema, cardiomegaly, and hepatomegaly.

**E. Hemodynamics.**

1. Acute hypovolemic shock.
   a. Internal hemorrhage resulting from birth trauma; intracranial hemorrhage.
   b. External hemorrhage resulting from placenta previa or abruptio placentae; cord accident; fetal–maternal or twin-to-twin transfusion.
   c. Respiratory distress, pallor, poor perfusion, hypotension, weak or absent pulses, anemia.
2. Polycythemia.
   a. Plethoric, cyanotic, or excessively flushed with crying.
   b. Hypoglycemia.
   c. CNS symptoms, including jitteriness, hypotonia, lethargy, and seizures.
3. Anemia.
   a. Acute or chronic blood loss.
   b. Hemolysis from sepsis or ABO/Rh blood group incompatibilities.
   c. Reduced red blood cell production, manifested by severe asphyxia, sepsis, and aplastic anemia.
   d. Pale skin, murmur, tachypnea, normal arterial blood pressure, signs of congestive heart failure, including hepatosplenomegaly and increased vascular markings on x-ray film.

**F. Metabolic problems.**

1. Hypoglycemia (Jain et al., 2013; McGowan et al., 2011).
   a. Observed in infants who are large or small for gestational age, infants of diabetic mothers, premature infants, and stressed infants such as those with sepsis, cold stress, or respiratory distress.
   b. Clinical findings:
      (1) Jitteriness, irritability.
      (2) Seizures.
      (3) Hypothermia, temperature instability.
      (4) Lethargy.
      (5) Poor feeding, emesis.
      (6) Apnea.
      (7) Cardiorespiratory distress, cyanosis, oxygen requirement.
      (8) Pallor.
      (9) Tachycardia.
      (10) Weak or high-pitched cry.
2. Adverse effects of maternal medications; maternal use of illicit drugs.
   a. Magnesium sulfate. Infants present with respiratory depression, decreased muscle tone, and decreased serum calcium concentration.
   b. Tocolytics. Infants may present with hypoglycemia.
   c. Narcotics. Infants present with apnea, respiratory depression, and periodic breathing.
   d. Cocaine. Infants may present with apnea, poor muscle tone initially and then irritability and agitation, tremors, and feeding difficulties.
   e. Marijuana or methadone. Infants present with hyperthermia, agitation, and diarrhea.
   f. Alcohol. Infants have fetal alcohol syndrome with dysmorphic and behavioral abnormalities.

**G. Infection (see also Chapter 32).**

1. Generalized bacterial or viral disease; acquired in utero or nosocomial.
2. Clinical findings. NOTE: Nearly 90% of neonates with early-onset group B streptococcus have signs of infection within 12 hours of birth (median age is 8 hours) (Ferrieri and Wallen, 2013).
   a. Temperature instability.
   b. Tachypnea, apnea.
   c. Respiratory distress, cyanosis.
   d. Tachycardia.
   e. Cool, mottled skin; weak pulses; capillary refill lasting longer than 2 seconds; and hypotension.
   f. Disseminated intravascular coagulation.
   g. Hepatosplenomegaly.
   h. Unexplained jaundice.
   i. Purpura, petechiae.
   j. Hypoglycemia or hyperglycemia.
   k. Poor feeding, emesis, and abdominal distention.
   l. Lethargy, poor muscle tone.
3. In-utero viral infection. Infant may be small for gestational age with microcephaly.

**H. Congenital anomalies (frequently obvious on gross examination).**

1. Diaphragmatic hernia.
   a. Immediate onset, at birth, of significant respiratory distress.
   b. Shift in heart tones, decreased or unequal breath sounds, bowel tones heard in chest, scaphoid abdomen, and cyanosis.
2. Esophageal atresia with or without tracheoesophageal fistula.
   a. Excessive amniotic fluid.
   b. Increased pooling of secretions in the oropharynx, respiratory distress, unable to place orogastric tube.
3. Abdominal wall defects: omphalocele and gastroschisis.
4. Limb anomalies: amniotic banding, talipes equinovarus, polydactyly, and syndactyly.
5. Neural tube defects.
6. Intestinal obstructions.
7. Chromosomal abnormalities such as trisomy 21 or trisomy 18.
8. Urogenital abnormalities: exstrophy of bladder, hypospadias, epispadias, and ambiguous genitalia.

## Initial Stabilization of the Sick Newborn Infant

**A. Short-term observation in transition nursery or intermediate nursery to monitor trends before the infant's transfer to a neonatal intensive care unit (NICU).**

1. The infant may be capable of resolving the problem on his or her own if given time (e.g., correction of mild acidosis from asphyxia, clearing of lung fluid, stabilization of blood glucose concentration, and stabilization of blood pressure).
2. Monitor and record trends (i.e., improvement of respiratory rate toward normal, improved perfusion, and normal glucose screens).

**B. Avoid excessive handling.**

1. Organize care and interventions to avoid frequent, unnecessary stimulation of an already stressed infant.
2. Use pulse oximeter or cardiorespiratory monitor to reduce hands-on determination of vital signs.
3. Reduce background stimulation such as loud noises or bright lights.
4. Use nonnutritive sucking to lower activity levels and reduce energy needs.
   a. Infant may be more comfortable in a prone position.
   b. Crying can be stressful and is similar to a Valsalva maneuver, with prolonged exhalation, obstructed venous return, quick inspiratory gasp, and right-to-left shunting at the foramen ovale.
   c. Crying depletes energy reserves and increases oxygen consumption.

C. **Provide a neutral thermal environment (refer to Chapter 6).**
   1. Observe infant for apnea and hypotension during warming.
   2. Avoid hyperthermia.

D. **Supply glucose.**
   1. Oral administration of glucose for a blood glucose level of less than 40 mg/dL in an otherwise healthy asymptomatic neonate; early, frequent feedings by nipple, gavage, or nursing.
      a. Give at least 0.5 to 1 ounce of formula by nipple or gavage if there are no contraindications to enteral feedings and the infant is free of symptoms (see Routine Care Considerations During Transition). If condition is stable, infant may be allowed to nurse 5 to 10 minutes on each breast.
      b. Begin maintenance formula at 50 to 70 kcal/kg/day or breastfeed on demand every 2 to 3 hours.
      c. Check blood glucose 30 minutes to 1 hour after feeding.
      d. Consider giving a formula designed for premature infants when treating hypoglycemia orally.
         (1) These formulas provide 50% of carbohydrate in the form of glucose polymers that are easily absorbed; salivary amylase retains its activity in the infant's stomach because of increased gastric pH and is effective in the digestion of glucose polymers (Blackburn, 2013).
         (2) Approximately 50% of the fats are provided as medium-chain triglycerides (MCTs). As MCTs are absorbed from the stomach, they may also increase the level of plasma ketones, which can be used as an alternative substrate to glucose for brain metabolism (Blackburn, 2013).
         (3) The process of absorbing fat (fatty acid oxidation and ketogenesis) spares glucose for brain energy needs; free fatty acids and ketones promote glucose production by providing essential gluconeogenic cofactors.
         (4) Healthy newborn infants respond to a protein meal by preferentially increasing glucagon, which elicits a glycemic response.
   2. Intravenous administration of glucose for hypoglycemia (see Routine Care Considerations During Transition, item D: Glucose Needs/First Feeding) is as follows:
      a. Provide bolus (2 mL/kg) of 10% dextrose in water ($D_{10}W$), followed by an infusion of 4 to 6 mg/kg/min; $D_{10}W = 100$ mg/mL.
      b. Monitor therapy with frequent glucose checks and titrate the infusion rate and concentration to meet the infant's needs. NOTE: Do not administer an IV bolus of glucose greater than $D_{10}W$ because of reactive hypoglycemia and hypertonicity of the solution. Always follow a glucose bolus with a continuous infusion of glucose.

E. **Supply oxygen:** Assess needs with a pulse oximeter or with arterial blood gas determinations and close observation.
   1. Extended oxygen use in the transition nursery requires notification of the physician and transfer to a level II or III setting.
   2. Provide warmed, humidified oxygen by oxygen hood, continuous positive airway pressure by nasal prongs, or assisted ventilation by endotracheal tube according to the infant's needs (refer to Chapter 26).
   3. Monitor oxygen provided with an oxygen analyzer. Oxygen should be provided via a blender to provide the least $FiO_2$ required. The percentage and liters per minute should be recorded. Record blow-by oxygen in liters per minute and as distance from the infant's face.

F. **Supply volume expanders, including blood and normal saline solution.**
   1. For hypotension and blood loss.
   2. Requires IV line placement and transfer to level II or III nursery for continued management and observation, including cardiorespiratory monitoring and blood pressure checks to adjust therapy as necessary.

G. **Naloxone hydrochloride (Narcan).**
   1. Administer drug for severe respiratory depression with a normal heart rate and color in the delivery room and history of maternal narcotic administration within the past 4 hours.
   2. Do not use naloxone if the mother has a history of opioid dependency: may precipitate acute withdrawal symptoms.

**H. Antibiotics.**

1. As indicated by history, current status of the infant, and initial results of sepsis evaluation.
2. Administer via peripheral IV or heparin-lock IV line.

## PARENT TEACHING

### Before Delivery

A. **History.** Review obstetric history; anticipate needs of the infant at delivery.

B. **Complications.** If there are expected complications (preterm delivery, congenital anomalies) and time permits, discuss the anticipated plan of care with the family.

1. Discuss plans for managing the infant, including plans for transfer to a level II or III nursery and any special equipment that may be used (oxygen hood, incubator, ventilator, monitors).
2. Allow the parents to tour the NICU if possible.

C. **Parental support.** Encourage parents to express their feelings, fears, and misgivings; involve support people.

### At Delivery

A. **After drying the neonate, place on the mother's chest or abdomen when possible with uncomplicated deliveries.** A warm blanket should be placed over the baby's back. Use the family's birth plan as much as possible.

B. **After delivery room assessment, return the infant to the family if the infant's condition is stable.**

C. **Answer questions regarding acrocyanosis, Apgar scores, and morphologic findings.**

D. **Allow parents time to visit, breastfeed, and see extended family.**

### During Transition

A. **"Introduce" the newborn to the family by noting unique features (dimples, long eyelashes, hair color).**

B. **Encourage the support person to touch and talk to the infant.**

C. **Discuss physical findings such as caput succedaneum, head molding, positional deformities, and birthmarks.**

D. **Discuss the infant's sensory capabilities, including sight, hearing, and smell.**

E. **Listen to the parents.** Allow them to express their reactions as they compare their "dream" infant with the real infant they now have (too tiny, not the right sex, deformed, or premature).

F. **After completion of admission procedures, the infant is returned to the family for feeding and visiting.**

G. **Allow the family to participate in the infant's care as permitted by the neonate's condition.**

### Postpartum Period (Early Discharge)

A. **Parental involvement.** Involve the parents in evaluation of their learning needs; begin teaching as soon as delivery occurs.

B. **Short hospital stays and family instruction.** With shorter hospital stays, there is less time available for teaching and an increased importance of teaching. This may be the only information many families receive on care of a newborn infant.

1. Classes; videotaped lectures.
   a. Cardiopulmonary resuscitation; safety.
   b. Breastfeeding.
   c. Developmental milestones.
2. Follow-up visits by the nurse to the home and phone calls from postpartum nurses. Encourage families to call the nursery if they have questions about their newborn's care.
3. Follow-up visit with the primary care provider within 48 to 72 hours. Encourage the family to select a primary care provider and assist in making an appointment for the first visit.
4. Return visit for newborn screening if needed.

## Transfer to Level II or III Setting

A. **Provide prenatal teaching—if possible, with visits to NICU.**
B. **Provide information booklets, with location, phone numbers, visiting regulations, parent-to-parent groups, and necessary support personnel.**
C. **Bring the mother to the infant's bedside if the infant is unable to return to the mother after delivery.** Allow family members to be near the infant as much as possible and encourage them to see past the equipment to the infant and his or her special needs (gentle touch, stroking, soft voice, a familiar person).
D. **When the infant is stable, allow family members to visit in the privacy of their postpartum room or a parent room if condition warrants; for example, an infant with a heparin lock for antibiotics can be taken to the mother's room to nurse.**
E. **Provide a picture and footprints of the infant for the family.** This is especially important if transfer to a level II or III nursery will be to another facility.
F. **Facilitate the family in keeping in contact with the transfer facility, and be available to explain information given to the family.**

## REFERENCES

Alden, K.R.: Nursing care of the newborn and family. In D.L. Lowdermilk, S.E. Perry, K. Cashion, and K.R. Alden (Eds.): *Maternity & women's health care* (10th ed.). St. Louis, 2012a, Elsevier Mosby, pp. 553–605.

Alden, K.R.: Physiologic and behavioural adaptations of the newborn. In D.L. Lowdermilk, S.E. Perry, K. Cashion, and K.R. Alden (Eds.): *Maternity & women's health care* (10th ed.). St. Louis, 2012b, Elsevier Mosby, pp. 528–552.

American Academy of Pediatrics: Policy Statement: Routine evaluation of blood pressure, hematocrit, and glucose in newborns (RE9322). *Pediatrics*, 92(3):474–476, 1993.

American Academy of Pediatrics and American College of Obstetricians and Gynecologists: *Guidelines for perinatal care:* (7th ed.). Elk Grove Village, IL, and Washington, DC, 2012, American Academy of Pediatrics and American College of Obstetricians and Gynecologists.

Anderson, M.S., Wood, L.L., Keller, J.A., and Hay, W W.: Enteral nutrition. In S.L. Gardner, B.S. Carter, M. Enzman-Hines, and J.A. Hernandez (Eds.): *Merenstein and Gardner's handbook of neonatal intensive care* (7th ed.). St. Louis, 2011, Elsevier Mosby, pp. 398–433.

Blackburn, S.T.: *Maternal, fetal, and neonatal physiology: A clinical perspective:* (4th ed.). St. Louis, 2013, Elsevier Saunders.

Bradshaw, W.T., and Tanaka, D.T.: Physiologic monitoring. In S.L. Gardner, B.S. Carter, M. Enzman-Hines, and J.A. Hernandez (Eds.): *Merenstein and Gardner's handbook of neonatal intensive care* (7th ed.). St. Louis, 2011, Elsevier Mosby, pp. 134–152.

Brown, V.D., and Landers, S.: Heat balance. In S.L. Gardner, B.S. Carter, M. Enzman-Hines, and J.A. Hernandez (Eds.): *Merenstein and Gardner's handbook of neonatal intensive care* (7th ed.). St. Louis, 2011, Elsevier Mosby, pp. 113–133.

Ferrieri, P., and Wallen, L.D.: Neonatal bacterial sepsis. In C.A. Gleason, and S.U. Devaskar (Eds.): *Avery's diseases of the newborn* (9th ed.). Philadelphia, 2013, Elsevier Saunders, pp. 538–550.

Gardner, S.L., Enzman-Hines, M., and Dickey, L.A.: Respiratory diseases. In S.L. Gardner, B.S. Carter, M. Enzman-Hines, and J.A. Hernandez (Eds.): *Merenstein and Gardner's handbook of neonatal intensive care* (7th ed.). St. Louis, 2011, Elsevier Mosby, pp. 581–677.

Gardner, S.L., and Hernandez, J.A.: Initial nursery care. In S.L. Gardner, B.S. Carter, M. Enzman-Hines, and J.A. Hernandez (Eds.): *Merenstein and Gardner's handbook of neonatal intensive care* (7th ed.). St. Louis, 2011, Elsevier Mosby, pp. 52–77.

Gauda, E.B., and Martin, R.J.: Control of breathing. In C.A. Gleason, and S.U. Devaskar (Eds.): *Avery's diseases of the newborn* (9th ed.). Philadelphia, 2013, Elsevier Saunders, pp. 584–597.

Hillman, N.H., Kallapur, S.G., and Jobe, A.H.: Physiology of transition from intrauterine to extrauterine life. *Clinics in Perinatology*, 39:769–783, 2012.

Jain, V., Chen, M., and Menon, R.K.: Disorders of carbohydrate metabolism. In C.A. Gleason, and S.U. Devaskar (Eds.): *Avery's diseases of the newborn* (9th ed.). Philadelphia, 2013, Elsevier Saunders, pp. 1320–1329.

Leone, T.A., and Finer, N.N.: Resuscitation in the delivery room. In C.A. Gleason, and S.U. Devaskar (Eds.): *Avery's diseases of the newborn* (9th ed.). Philadelphia, 2013, Elsevier Saunders, pp. 328–340.

Martin, R.J., and Crowley, M.A.: Respiratory problems. In A.A. Fanaroff, and J.M. Fanaroff (Eds.): *Klaus & Fanaroff's care of the high-risk neonate* (6th ed.). Philadelphia, 2013, Elsevier Saunders, pp. 244–269.

McGowan, J.E., Rozance, P.J., Price-Douglas, W., and Hay, W.W.: Glucose homeostasis. In S.L. Gardner, B.S. Carter, M. Enzman-Hines, and J.A. Hernandez (Eds.): *Merenstein and Gardner's handbook of neonatal intensive care* (7th ed.). St. Louis, 2011, Elsevier Mosby, pp. 353–377.

Moore, K.L., Persaud, T.V.N., and Torchia, M.G.: *The developing human: Clinically oriented embryology* (9th ed.). Philadelphia, 2013, Elsevier Saunders pp. 333-336.

Niermeyer, S., and Clarke, S.B.: Delivery room care. In S.L. Gardner, B.S. Carter, M. Enzman-Hines, and J.A. Hernandez (Eds.): *Merenstein and Gardner's handbook of neonatal intensive care* (7th ed.). St. Louis, 2011, Elsevier Mosby, pp. 52–77.

Phelps, C.M., Thrush, P.T., and Cua, C.L.: The heart. In A.A. Fanaroff, and J.M. Fanaroff (Eds.): *Klaus & Fanaroff's care of the high-risk neonate* (6th ed.). Philadelphia, 2013, Elsevier Saunders, pp. 368–409.

Rezaee, R.L., Lappen, J.R., and Gecsi, K.S.: Antenatal and intrapartum care of the high-risk neonate. In A.A. Fanaroff, and J.M. Fanaroff (Eds.): *Klaus & Fanaroff's care of the high-risk neonate* (6th ed.). Philadelphia, 2013, Elsevier Saunders, pp. 10–53.

Scher, M.S.: Brain disorders of the fetus and neonate. In A.A. Fanaroff, and J.M. Fanaroff (Eds.): *Klaus & Fanaroff's care of the high-risk neonate* (6th ed.). Philadelphia, 2013, Elsevier Saunders, pp. 476–524.

Scholz, T.D. and Reinking, B.E.: Congenital heart disease. In C.A. Gleason S.U. Devaskar (Eds.): *Avery's diseases of the newborn* (9th ed.). Philadelphia, 2013, Elsevier Saunders, pp. 762–788.

Taylor, J.A., Wright, J.A., and Woodrum, D.: Routine newborn care. In C.A. Gleason, and S.U. Devaskar (Eds.): *Avery's diseases of the newborn* (9th ed.). Philadelphia, 2013, Elsevier Saunders, pp. 300–315.

Venkatesh, M.P., Adams, K.M., and Weisman, L.E.: Infection in the neonate. In S.L. Gardner, B.S. Carter, M. Enzman-Hines, and J.A. Hernandez (Eds.): *Merenstein and Gardner's handbook of neonatal intensive care* (7th ed.). St. Louis, 2011, Elsevier Mosby, pp 553–580.

Verklan, M.T.: Physiologic variability during transition to extrauterine life. *Critical Care Nursing Quarterly*, 24(4):41–56, 2002.

Volpe, J.J.: *Neurology of the newborn:* (5th ed.). Philadelphia, 2008, Elsevier Saunders.

CHAPTER

# 5 Neonatal Delivery Room Resuscitation

BARBARA ELIZABETH PAPPAS AND DEANNA LYNN ROBEY

**OBJECTIVES**

1. Describe three anatomically unique features of the neonate that require special consideration during resuscitation.
2. Compare three physiologic characteristics of the neonate that make neonatal resuscitation different from adult resuscitation.
3. List three antepartum and intrapartum factors that indicate the neonate may be at risk for developing asphyxia.
4. Identify the equipment needed for neonatal resuscitation.
5. Review the components of neonatal resuscitation as outlined by the Neonatal Resuscitation Program (NRP) of the American Heart Association/American Academy of Pediatrics.
6. Recognize three neonatal disease states, congenital malformations, or special situations that may alter the resuscitation process.
7. Describe three potential complications of neonatal resuscitation.
8. Discuss the postresuscitative needs of the neonate.
9. Verbalize three risk factors that may leave the neonate at risk for cardiopulmonary arrest after the initial period of stabilization.
10. Discuss ethical considerations surrounding resuscitation of periviable or marginally viable neonates or those with unpredictable life expectancy.

Few neonates require resuscitation at birth. Approximately 10% of all newborn infants require some assistance at birth, but less than 1% require full resuscitative measures (Perlman et al., 2010). Most neonates only require basic stabilization, including thermal and airway management. Neonates requiring more advanced resuscitation often have respiratory insufficiency or depression.

Neonates at risk for resuscitation benefit from prompt, organized, and efficient interventions tailored to their needs and response. High-functioning resuscitation teams are optimal. Formalized education, hands-on experience with equipment, periodic review, and mock codes are all beneficial in promoting the resuscitation skills necessary for a smooth and coordinated resuscitation.

The risk for cardiopulmonary arrest does not stop once the neonate leaves the delivery environment. Physical and physiologic vulnerabilities continue to place the neonate at risk. Prevention is key, and although studies regarding neonatal rapid response teams are not available, rapid response teams should be considered as an avenue to reduce the need for resuscitation in the neonatal period.

## DEFINITIONS

**Newly born:** time of the infant's life from birth to the first hours after birth.
**Neonate:** refers to the first 28 days of the infant's life.
**Infant:** neonatal period extending through the first 12 months of life.

## ANATOMY AND PHYSIOLOGY

A. **Physiologic and anatomic characteristics.** Normal characteristics specific to the neonate differ from those specific to the adult, leaving the neonate at significant risk for compromise.

A thorough understanding of the uniqueness of the neonate often allows anticipation and intervention before the neonate is compromised to the point of cardiac failure. Unique characteristics specific to the neonate include the following.

1. Large head in proportion to body size. At risk for:
   a. Insensible water loss (IWL).
   b. Heat loss: no insulating fat layer.
   c. Minimal insulation and moisture retention from hair.
2. Large surface area/body size ratio. At risk for:
   a. IWL.
   b. Heat loss.
3. Decreased muscle mass. At risk for:
   a. Increased potential for heat loss through external gradient.
   b. Decreased ability to flex body to conserve heat, causing increased surface area in premature or ill neonate.
   c. Decreased ability to generate heat.
4. Decreased subcutaneous fat (premature birth, intrauterine growth restriction). At risk for:
   a. Decreased heat production (from brown fat metabolism).
   b. Increased heat loss (from lack of insulation and decreased flexion).
5. Thinner epidermal layer. At risk for:
   a. Increased IWL; the more premature, the greater the loss.
   b. Decreased support of internal gradient to maintain heat.
   c. Increased risk for breakdown and injury can contribute to increased IWL.
6. Immature systems.
   a. Central nervous system: impaired ability to regulate vasomotor stability, resulting in impaired perfusion and poor autoregulation of blood pressure and temperature regulation.
   b. Neuromuscular system: decreased ability to shiver and generate heat.
   c. Liver: ability to metabolize drugs and mobilize glucose stores is decreased.
   d. Kidneys: risk for decreased perfusion with compromise; ability to excrete drugs and fluids is impaired.
   e. Gastrointestinal tract: gastric distention and respiratory compromise related to decreased gastrointestinal motility and forced air entry with bag-and-mask ventilation.
   f. Metabolism: decreased stores, decreased ability to convert stored glucose, inefficient energy production from stored glucose, and increased utilization of glucose result in hypoglycemia.
   g. Respiratory system: decreased absorption of lung fluid if cesarean section without trial of labor, decreased surface area for gas exchange, decreased availability of surfactant, and increased risk for aspiration from gastric distention.
   h. Immune system: increased predisposition to infection, immature immune response despite adequate cell counts.
7. Glottis positioned anteriorly in the hypopharynx.
   a. Intubation may be difficult.
   b. The neonate is predisposed to airway compromise from positioning.
8. Short neck.
   a. Lack of clarity in identifying landmarks contributes to difficulty in intubation.
   b. Tendency for hyperextension and flexion of neck.
9. Preferential nasal breathing.
   a. Preferential nose breather; patency is essential to airway maintenance.
   b. Anatomic patency must be confirmed.
   c. Increased airway resistance with edema from nasal suctioning.
10. Venous access.
    a. Small and superficial veins: access is difficult, vessels fragile.
    b. Vasoconstriction associated with acidosis, hypothermia, hypoglycemia, and shock.
    c. Umbilical access. Normal cord includes two arteries and one vein. Inadvertent cannulization of the portal vein with umbilical vein catheterization can lead to liver damage with chemical resuscitation.

11. Unknown physical variations make resuscitation and stabilization challenging.
    a. Lack of adequate perinatal information (i.e., ultrasound, genetic testing).
    b. Gross physical assessment only.

## RISK FACTORS

Risk factors are warning signs that alert the perinatal team to the possibility of a crisis and the need for anticipatory preparation of neonatal resuscitation.

A. **Antepartum period:** conditions during pregnancy that predispose mother and fetus to stress and can interfere with successful transition of the fetus to extrauterine life.
   1. Maternal age less than 16 years or more than 35 years.
   2. Maternal diabetes.
   3. Hemorrhage, anemia.
   4. Maternal substance abuse.
   5. Maternal drug therapy such as magnesium sulfate, adrenergic blocking agents, over-the-counter or herbal medications.
   6. Maternal infection.
   7. No or late entry to prenatal care.
   8. Polyhydramnios or oligohydramnios.
   9. Maternal cardiac, renal, pulmonary, thyroid, endocrine, gastrointestinal, or neurologic disease.
   10. Premature rupture of membranes.
   11. Anatomic abnormalities of the uterus.
   12. Isoimmunization, Rh, or ABO (blood group) incompatibilities.
   13. Hypertension (pregnancy-induced hypertension, chronic).
   14. Multiple gestation.
   15. Post-term gestation.
   16. Discrepancy in size and dates.
   17. Previous pregnancy complication or fetal loss.
   18. Diminished or absent fetal activity.
   19. Fetal malformations or anomalies (i.e., fetal hydrops).

B. **Intrapartum period:** conditions that predispose the fetus to difficult transition to extrauterine life or signs that the fetus is not tolerating the stresses of labor. Unsuccessful transition may ensue.
   1. Abnormal fetal positioning or presentation (e.g., breech position).
   2. Cesarean delivery.
   3. Fetal heart rate abnormalities (e.g., bradycardia, tachycardia).
   4. Nonreassuring fetal heart rate patterns (category 2 or 3).
   5. Maternal or fetal intrapartum blood loss (e.g., abruptio placentae, placenta previa).
   6. Maternal sedation, anesthesia, or analgesia (e.g., narcotics in the previous 4 hours).
   7. Maternal fever or infection (e.g., chorioamnionitis).
   8. Prolonged labor (>24 hours or second stage >2 hours).
   9. Premature labor.
   10. Precipitous delivery.
   11. Prolonged rupture of membranes (>18 hours).
   12. Prolapse of the umbilical cord.
   13. Fetal malformations.
   14. Meconium-stained amniotic fluid.
   15. Uterine hyperstimulation and/or tachysystole with fetal heart rate pattern changes.
   16. Instrument-assisted delivery (e.g., vacuum or forceps).
   17. Macrosomia.

C. **Newly born period:** signs or conditions in the delivery room or during the transitional period that indicate the neonate is having difficulty making all the physiologic changes needed for successful adaptation from intrauterine to extrauterine life.
   1. Congenital malformations (e.g., cardiac, respiratory, gastrointestinal, neurologic, genitourinary).

2. Cardiac arrhythmia or murmur (e.g., tachycardia or bradycardia).
3. Extreme color change (e.g., cyanosis, plethora, pallor, mottling).
4. Prolonged or delayed capillary refill time.
5. Respiratory distress (e.g., apnea, tachypnea, grunting, altered breath sounds, excessive secretions).
6. Temperature instability.
7. Hypertonia/hypotonia.
8. Hypotension.
9. Seizures.
10. Hypoglycemia.
11. Prematurity.
12. Postmaturity.
13. Anemia or polycythemia.
14. Feeding difficulty or intolerance.
15. Seemingly well, then clinically deteriorates.

## ANTICIPATION OF AND PREPARATION FOR RESUSCITATION

Anticipation of and preparation for resuscitation require an evidence-based multidisciplinary approach. Internationally, the Neonatal Resuscitation Program (NRP) is recognized as the "gold standard" for neonatal resuscitation. Program content is based on the American Academy of Pediatrics and American Heart Association's "Neonatal Resuscitation: 2010 American Heart Association Guidelines for Cardiopulmonary Resuscitation and Emergency Cardiovascular Care" (Kattwinkel et al., 2010). The Guidelines are based on the International Liaison Committee on Resuscitation (2010) Consensus on Science statement regarding treatment recommendations for neonatal resuscitation (Perlman et al., 2010). All units and facilities caring for newborn infants and neonates must be adequately staffed, prepared, and equipped to deliver resuscitative care when anticipated or unexpected resuscitation needs arise.

**A. Education and competency development.**

1. Completion of educational program on neonatal resuscitation (e.g., NRP) does not equate to competency or confidence.
2. Development and implementation of regular mock code system for education and quality improvement.
3. Annual competency evaluation and review are recommended.
4. Establish a quality improvement process for reviewing neonatal codes (e.g., effectiveness of call system, response times, and drug doses).

**B. General preparation.**

1. Promote development of effective teams. Effective teams demonstrate clear communication and strong leadership and management.
2. Consider the development and utilization of a rapid response team.
3. Evaluate and update equipment frequently.
4. Arrange for periodic evaluation and maintenance of electrical equipment by the biomedical engineering department on a regularly scheduled basis.
5. Schedule periodic evaluation and maintenance of all respiratory equipment.
6. Formulate supply replacement procedures. Evaluate and replace supplies as quickly as possible after use (use equipment checklist).
7. Test alerting system for rapid, consistent response of personnel.

**C. Delivery room preparation.**

1. Anticipate the needs of the neonate by evaluation of gestational age, risk factors (e.g., meconium, infection), and immediate status at birth (e.g., crying, tone).
    a. Formulate a plan before anticipated need if possible (e.g., endotracheal tube size, drug doses, concentrations, and handling equipment).
    b. Promote effective communication between personnel, departments, and institutions that encourages identification and notification of high-risk situations and preparedness.

2. Prewarm room to minimize thermal losses in the newly born infant. Use a polyethylene plastic wrap or bag for neonate less than 29 weeks of gestation.
3. Assemble equipment in an organized, easily available system. Check function of equipment routinely and before use.
4. Ensure safety of team members and utilization of standard precautions.
5. Preheat warmer, hat, blankets, and nest (blanket rolls or bendable positioning device). Approximately 15 to 30 minutes (heat output set on high) is required to thoroughly warm the mattress on a radiant warmer bed. Assemble alternative heat sources (i.e., warming pad) at bedside as needed.
6. Identify and assemble available team members and designate roles.
7. Position resuscitation algorithms (Fig. 5-1) and charts easily within view of the resuscitative area.
8. Promote family-centered care through active family communication and involvement in decision making.

D. **Personnel roles.**
1. Personnel roles should be defined by institutional policies and job descriptions in addition to state laws, license regulations, and scope of practice definitions. The "resuscitative team" with identified member roles should be determined before delivery.
2. Preparedness for resuscitation should exist at every delivery. Every delivery should be attended by at least one person skilled in neonatal resuscitation who is immediately available and solely responsible for initiating resuscitation and stabilization of the neonate. Additional qualified personnel should be available for more complex situations. For multiple births, separate teams for each baby should be present.
3. A family-centered approach should include a designated support and communication liaison to the family. Family support should not be left unassigned. Family presence during resuscitation has not been shown to be detrimental to the outcome of the neonate.

E. **Behavioral skills of resuscitative team.** Teamwork, communication, and leadership are essential skills of a successful resuscitation. Team members may consist of a variety of provider levels, and experience working in stressful situations is critical. Key behavioral skills of an effective and efficient team include the following:
1. Knowledge of your environment.
2. Anticipation and planning.
3. Assuming leadership role.
4. Effective communication.
5. Optimal workload delegation.
6. Wise attention allocation.
7. Using all available information.
8. Using available resources.
9. Recruiting additional help when needed.
10. Professional behavior.

F. **Non–delivery room preparation.** As with delivery room resuscitation, being prepared for unforeseen events throughout the infant's entire hospitalization can facilitate success in a time of crisis. Unlike delivery room events, non–delivery room resuscitation is often unpredictable and risks ill preparedness. The following events may precipitate respiratory or circulatory compromise:
1. Apnea.
2. Choking or aspiration (i.e., feedings).
3. Unwitnessed cardiac arrest.
4. Seizure.
5. Hypoxia or airway obstruction.
6. Infection.
7. Postoperative period.
8. Air leak syndromes.
9. Severe anemia (i.e., subgaleal hemorrhage, abruption).
10. Shock.

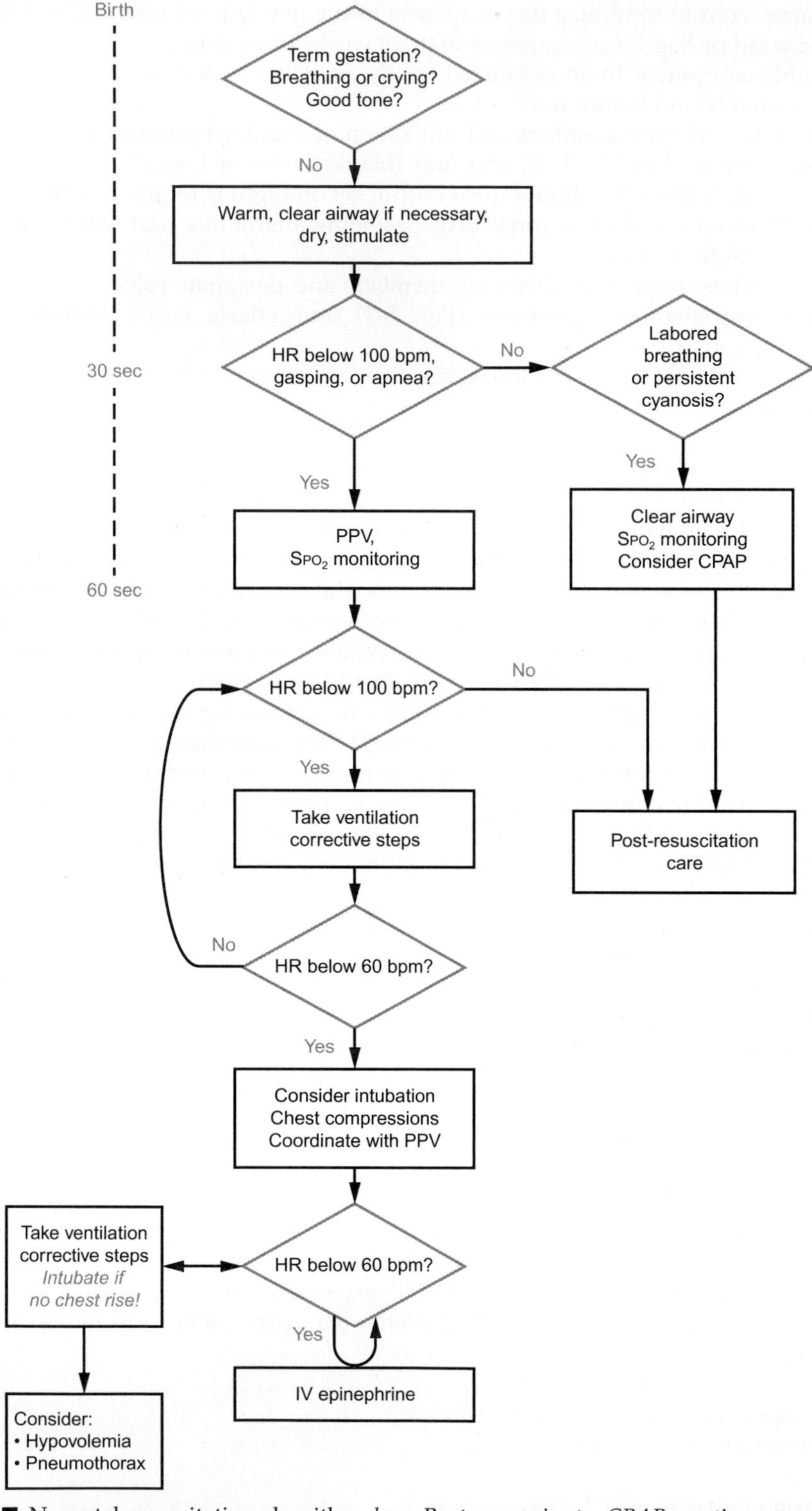


FIGURE 5-1 ■ Neonatal resuscitation algorithm. *bpm*, Beats per minute; *CPAP*, continuous positive airway pressure; *HR*, heart rate; *IV*, intravenous; *PPV*, positive pressure ventilation. (From Kattwinkel, J. [Ed.]: *Textbook of Neonatal Resuscitation* [6th ed.]. Elk Grove Village, Ill., 2011, American Academy of Pediatrics and American Heart Association).

## EQUIPMENT FOR NEONATAL RESUSCITATION

Not every item on the equipment list (Box 5-1) will be used, but it is important to have appropriate sizes and supply quantities to support a prolonged effort. Ensuring that equipment is functional and up to date is vital to a successful resuscitation. It is important that staff members be familiar with the equipment they will be using and practice with it frequently.

BOX 5-1

**NEONATAL RESUSCITATION EQUIPMENT LIST**

**Suction Equipment**

- Bulb syringe
- Mechanical suction with tubing
- Suction catheters: 5 F or 6 F, 8 F, 10 F, 12 F, and 14 F
- 8Fr feeding tube with 20-mL syringe
- Meconium aspiration device

**Bag-and-Mask Equipment**

- Oxygen source
- Compressed air source
- Oxygen blender with flowmeter (flow rate up to 10 L/min) and tubing
- Positive pressure ventilation device capable of delivering 90% to 100% oxygen
- Face mask (preterm and term) with cushioned rim
- Pulse oximeter and oximeter probe

**Airway**

- Laryngoscope with straight blades 00, 0, and 1 size
- Extra batteries and bulb for laryngoscope
- Endotracheal tubes: 2.5, 3, 3.5, and 4 mm
- Stylet (optional)
- Carbon dioxide detector
- Scissors
- Tape or securing device for endotracheal tube (latex-free preferred)
- Pectin-based skin preparation (approved for neonate)
- Oral airways: size 000, 00, and 0, or 30-, 40-, and 50-mm lengths
- Laryngeal mask airway, size 0.5, 1

**Medications**

- Epinephrine 1:10,000 (0.1 mg/mL)
- Isotonic crystalloid solutions (normal saline or Ringer's lactate)
- Surfactant (optional)
- Dextrose 10%
- Normal saline for flushes
- Umbilical vessel catheterization supplies (refer to procedure, Chapter 15)

**Miscellaneous**

- Radiant warmer bed and/or other heat source
- Warmed linen
- Blood gas syringes or supplies for blood gas evaluation
- Cardiac monitor
- Stethoscope—neonatal size
- Clock with second hand (timer optional)
- Standard precaution supplies: gloves and personal protection equipment

**Premature Neonate Supplies**

- Polyethylene wrap or plastic bag
- Chemically activated warming pad
- Transport incubator for transfer to nurse

## APGAR SCORING

The Apgar score (Table 5-1) is a descriptive tool for documenting the status of the newborn after birth. Generally scored during or after resuscitation and stabilization at 1 and 5 minutes, it describes the infant's physiologic condition in five categories: color, heart rate, reflex irritability, muscle tone, and respiratory effort. When the 5-minute score is less than 7, the Apgar score should be determined every 5 minutes until 20 minutes of age. The scores are not used for decision making during resuscitation. The scores are influenced by interventions, gestational age, maternal medications, and cardiorespiratory and neurologic conditions (e.g., malformations, hypoglycemia). An expanded Apgar score has been proposed by the American Academy of Pediatrics and American College of Obstetricians and Gynecologists (2006) to record the correlation of infant's status with resuscitative interventions. Narrative documentation detailing interventions (e.g., ventilation, medications, and oxygen) should accompany the scoring.

## DECISION-MAKING PROCESS

Decision making during resuscitation requires quick and frequent assessment, intervention, and evaluation. The initial steps to resuscitation should be preceded by three questions that facilitate determination of whether resuscitation measures are required. Ask the following questions:

- Is the baby term gestation?
- Is the baby breathing or crying?
- Is there good muscle tone?

At most deliveries, the following steps are the only interventions necessary. These initial steps should be initiated within a few seconds and completed as quickly as possible unless meconium is present and the neonate is not vigorous. Although these are noted as initial steps, they may be applied at any time during the process.

■ TABLE 5-1
■ ■ **Apgar Score** **Gestational Age: ________ Weeks**

| Sign | 0 | 1 | 2 | 1 Minute | 5 Minutes | 10 Minutes | 15 Minutes | 20 Minutes |
|---|---|---|---|---|---|---|---|---|
| Color | Blue or pale | Acrocyanotic | Completely pink | | | | | |
| Heart rate | Absent | <100/minute | >100/minute | | | | | |
| Reflex irritability | No response | Grimace | Cry or active withdrawal | | | | | |
| Muscle tone | Limp | Some flexion | Active motion | | | | | |
| Respiration | Absent | Weak cry: Hypoventilation | Good: Crying | | | | | |
| | | | Total | | | | | |
| | | | | **Resuscitation** | | | | |
| **Comments:** | | | | **1 Minute** | **5 Minutes** | **10 Minutes** | **15 Minutes** | **20 Minutes** |
| | | | Oxygen | | | | | |
| | | | PPV/NCPAP | | | | | |
| | | | ETT | | | | | |
| | | | Chest compressions | | | | | |
| | | | Epinephrine | | | | | |

*ETT*, Endotracheal tube; *NCPAP*, nasal continuous positive airway pressure; *PPV*, positive pressure ventilation.

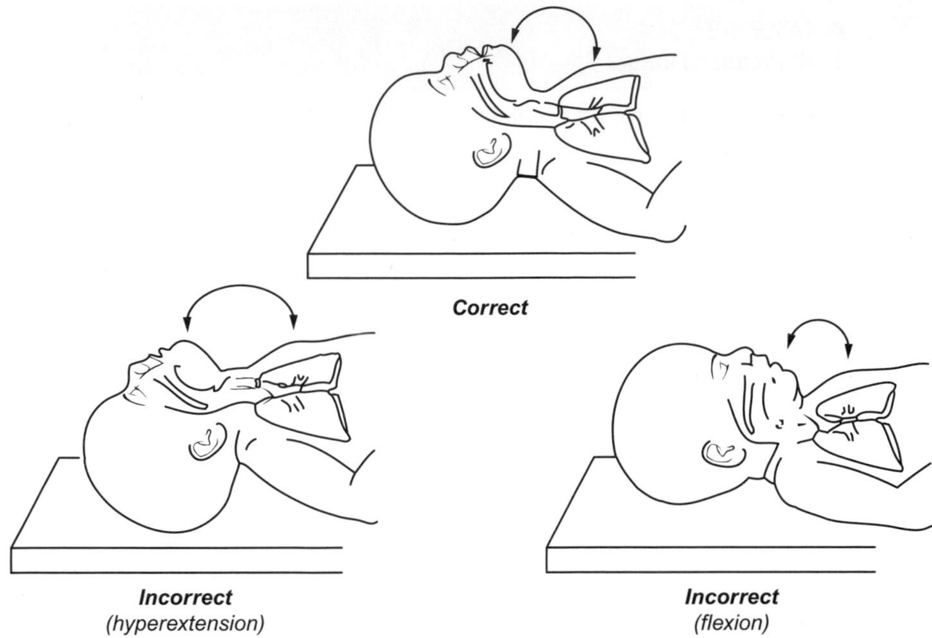


FIGURE 5-2 ■ Correct and incorrect head positioning for resuscitation. (From Kattwinkel, J. [Ed.]: *Textbook of Neonatal Resuscitation* [6th ed.]. Elk Grove Village, Ill., 2011, American Academy of Pediatrics and American Heart Association).

- Prevent hypothermia and hyperthermia, which may increase metabolic requirements and contribute to respiratory distress, metabolic acidosis, and hypoglycemia. If severe asphyxia is suspected, caution should be taken to not overheat the infant.
- Place and keep the neonate in a preheated environment (radiant warmer and/or other heat source). Stable neonates should be placed skin-to-skin on maternal chest if possible. Supplement environmental support with warmed cap and linens.
- Avoid drafts, for example, sidewalls up on radiant warmer; keep bed away from ventilation drafts, and outside walls and windows.

**A. Airway.**

1. Open the airway.
2. Position infant on the back or side with the neck slightly extended.
   - **a.** Care should be taken to avoid hyperextension or flexion of the neck (Fig. 5-2).
   - **b.** A shoulder pad may help maintain the correct airway position, especially for neonates with a large occiput.
   - **c.** When supine, the infant's head should be in the "sniffing" position.
3. Clear the airway.
   - **a.** Use the least invasive method possible. May wipe nose and mouth with towel, suction with bulb syringe, or use suction catheter to mechanical suction. The suction pressure should be approximately 100 mm Hg. Suction the mouth before the nose in order to prevent aspiration should the infant gasp.
   - **b.** Vigorous or prolonged deep suctioning can result in trauma, bradycardia, or apnea induced by stimulation of the posterior pharynx and vagus nerve.
   - **c.** When meconium-stained fluid is present and the neonate is not vigorous (heart rate less than 100 beats per minute [bpm], depressed respirations, and decreased muscle tone), suction the trachea with 12 F or 14 F suction catheter or endotracheal tube attached to suction device, prior to additional stimulation. Repeat intubation and suctioning until clear of meconium or heart rate indicates continued deterioration.
   - **d.** A vigorous neonate born through meconium-stained fluid should have mouth and nose cleared with bulb syringe or large-bore suction catheter. Clinical judgment must be used.

TABLE 5-2
**Preductal Target $Spo_2$**

| Targeted Preductal $Spo_2$ After Birth (in Percentage by Minutes) | |
|---|---|
| 1 minute | 60% to 65% |
| 2 minutes | 65% to 70% |
| 3 minutes | 70% to 75% |
| 4 minutes | 75% to 80% |
| 5 minutes | 80% to 85% |
| 10 minutes | 85% to 95% |

Adapted from Mariani, G., et al. Pre-ductal and post-ductal $O_2$ saturation in healthy term neonates after birth. *Journal of Pediatrics*, 150:418-421, 2007.

4. Dry, stimulate, reposition.
5. Maintain dry, warm environment.
   a. Dry thoroughly.
   b. Remove wet linen immediately after drying infant and replace with dry linen.
   c. Provide additional heat source as necessary. Do not use warm water gloves or microwaved heat source (e.g., blankets, saline bag).
6. Reposition airway.
7. Evaluate respirations and heart rate.
   a. If apneic, gently slap or flick the soles of the infant's feet.
   b. Gently rub the back, trunk, and extremities.
   c. Attempts to stimulate should be brief, no more than two attempts. If respirations do not begin, proceed to bag-and-mask ventilation (unless diaphragmatic hernia is suspected, in which case, intubate the trachea and ventilate the infant through the endotracheal tube with the resuscitation bag).
   d. Pulse oximetry should be available for all neonates and used to confirm cyanosis.
   e. Placement of oximeter should be preductal (right upper extremity), and trending levels may take more than 10 minutes to rise to 90% or more in the full-term, stable neonate (Table 5-2). Occasional dips in oxygen saturation ($Spo_2$) to a high 80% range may be considered normal in the first few days of life when unaccompanied by other changes in status.
8. Begin supplemental oxygen at any time if central cyanosis is present, heart rate is greater than 100 bpm, and respirations are adequate.
   a. Use oxygen with a flow of at least 5 L/min. Deliver oxygen by mask, cupped hand holding tubing over infant's face, flow-inflating bag and mask, or T-piece resuscitator. The closer the oxygen source to the face, the higher will be the oxygen concentration delivered.
   b. When using a flow-inflating bag and mask, allow some oxygen to escape the mask to prevent a buildup of pressure within the bag-and-mask system.
   c. Continue oxygen delivery until infant pinks and then slowly withdraw the oxygen per pulse oximeter and neonate status, ensuring adequate delivery for the infant to maintain oximeter at target saturations.
9. Evaluate frequently and simultaneously the following:
   a. Airway: for alignment, secretions.
   b. Respiratory effort: rate, breath sounds, work of breathing (grunting, flaring, retracting, depth), symmetry of chest movement.
   c. Heart rate: count for 6 seconds and multiply by 10. Obtain heart rate by:
      (1) Palpation at the base of the umbilical cord stump, and/or
      (2) Auscultation of the apical heartbeat with a stethoscope.

**B. Breathing.**

1. Positive pressure ventilation (PPV) should be initiated with bag and mask when:
   a. Infant has apnea or gasping respirations,
   b. Heart rate is less than 100 bpm even with breathing, and/or
   c. Saturation levels ($SpO_2$) continue below target range despite supplemental oxygen increased to 100%.

2. Resuscitation bags should not be larger than 750 mL and should be connected to oxygen and air source with blender attached.
   a. Self-inflating bags must have a reservoir to deliver high concentrations of oxygen, a pressure gauge and a pressure-release valve. Bag cannot be used to deliver free-flow oxygen or continuous positive airway pressure (CPAP).
   b. Flow-inflating (anesthesia) bags must have a gas source, pressure gauge, and flow control valve and can deliver free-flow oxygen of 21% to 100%. Positive end-expiratory pressure (PEEP) is controlled by the adjustable control valve.
   c. T-piece resuscitator requires compressed gas source and allows manual setting of inspiratory pressure and PEEP; can deliver up to 100% oxygen.
   d. Mask of proper size should be used to obtain adequate seal. Appropriate sizing should have the mask covering the chin, mouth, and nose, but not the eyes.
   e. Equipment should always be present and ready for use, preset, and checked before each use.
3. Procedure.
   a. Assemble, set, and test the equipment.
   b. Position and open airway as in "Airway."
   c. Apply mask and ensure proper seal. Be careful not to apply too much pressure to the neonate's face or neck.
   d. Observe for improvement of heart rate and oximeter saturation. Rate of ventilation is 40 to 60 breaths per minute with initial inspiratory pressure of 20 cm $H_2O$. Pressure increase to 30 cm $H_2O$ or more may be needed if no improvement.
   e. Effective ventilation and signs of improvement include increasing heart rate, improving oximeter saturations, spontaneous breathing, and improving breath sounds and chest movement.
   f. After 30 seconds of ventilation, pause to check 6-second heart rate. Continue ventilation and check for signs of improvement every 30 seconds until the neonate begins sustained spontaneous breathing, the heart rate is greater than 100 bpm, and $Spo_2$ is within target range, at which point PPV may be discontinued and supplemental oxygen weaned.
   g. If manual ventilation is ineffective or if there is a need for prolonged ventilation, endotracheal intubation should be performed.
4. Reassess airway. Use of acronym MR SOPA can assist in assessing ineffective ventilation.
   a. Mask adjustment on face.
   b. Reposition airway to "sniffing" position.
   c. Suction mouth and nose for secretions.
   d. Open mouth slightly with jaw lifted forward.
   e. Pressure increase gradually.
   f. Airway alternative with intubation or laryngeal mask airway.
5. Orogastric tube placement.
   a. Ventilation for more than several minutes (with or without compressions) can cause air to accumulate in the stomach.
   b. Ensure the tube is placed through the mouth rather than the nose to maximize ventilation through the nose.
   c. Aspirate contents, secure in place, and leave open to air.
6. Ventilation via endotracheal tube.
   a. Indications:
      (1) When meconium-stained fluid is present with depressed respirations, decreased heart rate, and diminished muscle tone, immediate intubation is indicated in order to perform tracheal suctioning.
      (2) The neonate does not respond to PPV, as evidenced by inadequate clinical improvement and decreased chest rise.
      (3) Suspected mechanical blockage or impaired lung function (e.g., diaphragmatic hernia).
      (4) Prolonged ventilation is required.
      (5) Extreme prematurity.
      (6) Surfactant administration.
      (7) Administration of chest compression to facilitate coordination of compressions and ventilation, maximize efficiency of ventilation.

b. Equipment (see Box 5-1).
c. Endotracheal intubation (see Chapter 15).
   (1) Should be a clean procedure.
   (2) Perform intubation.
   (3) Confirm placement of endotracheal tube as evidenced by increase in heart rate, breath sounds over both lung fields, "fogging" in endotracheal tube, and evidence of exhaled $CO_2$ on colorimetric $CO_2$ detector.
   (4) Secure tube.
   (5) Observe for dislocation of endotracheal tube or unplanned extubation (e.g., central cyanosis, oximeter desaturation, bradycardia, decreased or asymmetrical chest movement, breath sounds absent or diminished, $CO_2$ detector does not indicate presence of $CO_2$, distended abdomen, air noises audible over stomach, or no mist or fogging in tube).
d. Laryngeal mask airway (LMA).
   (1) Airway device useful when PPV ineffective or endotracheal intubation not feasible or unsuccessful.
   (2) May be helpful in infants with congenital anomalies of the mouth, lip, palate, tongue, pharynx, or neck. May be necessary with extremely small mandible and large tongue, such as Pierre Robin syndrome or trisomy 21.
   (3) Soft, inflatable mask inserted into mouth and guided along hard palate until mask covers larynx.
   (4) Limitations: LMA cannot be used to suction meconium from airway, leaks with high pressures, may be ineffective with chest compression, and results in prolonged ventilation and inability to deliver endotracheal medications.

**C. Chest compressions.**

1. Chest compressions should be initiated when the heart rate is less than 60 bpm after at least 30 seconds of effective PPV.
2. Should always be accompanied by ventilation, which requires a second provider.
3. Use one of the following two methods (Fig. 5-3):
   a. Thumb technique (preferred).
      (1) Place both thumbs side by side or, on small neonate, one over the other. Location is the lower third of the infant's sternum above the xiphoid process.
      (2) Flex thumbs at first joint and apply pressure vertically.
      (3) Encircle the infant's torso with hands and provide support for the back. If hands are too small, ensure that the infant is on a firm surface.
   b. Two-finger technique.
      (1) Place the tips of the middle finger and either the index finger or the ring finger of one hand over the lower third of the infant's sternum.

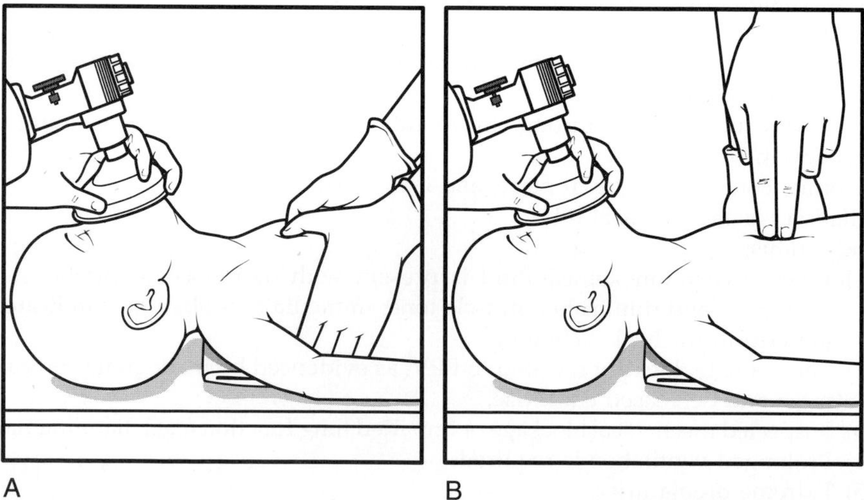


FIGURE 5-3 ■ Two techniques for providing chest compressions: **(A)** thumb (preferred technique) and **(B)** two-finger. (From Kattwinkel, J. [Ed.]: *Textbook of Neonatal Resuscitation* [6th ed.]. Elk Grove Village, Ill., 2011, American Academy of Pediatrics and American Heart Association.)

(2) Place the other hand under the infant's back to provide support.
(3) Compressions should squeeze the heart between the spinal column and the sternum.
  (a) Force of compression should be straight down to minimize rib or lung damage.
  (b) Depress the sternum approximately one third of the anterior–posterior diameter of the chest and release to allow heart to refill.
  (c) Fingers or thumbs should remain in contact with the chest at all times, during both compression and release. Lack of contact with chest wall increases the risk for complications and wastes time relocating landmarks for compression area.
(4) Compression/ventilation ratio of 3:1.
  (a) Provide three compressions, pause for a single ventilation. This will equal 90 compressions to 30 ventilations, or 120 events per minute.
  (b) Optimally, the neonate's trachea should be intubated during compressions.
  (c) Reevaluate heart rate after 45 to 60 seconds during compressions and ventilations.
(5) Indications for discontinuing chest compressions.
  (a) Heart rate greater than 60 bpm; continue ventilation at 40 to 60 breaths per minute.
  (b) After 10 minutes of asystole.

**D. Drugs.** Most neonatal resuscitations do not require medications or volume expanders. When medications are required, an umbilical venous catheter may be the fastest and most direct route. Intravenous (IV) administration of resuscitation medications is preferable whenever available. A peripheral IV line may also be used to administer medications or volume expanders (see Chapter 15). If unable to place umbilical venous catheter or IV line, intraosseous access may be an acceptable alternative.

1. Epinephrine, a cardiac stimulant, increases the heart rate and strength of contractions, causes peripheral vasoconstriction, and increases blood flow through coronary arteries and the brain.
   a. Indications for use: heart rate is less than 60 bpm despite 30 seconds of effective assisted ventilation and another 45 to 60 seconds of coordinated chest compression and ventilation.
   b. Dosing: IV route is preferred route, with recommended dose of 0.1 to 0.3 mL/kg of 1:10,000 concentration. Endotracheal dose of 0.5 to 1 mL/kg may be given while IV access is obtained.
   c. Response: the heart rate should increase to greater than 60 bpm within 1 minute of IV administration. If this does not happen, dosing may be repeated every 3 to 5 minutes, given intravenously if possible.
2. Volume expanders are fluids that increase the neonate's circulating blood volume to correct hypovolemia and facilitate tissue perfusion. Normal saline, Ringer's lactate, and O Rh-negative blood may be used; normal saline is the preferred fluid.
   a. Indicated when there is suspected shock (pallor, weak peripheral pulses, persistent bradycardia, and no improvement in respiratory status) and the neonate is not responding to resuscitative efforts or there is a known condition with associated fetal blood loss, such as placenta previa, twin-to-twin transfusion.
   b. Dose: 10 mL/kg given over 5 to 10 minutes intravenously.
   c. Dose may be repeated if no signs of improvement.
3. Sodium bicarbonate, a base buffer, raises the pH of the blood.
   a. Use during resuscitation is controversial. May be harmful if given too early in a resuscitation.
   b. Adequate ventilation required to remove by-product of $CO_2$.
   c. Indications for use: documented metabolic acidosis.
   d. Dose: 2 mEq/kg of 4.2% solution (0.5 mEq/mL) given intravenously at a rate no faster than 1 mEq/kg/min. Rapid administration of sodium bicarbonate may be associated with intraventricular hemorrhage in premature infants and thus it should be given slowly.
   e. Sodium bicarbonate can be very damaging to lung tissue and should never be given per endotracheal tube. It is caustic and hypertonic and must be administered in a large vein.

## UNUSUAL SITUATIONS

A. **Respiratory**

1. Choanal atresia/upper airway obstruction.
   a. Definition and characteristics:
      (1) Bony or soft tissue obstruction of the posterior nares; may be bilateral or unilateral.
      (2) Respiratory distress may be present immediately after birth because of blockage of the primary airway, the nose.
      (3) May present with cyanosis when quiet or at rest, pinks with crying.
      (4) Inability to pass small-gauge suction catheter or nasogastric tube through each nare may be an indicator of choanal atresia.
   b. Management:
      (1) Stimulate neonate to cry, thereby using the secondary airway (mouth) for ventilation.
      (2) Insert an oral airway or endotracheal tube as an oral airway into the posterior pharynx.
      (3) Infants with more complicated craniofacial malformations may require endotracheal intubation.
2. Pierre Robin sequence.
   a. Definitions and characteristics: small mandible causing displacement of the tongue posteriorly into the pharynx, causing partial or complete obstruction.
   b. Management:
      (1) Maintain patent airway by turning the neonate onto the stomach (prone), which should cause the tongue to fall forward and open the airway.
      (2) If this is not effective, insert an oral airway; or a large catheter (12 F) or small endotracheal tube (2.5 mm) nasally to the posterior pharynx. If these procedures are unsuccessful, placement of an LMA may also be effective.
3. Pulmonary hypoplasia.
   a. Definition and characteristics:
      (1) Underdeveloped lungs resulting from insufficient space within the thoracic cavity for normal development.
      (2) Associated with Potter sequence, dysplastic renal conditions, chronic oligohydramnios, and diaphragmatic hernia.
   b. Clinical presentation: deterioration may be acute.
      (1) Inability to ventilate lungs adequately exhibited by poor chest movement, decreased breath sounds, and cyanosis.
      (2) Very high pressures are required to expand small, stiff lungs.
      (3) High risk of pulmonary air leak.
      (4) Low and/or descending Apgar scores.
      (5) Poor perfusion.
      (6) Diminished muscle tone.
      (7) Respiratory and/or metabolic acidosis.
   c. Management:
      (1) Intubate.
      (2) Ventilate with as much pressure and oxygen necessary to expand the lungs (i.e., adequate chest rise and fall).
      (3) Transilluminate and auscultate chest frequently, assessing for pulmonary air leaks. Be prepared for emergency evacuation of air leak.
4. Congenital diaphragmatic hernia.
   a. Definition and characteristics (see Chapter 29):
      (1) Herniation of the abdominal contents into the chest cavity during gestational development.
      (2) Pulmonary hypoplasia arises secondary to compression from abdominal organs and limited capacity for growth in the thoracic cavity.
      (3) Most commonly occurs on the left.
      (4) May present with a scaphoid abdomen.

(5) Severity of symptoms is associated with the amount of lung compression and pulmonary hypoplasia. May present with respiratory distress shortly after birth and descending Apgar scores at the time of delivery or with later-onset respiratory distress.
(6) Lung sounds absent or decreased on the side of defect.
(7) Bowel sounds audible in the chest.
(8) Heart sounds may be audible on the right side if left-sided defect.
(9) Prenatal diagnosis possible through ultrasound. Polyhydramnios often present.

**b.** Management:
(1) Consider immediate endotracheal intubation and ventilation to minimize overdistention of the stomach resulting from bag-and-mask ventilation.
(2) Provide gastric decompression per 10 F orogastric tube, preferably, Replogle (double-lumen Salem sump).
(3) Systemic hypotension and respiratory or metabolic acidosis commonly occur. Aggressive management necessary to minimize pulmonary hypertension.
(4) Inhaled nitric oxide may be used for infants not responding to conventional therapies.

**5.** Persistent respiratory depression. After PPV has restored a normal heart rate and target $Spo_2$ saturation; this respiratory depression or decreased muscle activity may be related to:
**a.** Brain injury such as hypoxic–ischemic encephalopathy, severe acidosis, or a central nervous system or neuromuscular abnormality, or
**b.** Sedation related to a history of maternal narcotic administration within the 4 hours before delivery.
**c.** Naloxone hydrochloride, a short-acting narcotic antagonist, displaces narcotics from receptor sites and reverses the physiologic depressant effects of a narcotic drug.
(1) Not the first intervention for respiratory depression. Use should follow ventilatory support and other initial steps of resuscitation.
(2) Administration to neonate of a mother who is narcotic-addicted or on methadone maintenance may cause severe withdrawal, seizures, and/or cardiorespiratory arrest.
(3) Dose concentration is 1 mg/mL; the dose is 0.1 mg/kg given rapidly intravenously.
(4) Respiratory depression should decrease within seconds or minutes (depending on route) after administration. Duration of action is widely variable (1 to 4 hours). Monitor closely for return of respiratory depression and need for ongoing support.

**B. Multiple gestation.**
**1.** Characteristics:
**a.** May be small for gestational age or intrauterine growth restricted.
**b.** Compression deformations may be present.
**c.** Distress may be related to placental abnormalities, compromise of cord blood flow, or mechanical complications during delivery.

**2.** Management:
**a.** Delivery of multiples may be unexpected.
**b.** Separate resuscitation team for each neonate.
**c.** Twin-to-twin transfusion may require volume resuscitation of donor twin.
**d.** Premature delivery common.
**e.** Systematic and planned approach for mobilizing extra resuscitative teams is necessary to ensure appropriate resuscitation of unexpected multiples.
**f.** Ensure adequate supplies and equipment are available, in addition to backup supplies, to manage multiple prolonged resuscitative efforts.

**C. Prematurity.**
**1.** Definition and characteristics:
**a.** Multisystem immaturity.
**b.** Fragile skin, especially with very low birth weight (VLBW) infant.
**c.** Susceptible to trauma from resuscitative intervention.
**d.** Susceptible to infection.
**e.** Susceptible to hypovolemia.
**f.** Increased thermal instability.

**2.** Management:
**a.** Have additional trained personnel available for full resuscitation.

**b.** Thermal stability.
 (1) Increase the temperature of the delivery room to 77° to 79° F (25° to 26° C).
 (2) Use additional heat sources to maintain a neutral thermal environment.
 (3) Preheat radiant warmer.
 (4) Thermal wrapping with polyethylene plastic wrap or bag and portable warming pad for neonates less than 29 weeks of gestation. Portable warming pad should be below layers of warm linen. Monitor temperature closely.
 (5) Use a prewarmed transport unit during transfer.

**c.** Respiratory support.
 (1) Oxygen.
  (a) Use a pulse oximeter to maintain target $Spo_2$ range for gestational age.
  (b) Use a blender to titrate oxygen to achieve appropriate $Spo_2$ range using the same parameters as for term infants.
 (2) Ventilation.
  (a) Consider CPAP if heart rate greater than 100 bpm, spontaneous respirations with respiratory distress, decreased pulse oximetry, and cyanosis.
  (b) If PPV needed, the lowest pressures possible should be used to obtain adequate responses, starting with 20 to 25 cm $H_2O$.
  (c) If endotracheal intubation is necessary, use initial PEEP of 2 to 5 cm $H_2O$.
 (3) Administration of surfactant is shown to be beneficial in infants less than 30 weeks of gestation even without signs of respiratory distress. Indications for and timing of surfactant administration remain controversial.

**d.** Neuroprotection.
 (1) Be as gentle as possible with the tiny neonate (i.e., drying, ventilating, and cardiopulmonary resuscitation).
 (2) Maintain head in midline positioning as much as possible, preferably for the first 72 hours of life.
 (3) Maintain a neutral thermal environment.
 (4) Keep head of bed flat (avoid Trendelenburg's position).
 (5) Infuse fluids slowly and cautiously.
 (6) Avoid delivering excess positive pressure or CPAP.
 (7) Use pulse oximeter and blood gases to adjust ventilation and oxygen concentration gradually and appropriately.

**e.** Infection control.
 (1) Implement strategies to reduce nosocomial infection (i.e., ventilator-associated pneumonia, catheter-related bloodstream infections).
 (2) Use sterile supplies (i.e., sterile water) when possible for VLBW infants.
 (3) Minimize use of tape and adhesives.

**f.** Provide developmental care to promote physiologic stability.

**g.** If at all possible, the family and the primary care physician, along with the neonatal team, should explore viability issues and expected outcome before the birth.

## COMPLICATIONS OF RESUSCITATION

**A. Trauma.**
1. Skin: bruises and abrasions from chest compressions, handling, and tape application and removal.
2. Mucosa: laryngoscopy and intubation can cause trauma to and bleeding of the gums, lips, pharynx, and trachea.
3. Internal organ damage from chest compressions.

**B. Respiratory.**
1. Pulmonary hypertension.
2. Pneumonia.
3. Pulmonary air leaks, including pneumothorax, pneumomediastinum, pneumopericardium.
4. Surfactant deficiency or deactivation.
5. Meconium aspiration syndrome.

C. **Neurologic.**
  1. Hypoxic–ischemic encephalopathy.
  2. Apnea.
  3. Seizures.
  4. Intracranial hemorrhages such as subarachnoid, periventricular, intraventricular, subgaleal.

D. **Metabolic/Hematologic.**
  1. Hypothermia.
  2. Hypoglycemia.
  3. Electrolyte imbalance, especially calcium, sodium, potassium.
  4. Anemia.
  5. Thrombocytopenia.

E. **Gastrointestinal.**
  1. Ileus.
  2. Necrotizing enterocolitis.

## POSTRESUSCITATION CARE

The goal of postresuscitation care is to evaluate the infant's condition for complications, avoid intensifying conditions that may impair outcome (i.e., hypothermia, hypoglycemia), and help diagnose and treat underlying disease.

A. **Assess oxygenation, ventilation, and acid–base balance.**
  1. Check blood gas concentrations (capillary, arterial, and venous).
  2. Correlate findings with the neonate's clinical condition.
  3. Correlate findings with pulse oximetry and/or transcutaneous monitoring devices.
  4. Adjust the neonate's respiratory and oxygen support as needed. Assess for increase or return of respiratory distress, especially pulmonary hypertension and pneumonia.

B. **Monitor glucose concentrations to ensure normoglycemia.**
  1. Serial screening of blood glucose.
  2. Treat hypoglycemia and adjust maintenance dextrose infusion if IV fluids are required. Bolus infusions ($D_{10}W$, 2 mL/kg) may be required to elevate serum glucose in addition to maintenance infusion.
  3. Feeding may not be recommended depending on infant's status.

C. **Volume and electrolyte support.**
  1. Assess perfusion and evaluate for anemia, polycythemia, and hypovolemia.
  2. Calculate the fluid volume received during resuscitation and estimate volume deficiencies.
  3. Determine the amount needed (in milliliters per kilogram per day).
  4. Adjust IV rate as needed. Include all fluids in fluid calculations.
  5. Monitor the urine output. Keep an accurate account of the intake.

D. **Chest and abdominal x-ray examination for pneumothorax, pneumomediastinum, pneumopericardium, and pneumoperitoneum.**
  1. Assess endotracheal tube position.
  2. Assess the position of umbilical catheters.
  3. Evaluate for lung and cardiac disease.
  4. Rule out fractures and anomalies.

E. **Central nervous system assessment.**
  1. Assess neurologic status and reflexes.
  2. Monitor for seizure activity, unexplained apnea.
  3. Provide sedation as needed.
  4. Consider induced therapeutic hypothermia once infant meets protocol if available.

F. **Monitor vital signs.**
  1. Provide a neutral thermal environment to prevent the sequelae of hypothermia or hyperthermia.
  2. Continue the assessment of perfusion and capillary refill time.
  3. Monitor the blood pressure, preferably arterial.
  4. Continuous cardiorespiratory monitoring is recommended. Assess the heart rate and respiratory rate as needed.

**G. Screen for infection.**
1. Evaluate maternal history: titers, cultures, pretreatment, and risk factors.
2. Obtain a complete blood cell count, differential cell count, platelet count, and C-reactive protein.
3. Obtain blood and tracheal samples for cultures and for sensitivity testing as indicated.
4. If the index of suspicion is high and the neonate's condition is stable, lumbar puncture may be performed for cerebrospinal fluid analysis.

**H. Support family.**
1. Provide a family-centered approach to care. Actively collaborate with family regarding decision making.
2. Report the neonate's condition to mother and significant others.
3. Make appropriate referrals to ancillary support services.

**I. Documentation.**
1. Accurate charting, including descriptive and often minute-by-minute documentation, reveals the events, interventions, and infant responses to the resuscitative efforts.
2. Include pertinent perinatal factors, physical findings, procedures and care performed, infant response, and team communication.
3. Vital signs, medications, laboratory findings, and other factual data should also be included.
4. Developmental support and the infant's behavioral response to care should be integrated into resuscitation and stabilization documentation.

**J. Safety.**
1. Ensure the neonate is accurately identified.
2. Nurse-to-nurse communication should include a thorough history of resuscitation and stabilization.
3. Reconcile medications if the neonate is transferred to another unit or another hospital.

**K. Ethics (Sayeed, 2006).**
1. Collaboration with the family is essential with all decision making.
2. Noninitiation of resuscitation may be appropriate in the delivery room when:
   a. Confirmed less than 23 weeks of gestation and less than 400 g birth weight.
   b. Anencephaly.
   c. Confirmed lethal genetic anomaly.
   d. Data available to support extremely high index of death or severe disability.
3. Discontinuation of support may be appropriate after 10 minutes of resuscitative efforts with no heart rate. Gestational age, reason for arrest, involvement of other complications, whether therapeutic hypothermia is potential, and the expressed feeling and expectations of the parents need to be considered.
4. Information at or around the time of delivery is often incomplete. Resuscitative options may include initiation of therapy and reevaluation of treatment decision making after more information is available.
5. Involve resource supports, such as clergy, social services, and palliative care team.
6. Consult hospital ethics committee or legal counsel if needed.

## REFERENCES


American Academy of Pediatrics and American College of Obstetricians and Gynecologists: *Guidelines for perinatal care* (7th ed.). Elk Grove Village, IL, and Washington, DC, 2012, American Academy of Pediatrics and American College of Obstetricians and Gynecologists.

American Academy of Pediatrics and American College of Obstetricians and Gynecologists: The Apgar score. *Pediatrics*, 117(4):1444–1448, 2006.

Kattwinkel, J. (Ed.): *Textbook of neonatal resuscitation* (6th ed.). Elk Grove Village, IL, 2011, American Academy of Pediatrics and American Heart Association.

Kattwinkel, J., Perlman, J.A., Aziz, K., et al.: Neonatal resuscitation: 2010 American Heart Association guidelines for cardiopulmonary resuscitation and emergency cardiovascular care. *Pediatrics*, 126(5): e1400–e1413, 2010.

Mariani, G., Dik, P.B., Ezquer, A., et al.: Pre-ductal and post-ductal $O_2$ saturation in healthy term neonates after birth. *Journal of Pediatrics*, 150:418–421, 2007.

Perlman, J.M., Wyllie, J., Kattwinkel, J., et al.: Part 11: Neonatal resuscitation 2010 International Consensus on Cardiopulmonary Resuscitation and Emergency Cardiovascular Care Science with Treatment Recommendations. *Circulation*, 122(16 Suppl 2):S516–S538, 2010.

Sayeed, S.A.: The marginally viable newborn: Legal challenges, conceptual inadequacies, and reasonableness. *Journal of Law, Medicine, & Ethics*, Fall:600–610, 2006.

CHAPTER

# 6 Thermoregulation

M. COLLEEN BRAND AND HOLLY A. BOYD

**OBJECTIVES**

1. Discuss the importance of thermoregulation in the care of newborn infants.
2. Compare mechanisms of heat transfer involved in newborn thermoregulation.
3. Identify newborns at increased risk for thermal instability.
4. Recognize symptoms of hypothermia and hyperthermia in neonates.
5. Describe the physiologic processes involved in thermoregulation.
6. Apply strategies for managing the thermal environment.

## INTRODUCTION

Neonates are the most vulnerable population in regard to temperature control. The smallest and most premature are unable to protect themselves against fluctuations in environmental temperature. Nurses are the first line of defense for this population. It is important that nurses understand the physiology and management of thermoregulation and use their skill and expertise to provide the best environment for these at-risk patients.

**A. The importance of thermoregulation.**

1. There are adverse consequences associated with both hypothermia and hyperthermia. Hypothermia is the major temperature abnormality in neonates. An increase in mortality and morbidity associated with hypothermia is well documented and is recognized as a problem worldwide.
   a. In Europe during the mid to late 1800s, the use of an early crude form of incubator began and it was observed that more small babies survived.
   b. In the early 1900s, premature babies were displayed at world fairs and expositions in these devices to show small babies previously believed to have very little chance of survival now thriving in this new warmer environment.
   c. In the 1950s, Silverman demonstrated that hypothermia increased morbidity and mortality (Silverman et al., 1958). More recent studies confirm this finding (Costeloe et al., 2000; Laptook et al., 2007).
   d. The World Health Organization (WHO) recognizes thermoregulation of the newborn as a major threat to the health of newborns throughout the world (WHO, 1997).
   e. The term "golden hour" has been used recently in reference to strategies implemented in the delivery room to improve the outcome of neonates. A major focus during the "golden hour" is prevention of heat loss (Bissinger and Annibale, 2010).

**B. Mechanisms of heat transfer.**

1. Heat transfer infers the transfer of heat from warm to cool. There are four mechanisms of heat transfer that affect neonates: conduction, convection, radiation, and evaporation. Table 6-1 lists mechanisms of heat transfer and activities that are associated with heat loss and heat gain as well as strategies to prevent both loss and gain.
   a. Conduction is the transfer of heat via direct contact.
      (1) Heat is lost when the neonate comes in contact with a cold surface such as a mattress, x-ray plate, or scale.
      (2) Heat is gained when the neonate comes in contact with a warmer surface such as a chemical warming mattress or warm blankets.
      (3) The rate of heat transfer varies with the temperature gradient and the amount of skin in contact with the surface. Heat is transferred more readily from the skin to a metal object than from the skin to a cloth surface.

■ TABLE 6-1
■ ■ **Mechanisms of Heat Transfer**

| Mechanism | Heat Transfer | Situation | Strategies for Prevention |
|---|---|---|---|
| Conduction | Loss | Cold mattress | Prewarm bed or cover with several layers of warm blankets |
| | | Weighing scale | Cover scale with a prewarmed blanket |
| | | Extended posture | Position infant in a flexed/nested position |
| | Gain | Chemical mattress | No direct heat due to burn risk; place a blanket over mattress<br>Follow manufacturer's recommendations |
| | | Hot water bottle | Limit use due to inability to control temperature<br>No direct heat due to burn risk; place a blanket over bottle |
| | | Too many layers of clothing/blankets | Educate parents in thermoregulation |
| Convection | Loss | Cold air | Increase temperature in delivery room<br>Move away from air conditioning vents<br>Use radiant warmer |
| | Gain | Incubator | Monitor temperature frequently until neutral thermal conditions are established |
| Evaporation | Loss | Amniotic fluid | Place skin-to-skin with mother if condition allows<br>Dry with warm blankets<br>Wrap with warm blankets<br>VLBW: place in polyethylene bag |
| | | Bathing | Warm room<br>Warm water<br>Bathe quickly<br>Dry and dress |
| | | Vasodilation | Avoid overheating<br>Avoid rapid rewarming |
| | Gain | Humidified incubator | Maintain prescribed humidity |
| | | Vasoconstriction | Maintain neutral thermal environment<br>Avoid situations that contribute to cold stress |
| Radiation | Loss | Cold incubator wall | Prewarmed incubator<br>Double-walled incubator |
| | | Cold window | Move away from window or cover window<br>Radiant warmer with servo-control |
| | Gain | Direct sunlight | Position away from windows or close blinds |
| | | Radiant warmer | Always use in servo-control mode |
| | | Heat lamp | Use only as a last resort and monitor infant's temperature frequently |

*VLBW*, very low birth weight.

b. Convection is heat transfer due to air currents or drafts.
   (1) Incubators transfer heat to infants through the circulation of warm air (convective heat gain).
   (2) Heat loss will occur when an infant is exposed to cool air, such as air conditioning, or is placed into an incubator that has not been prewarmed.
   (3) Heat transfer increases with the temperature gradient between skin and air, with increased airflow, and with increased skin exposure.

c. Radiation is the transfer of heat from a warm object to a cooler object that is not in direct contact through infrared energy transfer. Think of standing near a sunny window in summer (heat gain) or a frosty window in winter (heat loss).
   (1) Radiant warmers provide this type of heat.
   (2) Heat transfer is affected by the temperature gradient and the distance and angle between the heat source and the skin surface. Radiant heat transfer is not affected by the ambient air temperature or circulating air.
   (3) If the walls of an incubator are cold, an infant may lose heat and be cold-stressed despite warm air circulating through the incubator (Blackburn, 2013).

d. Evaporation is heat transfer due to water vaporizing from the skin or respiratory tract into the drier surrounding air and, in the case of premature infants with thin permeable skin, through transepidermal water loss (TEWL).
e. In the delivery room, evaporation of amniotic fluid accounts for 25% of neonatal heat loss (Dahm and James, 1972).
f. High total body water, immature skin, and relatively large body surface area result in increased evaporative losses in premature infants. This is even more significant in very low birth weight (VLBW) and especially in extremely low birth weight (ELBW) infants.

**C. Thermal instability.**

1. Hypothermia.
   a. Nurses caring for neonates should be able to identify infants who are at high risk for thermal instability. Infants who have decreased brown fat and decreased glycogen stores, those with high TEWL, and those who lack muscle tone would be considered at increased risk for hypothermia.
   b. Infants at risk for hypothermia include premature and late preterm infants and infants who have intrauterine growth restriction, are critically ill, are sedated, or have neurologic problems. Infants with open skin defects that place them at risk for increased water loss, such as neural tube or abdominal wall defects, are also at increased risk (American Academy of Pediatrics [AAP] and American College of Obstetricians and Gynecologists [ACOG], 2007; Blackburn, 2013) (Box 6-1).

BOX 6-1
**INFANTS AT RISK FOR HYPOTHERMIA AND HYPERTHERMIA**

**Hypothermia**
- Cardiorespiratory abnormalities
- Central nervous system (CNS) abnormalities
- Critically ill
- Endocrine disorders
- Hypoglycemia
- Infection
- Large abdominal wall defects
- Large neural tube defects
- Premature
- Sedated infants/neuromuscular blockade
- Small for gestational age/growth restriction

**Hyperthermia**
- Cardiac defect
- CNS injury or malformation
- Dehydration
- Drug withdrawal
- Iatrogenic overheating
- Infection
- Maternal epidural anesthesia
- Maternal fever
- Medication side effects (prostaglandin)

Data from American Academy of Pediatrics and American College of Obstetricians and Gynecologists: *Guidelines for perinatal care* (6th ed.). Elk Grove Village, IL, and Washington, DC, 2007, American Academy of Pediatrics and American College of Obstetricians and Gynecologists; Baumgart, S.: Iatrogenic hyperthermia and hypothermia in the neonate. *Clinics in Perinatology*, 35(1):183-197, ix-x, 2008; Blackburn, S.: *Maternal, fetal, & neonatal physiology* (4th ed.). St. Louis: 2013, Elsevier Saunders; Knobel, R., and Holditch-Davis, D.: Thermoregulation and heat loss prevention after birth and during neonatal intensive-care unit stabilization of extremely low-birthweight infants. *JOGNN: Journal of Obstetric, Gynecologic and Neonatal Nursing*, 36(3):280-287, 2007; Lieberman, E., Lang, J., Richardson, D.K., et al.: Intrapartum maternal fever and neonatal outcome. *Pediatrics*, 105(1 Pt. 1):8-13, 2000; and Mance, M.J.: Keeping infants warm: Challenges of hypothermia. *Advances in Neonatal Care*, 8(1):6-12, 2008.

c. Symptoms of hypothermia include apnea, bradycardia, decreased cardiac output, poor oral feeding, feeding intolerance, hypoglycemia, hypotension, hypoxia, irritability, lethargy, weak cry, metabolic acidosis, peripheral vasoconstriction, pulmonary vasoconstriction, and respiratory distress (Box 6-2).

d. Poor weight gain may be a symptom of chronic hypothermia due to increased caloric use to attempt to maintain a normal temperature.

BOX 6-2

**SYMPTOMS OF THERMAL STRESS IN NEWBORNS**

**Hypothermia**

- Apnea
- Bradycardia
- Central cyanosis
- Central nervous system (CNS) injury
- Coagulation defects (i.e., pulmonary hemorrhage)
- Death
- Hypoglycemia
- Hypotension/decreased cardiac output
- Hypotonia
- Hypoxia
- Feeding intolerance (abdominal distention, emesis, increased residuals)
- Increased metabolic rate
- Irritability
- Lethargy
- Metabolic acidosis
- Peripheral vasoconstriction (pallor, decreased capillary refill time)
- Poor weight gain (chronic hypothermia)
- Pulmonary vasoconstriction (persistent pulmonary hypertension of the newborn)
- Respiratory distress (decreased surfactant synthesis and activity)
- Shivering (mature neonates in presence of severe hypothermia)
- Weak cry or suck

**Hyperthermia**

- Apnea
- CNS depression/injury
- Death
- Dehydration (increased insensible water loss)
- Flushed/red skin
- Hypernatremia
- Irritability
- Lethargy/weak cry
- Poor feeding
- Seizures
- Sweating (term neonates)
- Tachycardia
- Tachypnea
- Vasodilation
- Warm to touch

Data from Baumgart, S.: Iatrogenic hyperthermia and hypothermia in the neonate. *Clinics in Perinatology*, 35(1):183-197, ix-x, 2008; Blackburn, S.: *Maternal, fetal, & neonatal physiology* (4th ed.). St. Louis: 2013, Elsevier Saunders; Knobel, R., and Holditch-Davis, D.: Thermoregulation and heat loss prevention after birth and during neonatal intensive-care unit stabilization of extremely low-birthweight infants. *JOGNN: Journal of Obstetric, Gynecologic and Neonatal Nursing*, 36(3):280-287, 2007; and Mance, M.J.: Keeping infants warm: Challenges of hypothermia. *Advances in Neonatal Care*, 8(1):6-12, 2008.

e. In severe cases of hypothermia, coagulation defects and death may result (Blackburn, 2013). Although shivering is rare, it may be seen in term infants after prolonged cold stress (Bissinger and Annibale, 2010).

2. Hyperthermia.
   a. Infants are also at risk for hyperthermia because of the inability to dissipate heat. Close monitoring and attention to the thermal environment are indicated when caring for these infants.
   b. Infants at risk for hyperthermia include those with hypermetabolism, including sepsis, cardiac problems, and drug withdrawal, those with dehydration, and infants with central nervous system (CNS) injury or malformation (see Box 6-1).
   c. Symptoms of hyperthermia include apnea, CNS depression, hypernatremia from dehydration, irritability, lethargy, weak cry, poor oral feeding, seizures, tachycardia, and vasodilation (Brown and Landers, 2011) (see Box 6-2).
   d. Severe hyperthermia may be associated with seizures and death.
3. Monitoring temperature (Smith et al., 2013).
   a. Early detection and management of hypothermia and hyperthermia is essential to the well-being of neonates. Frequent temperature measurements and observation are key to early detection until the infant's temperature is stable.
   b. It is important to measure the neonate's temperature accurately in order to assure the temperature is within the normal range and to document the temperature in the medical record to provide data for following temperature trends.
   c. Axillary temperatures are commonly used in the nursery as they are easy to obtain, are minimally invasive, and correlate well with core temperature.
      (1) Normal axillary ranges are 36.5° to 37.5°C (97.7° to 99.5°F) for the term neonate and 36.3° to 36.9°C (97.3° to 98.6°F) for the preterm neonate (Brown and Landers, 2011).
      (2) Electronic or digital thermometers should be used according to the manufacturer's specifications.
   d. Rectal temperatures should not be used due to the risk of intestinal perforation and because the core temperature may not decrease until the neonate has totally decompensated.
      (1) Rectal thermistors may be used to provide continuous monitoring during therapeutic cooling for hypoxic–ischemic encephalopathy (HIE).
   e. Esophageal temperature monitoring may be used to monitor core temperature during therapeutic cooling for HIE or during surgery.
   f. Continuous skin monitoring is done when servo-controlled equipment is in use. The thermistor should be securely attached to an exposed area of skin with an insulated cover.
      (1) Avoid areas of brown adipose tissue (BAT) such as the axilla, as the temperature may be higher in these areas due to increased metabolic activity. BAT is discussed later in this chapter.
         (a) Desired skin temperatures range from 36° to 37.5°C (96.8° to 99.5°F) (Bissinger and Annibale, 2010; Brown and Landers, 2011; Gomella, 2009; Malin and Baumgart, 1987).
      (2) Abdominal temperatures greater than 36.5° C are associated with lower oxygen consumption in radiant warmers (Malin and Baumgart, 1987).
      (3) A study on temperature and heart rate suggests a target of 36.8° to 36.9° C might be more optimal during transition in ELBW infants (Knobel et al., 2010).
      (4) If both central (abdominal) and peripheral temperatures are monitored, the expected difference is 0.5° to 1° C (Turnbull and Petty, 2013). A difference of 2° C or greater has been associated with cold stress resulting in peripheral vasoconstriction in infants beyond the first day of life (Horns, 2002; Knobel et al., 2009; Lyon et al., 1997; Mok et al., 1991).
   g. Ear thermometers are fast and easy to use but may be too large for premature infants. If the probe is not placed correctly, the surface temperature may be measured rather than an approximation of core temperature.
   h. Infrared thermometers, also called temporal artery thermometers, measure the surface temperature without touching the infant by capturing heat radiated from the skin surface. More study is needed before these thermometers are used routinely in neonatal units.

## PHYSIOLOGY OF THERMOREGULATION

**A. In utero, the maternal temperature is the ambient environmental temperature for the fetus.** The neonate's temperature at birth will be reflective of the intrauterine temperature. If the mother has a fever, it is common for the neonate's temperature to be elevated. It is important to distinguish between environmental, iatrogenic, and infectious causes of elevations in neonatal temperatures.

1. The intrauterine temperature may be 0.8° C (1.3° F) greater than the maternal oral temperature (Banerjee et al., 2004).
2. Maternal temperature increases as labor progresses and may increase by an average of 1° C during labor due to physical activity and stimulation of the thermoregulatory center in the hypothalamus (Blackburn, 2013).
3. Epidural anesthesia may also increase the maternal temperature. Temperatures as high as 37.5° to 38°C (99.5° to 100.4° F) have been reported.
4. Neonatal symptoms associated with increased maternal temperature in noninfected women include lower Apgar scores, hypotonia, hypoxia, and an increased need for resuscitation and oxygen at birth (Kattwinkel, 2011).

**B. Once the infant is delivered, a number of physiologic conditions affect thermal stability, including the physical characteristics of the neonate, metabolic processes, and physical activity.**

1. Physical characteristics of the neonate affecting neonatal thermoregulation including thermal receptors in the skin, surface area–to–body mass ratio, skin permeability, body posture, and the type and amount of subcutaneous fat.
   a. Thermal receptors in the skin affect the infant's response to cold stimuli (Blackburn, 2013).
      (1) The most prominent and sensitive skin receptors are in the trigeminal area of the face.
      (2) Stimulation of thermal receptors leads to vasoconstriction as a measure to conserve heat.
      (3) ELBW infants are unable to respond to hypothermia with vasoconstriction during the first 12 hours after birth (Knobel et al., 2009).
   b. Neonates have a relatively large surface area–to–body mass ratio, which has an impact on thermoregulation.
      (1) In term neonates, the surface area–to–body mass ratio is three times greater than that of an adult (Blackburn, 2013).
      (2) In the preterm infant, the surface area–to–body mass ratio is five to six times greater than that of an adult. The surface area–to–body mass ratio in preterm infants increases as the gestation decreases.
   c. Premature infants have very thin skin, allowing greater loss of water and heat than seen in term neonates. Thin permeable skin allows water to evaporate from the skin surface.
      (1) Heat is lost by evaporation. This is known as TEWL (Sedin and Agren, 2006).
      (2) At 25 weeks of gestation, premature infants can lose 15 times more water through their skin than term neonates. This water loss is inversely proportional to gestational age until about 33 weeks of gestation, when TEWL is similar to that of a term infant (Agren et al., 2006; Sedin and Agren, 2006).
   d. Posture can affect body temperature by decreasing or increasing surface area for heat loss.
      (1) Term neonates may lie in a tucked position to conserve heat or extend their arms and legs to dissipate heat.
      (2) Preterm infants lack the muscle tone to maintain a flexed position and rely on caregivers to position them appropriately.
   e. Thermoregulation in neonates is affected by the type and amount of accumulated fat, which in turn is affected by both gestational age and birth weight.
      (1) Infants have less insulating subcutaneous fat than adults. Term neonates have only 16% of body fat compared to 30% to 35% in adults; preterm infants have even less.
      (2) BAT, also known as brown fat, generates more energy than any other tissue in the body and is very important in thermoregulation.
         (a) Heat production through the metabolism of BAT is regulated by uncoupling protein-1, norepinephrine, and triiodothyronine (Bissinger and Annibale, 2010; Blackburn, 2013).

(b) BAT is metabolized during nonshivering thermogenesis (NST) to produce heat.
(c) A heavy concentration of blood vessels gives BAT its characteristic brown color and serves to conduct heat into the circulation.
(d) Metabolism of BAT involves the breakdown of triglycerides into glycerol and fatty acids and is dependent on the availability of oxygen, glucose, and ATP. If these elements are not available, as is the case during hypoxia, acidosis, and hypoglycemia, heat production will suffer (Cypess and Kahn, 2010).
(e) BAT is found around the kidneys and adrenal glands, at the nape of the neck, between the scapulas, in the mediastinum, and around the trachea, heart, lungs, liver, and abdominal aorta.
(f) The amount of available BAT is dependent on gestational age (Blackburn, 2013).
   i. It begins to appear at 25 to 26 weeks, so only a minimal amount is available in VLBW infants.
   ii. Infants less than 32 weeks of gestation do not have enough BAT to produce significant amounts of heat by NST (Knobel and Holditch-Davis, 2007).
   iii. BAT increases significantly during the third trimester.
   iv. BAT continues to increase in the early weeks after birth and is thought to play a role in thermoregulation until a child is approximately 2 years of age.

2. Metabolic processes generate energy by metabolism of fat, including BAT (above), glucose, and protein (Blackburn, 2013).
   a. NST is the major method of heat production in the neonate.
   b. NST is triggered when skin temperature decreases to less than 35° to 36° C (95° to 96.8° F).
   c. NST relies on the availability of BAT and therefore is limited in ELBW infants.
   d. All metabolically active tissues can generate heat. The organs that generate the greatest amount of energy are the brain, heart, and liver.
   e. An increase in metabolic rate can produce heat but also leads to an increase in oxygen consumption. This may be a problem in critically ill neonates with borderline oxygenation.
   f. Term neonates can increase their metabolic rate by 200% to 300% through a combination of metabolic and physical responses (Blackburn, 2013).
   g. VLBW infants may only be able to increase their metabolic rate by 25%, while ELBW infants may not be able to respond at all.
   h. Critically ill neonates may not have the reserves of oxygen, glucose, or energy to mount an increase in metabolic rate and adapt to an unstable thermal environment.
   i. Hypothermia may lead to respiratory distress, hypoglycemia, and the production of lactic acid (see Box 6-2).
3. Physical activity can generate heat, but only late preterm and term infants have enough muscle tone to produce heat by this method and this may only be effective for a short time.
   a. Increased physical activity, such as feeding, crying, restlessness, or hyperactivity, increases the metabolic rate.
   b. Neonates receiving sedation, paralytics, or other medications leading to decreased activity or muscle tone may have a blunted response to environmental temperatures outside the normal range.
   c. Shivering is an involuntary method of heat production that is rarely seen in the neonatal population. The neonate only shivers after prolonged cold stress that leads to decreased spinal cord temperature (Blackburn, 2013).

## MANAGEMENT OF THE THERMAL ENVIRONMENT

A. **This aspect of neonatal care falls under the purview of the nurse.** All infants have thermal management challenges in the delivery room and during transition. Premature infants have ongoing needs that must be addressed until they are able to maintain their own core temperature without metabolic consequences such as poor weight gain. It is crucial for the nurse to understand the importance of this role and to be versed in the use of equipment available to manage the thermal environment of newborn infants whether they are in the delivery room, in the nursery, or during transport.

1. Delivery room management (Bissinger & Annibale, 2010).
   a. The primary challenge in thermal management of newborns is the prevention of hypothermia because the neonate is expected to transition from a warm, moist environment to a much colder, drier environment. Late preterm and preterm infants are at an increased risk of hypothermia, especially those who are less than 28 weeks of gestation at birth and/or weigh 1500 g or less at birth. A number of strategies have been described to maintain temperature at birth, including warming the room, drying the infant, providing skin-to-skin contact with the mother, utilization of heat loss barriers, use of external heat sources, and use of polyethylene plastic wrap or bag for neonates less than 29 weeks of gestation (Kattwinkel, 2011; McCall et al., 2010).
      (1) Room temperature.
         (a) A newborn's temperature may fall rapidly. The infant's temperature may drop 0.2° C to 1° C per minute due to evaporative losses from amniotic fluid, convective losses to cooler room air, and radiation to cooler structures in the room such as walls (Blackburn, 2013).
         (b) The gradient between the ambient room temperature in the delivery room and the infant's skin temperature promotes heat loss. The delivery room should be maintained above 25° to 26° C (77° to 78.8° F), or at least 26° to 27° C (78° to 80° F) for infants less than 29 weeks of gestation, to minimize convective heat loss (AAP & ACOG, 2012; Hammarlund et al., 1980; Kattwinkel, 2011; Knobel et al., 2005).
      (2) Dry the infant immediately and remove wet linen (unless using a polyethylene bag) to minimize evaporative heat loss (Bissinger & Annibale, 2010).
         (a) Use prewarmed absorbent towels to dry the infant gently, taking care not to damage the skin.
         (b) Use warm blankets and prewarm any surfaces that come in contact with the infant's skin during stabilization, routine delivery care, and weighing of the infant to minimize conductive heat loss.
      (3) Avoid drafts to minimize convective heat loss.
      (4) Skin-to-skin holding.
         (a) If condition of the infant allows, drying and placing the infant against the mother's bare skin, then covering with a warm blanket, allows heat from the mother to maintain the infant's temperature (McCall et al., 2010).
         (b) Skin-to skin holding can be used in the neonatal intensive care unit as well, even in VLBW infants. The conduction of heat from mother (or father) to the infant is high enough to compensate for increased heat loss through evaporation and convection while the infant is out of the humidified incubator (Karlsson et al., 2012).
      (5) Barriers to heat loss (Bissinger & Annibale, 2010; McCall et al., 2010).
         (a) Polyethylene bags or wraps should be used in infants less than 29 weeks of gestation to prevent evaporative heat loss and allow visualization, stabilization, and heat gain through radiation from the radiant warmer. The infant is placed in the wrap immediately and wrapped from the neck to the feet. Only the head is dried. Maintain the wrap until the infant's temperature is stable in a humidified environment for 1 hour (AAP and ACOG, 2012; Knobel et al., 2005; Trevisanuto et al., 2010; Vohra et al., 2004).
         (b) Use a polyethylene or insulated cap (not stockinette) after drying the baby's head to prevent evaporative heat loss (Trevisanuto et al., 2010).
         (c) Open skin defects (gastroschisis, myelomeningocele) present a major challenge to thermoregulation as the open defect presents a permeable surface for rapid fluid losses and increased evaporative heat loss. Cover the defect with sterile saline-soaked gauze and a sterile waterproof barrier to reduce evaporative losses. (See Chapter 29.)
      (6) External heat sources.
         (a) A radiant warmer or prewarmed incubator should be used in the delivery room to maintain the infant's temperature during routine care and stabilization. Radiant warmers should always be used with a servo-control to prevent overheating (AAP and ACOG, 2012).

(b) Chemical mattresses, also called transwarmers, may be used to improve thermal control in VLBW infants. These may be used in the delivery room or during transport and should be removed once the infant is warm and in a stable thermal environment. Because heat is provided by conduction, a blanket should be placed under the neonate to prevent skin burns (AAP and ACOG, 2007, 2012; Brown and Landers, 2011; McCall et al., 2010).

(c) Avoid overheating if perinatal asphyxia is suspected. In some cases providing hypothermia strategies to preserve brain function may be appropriate. (See Chapter 34.)

(d) Use a prewarmed transport incubator to transfer neonates to the nursery. A transport incubator uses batteries and continues to provide heat during transfer. The incubator usually has equipment built in or attached for monitoring, suctioning, and providing respiratory support and intravenous infusions.

**2.** Nursery (AAP and ACOG, 2012).

**a.** The temperature in the nursery should be maintained at 22° to 27° C (72° to 78° F) (Bissinger and Annibale, 2010).

**b.** Humidity in the nursery should be maintained at 30% to 60% (Blackfan and Yaglou, 1933).

**3.** Equipment.

**a.** Nurses should be familiar with equipment used in their nursery. Equipment should be used according to the manufacturer's directions and the unit's policies and procedures.

**b.** Incubators.

(1) Incubators warm infants using convective heat.

(a) Incubator covers can be used to decrease radiant heat loss from incubator walls (Fig. 6-1).

(b) Incubator covers can be used with transport incubators to decrease radiant loss in cold climates and to decrease radiant gain in hot climates, especially on sunny days (Fig. 6-2).

(2) Servo-control uses the infant's skin temperature to control the temperature inside the incubator (Sherman et al., 2006).

(a) It is essential that the skin probe is securely attached to the infant's skin to function correctly.

(b) Safety features to prevent overheating include the setting of upper limits of air temperature and alarms to alert the nurse to a detached probe.

(c) In this mode, the nurse must document the neonate's axillary temperature, the incubator set point, the skin temperature, and the air temperature.

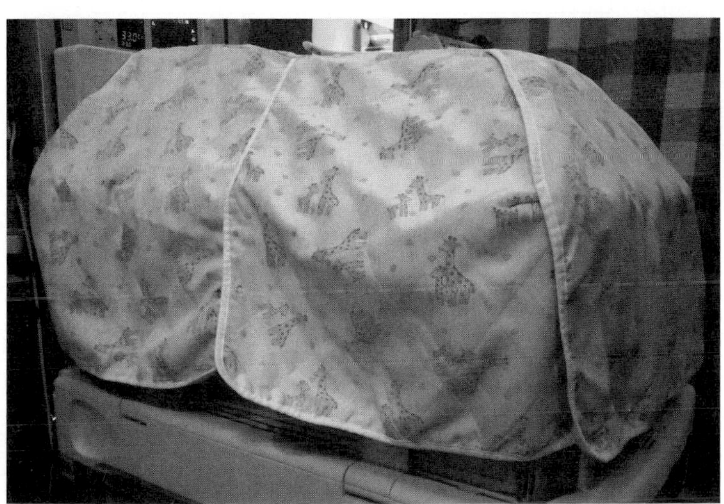

FIGURE 6-1 ■ Incubator with cover. (Courtesy Allen S. Kramer, Texas Children's Hospital, Houston, Tex.)

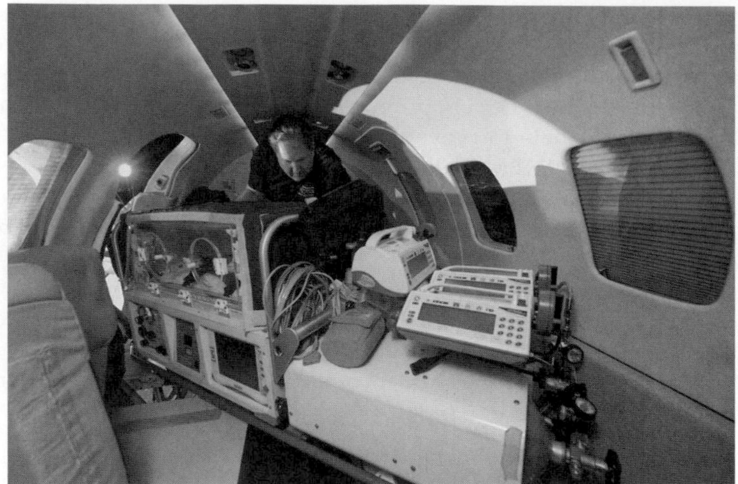

FIGURE 6-2 ■ Transport incubator with cover. (Courtesy Allen S. Kramer, Texas Children's Hospital, Houston, Tex.)

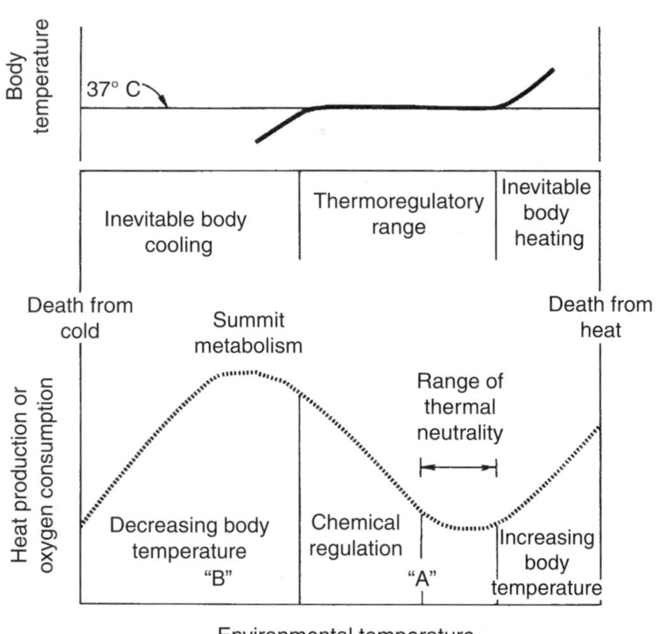


FIGURE 6-3 ■ Temperature versus oxygen consumption. (From Fanaroff A.A. and Fanaroff J.M.: *Klaus & Fanaroff's care of the high-risk neonate* [6th ed.]. Philadelphia, 2013, Elsevier Saunders.)

(3) Manual or air control uses the air temperature to control heater output.
  (a) There is less variability in air temperatures when manual control is used compared to when servo-control is used.
  (b) In this mode, the nurse must document the neonate's axillary temperature, the set point, and the air temperature.
  (c) The goal of incubator care is to provide a neutral thermal environment (NTE). This is the temperature that is required to maintain the core temperature while minimizing metabolic needs and oxygen consumption (Fig. 6-3).
    i. The use of an NTE chart to select the initial incubator setting may be helpful (Table 6-2), although some incubators have a built-in feature that uses age and birth weight to recommend a starting temperature. The initial temperature setting is then adjusted for an individual infant's needs.

■ TABLE 6-2
■ ■ **Neutral Thermal Environmental Temperatures**

| Age and Weight | Range of Temperature (° C) | Age and Weight | Range of Temperature (° C) |
|---|---|---|---|
| 0 to 6 hours | | 72 to 96 hours | |
| <1200 g | 34 to 35.4 | <1200 g | 34 to 35 |
| 1200 to 1500 g | 33.9 to 34.4 | 1200 to 1500 g | 33 to 34 |
| 1501 to 2500 g | 32.8 to 33.8 | 1501 to 2500 g | 31.1 to 33.2 |
| >2500 g | 32 to 33.8 | >2500 g | 29.8 to 32.8 |
| 6 to 12 hours | | 4 to 12 days | |
| <1200 g | 34 to 35.4 | <1500 g | 33 to 34 |
| 1200 to 1500 g | 33.5 to 34.4 | 1501 to 2500 g | 31 to 33.2 |
| 1501 to 2500 g | 32.2 to 33.8 | >2500 g | |
| >2500 g | 31.4 to 33.8 | 4 to 5 days | 29.5 to 32.6 |
| 12 to 24 hours | | 5 to 6 days | 29.4 to 32.3 |
| <1200 g | 34 to 35.4 | 6 to 8 days | 29 to 32.2 |
| 1200 to 1500 g | 33.3 to 34.3 | 8 to 10 days | 29 to 31.8 |
| 1501 to 2500 g | 31.8 to 33.8 | 10 to 12 days | 29 to 31.4 |
| >2500 g | 31 to 33.7 | 12 to 14 days | |
| 24 to 36 hours | | <1500 g | 32.6 to 34 |
| <1200 g | 34 to 35 | 1501 to 2500 g | 31 to 33.2 |
| 1200 to 1500 g | 33.1 to 34.2 | >2500 g | 29 to 30.8 |
| 1501 to 2500 g | 31.6 to 33.6 | 2 to 3 weeks | |
| >2500 g | 30.7 to 33.5 | <1500 g | 32.2 to 34 |
| 36 to 48 hours | | 1501 to 2500 g | 30.5 to 33 |
| <1200 g | 34 to 35 | 3 to 4 weeks | |
| 1200 to 1500 g | 33 to 34.1 | <1500 g | 31.6 to 33.6 |
| 1501 to 2500 g | 31.4 to 33.5 | 1501 to 2500 g | 30 to 32.7 |
| >2500 g | 30.5 to 33.3 | 4 to 5 weeks | |
| 48 to 72 hours | | <1500 g | 31.2 to 33 |
| <1200 g | 34 to 35 | 1501 to 2500 g | 29.5 to 32.2 |
| 1200 to 1500 g | 33 to 34 | 5 to 6 weeks | |
| 1501 to 2500 g | 31.2 to 33.4 | <1500 g | 30.6 to 32.3 |
| >2500 g | 30.1 to 33.2 | 1501 to 2500 g | 29 to 31.8 |

Adapted from Scopes, J.W. and Ahmed, I.: Range of critical temperatures in sick and premature babies. *Archives of Disease in Childhood*, 41:417, 1966. In Fanaroff A.A. and Fanaroff J.M.: *Klaus & Fanaroff's care of the high-risk neonate* (6th ed.). Philadelphia, 2013, Elsevier Saunders.

For their table, Scopes and Ahmed had the walls of the incubator 1° to 2° C warmer than the ambient air temperatures.

ii. A number of factors affect the temperature needed to maintain thermal stability, including gestational age, birth weight, chronologic age, humidity, proximity to outside walls and windows, and the use of positioning devices, clothing, or swaddling.

(4) Double-walled incubators direct warm air between inner and outer incubator walls. The use of double-walled incubators decreases heat loss and reduces oxygen consumption (Bissinger and Annibale, 2010; Laroia et al., 2007).

(a) Avoid placing objects on top of incubators as this increases sound levels inside the incubator. Open and close portholes gently to minimize noise associated with this activity.

c. Humidity should be used with VLBW infants to reduce evaporative heat loss through TEWL. Evaporative heat loss is the major source of thermal instability in the first few weeks of life due to increased body surface area, increased skin permeability, and increased extracellular fluid (Agren et al., 2006; Bissinger and Annibale, 2010; Fidler, 2011; Karlsson et al., 2012; Lund et al., 2013).

(1) Use of humidity can reduce the infant's fluid needs (Kim et al., 2010; Sherman et al., 2006).
  (a) Start humidity at 70% or greater for the first 7 days of life. Avoid condensation inside the incubator (Lund et al., 2013).
  (b) Gradually decrease humidity to 50% until the infant is 28 days old or 30 to 32 weeks postmenstrual age (Lund et al., 2013).
    i. There is less need for humidity after the first week of life due to maturation of the infant's skin and decreased insensible water loss from TEWL. Barrier maturation usually develops in 2 to 4 weeks. This may take longer in extremely premature infants. Continuing high humidity beyond the first week may slow skin maturation (Agren et al., 1998).
  (c) Humidity can be provided while the infant is under a radiant warmer through the use of a polyethylene tent coupled with a device that provides constant humidity heated to body temperature (2001).
  (d) High-absorbency cellulose/polyacrylate diapers absorb moisture in a high-humidity environment and may interfere with assessment of accurate urine output (Amey et al., 2008; Fidler, 2011).
(2) Current humidification systems are designed to heat the water to a temperature that kills most organisms. The humidity is then introduced into the environment as a vapor to avoid droplet formation as droplets can serve as vectors for bacteria. Cleaning and water changes should be done according to manufacturer's recommendations (Sherman et al., 2006).
(3) Weaning from an incubator to an open crib is considered once the infant is medically stable and weighs 1600 g or greater (New et al., 2011, 2012; Turnbull and Petty, 2013; Zecca et al., 2010).
  (a) The incubator is slowly weaned to 28° to 29° C as a thermal challenge before transferring the infant to a crib or bassinet.
  (b) Swaddling, caps, and avoiding drafts are important in maintaining thermal stability.
  (c) Monitor temperature and weight gain in infants who have been weaned from the incubator. Infants who are not able to maintain an axillary temperature greater than or equal to 36.5° C should be returned to the incubator.
  (d) Reports vary regarding the impact of early weaning on length of stay (New et al., 2012; Zecca et al., 2010).
  (e) Benefits of incubator weaning include positive maternal perception, potential impact on breastfeeding and infant development, and increased discharge teaching and planning by nursing staff (Schneiderman et al., 2009).

**d.** Radiant warmer.
(1) Provides radiant heat to maintain temperature while providing improved access to the infant for assessment and procedures when compared to an incubator.
(2) Manual control is used for prewarming.
(3) Servo-control is used when caring for an infant on a warmer and provides a feedback loop regarding the infant's skin temperature to regulate heater output. This is important due to the risk of under- or overheating when on manual control.
(4) An increase in insensible water loss occurs when infants are cared for in radiant warmers. This increased fluid loss poses a risk for fluid and electrolyte imbalance. Careful documentation of intake, output, and weight are essential in managing infants cared for in radiant warmers (Sherman et al., 2006).
(5) Convective losses are also increased in a radiant warmer. Care should be taken to minimize drafts.

**e.** Hybrid incubators.
(1) Hybrid incubators function as either incubators or radiant warmers.
  (a) Rapid conversion from one mode of thermal support to the other avoids having to move patients during emergent events and procedures, reducing the risk for heat loss during transfer or dislodging indwelling lines or tubes (Greenspan et al., 2001; Sherman et al., 2006) (Fig. 6-4).

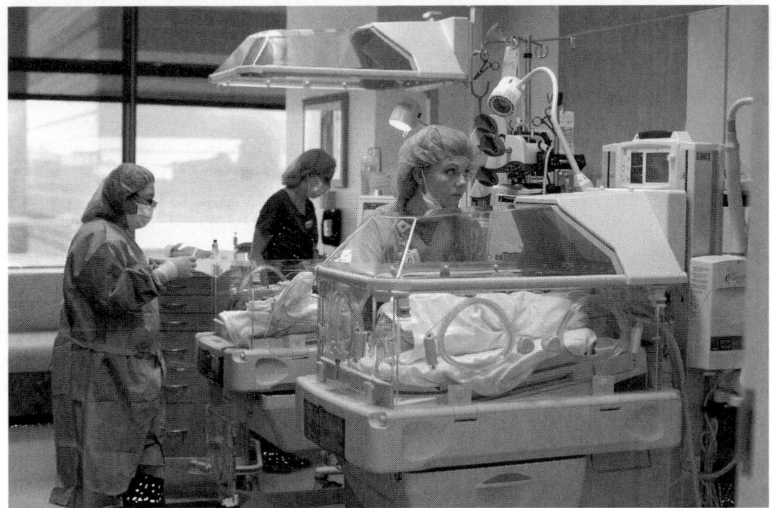

FIGURE 6-4 ■ Hybrid incubators can be used closed with porthole access to the infant or can be used as an overhead warmer with full access for procedures and emergencies without moving the infant. (Courtesy Allen S. Kramer, Texas Children's Hospital, Houston, Tex.)

f. Caution should be used when rewarming infants who are hypothermic as rewarming may be associated with apnea, hypotension secondary to vasodilation, and increased oxygen consumption (Gomella, 2009; Kaplan and Eidelman, 1984; Mathur et al., 2006).

## SUMMARY

Managing the thermoregulation needs of the newborn is an essential role of the neonatal nurse. The most vulnerable infants present a complex challenge requiring a nurse with knowledge and clinical expertise to provide an appropriate environment in which they can heal and grow.

## REFERENCES

Agren, J., Sjors, G. and Sedin, G.: Ambient humidity influences the rate of skin barrier maturation in extremely preterm infants. *Journal of Pediatrics*, 148 (5):613–617, 2006.

Agren, J., Sjors, G. and Sedin, G.: Transepidermal water loss in infants born at 24 and 25 weeks of gestation. *Acta Paediatric*, 87:1185–1190, 1998.

American Academy of Pediatrics and American College of Obstetricians and Gynecologists: *Guidelines for perinatal care* (7th ed.). Elk Grove Village, IL, and Washington, DC, 2012, American Academy of Pediatrics and American College of Obstetricians and Gynecologists.

American Academy of Pediatrics and American College of Obstetricians and Gynecologists: *Guidelines for perinatal care* (6th ed.). Elk Grove Village, IL, and Washington, DC, 2007, American Academy of Pediatrics and American College of Obstetricians and Gynecologists.

Amey, M., Butchard, N., Hanson, L., et al.: Cautionary tales from the neonatal intensive care unit: Diapers may mislead urinary output estimation in extremely low birthweight infants. *Pediatric Critical Care Medicine*, 9(1):76–79, 2008.

Banerjee, S., Cashman, P., Yentis, S.M. and Steer, P.J.: Maternal temperature monitoring during labor: Concordance and variability among monitoring sites. *Obstetrics and Gynecology*, 103(2):287–293, 2004.

Baumgart, S.: Iatrogenic hyperthermia and hypothermia in the neonate. *Clinics in Perinatology*, 35 (1):183–197, ix-x, 2008.

Bissinger, R.L. and Annibale, D.J.: Thermoregulation in very low-birth-weight infants during the golden hour: results and implications. *Advances in Neonatal Care*, 10(5):230–238, 2010.

Blackburn, S.: *Maternal, fetal, & neonatal physiology* (4th ed.). St. Louis: 2013, Elsevier Saunders.

Blackfan, K.D. and Yaglou, C.P.: The premature infant. *American Journal of Diseases of Children*, 46 (5):1175–1236, 1933.

Brown, V. and Landers, S.: Heat balance. In S.L. Gardner, B.S. Carter, M.E. Hines, and J.A. Hernandez (Eds.): *Merenstein & Gardner's handbook of neonatal intensive care* (7th ed.). St. Louis, 2011, Elsevier Mosby.

Costeloe, K., Hennessy, E., Gibson, A.T., et al.: The EPICure study: Outcomes to discharge from hospital for infants born at the threshold of viability. *Pediatrics*, 106(4):659–671, 2000.

Cypess, A.M. and Kahn, C.R.: The role and importance of brown adipose tissue in energy homeostasis. *Current Opinion in Pediatrics*, 22(4):478–484, 2010.

Dahm, L.S. and James, L.S.: Newborn temperature and calculated heat loss in the delivery room. *Pediatrics*, 49 (4):504–513, 1972.

Fidler, H.L.: Incubator humidity: More than just something to sweat about!! *Advances in Neonatal Care*, 11 (3):197–199, 2011.

Gomella, T.L.: Diseases and drugs. In T.L. Gomella, M.D. Cunningham, and F.G. Eyal (Eds.): *Neonatology: Management, procedures, on-call problems, diseases and drugs* (7th ed.): New York City, McGraw-Hill, 2009.

Greenspan, J.S., Cullen, A.B., Touch, S.M., et al.: Thermal stability and transition studies with a hybrid warming device for neonates. *Journal of Perinatology*, 21(3):167–173, 2001.

Hammarlund, K., Nilsson, G.E., Oberg, P.A. and Sedin, G.: Transepidermal water loss in newborn infants. V. Evaporation from the skin and heat exchange during the first hours of life. *Acta Paediatrica Scandinavica*, 69(3):385–392, 1980.

Horns, K.M.: Comparison of two microenvironments and nurse caregiving on thermal stability of ELBW infants. *Advances in Neonatal Care*, 2(3):149–160, 2002.

Kaplan, M. and Eidelman, A.I.: Improved prognosis in severely hypothermic newborn infants treated by rapid rewarming. *Journal of Pediatrics*, 105 (3):470–474, 1984.

Karlsson, V., Heinemann, A.B., Sjors, G., et al.: Early skin-to-skin care in extremely preterm infants: Thermal balance and care environment. *Journal of Pediatrics*, 161(3):422–426, 2012.

Kattwinkel, J. (Ed.): *Textbook of neonatal resuscitation* (6th ed.). Elk Grove Village, IL, 2011, American Academy of Pediatrics and American Heart Association.

Kim, S.M., Lee, E.Y., Chen, J. and Ringer, S.A.: Improved care and growth outcomes by using hybrid humidified incubators in very preterm infants. *Pediatrics*, 125(1):e137–e145, 2010.

Knobel, R. and Holditch-Davis, D.: Thermoregulation and heat loss prevention after birth and during neonatal intensive-care unit stabilization of extremely low-birthweight infants. *JOGNN: Journal of Obstetric, Gynecologic and Neonatal Nursing*, 36(3):280–287, 2007.

Knobel, R.B., Holditch-Davis, D. and Schwartz, T.A.: Optimal body temperature in transitional extremely low birth weight infants using heart rate and temperature as indicators. *JOGNN: Journal of Obstetric, Gynecologic and Neonatal Nursing*, 39(1):3–14, 2010.

Knobel, R.B., Holditch-Davis, D., Schwartz, T.A. and Wimmer, J.E. Jr.: Extremely low birth weight preterm infants lack vasomotor response in relationship to cold body temperatures at birth. *Journal of Perinatology*, 29(12):814–821, 2009.

Knobel, R.B., Wimmer, J.E., Jr., and Holbert, D.: Heat loss prevention for preterm infants in the delivery room. *Journal of Perinatology*, 25(5):304–308, 2005.

Laptook, A.R., Salhab, W. and Bhaskar, B.: Admission temperature of low birth weight infants: Predictors and associated morbidities. *Pediatrics*, 119(3): e643–e649, 2007.

Laroia, N., Phelps, D.L. and Roy, J.: Double wall versus single wall incubator for reducing heat loss in very low birth weight infants in incubators. *Cochrane Database of Systematic Reviews*, (2):CD004215, 2007.

Lieberman, E., Lang, J., Richardson, D.K., et al.: Intrapartum maternal fever and neonatal outcome. *Pediatrics*, 105(1 Pt. 1):8–13, 2000.

Lund, C.H., Kuller, J., Raines, D.A., et al.: Neonatal skin care: Evidence-based clinical practice guidelines (3rd ed.). Washington, DC, 2013, AWHONN.

Lyon, A.J., Pikaar, M.E., Badger, P. and McIntosh, N.: Temperature control in very low birthweight infants during first five days of life. *Archives of Disease in Childhood: Fetal and Neonatal Edition*, 76(1):F47–F50, 1997.

Malin, S.W. and Baumgart, S.: Optimal thermal management for low birth weight infants nursed under high-powered radiant warmers. *Pediatrics*, 79 (1):47–54, 1987.

Mance, M.J.: Keeping infants warm: Challenges of hypothermia. *Advances in Neonatal Care*, 8(1):6–12, 2008.

Mathur, N.B., Krishnamurthy, S. and Mishra, T.K.: Estimation of rewarming time in transported extramural hypothermic neonates. *Indian Journal of Pediatrics*, 73 (5):395–399, 2006.

McCall, E.M., Alderdice, F., Halliday, H.L., et al.: Interventions to prevent hypothermia at birth in preterm and/or low birthweight infants. *Cochrane Database of Systematic Reviews*, (3):CD004210, 2010.

Mok, Q., Bass, C.A., Ducker, D.A. and McIntosh, N.: Temperature instability during nursing procedures in preterm neonates. *Archives of Disease in Childhood*, 66(7 Spec. No):783–786, 1991.

New, K., Flenady, V. and Davies, M.W.: Transfer of preterm infants from incubator to open cot at lower versus higher body weight. *Cochrane Database of Systematic Reviews*, (9):CD004214, 2011.

New, K., Flint, A., Bogossian, F., et al.: Transferring preterm infants from incubators to open cots at 1600 g: A multicentre randomised controlled trial. *Archives of Disease in Childhood: Fetal and Neonatal Edition*, 97(2): F88–F92, 2012.

Schneiderman, R., Kirkby, S., Turenne, W. and Greenspan, J.: Incubator weaning in preterm infants and associated practice variation. *Journal of Perinatology*, 29(8):570–574, 2009.

Sedin, G. and Agren, J.: Water and heat—the priority for the newborn infant. *Upsala Journal of Medical Sciences*, 111(1):45–59, 2006.

Sherman, T.I., Greenspan, J.S., St Clair, N., et al.: Optimizing the neonatal thermal environment. *Neonatal Network*, 25(4):251–260, 2006.

Silverman, W.A., Fertig, J.W. and Berger, A.P.: The influence of the thermal environment upon the survival of newly born premature infants. *Pediatrics*, 22 (5):876–886, 1958.

Smith, J., Alcock, G. and Usher, K.: Temperature measurement in the preterm and term neonate: A review of the literature. *Neonatal Network*, 32(1):16–25, 2013.

Trevisanuto, D., Doglioni, N., Cavallin, F., et al.: Heat loss prevention in very preterm infants in delivery rooms: A prospective, randomized, controlled trial of polyethylene caps. *Journal of Pediatrics*, 156 (6):914–917, 2010.

Turnbull, V. and Petty, J.: Evidence-based thermal care of low birthweight neonates. Part one. *Nursing Children and Young People*, 25(2):18–22, 2013.

Vohra, S., Roberts, R.S., Zhang, B., et al.: Heat Loss Prevention (HeLP) in the delivery room: A randomized controlled trial of polyethylene occlusive skin wrapping in very preterm infants. *Journal of Pediatrics*, 145(6):750–753, 2004.

World Health Organization: Thermal protection of the newborn: A practical guide. 1997. Retrieved August 22, 2008, from http://www.who.int/reproductive-health/publications/MSM_97_2_Thermal_protection_of_the_newborn/thermal_protection_newborn2.pdf.

Zecca, E., Corsello, M., Priolo, F., et al.: Early weaning from incubator and early discharge of preterm infants: Randomized clinical trial. *Pediatrics*, 126(3): e651–e656, 2010.

CHAPTER

# 7 Physical Assessment

KATHLEEN BENJAMIN AND SUSAN ARANA FURDON

**OBJECTIVES**

1. Review key aspects of the perinatal history as it relates to physical assessment of the newborn.
2. Describe methods of determining gestational age (GA).
3. Relate growth pattern and maturity to classification of newborns by GA and weight.
4. Describe a systematic approach in the examination of the newborn infant.

A comprehensive newborn physical examination requires a synthesis of perinatal and neonatal risk factors with a systematic approach to the examination. An understanding of growth, maturity, and GA risk factors provides a framework for defining wellness or subsequent problems. The nurse is in a unique position of providing a detailed observation and description within the context of these factors.

## PERINATAL HISTORY (SEE CHAPTERS 1, 2, 3, AND 4)

Elements of a perinatal history focus on the relationship of maternal medical condition and the overall growth and maturity of the infant. Communication from obstetric staff to pediatric staff of fetal anomalies and risk factors for abnormal growth or fetal well-being is essential.

A. **Family history.**
   1. Known inherited diseases/conditions: http://www.nlm.nih.gov/medlineplus/geneticdisorders.html.
      a. Cystic fibrosis, Down syndrome (translocation only), fragile X syndrome, cleft lip/palate, neural tube defects, dwarfism and osteogenesis imperfecta, muscular dystrophy.
      b. Hereditary anemia/coagulation disorders: sickle cell anemia, thalassemia, Von Willebrand's disease, hemophilia.
      c. Genetic brain disorder: leukodystrophy, phenylketonuria, Tay–Sachs disease, Wilson's disease.
   2. Chronic disorders or disabilities: diabetes, hypertension, mental retardation, cardiac lesions, renal disease, and seizures.

B. **Maternal medical history.**
   1. General health: age, body mass index, physical activity, diet, and exposure to potential teratogens.
   2. Chronic illness: diabetes, cardiac disease, hypertension, asthma, thyroid disorder, systemic lupus erythematosus, herpes simplex virus, addiction, and anxiety/depression disorder.
   3. Surgical procedures and hospitalizations.
   4. Medications before and during pregnancy inclusive of prescribed opiates, medical marijuana/illicit substance use.

C. **Obstetric history.**
   1. History of infertility: abnormal uterine structure, hormonal imbalance, infertility tests, and assisted reproductive technology.
   2. Previous pregnancies (gravida): number of live born, term versus preterm, spontaneous or elective abortions.
   3. Birth weight(s) of live born and neonatal problems identified.
   4. Previous fetal demise or neonatal death(s): age of infant and reason for death.

D. **Social history:** early identification of family stressors or support and barriers to teaching.
   1. Marital status and consanguinity.
   2. Financial support, socioeconomic status, and education level.

3. Tobacco, alcohol, and illicit drug use.
4. History of depression.
5. Domestic violence.
6. Religious and cultural considerations.
7. Factors affecting teaching.
   a. Primary language.
   b. Sensory deficits.

E. **Pregnancy history.**
   1. Prenatal care: timing of first visit, compliance with follow-up.
   2. Estimated date of confinement.
      a. Last menstrual period.
      b. Ultrasound dating.
      c. Birth date calculator (wheel).
   3. Single versus multiple gestation.
   4. Weight gain and nutritional status.
   5. Blood group incompatibility and risk for isoimmunization: maternal blood type and Rh status.
      a. Antepartum administration of $Rh_o$(D) immunoglobulin prophylaxis for D-negative blood group.
      b. Positive antibody screen (examples: Cc, Ee, Kell, and Duffy).
      c. Serial fetal surveillance for positive isoimmunization status: antibody titers, ultrasounds, amniocentesis, fetal transfusion.
   6. Maternal serum screening: triple or quad screen.
   7. Group B streptococcus (GBS) culture at 35 to 37 weeks of gestation.
   8. Congenital infection: rubella, syphilis, cytomegalovirus, hepatitis, human immunodeficiency virus, herpes simplex virus, human papillomavirus, chlamydia, gonorrhea, and parvovirus. Congenital West Nile virus has also been reported (O'Leary et al., 2006).
   9. Maternal diabetes.
      a. Gestational or type 1.
      b. Classification.
      c. Glucose control.
   10. Hypertensive disorders.
      a. Gestational hypertension (formerly called pregnancy-induced hypertension).
      b. Preeclampsia/eclampsia.
      c. Chronic hypertension.
      d. *H*emolysis, *e*levated *l*iver enzymes, and *l*ow *p*latelet count (HELLP syndrome).
   11. Abnormal fetal growth: fundal height, serial ultrasounds.
      a. Intrauterine growth restriction (IUGR) factors: multiple maternal, placental, uterine, and fetal factors limit intrauterine growth potential (Breeze and Lees, 2007; Lawrence, 2006).
         (1) Previous small-for-gestational-age (SGA) or IUGR baby.
         (2) Age greater than 35 or less than 16 years, single marital status, low socioeconomic status.
         (3) Malnutrition, low pregnancy weight gain, active Crohn's disease, untreated celiac disease.
         (4) Unexplained history of miscarriage or stillbirth (fetal loss at >20 weeks of gestation).
         (5) Multiple gestation.
         (6) Tobacco exposure.
            (a) Nicotine releases catecholamines, reduces prostacyclin synthesis.
            (b) Vasoconstriction and increased vascular resistance decrease placental delivery of nutrients and oxygen.
            (c) Associated with placental abruption and late fetal death.
            (d) IUGR rates 3 to 4.5 times those for nonsmokers.
         (7) Hypertensive/vascular disorders causing placental insufficiency.
            (a) Chronic hypertension. Incidence 4 times greater, with severe versus mild hypertension.
            (b) Preeclampsia.

(c) Advanced diabetes mellitus.
(d) Placental or umbilical cord abnormalities or disruption.
(8) Chronic renal failure.
(9) Congenital infections: *t*oxoplasmosis, *o*ther infections, *r*ubella, *c*ytomegalovirus, and *h*erpesvirus (TORCH); cytomegalovirus most common association.
(10) Congenital malformations and chromosomal abnormalities.

**b.** Large-for-gestational-age (LGA) infant (Lawrence, 2007).
(1) Maternal race.
(2) Maternal diabetes.
(3) Obesity.
(4) Previous LGA infant.

**12.** Fetal anomaly: ultrasound, fetal echocardiography, and amniocentesis.

**13.** Placental or vascular abnormality:
**a.** Abnormal cord insertion: velamentous.
**b.** Abnormal umbilical artery Doppler studies: reverse end-diastolic flow, increased middle cerebral flow velocity.
**c.** Twin-to-twin transfusion.

**14.** Amniotic fluid volume: polyhydramnios, oligohydramnios.

**15.** Recurrent urinary tract infections.

**F. Labor and delivery.**

**1.** History of presenting problem.
**a.** Labor: preterm labor, post-dates.
**b.** Bleeding.
**c.** Acute abdominal pain.
**d.** Hypertension.
**e.** Medically indicated elective delivery conditions: maternal conditions and/or poor fetal growth/status.
**f.** Trauma.

**2.** Infection risks:
**a.** Symptoms of chorioamnionitis: maternal or fetal tachycardia, maternal fever $\geq$100.4° F, uterine tenderness, elevated maternal white blood cell count.
**b.** GBS: revised Centers for Disease Control and Prevention (CDC) guidelines (Verani et al., 2010).

**3.** Risk factors that increase neonatal early-onset GBS infection: preterm premature rupture of membranes, prolonged rupture of membranes greater than 18 hours (Baker et al., 2011).

**4.** Intrapartum chemoprophylaxis for GBS colonization.
**a.** Preterm labor with intact membranes is associated with occult intra-amniotic infection (American Academy of Pediatrics and American College of Obstetricians and Gynecologists [AAP and ACOG], 2012).

**5.** Fetal lung maturity.
**a.** Less than 5% risk of respiratory distress syndrome if mature fetal lung maturity test after 34 weeks of gestation.
**b.** Antenatal corticosteroids administered for anticipated preterm delivery at less than 34 weeks of gestation are effective in decreasing neonatal morbidity and mortality (AAP and ACOG, 2012).
**c.** Optimal benefit of glucocorticosteroid: 24 hours after administration for up to 7 days; may be beneficial at less than 24 hours of treatment (Surbek et al., 2012).

**6.** Spontaneous versus induced labor, indication for induction of labor.

**7.** Cord prolapse.

**8.** Fetal distress and nonreassuring fetal heart tracing (Macones et al., 2008).

**9.** Analgesic and anesthetic prior to and at delivery.

**10.** Mode of delivery: vaginal, cesarean, assisted (forceps and vacuum); indication for cesarean.

**11.** Presentation: vertex, breech, brow, chin, and arm.

**12.** Appearance of amniotic fluid.
**a.** Clear: normal.
**b.** Green: meconium stained.

c. Yellow: old meconium, old blood, and sepsis.
d. Cloudy: sepsis.

13. Shoulder dystocia (Benjamin, 2005).
  a. Multifactorial:
    (1) Maternal risk factors: uterine abnormalities, diabetes, maternal body proportions.
    (2) Infant risk factors: macrosomia, transverse lie, poor tone, 5-minute Apgar score less than 5.
  b. Intrapartum events:
    (1) Mechanical forces of labor alone.
    (2) Vaginal breech delivery/operative vaginal delivery.
    (3) Prolonged duration of labor.
    (4) Precipitous delivery.
    (5) Prolonged head-to-body interval at delivery.

**G. Newborn resuscitation (see Chapter 5).**

## GESTATIONAL-AGE INSTRUMENTS

The principal basis for use of GA instruments is that fetal maturity follows a predictable, organized course and that physical and neurologic characteristics are common to a given GA. An accurate GA is critical for counseling families and making treatment decisions based on known GA morbidity and mortality risks for a specific GA and birth weight.

**A. General considerations.**
1. Use neonatal assessment tools from birth to 5 days, before physical characteristics change.
2. Perform within 48 hours of birth for highest accuracy.
3. Consider problems with accuracy of GA assessments when using GA-based treatment guidelines for extremely preterm treatment or withdrawal-of-care decisions (Parikh et al., 2010).
4. Neurologic findings may be influenced by prematurity and disease processes.

**B. Most common tools.**
1. Dubowitz: clinical assessment of GA (Dubowitz et al., 1970).
  a. Scores criteria: 10 neurologic and 11 external (physical).
  b. Combined total score correlated to weeks of gestation.
  c. Combined score has higher correlation ($\pm 2$ weeks, 95% confidence) than either component separately.
  d. SGA infants: external signs underscored and neurologic signs overscored; combined score reliable.
  e. Overestimates GA in premature infants.
  f. Widely used before development of Ballard score.
2. Ballard: newborn maturity rating.
  a. Simplified system based on Dubowitz's method, less time to use.
  b. Eliminates active tone scoring, passive tone more useful than active tone.
  c. Six neurologic and six physical criteria, scores totaled.
  d. GA maturity rating assigned using form chart.
3. New Ballard Score (Ballard et al., 1991).
  a. Modified to assess GA of 20 to 44 weeks.
  b. Accurate within 2 weeks of gestation; sick or well infants.
  c. For 20 to 26 weeks of gestation: most accurate when scored within first 12 hours of life.
  d. Limitations.
    (1) Examination should be done twice by two different examiners for objectivity.
    (2) Infant must be in a quiet, alert state.
    (3) Scoring affected by:
      (a) Breech and positional deformities,
      (b) Neurologic disorders and asphyxia, and
      (c) Infants affected by maternal medications.
4. Eye examination: anterior vascular lens capsule evaluation (Fig. 7-1).

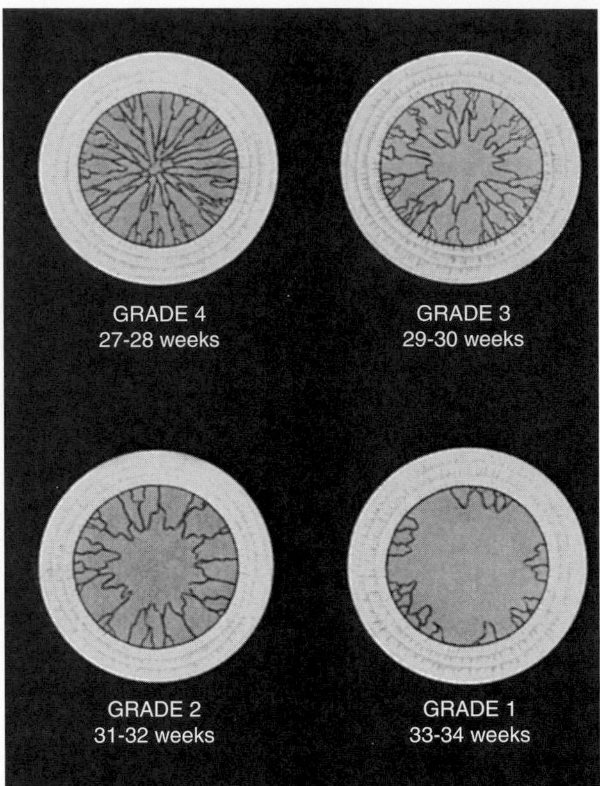


FIGURE 7-1 ■ Grading system for assessment of gestational age by examination of anterior vascular capsule of lens. (From Hittner, H.M., Hirsch, N.J., and Rudolph, A.J.: Assessment of gestational age by examination of the anterior vascular capsule of the lens. *Journal of Pediatrics*, 91[3]:455-458, 1977.)

a. Based on timing of embryonic lens vessels development and atrophy; disappear at 27 to 34 weeks of gestation.
b. Limitations: requires direct ophthalmoscopic exam, cannot be used at less than 27 weeks of gestation, and must be done in first 24 to 48 hours of life. Not used routinely.

C. **GA examination technique:** Use published New Ballard chart for scoring each criterion.
1. Neurologic criteria features.
a. Posture.
(1) Evaluates degree of arm and leg flexion and extension and leg abduction.
(2) Flexion and hip adduction increase with increasing GA.
(3) Early in gestation, the infant's resting posture is hypotonic.
(4) Observe infant's posture while supine and quiet.
b. Square window.
(1) Evaluates flexion when the wrist is at a right angle to the forearm.
(2) Angle decreases with increasing GA because of the influence of maternal hormones at the end of pregnancy.
(3) Findings do not change after birth.
(4) Flex infant's hand on the forearm between examiner's thumb and index finger. Use sufficient pressure to get full flexion. Visually measure angle between hypothenar eminence and ventral aspect of forearm.
c. Arm recoil.
(1) Evaluates degree of arm flexion and the strength of recoil.
(2) Place infant supine, flex arms for 5 seconds, then fully extend arms by pulling the hands downward, then release.
d. Popliteal angle.
(1) The angle decreases with increasing GA.

(2) Position infant supine, pelvis flat on surface; hold thigh in knee–chest position with left index finger and thumb. Place right index finger behind infant's ankle and extend leg with gentle pressure.
(3) Measure the angle between the lower leg and thigh, posterior to the knee.

**e.** Scarf sign.
(1) Position infant supine; take hand and pull across chest and around neck as far posterior as possible toward the opposite shoulder. Assist maneuver by lifting elbow across body.
(2) Observe the position of the elbow relative to the midline of the infant's body.

**f.** Heel to ear.
(1) Position infant supine, pelvis flat on the bed. Draw foot to head as near as it will extend without force.
(2) Observe distance between the foot and head and the degree of knee extension. Knee is left free and may draw down alongside abdomen.

**2.** Physical examination criteria: observe and grade according to Figure 7-2.

**a.** Skin.
(1) With increasing GA, transparency decreases and more texture develops, vessels become obscured.
(2) As gestation progresses beyond 38 weeks, subcutaneous tissue decreases, causing wrinkling and desquamation.

**b.** Lanugo.
(1) Fine, downy hair that covers the body of the fetus from 20 to 28 weeks.
(2) At 28 weeks, it begins to disappear around the face and anterior aspect of the trunk.
(3) At term, a few patches may be present over the shoulders.

**c.** Plantar creases.
(1) Creases first appear on the anterior portion of the foot, between 28 and 30 weeks of gestation, and extend toward the heel as gestation progresses.
(2) An infant with IUGR and early loss of vernix caseosa may have more plantar creases than expected for size.
(3) After 12 hours, the skin begins to dry and plantar creases are no longer a valid indicator of GA.

**d.** Breast development.
(1) Nipple size and amount of breast tissue are examined.
(2) A 1- to 2-mm nodule of breast tissue is palpable by about 36 weeks and grows to approximately 10 mm by 40 weeks of gestation.

**e.** Eyes and ears.
(1) Evaluate for fused eyelids.
(2) At 26 to 28 weeks of gestation, fused eyelids open.
(3) Assess ear formation and amount of pinna cartilage.
(4) Inward curving of the upper pinna usually begins by 34 weeks of gestation and by 40 weeks extends to the lobe.
(5) Before 34 weeks, the pinna has little cartilage and will stay folded on itself.
(6) By 36 weeks there is some cartilage, and the pinna will spring back from being folded.

**f.** Genitalia.
(1) Female infant: evaluate development of the labia minora and majora and prominence of the clitoris.
(a) Early in gestation the clitoris is prominent, with small, widely separated labia.
(b) By 40 weeks, fat deposits have increased in size in the labia majora, so that the labia majora completely cover the labia minora.
(2) Male infant: evaluate presence of testes, degree of descent into scrotum, and development of rugae on the scrotum.
(a) The testes begin to descend from the abdomen at 28 weeks.
(b) At 37 weeks, the testes can be palpated high in the scrotum.
(c) At 40 weeks, the testes are completely descended and scrotum is covered with rugae.
(d) As gestation progresses, the scrotum becomes more pendulous.

NEUROMUSCULAR MATURITY

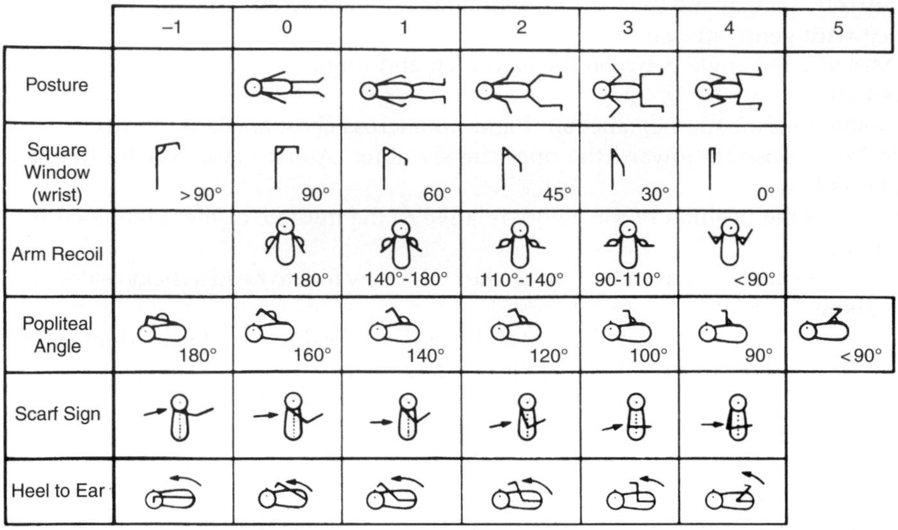

| | −1 | 0 | 1 | 2 | 3 | 4 | 5 |
|---|---|---|---|---|---|---|---|
| Posture | | | | | | | |
| Square Window (wrist) | >90° | 90° | 60° | 45° | 30° | 0° | |
| Arm Recoil | | 180° | 140°-180° | 110°-140° | 90-110° | <90° | |
| Popliteal Angle | 180° | 160° | 140° | 120° | 100° | 90° | <90° |
| Scarf Sign | | | | | | | |
| Heel to Ear | | | | | | | |

SCORE

Neuro-muscular ______

Physical ______

Total ______

PHYSICAL MATURITY

| Skin | Sticky friable transparent | Gelatinous red, translucent | Smooth pink, visible veins | Superficial peeling &/or rash, few veins | Cracking pale areas rare veins | Parchment deep cracking no vessels | Leathery cracked wrinkled |
|---|---|---|---|---|---|---|---|
| Lanugo | None | Sparse | Abundant | Thinning | Bald areas | Mostly bald | |
| Plantar Surface | Heel–toe 40-50 mm: −1 <40 mm: −2 | >50 mm no crease | Faint red marks | Anterior transverse crease only | Creases ant. 2/3 | Creases over entire sole | |
| Breast | Imperceptible | Barely perceptible | Flat areola no bud | Stippled areola 1-2 mm bud | Raised areola 3-4 mm bud | Full areola 5-10 mm bud | |
| Eye/Ear | Lids fused loosely: −1 tightly: −2 | Lids open pinna flat stays folded | Sl. curved pinna; soft; slow recoil | Well-curved pinna; soft but ready recoil | Formed & firm instant recoil | Thick cartilage ear stiff | |
| Genitals, male | Scrotum flat, smooth | Scrotum empty faint rugae | Testes in upper canal rare rugae | Testes descending few rugae | Testes down good rugae | Testes pendulous deep rugae | |
| Genitals, female | Clitoris prominent labia flat | Prominent clitoris small labia minora | Prominent clitoris enlarging minora | Majora & minora equally prominent | Majora large minora small | Majora cover clitoris & minora | |

MATURITY RATING

| Score | Weeks |
|---|---|
| −10 | 20 |
| −5 | 22 |
| 0 | 24 |
| 5 | 26 |
| 10 | 28 |
| 15 | 30 |
| 20 | 32 |
| 25 | 34 |
| 30 | 36 |
| 35 | 38 |
| 40 | 40 |
| 45 | 42 |
| 50 | 44 |

FIGURE 7-2 ■ New Ballard Score, expanded to include extremely premature infants. (From Ballard, J.L., Khoury, J.C., Wedig, K., et al.: New Ballard Score, expanded to include extremely premature infants. *Journal of Pediatrics*, 119[3]:417-423, 1991.)

**D. Clinical estimate of GA (AAP, 2004; AAP and ACOG, 2012).**

1. Document GA on all newborns.
2. Use standard terminology.
   a. GA is the time between the last menstrual period and the day of delivery.
   b. Use obstetric estimated GA when the physical exam approximates the GA by estimated date of confinement within 2 weeks (Thilo and Rosenberg, 2012).
   c. Express in completed weeks of gestation.
3. Document marked discrepancy between obstetric and physical data.

4. Assign GA using assessment of all obstetric, pediatric, and nursing data (AAP and ACOG, 2012).
5. Classify maturity.
   a. Preterm: infant born on or before the end of the 37th week of gestation.
      (1) Subcategory: "late preterm" defined as between $34^{0/7}$ and $36^{6/7}$ weeks of gestation (Engle, 2006).
      (2) Replaces the phrase *near term*, emphasizes the higher morbidity and mortality of premature infants.
   b. Term: infant born from the first day of the 38th week to the last day of the 42nd week.
   c. Post-term: infant delivered from the first day of the 43rd week.

## CLASSIFICATION OF GROWTH AND MATURITY

The intrauterine growth pattern reflects fetal well-being. This pattern is influenced by race, maternal health or disease, placental function, medications, socioeconomic factors, nutrition, altitude, substance abuse, and smoking. There are multiple reasons to classify growth and maturity of the newborn infant:

- Assist in identification of the most commonly occurring problems in the newborn period.
- Estimate dating if there is no prenatal care.
- Examine discrepancy between weight and GA.
- Standardize reports of health statistics.

**A. Measurement.**
   1. Comparison of newborn's measurements should be of population-based growth data, representing the patient in gender, race, geographic region for altitude, and other environmental variances.
   2. Growth curves should be GA- and gender-specific for weight, length, and head circumference.

**B. Obtain measurements.**
   1. Type.
      a. Normal-appearing infants: weight, length, and head circumference.
      b. Dysmorphic appearance: may require more extensive measurements.
   2. Birth weight.
      a. Obtain as soon as possible after delivery.
      b. Express in grams.
      c. Weigh unclothed infant when quiet (weight can be falsely increased with significant motion).
      d. Classifications (regardless of GA) (AAP and ACOG, 2012).
         (1) Low birth weight: less than 2500 g birth weight.
         (2) Very low birth weight: less than 1500 g birth weight.
         (3) Extremely low birth weight: less than 1000 g birth weight.
   3. Length: crown-to-heel measurement.
      a. Most variable measurement: requires full extension of normally flexed infant.
      b. Measure length with infant supine and leg extended, head to heel.
      c. Accuracy facilitated by use of measurement board.
      d. Use crown-to-rump measurement to establish proportionality when length falls below norms (referenced data in *Smith's Recognizable Patterns of Human Malformation* [Jones, 2006]).
         (1) Congenital bone disorders.
         (2) When lower extremity anomalies make crown-to-heel measurement unreliable.
   4. Head circumference (HC): indication of normal brain growth.
      a. Measurement of largest occipitofrontal circumference.
      b. Apply paper measurement tape firmly around head above the eyebrow ridges, from most prominent frontal to occipital areas.
      c. Occipitofrontal circumference as measured may be erroneous: significant cranial molding, craniosynostosis, caput succedaneum, and cephalohematoma need to be noted along with the measurement.
      d. Consider parent head size versus intracranial pathology when head size is of concern.

**C. Plot newborn's weight, length, and head circumference by GA on standardized growth charts.**

1. CDC national reference for term infants.
   a. Recommend use of World Health Organization growth charts for ages 0 to 24 months (Grummer-Strawn et al., 2010).
   b. Growth below the 2nd percentile and above the 97th percentile indicates growth 2 standard deviations from median and should be investigated.
   c. Available at www.cdc.gov/growthcharts.
2. Colorado Intrauterine Growth Chart (Fig. 7-3) (Lowdermilk and Perry, 2007).
   a. Colorado growth charts developed in 1960s.
   b. Other limitations of Lubchenco data (Thomas et al., 2000).
      (1) Charts developed at mile-high elevation (Denver); 10th percentile is lower than data from centers at sea level.

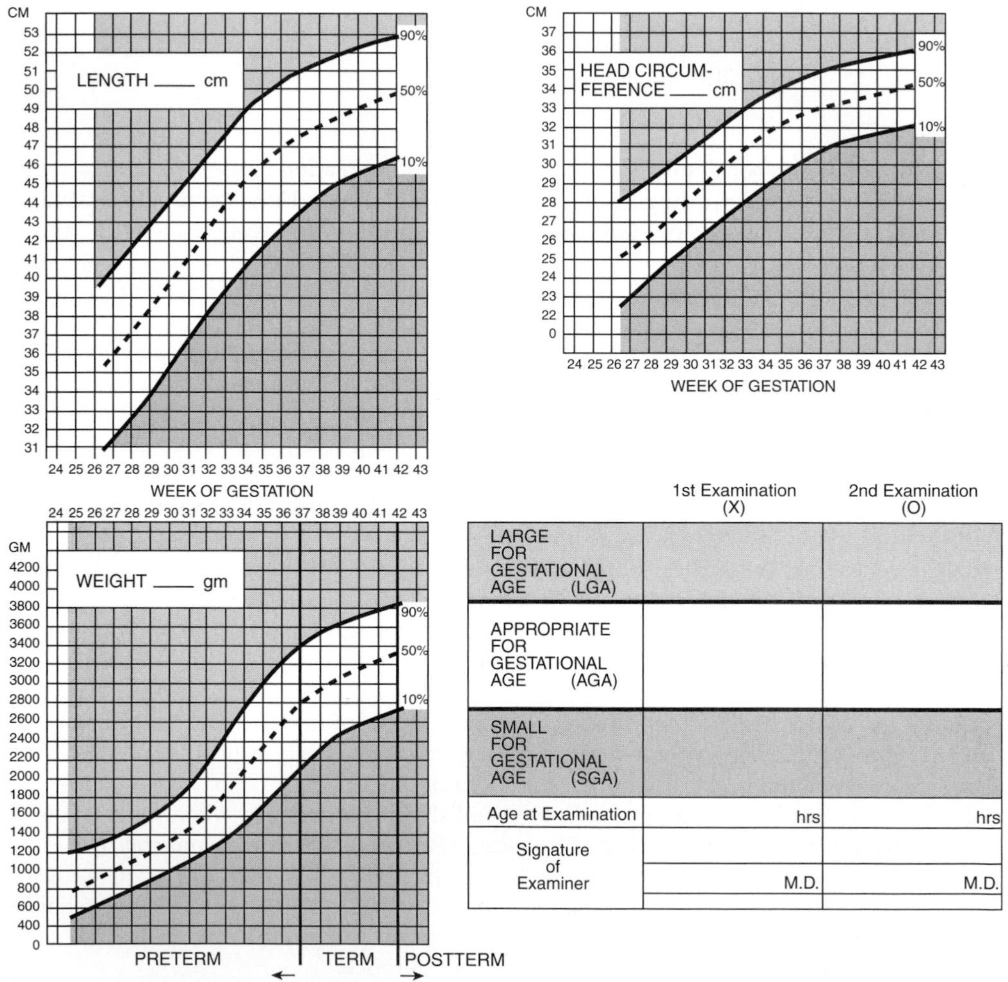


FIGURE 7-3 ■ Estimating gestational age: Newborn classification based on maturity and intrauterine growth. (From Lowdermilk, D.L. and Perry, S.E.: *Maternity & women's health care* [9th ed.]. St. Louis, 2007, Elsevier Mosby; modified from Lubchenco, L., Hansman, C., Boyd, E.: Intrauterine growth in length and head circumference as estimated from live births at gestational ages from 26 to 42 weeks. *Journal of Pediatrics*, 37:403, 1966; Battaglia, F. and Lubchenco, L.: A practical classification of newborn infants by weight and gestational age. *Journal of Pediatrics*, 71[2]:159-163, 1967.)

(2) Overestimates number of infants greater than 90th percentile and less than 10th percentile.
(3) Population sampled only whites and primarily low socioeconomic groups.
c. Leads to inaccurate classification of SGA and LGA.
3. Babson and Benda fetal–infant growth graph (Fenton, 2003).
a. Allows evaluation of catch-up growth by extending intrauterine growth from 22 weeks to 10 weeks post-term.
b. CDC growth charts could be used after 50 weeks.
c. Original 1976 chart updated in 2003 with growth data from the National Institute of Child Health and Human Development Neonatal Research Network.
d. Useful in neonatal intensive care units as it reflects preterm infants' postnatal weight and length delay in comparison to head growth.
e. Open access with credit given, available online at http://www.biomedcentral.com/1471-2431/3/13.
4. Pediatrix Medical Group Inc. Growth Chart (Thomas et al., 2000) (Fig. 7-4).
a. GA had largest influence on each growth parameter.
b. Infants less than 30 weeks of GA: overall lower growth parameters compared to Lubchenco chart.
c. Infants greater than 36 weeks of GA: larger and heavier.
d. Updated intrauterine growth curves using large, racially and geographically diverse sample from Pediatrix Medical Group NICU's (Olsen et al., 2010).

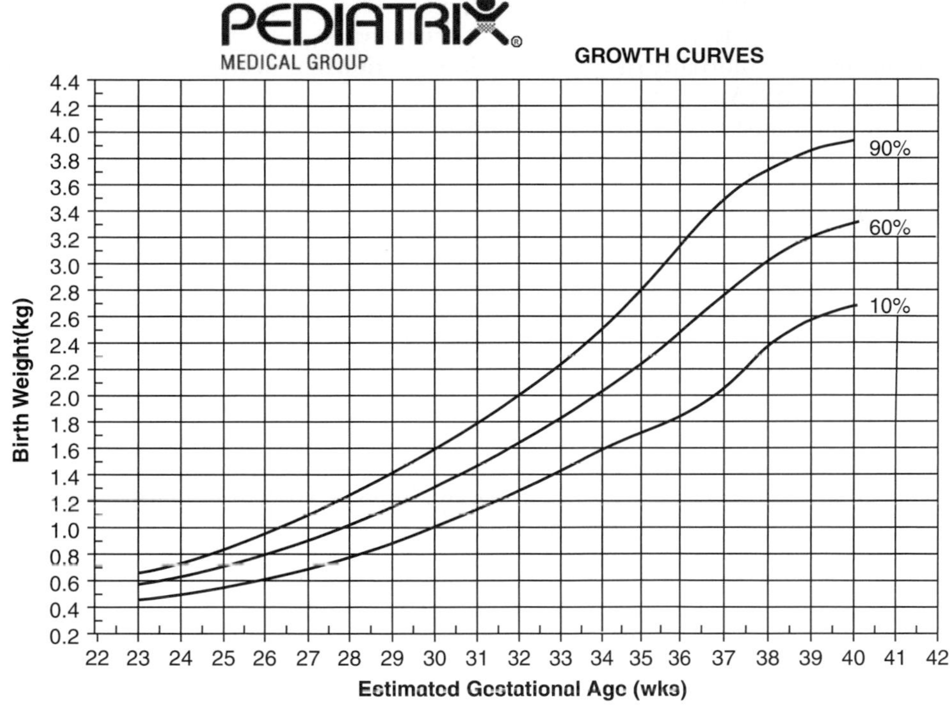


FIGURE 7-4 ■ These growth curves represent an estimate of intrauterine growth based on data from 80,011 neonates admitted to 114 neonatal intensive care units (birth weight above 250 g and gestational age of 22 to 42 weeks). Gender, race, and multiple births had a small but significant effect on each parameter (see the Clinical Research Center at Pediatrix U, www.pediatrixu.com/clinical_research_center.asp). These curves are a reference for the clinician to assess neonates' intrauterine and postnatal growth. The CDC national references (http://www.cdc.gov/growthcharts/) may also be used for term infants. (Copyright 2001 Pediatrix Medical Group, Inc. Reproduction of this material by any means without the express written permission of Pediatrix Medical Group, Inc., is prohibited. Please see www.pediatrix.com for updated information.)

**D. Compare weight with GA to determine size classification (weight compared with established norm).**

1. SGA: birth weight less than 10th percentile.
2. Appropriate for gestational age (AGA): birth weight within 10th and 90th percentiles.
3. LGA: birth weight greater than 90th percentile.

**E. Compare all growth parameters (head circumference, birth weight, and length) with GA.**

1. IUGR/SGA.
   a. Process of slowing of intrauterine growth rate.
   b. IUGR infants may or may not be SGA.
   c. Below expected norms for weight and length at birth based on GA, race, and gender.
2. Classifications.
   a. Symmetrical.
      (1) Proportional decreased growth.
      (2) Measurements for weight, length, and HC all within the same growth curve, all less than 10th percentile.
      (3) Etiology: decreased growth potential or reduced fetal cells (see Pregnancy History).
         (a) Intrauterine congenital infection.
         (b) Congenital malformation.
         (c) Chromosomal disorder.
   b. Asymmetrical (head-sparing).
      (1) Disproportionate reduction in weight and length at birth compared with head circumference.
      (2) Weight below expected norms for GA, race, and gender.
      (3) Etiology: normal number of cells; reduced cell size.
         (a) Uteroplacental insufficiency.
         (b) Maternal malnutrition.
         (c) Extrinsic factors occurring late in pregnancy.

**F. Determine neonatal mortality risk based on classification of newborns by standardized birth weight norms and GA.**

1. Morbidity and mortality statistics: standardized reporting of reproductive health statistics.
2. Establishment of level of risk for short- and long-term complications.
3. Mortality risk (Fig. 7-5).
4. Morbidity risk by birth weight and GA (Fig. 7-6).

**G. Identify infants at risk for respiratory disease, hypoglycemia, and thermal instability based on classification(s):**

1. Preterm: problems with immaturity of body systems: respiratory distress syndrome, necrotizing enterocolitis, and patent ductus arteriosus.
2. Late preterm (Engle, 2006; McIntire and Leveno, 2008).
   a. Subgroup of later-gestation preterm infants with increased morbidity and mortality compared with term infants.
   b. GA $\geq$34 and less than 37 weeks.
   c. Potential problems: temperature instability, hypoglycemia, respiratory distress, apnea, bradycardia, feeding difficulty, and hyperbilirubinemia.
3. Post-term: problems associated with placental insufficiency—asphyxia and meconium aspiration.
4. IUGR (Doctor et al., 2001; Rosenberg, 2008).
   a. Focus initial exam on identification of congenital anomalies and dysmorphic features.
   b. Associated with chromosomal syndromes, intrauterine drug exposure, and viral infections.
   c. Typical appearance of asymmetrically growth-restricted infant.
      (1) Head disproportionately large for trunk.
      (2) Extremities appear wasted.
      (3) Facial appearance of "old man."
      (4) Large anterior fontanelles with cranial sutures wide or overlapping.
      (5) Thin umbilical cord, diminished Wharton's jelly.
      (6) Scaphoid abdomen.

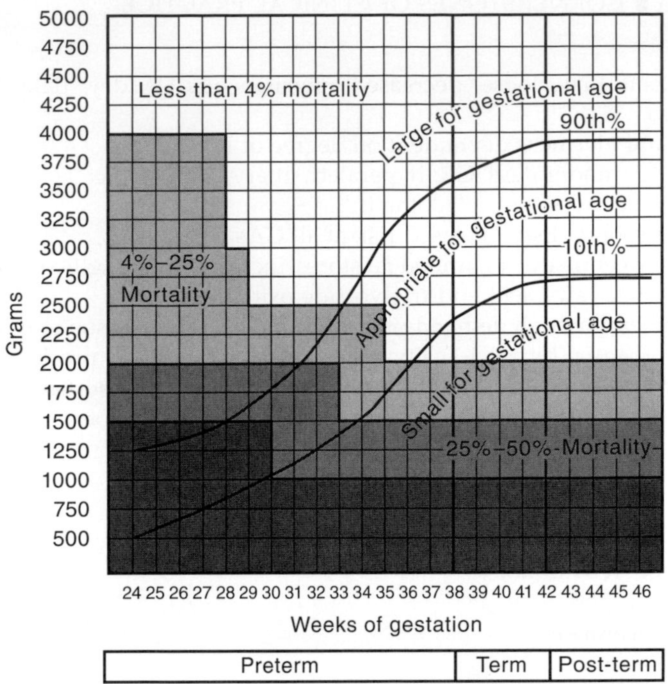


FIGURE 7-5 ■ University of Colorado Medical Center classification of newborns by birth weight and gestational age and by neonatal mortality risk. (From Battaglia, F. and Lubchenco, L.: A practical classification of newborn infants by weight and gestational age. *Journal of Pediatrics*, 71[2]:159-163, 1967.)

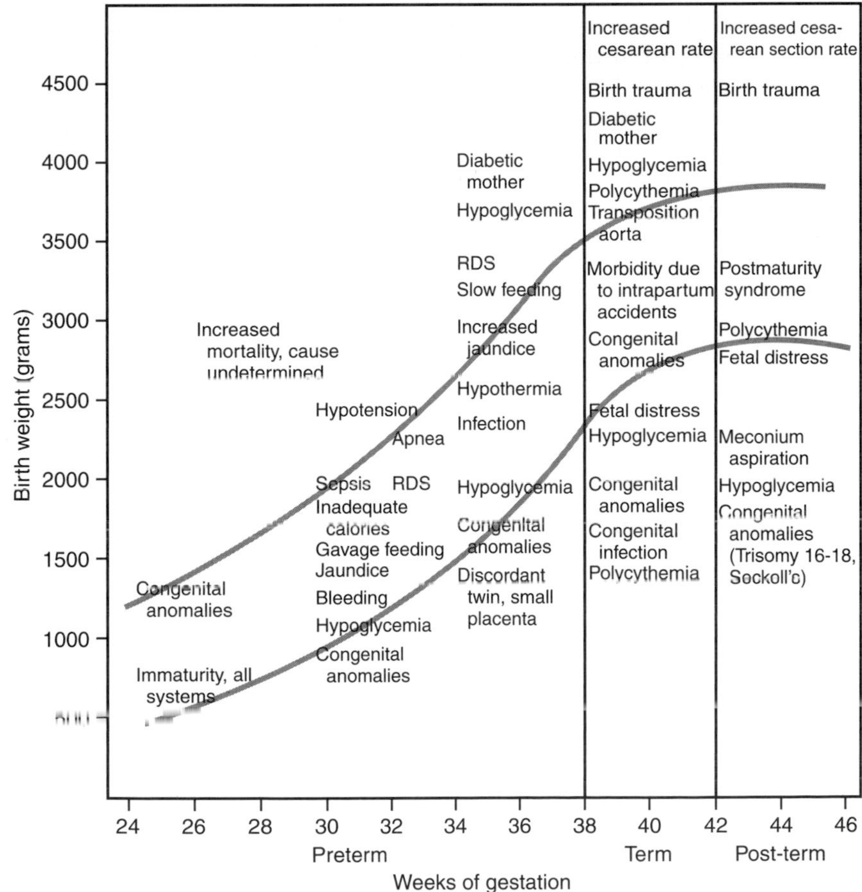


FIGURE 7-6 ■ Specific neonatal morbidity by birth weight and gestational age. *RDS*, respiratory distress syndrome. (From Lubchenco, L.O.: *The high-risk infant*. Philadelphia, 1976, W.B. Saunders.)

(7) Skin: petechiae, loose, decreased subcutaneous fat, dry, flaky, little or no vernix caseosa.
(8) Tone and alertness dependent on degree of IUGR.
(a) Mild/moderate IUGR: hyperalert, jittery, hypertonic.
(b) Severe: hypotonic, "apathetic."

**d.** Potential problem list; increased risk at all GAs with IUGR.
(1) Hypoglycemia due to limited fat stores, increased tissue glucose utilization, and ineffective free fatty acid and triglyceride oxidation.
(2) Hypothermia: high demand plus inadequate adipose tissue to maintain temperature.
(3) Polycythemia/hyperviscosity: increased red blood cell production in utero caused by chronic hypoxia or endocrine/metabolic or chromosomal disorder.
(4) Hypoxia: birth asphyxia, persistent pulmonary hypertension, and meconium aspiration.
(5) Infection.
(6) Problems related to etiology of growth restriction.
(7) Long-term morbidity and mortality dependent on etiology: 10 to 20 times perimortality of AGA infants.

**5.** LGA infant.

**a.** Typical appearance.
(1) Macrosomia.
(2) Infant of diabetic mother.
(a) Hairy ear (Clark, 2000).
(b) Characteristic large body with head circumference within normal limits for GA (insulin does not cross the blood–brain barrier).

**b.** Potential problem list (Lawrence, 2007).
(1) Abnormal glucose metabolism after birth, hyperinsulinemia, and hypoglycemia.
(2) Birth trauma from difficult extraction (fractured clavicle, brachial plexus injury) or asphyxia.
(3) Complications from operative or assisted delivery: respiratory distress, adverse effects of anesthesia.
(4) Iatrogenic prematurity: overestimation of fetal GA.
(5) Association with other problems related to infant of diabetic mother: respiratory distress syndrome, hypoglycemia, hypocalcemia, polycythemia, hyperbilirubinemia, and congenital anomalies.
(6) Pulmonary hypertension.
(7) Poor feeding.
(8) Thermal instability as a result of central nervous system (CNS) trauma or infection.
(9) Beckwith–Wiedemann syndrome, LGA, macroglossia, hypoglycemia, umbilical hernia, undescended testes.

## PHYSICAL EXAMINATION

A systematic approach to the physical examination of the newborn should be performed in the first 12 to 18 hours of life after successfully transitioning. This prevents pertinent omissions and provides a detailed description that can be utilized in communication of alterations in anatomic structure or changes in physiology or function. These observations ultimately must be made within the context of the patient's history and GA. Communication to the primary care provider is essential for further evaluation and prompt treatment.

**A. Assessment techniques.**

**1.** Examine in well-lit room; direct light should not be in infant's face.
**2.** Warm hands and equipment.
**3.** Keep infant warm by using overhead heat source or uncovering small areas at a time to prevent hypothermia.
**4.** Complete detailed observations prior to physical contact.
**5.** Order of examination:

a. Depends on the purpose of the examination and the current state of the infant (Fletcher, 1998).
b. Generally: least invasive observations to most disturbing techniques.
c. Observe skin throughout the examination.
d. Evaluate neurobehavior within the context of the infant's behavioral state.
6. Document physical examination in patient care record inclusive of description of abnormalities and vital signs.

**B. Timing of examinations (AAP and ACOG, 2012).**
1. Recognize life-threatening symptoms and address those prior to a comprehensive examination.
2. Modify elements of examination based on infant's state or illness.
a. Initial examination in delivery room.
b. Apgar scoring.
c. Inspection for birth injury or major congenital malformation.
d. Evaluation of pulmonary and cardiovascular adjustment to extrauterine life.
e. Notification of primary care provider.
(1) Apgar score less than 5.
(2) Maternal fever.
(3) Abnormal examination findings.
(4) Evidence of and/or suspected substance abuse.
3. Comprehensive newborn examination.
a. Within 12 to 18 hours of life: evaluation of size, growth, and GA; transition to extrauterine life; and congenital anomalies.
b. Discharge examination: focus on problem(s) during hospitalization, problems with feeding and weight gain, and ability of parent(s) to meet infant's needs.

**C. General appearance: initial impression.**
1. State: indicator of well-being.
a. Sleep states: deep sleep and light sleep.
b. Awake states: quiet alert, actively alert, and crying.
2. Color.
a. Most reliable indicator of color: mucous membranes. Other areas include conjunctiva, nail beds, lips, buccal mucosa, earlobes, and soles of feet.
b. Lighting and color of blankets can affect perception of color.
c. Central cyanosis; always abnormal.
(1) Recognition influenced by hematocrit, temperature, and environmental factors.
(2) Central cyanosis: superficial capillaries exceed 5 g/dL unsaturated hemoglobin (Park, 2008).
(3) Variety of etiologies: cardiac, pulmonary, infection, metabolic, neurologic, and hematologic.
d. Acrocyanosis.
(1) Suggests instability of peripheral circulation.
(2) Cyanosis limited to hands, feet, and circumoral area (lips).
(3) May be a result of cold, stress, shock, and polycythemia.
(4) Normal finding for 24 to 48 hours after birth.
e. Pallor: pale, white appearance.
(1) Reflects poor perfusion and circulatory failure or acidosis.
(2) With bradycardia, indicates anoxia or vasoconstriction found in shock, sepsis, or severe respiratory distress.
(3) With tachycardia, can indicate anemia.
f. Plethora: ruddy or red appearance.
(1) May indicate polycythemia.
g. Jaundice: yellow pigmentation in skin or conjunctivae due to deposition of bilirubin.
(1) Abnormal in the first 24 hours of life. Needs immediate investigation.
(2) Cephalocaudal progression.
h. Mottling: checkerboard red-and-white pattern.
(1) May be normal in neonatal period, especially in preterm infants. Reflects vasomotor instability and unequal capillary blood to cutaneous tissue.

(2) May be seen in cold stress, hypovolemia, and sepsis.
(3) Cutis marmorata: exaggerated marbling greatest on extremities but also present on trunk (Fletcher, 1998).

**i.** Harlequin sign: distinct midline demarcation.
(1) Pale on one side and red on the opposite side.
(2) Owing to immature autoregulation of blood flow.

**3.** Respiratory effort.
**a.** Rate.
(1) Normal 40 to 60 respirations per minute.
(2) Rate can vary with activity of infant.
**b.** Quality: absence of "work of breathing."
(1) Retractions: occur more often in premature infant as a result of highly compliant chest wall.
(2) Nasal flaring: diameter of nares increased as mechanism to decrease airway resistance.
(3) Expiratory grunting: increase in intrathoracic pressure to prevent volume loss during expiration as a result of alveolar collapse.

**4.** Wheezing: due to increased airway resistance. High-pitched rhonchi heard more loudly on expiration.

**5.** Stridor: partially obstructed airway.

**6.** Nutritional status.
**a.** Well nourished: increased subcutaneous fat, without loose skin.
**b.** Growth restricted: thin and wasted appearance, no subcutaneous fat, loose skin.

**7.** Tone.
**a.** Based on GA expectations.
**b.** Initial position reflects intrauterine position and may reflect limitation of movement or increased pressure on head, trunk, or extremities.
**c.** Degree of flexion and amount of resistance demonstrated with examiner's extension of extremities.
**d.** Decreased flexion (hypotonia) or increased flexion (hypertonia) should be evaluated further.

**8.** Congenital defects.
**a.** Determine if malformation (abnormal shape or structure) or deformation (fully formed but influenced by in utero environment).
**b.** Describe anatomic structures fully: size, number, shape, position, color, texture, continuity, and alignment.

**9.** Temperature (see Chapter 6).

**D. Skin (see Chapter 36).**

**1.** General considerations.
**a.** Findings differ with GA, especially with extremely low birth weight.
**b.** Indicators of underlying illness: petechiae, pigmentation, rashes, and pustules.
**c.** Congenital lesions may not be apparent at birth; influenced by maternal hormones.
**d.** Differentiate between findings at birth versus injury after birth (medical interventions).
**e.** Use basic descriptors: color, quantity, size, shape, pattern of distribution, and texture.

**2.** Skin is soft, smooth, and opaque and should be warm to the touch; cold, clammy skin may indicate shock.

**3.** Inspect lesions, rashes, bruises, and birthmarks. Differentiate between benign findings and those suspicious of infection or hematologic or neurologic disturbance.

**4.** Palpate for texture (raised, flat) unless lesion is open.

**5.** Vernix caseosa.
**a.** White or yellow material on the skin; discolored with postmaturity, hemolytic disease, and meconium staining.
**b.** Sebaceous gland secretions and exfoliated skin cells.
**c.** Presents during third trimester and decreases with increasing GA.

**6.** Lanugo: fine soft hair covering face, trunk.
**a.** Amount and distribution are GA dependent.

b. Covers entire body in preterm, disappears at 32 to 37 weeks from face and lower back.
c. At term, present on upper back and limbs.
7. Erythema toxicum (newborn rash).
a. Erythematous macules, each containing a central papule (yellow or white).
b. Papules contain eosinophils in a fluid that is sterile.
c. Persist for several days and then resolve spontaneously.
d. Most often located on trunk, arms, and perineal areas.
e. Never located on soles of feet or palms of hands.
8. Pustular melanosis.
a. Benign, transient, nonerythematous pustules and vesicles.
b. Single or clusters, rupture leaves scaly white lesion.
9. Ecchymosis: nonblanching blue or black area.
a. Extravasation of blood into tissue.
b. Related to trauma of blood vessels.
10. Petechiae.
a. Tiny red or purple nonblanching pinpoint macules.
b. Benign when found on presenting part; result from areas of compression during delivery.
c. More diffuse distribution suggests general thrombocytopenia.
d. Require further evaluation when progressive.
11. Vascular nevi.
a. Common cutaneous malformation(s) that can occur anywhere on body.
b. May present at birth or may develop in early infancy.
c. Types.
(1) Nevus simplex or capillary hemangiomas (stork bite).
(a) Macular patches with diffuse borders.
(b) Found on forehead, nape of neck, glabella, and eyelids.
(c) Blanch when pressure is applied.
(d) Resolve spontaneously.
(2) Nevus flammeus (port wine stain).
(a) Flat, sharply defined lesion.
(b) Most common on back of neck.
(c) If present over the face following branches of trigeminal nerve (forehead and upper eyelid), may be associated with Sturge–Weber syndrome.
(d) Will not blanch with pressure.
(e) May fade with time but will not resolve.
12. Café-au-lait spots.
a. Light tan or brown macules with well-defined borders.
b. Deeper pigmentation than surrounding skin.
c. Six or more may be pathologic.
13. Strawberry hemangioma(s).
a. Red, raised, circumscribed, and compressible.
b. Can occur anywhere on the body.
c. Proliferate: increase in size and number.
d. Most involute spontaneously.
e. No treatment is required unless they affect vital function.
f. Occur with increasing frequency with decreased GA.
14. Epidermolysis bullosa.
a. Blistering internally and externally.
b. May be either autosomal dominant or recessive.
15. Staphylococcal scalded skin syndrome.
a. Skin response to *Staphylococcus aureus*.
b. Scalded skin appearance.
16. Sucking blisters: skin erosion on thumbs, index fingers, wrist, or forearm from intrauterine sucking.

E. Head.
1. General considerations.

a. Up to 90% of the congenital malformations present at birth are apparent on the head and neck (Jones, 2006).
b. Review perinatal history, abnormal ultrasound findings, and mode of delivery.
c. Many variations are transient or racial, sexual, or familial traits.

2. Obtain head circumference (HC measurements).
   a. Measurement reflects brain growth.
   b. Predictable measurement: follows norms for GA and weight.
   c. Usually HC falls on same percentile curve as length. Determine etiology of abnormal growth if length and HC differ by greater than one quartile.
   d. Normal HC 32 to 38 cm for full-term AGA.
      (1) Microcephalic: poor brain growth, atrophy, or premature cranial synostosis.
      (2) Macrocephalic: familial (follows persistently higher but consistent growth curve) and pathologic (hydrocephalus: increase in cerebrospinal fluid results in increasing HC).
3. Observe shape and symmetry; may reflect effect of birth process or in utero position or significant anatomic defect.
   a. Molding.
      (1) Occurs with vaginal delivery from a vertex position; adaptive mechanism to facilitate passage through birth canal.
      (2) Elongation of head with prominence of occiput and overriding sagittal suture line.
      (3) Resolution in first week of life.
      (4) Not uncommon for overriding sutures to persist longer than 1 week in the extremely low birth weight infant.
   b. Rounded head occurs with delivery by cesarean section without labor; flat head with increased occipital–frontal diameter occurs with breech delivery.
   c. Abnormal prominence, depressions, or flattening.
   d. Abnormal shape of skull.
      (1) Plagiocephaly: asymmetrical appearance of head, flattened on one side.
      (2) Craniosynostosis: premature closing of one or more of cranial sutures.
      (3) Anencephaly: failed closure of neural tube without skull formation.
4. Palpate sutures and fontanelles (Fig. 7-7).
   a. Sutures: check for mobility of sutures by placing thumb on opposite sides of suture and alternately pushing (gently).
      (1) Well approximated.
      (2) Overriding.
         (a) Molding.
         (b) Fused suture: premature synostosis.
      (3) Wide sutures.
         (a) May be wide in the absence of increased intracranial pressure.
         (b) Widened lambdoid suture: indicates increased pressure.
         (c) Sagittal and metopic sutures normally wider in black infants (Fletcher, 1998).
      (4) Craniotabes: soft demineralized area typically found in parietal and occipital regions along the lambdoidal suture line.
         (a) Under gentle pressure, the area will collapse and then recoil.
         (b) Infant engaged in the vertex position for a prolonged period.
         (c) Pressure of skull against maternal pelvis results in delayed ossification or reabsorption of bone.
   b. Anterior fontanelle.
      (1) Location: junction of sagittal and coronal sutures.
      (2) Shape: diamond.
      (3) Size: measures 4 to 6 cm at the largest diameter (bone to bone).
      (4) Normally closes at 18 months.
   c. Posterior fontanelle.
      (1) Location: junction of lambdoidal and sagittal sutures.
      (2) Shape: triangular.
      (3) Size: usually fingertip.
      (4) Normally closes by 2 months of age.

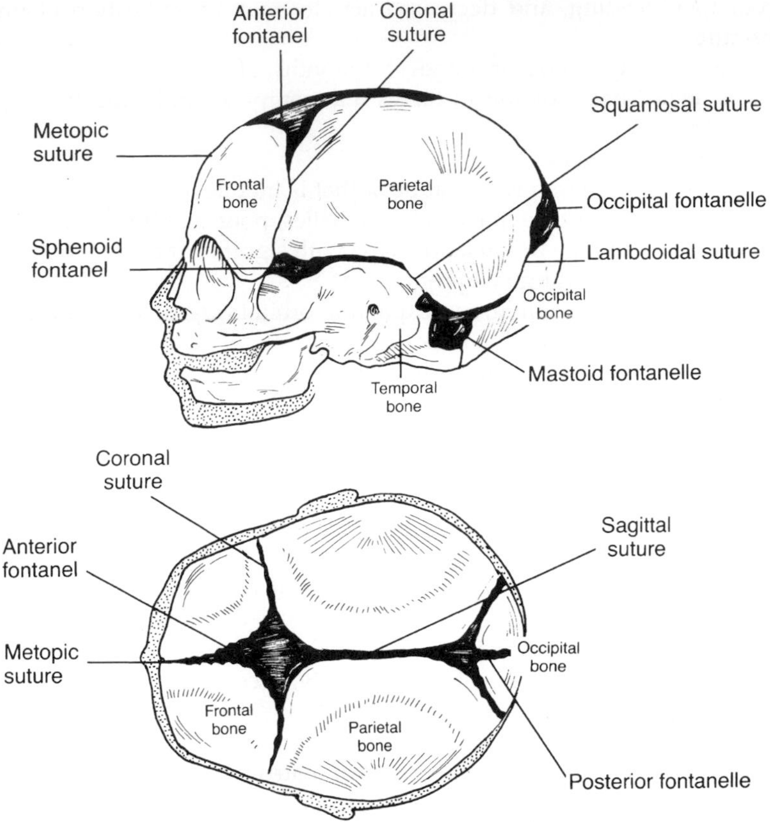


FIGURE 7-7 ■ Two views of skull, showing fontanelles and sutures.

**d.** Abnormal findings.
   (1) Third fontanelle: between anterior and posterior fontanelles along the sagittal suture (may be associated with congenital anomalies).
   (2) Size: large fontanelle, considerable racial variations; not pathognomonic for any condition (Fletcher, 1998).
   (3) Closed fontanelles with immobile, rigid sutures suggest premature synostosis.
   (4) Bruit over temporal, frontal, or occipital area associated with high-output cardiac failure and arteriovenous malformation.
   (5) Abnormal tension.
      (a) Bulging, tense, full fontanelle: associated with increased intracranial pressure secondary to hydrocephalus, birth injury, bleeding, or infection.
      (b) Depressed fontanelle: associated with dehydration.

**5.** Palpate soft tissue findings on scalp, face, and neck (Furdon and Clark, 2001).
   **a.** Caput succedaneum: common finding in infants born in the vertex position as a result of compression of local blood vessels.
      (1) Maximal swelling present at birth.
      (2) Edema extends across suture lines and has poorly defined borders.
      (3) Edema can shift to dependent position.
      (4) $\pm$ Ecchymosis, petechiae, or purpura.
      (5) Disappears within 24 to 48 hours.
   **b.** Cephalohematoma: subperiosteal hemorrhage due to delivery trauma.
      (1) Typically not present at birth, increases in size over the first day of life.
      (2) Unilateral; fixed, firm, and palpable mass.
      (3) Swelling does not cross suture lines.
      (4) Often no ecchymosis.

(5) Poor tone, feeding, and decreased activity may be indication of underlying skull fracture.
(6) Resolution may not occur for several months, often leaving a calcified "knot."

c. Subgaleal hemorrhage: owing to forces that compress and drag the head through the pubic outlet.
(1) Is a clinical emergency.
(2) Ballotable scalp mass present at birth that is mobile, not fixed.
(3) Swelling crosses suture lines and fontanelles, poorly defined margins.
(4) Rapidly can increase in size and shape with significant acute blood loss, resulting in shock as the presenting symptom.
(5) Bleeding, seen as swelling, can expand to orbital ridges, around the ears and dissect along tissue planes into the neck.
(6) Least common of the birth injuries; however, has the greatest potential for complications.

6. Inspect the scalp.
a. Intact skin.
b. Normal hair pattern (direction of growth) and distribution (Furdon and Clark, 2003).
(1) Color concordant racially with parents; genetic disorders can present with hypopigmentation of scalp hair.
(2) Localized patches of hypopigmentation (e.g., white forelock: Waardenburg's syndrome).
(3) Areas of diffuse or localized absence or abundance of hair.
(4) Hair texture: brittle, fragile, twisted, wooly, excessively kinky.
(5) Anterior and posterior hair margins.
c. Abnormal findings.
(1) Lacerations or abrasions as the result of instruments at delivery or scalp electrode.
(2) Vesicles: electrode site and behind the ears.
(3) Cutis aplasia: localized absence of skin associated with trisomy 13.
(4) Hair whorls: spiral hair growth pattern; multiple hair whorls or abnormal placement may represent abnormal brain growth or development.
(5) Anterior hairline well onto the forehead.

7. Note position in which infant holds head at rest.
a. Reflects fetal position.
b. Usual position: anterior neck flexion.
c. Observe for full range of motion.

**F. Face.**

1. Observe for symmetry and location of eyes, nose, and mouth.
a. Divide the face into thirds for inspection: one third, forehead; one third, eyes and nose; and one third, mouth and chin.
b. At rest and with crying or sucking.
(1) Asymmetry when infant crying:
(a) Facial nerve compression from in utero positioning or forceps pressure; most resolve spontaneously.
(b) Congenital hypoplasia of depressor anguli oris muscles; most evident with crying; localized paralysis of one corner of mouth with rest of facial movement intact.
(2) Symmetrical: Möbius sequence; mask-like facies due to sixth and seventh cranial nerve palsy (Jones, 2006).

2. Observe relationship and location of eyes, nose, and mouth.
a. Eyes.
(1) Open spontaneously with upright position and gentle forward and backward motion.
(2) Space between inner and outer canthus of one eye approximates the width between the two inner canthi.
(a) Hypertelorism (widened distance between orbits); hypotelorism (decreased distance between orbits) associated with various syndromes.
(3) Number: anophthalmos (absent); cyclopia (one).
(4) Conjunctiva and sclera.

(a) Subconjunctival hemorrhage: results from pressure on fetal head during delivery.
(b) Sclera color usually white.
(c) Blue sclera: extreme prematurity, osteogenesis imperfecta, other chromosomal associations.
(d) Yellow sclera: jaundiced.

(5) Cornea, iris, and pupils.
(a) Cornea relatively cloudy at birth:
i. Term infant: cloudiness resolves within a few days.
ii. Asymmetrical or dense cloudiness abnormal.
iii. Infantile cataracts: rubella, cytomegalovirus, familial association, and chromosomal defect.
iv. Congenital glaucoma: cornea size greater than 1 cm diameter with tearing and light sensitivity. Need immediate ophthalmology consult (Carlo, 2011).
(b) Iris: dark blue until 3 to 6 months of age, then eye color may change.
i. Brushfield's spots: speckled appearance; occurs in 75% of infants with trisomy 21; also normal variant (Fletcher, 1998).
ii. Coloboma: cleft-shaped fissure (keyhole shape); can be sporadic or in association with trisomy 13 or CHARGE sequence (posterior *c*oloboma, *h*eart defect, choanal *a*tresia, *r*etardation, *g*enital and *e*ar abnormalities).
(c) Pupils.
i. PERRL (*p*upils *e*qual, *r*ound, and *r*eactive to *l*ight).
ii. Pupillary reflexes present after 28 to 30 weeks.
(d) Red reflex: reflection of ophthalmoscope's light on the retina.
i. Color range: normal red (light-skinned infant) to yellow (dark-skinned infant).
ii. White (leukokoria): congenital cataracts, tumor, chorioretinitis.
iii. Absence: retinoblastoma, glaucoma, or hemorrhage.

(6) Symmetry of eye movements.
(a) Eyelids.
i. Should open to above midpoint of pupil when the eye is in a neutral position.
ii. Edema: related to birth process or chemical irritation with eye prophylaxis.
iii. Fused eyelids: extreme prematurity; generally not fused by 28 weeks of gestation; should not be used as an indicator of viability or nonviability.
iv. Ptosis: abnormal drooping of one or both eyelids.
(b) Palpebral fissures.
i. Slant is primarily racially determined.
ii. Variations typical of several syndromes.
(c) Epicanthal folds.
i. Vertical fold of skin at inner canthus of eye on either side of the nose.
ii. Common in trisomy 21.
iii. Manifestation of in utero compression (Potter facies).
(d) Eyelashes, eyebrows.
i. Appear at 20 to 23 weeks.
ii. Abnormalities.
1. Absent lashes or long lashes.
2. High-arched eyebrows or synophrys (meeting of eyebrows in middle).

**b.** Nose.
(1) Shape and size.
(a) Positional deformities often due to birth process; resolve without treatment.
(b) Abnormal shape: may be associated with a congenital syndrome.
(c) Abnormal: flat, broad nasal bridge.
(2) Patency of nostrils.
(a) The neonate is an obligate nose breather. If blockage is suspected, alternately occlude each nare and observe for distress.
(b) Causes of nasal obstruction.
i. Choanal atresia or stenosis: membranous or bony obstruction; unilateral or bilateral.

ii. Iatrogenic: swollen mucosa from suction catheters.
iii. Inflammation and secretions.
iv. Nares deformity: Differentiate nasal compression from true septal deviation. Gently compress naris on side of asymmetrical naris.
v. Nasal compression will correct; dislocated septum remains angled at base. Consult ear, nose, and throat physician for septal dislocation: relocation of dislocated septum should be done within a few days of birth for best outcome (MacDonald, 2013).

**c.** Mouth, tongue, and perioral region.
(1) Mouth should be symmetrical and positioned in the midline:
(a) Microstomia: very small mouth; may be associated with trisomy 18.
(b) Macrostomia: large mouth; often associated with mucopolysaccharidosis, Beckwith–Wiedemann syndrome, or hypothyroidism.
(c) Suck-and-swallow reflex develops at 32 to 34 weeks, and root and gag response at 36 weeks. They should be elicited during the examination.
(2) Cleft upper lip: can vary from a niche in the lip to a complete separation extending up onto the floor of the nose.
(3) Thin upper lip in association with flat philtrum: fetal alcohol syndrome.
(4) Soft and hard palate should be visually inspected, then palpated (Merritt, 2005):
(a) Presence of submucous or membranous clefts.
(b) Narrow or high-arched palate may indicate a decrease in neuromotor activity or sucking in utero.
(5) Mucosal cysts.
(a) Epithelial or Epstein's pearls: small, white epidermal cysts commonly found on the hard and soft palates and on gum margins; disappear after a few weeks.
(b) Bohn's nodule: equivalent to milia on the skin.
(c) Gingival or alveolar cysts.
(6) Dental eruptions and neonatal teeth.
(a) If mobile or poor root formation: generally removed.
(b) Consult with pediatric dentist; may be primary teeth.
(7) Frenulum.
(a) Small lingual frenulum normal.
(b) Ankyloglossia (tongue-tied): short frenulum that limits tongue movement. Abnormal; tip of tongue will form an inverted V shape. Rarely problematic. If persistent feeding problems, frenotomy may be indicated (Carlo, 2011).
(8) Tongue.
(a) Large tongue (macroglossia): generally part of syndrome (Beckwith–Wiedemann).
(b) Large tongue can obstruct the airway.
(c) Protruding tongue: trisomy 21 and Beckwith–Wiedemann syndrome.
(9) Thrush: oral moniliasis: usually contracted from mothers with vaginal moniliasis at time of delivery.
(a) Lacy white material present on surface of oral mucous membranes.
(b) Does not wipe away with a cotton-tipped swab.

**3.** Observe other facial features.
**a.** Nasolacrimal ducts.
(1) Tears are rare until 2 to 4 months of age.
(2) Obstruction: visible mass.

**4.** Inspect facial skin.
**a.** Milia: 1-mm white or yellow papules without erythema; resolve spontaneously within first weeks of life.
**b.** Miliaria: clear, thin vesicles (1 to 2 mm) that develop in sweat glands; primarily seen on forehead, scalp, and creases.
**c.** Lacerations, ecchymosis, abrasions from forceps.
**d.** Petechiae over head and neck: typically from nuchal cord, rapid second stage of labor.
**e.** Pits or sinus: facial cleft syndromes.

5. Observe for size of jaw and relationship to maxilla.
   a. Micrognathia: abnormally small jaw with normal-sized tongue.
      (1) May present serious airway problem.
      (2) Seen in Pierre Robin, Treacher Collins, and de Lange's syndromes.

**G. Ears (Spilman, 2002).**

1. Note presence or absence of external ear.
2. Determine position and rotation.
   a. Helix attaches to scalp at a point horizontal to the inner canthus of the eye.
   b. Normal: 30% of pinna above imaginary line drawn from the inner canthi of the eyes toward the occiput and tragus (cartilaginous projection in front of the external meatus of the ear).
   c. Cranial molding may distort landmarks; ears may appear low-set.
   d. Low-set ears may be associated with various syndromes and chromosomal abnormalities.
3. Check for presence of ear canals; visualization of eardrums not typically necessary.
4. Examine for abnormal findings.
   a. Microtia: disorganized or dysplastic ear.
      (1) Associated with atresia of auditory meatus and conductive hearing loss.
      (2) Variations.
         (a) Lop ear: helix folded downward because of inadequate development of the antihelix.
         (b) Cup ear: small cup-shaped ear.
   b. Preauricular pits and sinus.
      (1) Pinpoint openings at base of helix or front of tragus.
      (2) Increased risk of congenital deafness and renal abnormalities.
   c. Preauricular ear appendages (tags).
      (1) Single or multiple; vary in size.
      (2) Differentiate from accessory auricle or tragus.
      (3) Consistently seen in Goldenhar's syndrome: syndrome with wide range of facial, ear, and vertebral defects (Jones, 2006).
      (4) Associated with other brachial arch abnormalities: cleft lip, cleft palate, and hypoplasia of mandible.
      (5) Isolated skin tags not associated with significant renal anomalies unless found with other systemic abnormalities such as CHARGE or with diabetic embryopathy (Deshpande and Watson, 2006).

**H. Neck and clavicles.**

1. Inspect and palpate neck.
   a. Mass: note location.
      (1) Most common: cystic hygroma.
         (a) Multiloculated cyst arising from lymphatic channels typically located posterior to the sternocleidomastoid muscle and extending into the scapula and axillary and thoracic compartments.
         (b) Can distort the anatomy of the airway.
      (2) Thyroglossal duct cyst or branchial cleft cyst.
   b. Webbing.
      (1) Excessive skinfold extending from the mastoid process to the shoulders.
      (2) Associated with Turner's and Noonan's syndromes and trisomy 21.
   c. Torticollis: rotation limited due to constant position of head to one side.
2. Gently palpate neck and clavicles.
   a. Crepitus: due to fractured bone ends rubbing together.
      (1) Swelling, discoloration, or tenderness associated with fractured clavicle.
      (2) Observe for asymmetrical arm movement with the Moro reflex or signs of pain with manipulation.

**I. Chest and lungs.**

1. Review influencing factors: GA, timing of examination, intrapartum and delivery history, maternal drugs, and cool environment.

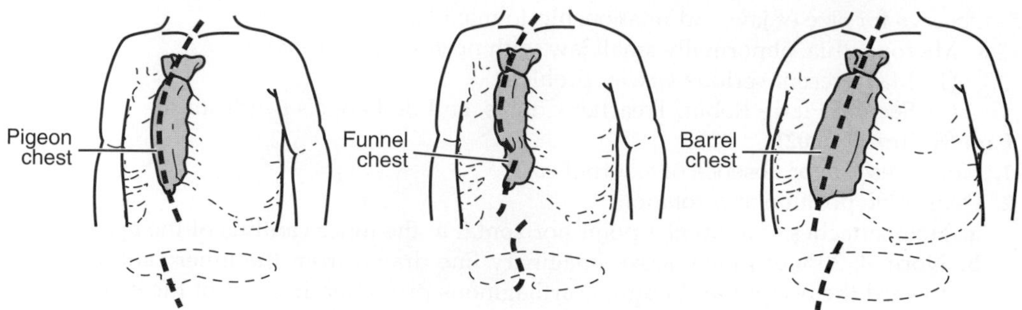


FIGURE 7-8 ■ Different chest shapes. (Adapted from Alexander, M.M. and Brown, M.S.: *Pediatric history taking and physical diagnosis for nurses* [2nd ed.]. St. Louis, 1979, Mosby.)

2. Inspect the shape and size of the chest (Fig. 7-8).
   a. Compare size relationship of the thorax and abdomen.
   b. Normal: round symmetrical shape with the anterior–posterior diameter approximately the same as the transverse diameter.
   c. Large or barrel-shaped chest: associated with air trapping and hyperinflation.
   d. Pigeon chest or protrusion of sternum: associated with Marfan syndrome.
   e. Chest wall itself depressed or funnel-shaped: pectus excavatum; no clinical significance.
   f. Short sternum: associated with trisomy 18.
   g. Rib margins apparent in premature infants: thinner layers of muscle and fat.
3. Observe.
   a. Color: refer to C. General Appearance: Initial Impression.
   b. Respiratory rate and pattern.
      (1) Should be evaluated at rest and before any manipulation.
      (2) Rate: normal—40 to 60 breaths per minute, easy, unlabored, and typically abdominal or diaphragmatic.
      (3) Tachypnea: rate greater than 60 breaths per minute—lung pathology, cardiac disease, infection, overheating, fever, and pain.
      (4) Bradypnea or shallow respirations: CNS depression.
      (5) Periodic breathing: 5- to 20-second pauses without changes in color, tone, or heart rate.
      (6) Apnea: cessation of breathing for more than 20 seconds. May be accompanied by bradycardia, change in muscle tone, or color change; apnea of prematurity, infection, respiratory insufficiency, gastroesophageal reflux.
      (7) Slow, gasping respirations: respiratory failure and acidosis.
   c. Depth and ease of respirations.
      (1) Normal: irregular and varying depth.
      (2) Chest pulled inward as abdomen rises with inspiration as a result of normal diaphragmatic excursion.
      (3) Retractions: accessory muscles used.
         (a) Note depth (minimal, marked).
         (b) Subcostal, substernal: common after birth. Persistence may indicate respiratory problems.
         (c) Intercostal.
      (4) Nasal flaring retractions, tachypnea, and grunting—symptomatic of respiratory distress.
4. Auscultate breath sounds.
   a. Compare and contrast each side of chest.
   b. Presence of air entry: normal, fair, or poor.
   c. Asymmetrical breath sounds: pneumothorax, cystic adenomatoid malformation, or congenital diaphragmatic hernia (CDH).
   d. Normal breath sounds: clear and equal, little differentiation between inspiration and expiration.
   e. Adventitious breath sounds.

(1) Crackles: fine or coarse, lower pitched, fine crackles heard on inspiration, often present after birth due to clearing lung fluid.
(2) Wheeze: high pitched, usually heard on exhalation, reactive airway.
(3) Rhonchi: low pitched, arise from partial obstruction by mucus or secretions.
(4) Stridor: rough, harsh sound worse during inspiration, caused by reduced airway diameter (edema, mass, vascular ring).
(5) Diminished breath sounds: atelectasis, effusion, decreased air entry, poor respiratory effort.
(6) Peristaltic sounds: bowel sounds indicate CDH.
(7) Friction rub: pleural effusion.

**5.** Inspect breasts and nipples.

**a.** Size.
(1) Based on GA.
(2) Enlarged breasts: effects of maternal estrogen, transient.
(3) Unilateral redness or firmness indicates sepsis.

**b.** Location and symmetry: widespread nipples—distance between nipples more than 25% of full chest circumference; may indicate variety of conditions.

**c.** Number: supernumerary nipples; small, raised, pigmented areas vertical with main nipple line 5 to 6 cm below normal nipple; familial.

**d.** Discharge.
(1) Witch's milk.
(a) Milky discharge produced in response to maternal hormones.
(b) Lasts for several weeks to months.
(2) Purulent: mastitis due to staphylococcal infection.

**J. Heart and cardiovascular system.**

**1.** General considerations: congenital heart defects are associated with other congenital malformations, chromosomal defects, maternal medication or substance use (phenytoin [Dilantin], alcohol), maternal health or illness (diabetes), viral illness, and familial association.

**2.** Observe color.

**3.** Heart rate: normal range 120 to 160 beats per minute (bpm), varies with infant behavioral state.

**a.** Bradycardia: rate less than 80 bpm in newborn (Park, 2008).
(1) May be associated with apnea, cerebral defects, vagal response, congenital heart block.
(2) Term infant in deep sleep can have heart rate of 80 to 90 bpm; should increase as infant awakens.

**b.** Tachycardia: more than 160 bpm sustained.
(1) May be associated with respiratory distress, anemia, congestive heart failure, hyperthermia, shock, and supraventricular tachycardia.

**c.** Brief irregularities are common; identification of abnormality cannot be made by auscultation alone.

**4.** Location of point of maximal intensity.

**a.** Normal: lateral to midclavicular line at the fourth intercostal space.

**b.** Shift in location can indicate tension pneumothorax.

**c.** Right-side location: dextrocardia, CDH.

**d.** Observe precordial activity.
(1) Within first hours of birth, may be visible along left sternal border due to normal right ventricle dominance at birth.
(2) Visible for longer periods in premature infants.
(3) Associated with congestive heart failure, heart disease, and fluid overload when seen after postnatal transition.

**5.** Auscultate heart sounds.

**a.** First heart sound.
(1) Accentuated at birth.
(2) Increase in intensity: patent ductus arteriosus, ventricular septal defect, tetralogy of Fallot, anemia, hyperthermia, and arteriovenous fistula.

**b.** Second heart sound.

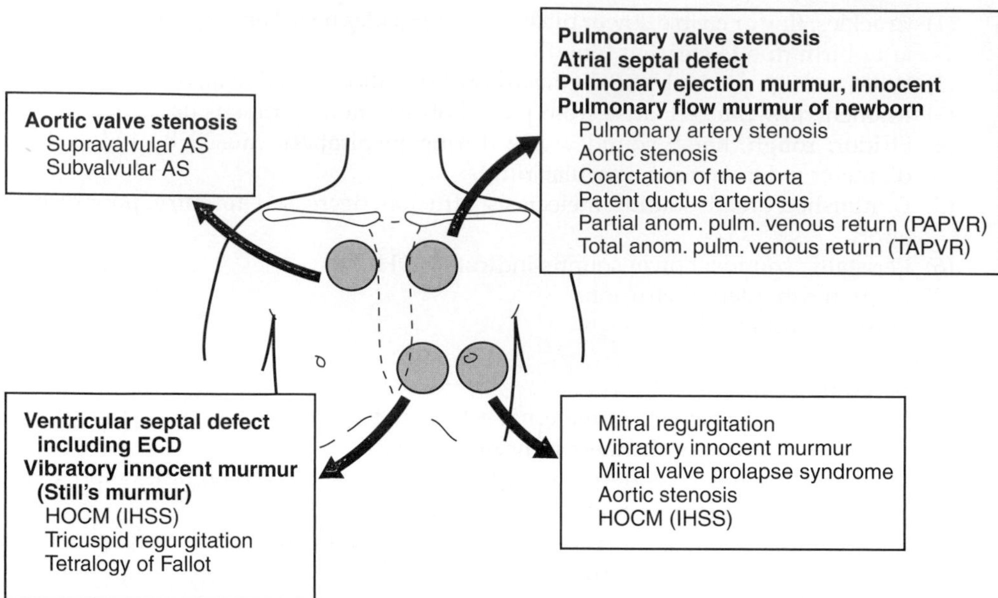


FIGURE 7-9 ■ Diagram showing systolic murmurs audible at various locations. Less common conditions are shown in lighter type. *AS*, Aortic stenosis; *ECD*, endocardial cushion defect; *HOCM*, hypertrophic obstructive cardiomyopathy; *IHSS*, idiopathic hypertrophic subaortic stenosis. (From Park, M.K.: *Pediatric cardiology for practitioners* [5th ed.]. St. Louis, 2008, Elsevier Mosby.)

(1) Sound produced by closure of aortic and pulmonary valves.
(2) No splitting of heart sound: pulmonary atresia, transposition of the great artery, or truncus arteriosus.

c. Muffled heart sounds: may indicate pneumopericardium, pneumomediastinum, or CDH.

6. Auscultate murmur: turbulence in blood flow (Fig. 7-9).
   a. Can be innocent or pathologic (underlying cardiovascular disease).
   b. Timing of appearance.
      (1) First 48 hours of life: can be related to cardiovascular transition; should be followed up.
      (2) Audible after transition complete: ventricular septal defect, turbulence in pulmonary arteries secondary to obstruction; severe outflow tract obstruction.
   c. Location and radiation.
      (1) Describe as interspace, midclavicular, midsternal, or axillary.
      (2) Transmission: auscultate back or axilla.
   d. Timing within cycle.
      (1) Continuous: extends beyond second heart sound into diastole.
      (2) Systolic ejection murmur: occurs before the first heart sound; ends at or before second heart sound; flow across pulmonary valve.
   e. Loudness or quality.
      (1) Grade 1: barely audible.
      (2) Grade 2: soft but easily audible.
      (3) Grade 3: moderately loud but no thrill.
      (4) Grade 4: loud with thrill.
      (5) Grade 5: loud; audible with stethoscope placed lightly on chest.
      (6) Grade 6: loud; audible with stethoscope placed near chest.
7. Palpate pulses: strength and equality (upper to lower and side to side).
   a. Brachial, radial, and palmar.
   b. Femoral, popliteal, posterior tibial, and dorsalis pedis.
   c. Grading scale.
      (1) 0: Not palpable.
      (2) +1: Very difficult to palpate; weak, thready, easily obliterated with pressure.
      (3) +2: Difficult to palpate; may be obliterated with pressure.

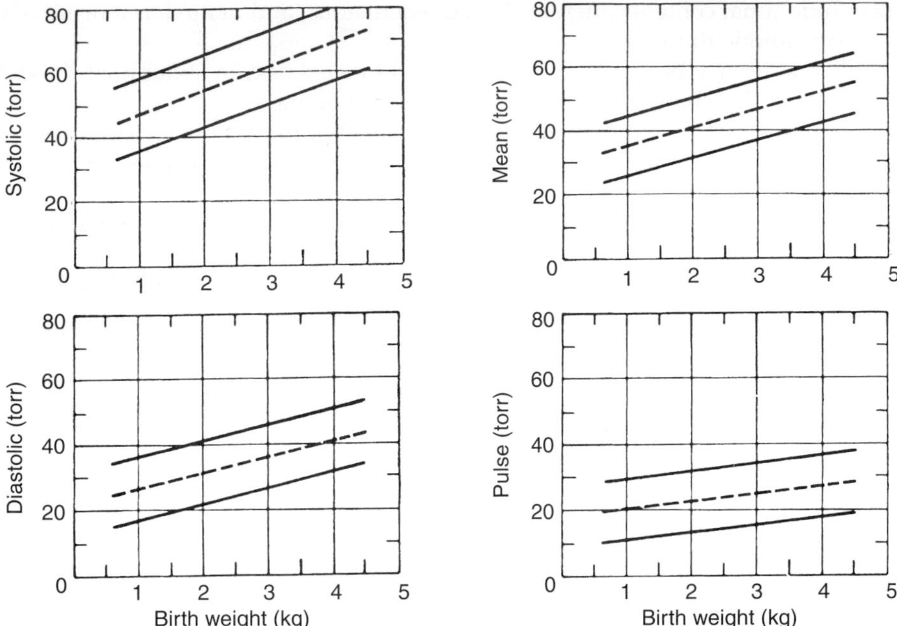


FIGURE 7-10 ■ Blood pressure by birth weight. (From Versmold, H.T., Kitterman, J.A., Phibbs, R.H., et al.: Aortic blood pressure during the first 12 hours of life in infants with birth weight 610 to 4200 grams. *Pediatrics*, 67[5]:607-613, 1981.)

(4) +3: Easy to palpate; not easy to obliterate with pressure; found in normal pulses.
(5) +4: Strong and bounding; not obliterated with pressure; associated with patent ductus arteriosus.

**d.** Absent femoral: associated with coarctation of aorta.

**8.** Assess capillary refill or perfusion.

**a.** Press and release skin over abdomen until area blanches.
**b.** Count number of seconds until color returns to area.
**c.** Normal: ≤3 seconds.

**9.** Blood pressure (BP) (Fig. 7-10).

**a.** Depends on GA and chronologic age.
**b.** Differential greater than 20 mm Hg between upper and lower extremity BP indicates obstruction (coarctation of aorta).
**c.** BP in lower extremities should be slightly higher than in the upper extremities.

**K. Abdomen.**

**1.** General considerations: review history for feeding intake, emesis, stooling, maternal medications affecting bowel function, maternal blood type, and intrauterine infection.

**2.** Observe abdomen: slightly rounded, soft, and symmetrical.

**a.** Scaphoid abdomen: abdominal contents in chest (diaphragmatic hernia). May appear slightly concave at birth, but will become distended as bowel fills with air.
**b.** Decreased abdominal tone or muscles in abdominal wall, with visible bowel loops and margins of spleen and liver (prune-belly syndrome) (Woods and Brandon, 2007).
**c.** Distention: obstruction, infection, masses, or enlargement of an abdominal organ.

**3.** Observe for abdominal wall defect.

**a.** Etiology: disruption in migration of abdominal contents from the umbilical cord and defect in the development of abdominal wall musculature.
**b.** Omphalocele: abdominal contents usually covered with a membrane; umbilical cord inserts into sac; commonly associated with cardiac lesions, trisomy 13, trisomy 18, Beckwith–Wiedemann syndrome.
**c.** Gastroschisis: abdominal wall defect resulting in protrusion of abdominal contents not covered with a membrane.

(1) Typically located to the right of midline.

(2) Abdominal contents often thickened, edematous, and matted as a result of exposure to amniotic fluid.

d. Umbilical hernia: bulge at umbilicus related to weakness in abdominal muscle.

4. Palpate gently for enlargement in liver or presence of masses.
   a. Normal: liver edge 1 to 2 cm below right costal margin in midclavicular line.
   b. Begin palpation in right lower quadrant and progress upward so liver edge will not be missed.
   c. Enlarged liver: congenital heart disease, infection, hemolytic disease, and arteriovenous malformation.
   d. A normal spleen is rarely palpable; palpable spleen more than 1 cm below left costal margin is abnormal.
   e. Abdominal mass: most often of urinary tract origin.
5. Palpate kidneys and bladder.
   a. Place one hand under the flank and palpate gently from above with the fingertips of the other hand.
   b. Normal kidney in term infant is 4.5 to 5 cm from pole to pole.
   c. Further evaluation needed: absence of palpable kidney or enlarged kidneys.
   d. Bladder can be palpated 1 to 4 cm above pubic symphysis when urine present.
6. Auscultate for bowel sounds.
   a. Absent or hyperactive bowel sounds may indicate obstruction.
7. Inspect the umbilical cord (Donlon et al., 2002).
   a. Important clues to fetal growth, development, and well-being.
   b. Normal: bluish white, moist, and gelatinous.
   c. Diameter of cord varies and is related to Wharton's jelly.
      (1) Supportive covering protecting the cord vessels from compression or occlusion.
      (2) Increases with GA.
      (3) Thin cord may reflect placental insufficiency and IUGR.
   d. Total length of cord: normal 30 to 90 cm.
      (1) Length determined by intrauterine space and fetal activity.
      (2) Infants with limited fetal activity (Down syndrome, congenital neuromuscular disorders) have short cords.
   e. Presence of knots.
   f. Color: green or yellow (meconium); red (blood); depth of staining correlates with duration of exposure.
   g. Number of vessels.
      (1) Normally contains two arteries and one vein.
      (2) Single umbilical artery: associated with fetal growth restriction; no increased chromosomal anomalies if an isolated finding (Mu et al., 2008); may be associated with other renal (hydronephrosis) or cardiac anomalies (Hua et al., 2010).
   h. Urine draining from umbilicus: patent urachus (embryologic communication between bladder and umbilicus).

**L. Genitalia and anus.**

1. General considerations.
   a. Review pertinent history.
      (1) GA; appearance changes with GA.
      (2) Oligohydramnios or polyhydramnios: possible renal/urinary or gastrointestinal/pulmonary anomaly.
      (3) Family history: associated genetic predisposition.
   b. Congenital defects are relatively rare but highly stressful to parents.
   c. Normal variations are more common than pathologic conditions.
   d. Genitourinary anomalies are highly associated with other system disorders (see Chapter 33).
   e. Breech deliveries can cause significant bruising and edema of genitalia and perineum.
   f. No circumcision should be done in infants with epispadias, hypospadias, or chordee.
2. General inspection and palpation: position infant supine for examination.

a. Gender identification: if not clearly distinguishable, do not assign sex until further evaluation. Inform parents of ambiguity and need for further testing.
b. Anus: locate position in relation to genitalia and determine patency.
   (1) Anal opening: approximately midline.
   (2) Slightly more anterior to genitalia in females.
   (3) Check for anal wink in any infant suspected of neural tube defect; stroke anal opening lightly; observe positive constriction.
c. Passage of meconium; ensures open communication only.
   (1) Fistulas: anteriorly or posteriorly placed; may be accompanied with bowel distention.
      (a) Rectovaginal fistula (female) or rectoperineal fistula (male).
   (2) Constant dribbling of loose stool: suspect neural tube defect.
d. Inguinal area.
   (1) Assess for hernia(s) when inguinal mass observed.
   (2) Groin bulge: may be unilateral or bilateral; increases in size with crying or straining, or spontaneously reduces.
   (3) Palpate from lower abdomen along the inguinal canal to the labia or scrotum.
   (4) Attempt to gently compress bowel back toward abdomen. Irreducible hernias are at high risk for incarceration and subsequent necrosis.

3. Male.
   a. Penis: inspect size, appearance, and foreskin.
      (1) Normal.
         (a) Straight, may be erect.
         (b) Size proportionate to body, average term length 2.5 to 3.5 cm from pubic bone to glans tip (Fletcher, 1998).
         (c) Glans covered by prepuce (foreskin) in uncircumcised infant.
         (d) Physiologic phimosis: tight, nonretractable foreskin; does not retract until 2 to 3 years of age.
         (e) Prepuce: foreskin or fold of skin over the glans.
            i. Amount and distribution: hooded (appearance of distal foreskin).
            ii. Small, white epithelial cysts on distal prepuce.
      (2) Abnormal.
         (a) Chordee: curving or bowing of penis; sometimes occurs in conjunction with hypospadias.
         (b) Micropenis: less than 2.5 cm in the term neonate.
   b. Determine position of urinary meatus.
      (1) Normal: midline at the glans tip.
      (2) Abnormal.
         (a) Hypospadias (Stokowski, 2004):
            i. Urethral opening located at the ventral surface of the penis; associated with chordee, meatal stenosis, inguinal hernia, and undescended testes.
            ii. May be blind dimple or pit in the glans at expected location of meatus.
         (b) Epispadias: urethral opening located on the dorsal surface of the penis.
   c. Urine: observe strength, direction of stream, and color.
      (1) Normal.
         (a) Straight, forceful, and continuous stream.
         (b) Most newborns void within first 24 hours of birth.
         (c) Uric acid crystals (flaky, rust-colored) are a normal variant.
      (2) Abnormal.
         (a) Altered stream direction may indicate urinary obstruction; urine from perineum or abdomen indicates urinary fistula.
         (b) Abnormal color: red (hemoglobin or myoglobin), brown (bilirubin), brown-yellow (concentrated).
   d. Scrotum and testes: inspect for size, symmetry, color, presence of rugae, and location of testes.
      (1) Normal.

(a) Firm, smooth testes of equal size palpable in scrotal sac; undescended testes in inguinal canal normal for preterm infants.
(b) Darker skin pigmentation.
(2) Abnormal: scrotal swelling or discoloration, nonpalpable testes.
(a) Cryptorchidism, extrascrotal testes position—needs further investigation with ultrasound and karyotyping.
(b) Nonpalpable testes (cryptorchidism): if not detected in phenotypic male, evaluate for virilizing adrenal hyperplasia. Ultrasound evaluation unreliable (Tasian and Copp, 2011).
(c) Bifid scrotum: deep midline cleft in the scrotum.
(d) Hydrocele: unilateral or bilateral fluid collection in scrotal sac, positive transillumination.
(e) Testicular torsion: blue discoloration, palpable firm mass, tender or nontender, negative transillumination. May be surgical emergency.

**4.** Female.

**a.** Labia and clitoris: separate labia and exert gentle downward traction to evaluate structures.
(1) Normal: smooth, wrinkling with weight loss, hyperpigmented from hormonal influence.
(2) Edematous at birth due to maternal hormones.
(3) Perineum is smooth, no dimpling; fingertip width.
(4) Abnormal.
(a) Labial bulge may indicate inguinal hernia or ectopic ovary.
(b) Labioscrotal fusion, female virilization.
(c) Clitoromegaly, pseudohermaphroditism.
(d) Genitourinary anomalies: abnormal spacing between orifices.
(e) Rugae: ambiguous genitalia.

**b.** Vagina.
(1) Normal: pink, patent.
(a) White or blood-tinged discharge due to hormonal influence (pseudomenstruation); can persist 2 to 4 weeks.
(b) Redundant hymen tissue and vaginal skin tags are common.
(2) Abnormal.
(a) Rectovaginal fistula: feces from vagina, indicates rectovaginal fistula.
(b) Imperforate hymen: secretions pool in vagina; can be confused with enlarged Bartholin cysts.
(c) Hydrometrocolpos: membrane covering vaginal opening causes uterine enlargement and pooling of vaginal secretions; seen as perineal or suprapubic mass.

**c.** Urethral meatus.
(1) Normal position: below clitoris; often obscured by hymen.
(2) Abnormal: anterior displacement.

**5.** Intersex conditions.

**M. Back, spine, and extremities.**

**1.** General considerations.

**a.** Influencing factors: GA, maternal hormones, in utero position, delivery mode/history, and timing of examination.

**b.** Many abnormalities are deformations from compression and contracture in utero rather than congenital defects.

**c.** Review for relevant history (Brand, 2007).
(1) Elevated maternal $\alpha$-fetoprotein (neural tube defects).
(2) Maternal diabetes mellitus (sacral agenesis).
(3) Maternal deficiency of folic acid or zinc; use of anticonvulsant medication.
(4) Decreased fetal movement (congenital neuromuscular disorders).
(5) Postnatal *S. aureus* sepsis (risk for osteomyelitis).
(6) Family history (hip dysplasia).

2. Observe infant at rest: appropriate number of limbs and digits; size and symmetry of upper and lower extremities; movement, position of comfort, range of motion, and trauma.
3. Palpate for joint or bone swelling, tenderness, or crepitus.
4. Back: position infant prone.
   a. Inspect for symmetry of sides, scapula position and symmetry, spine alignment and integrity, and presence of dermal lesions over spine or masses.
   b. Inspect skin.
      (1) Mongolian spots.
         (a) Normal variant; macular gray-blue lesions from melanocyte concentration in dermis.
         (b) Most commonly in lumbosacral region but can be found on legs, back, and shoulders.
         (c) Occurs more often in African American, Hispanic, Asian, and Native American infants.
         (d) Benign; fade during childhood.
      (2) Subtle cutaneous findings can indicate hidden spinal defects; observe for sacral pits or dimples, sacral tracts (pilonidal cysts), skin tags, abnormal hair distribution or hair tufts, unusual pigmentation, hemangiomas, or lipomas (Brand, 2007).
      (3) Asymmetry of gluteal fold: suggests underlying mass (lipoma) or tethered cord (Brand, 2007).
   c. Congenital spine defects.
      (1) Closed spinal dysraphism (Brand, 2007).
         (a) Spinal lipoma.
         (b) Dermoid tumor.
         (c) Tethered cord.
         (d) Split cord malformation.
         (e) Skin tags and appendages, human tail.
         (f) Dermal sinus tract.
      (2) Neural tube defect.
         (a) Failure of posterior neural tube closure (see Chapters 34 and 35).
         (b) Defect can be open, with spine and nerves exposed, or covered with skin or tissue.
      (3) Sacrococcygeal teratoma: tumor (mainly benign).
      (4) Scoliosis: lateral spine curvature; evaluate for associated genitourinary tract anomalies.
5. Extremities.
   a. Upper extremities.
      (1) Absent humerus, radius, or ulna: associated with syndromes.
      (2) Clavicle or humerus fractures: associated with birth injury or osteogenesis imperfecta.
      (3) Blisters on hands or forearms: in utero sucking.
      (4) Brachial plexus injury: stretching or tearing of nerve roots by lateral traction on shoulder during birth (Volpe, 2008); or pressure from the maternal sacral promontory during fetal descent (Benjamin, 2005).
         (a) Erb's palsy ("waiter's tip"): paralysis of arm with intact grasp; asymmetrical Moro reflex.
         (b) Klumpke's paralysis: forearm paralysis with absent grasp.
         (c) Total brachial plexus injury; because the neonate cannot move the shoulder, the arms remain extended and turned inward, with the flaccid hand suggesting a "waiter's tip" hand.
      (5) Observe the shape of hands and digits.
         (a) Syndactyly: webbing between adjacent digits of hands.
         (b) Polydactyly: supernumerary digits.
         (c) Clinodactyly: congenital deviation of digits.
         (d) Brachydactyly: shortened digit from shortened finger joint; normal variant; associated with achondroplasia and trisomy 21.

(6) Simian crease: single palmar crease; normal variant, positive finding in less than 50% of trisomy 21 infants (Jones, 2006).
(7) Nails: yellowing from meconium or postmaturity; dysplasia with chromosomal defects.

**b.** Buttocks.
(1) Observe for blanching or cyanosis of extremities or buttocks while umbilical catheters in use; indicates circulation compromise and potential necrosis.
(2) Dimple on buttocks can indicate congenital anomaly of femur (Fletcher, 1998).

**c.** Hips.
(1) Positional hip abduction: persistent joint flexion or contraction with knee extension resulting from prolonged breech position in utero.
(2) Developmental dysplasia of the hip (Witt, 2003).
(a) Asymmetrical creases of buttocks and thighs due to shortened adductor muscles.
(b) Uneven knee level (positive Galeazzi sign) when positioned prone with feet level and knees at a 90-degree angle.
(c) Ortolani maneuver: detects dislocated hips.
(d) Barlow maneuver: determines dislocatable hips (Fig. 7-11).

**d.** Lower extremities.
(1) Legs normally slightly bowed with everted feet.
(2) Genu recurvatum: knee hyperextension; related to in utero position.
(a) Usually found in breech position, females more often than males.
(b) Associated with Ehlers-Danlos, Marfan, Klinefelter's, and Turner's syndromes.
(c) Mild cases are benign; severe cases may require splinting/casting.
(3) Limb or digit amputation (amniotic band syndrome).
(a) Strands of amnion can wrap around any digit or, more frequently, a limb.
(b) Causes constriction and amputation.
(4) Metatarsus adductus (Furdon and Reu Donlon, 2002).
(a) May be positional or structural.
(b) Convex shape to lateral border of foot (C-shaped).
(c) Adduction at tarsal–metatarsal joint; wider space between first and second toes.
(5) Talipes equinovarus; club foot.
(a) May be positional or structural.
(b) Inversion deformity of heel (sole points medially), forefoot incurving and ankle in equinus posture (toes pointing down and heel pointing up).
(6) Talipes calcaneovalgus: related to intrauterine position; sole of foot is flattened against uterine wall.
(7) Rocker-bottom foot: arch looks like rocker bottom.

**N. Neurologic examination.**

1. General considerations.
**a.** Repeat examination of abnormal findings; assess changes over time.
**b.** Review history: familial, genetic, or neurologic diagnosis; birth trauma; difficult delivery; perinatal depression; maternal medication, alcohol, and/or drugs.
**c.** GA is an important consideration; responses of preterm infant are immature.
**d.** Timing and sequence of examination may alter the neurologic examination (Volpe, 2008).
(1) Optimal timing for older newborns is about two thirds of time between feedings.
(2) Clinical condition may necessitate exclusion of parts of examination.

2. Observe for skin lesions related to neurologic disorders (Jones, 2006).
**a.** Neurofibromatosis: café-au-lait spots, greater than 1.5 cm in length or in numbers of six or greater.
**b.** Sturge–Weber syndrome: nevus flammeus noted unilaterally, following the trigeminal nerve tract on the face and possibly involving the upper trunk.
**c.** Tuberous sclerosis: areas of hypopigmented (white) macules on the skin.

3. Assess posture: assess infant in quiet awake, quiet active, or light sleep state(s); unswaddled; position supine with head midline.

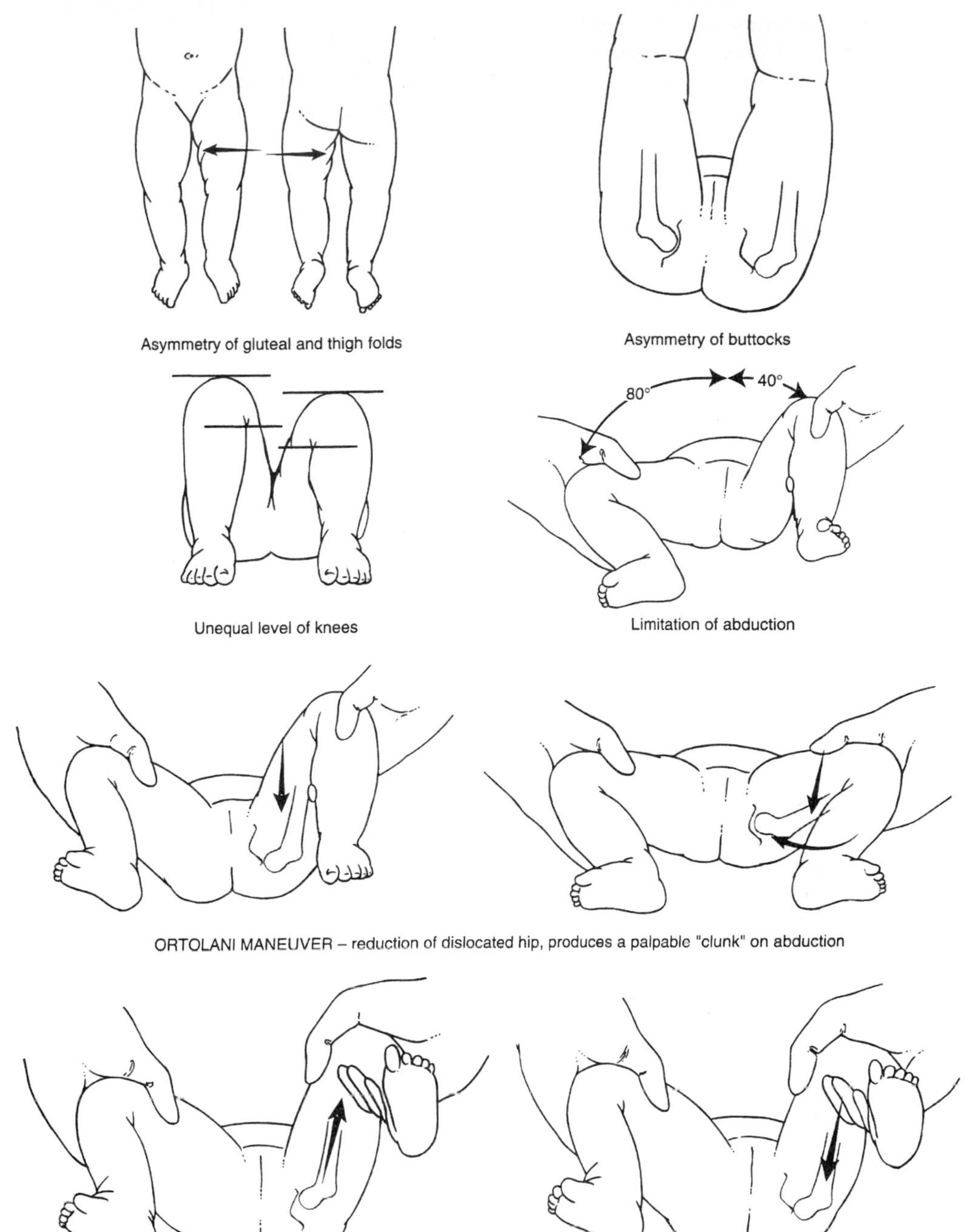
Asymmetry of gluteal and thigh folds
Asymmetry of buttocks
80°
40°
Unequal level of knees
Limitation of abduction
ORTOLANI MANEUVER – reduction of dislocated hip, produces a palpable "clunk" on abduction
BARLOW MANEUVER – dislocation of unstable hip, produces a palpable "clunk" on adduction with gentle downward pressure

FIGURE 7-11 ■ Assessment of newborn infant for dislocated or unstable hip includes gluteal and thigh folds, buttocks, knees, abduction, Ortolani maneuver, and Barlow maneuver. (From Nichols, F.H. and Zwelling, E.: *Maternal-newborn nursing: Theory and practice.* Philadelphia, 1997, W.B. Saunders.)

**a.** Term infant lies with arms adducted, hips abducted and partially flexed, moderate flexion of all extremities, and with loosely clenched fists.

**b.** Preterm infant becomes more hypotonic with decreasing GA.

**c.** Abnormal.

(1) Persistent neck extension (opisthotonus).

(2) Obligate thumb flexion (cortical thumb).

(3) Elbow flexion with dorsum of hands on bed.

(4) Frog-leg position at greater than 36 weeks of gestation.

4. Observe spontaneous movement.
   a. Term infant moves limbs smoothly.
   b. Preterm infant's movements may be jittery and jerky, with tremors.
   c. Environmental stimuli or discomfort produces mass movements.
   d. Coarse tremors and brief chin trembling are normal.
   e. Jittery: rhythmic movements of equal intensity.
      (1) Occurs more after startle or crying.
      (2) Distinguish between tonic and clonic seizures using gentle restraint: tremors will stop; seizures will continue.
5. Cry.
   a. Lusty, with normal pitch: normal term infant.
   b. Weak or monotonous cry: depressed, ill, or preterm infant.
   c. High-pitched cry: neurologic or metabolic abnormalities, drug withdrawal.
6. Tone.
   a. With decreasing GA, it may be more difficult to distinguish between random movement and true recoil.
   b. Note weak, absent, or unequal responses.
   c. Assess resistance to movement (passive tone).
      (1) Limb recoil, heel-to-ear, scarf sign.
      (2) Tendon reflex: only patellar reflex is reliable at birth; note sustained clonus.
   d. Assess resistance to gravity (active tone).
      (1) Traction response: pull-to-sit, ventral suspension; note degree of resistance.
      (2) Ventral and horizontal suspension.
7. Reflexes.
   a. Developmental reflexes (primitive reflexes): should be elicited in the normal term infant. Note any exaggerated or absent responses.
      (1) Sucking reflex: gently stimulate lips; infant opens mouth and begins to suck.
         (a) Evaluate the coordination and strength of the suck with a gloved finger.
         (b) Present at birth even in the premature infant, although it is not as strong as at term.
      (2) Rooting reflex: stroke cheek; infant turns head and opens mouth toward the stimulated side.
      (3) Palmar grasp: stroke the infant's palm with finger; infant will grasp the finger.
         (a) Attempts to remove the finger will elicit a tighter grasp.
         (b) Grasp should be equal bilaterally.
      (4) Tonic neck reflex (fencing position).
         (a) Position the infant supine. Turn the infant's head to one side.
         (b) The infant will extend the upper extremity on the side where the head is turned and flex the opposite upper extremity.
      (5) Moro reflex (startle reflex): "head drop" method preferred depending on the infant's condition. The high-risk neonate can be startled by making a loud noise close to the ear and noting the response.
         (a) Hold infant supine in a neutral position several inches off the bed.
         (b) Hold one hand behind the upper back and other supporting head. Infant's arms should cover the chest.
         (c) Head is held midline and dropped back 1 cm with supportive hand.
         (d) Infant will partially abduct shoulder, extend, and then smoothly adduct arms.
            i. Evaluate arm responses only.
            ii. Repeat two or three times as needed for detailed observation.
            iii. Asymmetrical response may indicate brachial plexus injury.
      (6) Stepping reflex: hold the infant upright, allowing the soles of the feet to touch a flat surface; infant will alternate stepping movements.
      (7) Babinski's reflex.
         (a) Stimulate sole of foot; infant will either flex or extend toes.
         (b) Persistent absence of reflex can indicate CNS depression or spinal nerve dysfunction.

b. Spinal reflexes.
   (1) Truncal incurvation reflex (Galant reflex).
      (a) Hold infant in ventral suspension.
      (b) Apply firm pressure along the side parallel to spine.
      (c) Infant should flex pelvis toward the stimulated side.
      (d) Indicates T2–S1 innervation.
   (2) Anocutaneous reflex (anal wink).
      (a) Stimulate perianal skin.
      (b) External sphincter constricts.
      (c) Indicates S4-5 innervation.

8. Cranial nerves.
   a. Olfactory (I).
      (1) Not usually assessed in newborns.
      (2) Can attempt in infants with strong scents such as clove or peppermint placed under nose; evaluate for sniffing, grimace, or startle reflex.
   b. Optic (II).
      (1) Evaluate visual acuity and fields by using tracking methods.
      (2) Watch for wandering or persistent nystagmus.
      (3) Check pupils for size and constriction in response to light.
   c. Oculomotor (II), trochlear (IV), and abducens (VI) nerves: supply pupils and extraocular muscles.
      (1) Observe pupil response to light.
      (2) Evaluate eye size and symmetry.
      (3) Doll's eye reflex (vestibular response): move infant's head from side to side, eyes should move away from the direction of rotation.
      (4) Fixed position or movement in same direction may indicate brainstem or oculomotor dysfunction.
   d. Trigeminal nerve (V): supplies sensory nerves of jaw and face.
      (1) Touch the cheek; infant will demonstrate rooting reflex.
      (2) Place a gloved finger in the infant's mouth to evaluate sucking and biting reflex.
   e. Facial nerve (VII): controls facial expression.
      (1) Observe for symmetrical movement of the face.
      (2) Inability to wrinkle brow or close eyes with crying indicates injury.
   f. Auditory nerve (VIII): tested only grossly without proper auditory equipment (see 9, Sensory Function Responses).
   g. Glossopharyngeal nerve (IX): evaluate and inspect tongue movements and elicit gag reflex.
   h. Vagus nerve (X): supplies the soft plate, pharynx, and larynx.
      (1) Listen to cry: determine the presence or absence of stridor, hoarseness, or aphonia.
      (2) Evaluate infant's ability to swallow.
   i. Accessory nerve (XI): supplies neck muscles (sternocleidomastoid and trapezius).
      (1) Turn infant's head from midline to one side.
      (2) Infant should attempt to bring head back to midline.
   j. Hypoglossal nerve (XII): supplies tongue muscles. Evaluate suck, swallow, and gag reflexes.

9. Sensory function responses.
   a. Touch.
      (1) Painful stimulus to a foot elicits a withdrawal reflex.
      (2) Touch sole of the foot with a pin to provoke flexion of the limb and extension of the contralateral limb.
      (3) Absence of flexion in the stimulated leg is abnormal.
   b. Light: shining a penlight into the infant's eye results in eyelid closure.
   c. Sound.
      (1) Ring a bell sharply within a few inches of the infant's ear while the infant is lying supine.
      (2) Response is based on observable attentiveness to the sound.
      (3) A brainstem auditory evoked response is recommended in the newborn period for all infants.

## REFERENCES


American Academy of Pediatrics: Policy statement: Age terminology during the perinatal period. *Pediatrics*, 114(5):1362–1364, 2004.

American Academy of Pediatrics and American College of Obstetricians and Gynecologists: *Guidelines for perinatal care* (7th ed.). Elk Village Grove, IL, and Washington, DC, 2012, American Academy of Pediatrics and American College of Obstetricians and Gynecologists.

Baker, C.J., Byington, C.L. and Polin, R.A.: Policy statement—Recommendations for prevention of perinatal group B streptococcal disease. Committee on Infectious Diseases, Committee on Fetus and Newborn. *Pediatrics*, 128(3):611–616, 2011.

Ballard, J.L., Khoury, J.C.Wedig, K., et al.: New Ballard Score, expanded to include extremely premature infants. *Journal of Pediatrics*, 119(3): 417–423, 1991.

Benjamin, K.: Part I Injuries to the brachial plexus: Mechanism of injury and identification of risk factors. *Advances in Neonatal Care*, 5(4):181–189, 2005.

Brand, M.C.: Part 3: Examination of the newborn with closed spinal dysraphism. *Advances in Neonatal Care*, 7(1):30–40, 2007.

Breeze, A.C.G. and Lees, C.C.: Prediction and perinatal outcomes of fetal growth restriction. *Seminars in Fetal and Neonatal Medicine*, 12:383–397, 2007.

Carlo, W.A.: The newborn infant. In R.M. Kliegman, B.F. Stanton, and J.W. Gemell, et al. (Eds.): *Nelson textbook of pediatrics* (19th ed.). Philadelphia, 2011, Elsevier Saunders.

Clark, D.A.: Atlas of neonatology. Philadelphia, 2000, W.B. Saunders.

Deshpande, S.A. and Watson, H.: Renal ultrasonography not required in babies with isolated minor ear anomalies. *Archives of Disease in Childhood: Fetal and Neonatal Edition*, 91:F29–F30, 2006.

Doctor, B.A., O'Riordan, M.A.Kirchner, H.L., et al.: Perinatal correlates and neonatal outcomes of small for gestational age infants born at term gestation. *American Journal of Obstetrics and Gynecology*, 185 (3):652–659, 2001.

Donlon, C.R., Furdon, S.A. and Clark, D.A.: Look before you clamp: Delivery room examination of the umbilical cord. *Advances in Neonatal Care*, 2(1): 19–26, 2002.

Dubowitz, L.M.S., Dubowitz, V. and Goldberg, C.: Clinical assessment of gestational age in the newborn infant. *Journal of Pediatrics*, 77(1):1–10, 1970.

Engle, W.A.A.: A recommendation for the definition of "late preterm" (near-term) and the birth weight—gestational age classification system. *Seminars in Perinatology*, 30:2–7, 2006.

Fenton, T.R.: A new growth chart for preterm babies: Babson and Benda's chart updated with recent data and a new format. *BMC Pediatrics*, 3:13, 2003.

Fletcher, M.A.: Physical diagnosis in neonatology. Philadelphia, 1998, Lippincott-Raven.

Furdon, S.A. and Clark, D.A.: Scalp hair characteristics in the newborn infant. *Advances in Neonatal Care*, 3 (6):286–296, 2003.

Furdon, S.A. and Clark, D.A.: Differentiating scalp swelling in the newborn. *Advances in Neonatal Care*, 1:22, 2001.

Furdon, S.A. and Reu Donlon, C.: Examination of the newborn foot: Positional and structural abnormalities. *Advances in Neonatal Care*, 2(5):248–258, 2002.

Grummer-Strawn, L.M., Reinold, C. and Krebs, N.F.: Use of World Health Organization and CDC growth charts for children aged 0-59 months in the United States. Centers for Disease Control and Prevention. *MMWR Recommendations and Reports*, 59(RR-9):1–15, 2010.

Hua, M., Odibo, A.O.Macones, G.A., et al.: Single umbilical artery and its associated findings. *Obstetrics and Gynecology*, 115:930–934, 2010.

Jones, K.L.: Facial features as major feature. In K.L. Jones (Ed.): *Smith's recognizable patterns of human malformation* (6th ed.). Philadelphia, 2006, Elsevier Saunders.

Lawrence, E.J.: A matter of size: Part 2. Evaluating the large-for-gestational-age neonate. *Advances in Neonatal Care*, 7(4):187–197, 2007.

Lawrence, E.J.: Part 1. A matter of size: Evaluating the growth-restricted neonate. *Advances in Neonatal Care*, 6(6):313–322, 2006.

Lowdermilk, D.L. and Perry, S.E.: *Maternity & women's health care* (9th ed.). St. Louis, 2007, Elsevier Mosby.

MacDonald, M.G.: Relocation of a dislocated nasal septum. In M.G. MacDonald, J. Ramasethu, and K. Rais-Bahrami (Eds.): *Atlas of procedures in neonatology* (5th ed.). Philadelphia, 2013, Lippincott Williams & Wilkins, pp. 390–392.

Macones, G.A., Hankins, G.D.Spong, C.Y., et al.: The 2008 Institute of Child Health and Human Development workshop report on electronic fetal monitoring: Update on definitions, interpretation and research guidelines. *Journal of Obstetric, Gynecologic and Neonatal Nursing*, 37(5):510–515, 2008.

McIntire, D.D. and Leveno, K.J.: Neonatal mortality and morbidity rates in late preterm births compared with births at term. *Obstetrics and Gynecology*, 111(1):35–41, 2008.

Merritt, L.: Part 2. Physical assessment of the infant with cleft lip and/or palate. *Advances in Neonatal Care*, 5 (3):125–134, 2005.

Mu, S-C., Lin, C-H., Chen, Y-L., et al.: The perinatal outcomes of asymptomatic isolated single umbilical artery in full-term neonates. *Pediatric Neonatology*, 49 (6):230–233, 2008.

O'Leary, D.R., Kuhn, S.Kniss, K.L., et al.: Birth outcomes following West Nile Virus infection of pregnant women in the United States: 2003-2004. *Pediatrics*, 117(3):e537–e545, 2006.

Olsen, I.E., Groverman, M.S., Clark, R.H. and Zemel, B.S.: New intrauterine growth curves based on United States data. *Pediatrics*, 125:e214–e224, 2010.

Parikh, N.A., Cody, A., Langer, J. and Tyson, J.E.: Evidence-based treatment decisions for extremely preterm newborns. *Pediatrics*, 125:813, 2010.

Park, M.K.: *Pediatric cardiology for practitioners* (5th ed.). Philadelphia, 2008, Elsevier Mosby.

Rosenberg, A.: The IUGR newborn. *Seminars in Perinatology*, 32:219–224, 2008.

Tasian, G.E. and Copp, H.L.: Diagnostic performance of ultrasound in nonpalpable cryptorchidism: A systematic review and meta-analysis. *Pediatrics*, 127:119–128, 2011.

Thilo, E. and Rosenberg, A.: The newborn infant. In W.W. Hay, M.J. Levin, and R.R. Deterding (Eds.) *Current diagnosis and treatment in pediatrics* (21st ed.). New York, 2012, McGraw-Hill.

Spilman, L.: Examination of the external ear. *Advances in Neonatal Care*, 2(2):72–80, 2002.

Stokowski, A.A.: Hypospadias in the neonate. *Advances in Neonatal Care*, 4(4):206–215, 2004.

Surbek, D., Drack, G.Irion, O., et al.: Antenatal corticosteroids for fetal lung maturation in threatened preterm delivery: Indications and administration. *Archives of Gynecology*, 286(2):277–281, 2012.

Thomas, P., Peabody, J., Turnier, V. and Clark, R.H.: A new look at intrauterine growth and the impact of race, altitude, and gender. *Pediatrics*, 106(2):e21, 2000. Retrieved March 5, 2003, from www.pediatrics.org/cgi/content/full/106/2/e21.

Verani, J.R., McGee, L. and Schrag, S.J.: Prevention of perinatal group B streptococcal disease—revised guidelines from CDC, 2010. *MMWR Recommendations and Reports*, 59(RR-10):1–36, 2010.

Volpe, J.H.: *Neurology of the newborn* (5th ed.). Philadelphia, 2008, Elsevier Saunders.

Witt, C.: Detecting developmental dysplasia of the hip. *Advances in Neonatal Care*, 3(2):65–75, 2003.

Woods, A.G. and Brandon, D.H.: Prune belly syndrome: A focused physical assessment. *Advances in Neonatal Care*, 7(3):132–143, 2007.

CHAPTER 8

# Fluid and Electrolyte Management

BRENDA HUESKE HALBARDIER

**OBJECTIVES**

1. Identify the influences on fluid and electrolyte homeostasis in the newborn infant.
2. Describe fluid and electrolyte management in the neonate.
3. Compare fluid and electrolyte management of the full-term infant and the prematurely born newborn.
4. Discuss acid–base balance in the neonatal period.

An essential part of the successful transition to extrauterine life is the achievement of fluid, electrolyte, and acid–base homeostasis and control. Because mature control of these processes may not occur for days to weeks after birth, premature and other stressed neonates can have transient disturbances of fluid, electrolyte, and acid–base balance.

## FLUID BALANCE

### Physiologic and Assessment Considerations

A. **Fluid homeostasis in the fetus and neonate.**
  1. Body water distribution. Water, the most abundant component of the body, is distributed in two main compartments: intracellular fluid (ICF) and extracellular fluid (ECF); the latter is composed of intravascular and interstitial spaces. As gestation progresses, the fetus undergoes changes in total body water (TBW) content and its distribution (Fig. 8-1):
    a. Early in gestation, water makes up 95% of total body weight, with the majority in ECF compartments.
    b. By term, water makes up 75% of body weight and a greater proportion has shifted from ECF to ICF compartments. These changes are largely due to increases in body fat content.
  2. Fluid adjustments after birth.
    a. An acute increase in intravascular volume occurs after birth. Timing of cord clamping can influence the volume increase.
    b. A physiologic contraction of ECF volume occurs with diuresis in the first week of life, resulting in postnatal weight loss. This is reflected in a weight loss of 5% to 10% in term infants and up to 20% in preterm infants. This may be related to levels of circulating atrial natriuretic peptide (Blackburn, 2013; Modi et al., 2000).

B. **Regulation of fluid balance.**
  1. Renal mechanisms.
    a. Because water and electrolyte balance is regulated by the placenta, the role of the fetal kidneys is primarily to maintain amniotic fluid volume. Fetal nephrons are functional but immature until 34 weeks. Renal blood flow, renal tubular function, and glomerular filtration rate (GFR) are all immature in the fetus and in the extremely premature infant (Kenagy and Vogt, 2013).
    b. After birth, renal blood flow increases as renal vascular resistance falls. Improved renal function in the days after birth from increased GFR is more pronounced in the term than in the preterm infant.
    c. Both term and preterm infants can dilute urine; however, when faced with a rapid fluid load, the preterm infant may have a delayed response, resulting in fluid retention.
    d. Reabsorption of sodium, bicarbonate, and glucose is limited in the newborn infant.

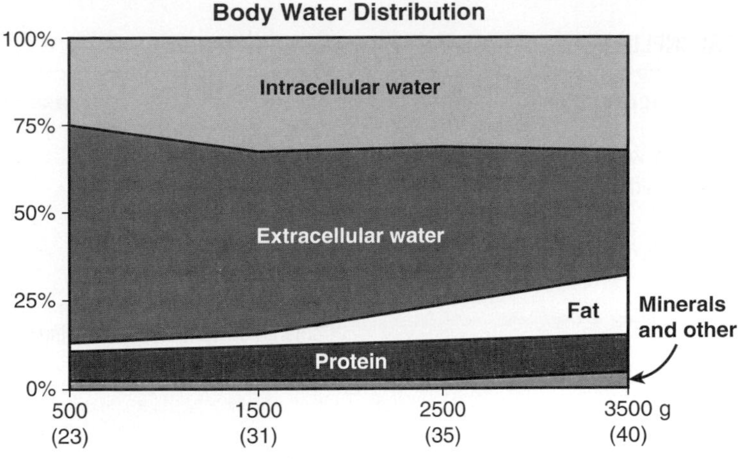


FIGURE 8-1 ■ Body composition in relation to fetal weight and gestation age. (From Dweck, H.S.: Feeding the prematurely born infant: Fluids, calories, and methods of feeding during the period of extrauterine growth retardation. *Clinics in Perinatology*, 2:183-202, 1975. Data from Widdowson, E.M.: Growth and composition of the fetus and newborn. In N.S. Assali [Ed.]: *Biology of gestation* [Vol. 2]. New York, 1968, Academic Press.)

2. Hormonal mechanisms.
   a. Antidiuretic hormone (ADH) is released by the posterior pituitary in response to a variety of stimuli, including hypotension and hyperosmolality. ADH influences water balance by stimulating the kidneys to conserve water. In the absence of ADH, the distal tubules remain impermeable to water, which is excreted as urine.
   b. Because of decreased responsiveness to ADH, neonates cannot efficiently concentrate urine in response to fluid deprivation.

**C. Fluid losses in the neonatal period.**

1. Renal losses: Urine output ranges from 1 to 4 mL/kg/hr. Highest flow rates occur during the physiologic reduction in ECF.
2. Insensible water losses (IWLs): These are the nonmeasurable losses that occur through the skin and respiratory system. Factors influencing IWLs are summarized in Box 8-1.
   a. Transepidermal water loss (TEWL): TEWL occurs as body water diffuses through the immature epidermis and is lost to the atmosphere. Skin features such as poor keratinization, high water content, low subcutaneous fat, large surface area, and high degree of skin vascularity all predispose the premature infant to high evaporative losses.
      (1) TEWL increases with decreasing gestational age (Lund and Kuller, 2007).
      (2) TEWL is the major source of IWL in very premature infants.
      (3) TEWL is highest on the first day after birth, decreasing on subsequent days as the barrier function of the skin improves. This improvement slows with decreasing gestational age, taking several weeks for the development of a fully functional stratum corneum in the extremely premature infant (Lund and Kuller, 2007).
      (4) TEWL is closely related to ambient relative humidity. TEWL increases with decreasing ambient humidity.
      (5) TEWL does not appear to be influenced by antenatal steroids or gender (Jain et al., 2000).
      (6) Failure to account for TEWL increases the possibility of inaccurate estimates of fluid needs, with resultant fluid and electrolyte imbalances.
      (7) Caring for very premature infants in an incubator capable of providing measured humidity has been shown to decrease TEWL.
   b. Respiratory losses: roughly 0 to 10 mL/kg/day; related to the temperature and humidity of inspired gases and to minute ventilation.

■ BOX 8-1
■ **ENVIRONMENTAL INFLUENCES ON INSENSIBLE WATER LOSS (IWL)**

| Factors That May Increase IWL: | Factors That May Decrease IWL: |
|---|---|
| Extreme prematurity | Increasing gestation |
| Postnatal age less than 1 week | Increasing postnatal age |
| Low relative ambient humidity | High relative ambient humidity |
| Radiant warmer use | Double-walled incubator use |
| High ambient temperature | Neutral thermal environment |
| Hyperthermia | Heat shields/plastic blankets |
| Convection; drafts | Humidification of inspired gases |
| Ventilation with dry gases | Ointments or transparent dressings on skin |
| Tachypnea | Clothing |
| High minute ventilation | |
| Phototherapy | |
| Activity | |

3. Stool losses: estimated to be 5 mL/kg/day in the first week of life, increasing to 10 mL/kg/day thereafter.
4. Other losses are possible. These include but may not be limited to gastric drainage, enterostomies, surgical wounds, and pleural fluid drainage.

D. **Fluid therapy.**
1. Goal of fluid therapy: The goal is to permit physiologic, adaptive fluid, and electrolyte changes to occur appropriately (Jones et al., 2011).
2. General principles guiding fluid volume decisions. No fixed fluid administration schedules are appropriate for all infants. Lower fluid administration rates are associated with lower incidence of morbidity such as patent ductus arteriosus (PDA) and necrotizing enterocolitis (Bell and Acarregui, 2008).
   a. During the first 3 to 5 days after birth, fluid intake should be at a level that allows a reasonable weight loss yet avoids intracellular dehydration. Provision of 60 to 100 mL/kg/day, depending on the degree of control over IWL, is a typical starting point. Extremely premature infants require more fluid relative to body weight because of a larger IWL. Fluids given to correct shock, hypoglycemia, or acidosis must be taken into account.
   b. Fluid intake is gradually increased on subsequent days to 150 to 175 mL/kg/day, although fluids may be restricted longer for infants with severe cardiorespiratory disorders, renal failure, and postasphyxial syndrome.
   c. Infants with ongoing fluid losses (chest tube drainage, gastric drainage, enterostomy drainage, diarrhea) may need replacement of these volumes with appropriate fluids.
   d. It is generally recommended to use birth weight, rather than current body weight, to calculate fluids on a per-kilogram basis until birth weight is regained.
3. Fluid constituents.
   a. Dextrose 10% in water is most commonly used for initial fluid therapy. Decreasing dextrose concentrations may be prescribed initially for infants who weighed less than 1 kg at birth, because of the incidence of hyperglycemia in this population.
   b. Electrolytes are not usually added to maintenance intravenous (IV) fluids for the first 24 to 48 hours after birth. Serum electrolyte levels and urine output are used to determine when to add these electrolytes to IV fluids.

E. **Assessment of fluid balance:** Quantifying fluid requirements in extremely preterm infants is difficult. Fluid restriction places the infant at risk for dehydration, whereas fluid excess places the infant at risk for intravascular fluid overload (Jones et al., 2011). Close monitoring of hydration status is imperative, with some infants requiring assessment of their fluid balance as often as every 6 to 8 hours.

1. Body weight: Weight changes with alterations in fluid balance only if there is a net change in TBW; internal shifts of body fluid may not be detected by weight alone. Because the procedure for weighing the extremely low birth weight (ELBW) infant is prone to errors and a significant source of stress for the infant, some neonatal intensive care units have abandoned weighing these infants in the first few days after birth. In-bed electronic scales may be used; however, weights obtained in this manner can be affected by the amount of equipment attached to the infant and how the neonate is handled during weighing.
2. Urine volume: For greatest possible accuracy, urine output must be measured right after it occurs; urine collected onto diapers lying under radiant warmers may evaporate before the diapers are weighed for determination of output.
3. Specific gravity of urine: an indirect measure of urine osmolality. Normal values (1.002 to 1.012) reflect a normal urine osmolality (100 to 300 mOsm/L). Specific gravity is an unreliable predictor of urine osmolality if glucose, blood, or protein is present.
4. Assessment parameters:
   a. Physical assessment: quality of skin turgor, mucous membranes, presence of edema, appearance of eyes, and level of anterior fontanelle.
   b. Hemodynamic assessment: pulse quality, blood pressure, and perfusion (capillary refill time, temperature, and acid–base balance).
5. Laboratory evaluation of hydration status: serum sodium level, osmolality, blood urea nitrogen (BUN), creatinine, and/or hematocrit.

## DISORDERS OF FLUID BALANCE

Disorders of fluid balance in the newborn infant do not always fit neatly into categories such as "fluid depletion" or "fluid excess"; some involve elements of both. One such disorder is septic shock, in which low intravascular volume (a fluid deficit) can coexist with interstitial and cellular edema (a fluid surplus). For simplicity, an attempt is made here to group clinical conditions according to the primary effect on TBW (e.g., decreased, as in dehydration, or increased, as in congestive heart failure), even though there may be an overlap.

### Fluid Depletion

A. **Pathophysiology:** Fluid can be lost from the body acutely or gradually. Sudden loss of body fluid can result in signs and symptoms of shock. If lost fluid is not restored, the body will attempt to compensate by retaining sodium and water. Gradual or chronic fluid loss, even though central blood pressure may be maintained, can result in serious metabolic disturbances.

B. **Causes and precipitating factors.**
   1. Extreme prematurity (<28 weeks of gestation, <800 g). The large TEWL and rapid contraction of the ECF result in a sodium excess that cannot be excreted efficiently by the kidneys. If fluid intake is inadequate, hyperosmolar hypernatremic dehydration ensues.
   2. Acute blood loss/hypovolemia: hemorrhagic losses at birth, postnatal internal hemorrhage, surgical blood loss, or the removal of large volumes for laboratory tests.
   3. Diarrhea.
   4. Diabetes insipidus (pure renal water loss from failure to secrete or respond to ADH). This condition is treated with intranasally administered arginine vasopressin (DDAVP).
   5. Abdominal or pleural cavity exposure during surgery.
   6. Unreplaced losses from gastric suction.
   7. Medications that may cause diuresis: caffeine and theophylline.
   8. Breastfeeding malnutrition: inadequate intake in a breastfed infant with a cycle of reduced milk production and decreasing demand, resulting in severe malnutrition, dehydration, and hypernatremia.

C. **Clinical presentation and assessment.**
   1. Weight loss if net reduction in TBW.
   2. Low urine output (<0.5 mL/kg/hr); possibly high specific gravity. Urine output may be normal or even high in the ELBW infant during postnatal diuresis.

3. Poor skin turgor (gently pinched skin is slow to retract) and dry skin and mucous membranes.
4. Hemodynamic changes: tachycardia or decreased pulses with peripheral vasoconstriction (pale, cool, mottled skin with prolonged capillary filling time), increased core–peripheral temperature differential, central blood pressure either normal or low.
5. In breastfeeding malnutrition, possible excessive sleepiness, disinterest in feeding, or irritability.

D. **Diagnostic studies.**
1. Serum sodium can be low, normal, or high, depending on the cause of dehydration/fluid loss.
2. With dehydration, BUN and creatinine levels may be elevated.
3. Hematocrit levels may be increased or decreased with blood loss.
4. Blood gas values may reveal metabolic acidosis in the infant with hypovolemia.

E. **Patient care management.**
1. Hypovolemic states (shock, hemorrhage) are managed acutely with volume replacement and vasoactive inotropic agents (see Chapter 28).
2. The type of fluid given to replace other fluid deficits depends on the constituents of lost fluid (e.g., free water loss, electrolyte loss) and the infant's electrolyte levels. Determination of the fluid constitution can be guided by evaluating the electrolyte composition of the fluid being lost.
3. Management of severe dehydration involves replacing the free water deficit slowly over several days to avoid a rapid fall in serum osmolality.

F. **Fluid management of hypernatremic hyperosmolar dehydration in the preterm infant.**
1. Prevention of TEWL is more effective than replacing these losses. This is because the fluid lost is mostly solute free, whereas replacement fluids contain solutes that can aggravate hyperosmolality.
2. The single method or combination of methods most effective in reducing TEWL has yet to be proved. Each of the following strategies will decrease TEWL to some degree.
   a. Use of incubators rather than radiant warmers. TEWL is higher under radiant warmers because of the lower ambient relative humidity and increased air currents the neonate is exposed to when on a radiant warmer.
   b. Supplemental humidity. Devices to saturate the air immediately surrounding the infant can be used with both incubators and radiant warmers. Humidifier temperature, airflow setting, and seasonal ambient relative humidity variations can significantly affect the achievable humidity level.
   c. Heat shields or plastic film "blankets" increase ambient humidity by using the infant's own trapped evaporative losses.
   d. Semipermeable dressings (adhesive or nonadhesive) may help reduce TEWL.
3. Reduce respiratory water losses by using humidified gas mixtures.
4. Even with maximal reductions in IWL, fluid intake must occasionally be increased, especially in ELBW infants. Giving too much fluid in response to hypernatremic dehydration can aggravate hyperglycemia and increase the risk of heart failure, pulmonary edema, and central nervous system (CNS) injury. It is usually recommended to give just enough fluid to maintain the serum sodium in the high normal range (145 to 150 mEq/L) during the first 24 to 72 hours of life (Jones et al., 2011).
5. Restrict sodium (unless the infant is hyponatremic), adding gradually when serum sodium level decreases and diuresis begins.
6. Monitor hydration closely. Weight loss may be accepted if other parameters indicate adequate hydration.

G. **Complications.**
1. Excessive weight loss.
2. Hypotension, tissue damage, or metabolic acidosis from hypoperfusion.
3. Impaired excretion of drugs when urine output is minimal.
4. Electrolyte imbalances from slow excretion of daily solute load.
5. Renal failure and vascular thrombosis: possible result of severe dehydration.

## Fluid Excess

A. **Pathophysiology:** The spectrum of disease that can cause body fluid excess in the neonate is broad. Many of the disorders are characterized by edema, which is the abnormal accumulation of ECF within the interstitial spaces. Edema can be caused by the following:
   1. Low colloid osmotic pressure (decreased plasma protein concentration).
   2. Increased capillary permeability to water and protein (may be secondary to tissue hypoxia).
   3. Increased hydrostatic pressure within the capillaries.
   4. Impaired lymphatic drainage of interstitial fluids and proteins.

With some of the disorders associated with these pathologic processes, a combination of venous congestion, renal failure, and edema suggests a state of fluid overload even when circulating blood volume is low.

B. **Etiologies and precipitating factors.**
   1. Cardiac dysfunction: congenital heart disease, congestive heart failure, PDA.
   2. Respiratory distress syndrome and bronchopulmonary dysplasia (BPD). Therapeutic use of oxygen and positive pressure ventilation causes endothelial injury with subsequent fluid leakage. In the first few days after birth, increased lung fluid complicates the picture of respiratory distress and failure to clear the fluid adds to the possibility of developing BPD (Blackburn, 2013; Martin and Crowley, 2013).
   3. Perinatal asphyxia.
   4. Sepsis, necrotizing enterocolitis.
   5. Hydrops fetalis.
   6. Renal failure.
   7. Miscalculation of fluid needs or provision of too much fluid (possibly from failure to account for all sources of fluid, such as flush solutions, medications, and colloids).
   8. Use of neuromuscular blocking agents.
   9. Syndrome of inappropriate antidiuretic hormone (SIADH): usually associated with CNS infection or injury. ADH secretion is inappropriate to usual osmotic and volume stimuli. The result is fluid retention with hyponatremia, low serum osmolality, and high urinary sodium loss.

C. **Clinical presentation and assessment.**
   1. Weight gain, if there is a net increase in TBW.
   2. Urine output: possible decrease.
   3. Edema: peripheral, generalized, pulmonary.
   4. Hemodynamic changes: dependent on intravascular volume status. When increased, there may be symptomatic PDA, tachycardia, and increased pulses or blood pressure. With congestive heart failure, venous filling pressure is high.

D. **Diagnostic studies.**
   1. Serum osmolality is low (<280 mOsm/L); urine osmolality is normal.
   2. In SIADH, osmolalities and sodium levels of urine and serum are diagnostic (urine output is low with high specific gravity and high sodium levels; serum has low sodium level and low osmolality).

E. **Patient care management:** In addition to therapy aimed at the underlying disease process:
   1. Precise fluid management with fluid restriction is necessary. Daily fluid calculations must take into account renal function and the extra fluids given to administer medications and flush intravascular catheters.
   2. Diuretics may be useful.
   3. Infants with severe edema and low intravascular volume (shock) present a challenge. Maintenance of an adequate circulating blood volume may require volume expansion and vasoactive agents while minimizing maintenance fluid administration.
   4. Edema may predispose the infant to necrotic injury of the skin. The skin must be protected from pressure with careful repositioning, support, and the use of a nonrigid sleeping surface, such as a gel- or water-filled mattress.

F. **Complications.**
   1. Fluid sequestration in static body fluid compartments ("third spacing") can result in a loss of effective blood volume, compromising the delivery of oxygen and nutrients to tissues

throughout the body. This can lead not only to serious metabolic imbalances but also to permanent tissue damage.

2. Excessive fluid administration early in life has been associated with worsening of respiratory distress syndrome and development of BPD, symptomatic PDA, and necrotizing enterocolitis.

## ELECTROLYTE BALANCE AND DISORDERS

### Sodium

A. **Sodium homeostasis:** Reference ranges vary slightly between laboratories. In general, a range of 135 to 145 mEq/L is acceptable.

1. Functions of sodium (Na). Na, the major extracellular cation, is closely involved in water balance. Na and other electrolytes are found in varying concentrations in all body fluid compartments. Electrolytes determine the tonicity of the fluid compartment and influence the passage of water through the vascular and cell membranes, thereby controlling the osmotic equilibrium between compartments. With a surplus of Na, blood becomes hypertonic, causing a shift of fluid from intracellular to extracellular spaces, which results in cellular dehydration. A deficit of Na causes hypotonicity and fluid shifts into the cells (cellular edema).
2. Regulation of Na. Cellular transport of Na is achieved by the sodium–potassium pump, which maintains the electrochemical Na and potassium gradients across the cell membrane. Renal (GFR, tubular function) and hormonal (aldosterone, ADH) mechanisms influence the body content of Na. Although preterm infants can excrete Na, a low GFR early in life may hamper this ability. In addition, minimal responsiveness to aldosterone and ADH contributes to a baseline salt-wasting tendency.
3. Positive Na balance. Na intake greater than Na losses. This is a prerequisite for the growth of new tissue.

B. **Hyponatremia.**

1. Pathophysiology: A serum Na below 130 mEq/dL. Reflects either an excess of body water relative to normal body Na content or a primary Na depletion. When urinary Na wasting occurs, a proportionate loss of water (isotonic dehydration) can reduce ECF volume and lead to oliguria.
2. Causes and precipitating factors.
   a. Prematurity (renal and hormonal immaturity, with tendency to excrete Na). Preterm infants are most vulnerable to hyponatremia just after the period of postnatal extracellular volume contraction (Guignard and Sulyok, 2013; Jones et al., 2011).
   b. Conditions associated with low intravascular volume (e.g., shock). Baroreceptor stimulation of ADH results in reduced renal water excretion and a dilutional hyponatremia.
   c. Dilutional hyponatremia from excessive free water intake.
   d. Renal losses related to prematurity or medications (furosemide, methylxanthines). Urine Na excretion rate should be measured to rule out excessive Na losses.
   e. Inadequate Na intake during period of rapid growth, especially in preterm infants fed exclusively human milk. Called *late hyponatremia* because it occurs after the first week of life.
   f. Serum Na can be factitiously low in the presence of hyperlipidemia.
3. Clinical presentation and assessment.
   a. Usually asymptomatic, but apnea, irritability, twitching, or seizures can occur if Na drops acutely or falls to less than 115 mEq/L.
   b. Infants with late hyponatremia may fail to gain weight.
4. Patient care management.
   a. Provide Na supplementation after postnatal diuresis begins (usually on day 2). Maintenance Na requirement is 1 to 4 mEq/kg/day and is usually given as sodium chloride (NaCl), though sodium acetate or sodium bicarbonate ($NaHCO_3$), may be used if the infant has metabolic acidosis. In very small infants, early Na supplementation has been associated with increased risk of BPD (Posencheg and Evans, 2013).
   b. A chronic hyponatremic state is corrected gradually over 48 to 72 hours to prevent injury to brain cells (Posencheg and Evans, 2013).
   c. Monitor weight, urine output, parameters of hydration, and adequacy of intravascular volume (monitoring of central venous pressure, capillary refill time, and core–peripheral temperature differential).

d. When hyponatremia is associated with an excess of body water, fluids are restricted. True SIADH is managed with fluid restriction and monitoring of Na, osmolality, and urine output.

e. Commercial preparations designed to fortify human milk supply additional dietary Na for this population.

5. Complications.

a. Acute drops in the serum Na can lead to a shift of fluid into brain cells and cellular edema. This may result in apnea and seizures.

b. The degree to which the infant's brain may be able to adapt to chronic hyponatremia is not known; however, chronic hyponatremia does impair skeletal and tissue growth.

C. **Hypernatremia.**

1. Pathophysiology: A serum Na level greater than 150 mEq/L. Usually reflects a deficiency of water relative to total body Na content and thus is actually a disorder of water balance rather than one of Na balance.

2. Causes and precipitating factors.

a. Excessive IWL with insufficient fluid intake (even without added Na).

b. High inadvertent Na intake (saline infusions in arterial catheters, $NaHCO_3$, medications) or early addition of maintenance NaCl.

c. Breastfeeding malnutrition in term infants. Elevated human milk Na content accompanying insufficient lactation and decreased amount of free water contribute to the hyperosmolar state.

d. Diabetes insipidus: deficiency of pituitary-secreted ADH, causing loss of water in excess of loss of Na.

3. Clinical presentation and assessment.

a. Signs of dehydration may be present.

b. In severe hypernatremia, high-pitched cry, lethargy, irritability, and apnea can progress to seizures and coma.

4. Patient care management.

a. Gradually restrict Na to avoid sudden fall in plasma osmolality. If maintenance Na administration has not been started, it is usually delayed.

b. Recalculate fluid intake. Fluids may have been restricted too much in light of insensible losses.

c. Prevent hypernatremia in ELBW infants. Na supplementation may be withheld longer than usual after birth if serum Na level remains normal. In addition, measures to reduce TEWL will aid in the prevention of hypernatremia (Jones et al., 2011; Posencheg and Evans, 2013).

d. The need for saline solutions to maintain catheter patency presents a dilemma. Attempts to lower the infused Na concentration too far result in administration of hypotonic solutions, with risk of hemolysis.

5. Complications: As hypernatremia develops, intracellular water can be drawn out, causing cells to shrink. If this process is rapid, this can affect the brain. Sudden increases in plasma osmolality can also contribute to intraventricular hemorrhage.

## Potassium

A. **Potassium homeostasis:** A generally accepted reference range is 3.5 to 5.5 mEq/L.

1. Functions of potassium (K): The major cation in ICF, K contributes to intracellular osmotic activity and in part determines ICF volume. K plays a fundamental role along with Na in regulating cell membrane potential.

2. Regulation: K is distributed both intracellularly and extracellularly. The distribution of K between ICF and ECF is regulated by the sodium–potassium pump and is influenced by acid–base balance, insulin, and glucagon. The excretion of K from the body depends on kidney function, GFR, urine flow rate, and aldosterone sensitivity.

B. **Hypokalemia:** Serum K less than 3.5 mEq/L.

1. Pathophysiology: Because K is 90% intracellular, it is assessed indirectly by measuring the quantity in the serum. A subnormal serum K implies insufficient K within the cells, which

may impede their function. Muscle cells of the gastrointestinal system and the heart can be affected.

2. Causes and precipitating factors.
   a. Loss of K in the urine (kaliuresis) during postnatal diuresis, before K supplementation is begun.
   b. Inadequate K intake.
   c. Increased gastrointestinal losses from an enterostomy or nasogastric tube output or vomiting.
   d. Metabolic alkalosis. A high serum pH drives K into cells, resulting in a low serum K.
   e. Medications including bicarbonate, diuretics, and insulin. Insulin increases cellular uptake of K through stimulation of activity of the sodium–potassium pump.
3. Clinical presentation and assessment: cardiac effects (flattened T waves, prominent U waves, ST segment depression), hypotonia, abdominal distention, and ileus.
4. Patient care management.
   a. Begin K supplementation when urine output is well established, usually on the second or third day of life. The maintenance K requirement is 2 to 3 mEq/kg/day.
   b. Correction of hypokalemic states must be done cautiously, with continuous cardiac monitoring.
5. Complications.
   a. Rapid administration of K to correct hypokalemia can lead to fatal arrhythmias.
   b. Hypokalemia potentiates digitalis toxicity.

C. **Hyperkalemia:** Serum K greater than 6.5 mEq/L.
1. Pathophysiology: Heel-stick samples are often hemolyzed, rendering results unreliable. Venipuncture or arterial line sample must be obtained to determine level. In the ELBW infant, the normal postnatal shift of K from the intracellular to the extracellular compartment is intensified. During the prediuretic phase, this excess K is not efficiently excreted secondary to a low GFR and a low Na excretion rate (Eichenwald, 2013).
2. Causes and precipitating factors.
   a. Extreme prematurity. Nonoliguric hyperkalemia (hyperkalemia in the absence of renal failure) most likely secondary to shift in K from intracellular space to extracellular space.
   b. Endogenous release of K from tissue destruction, hypoperfusion, hemorrhage, and bruising.
   c. Metabolic acidosis. A low serum pH shifts K out of cells.
   d. Renal failure, with decreased K clearance. Tests of renal function: BUN, creatinine should be measured concomitantly.
   e. Adrenal insufficiency.
   f. Transfusion with blood stored longer than 3 days.
3. Clinical presentation and assessment: Cardiac effects may be seen—ventricular tachycardia, peaked T wave, or a widened QRS complex. An electrocardiogram should be obtained to detect cardiac arrhythmias. Serum ionized calcium should also be assessed as hypocalcemia may potentiate cardiac toxicity from hyperkalemia.
4. Patient care management.
   a. For prevention of hyperkalemia, K is withheld from early IV fluids. Serum K is monitored as diuresis (and K excretion) begins; K is added when serum K stabilizes in the 4- to 4.5-mEq/L range.
   b. Acidosis is corrected.
   c. Diuretics and low-dose dopamine therapy may improve renal excretion of K. Dopamine also enhances K uptake by stimulation of activity of the sodium–potassium pump.
   d. Temporary measures may be needed to reduce the effects of circulating K until the total body K level can be reduced.
      (1) Administration of calcium gluconate will lower the cell membrane threshold transiently, antagonizing the effects on the heart muscle.
      (2) Glucose/insulin infusion to enhance cellular uptake of K. Close monitoring of serum glucose is imperative with this strategy, and the clinician should anticipate the need for increasing the glucose infusion rate. The insulin infusion tubing must be primed to ensure delivery of the drug once the infusion is begun.
      (3) $NaHCO_3$ (metabolic alkalosis shifts K into cells).

e. When other measures fail to normalize K:
   (1) Cation exchange resins are not the preferred treatment for neonates and should be used only in those infants with refractory hyperkalemia. Oral administration is not recommended in infants. Sodium polystyrene sulfonate (Kayexalate) exchanges Na for K in the intestine to increase the excretion of K. Because the onset of action is within 2 to 24 hours, treatment with this medication alone may not be sufficient to rapidly correct severe hyperkalemia (Taketamo et al., 2012).
   (2) Exchange transfusion.
   (3) Peritoneal dialysis or continuous arteriovenous hemofiltration for severe, intractable hyperkalemia.

5. Complications.
   a. Hyperkalemia is life threatening because of the risk of cardiac arrest.
   b. Sodium polystyrene sulfonate (Kayexalate) can cause hypocalcemia, hypomagnesemia, and hypernatremia.

## Calcium

A. **Calcium homeostasis:** A reference range of 8.5 to 10.2 mg/dL is generally used for serum calcium (Ca). Some care providers prefer to follow the ionized calcium (iCa). An acceptable reference range for iCa is 4.4 to 5.3 mg/dL.
   1. Functions of Ca: Ca plays a central role in many physiologic processes, maintaining cell membrane permeability and activating enzyme reactions for muscle contraction, nerve transmission, and blood clotting. Ca is vital for normal cardiac function and development of the skeleton, where 99% of the body's Ca is stored.
   2. Regulation:
      a. Parathyroid hormone (PTH) increases serum Ca by mobilizing Ca from the bone and intestines and reducing renal excretion of Ca. PTH is stimulated by low serum Ca and magnesium (Mg) levels and is suppressed by high Ca and Mg levels.
      b. Vitamin D acts with PTH to restore Ca to normal levels by increasing absorption of Ca and phosphorus from the intestines and bone.
      c. Calcitonin, a Ca counterregulatory hormone secreted from thyroid C cells, lowers Ca levels primarily by inhibiting bone resorption.
      d. Phosphorus (P) also inhibits the absorption of Ca (the higher the P, the lower the absorption of Ca).
   3. Serum Ca is transported in three forms:
      a. Protein-bound Ca, accounting for 40% of total serum Ca.
      b. Inactivated Ca (complexed with anions such as bicarbonate, lactate, and citrate), accounting for 10% of total serum Ca.
      c. Free ionized calcium (iCa), the physiologically active form that can cross the cell membrane, accounting for 50% of the total serum Ca. Blood pH influences the amount of iCa: acidosis increases iCa, and alkalosis decreases iCa.

B. **Fetal Ca metabolism:** Fetal Ca needs are met by active transport of Ca across the placenta. Ca accretion increases during the last trimester as Ca is incorporated into newly forming bones. Because maternal PTH and calcitonin do not cross the placenta, the fetus is relatively hypercalcemic, which suppresses fetal PTH and stimulates fetal calcitonin.

C. **Neonatal Ca metabolism:** When the supply of Ca ceases at birth, the neonate depends on stored and dietary Ca to avoid hypocalcemia. After birth, the Ca level declines to its nadir by 24 hours of age, but PTH activity remains low. By 48 to 72 hours, PTH and vitamin D levels rise and the calcitonin level declines, allowing Ca to be mobilized. The serum Ca level returns to normal despite a low Ca intake. Approximately 16% of infants born less than 32 weeks of gestation develop nephrocalcinosis in the face of normal serum Ca levels (Kenagy and Vogt, 2013). Development is multifactorial but is associated with increased furosemide use, increased gentamicin levels, and extreme prematurity.

D. **Hypocalcemia:** Serum Ca less than 7 mg/dL or iCa less than 4.4 mg/dL.
   1. Pathophysiology: Failure to achieve Ca homeostasis after birth can result from inadequate Ca stores, immature hormonal control, inability to mobilize Ca, or interference with Ca use.

Hypocalcemia increases cellular permeability to Na ions and increases cell membrane excitability.

2. Causes and precipitating factors.
   a. "Early" hypocalcemia.
      (1) Prematurity: reduced Ca stores and relative hypoparathyroidism (blunted PTH response to hypocalcemia).
      (2) Infant of a diabetic mother (IDM): prolonged delay in PTH production by infant after birth.
      (3) Placental insufficiency: reduced Ca stores.
      (4) Perinatal asphyxia and stress, which precipitate a surge in calcitonin that suppresses Ca. In addition, tissue damage and glycogen breakdown release phosphorus into the circulation, which decreases Ca uptake.
      (5) Maternal anticonvulsant therapy, which affects hepatic enzymes involved in vitamin D metabolism.
      (6) Low intake of Ca.
      (7) Factors that may decrease iCa even when the total serum Ca is normal: exchange transfusion, IV administration of lipid emulsion, alkalosis, or alkali therapy for acidosis.
   b. "Late" hypocalcemia.
      (1) Hypomagnesemia.
      (2) Transient congenital hypoparathyroidism or secondary hypoparathyroidism from maternal hyperparathyroidism. An increased PTH level in the mother raises the fetal Ca level and suppresses the fetal parathyroid gland. After birth, the suppressed gland cannot maintain a normal Ca level.
      (3) DiGeorge syndrome: absence of thymus and parathyroid glands.
      (4) High-phosphate formulas or cereals. The neonate cannot excrete the excess phosphate; the hyperphosphatemia suppresses Ca.
      (5) Intestinal malabsorption.
3. Clinical presentation and assessment.
   a. Early hypocalcemia is usually asymptomatic; signs of neuromuscular excitability (jitteriness, twitching) may be present.
   b. Severe hypocalcemia (neonatal tetany) is rare and presents with jitteriness, seizures, high-pitched cry, laryngospasm, stridor, and a prolonged Q–T interval.
4. Patient care management.
   a. Monitor serum Ca of infants at risk: premature, IDM, asphyxiated.
   b. Early, mild hypocalcemia often resolves without treatment.
   c. Serious hypocalcemia is treated with boluses and/or continuous infusions of calcium gluconate (can also be given orally).
   d. Treatment of late hypocalcemia depends on the underlying cause.
5. Complications.
   a. Rapid infusion of Ca can cause bradycardia or cardiac arrest. Infusions for rapid correction of hypocalcemia should be administered slowly, over 20 to 30 minutes by syringe pump, while the heart rate is monitored.
   b. Tissue necrosis and calcifications can result from extravasated Ca infusions.
   c. Intestinal necrosis and liver necrosis have been reported with Ca infusion given via incorrectly placed umbilical catheters.

**E. Metabolic bone disease.**

1. Pathophysiology: Infants born prematurely can miss all or most of the period of greatest intrauterine mineral accretion, which places them at risk of having inadequate postnatal bone mineralization. The primary cause of metabolic bone disease (MBD) is inadequate Ca and P intake, rather than vitamin D deficiency.
2. Causes and precipitating factors.
   a. Prematurity: the more immature the infant, the higher the MBD rate.
   b. Parenteral nutrition: low Ca and P intakes.

c. Unsupplemented human milk feeding (inadequate Ca and P content) or use of formulas not designed for the preterm infant.
d. BPD secondary to fluid restriction and use of diuretics, with renal Ca wasting.
3. Clinical presentation and assessment.
a. MBD is asymptomatic; it is often detected initially on routine x-ray examination.
b. Skeletal fractures may be seen in the thoracic cage or extremities.
c. Other reported presentation is late-onset respiratory distress from "softening" of the ribs.
d. Pain may occur with handling; close monitoring of response is necessary.
4. Diagnostic tests.
a. Serum: normal Ca, low P, high alkaline phosphatase, and high 1,2,5-dihydroxyvitamin D levels. Ca and P levels alone are not good indicators of MBD.
b. Urine: low or absent P excretion; increased urinary Ca.
c. Radiologic bone examinations; wrist x-ray films at age 6 to 8 weeks may be used to monitor for MBD. Early evidence can be difficult to discern because bone mineral content must decrease by 30% to be visible. Photon absorptiometry may be done in centers where the necessary equipment is available.
d. X-ray examination; findings may include "washed out" (undermineralized) bones, known as osteopenia, or epiphyseal dysplasia and skeletal deformities, known as rickets (Rubin, 2013).
5. Patient care management and prevention of MBD.
a. Maintain Ca/P ratio in parenteral nutrition at 1.3:1 to 1.7:1.
b. For enteral feeding, use preterm formulas or human milk supplementation.
c. Direct supplementation of Ca and P may be needed. Ca given without P will be inadequately used, resulting in hypercalciuria and possibly nephrocalcinosis.
d. Gentle handling of infants at risk and avoidance of chest physiotherapy are warranted to prevent fractures.

F. **Hypercalcemia:** Serum Ca greater than 11 mg/dL or iCa greater than 5.8 mg/dL.
1. Pathophysiology: A rise in the serum Ca level can rapidly overwhelm the infant's compensatory mechanisms for Ca equilibrium. An excess supply of Ca has multiple effects and is potentially lethal.
2. Causes and precipitating factors.
a. Iatrogenic: overtreatment with Ca or vitamin D.
b. Hyperparathyroidism: primary neonatal disorder or secondary to maternal hypoparathyroidism, with chronic stimulation of the fetal parathyroid gland. In hyperparathyroidism the serum Ca level is high, phosphate levels may be low, and urinary Ca and phosphate excretion are high.
c. Phosphate depletion: caused by low dietary intake; may be associated with low phosphate content in human milk.
d. Subcutaneous fat necrosis: found over the back and limbs; associated with difficult delivery, hypothermia, and maternal diabetes. Pathogenic mechanism is unknown.
e. Familial infantile hypercalcemia.
f. Hypervitaminosis D: excessive maternal intake of vitamin D.
3. Clinical presentation and assessment.
a. Hypotonia, weakness, irritability, and poor feeding, all from a direct effect of Ca on the CNS.
b. Bradycardia.
c. Constipation.
d. Polyuria, dehydration (associated with severe hypercalcemia).
4. Patient care management.
a. Hydrate infant and promote excretion of Ca (furosemide has calciuretic action).
b. Restrict Ca and vitamin D intake; increase phosphate intake.
5. Complications.
a. Nephrocalcinosis from hypercalciuria, but may be seen with normal serum Ca levels.
b. Metastatic calcification of damaged cells or tissues throughout the body, including the brain.
c. Cardiac effects: bradycardia and arrhythmias.

## Magnesium

A. **Magnesium (Mg) homeostasis.** A reference range of 1.5 to 2.5 mg/dL is usually accepted.
   1. Functions: Magnesium (Mg) is a catalyst for many intracellular enzyme reactions, including muscle contraction and carbohydrate metabolism, and is critical for normal parathyroid function and bone–serum Ca homeostasis. Mg is regulated primarily by the kidneys.
   2. Fetal and neonatal Mg homeostasis: The fetus receives its supply of Mg by active transport across the placenta. Maternal health and diet can influence the amount of Mg accrued by the fetus. After birth, Mg level falls along with Ca level, then rises to normal within 48 hours.
   3. Serum total Mg versus the ionized form: Ionized Mg (iMg) is the biologically active fraction of Mg. Total Mg concentration in the serum does not necessarily reflect iMg activity.
   4. Concurrent use of Mg and gentamicin potentiates the neuroblocking effect of the Mg, which may result in apnea. Clinical status must be monitored closely. Slow infusion times for gentamicin are indicated (Taketamo et al., 2012).

B. **Hypomagnesemia:** Serum Mg level less than 1.5 mg/dL.
   1. Pathophysiology: A low neonatal Mg level is directly related to the maternal level before birth. Although an acute decline in Mg stimulates PTH release, chronic Mg deficiency suppresses PTH and blocks the hormone's actions on the bone and kidneys. Hypocalcemia ensues.
   2. Causes and precipitating factors.
      a. Decreased Mg supply: prematurity, placental insufficiency and intrauterine growth restriction, low dietary intake.
      b. Increased Mg losses: renal and intestinal disorders, including renal tubular acidosis, diarrhea, short bowel syndrome.
      c. Endocrine causes: neonatal hypoparathyroidism, maternal hyperparathyroidism.
   3. Clinical presentation and assessment.
      a. Tremors, irritability, and hyperreflexia, progressing to seizures.
      b. Failure to respond to therapy for hypocalcemia: hypomagnesemia a possibility.
   4. Patient care management.
      a. If hypomagnesemia is severe, administration of magnesium sulfate may be necessary to relieve symptoms until Ca balance is restored.
      b. Seizures are usually unresponsive to anticonvulsant agents.
   5. Complications: Overtreatment with magnesium sulfate can result in hypotonia and respiratory depression, hypotension, and cardiac arrhythmias.

C. **Hypermagnesemia:** Serum Mg greater than 2.5 mg/dL.
   1. Pathophysiology: Excess Mg is slow to be excreted by the neonatal kidneys. Very high Mg levels can cause CNS and neuromuscular depression.
   2. Causes and precipitating factors.
      a. Excessive Mg load: magnesium sulfate treatment in labor, excess administration of Mg to neonate.
      b. Reduced excretion of Mg: renal failure, oliguria.
   3. Clinical presentation and assessment (may be asymptomatic).
      a. Respiratory depression, apnea.
      b. Neuromuscular depression: lethargy, poor suck, loss of reflexes, flaccidity, hypotonia.
      c. Gastrointestinal hypomotility, abdominal distention.
   4. Patient care management.
      a. Prepare to resuscitate infants born to mothers receiving large doses of magnesium sulfate.
      b. Hypermagnesemia usually resolves with adequate hydration and urine output. Mg excretion can be increased with furosemide.
      c. If infant is unresponsive to treatment, exchange transfusion may be necessary.
   5. Complications: Cardiac arrest and respiratory failure are possible.

# ACID–BASE BALANCE AND DISORDERS

## Acid–Base Physiology

A. **pH:** Acid–base balance is normal when the pH of the blood is between 7.35 and 7.45. The pH is determined by the hydrogen ion ($H^+$) concentration in the ECF. An acid is an $H^+$ donor; a base is an $H^+$ receptor. A complex system of buffers, compensation, and excretion regulates the $H^+$ concentration, thus keeping the pH in the normal range. Note that normal fetal pH is between 7.25 and 7.35 and the clinician should expect values obtained during the early transition period to reflect this lower pH.

B. **Buffering system:** This is the first line of defense against excess $H^+$ concentration. Buffers, including bicarbonate ($HCO_3^-$), plasma proteins, and hemoglobin, act rapidly to pick up excess $H^+$. The major buffer, $HCO_3^-$, teams with $H^+$ to form carbonic acid, which dissociates into water and $CO_2$ to be eliminated. The normal $HCO_3^-$ level in the neonate is 22 to 26 mEq/L, lower than in the adult.

C. **Lung regulation:** The lungs act to lower the $H^+$ level in the blood by removing $CO_2$, which is produced as a waste product of cellular metabolism. It is then transported to the lungs, where it is removed from the body by ventilation. The rate of $CO_2$ removal can be increased or decreased by altering minute ventilation.

D. **Kidney regulation:** The kidney acts to maintain equilibrium between acids and bases in the body by reabsorbing $HCO_3^-$ and other buffers and by excreting $H^+$ and other acids. In this way, the body eliminates the daily load of nonvolatile acids produced by normal metabolism.

E. **Compensation:** When one or more of the body's regulatory systems fail, other systems have a limited ability to maintain the acid–base equilibrium. When the pH is outside the normal range ($<7.35$ or $>7.45$), compensation has failed.
   1. An acid–base deviation is respiratory if it is due to an abnormal $P_{CO_2}$ and metabolic if it is due to an abnormal level of plasma $HCO_3^-$.
   2. The lungs attempt to compensate for a metabolic aberration, and the kidneys for a respiratory aberration. The result is a change in pH toward normal despite an abnormal blood $P_{CO_2}$ or $HCO_3^-$. The lungs compensate much more quickly than the kidneys; however, neither can totally normalize the pH unless the underlying disorder is corrected.

## Disorders of Acid–Base Balance

Only those disorders classified as primary metabolic problems are discussed here.

A. **Metabolic acidosis.**
   1. Pathophysiology: A pH of less than 7.35 or serum $HCO_3^-$ of less than 22 mEq/L can result from the loss of $HCO_3^-$ (buffering capacity) or from excess acid production. The immature kidneys contribute to acidosis by failing both to reabsorb $HCO_3^-$ and to excrete $H^+$ when faced with an acid load. When cells do not receive enough oxygen (because of low blood oxygen levels or diminished perfusion), they must use anaerobic metabolism to meet energy needs. This results in the accumulation in the body of lactic acid (lactate), the level of which reflects the severity of tissue oxygen deficiency. Blood lactate may be a more sensitive indicator of tissue hypoxia than pH and base-excess values (Volpe, 2008). Calculation of the anion gap (difference between positive and negative ions) can be a useful tool to differentiate between excess acid and insufficient $HCO_3^-$ as cause of acidosis. Anion gap = (serum $Na^+$ + $K^+$) − (serum $Cl^-$ + $HCO_3^-$ [*or serum* $CO_2$]). Usual range is 8 to 16 mEq/L. If high ($>20$ mEq/L), acidosis is due to excess acid. If normal with elevated chloride level, acidosis is due to loss of $HCO_3^-$.
   2. Causes and precipitating factors.
      a. Loss of $HCO_3^-$: normal anion gap.
         (1) Prematurity: poor renal conservation of $HCO_3^-$.
         (2) Renal tubular acidosis: decreased proximal reabsorption.
         (3) Severe diarrhea or ileal drainage.
      b. Excess acid load: ingestion or endogenous production of acid, greater than the ability to excrete it; increased anion gap.
         (1) Lactic acidosis from conditions resulting in hypoxia or hypoperfusion: respiratory distress, congenital heart disease, PDA, sepsis, asphyxia, or shock/hypovolemia. Plasma lactate level greater than 2.5 mmol/L; may be elevated in some conditions, such as early sepsis, even when the pH is normal.
         (2) Inborn errors of metabolism: disorders of organic acid and carbohydrate metabolism.
         (3) Caloric deprivation: catabolism of protein or fat for energy.

(4) Parenteral amino acid solutions.
(5) "Late metabolic acidosis" of prematurity, caused by intolerance of cow's milk protein.

3. Clinical presentation and assessment.
   a. Metabolic acidosis occurring early in life is primarily related to systemic illness (e.g., respiratory, cardiac); thus the signs and symptoms are those of the underlying condition(s).
   b. Late metabolic acidosis may present at 1 to 3 weeks of age with poor growth, hyponatremia, and persistent renal acid excretion (urinary pH $<5$). Urinary pH greater than 7 with systemic acidosis suggests renal tubular acidosis.
   c. Infants with profound acidosis (metabolic defects such as congenital lactic acidosis) may have respiratory compensation (tachypnea, hyperpnea) or neurologic depression (seizures, coma) reflecting CNS acidosis.
4. Patient care management.
   a. Treat the underlying cause of acidosis.
   b. Correction of severe acidosis (pH $<7.2$) is usually with $NaHCO_3$ (concentration of 0.5 mEq/mL), in a 1- to 2-mL/kg dose. Administer slowly (over 1 to 2 hours) by syringe pump or continuous drip; rapid increase in osmolality and pH may be dangerous.
   c. Late metabolic acidosis, if not self-correcting, is sometimes treated with oral $NaHCO_3$.
5. Complications.
   a. Severe acidosis: may depress myocardial contractility and cause arteriolar vasodilation, hypotension, and pulmonary edema.
   b. Impaired surfactant production.
   c. Electrolyte imbalance: decreased iCa, hyperkalemia.
   d. Adverse effects of $HCO_3^-$: cerebral hemorrhage or edema related to wide swings in plasma osmolality. Increased cerebral blood flow, more pronounced when infused rapidly (van Alfen-van der Velden et al., 2006). $NaHCO_3$ can also worsen acidosis by rapidly increasing $CO_2$ if lung disease is present and ventilation is inadequate. $NaHCO_3$ can aggravate hypernatremia and cause tissue injury in extravasation.
6. Outcome: In follow-up studies, metabolic acidosis was correlated with poor developmental outcome in VLBW infants (van Alfen-van der Velden et al., 2006).

**B. Metabolic alkalosis.**

1. Pathophysiology: Metabolic alkalosis (pH $>7.45$ or $HCO_3^-$ $>26$ mEq/L) results from an excess of $HCO_3^-$ or from a loss of acid.
2. Causes and precipitating factors.
   a. Gain of $HCO_3^-$ from overcorrection of acidosis with $NaHCO_3$.
   b. Loss of $H^+$ during vomiting or nasogastric suction.
   c. Increased renal acid loss from diuretic therapy.
   d. Rapid ECF reduction (contraction alkalosis).
3. Patient care management.
   a. Decrease $NaHCO_3$ intake if alkali therapy is the cause of alkalosis.
   b. Restoring fluid and electrolyte balance is critical.
4. Complications: Severe alkalosis causes tissue hypoxia, neurologic damage, and electrolyte disturbances (increased iCa, hypokalemia).

(Please refer to Chapter 26 for discussion of respiratory acidosis and respiratory alkalosis.)

## REFERENCES

Bell, E.F. and Acarregui, M.J.: Restricted versus liberal water intake for preventing morbidity and mortality in preterm infants. *Cochrane Database of Systematic Reviews,* (1):CD000503, 2008.

Blackburn, S.T.: *Maternal, fetal, and neonatal physiology: A clinical perspective* (4th ed.). St. Louis, 2013, Elsevier Saunders.

Eichenwald, E.C.: Care of the extremely-low-birth-weight infant. In C.A. Gleason and S.U. Devaskar (Eds.): *Avery's diseases of the newborn* (9th ed.). Philadelphia, 2013, Elsevier Saunders, pp. 390–404.

Guignard, J.P. and Sulyok, E.: Renal morphogenesis and development of renal function. In C.A. Gleason, and S.U. Devaskar (Eds.): *Avery's diseases of the newborn*

(9th ed.). Philadelphia, 2013, Elsevier Saunders, pp. 1165–1175.

Jain, A., Rutter, N. and Cartlidge, P.: Influence of antenatal steroids and sex on maturation of the epidermal barrier in the preterm infant. *Archives of Disease in Childhood: Fetal and Neonatal Edition*, 83(2): F112–F116, 2000.

Jones, J.E., Hayes, R.D., Starbuck, A.L. and Porcelli, P.J.: Fluid and electrolyte management. In S.L. Gardner, B.S. Carter, M. Enzman-Hines, and J.A. Hernandez (Eds.): *Merenstein and Gardner's handbook of neonatal intensive care* (7th ed.). St. Louis, 2011, Elsevier Mosby, pp. 333–352.

Kenagy, D.N. and Vogt, B.A.: The kidney. In A.A. Fanaroff, and J.M. Fanaroff (Eds.): *Klaus & Fanaroff's care of the high-risk neonate* (6th ed.). Philadelphia, 2013, Elsevier Saunders, pp. 410–431.

Lund, C.H. and Kuller, J.M.: Integumentary system. In C. Kenner, and J.W. Lott (Eds.): *Comprehensive neonatal care: An interdisciplinary approach* (4th ed.). St. Louis, 2007, Elsevier Saunders, pp. 65–91.

Martin, R.J. and Crowley, M.A.: Respiratory problems. In A.A. Fanaroff and J.M. Fanaroff (Eds.): *Klaus & Fanaroff's care of the high-risk neonate* (6th ed.). Philadelphia, 2013, Elsevier Saunders, pp. 244–269.

Modi, N., Betremieux, P., Midgley, J. and Hartnoll, G.: Postnatal weight loss and contraction of the extracellular compartment is triggered by atrial natriuretic peptide. *Early Human Development*, 59(3):201–208, 2000.

Posencheg, M.A. and Evans, J.R.: Acid-base, fluid and electrolyte management. In C.A. Gleason, and S.U. Devaskar (Eds.): *Avery's diseases of the newborn* (9th ed.). Philadelphia, 2013, Elsevier Saunders, pp. 367–389.

Rubin, L.P.: Disorders of calcium and phosphorus metabolism. In C.A. Gleason and S.U. Devaskar (Eds.): *Avery's diseases of the newborn* (9th ed.). Philadelphia, 2013, Elsevier Saunders, pp. 1255–1273.

Taketamo, C.K., Hodding, J.H. and Kraus, D.M.: Pediatric Lexi-Comp Drugs [online]. 2012. Available at www.lexi.com; accessed July 15, 2013.

Van Alfen-van der Velden, A.A.E.M., Hopman, J.C.W. Klaessens, J.H.G.M., et al.: Effects of rapid versus slow infusion of sodium bicarbonate on cerebral hemodynamics and oxygenation in preterm infants. *Biology of the Neonate*, 90:122–127, 2006.

Volpe, J.J.: Hypoxic-ischemic encephalopathy: Biochemical and physiological aspects. In J.J. Volpe (Ed.): *Neurology of the newborn* (5th ed.). Philadelphia, 2008, Elsevier Saunders, pp. 247–324.

CHAPTER

# 9 Glucose Management

DEBRA ARMENTROUT

**OBJECTIVES**

1. Describe the mechanisms of glucose homeostasis in the fetus and newborn.
2. Discuss hypoglycemia and hyperglycemia in the neonate.
3. Discuss infants of diabetic mothers.
4. Differentiate neonatal diabetes from hyperglycemia.

Organ systems, especially the human brain, are primarily dependent on glucose as their major energy source. Compared with adults, infants have a higher brain-to-body-weight ratio, resulting in a higher glucose demand in relation to glucose production capacity. Cerebral glucose utilization accounts for 90% of the neonate's total glucose consumption. Continuous glucose and energy delivery to the fetus is provided from the maternal circulation via the placenta so there is no need for fetal glucose production in utero. An essential part of the neonate's successful transition to extrauterine life therefore is the maintenance of euglycemia. Whereas most infants are indeed able to readily adapt to the metabolic demands of extrauterine life, newborns in general remain extremely susceptible to any condition that may impair their ability to establish normal glucose homeostasis during this transition process (Hume et al., 2005; Jain et al., 2012; Kalhan and Devaskar, 2011).

## GLUCOSE HOMEOSTASIS

Glucose is vital for cellular metabolism throughout the body. Blood glucose concentration is determined by the balance between intake/production of glucose and glucose use by the body.

A. **Glucose production.**
   1. Glucose taken in but not used for immediate energy needs is converted to glycogen via glycogenesis and stored in the liver, heart, and skeletal muscles. During fasting, glycogen is broken down to re-form glucose that is then released from the liver in a process known as glycogenolysis. The infant's ability for glycogenolysis varies according to fetal growth and maturity.
   2. The other main source of glucose is gluconeogenesis: production of glucose and glycogen in the liver by means of nonglucose precursors such as lactate, pyruvate, glycerol (fat), and amino acids (Hume et al., 2005; Kalhan and Devaskar, 2011).

B. **Glucose metabolism (Blackburn, 2013; Ogata, 2005).**
   1. Glucose can be metabolized in the body in several ways: production of energy, storage as glycogen, and conversion to gluconeogenic precursors.
   2. In the brain, oxidized glucose provides 99% of the cerebral energy production, a process dependent on a number of important enzymes and reactions.
      a. Glucose molecules are transported across the blood–brain barrier and into the brain cells by glucose transporter proteins.
      b. Within the cytoplasm, glucose is metabolized by glycolysis to pyruvate. Pyruvate is then oxidized to acetyl-coenzyme A (acetyl-CoA), which is transported to the mitochondrion for entry into the citric acid cycle. The end products are carbon dioxide, water, and energy released in the generation of adenosine triphosphate (ATP).
      c. Of importance to the neonate is that during hypoglycemia other substrates (ketone bodies, lactate, glycerol, and amino acids) can also be converted to pyruvate, enter the citric acid cycle, and produce ATP, thus serving as a source of energy for the brain.

**C. Hormonal regulation of glucose homeostasis (Blackburn, 2013; Ogata, 2005).**

1. Insulin: Secreted by the pancreatic beta cells in response to an increase in plasma glucose, insulin decreases the blood glucose level by promoting glycogen formation, suppressing hepatic glucose release, and driving the peripheral uptake of glucose. Insulin does not control the entry of glucose into the brain or liver.
2. Glucagon: Secreted by the pancreatic beta cells when blood glucose levels decrease, glucagon promotes glycogenolysis and gluconeogenesis. Glucagon is called a counterregulatory hormone because it opposes the effect of insulin by raising the blood glucose level. Other counterregulatory hormones include catecholamines, cortisol, and growth hormone. Although these hormones may not be important regulators in the fast-feed cycle of healthy neonates, minimum basal levels may be needed to maintain euglycemia.

**D. Fetal glucose homeostasis.**

1. Glucose reaches the fetus by carrier-facilitated diffusion across the placenta at a concentration of about 70% to 80% of the maternal glucose concentration (Kalhan and Devaskar, 2011).
2. Glycogen storage for postnatal energy needs begins early in gestation, with most glycogen accumulating during the third trimester.
3. Fetal insulin is detectable by 8 to 11 weeks of gestation, but the response to a glucose load is not fully developed even at term (Blackburn, 2013; Stokowski, 2007).
4. The fetus is capable of gluconeogenic activity, using substrates such as lactate if needed to meet metabolic demands in utero.

**E. Neonatal glucose homeostasis.**

1. After cord clamping, the neonate's blood glucose concentration falls, reaching a nadir at 1 to 2 hours of age.
2. In the first postnatal hours, the neonatal brain metabolizes lactate, which is abundant, so that even though the glucose concentration is low, the brain is not fuel deficient.
3. The neonate gradually mobilizes glucose to meet energy needs by secreting glucagon and catecholamines and suppressing insulin release. Thus, even if a healthy term newborn infant is not fed soon after birth, blood glucose levels rise at 3 to 4 hours of age.
4. Hepatic glycogen, however, is rapidly depleted if feeding is not established early and the infant is dependent on gluconeogenesis and lipolysis as the primary modes of maintaining euglycemia (Hume et al., 2005; Kalhan and Devaskar, 2011).

## HYPOGLYCEMIA

**A. Definition of hypoglycemia (Adamkin and Committee on Fetus and Newborn, 2011; Blackburn, 2013; Rozance and Hay, 2006).**

1. Most clinicians believe that, rather than a specific value, neonatal hypoglycemia lies on a continuum of low blood glucose values of varied duration and severity that is influenced by a number of different factors:
   a. Conceptual and postmenstrual age.
   b. Adequacy of gluconeogenic pathways.
   c. General health status.
   d. Presence or absence of symptoms.
2. A widely used cutoff point for plasma glucose concentration is 40 mg/dL as the typical threshold for intervention in both premature and term neonates, with some authors advocating 55 to 70 mg/dL (Rozance and Hay, 2006; Steinkrauss et al., 2005).
3. The optimal range for plasma glucose is 70 to 100 mg/dL, and there is no evidence that neonates have a lower requirement for glucose concentrations, or that the neonatal brain can better tolerate hypoglycemia when compared to older infants and adults (Jain et al., 2012).

**B. Incidence.**

1. Overall incidence is 1 to 5 per 1000 live births.
2. The incidence in at-risk infants may be as high as 30%, occurring in 8% of large-for-gestational-age (LGA) infants and in 15% of premature and small-for-gestational-age (SGA) infants (McGowan, 1999).

**C. Pathophysiology (Blackburn, 2013; Jain et al., 2012; Ogata, 2005).**

1. The immediate postnatal drop in the blood glucose concentration is physiologic. Failure to increase glucose concentrations after 4 hours is pathologic. Subsequently, hypoglycemia is usually a result of inadequate hepatic glucose production that cannot meet peripheral demand or excessive insulin production.
2. Glucose delivery is dependent on blood glucose concentration and blood flow rate. During hypoglycemia, the brain increases blood flow to improve glucose delivery that may predispose the neonatal brain to hemorrhagic and hyperoxic injury if there is diminished cerebral autoregulatory ability.
3. When glucose consumption exceeds delivery, the brain uses alternate fuels such as ketone bodies, lactic acid, free fatty acids, and glycerol if they are available. The production of energy from these sources involves the use of brain structural components such as proteins and phospholipids that may play a contributory role in neuronal damage.
4. Lactic acid becomes elevated in late fetal and early postnatal life and healthy term infants produce ketones effectively on days 2 and 3 of life, thus protecting their brains from fuel deficiency if the blood glucose level falls while feeding becomes established. However, the ability of preterm infants and of infants who are SGA to mount a counterregulatory ketogenic response at any time is severely limited, so these infants are heavily dependent on an adequate glucose supply (Rozance and Hay, 2006).
5. Prolonged hypoglycemia, when not compensated by a supply of alternative fuels, induces biochemical changes at the cellular level that may damage the neuronal and glial cells of the brain. It is thought that an accumulation of excitatory amino acids, especially glutamate, during hypoglycemia leads to prolonged cellular depolarization with entry of water and calcium into the cell, first impairing neuronal growth and eventually causing cell death. In addition, the hypoglycemic brain may be more vulnerable to the damaging effects of ischemia. Degrees of ischemia and hypoglycemia that alone would not result in brain injury might do so in combination (Volpe, 2008).

D. **Etiologies and precipitating factors.**
1. Inadequate production or supply of glucose accounts for the more common causes of neonatal hypoglycemia. These conditions involve decreased substrate (glycogen, lactate, glycerol, amino acids) availability, immature or altered enzyme pathways, or altered responses to neural or hormonal factors (Blackburn, 2013; Jain et al., 2012; Ogata, 2005).
   a. Prematurity: possible diminished oral and parenteral intake, immature counterregulatory response to low glucose concentration, and insufficient glycogen stores and release.
   b. Intrauterine growth restriction: low glycogen and fat stores, increased substrate utilization.
   c. Delayed feedings, insufficient breastfeeding, or fluid restriction.
   d. Inborn errors of metabolism: defective gluconeogenesis and/or glycogenolysis (e.g., galactosemia, amino acid disorders, organic acid deficiencies, fatty acid oxidation disorders).
   e. Glycogen storage disease: autosomal recessive defects characterized by a deficient or abnormally functioning enzyme involved with formation or degradation of glycogen in the liver.
   f. Perinatal stress/hypoxia, respiratory distress, hypothermia, polycythemia/hyperviscosity, infection, adrenal hemorrhage, congestive heart failure.
2. Increased uptake of glucose related to hyperinsulinism (De Leon and Stanley, 2007; Steinkrauss et al., 2005).
   a. Infant of diabetic mother (IDM).
   b. Persistent neonatal hyperinsulinism and nesidioblastosis: autosomal recessive disorders thought to be caused by regulatory defects in beta cell function. Surgical exploration may be necessary for definitive diagnosis, with subtotal pancreatectomy the required therapeutic measure.
   c. Beckwith–Wiedemann syndrome: possibly genetic as majority of cases, but not all, involve a defect in the short arm of chromosome 11; characterized by omphalocele, macroglossia, visceromegaly, and hypoglycemia. Pancreatic islet cell hyperplasia is

noted. The resultant hypoglycemia may be quite profound and difficult to treat (Blackburn, 2013; Kalhan and Devaskar, 2011).

**d.** Rh incompatibility: severe cases can have associated beta cell hypertrophy and hyperinsulinemia.

**e.** High glucose infusion and tocolytics used before delivery. β-Adrenergic agonists such as terbutaline can stimulate fetal pancreatic beta cells.

**f.** Iatrogenic: position of tip of umbilical artery catheter near the pancreas can cause glucose to be directly delivered to the pancreas via the celiac artery, resulting in excessive insulin secretion.

**E. Clinical presentation and assessment (Blackburn, 2013; Jain et al., 2012; Ogata, 2005; Volpe, 2008).**

**1.** Clinical signs of hypoglycemia are nonspecific and may be present at varying blood glucose concentrations in different infants, or symptoms may not be evident at all even though the infant is experiencing severe hypoglycemia. In addition, signs often linked with hypoglycemia may occur in conjunction with other clinical conditions.

**a.** Tremors, jitteriness, irritability, exaggerated Moro reflex.

**b.** Abnormal cry: high-pitched or weak.

**c.** Respiratory distress: apnea, irregular respirations, tachypnea, cyanosis.

**d.** Stupor, hypotonia, lethargy, refusal to feed.

**e.** Hypothermia, temperature instability.

**f.** Seizures.

**F. Diagnostic studies.**

**1.** Point-of-care blood glucose screening.

**a.** Enzymatic reagent strips. Their reliability is questioned because they:

(1) May underestimate the true glucose level as whole blood gives a reading 10% to 15% lower than the plasma value;

(2) May fail to detect clinically important hypoglycemia because of unpredictable measurement errors; and

(3) Are sensitive to error from technical and operator variables such as timing, blotting, and distribution of blood droplets (Adamkin and Committee on Fetus and Newborn, 2011).

**b.** Absorption photometry and electrochemical glucose meters.

**c.** Subcutaneous microdialysis (Jain et al., 2012; Kalhan and Devaskar, 2011).

(1) Decreases the need for frequent blood sampling.

(2) Enables long-term glucose monitoring.

(3) Cannot measure glucose levels below 45 mg/dL with accuracy; large variance seen with high glucose values.

**2.** All current techniques require laboratory confirmation for establishing a diagnosis of neonatal hypoglycemia; however, appropriate interventions should be initiated promptly and not wait on laboratory confirmation (Adamkin and Committee on Fetus and Newborn, 2011).

**3.** In suspected hyperinsulinism, additional testing may include concurrent insulin and glucose levels, ketone and free fatty acid levels, and cortisol and growth hormone levels.

**G. Patient care management (Adamkin and Committee on Fetus and Newborn, 2011; McGowan et al., 2011).**

**1.** Identify infants at risk.

**2.** Prevent hypoglycemia by providing glucose substrate.

**a.** Early enteral feedings.

**b.** Intravenous (IV) glucose at 4 to 6 mg/kg/min.

**3.** Assess glucose status with blood glucose screening.

**a.** Perform blood glucose screening test on infants at risk on admission, frequently during the first 4 hours of life, and then at 4-hour intervals until the risk period has passed (Ogata, 2005).

**b.** Clinically unstable infants and any infant with signs of a possible low blood glucose concentration require regular monitoring.

c. Early and exclusive breastfeeding will meet the nutritional and energy needs of healthy full-term infants, and routine blood glucose screening of these infants is not presently recommended.

4. If hypoglycemia persists despite feeding, correction is with IV glucose infusion. A minibolus (dextrose 10% in water, 2 mL/kg), followed by continuous infusion at a rate of 6 to 8 mg/kg/min, rapidly raises the blood glucose level but does not treat the underlying hormonal and metabolic causes of the hypoglycemia.
5. Monitoring of blood glucose levels must then continue, for documentation of the resolution of hypoglycemia with IV therapy and subsequently during the transition to full enteral feedings. Oral feedings should be initiated once clinical symptoms have resolved (Rozance and Hay, 2006).
6. Persistent hypoglycemia raises the possibility of hyperinsulinism, although some infants without biochemical hyperinsulinism also have transiently high glucose requirements. Those with true hyperinsulinism may require the following:
   a. High IV glucose infusion rates (12 to 16 mg/kg/min). Delivery of concentrated glucose (>12.5%) requires a central line for safe administration.
   b. Hormonal therapy, which may include the following (Kalhan and Devaskar, 2011):
      (1) Glucagon: stimulates glycogen release from the liver. Glucagon, however, may also stimulate insulin release, so its use requires the presence of an IV glucose infusion. Mainly used to diagnose hepatic glycogen storage disease.
      (2) Diazoxide: suppresses pancreatic insulin secretion. Its use is reserved for situations of profound hyperinsulinism that have failed other therapies. It has been used for prolonged periods (years) without significant side effects noted. Usual dose 5 to 20 mg/kg/day administered orally 2 to 3 times per day.
      (3) Somatostatin: suppresses insulin and glucagon secretion; however, its use is limited by its extremely short half-life and short duration of action.
   c. Corticosteroids, which stimulate gluconeogenesis from noncarbohydrate (protein) sources (McGowan et al., 2011).
      (1) Hydrocortisone or prednisone may be used when parenteral glucose therapy is greater than 15 mg/kg/min.
      (2) Gradual decreases in corticosteroid dosage and decreases in parenteral glucose concentrations are required as oral intake is increased.
   d. Subtotal or total pancreatectomy if severe, persistent hyperinsulinism is unresponsive to medical therapy (De Leon and Stanley, 2007; Lindley and Dunne, 2005).

**H. Complications.**

1. Hypoglycemia will often recur when a bolus of glucose is not followed by a continuous infusion.
2. Extravasations of peripheral glucose infusions may cause necrosis of skin and other tissue (Lund and Kuller, 2007).
   a. Hyaluronidase can be injected subcutaneously around the periphery of any extravasation site to prevent or limit tissue injury.
   b. Skin injury can be prevented by making multiple puncture holes using an aseptic technique over the involved area and allowing the fluid to be infiltrated.
   c. Elevation of the affected area, if an extremity, may limit the leakage of the exudate.
   d. Use of an occlusive dressing (hydrocolloid dressing; hydrogel sheets, and amorphous gel) will provide for exudate management, adherence without damaging the surrounding tissue, and a microbial barrier; débridement and compression should be used.
3. Reactive hypoglycemia with return of symptomatology may occur if the IV glucose infusion infiltrates or is stopped abruptly.

**I. Outcome.**

1. Potential long-term sequelae remain unclear since there often are coexisting medical conditions that also predispose to brain injury (Ogata, 2005).
2. In general, outcome studies show that transient hypoglycemia in an otherwise healthy neonate has a good prognosis while neonates with seizure-associated and/or persistent hyperinsulinemic hypoglycemia have the worst neurologic prognosis (Kalhan and Devaskar, 2011; Rozance and Hay, 2006; Volpe, 2008).

## INFANT OF DIABETIC MOTHER

A. **Incidence:** 20% of infants of women with gestational diabetes mellitus and 35% of infants of mothers with other forms of diabetes (Blackburn, 2013).

B. **Pathophysiology:** The hormonal and metabolic changes that complicate diabetic pregnancy can adversely affect the developing fetus and neonate in a number of ways (Blackburn, 2013; Stokowski, 2007).

1. Early in gestation during organogenesis, the abnormal metabolic milieu is teratogenic, resulting in a higher incidence of congenital malformations.
2. Throughout pregnancy and particularly in the third trimester, the pregnant diabetic woman is increasingly insulin resistant and often has hyperglycemia and hyperaminoacidemia. Excess glucose and amino acids are freely delivered to the fetus, but maternal insulin is not. These nutrients stimulate the fetal pancreas to produce insulin to use the excess fuels, resulting in beta cell hyperplasia and hyperinsulinemia. This fetal hyperinsulinemia, in turn, stimulates protein, lipid, and glycogen synthesis, causing a high rate of fetal growth, increased deposition of fat and visceral enlargement (especially heart and liver), and subsequent macrosomia. This fetal macrosomia does not involve the brain or kidneys.
3. After birth, the neonate's pancreas continues to produce insulin, and available glucose is rapidly used. The infant's ability to mobilize glycogen stores is decreased. The IDM may exhibit an exaggerated and persistent hypoglycemia. Maternal glucose homeostasis during pregnancy as well as maternal glycemia during delivery influences the degree of neonatal hypoglycemia.
4. The IDM is at risk of having neural impairment because, even with plentiful adipose tissue, ketogenesis and lipolysis are suppressed by hyperinsulinemia, leaving the brain without a supply of alternative fuels for metabolism during hypoglycemia.

C. **Clinical presentation and assessment (McGowan et al., 2011).**

1. Hypoglycemia: It may occur immediately after birth without symptoms. In one large retrospective series, hypoglycemia (defined as serum glucose <40 mg/dL) occurred in about one third of IDMs. The majority of those responded rapidly to treatment, but 10% had persistent hypoglycemia despite treatment.
2. Macrosomia/LGA (approximately 35% of IDMs): Some infants are SGA because of placental insufficiency in advanced stages of the maternal diabetes.
3. Increase in preterm births in association with diabetic pregnancy: Hyperbilirubinemia in IDMs may be secondary to prematurity.
4. Respiratory distress syndrome and other conditions such as transient tachypnea of the newborn infant: Fetal hyperinsulinemia may delay the maturation of various aspects of the pulmonary surfactant system and not just inhibit surfactant production, delaying lung maturation.
5. Polycythemia (venous hematocrit >65%): The insulin-induced high glucose uptake and high metabolic rate cause a cellular hypoxia, leading to an elevated erythropoietin level (Ogata, 2005). Newborns with polycythemia do not always look plethoric, so the hematocrit level must be measured.
6. Hypocalcemia, hypomagnesemia thought to result from a functional hypoparathyroidism due to maternal magnesium loss (Jain et al., 2012).
7. Cardiomyopathy, visceromegaly possibly related to maternal diabetes control and to fetal/neonatal hyperinsulinemia.
8. Congenital malformations: Cardiac defects (especially transposition), neural tube defects, sacral agenesis, and caudal regression are 2 to 4 times more frequent than in the general population. The anomalies are thought to be due to the diabetic intrauterine environment during organogenesis, frequently before the pregnancy is recognized and prenatal diabetic treatment initiated.

D. **Diagnostic studies.**

1. Blood glucose screening with laboratory confirmation of plasma glucose.
2. Other laboratory analyses, including calcium and magnesium levels and venous hematocrit.
3. X-ray examination if fractures from traumatic delivery are suspected.
4. Echocardiography.

E. **Patient care management (McGowan et al., 2011; Stokowski, 2007).**
   1. The main goal of the treatment of gestational diabetes is to achieve and maintain euglycemia. Tight control of intrapartum glucose levels may reduce the incidence of neonatal complications.
   2. Anticipate problems of IDM before delivery; prompt recognition and treatment of neonatal morbidities postdelivery.
   3. Provide early feeding of human milk or formula, orally or via gavage tube if the infant does not feed well. IV administration of glucose is necessary for infants too small or sick to tolerate enteral feeding.

F. **Complications.**
   1. Seizures resulting from cerebral fuel deficiency.
   2. Shoulder dystocia: Macrosomic infants delivered with forceps or vacuum extraction may have brachial plexus injury (Erb's palsy) or fractures.
   3. Renal vein thrombosis (secondary to polycythemia/hyperviscosity).
   4. Development of juvenile insulin-dependent diabetes with a 2% transmission risk for female IDM and 6% for male IDM (Jain et al., 2012).

G. **Outcome (McGowan et al., 2011; Stokowski, 2007).**
   1. Increased perinatal mortality rate results from relatively high rates of congenital malformations, stillbirths, and premature delivery.
   2. Morbidities associated with IDM include neurologic sequelae, developmental delay, behavioral differences, obesity, and diabetes.
   3. Maternal complications, including poor glycemic control, vascular disease, infection, and pregnancy-induced hypertension, are associated with poorer perinatal outcome. Improved outcomes are seen in IDMs when maternal diabetes is metabolically controlled.
   4. The outcomes for SGA infants born to women receiving intensive therapy for gestational diabetes may be worse than those of appropriate-for-gestational-age or LGA infants.

## HYPERGLYCEMIA

A. **Definition:** Whole blood glucose concentration greater than 120 to 125 mg/dL or a plasma glucose concentration greater than 150 mg/dL.

B. **Incidence:** Prevalence of 29% to 86% in low birth weight infants overall; 2% of infants weighing more than 2000 g; 45% of infants less than 1000 g; and up to 80% of infants weighing less than 750 g (Jain et al., 2012; Le Compte et al., 2012; McGowan et al., 2011).

C. **Pathophysiology.**
   1. Normally an infant responds to an exogenous glucose supply with a rise in insulin, suppressing endogenous glucose production and enhancing peripheral uptake of glucose. Though clinically stable, extremely low birth weight (ELBW) infants may be able to regulate glucose in this manner; however, many of them become hyperglycemic.
   2. Hepatic glucose production in this latter group continues in the presence of hyperglycemia and circulating insulin. This represents a failure of glucose autoregulation involving both the pancreas and liver of infants with hyperglycemia.
   3. Corticosteroid therapy stimulates glycogenolysis and gluconeogenesis and may block insulin secretion as well as inhibit its peripheral action.

D. **Etiologies and precipitating factors.**
   1. Low birth weight, extreme prematurity, and intrauterine growth restriction (IUGR).
   2. Excessive glucose load (>6 to 8 mg/kg/min), with 50% of infants receiving a glucose infusion rate (GIR) of 11 mg/kg/min and all infants receiving a GIR of 14 mg/kg/min developing hyperglycemia.
   3. Stress related to clinical problems such as sepsis or infection.
   4. Transient or permanent neonatal diabetes mellitus (see "Transient or Permanent Neonatal Diabetes").
   5. Side effects of medications such as corticosteroids.
   6. Lipid infusion, which may contribute to hyperglycemia.
   7. Release of catecholamines secondary to surgery/anesthesia.

E. **Clinical presentation and assessment.**
   1. Onset can be as early as 24 hours of age; usually before 3 days of life.
   2. No characteristic clinical presentation.
   3. Symptoms may include glycosuria, dehydration, weight loss, fever, ketosis, metabolic acidosis and failure to thrive.

F. **Diagnostic studies.**
   1. Serum or plasma blood glucose levels greater than 125 mg/dL or 150 mg/dL, respectively.
   2. Urinary glucose. Very low birth weight (VLBW) infants have a low renal threshold for glucose and may spill sugar at blood glucose levels as low as 80 to 100 mg/dL.
   3. Investigation for possible underlying cause (sepsis workup to rule out infection or insulin level to rule out neonatal diabetes mellitus).

G. **Patient care management.**
   1. Monitor blood glucose of infants at risk for developing hyperglycemia, particularly when fluid intake is increased on day 2 or 3 of life.
   2. Decrease glucose load as much as possible to allow the blood glucose level to stabilize in a normal range (<125 mg/dL, or plasma glucose <150 mg/dL).
   3. Monitor weight, urine output, fluid intake, GIR, electrolytes, and acid–base balance.
   4. Insulin is sometimes administered to ELBW infants along with parenteral nutrition in an attempt to normalize blood glucose levels without reducing the caloric intake. Insulin is also used to treat transient neonatal diabetes. Insulin normalizes blood glucose by suppressing hepatic glucose production and by increasing peripheral glucose utilization. However, premature infants have a very small mass of insulin-dependent tissue, with only 10% of their glucose utilization being insulin dependent. Severe hyperglycemia may occur in the VLBW infant despite decreased glucose infusion rates. Continuous insulin infusion may be used, although routine use not advised because of adverse effects (Alsweiler et al., 2012).
   5. Begin enteral feedings when feasible because the subsequent release of gut hormones may promote insulin secretion, allowing for improved blood glucose control.

H. **Complications.**
   1. Neonatal hyperglycemia may be accompanied by urinary loss of glucose and an osmotic diuresis with its risk of dehydration. In addition, possible resultant hyperosmolarity of extracellular fluid in the brain may increase the premature infant's chance for intraventricular hemorrhage (IVH) (Jain et al., 2012).
   2. Insulin management may be difficult in the ELBW infant; blood glucose levels can fluctuate widely. A precisely controlled continuous-infusion pump is essential. Priming of the tubing is required because insulin tends to adhere to the catheters. Whether insulin therapy promotes linear growth or just converts glucose into fat is not yet fully understood (Alsweiler et al., 2012).
   3. Electrolyte abnormalities, elevated $CO_2$ retention, and an elevated triglyceride level.

I. **Outcome.**
   1. Controversy exists concerning the outcome of neonatal hyperglycemia.
      a. Hypothesized that hyperglycemia in the premature neonate may increase the risk of IVH because rapid fluctuations in osmolarity negatively impact the germinal matrix.
      b. There is a strong association between neonatal hyperglycemia and increased mortality rates or poor neurodevelopmental outcomes among survivors (Hays et al., 2006; Kao et al., 2006).
      c. Neonatal hyperglycemia is usually self-limiting and not associated with adverse outcomes.
      d. Possible association between hyperglycemia and severe retinopathy of prematurity in ELBW infants (Ertl et al., 2006).

## TRANSIENT OR PERMANENT NEONATAL DIABETES

A. **Definition:** Hyperglycemia requiring insulin therapy occurring within the first month of life and lasting at least 2 weeks to several months can be lifelong (Ozlu et al., 2006).

B. **Incidence:** 1:500,000. Predominantly occurring in SGA infants, with 46% developing permanent diabetes in the neonatal period, 23% in childhood or adolescence; 31% are resolved in the neonatal period (Ogata, 2005).

1. Appears in the first week of life and persists for greater than 2 weeks (Stokowski, 2007).
2. Etiology is variable, including dysfunctional insulin molecule or receptor deficiencies and activating mutations of the $K_{ATP}$ channel (Stokowski, 2007).
3. Instances of transient neonatal diabetes are associated with abnormalities of an imprinted region on chromosome 6q24. Mutations in encoder genes have been attributed to instances of permanent and transient neonatal diabetes (Babenko et al., 2006).

C. **Pathophysiology.**
1. Both transient and permanent neonatal diabetes mellitus are due to a failure of pancreatic beat cells causing an endogenous insulin deficiency, with the exact pathogenesis involved not yet fully understood (Ozlu et al., 2006; Stokowski, 2007).
2. The IUGR commonly seen with affected infants is due to insufficient insulin secretion (Stokowski, 2007).

D. **Clinical presentation.**
1. The transient form appears within the first week of life, resolves within weeks or months, and reappears in late childhood. The permanent form appears within days or months of birth and persists throughout life (Stokowski, 2007).
2. Hyperglycemia (frequently >600 mg/dL), polyuria, glycosuria, weight loss, dehydration, fever, failure to thrive, ketosis, metabolic acidosis (may or may not be evident), and low levels of C-peptide and plasma insulin (Ozlu et al., 2006; Stokowski, 2007).

E. **Patient care management.**
1. Restore intravascular volume.
2. Replace fluid and electrolyte losses as indicated and provide for ongoing needs.
3. Correct the hyperglycemia; monitor glucose levels.
4. Provide adequate nutrition for growth and development.
5. Usually a daily dose of 0.2 to 3 units/kg/day of insulin is necessary to achieve plasma glucose levels of 100 to 180 mg/dL; however, individualization of insulin requirement is needed.
6. Average length of insulin therapy varies from 2 weeks to 18 months. Tapering of insulin dose as requirement decreases lessens the risk of recurrent hyperglycemia (Ozlu et al., 2006; Stokowski, 2007).

F. **Complications:** See Hyperglycemia section above.

G. **Outcome.**
1. Course of disease is highly variable.
2. Close follow-up is recommended after remission because of a high rate of recurrence later in childhood.

## REFERENCES


Adamkin, D.H. and Committee on Fetus and Newborn: Postnatal glucose homeostasis in late-preterm and term infants. *Pediatrics*, 127(3):575–579, 2011.

Alsweiler, J.M., Harding, J.E. and Bloomfield, F.H.: Tight glycemic control in very low birth weight infants. *Pediatrics*, 129(4):639–647, 2012.

Babenko, A.P., Polak, M.Cavé, H., et al.: Activating mutations in the ABCC8 gene in neonatal diabetes mellitus. *New England Journal of Medicine*, 355(5): 456–466, 2006.

Blackburn, S.T.: *Maternal, fetal, & neonatal physiology: A clinical perspective* (4th ed.). St. Louis, 2013, Elsevier Saunders, pp. 560-585.

De Leon, D.D. and Stanley, C.A.: Mechanisms of disease: Advances in diagnosis and treatment of hyperinsulinism in neonates. *Nature Clinical Practice Endocrinology and Metabolism*, 3(1):57–68, 2007.

Ertl, T., Gyarmati, J.Gaal, V., et al.: Relationship between hyperglycemia and retinopathy of prematurity in very low birth weight infants. *Biology of the Neonate*, 89:56–59, 2006.

Hays, S., O'Brian Smith, E. and Sunehag, A.: Hyperglycemia is a risk factor for early death and morbidity in extremely low birth-weight infants. *Pediatrics*, 118 (5):1811–1818, 2006.

Hume, R., Burchell, A.Williams, F., et al.: Glucose homeostasis in the newborn. *Early Human Development*, 81:95–101, 2005.

Jain, V., Chen, M. and Menon, R.K.: Disorders of carbohydrate metabolism. In C.A. Gleason and S.U. Devaskar (Eds.): *Avery's diseases of the newborn* (9th ed.). Philadelphia, 2012, Elsevier Saunders, pp. 1320-1329.

Kalhan, S.C. and Devaskar, S.U.: Metabolic and endocrine disorders. In R.J. Martin, A.A. Fanaroff, and M.C. Walsh (Eds.): *Fanaroff and Martin's neonatal-perinatal medicine: Diseases of the fetus and infant* (9th ed.). St. Louis, 2011, Elsevier Mosby, pp. 1497–1620.

Kao, L.S., Morris, B.H.Lally, K.P., et al.: Hyperglycemia and morbidity and mortality in extremely low birth weight infants. *Journal of Perinatology*, 26 (12):730–736, 2006.

Le Compte, A.J., Lyn, A.M., Lin, J., et al.: Pilot study of a model-based approach to blood glucose control in very-low-birthweight neonates. *BMC Pediatrics*, 117, 2012. Retrieved February 7, 2013, from http://www.biomedcentral.com/1471-2431/12/117.

Lindley, K.J. and Dunne, M.J.: Contemporary strategies in the diagnosis and management of neonatal hyperinsulinaemic hypoglycemia. *Early Human Development*, 81:61–72, 2005.

Lund, C.H. and Kuller, J.M.: Assessment and management of the integumentary system. In C. Kenner, and J.W. Lott (Eds.): *Comprehensive neonatal nursing: A physiologic perspective* (3rd ed.). Philadelphia, 2007, Elsevier Saunders, pp. 700–724.

McGowan, J.E.: Neonatal hypoglycemia. *Pediatrics in Review*, 20(7):E6–E15, 1999. Retrieved August 10, 1999, from www.pedsinreview.org.

McGowan, J.E., Rozance, P.J., Price-Douglas, W. and Hay, W.W. Jr.: Glucose homeostasis. In G.B. Merenstein and S.L. Gardner (Eds.): *Merenstein & Gardner's handbook of neonatal intensive care* (7th ed.). St. Louis, 2011, Elsevier Mosby, pp. 353–377.

Ogata, E.S.: Carbohydrate homeostasis. In M.G. MacDonald, M.D. Mullet, and M.M.K. Seshia (Eds.): *Avery's neonatology: Pathophysiology and management of the newborn* (6th ed.). Philadelphia, 2005, Lippincott Williams & Wilkins, pp. 876–891.

Ozlu, F., Tyker, F. and Yuksel, B.: Neonatal diabetes mellitus. *Indian Pediatrics*, 43:642–645, 2006.

Rozance, P.J. and Hay, W.W.: Hypoglycemia in newborn infants: Features associated with adverse outcomes. *Biology of the Neonate*, 90:74–86, 2006.

Steinkrauss, L., Lipman, T.H.Hendell, C.D., et al.: Effects of hypoglycemia on developmental outcome in children with congenital hyperinsulinism. *Journal of Pediatric Nursing*, 20(2):9–17, 2005.

Stokowski, L.: Endocrine system. In C. Kenner and J.W. Lott (Eds.): *Comprehensive neonatal care: An interdisciplinary approach* (4th ed.). St. Louis, 2007, Elsevier Saunders, pp. 155–174.

Volpe, J.H.: *Neurology of the newborn* (5th ed.). Philadelphia, 2008, Elsevier Saunders.

CHAPTER

# 10 Nutritional Management

GEORGIA R. DITZENBERGER

**OBJECTIVES**

1. Describe the effects of prematurity on the gastrointestinal (GI) physiology of digestion and absorption.
2. Identify nutritional store deficiencies most common in premature and term infants.
3. Describe basic nutritional requirements for premature and high-risk term infants and factors that influence these requirements.
4. Identify nutritional components, uses, methods of delivery, complications, and nursing care issues for parenteral nutrition (PN).
5. Review the use of commercial preterm and full-term infant formulas for enteral nutrition management.
6. Review human milk feedings for premature and high-risk term infants and related nursing care issues.
7. Review the use of human milk supplements in enteral nutrition management for premature infants.
8. Describe the various methods of providing enteral feedings and the advantages and disadvantages of each.
9. Describe minimal enteral feedings and application in initiating enteral nutrition for premature infants.
10. Describe risks and interventions for feeding intolerances and nutritional deficiency states in premature infants.
11. Describe assessment of an infant's readiness for enteral nutrition.
12. Describe assessments used to determine premature and high-risk infant nutritional status.
13. Describe the standards used to assess growth in term and premature infants.

Neonatal nurses face challenges in helping to meet the basic nutritional requirements and support the growth needs of premature and high-risk infants. Tremendous advances in technology and pharmacology permit the survival of very premature infants who require intensive and specialized care and support for immature body systems. Nutritional care is of vital importance for premature infants, who are deprived of transplacentally acquired nutrient stores and have rapid extrauterine growth rates. Other high-risk infants have special needs related to illness-associated metabolic demands and physiologic instability.

Neonatal nurses with knowledge of the effects of prematurity on GI functioning, the special nutritional needs of premature and high-risk infants, and methods of delivering nutritional support can better assess infant status and contribute to nutritional management. This chapter reviews the nutritional requirements of premature and high-risk infants, methods for providing parenteral and enteral nutrition, and nursing interventions for optimal nutritional support.

## ANATOMY AND PHYSIOLOGY OF THE PREMATURE INFANT'S GI TRACT

A. **Anatomic and functional development of the GI tract.**
   1. Anatomic development (Berseth, 2006; Blackburn, 2013; Dimmitt and Sibley, 2012).
      a. Pylorus and fundus of stomach defined and gastric glands formed by 14 weeks of gestation.
      b. Esophageal sphincter present by 28 weeks of gestation.
      c. GI tract resembles that of a term newborn infant by 20 weeks of gestation.
      d. Gut lengthens to 250 to 300 cm by term; gastric capacity is about 30 mL.
   2. Functional development (Berseth, 2006; Blackburn, 2013; Dimmitt and Sibley, 2012).
      a. Premature infants have limited production of gut digestive enzymes and growth factors.

b. By 28 weeks, biochemical and physiologic capacities for limited digestion and absorption are present.
c. Major gut-regulating polypeptides—gastrin, motilin, cholecystokinin, pancreatic polypeptide, and somatostatin—are present in limited amounts by the end of the first trimester; act locally to regulate growth and development of the gut; reach adult distribution by term gestation.
d. Intestinal transport of amino acids seen by 14 weeks, glucose by 18 weeks, and fatty acid by 24 weeks of gestation.
e. Lactose is a predominate source of carbohydrate in breast milk and formula. Lactase reduces lactose to glucose.
f. Lactase activity is first seen at 9 weeks of gestation; at 24 weeks of gestation, less than one fourth the activity level of term infant; dramatically increases between 32 and 34 weeks of gestation to the activity level of term infant.
g. Disaccharidases, such as salivary amylase and mucosal glucoamylase, are functionally active after 27 to 28 weeks of gestation. Some formulas contain glucose polymers, likely hydrolyzed by salivary amylase or absorbed directly at the mucosal level via mucosal glucoamylase.
h. Fat (lipid) emulsification and hydroxylation to free fatty acids and monoglycerides result from lipase and bile acid activity.
i. Lingual and gastric lipases present by 26 weeks of gestation; limited in volume and function. Additional lipases also in breast milk; function well in conditions with low bile acid synthesis and stores such as seen in premature infants.
j. Bile acid secretion observed by 22 weeks of gestation.
k. Bile acid synthesis and stores of premature infant decreased when compared to term infant synthesis and stores, which is in turn one half that seen in adult synthesis and stores.
l. Gastric gland secretion activity seen by 20 weeks of gestation; gastric acid secretion lower than adult levels even at term gestation; activated with introduction of enteral feeding.
m. Ingested proteins are denatured by gastrin and cleaved by pepsin; further reduced by pancreatic proteolytic enzymes into oligopeptides and amino acids. Pepsin activity induced by increased gastric acid resulting from initiation of enteral feedings.
n. GI motility refers to the coordinated facilitation of mechanical digestion, the movement of food from injection to elimination; includes suck–swallow and esophageal, stomach, and intestinal peristalsis. Immature GI motility is a major limitation to enteral digestion; presence of disorganized, random contractions between 25 and 30 weeks of gestation; motility improves after 30 to 32 weeks of gestation, gradually becomes more organized closer to term gestation (Berseth, 2006; Blackburn, 2013; Dimmitt and Sibley, 2012).

**B. Postnatal development of the GI tract.**

1. GI motility is a major limitation in providing enteral nutrition for premature infants (Berseth, 2006; Dimmitt and Sibley, 2012).
   a. Nonnutritive suck coordination present around 28 weeks of gestation; suck–swallow coordination for adequate expression of milk from breast or nipple develops closer to 34 to 36 weeks of gestation; appears to be dependent on neuromaturation related to postmenstrual age rather than chronologic age (age in days since birth) (Berseth, 2006; Blackburn, 2013).
   b. Well-developed tone and swallow-related relaxation in the lower esophageal sphincter (LES), allowing food passage into the stomach from the esophagus; transient LES relaxation related to immaturity, allowing gastric contents to reenter the esophagus (gastroesophageal reflux [GER]); diminishes closer to term gestation (Horvath et al., 2008; Jadcherla, 2006).
   c. Delayed gastric emptying related to disorganized, random peristalsis contractions with immature duodenal response to food; duodenal contractions of premature infants cease rather than increase in response to food, delaying gastric emptying. Peristalsis becomes more organized, duodenal responses and gastric emptying time improves with increasing gestational age; regular enteral feeding for at least 10 days seems to have positive maturational effect on duodenal response for premature infants (Berseth, 2006; Blackburn, 2013; Dimmitt and Sibley, 2012; Jadcherla, 2006).

2. Influences on postnatal development of GI function include genetic endowment, gut trophic factors, and hormonal regulatory mechanisms, as well as enteral feeding initiation and feeding type (Blackburn, 2013).
   a. Gut trophic factors include nutrients, hormones, and peptides; principal nutrients: iron, zinc, vitamin $B_{12}$, vitamin A, and folate; principal hormones: insulin and growth factor; principal peptides: epidermal growth factor, transforming growth factor, insulin-like growth factors, and somatostatin.
   b. Hormonal regulatory mechanisms have a critical role in mediating gut development after birth. Gut development stimulated by increases in specific GI hormones and enteric neuropeptides such as enteroglucagon, promoting intestinal mucosa growth; gastrin, stimulating gastric mucosa and exocrine pancreas growth; motilin and neurotensin, stimulating development of gut motility; and gastric inhibitory peptide, promoting glucose tolerance.
   c. Initiation of enteral feeding is a major stimulus for hormonal regulatory mechanisms in both premature and term infants; response delayed in premature and high-risk infants receiving only PN without enteral feedings.
   d. Type of enteral feeding has an influence on gut maturation; breast milk contains high levels of GI trophic factors, which enhance the postnatal maturation of gut.
   e. Minimal enteral feeding, also known as trophic feeding, or gut or GI priming feeding, appears to stimulate hormonal regulatory mechanisms, with subsequent gut development; as little as 0.5 to 1 mL/kg/hr seems beneficial (Berseth, 2006; Blackburn, 2013).

C. **Nutrient deficiencies of premature infants:** cessation of transplacental transfer of nutrients during the third trimester, a critical period for somatic and brain growth (Limperopoulos et al., 2005).
1. Carbohydrate, lipid, and protein.
   a. Glucose is a primary source of carbohydrate; during the third trimester, glucose is stored as glycogen in the liver and cardiac and skeletal muscle, and to a lesser extent in the kidneys, intestines, and brain; glycogen stores of term infants are significantly greater than those of adults (Blackburn, 2013).
      (1) Glucose is the primary fetal energy source; accounts for 80% of fetal energy.
      (2) Carbohydrate in the form of lactose and glucose provides 40% of the postnatal caloric intake (Blackburn, 2013; Kleinman and American Academy of Pediatrics [AAP] Committee on Nutrition, 2009; Tudehope, 2013; Tudehope et al., 2013).
   b. Lipid stores; significant lipid accretion and increased adipose tissue deposition occur in the fetus between 24 and 40 weeks. At 26 to 28 weeks, fat stores account for approximately 3.5% of body composition, 30 to 34 weeks 8%, and by 35 to 38 weeks 16%; weight gain due to fat deposition is about 14 g/day (Moore et al., 2013).
      (1) Adipose tissue: white and brown (Blackburn, 2013; Moore et al., 2013; Nedergaard and Cannon, 2011).
         (a) White adipose tissue: subcutaneous tissue; acts as a heat insulator, shock absorber, and calorie storage unit.
         (b) Brown adipose tissue: accumulates in the neck, scapulae, axillae, mediastinum, and perirenal tissues; critical for nonshivering thermogenesis, a major method of neonatal heat production.
      (2) Lipids contribute minimally to fetal energy needs; critical component of brain development (neuronal and glial membranes, and myelin sheath), retinal development, cell membrane formation, synthesis of surfactant and other phospholipids, bile, serum lipoprotein, and adipose tissue deposition (Blackburn, 2013; Kashyap and Putet, 2011).
      (3) Lipids provide approximately 50% of the postnatal caloric intake; major postnatal energy source (Bhatia et al., 2013; Blackburn, 2013; Kashyap, 2007; Kashyap and Heird, 2011; Tudehope, 2013; Tudehope et al., 2013).
   c. Protein stores; major structural and functional components of all cells of the body; during the third trimester, fetal accretion rate is 3.6 to 4.8 g/kg/day (Berseth, 2006; Blackburn, 2013; Hay et al., 2011).

(1) Amino acids and lactate secondary fetal energy source; critical in all organ development, growth, and function.
(2) Protein catabolism contributes approximately 10% of postnatal caloric intake.

**d.** Premature infants have minimal adipose tissue and glycogen stores at birth; stores decrease with decreasing gestational age; at birth sources will be quickly exhausted if sufficient exogenous sources to meet energy needs are not provided (Blackburn, 2013).

**e.** Stable term infants have sufficient glycogen and fat stores to provide for energy demands during the relative state of low nutrient intake that normally occurs during the first few days of life (Blackburn, 2013).
(1) Estimated 90% of liver and 50% to 80% of cardiac and skeletal muscle glycogen stores used within the first 24 hours post birth.
(2) Fat is a major source of stored calories for term infant; preferred energy source for high energy demands of such tissues as the heart and the adrenal cortex.

**2.** Vitamins and minerals.

**a.** Fat-soluble vitamins A and E; stored in body fat and organs (Greer, 2006, 2008; Hambidge, 2006; Johnson and Bhutani, 2011; Shenai, 2011).
(1) Vitamin A transferred throughout pregnancy, increases in the third trimester, adequate fetal level maintained despite variations in maternal diet; essential for epithelial cell growth and differentiation, vision, healing, reproduction, and immune competency; stored primarily in liver.
(2) Vitamin E gradually increases throughout pregnancy with direct correlation between vitamin E level and body weight and adipose tissue; stored primarily in liver, adipose tissue, and skeletal muscle; at low levels after birth and through infancy, dependent on diet (breast milk, formula) for adequate supply; provides protection from oxidant free-radical damage.

**b.** Calcium, phosphorus, and magnesium (Husain et al., 2011; Itani and Tsang, 2006).
(1) Two thirds of the calcium accumulated in a term infant transplacentally transferred to fetus during the third trimester; allows for rapid fetal bone mineralization.
(2) Fetal phosphorus levels higher than maternal levels during the third trimester; important role in fetal intermediary metabolism and bone mineralization.
(3) Eighty percent of the magnesium in term infants is accrued in the third trimester; important to plasma membrane excitability, regulatory role in numerous biological processes involved in energy storage, transfer, and production, significant in calcium and bone homeostasis.

**c.** Trace elements: copper, selenium, chromium, manganese, molybdenum, cobalt, fluoride, iodine, iron, and zinc provided during pregnancy; essential for various metabolic processes, cell and organ function and development (Hambidge, 2006; Hambidge and Krebs, 2011).
(1) Iron has a prominent role in oxygen transport, principally in the hemoglobin; a 28-week fetus has 64 mcg iron per gram of fat-free tissue, and a term infant has 94 mcg; in term infants, almost 80% of the iron is stored in the hemoglobin; required by virtually all cells for normal growth and metabolism; rapidly growing and differentiating cells have particularly high iron requirements; necessary for the development and functional integrity of the immune system (deRegnier and Georgieff, 2011; Greer, 2008; Kleinman and AAP Committee on Nutrition, 2009).
(2) Fetal zinc levels markedly increase midpregnancy, then decrease gradually over the third trimester; zinc has important biological role in protein structure and function, enzymes, transcription factors, hormonal receptor sites, and cell membranes; and numerous central roles in DNA and RNA metabolism.

## NUTRITIONAL REQUIREMENTS

**A. Term infants (Table 10-1).**

**1.** Fluid requirements (Blackburn, 2013; Dell, 2011).

**a.** Parenteral: 100 to 120 mL/kg/day.

**b.** Enteral: 120 to 150 mL/kg/day.

■ TABLE 10-1
■ ■ **Daily Nutritional Requirements for Term Infants**

| Nutrient | Parenteral | Enteral |
|---|---|---|
| Fluid (mL/kg/day)* | 100 to 120 | 120 to 150 |
| Energy (kcal/kg/day)† | 80 to 90 | 100 to 120 |
| Protein (g/kg/day)‡ | 2 to 2.5 | 2 to 2.5 |
| Carbohydrate (g/kg/day) | 10 to 15 | 8 to 12 |
| Fat (g/kg/day) | 2 to 4 | 3 to 4 |
| Sodium (mEq/kg/day) | 2 to 3 | 2 to 3 |
| Potassium (mEq/kg/day) | 2 to 3 | 2 to 3 |
| Chloride (mEq/kg/day) | 2 to 3 | 2 to 3 |
| Calcium (mg/kg/day)§ | 60 to 80 | 130 |
| Phosphorus (mg/kg/day)§ | 40 to 45 | 45 |
| Magnesium (mg/kg/day) | 5 to 7 | 7 |
| Iron (mg/kg/day)‖ | 0.1 to 0.2 | 1 to 2 |
| Vitamin A (IU/day)¶ | 2300 | 1250 |
| Vitamin D (IU/day) | 400 | 300 |
| Vitamin E (IU/day)** | 7 | 5 to 10 |
| Vitamin K (mg/day) | 0.05 | 0.2 |
| Vitamin C (mg/day) | 80 | 30 to 50 |
| Vitamin $B_1$ (mg/day) | 1.2 | 0.3 |
| Vitamin $B_2$ (mg/day) | 1.4 | 0.4 |
| Vitamin $B_6$ (mg/day) | 1 | 0.3 |
| Vitamin $B_{12}$ (mcg/day) | 1 | 0.3 |
| Niacin (mg/day) | 17 | 5 |
| Folate (mcg/day)†† | 140 | 25 to 50 |
| Biotin (mcg/day) | 20 | 10 |
| Zinc (mcg/kg/day)‡‡ | 250 | 830 |
| Copper (mcg/kg/day)‡‡,§§ | 20 | 75 |
| Manganese (mcg/kg/day)§§ | 1 | 85 |
| Selenium (mcg/kg/day)¶¶ | 2 | 1.6 |
| Chromium (mcg/kg/day) | 0.2 | 2 |
| Molybdenum (mcg/kg/day) | 0.25 | 2 |
| Iodine (mcg/kg/day) | 1 | 7 |

Adapted from Blackburn, S.T.: *Maternal, fetal, & neonatal physiology: A clinical perspective* (4th ed.). St. Louis, 2013, Saunders.
*After immediate postnatal initiation of fluid therapy.
†Adjust according to weight gain and stress factors.
‡Requirements increase with increasing degree of prematurity.
§Inadequate amount in total parenteral nutrition solutions because of risk of precipitation.
‖Initiate between 2 weeks and 2 months of age. Delay initiation in preterm infants with progressive retinopathy.
¶Supplementation might reduce the incidence of bronchopulmonary dysplasia.
**Supplementation might reduce the severity of retinopathy of prematurity.
††Not present in oral multivitamin supplements.
‡‡Increased requirement in patients with excessive ileostomy drainage or chronic diarrhea.
§§Removed from total parenteral nutrition solutions in patients with cholestatic liver disease.
¶¶Not present in standard trace element solution for neonates.

2. Energy (caloric) intake requirements.
   a. Parenteral: 80 to 90 kcal/kg/day.
   b. Enteral: 100 to 120 kcal/kg/day.
3. Carbohydrate, fat, and protein (Blackburn, 2013).
   a. Total caloric intake should be represented by the following:
      (1) Carbohydrate: approximately 40%; 8 to 12 g/kg/day.
      (2) Fat.
         (a) Parenteral: 2 to 4 g/kg/day; 20% intravenous (IV) lipid emulsion preferred over 10%, and has less phospholipid per gram of fat. High phospholipid levels

associated with increased triglyceride, cholesterol, and low-density lipoprotein levels in neonates (Haumont et al., 1989).

(b) Enteral: 3 to 4 g/kg/day.

(3) Protein: both parenteral and enteral: 2 to 2.5 g/kg/day.

**b.** Human milk and standard commercial infant formulas supply these nutrients within acceptable ratios (AAP, Section on Breastfeeding, 2012; Blackburn, 2013; Kleinman and AAP Committee on Nutrition, 2009; Neville and McManaman, 2006).

**4.** Vitamins, minerals, and trace elements.

**a.** Dietary reference intakes for enteral and parenteral nutrition are summarized in Table 10-1.

**b.** Pediatric parenteral vitamin, mineral, and trace element solutions, human milk, and commercial infant formulas provide adequate amounts of most vitamins to meet the needs of infants (Greer, 2006, 2008; Kleinman and AAP Committee on Nutrition, 2009).

**c.** Newborn deficiencies in fat-soluble vitamins A, D, E, and K well described; countermanded with human milk and formulas; significant vitamin deficiency rare (Greer, 2006, 2008; Kleinman and AAP Committee on Nutrition, 2009).

(1) Vitamin K is the only vitamin routinely given at the time of birth, seems to sustain sufficient levels for the first 3 months of life for exclusively breastfeeding infants even though human milk does not meet dietary reference intakes; formulas have sufficient vitamin K to meet dietary reference intakes; oral forms of vitamin K not recommended, may not provide adequate vitamin K necessary to prevent hemorrhage later in infancy unless repeated doses given in the first 4 months of life.

(2) AAP recommends vitamin D supplementation for breastfed or formula-fed infants unless taking at least 500 mL/day of vitamin D–fortified formula or milk, beginning in the first 2 months of life (AAP Section on Breastfeeding, 2012).

(3) Fluoride supplements should not be provided for the first 6 months of life for any infant; after 6 months, fluoride supplementation recommended only if the fluoride level in drinking water supply is less than 0.3 parts per million (ppm); consideration should include other fluoride sources: food, toothpaste, other fluid sources (AAP Section on Breastfeeding, 2012).

(4) Iron supplements may be needed for healthy term infants before 6 months to support iron stores; recommended in the first 6 months of life for infants with hematologic disorders, or infants with inadequate iron stores at birth (AAP Section on Breastfeeding, 2012).

(5) Vitamin $B_{12}$ supplementation recommended for infants of vegan mothers with inadequate $B_{12}$ intake.

**B. Premature infants (Blackburn, 2013; Kleinman and AAP Committee on Nutrition, 2009; Lapillonne et al., 2013; Tudehope, 2013; Tudehope et al., 2013).**

**1.** General considerations.

**a.** Recommendations for nutritional requirements and advisable intakes are used as guidelines.

**b.** Individual premature infant nutritional needs vary with gestational age and health status.

**c.** Recommendations for parenteral and enteral nutritional needs are summarized in Table 10-2.

**2.** Fluid requirements.

**a.** Parenteral: 120 to 150 mL/kg/day.

**b.** Enteral: 150 to 200 mL/kg/day.

**c.** Varies with hydration state (e.g., dehydration to overhydration/edematous states), estimated insensible water losses, gestational age, postmenstrual age, generalized health status, and underlying disease state of the infant (e.g., presence of patent ductus arteriosus, bronchopulmonary disease, postrecovery phase of necrotizing enterocolitis [NEC], and short bowel syndrome).

**3.** Energy (caloric) intake requirements.

**a.** Based on an estimation of the caloric need of 90 to 120 kcal/kg/day for premature infants as summarized in Table 10-3.

**b.** Parenteral: 80 to 100 kcal/kg/day.

■ TABLE 10-2
## ■ ■ Daily Nutritional Requirements for Premature Infants

| Nutrient | Parenteral | Enteral |
|---|---|---|
| Fluid (mL/kg/day)* | 120 to 150 | 150 to 200 |
| Energy (kcal/kg/day)† | 80 to 100 | 110 to 130 |
| Protein (g/kg/day)‡ | 3 to 4 | 3 to 4.3 |
| Carbohydrate (g/kg/day) | 10 to 15 | 8 to 12 |
| Fat (g/kg/day) | 2 to 3.5 | 3 to 4 |
| Sodium (mEq/kg/day) | 2 to 3.5 | 2 to 4 |
| Potassium (mEq/kg/day) | 2 to 3 | 2 to 3 |
| Chloride (mEq/kg/day) | 2 to 3 | 2 to 3 |
| Calcium (mg/kg/day)§ | 60 to 90 | 210 to 250 |
| Phosphorus (mg/kg/day)§ | 40 to 70 | 112 to 125 |
| Magnesium (mg/kg/day) | 4 to 7 | 8 to 15 |
| Iron (mg/kg/day)‖ | 0.0 to 0.2 | 1 to 2 |
| Vitamin A (IU/day)¶ | 700 to 1500 | 700 to 1500 |
| Vitamin D (IU/day) | 120 to 260 | 400 |
| Vitamin E (IU/day)** | 2 to 4 | 6 to 12 |
| Vitamin K (mg/day) | 0.06 to 0.1 | 0.05 |
| Vitamin C (mg/day) | 35 to 50 | 20 to 60 |
| Vitamin $B_1$ (mg/day) | 0.3 to 0.8 | 0.2 to 0.7 |
| Vitamin $B_2$ (mg/day) | 0.4 to 0.9 | 0.3 to 0.8 |
| Vitamin $B_6$ (mg/day) | 0.3 to 0.7 | 0.3 to 0.7 |
| Vitamin $B_{12}$ (mcg/day) | 0.3 to 0.7 | 0.3 to 0.7 |
| Niacin (mg/day) | 5 to 12 | 5 to 12 |
| Folate (mcg/day)†† | 40 to 90 | 50 |
| Biotin (mcg/day) | 6 to 13 | 6 to 20 |
| Zinc (mcg/kg/day)‡‡ | 400 | 800 to 1000 |
| Copper (mcg/kg/day)‡‡,§§ | 20 | 100 to 150 |
| Manganese (mcg/kg/day)§§ | 1 | 10 to 20 |
| Selenium (mcg/kg/day)¶¶ | 1.5 to 2 | 1.3 to 3 |
| Chromium (mcg/kg/day) | 0.2 | 2 to 4 |
| Molybdenum (mcg/kg/day) | 0.25 | 2 to 3 |
| Iodine (mcg/kg/day) | 1 | 4 |

Adapted from Blackburn, S.T.: *Maternal, fetal, & neonatal physiology: A clinical perspective* (4th ed.). St. Louis, 2013, Elsevier Saunders; and Adamkin, D.H., Radmacher, P. G,. and Lewis S. Nutrition and selected disorders of the gastrointestinal tract. In A. A. Fanaroff and J. M. Fanaroff (Eds.): *Klaus & Fanaroff's care of the high risk neonate* (6th ed.). Philadelphia, 2013, Elsevier Saunders, pp. 151-200.
*After immediate postnatal initiation of fluid therapy.
†Adjust according to weight gain and stress factors.
‡Requirements increase with increasing degree of prematurity.
§Inadequate amount in total parenteral nutrition solutions because of risk of precipitation.
‖Initiate between 2 weeks and 2 months of age. Delay initiation in preterm infants with progressive retinopathy.
¶Supplementation might reduce incidence of bronchopulmonary dysplasia.
**Supplementation might reduce severity of retinopathy of prematurity.
††Not present in oral multivitamin supplement.
‡‡Increased requirement in patients with excessive ileostomy drainage or chronic diarrhea.
§§Removed from total parenteral nutrition solutions in patients with cholestatic liver disease.
¶¶Not present in standard trace element solution for neonates.

c. Enteral: 110 to 130 kcal/kg/day.

d. Varies depending on day of life, fluid intake, thermal environment, activity, maturation, health status, underlying disease state, and growth rate.

4. Carbohydrate, fat, and protein (Bhatia et al., 2013; Blackburn, 2013; Kashyap, 2007; Kleinman and AAP Committee on Nutrition, 2009; Torowicz et al., 2012).

a. Carbohydrate.

(1) Parenteral: 10 to 15 g/kg/day; glucose IV infusion.

■ TABLE 10-3
■ ■ **Estimation of Caloric Requirements for the Low Birthweight Infant (kcal/kg/day)**

| Physiologic Activity | kcal/kg/day |
|---|---|
| Energy expended | 40 to 60 |
| Resting metabolic rate | 40 to 50 |
| Activity | 0 to 5 |
| Thermoregulation | 0 to 5 |
| Synthesis | 15 |
| Energy stored | 20 to 30 |
| Energy excreted | 15 |
| *Total energy intake* | 90 to 120 |

Adapted from Kleinman, R.E., and American Academy of Pediatrics Committee on Nutrition: *Pediatric nutrition handbook* (6th ed.). Elk Grove Village, IL, 2009, American Academy of Pediatrics, p. 26.

(2) Enteral: 8 to 12 g/kg/day; primarily lactose.
(3) Glucose intake must be adequate to maintain serum levels greater than 45 mg/dL.
(4) Premature infants rapidly become hypoglycemic with inadequate glucose intake. Hyperglycemia can also be a problem with extremely premature infants. Hyperglycemia contributes to hyperosmolality and may be a risk factor for intracranial hemorrhage in those infants.

**b.** Fat.
(1) Parenteral: 2 to 3.5 g/kg/day.
(2) Enteral: 3 to 4 g/kg/day.
(3) Medium-chain triglycerides are easier to absorb than long-chain triglycerides; medium-chain triglycerides are absorbed by passive diffusion and do not require bile salts.
(a) Premature infant formulas use a combination of medium-chain triglycerides and shorter-chain vegetable fatty acids.
(b) Linoleic acid is an essential fatty acid and should account for at least 3% of total calories; achieved with adequate intake of human milk and commercial premature infant formulas.
(c) Very-long-chain fatty acids—arachidonic acid and docosahexaenoic acid—are derivatives of linoleic and linolenic acids and are found in human milk but not cow's milk; associated functionally with cognition and vision.

**c.** Protein (Adamkin et al, 2013; Kashyap, 2007; Kashyap and Heird, 2011; Lapillonne et al., 2013; Moya et al., 2012; Tudehope, 2013; Tudehope et al., 2013).
(1) Parenteral: 3 to 4 g/kg/day
(a) Extremely low birth weight (ELBW) infants, that is, less than 1000 g birth weight: 3.5 to 4.0 g/kg/day.
(b) Very low birth weight (VLBW) infants, that is, 1000 to 1500 g birth weight: 3.0 to 3.5 g/kg/day.
(2) Enteral: 3.0 to 4.3 g/kg/day; higher protein amounts for low birth weight (LBW) infants.
(3) Protein requirements for VLBW infants controversial owing to uncertainty related to ability to tolerate protein and what is actually needed to provide for growth and development.
(a) Protein losses can be significant for VLBW infants when not receiving amino acids; ELBW infants lose 1.5 g/kg/day body protein, equaling approximately 1.5% body protein, when they should be accumulating at a rate of 2% per day; 3 days of no protein intake results in 10% body protein deficit.
(b) Good evidence that early amino acid intake compensates for potential protein losses; 1.5 to 2 g/kg/day as soon as possible after birth preserves limited body protein stores in ELBW infants even at low caloric intakes; increasing caloric intake will improve protein accretion.

(c) Ultimate goal of parenteral amino acid administration is to achieve a rate of fetal protein accretion; recent evidence shows that 3.5 to 4.0 g/kg/day are tolerated for ELBW infants.

(d) Protein and energy intakes should be determined concurrently to optimize nitrogen retention and promote proportionate body composition (lean-to-fat mass ratio) growth; protein-to-energy intake ratio recommendations for VLBW infants range from 2.25 to 3.6 g/100 kcal.

(e) In addition to the eight essential amino acids necessary for cell growth, premature infants require four conditionally essential amino acids: histidine, taurine, cysteine, and tyrosine.

**5.** Vitamins, minerals, and trace elements (deRegnier and Georgieff, 2011; Greer, 2006, 2008; Hambidge, 2006; Hambidge and Krebs, 2011; Hay et al., 2011; Heird, 2006; Tudehope et al., 2013).

**a.** Dietary reference intakes for enteral and parenteral nutrition are summarized in Table 10-2.

**b.** Pediatric parenteral vitamin, mineral, and trace element solutions, and commercial premature infant formulas provide adequate amounts of most vitamins; premature infants on primarily human milk intake will require oral multivitamin supplement (Kleinman and AAP Committee on Nutrition, 2009).

**c.** Newborn deficiencies in fat-soluble vitamins A, D, E, and K are well described, countermanded with human milk and formulas; significant vitamin deficiency rare even for premature infants.

(1) Vitamin K per intramuscular injection at birth; oral forms not recommended (AAP Section on Breastfeeding, 2012).

(2) Vitamin D supplementation for breastfed or formula-fed infants until intake of vitamin D–fortified formula exceeds 500 mL/day (AAP Section on Breastfeeding, 2012).

**d.** Iron supplements recommended for premature infants, owing to inadequate iron stores at birth and iatrogenic blood losses, unless received multiple blood transfusions; required for erythropoietin treatment if given for early physiologic anemia of prematurity (AAP Section on Breastfeeding, 2012; Bhatia et al., 2013; Blackburn, 2013).

**6.** Electrolytes (Blackburn, 2013; Dell, 2011).

**a.** Sodium, potassium, and chloride: necessary for growth; significant role in water and acid–base balance.

**b.** Premature infants, especially VLBW infants, have increased urine sodium and obligatory water loss during the transitional neonatal period.

**c.** After reduction of the extracellular fluid, loss of body weight slows and urinary excretion of sodium chloride decreases. VLBW infants may require sodium supplements until renal tubular function matures.

**d.** Premature infant formulas provide higher amounts of sodium, potassium, and chloride than term infant formulas; milk from mothers of premature infants (premature human milk) has higher sodium and chloride levels than that from mothers of term infants (mature human milk) (after 4 weeks); may still need to supplement until renal tubular function matures.

## PARENTERAL NUTRITION (KLEINMAN AND AAP COMMITTEE ON NUTRITION, 2009; POINDEXTER AND DUNNE, 2012)

Parenteral nutrition (PN) is indicated for initiation of nutritional support for premature and high-risk neonates; provides nutritional support when enteral intake is not possible or does not provide sufficient caloric requirements. The initial goal of PN is to minimize losses and preserve existing body stores; it progresses to provide nutrition to promote growth and development.

**A. Indications for PN in the neonatal period.**

**1.** Congenital and/or surgical GI disorders: gastroschisis, tracheoesophageal fistula, malrotation, and intestinal obstruction.

**2.** Short bowel syndrome.

**3.** Acute GI conditions, such as NEC or intestinal perforation.

**4.** Renal failure.

5. Insufficient caloric or nitrogen (protein) content of enteral feeds.
6. Severe respiratory or cardiac disease.

**B. PN administration.**

1. Peripheral route.
   a. IV access may become problematic for prolonged PN use; limit dextrose concentrations to 12.5% or less to prevent irritation of small peripheral veins.
   b. Provides up to 90 kcal/kg/day with dextrose and lipid emulsions and adequate fluid intake.
2. Central route.
   a. Prolonged dwell time for central catheters, decreases IV access problems; dextrose concentrations not restricted except by desired glucose infusion rate (GIR).
   b. Complications of central catheters: sepsis; thrombosis of large vessels; pleural or pericardial effusions due to malposition outside the vessel; hemorrhage associated with erosion of central vessels; thrombophlebitis.
   c. Peripherally inserted central catheters provide prolonged venous access; inserted at the bedside with a strictly aseptic technique by qualified personnel.
   d. Surgically placed central venous catheters (i.e., Broviac or Hickman) provide long-term venous access; require anesthesia; and are recommended for home PN use.
   e. All central venous catheters require radiographic confirmation for placement prior to initiation of PN.

**C. Guidelines for determining appropriate intake, compositions of available preparations, and guidelines for IV administration (Poindexter and Dunne, 2012).**

1. Fluid
   a. Minimum requirement approximately 100 to 150 mL/kg/day.
   b. Varies with gestational and postnatal age and environmental conditions, such as incubator versus radiant heat source and phototherapy. Incubators and heat shields can reduce insensible water losses, whereas radiant warmers and phototherapy increase these losses.
2. Calories
   a. Parenteral requirements are about 20% less than enteral intake, 80 to 100 kcal/kg/day.
      (1) Caloric values must be adjusted to meet activity levels, body temperature, and degree of stress.
      (2) Activity and catabolic states can cause a 25% to 75% increase in metabolic demands.
3. Nutrients (Blackburn, 2013; Decaro and Vain, 2011; Ditzenberger et al., 1999; Kashyap and Heird, 2011; Ogilvy-Stuart and Beardsall, 2010; Poindexter and Dunne, 2012; Sinclair et al., 2009; Tudehope et al., 2013).
   a. Carbohydrates: glucose monohydrate (dextrose), 3.4 kcal/g.
      (1) Dextrose preparations are made according to the infant's tolerance; standard dextrose concentrations are available in 5% or 10% solutions (percentage: grams of dextrose per deciliter of solution). Other concentrations may be tailored to the individual needs of the infant.
      (2) Guidelines for carbohydrate administration:
         (a) GIR of 4 to 6 g/kg/day (2.5 to 4 mg/kg/min) is the starting point; provides for minimal caloric intake, protein metabolism, and growth; serves to preserve limited neonatal carbohydrate stores.
         (b) Gradual increase in GIR to 13 to 17 g/kg/day (9 to 12 mg/kg/min) over 2 to 7 days usually tolerated in the presence of amino acid administration; maintain serum glucose 40 to 150 mg/dL; maximum GIR recommended: 18 g/kg/day (12.5 mg/kg/min); higher rates exceed glucose oxidative capacity, cause extensive lipogenesis.
         (c) In some VLBW infants, severe hyperglycemia may present and continue despite reduced carbohydrate intakes; continuous insulin infusion may be used; routine use not advised because of side effects. The usual infusion of insulin is 0.01 to 0.1 unit/kg/hr to maintain blood glucose levels between 100 and 200 mg/dL.
   b. Fat: 20% lipid preparations, 2.2 kcal/mL.
      (1) In United States, all IV lipid emulsions are derived from soybean oil or a combination of soybean and safflower oils, contain long-chain triglycerides.

(2) IV lipid emulsions have a fatty acid profile substantially different from human milk.

(3) Lipid emulsions of 0.5 to 1 g/kg/day prevent deficiency of essential fatty acids; should be introduced as a component of PN by 24 to 48 hours of age; increase by 0.5 to 1 g/kg/day to 3 g/kg/day.

(4) Premature infants less than 28 weeks of gestational age have limited lipoprotein lipase activity and triglyceride clearance; may require slower advances in IV lipid infusion rate to improve tolerance.

(5) Although heparin releases lipoprotein lipase from the endothelium into circulation, there is no evidence that this increases lipid utilization in premature infants; therefore, routine addition of heparin into lipid infusion is not recommended.

**c.** Protein: amino acids, 4 kcal/g. Recommended intake: 2.25 to 4 g/kg/day.

(1) The smaller and less mature the infant, the higher the protein intake recommended; for example, infants weighing less than 1000 g may receive 4 g/kg/day protein intake (refer to the Nutritional Requirements, B. Premature Infants section).

(2) Pediatric amino acid solutions designed to mimic plasma amino acid concentrations in healthy 20-day-old breastfed infant (Trophamine) or fetal or neonatal cord blood amino acid concentrations (Primine); no evidence to support superiority of one solution over the other.

(a) Glutamine, an amino acid abundant in breast milk, not included in available amino acid solutions owing to issues of stability.

(b) Tyrosine has limited solubility, and so a small amount is included; Trophamine contains a soluble derivative of tyrosine but appears to have poor bioavailability; current research suggests that tyrosine supply in amino acids is suboptimal for VLBW infants.

(c) Cysteine unstable for long periods; cysteine hydrochloride supplement can be added to PN just prior to administration; there is conflicting evidence as to whether cysteine improves protein accretion.

**d.** Calcium and phosphorus.

(1) PN preparations for infants receiving 100 to 150 mL/kg/day should contain 50 to 60 mg/dL (12.5 to 15 mmol/L) elemental calcium and 40 to 47 mg/dL (12.5 to 15 mmol/L) phosphorus; provides 50 to 90 mg/kg/day calcium and 40 to 70 mg/kg/day phosphorus; a calcium-to-phosphorus ratio of 1.7:1 by weight (1.3:1 by molar ratio) maintains optimal bone mineralization.

(2) Precipitation of calcium and phosphorus remains an issue in the United States owing to commercially available solutions; not possible to supply VLBW infants with adequate amounts of parenteral calcium and phosphorus to support optimal bone mineralization.

**e.** Vitamins and trace elements are summarized in Tables 10-1 and 10-2.

**f.** Suggestions for monitoring growth and biochemical laboratory tests during PN use are summarized in Table 10-4.

**D. Complications associated with PN administration (Blackburn, 2013; Davis and Andres, 2008; Poindexter and Dunne, 2012)**

**1.** Increased risk of metabolic derangements (e.g., hyperglycemia, hypoglycemia, azotemia, acidosis, alkalosis), electrolyte imbalances: require close blood chemistry monitoring; alleviated with manipulation of PN constituents.

**2.** Cholestasis and cholestatic jaundice as a result of hepatic dysfunction: initial intracellular and intracanalicular cholestasis, followed by portal inflammation; progressing to bile duct proliferation after several weeks of PN administration; may progress to portal fibrosis and cirrhosis. Most often resolves gradually with cessation of PN use when on full enteral nutrition; rare instances of irreversible liver failure documented after several months of continuous PN.

**a.** Very little recent information regarding incidence of cholestasis; older studies suggest increased prevalence in ELBW infants; occurs predominantly in critically ill premature infants with prolonged PN administration who potentially experienced a variety of insults (e.g., hypoxia, hemodynamic instability, and/or infection); higher incidence of sepsis reported in infants with cholestasis.

■ TABLE 10-4
■ ■ **Suggested Monitoring Schedule for Infants Receiving Parenteral Nutrition**

| Parameter | Suggested Frequency Per Week | |
|---|---|---|
| | Initial Period* | Later Period* |
| **ANTHROPOMETRIC** | | |
| Weight | 7 | 7 |
| Length | 1 | 1 |
| Head circumference | 1 | 1 |
| **METABOLIC (BLOOD OR PLASMA)** | | |
| Electrolytes | 2 to 4 | 1 |
| Calcium, magnesium, and phosphorus | 2 | 1 |
| Acid–base status | 2 | 1 |
| Blood urea nitrogen/creatinine | 2 | 1 |
| Albumin | 2 | 1 |
| Liver function tests | 1 | 1 |
| Hemoglobin/hematocrit | 2 | 1 |
| **PREVENTION AND DETECTION OF INFECTION** | | |
| Clinical observations (e.g., activity, temperature) | Daily | Daily |
| White blood cell count, differential | As indicated | As indicated |
| Cultures | As indicated | As indicated |

Adapted from Heird, W.C.: Intravenous feeding. In P.J. Thureen and W.W. Hay (Eds.): *Neonatal nutrition and metabolism* (2nd ed.). New York, 2006, Cambridge University Press, p. 325.

*Initial period refers to the time before full intake is achieved as well as any period during which metabolic instability is present or suspected (postoperative, symptoms of sepsis). Later period refers to any time there is metabolic stability.

b. Precise cause unknown; probably multifactorial; growing body of evidence of association with prolonged lack of enteral nutrition; research evidence suggests that enteral feedings even at low caloric intakes can reduce the incidence of cholestasis.

c. Clinical features: hyperbilirubinemia and jaundice.
   (1) Direct bilirubin (DB) level greater than 1 mg/dL (17.1 μmol/L) and total serum bilirubin (TB) ≤5 mg/dL (85.5 μmol/L), or DB equal to 20% TB with TB greater than 5 mg/dL.
   (2) Sensitive, nonspecific early indicator: increase in γ-glutamyltransferase.
   (3) Later: increase in aspartate transaminase (serum glutamic-oxaloacetic transaminase) and alanine transaminase (serum glutamate-pyruvate transaminase).

3. PN-induced osteopenia: long-term PN associated with osteopenia and bone demineralization (Greer, 2008; Pieltain et al., 2013; Poindexter and Dunne, 2012; Williford et al., 2008).
   a. Hypercalciuria; several factors implicated in hypercalciuria: cyclic PN infusion, sulfur-containing amino acids, hypertonic dextrose infusions causing hyperinsulinemia and decreased tubular calcium resorption, acidosis, and low phosphate in PN.
   b. Aluminum-containing PN solutions; metabolic bone disease characterized by reduced bone formation and aluminum accumulation in bone correlating with decreased bone formation.
   c. Decreased mineral retention; inappropriate mineral ratio; suboptimal minerals in PN during periods of rapid growth rate.
   d. Vitamin D deficiency rare in infants receiving PN containing pediatric IV vitamins; does not contribute to PN-related metabolic bone disease.

4. Sepsis: infection is a major complication of PN; incidence higher in VLBW infants; increases with longer PN duration.
   a. Two most common bacterial pathogens: *Staphylococcus epidermidis* and *Staphylococcus aureus*.
   b. Two most common fungal pathogens: *Candida albicans* and *Malassezia furfur*.

5. Measures to prevent or minimize complications associated with PN.
   a. Standardized procedures/policies to facilitate a consistent methodology to prevent and/or minimize complications.
   b. Record intake and assess IV insertion site hourly.
   c. Readjust fluid volume, dextrose concentration, protein and/or fat intake, electrolytes, and minerals as needed in response to blood chemistry results.
   d. Initiate enteral feedings as soon as possible.
   e. Pharmacy preparation of PN under laminar airflow hood; nothing should be added to PN solution once it leaves the pharmacy; filter central PN with an in-line filter.
   f. Wash hands scrupulously before handling any PN tubing or IV sites; use sterile techniques for dressing changes.

## ENTERAL FEEDINGS: HUMAN MILK AND COMMERCIAL FORMULAS FOR TERM, SPECIAL-NEEDS, AND PREMATURE INFANTS

A. **Comparison of human milk, donor milk, and commercial infant formulas (AAP Section on Breastfeeding, 2012; Arslanoglu et al. and WAPM Working Group on Nutrition, 2010; Bertino et al., 2009; Bhatia and Greer, 2008; Blackburn, 2013; Kleinman and AAP Committee on Nutrition, 2009; Tudehope, 2013; Underwood, 2013; Wojcik et al., 2009; Young et al., 2012).**
   1. Human milk: host resistance factors and antimicrobial properties (e.g., lactoferrin, lysozyme, and secretory immunoglobulin A [IgA]), hormones (e.g., cortisol, somatomedin-C, insulin-like growth factors, insulin, thyroid hormone), and growth factors (e.g., epidermal and nerve growth factors); increased bioavailability of fat, amino acid, and carbohydrate with enhanced absorption, digestion, gastric motility, and gastric emptying; very-long-chain fatty acids (may be important for cognition, growth, and vision); increased absorption of zinc and iron; low renal solute load; optimal distribution of calories (7% protein, 55% fat, 38% carbohydrate); provides variability in nutrient amounts between feeds and/or time of day, which may enhance sensory development, acceptance of new flavors and foods later. A comparison of term and premature human milk summarized in Table 10-5.

■ TABLE 10-5

■ ■ **Composition of Premature and Mature Human Milk**

| Component | Premature Human Milk (1 Week) | Mature Human Milk (1 Month) |
|---|---|---|
| Volume (mL) | 100 | 100 |
| Energy (kcal) | 67 | 70 |
| Protein (g) | 2.4 | 1.8 |
| % Whey/casein | 70/30 | 70/30 |
| Fat (g) | 3.8 | 4 |
| % MCTs/LCTs | 2/98 | 2/98 |
| Carbohydrate (g) | 6.1 | 7 |
| % Lactose | 100 | 100 |
| Calcium (mg) | 25 | 22 |
| Phosphorus (mg) | 14 | 14 |
| Magnesium (mg) | 3.1 | 2.5 |
| Sodium (mg) | 50 | 30 |
| Potassium (mg) | 70 | 60 |
| Chloride (mg) | 90 | 60 |
| Zinc (mcg) | 500 | 320 |
| Copper (mcg) | 80 | 60 |
| Vitamin A (IU) | 560 | 400 |
| Vitamin D (IU) | 4 | 4 |
| Vitamin E (mg) | 1 | 0.3 |
| Vitamin C (mg) | 5.4 | 5.6 |

Adapted from Blackburn, S.T.: *Maternal, fetal, & neonatal physiology: A clinical perspective* (4th ed.). St. Louis, 2013, Saunders.
*LCTs*, Long-chain triglycerides; *MCTs*, medium-chain triglycerides.

a. Contraindications for human milk consumption: relatively few true contraindications exist.
   (1) Galactosemia; cannot ingest lactose-containing milk (e.g., human milk and commercial cow's milk–based formulas).
   (2) Human immunodeficiency virus (HIV): in the United States, counseled regarding risks to infant of breastfeeding, recommend not breastfeeding. Globally, health risks of the infant need to be balanced against the risk for acquiring HIV.
   (3) Human T-cell lymphotropic virus: no breastfeeding.
   (4) Miliary tuberculosis: no breastfeeding while contagious (needs documentation, generally approximately 2 weeks).
   (5) Herpetic lesions: if localized to breast, no breastfeeding; vaginal herpetic lesions not a barrier to breastfeeding.
   (6) Varicella lesions on breast: provide expressed human milk until completely crusted over; infant should receive varicella immune globulin.
   (7) Breast cancer; treatment should not be delayed; no breastfeeding with antimetabolite chemotherapy.
   (8) Maternal use of prescription and/or over-the-counter medications; direct contraindications for breastfeeding include cytotoxic drugs; some drugs have strong associations with adverse effects in infants; need extra caution with premature infants.
   (9) Illicit drug abuse: recommend counseling; no breastfeeding until free of abused drug(s).

2. Commercial infant formulas for term infants are cow's milk or soy based; available in powder, concentrate, and ready-to-feed forms; all should be iron fortified. Both types support adequate weight gain for term infants.
   a. Cow's milk–based formulas recommended except for infants with galactosemia, primary lactase deficiency, immunoglobulin E–mediated reaction to cow's milk–based formulas, or parents seeking vegan-based diet for term infant.
   b. Extensively hydrolyzed protein formula should be considered for infants with documented cow's milk protein allergy; 10% to 14% of these infants also have a soy protein allergy.
   c. Soy-based formulas not recommended for premature infants.

**B. Term infants (AAP Section on Breastfeeding, 2012; Bhatia and Greer, 2008; Neville and McManaman, 2006).**

1. Human milk is the ideal food for term infants. Exclusive breastfeeding should be encouraged for the first 6 months of life, at which time complementary foods are introduced; breastfeeding should be encouraged for at least the first year of infant's life and beyond for as long as mutually desired by mother and child.
2. Commercial term infant formulas used primarily when breastfeeding is contraindicated, as a supplement to breastfeeding during inadequate human milk supply or poor infant growth, or maternal preference not to breastfeed.

**C. Infants with special nutritional requirements.**

1. Infants with inborn errors of metabolism (IEM); also referred to as inherited metabolic disorders; disorders resulting from genetically inherited disruption of enzymatic activities that occur in normal metabolic processes (Thomas et al., 2006).
   a. Nutrition plays an important role in the management of treatable IEM disorders; modification of diet can alter biochemical imbalances to improve mental and physical development.
   b. Goals for nutritional support: provide all essential nutrients and supply the optimal amount of any nutrient that is restricted as a result of IEM to promote growth and correct metabolic imbalances.
   c. Management depends on the specific biochemistry and pathophysiology of the diagnosed IEM; includes restriction of any compound or precursor of metabolites that could accumulate as a result of the missing or defective enzyme(s) and/or supplement deficient end products and cofactors not produced as a result of the missing or defective enzyme(s).
   d. Premature infants have the same risk for IEM as term infants; may not be suspected when symptoms resemble more common problems expected in premature infants; diagnostic tests may be altered by common treatments (e.g., early blood transfusions producing false-negative newborn screen testing for galactosemia).

e. Examples of IEM with dietary restrictions, supplements requiring specialty formula compositions:
(1) Phenylketonuria: restriction of the amino acid phenylalanine; supplement with tyrosine.
(2) Maple syrup urine disease: restriction of branched-chain amino acids; supplement with valine and isoleucine.
(3) Galactosemia: restriction of galactose/lactose; supplement with calcium.
(4) Glycogen storage disease, type I (glucose-6-phosphatase deficiency): restriction of galactose/fructose; modified fat and moderate protein; frequent feedings, nocturnal continuous feedings; cornstarch in feedings.
(5) Urea cycle disorders: low-protein diet with nonessential amino acid restriction; supplement with carnitine, biotin, folate, and pyridoxine.

2. Infants with altered fluid and/or caloric intake requirements.
a. Bronchopulmonary disease (BPD): may have increased metabolic demands, respiratory workload, oxygen consumption; energy needs may increase by 20% to 40% above that of healthy infants. Postnatal growth failure common, extends beyond early neonatal life for several years; multifactorial causes of feeding difficulties related to fluid restriction, long-term PN, oral feeding intolerance, and GER; recover more quickly if given adequate caloric intake, yet metabolism of this energy results in increased $CO_2$ production and oxygen consumption in infants with compromised respiratory function (Atkinson, 2006; Blackburn, 2013; Botet et al., 2012; Dani and Poggi, 2012; Groothuis and Makari, 2012; Jobe, 2011; McCain et al., 2012).
(1) Relative fluid restriction to reduce pulmonary edema, appears to complicate the pathology of BPD.
(2) Infants with BPD may have higher caloric requirements to meet the demands of healing tissue and growth requirements.
(3) May benefit from specially developed nutritional products to allow for fluid restriction and support optimal growth; currently use increased caloric density formula and/or fortified human milk mixtures with variable results.
(4) May require special approaches to transition from gavage feeds to bottle or breast feeds in keeping with feeding readiness cues, ability to regulate frequency, duration of feed and volume tolerated per feed based on respiratory and energy status.

b. Cardiac problems: poor growth may result from increased metabolic demands, higher metabolic rate and oxygen consumption secondary to increased cardiac and respiratory workload; tissue hypoxia, protein loss, increased associated frequency of infections, and decreased nutrient absorption owing to diminished splenic blood flow; might be fluid and sodium restricted to reduce overcirculation; infant may be easily fatigued and become tachypneic and stressed with feeding (Barry and Thureen, 2006; Blackburn, 2013; Hartman and Medoff-Cooper, 2012; Pye and Green, 2004).
(1) Caloric requirements to improve growth may be met with increased caloric density of formula and/or breast milk mixtures.
(2) Often described as poor feeders, give fewer cues, and are less responsive to caregivers during feeds.
(3) Formula and/or breast milk may be fortified to meet higher caloric needs and not exceed possible fluid restriction or normal fluid intakes with increased caloric densities.
(4) Osmolarity of formulas and breast milk mixtures increases by approximately the same percentage as the caloric increase; strict attention must be paid to the renal solute load and osmolarity when concentrating formulas and adding calories to breast milk beyond 24 cal/ounce.

3. Infants with short bowel syndrome: intestinal length (normal small bowel length not clearly established; estimated 250 to 270 cm at term) reduced because of surgical resection resulting from congenital anomaly (e.g., gastroschisis, midgut volvulus, intestinal atresias) or NEC; results in reduction of the intestinal absorptive surface area; remaining sections of bowel may have been ischemic, resulting in villous atrophy; full enteral feedings might be achieved if at least 25 cm of the small bowel with ileocecal valve or 40 cm without ileocecal valve remains after surgical resection (Blackburn, 2013; Gutierrez et al., 2011; Soundheimer, 2006).

a. Depending on the length of the intestine, may need PN for prolonged period until linear growth occurs.
b. Slow initiation of enteral feedings, similar to minimal feeding regimen of premature infants, may be beneficial.

**D. Premature infants.**

1. Human milk from mothers of premature infants contains slightly higher concentrations of protein, sodium, and chloride; more lipid, energy, vitamins, and trace elements; lower concentrations of phosphorus and calcium; and has lower osmolality than breast milk from mothers of term infants; differences decline as lactation progresses, becoming similar in composition between 2 and 4 weeks. A comparison of premature and mature human milk is summarized in Table 10-5 (Blackburn, 2013; Neville and McManaman, 2006; Underwood, 2013).
   a. The significant benefits of human milk for premature infants warrant encouraging and actively supporting mothers to pump and provide milk for their infants.
      (1) Importance of human milk for premature infants should be discussed during the first visit with parents; counseling as early as possible increases the incidence of lactation initiation and does not seem to increase maternal stress and/or anxiety.
      (2) Important to begin expressing human milk at the earliest possible moment following delivery.
      (3) Initial volume may be few drops of colostrum for the first 24 to 48 hours postpartum; may have considerable delay before substantial production begins; increases from about 50 mL/day to 500 to 600 mL/day in subsequent 36 hours (the "coming in" period of milk).
      (4) Encourage expressing milk at least 8 times in 24 hours; break in frequency while establishing milk supply may seriously compromise potential of maximum production.
      (5) Goal of 600 to 750 mL/day by day 10 to 14; milk production typically plateaus by 14 days postpartum.
      (6) Once milk production is established, it can be maintained with greater than 6 pumps per day (at least 45 pumping times per week); needs to be monitored for ongoing success.
      (7) Optimal milk expression technique includes the following:
         (a) Supportive environment for mother.
         (b) Regular breast massage with good technique.
         (c) Simultaneous pumping of both breasts with high-quality breast pump and properly fitting milk expression shield.
      (8) Donor human milk: procurement recommended from human milk banks for safe use; differs from individual mother's mature human milk in nutrient content and energy value; pasteurizing recommended to decrease transmission of HIV, cytomegalovirus, hepatitis B and C; pasteurizing reduces secretory IgA, lactoferrin, lysozyme, insulin-like growth factors, hepatocyte growth factor, water-soluble vitamins, bile salt–stimulated lipase, lipoprotein lipase, and antioxidant activity; does not decrease oligosaccharides, long-chain polyunsaturated fatty acids, gangliosides, lactose, fat-soluble vitamins, or epidermal growth factor; increasingly preferred for premature infants in particular over commercial formulas when mother's own milk is not available.
   b. Storage, handling of human milk: needs to be collected, processed, and stored to ensure microbiological safety and nutrition quality (AAP Section on Breastfeeding, 2012; Ramírez-Santana et al., 2012; Slutzah et al., 2010; Vieira et al., 2011).
      (1) Wash hands with soap and warm water.
      (2) Collection kits should be rinsed, cleaned with hot soapy water, and air-dried.
      (3) Glass or hard plastic containers for storage.
      (4) Freeze milk that is not to be used within 48 hours; single milk expressions in each container, labeled with name, date, and time of pumping; keeps from 3 to 6 months in the rear of freezer compartment.
         (a) Freezing preserves many of the nutritional and immunologic benefits of human milk.

(b) Thaw completely with tepid running (not hot) water or commercial human milk thawing machine; never thaw or warm in microwave oven; once thawed, do not refreeze; use completely within 24 hours refrigerated at 4 ° C; recent evidence suggests human milk may be stored at 4 ° C in refrigerator for up to 96 hours with minimal change in macronutrients, IgA, lactoferrin, total fat and protein and no increase in bacterial count.

2. Human milk fortifiers, powdered and liquid forms, provide additional protein, fat, carbohydrate, sodium, potassium, phosphorus, and calcium; 4 packets added to 100 mL human milk averages 24 cal/oz, 2.7 g protein, 4.5 g fat, and 7.5 g carbohydrate (AAP Section on Breastfeeding, 2012; Arslanoglu et al., 2012; Blackburn, 2013; Moya et al., 2012).
3. Commercial premature infant formulas, 24 cal/oz, have increased amounts of protein, carbohydrate, fat, sodium, potassium, calcium, and phosphorus; supply these nutrients within acceptable ratios similar to breast milk with added human milk fortifier (Blackburn, 2013; Kleinman and AAP Committee on Nutrition, 2009).
4. Transitional premature infant formulas provide 22 cal/oz and more calcium, phosphorus, and magnesium than term infant formulas but less than premature infant formulas, and are designed for use after hospital discharge; studies vary as to how long to continue using the transitional formulas (Blackburn, 2013; Kashyap, 2007; Kleinman and AAP Committee on Nutrition, 2009; Lapillonne and Griffin, 2013; Natarajan et al., 2013; Tudehope, 2013; Underwood, 2013; Young et al., 2012).

## ENTERAL FEEDING METHODS

Enteral feedings are achieved via several routes, including nasogastric, orogastric, transpyloric, and gastrostomy tubes, and orally by bottle or breast. Decisions regarding enteral feeding are dependent on gestational age, birth weight, and clinical condition of the infant. When to initiate feeding, type of feeding, method of delivery, feeding frequency, concentration of feeding, and rate of advancement may vary according to unit practices (Blackburn, 2013; Kleinman and AAP Committee on Nutrition, 2009).

A. **Minimal enteral feedings or trophic feeding (Blackburn, 2013; Kleinman and AAP Committee on Nutrition, 2009; Thureen and Hay, 2009).**
   1. Have benefit without adverse consequences for most VLBW infants.
   2. Defined as ≤25 mL/kg/day of human milk or premature infant formula.
   3. Not intended for primary source of nutrition.
   4. Given concurrently with PN as primary nutrition.
   5. Intended to provide physiologic effects, including stimulating and maintaining digestive–absorptive, immunologic, and neuroendocrine functions of the GI tract.
      a. Promotion of gut mucosal development.
      b. Stimulation of intestinal motor activity.
      c. Increased secretion of GI hormones and peptides.
      d. Colonization of the gut with normal flora, limiting colonization by other pathogenic organisms, helps development of the innate immune system of the GI tract.
   6. Does not increase the incidence of NEC.
   7. Dilute formula or breast milk or sterile water does not stimulate GI motor activity as well as full-strength formula or breast milk.
   8. Recommended length of minimal enteral nutrition: 1 to 5 days; longer period for more immature infants.

B. **Potential contraindications for initiation of feedings, advancing feeds, and feeding tolerance/intolerance for VLBW infants (Blackburn, 2013; Gomella, 2013; Jacobi and Odle, 2012; Kleinman and AAP Committee on Nutrition, 2009; Lucchini et al., 2011; Moore, 2011; Neu et al., 2013; Thureen and Hay, 2009).**
   1. Perceived contraindications for initiating and/or continuing feeds: hypoxic–ischemic insults at birth (low Apgar scores), apnea and/or bradycardia, sepsis, umbilical arterial catheters, indomethacin administration, inotropic agents (dopamine), heme-positive stools.

a. Presence of apnea and/or bradycardia: one reason given to not feed infant is that apnea causes transient ischemia to the intestine, may lead to NEC; epidemiologic investigations did not find this to be an increased risk.
b. Presence of umbilical arterial catheters (UAC): variable evidence to suggest safety of feeding with UACs; have been implicated as a risk factor for NEC because of potential for thrombi; frequent blood draws and flushes may compromise the hemodynamics of the intestine; however, these possibilities exist but true cause-and-effect relationships or strong associations between the UAC and NEC have not been demonstrated.
c. Minimal enteral nutrition does not appear to increase the incidence of NEC in the presence of apnea and/or bradycardia, UACs, indomethacin; caution must be used in advancing feedings while in the presence of these situations.

2. Evidence that advancing enteral feedings faster than 20 mL/kg/day is associated with increased incidence of NEC.
3. Assessing for feeding tolerance/intolerance: feeding intolerance has no uniform definition, in premature infants refers to not digesting formula or breast milk rather than intolerance to the carbohydrate source of formulas (e.g., lactose intolerance). Manifestations of intolerance vary, based on pre-feed gastric residual volume, color, and associated clinical manifestations such as abdominal distention, emesis, and/or presence of blood in stools, apnea, and bradycardia.
   a. Gastric aspirates; pre-feed gastric residuals.
      (1) Fasting basal gastric residuals average 3 mL every 4 hours found in infants of 28 to 36 weeks of gestational age; greater than 2 mL in less than 760-g infants and 3 mL in greater than 750-g infants; volume of greater than 30% of the milk given during previous feedings may be abnormal and requires more extensive evaluation; greater than 10 to 15 mL is considered excessive.
      (2) Bile-stained aspirate may not be sufficient reason to withhold feeds; may be due to immature gut motility, leading to periodic antiperistalsis.
      (3) Determination of significance of gastric aspirate may need to rely on what volume is reasonably expected at the infant's gestational age or what is "normal" for an individual infant, and the presence of clinical manifestations.
      (4) Clinical manifestations: abdominal distention, emesis, blood in stools, apnea, and bradycardia.
         (a) Abdominal distention: visual examination for visible bowel loops, erythema, auscultate for bowel tones, palpate to assess whether soft, firm, and for tenderness; ascertain when last stool occurred.
         (b) Emesis: may be result of LES or increased abdominal pressure resulting from NEC, obstruction, undigested milk feeding.
         (c) Blood in stools: trauma from nasogastric tube; swallowed maternal blood (if soon after delivery), bleeding disorder (such as vitamin K deficiency, disseminated intravascular coagulation, congenital coagulopathy); stress ulcer; severe fetal asphyxia; NEC; medications (such as indomethacin, corticosteroids).
         (d) Apnea and bradycardia: generalized response to change in condition, sepsis, NEC.

**C. Nasogastric and orogastric tube feeding (Blackburn, 2013; Gomella, 2013; Kleinman and AAP Committee on Nutrition, 2009).**

1. Most commonly used method in the neonatal intensive care unit (NICU) environment; used for very premature or critically ill infants to reduce risk of aspiration and conserve energy; determined by infant's lack of ability to coordinate a suck–swallow–breathe feeding pattern.
2. Procedure for gastric (nasal or oral) insertion:
   a. Gather equipment: infant feeding tube, stethoscope, sterile water (lubricant), syringe (5 to 10 mL), transparent dressing, gloves, suctioning equipment.
   b. Monitor heart rate and respiratory function throughout the procedure.
   c. Place infant supine; head of bed may be elevated.
   d. Choose size of gastric tube: general guideline—for infants less than 1000 g, No. 5 French gastric tube; $\geq$1000 g, No. 6 to 8 French gastric tube.

e. Determine the length of tubing required to reach the stomach: measure the distance from the nose to the earlobe to the midumbilicus, mark the tube at the appropriate length (Cirgin-Ellett et al., 2011).

f. Moisten the tip of the tube with sterile water and insert via mouth or nare.
   (1) Oral insertion: push the tongue down and insert the tube into the oropharynx; advance as tolerated to desired length. The oral route is preferable because neonates are obligate nose breathers, and use of the nasal route increases airway resistance.
   (2) Nasal insertion: flex neck, push nose up, insert the tube straight back into the nares, and advance as tolerated to desired length.

g. Verify correct positioning in the stomach.
   (1) Aspirate contents from the tube with a syringe; assess color and consistency of aspirate to determine stomach contents.
   (2) Inject small amounts of air into the tube with a syringe; listen with a stethoscope for rush of air into the stomach. May be unreliable because rush of air can be auscultated as if entering the stomach when the tip of the tube is actually positioned in the distal esophagus; recommended to use concurrently with other methods of determination.
   (3) Definitive verification of tube placement with chest/abdominal radiographic imaging.

h. Complications.
   (1) Apnea and bradycardia: vagal response; usually resolve without specific treatment beyond stimulation.
   (2) Hypoxia: resolves with correction of apnea and bradycardia response; may require oxygen to resolve; if severe, may need positive pressure ventilation with bag and mask. If this continues, suspect misplacement of tube into the trachea and remove the tube immediately.
   (3) Perforation of the esophagus, posterior pharynx, stomach, or duodenum (rare): the tube should never be forced during the insertion procedure.
   (4) Aspiration: complication of misplacement into the trachea, esophagus, or hypopharynx; results from stomach distention or failure of feeding to continue through the GI tract. Verify position of tube and the presence of residuals prior to every bolus feeding or periodically with continuous feeding infusion.

3. Feeding may be accomplished by bolus or continuous infusion of human milk or formula (Blackburn, 2013; Gomella, 2013; Kleinman and AAP Committee on Nutrition, 2009).
   a. Bolus feeds every 2 to 3 hours similar to feeding pattern when bottle- or breast-feeding; associated with improved nutrient absorption and growth.
   b. Continuous infusions associated with increased feeding intolerance, reduced nutrient absorption, and decreased growth in premature infants; may be perceived to be necessary with early feeding initiation; should transition to bolus feeds as tolerated. Human milk fat and medium-chain triglyceride additives adhere to feeding tube surfaces, and nutrient loss from human milk fortifiers further reduces nutrient intake and energy density provided by continuous enteral tube feeding.

**D. Transpyloric and gastrostomy tube feeding (Blackburn, 2013; Gomella, 2013; Kleinman and AAP Committee on Nutrition, 2009).**

1. Transpyloric tube feeding bypasses the stomach and reduces the digestive capability of the GI tract.
   a. Feeds can only be by continuous infusion; placement confirmed with radiographic imaging.
   b. Associated with significant risks: abdominal distention, gastric bleeding, bilious vomiting, and mortality.
   c. Does not improve energy intake or growth.
   d. Should be used only in rare instances of prolonged gastroparesis or dysmotility.
   e. Gastric feedings should be resumed as soon as possible.
2. Gastrostomy tube feeding via a surgically placed tube through the abdominal wall directly into the stomach; can be bolus or continuous infusion; used primarily for infants unable to sustain full oral feeds or maintain sufficient caloric intake to promote growth, such as abnormal neurologic status, congenital anomalies of the GI tract (e.g., esophageal atresia), or other conditions requiring long-term gavage feedings.

E. **Oral feeding, breast or bottle:** Determined by the infant's ability to coordinate a suck–swallow–breathe pattern, sustain an alert–awake behavior, and maintain cardiorespiratory stability; premature infants limited by weaker flexor control and immature musculature (Blackburn, 2013; Boiron et al., 2007; Jones, 2012; McCain et al., 2012; Nye, 2008; Puckett et al., 2008).
   1. Oral feeding readiness.
      a. Infant should be free of signs and/or symptoms of respiratory distress (e.g., respiratory rate <60 breaths per minute; blood gas values within normal limits); criteria may be modified for infants with BPD or congenital heart disease.
      b. Infant demonstrates suck–swallow–breathe coordination with an intact gag reflex.
         (1) Swallow reflex well developed by 28 to 30 weeks, easily exhausted; matures by 34 weeks.
         (2) Gag reflex matures by 34 weeks.
         (3) Suck maturation related to gestational not postnatal age; nonnutritive suck present at less than 32 to 33 weeks of gestation; nutritive suck appears by 32 to 33 weeks; matures by 37 weeks of gestation.
         (4) Suck–swallow reflexes are present by 28 weeks; synchrony of suck–swallow appears by 32 to 34 weeks; complete coordination develops by 36 to 37 weeks of gestation.
   2. Oral feeding initiation: major goal of nurses and families: assist VLBW infants to develop safe and effective early oral feeding skills, improve breastfeeding outcomes.
      a. Healthy infants ≥34 weeks of gestation may have oral feedings initiated as soon after birth as indicated. Factors to be considered include infant behavior and maternal preference for breastfeeding or bottle-feeding (Blackburn, 2013).
      b. Transition from gastric tube feeding to oral feeding (breast or bottle) may be dependent on infant behavior, unit-specific feeding policy, and/or gestational age or weight criteria (Jones, 2005; Kirk et al., 2007).
         (1) Use of infant state assessment and feeding cues shown to facilitate improved progression to full oral feedings.
         (2) Careful monitoring must take place during feedings to ensure safe intake without complications of aspiration, desaturation (or increased requirement for fractional inspired oxygen), apnea, and bradycardia; reported to occur less frequently during breastfeeding than bottle-feeding.
      c. Increasing number of VLBW infants are referred for treatment of significant, persistent feeding problems after discharge; during hospitalization, provide positive feeding experiences and identify feeding problems at an early stage when most amenable to change.

## NURSING INTERVENTIONS TO FACILITATE TOLERANCE OF ENTERAL FEEDINGS

A. **Sensory–motor–oral stimulation and nonnutritive sucking provided during gavage feedings (Jones, 2012; Nye, 2008; Puckett et al., 2008).**
   1. May promote earlier oral feeding and decrease length of stay.
   2. May enhance sucking patterns and coordination.
   3. May support maturation of neural structures, which, in turn, may result from influences of learned experiences.

B. **Assessment of infant readiness.**
   1. May be defined in terms of readiness for the initiation of oral feedings in general and in terms of a specific feeding time in particular.
   2. May enhance oral feeding initiation and success.
   3. May promote infant engagement during bottle-feeding.
   4. May promote successful breastfeeding of premature infants.
      a. Premature infants have been able to breastfeed successfully as early as 32 weeks of gestation and may establish mature suck–swallow–breathe coordination earlier with breastfeeding than with bottle-feeding.
      b. Higher birth weight, less need of ventilator and oxygen, higher hemoglobin, no bottle-feeding, minimal apnea of prematurity, and no signs and symptoms of infection are associated with successful breastfeeding.

c. Test-weighing of infants (before and after breastfeeding) with an electronic scale is a relatively reliable method of determining infant intake of human milk from the breast for in-hospital assessment.

**C. Position of infant during and after feedings (Corvaglia et al., 2007; Elser, 2012; Fanaro, 2012; Nye, 2008).**

1. Kangaroo care (skin-to-skin positioning of infant on mother's chest) during gavage feeding is associated with improved breast milk production and may improve breastfeeding rates.
2. Prone or left lateral positions with 30-degree elevation are associated with fewer GER-like episodes, improved gastric emptying.

## NUTRITIONAL ASSESSMENT AND STANDARDS FOR ADEQUATE GROWTH

Nutritional management is meant to improve growth and minimize harm; requires nutritional assessment tools to provide for growth in an efficacious and safe manner (Auron and Mhanna, 2006; Bhatia, 2013; Blackburn, 2013; Gomella, 2013; Kleinman and AAP Committee on Nutrition, 2009; Moyer-Mileur, 2007; Olsen et al., 2010; Roggero et al., 2010; Williford et al., 2008).

**A. Nutritional intake: ascertain whether the prescribed nutritional intake is provided.**

1. Monitor volume and caloric intakes daily: follow current recommended intakes for gestational age and condition of infant; adjust intake accordingly to maintain nutritional goals.
2. Periodically review all dietary intakes from birth; early nutrition has a profound impact on long-term growth and development.

**B. Laboratory assessment: serves a key role in the assessment of nutritional adequacy and toxicity.**

1. Electrolytes, sodium ($Na^+$), potassium ($K^+$), chloride ($Cl^-$), bicarbonate ($NaCO_3^-$).
   a. Provide information on renal function and fluid status.
   b. Results need to be assessed in relation to an infant's fluid status (intake and output), condition and previous trends in electrolyte results.
2. Blood urea nitrogen (BUN) and creatinine (Cr).
   a. BUN may not be a good indicator of protein intake and/or tolerance in the first weeks of life for VLBW infants; should not be considered as a biochemical marker during this period; reflects more the fluid status.
   b. BUN level has improved validity for protein intake with serial levels in stable, older VLBW infants who are receiving enteral nutrition, if taken into consideration with GFR and renal function indicators (creatinine level) and anthropometric growth parameters; may have increased sensitivity and specificity for protein tolerance during this period.
   c. Creatinine and creatinine clearance are valid biochemical markers for renal function assessment for VLBW infants.
3. Calcium ($Ca^+$), magnesium ($Mg^+$), phosphorus ($PO_4^-$), and alkaline phosphatase (alk phos).
   a. Followed for management and surveillance of metabolic bone disease, assessment of bone mineralization status. Decreased calcium and phosphorus levels or increased alkaline phosphatase levels may indicate bone demineralization; alkaline phosphatase levels greater than 500 to 700 mg/dL or radiologic evidence of rickets indicates need for increased calcium and phosphorus intake. Hypophosphatemia (serum concentration <4 mg/dL) considered an early warning sign of decreased bone mineralization.
   b. Calcium levels may remain within the normal range, preserved at the expense of bone calcium stores; serum alkaline phosphatase concentration is a more direct method to assess increased bone turnover.
   c. Medications that have a negative effect on calcium and phosphorus stores: furosemide, caffeine citrate, and glucocorticosteroids.

**C. Anthropometric measurements.**

1. Daily approximate weight gains with recommended caloric intake.
   a. 24 to 32 weeks: 15 to 20 g/kg/day.
   b. 33 to 36 weeks: 14 to 15 g/kg/day.
   c. 37 to 40 weeks: 7 to 9 g/kg/day.
   d. 40 weeks to 3 months: 30 g/day.

2. Weekly length and head circumference measurements. Although it is common to discuss growth expectations of VLBW infants in terms of weight gain, gains in head circumference and lengths are just as necessary to determine optimal growth. Head circumference has a close relationship with the growth of brain volume. Length in comparison with weight gives good indication of body composition, if accurately measured.
   a. Length measurement.
      (1) Typically crown to heel of naked infant.
      (2) For accurate measurement, two people perform the procedure with length board specific for premature infants (e.g., Premie Length Board [O'Leary, Ellard Instrumentation, Seattle, WA]); one person holding the head in place against board top and another providing gentle straightening of body and lower extremities with one hand while pushing the moveable footrest into place with the other hand; average of two to three measurements.
      (3) Average gain in length from 24 to 40 weeks of gestation: 0.69 to 0.75 cm/wk.
   b. Head circumference, also known as occipital–frontal circumference.
      (1) Determined by applying paper or plasticized paper measurement tape firmly around the head above the supraorbital ridges, over the most prominent part of the frontal bulge anteriorly, and the part of the occiput that gives the maximum circumference; average of two to three measurements.
      (2) Average gain in head circumference from 24 to 40 weeks of gestation: 0.1 to 0.6 cm/wk.
3. Plot weight, head circumference, and length on growth chart weekly.

**D. Growth Charts (Kleinman and AAP Committee on Nutrition, 2009).**

1. Term infant growth charts include incremental growth curves and percentiles of weight, length, and head circumference; developed by the National Center for Health Statistics and the National Center for Chronic Disease Prevention and Health Promotion; available at http://www.cdc.gov/growthcharts.
2. Premature infant growth charts include incremental growth curves and percentiles of weight, length, and head circumference (Bhatia, 2013; Blackburn, 2013; Olsen et al., 2010).
   a. Adequate growth to genetic potential for premature infants implies lean mass accumulation, brain volume development, and somatic growth to maintain body composition comparable to that of a fetus of similar gestation.
   b. Typical growth curve charts with weight, length, and head circumference, used in the NICU to establish growth patterns and in current research, based on fetal and newborn growth and less frequently on the growth of former VLBW infants.
3. Postnatal growth curves for premature infants based on actual growth of premature infants; controversy over appropriateness of using growth curves based on the actual postnatal growth of VLBW infants of the 1990s as references for assessment of current VLBW infants.
   a. Postnatal growth curves reflect a slower growth velocity than is seen with growth curves based on intrauterine and newborn growth curves.
   b. Postnatal growth curves are a reflection of longitudinal growth for VLBW infants of the 1990s; recent studies of premature infants with similar postnatal growth restriction followed through to school age reflect neurologic and physical deficits that had been reported for VLBW infants of the 1980s; postnatal growth restriction is associated with poorer outcomes (Belfort et al., 2011; Biasini et al., 2012; Franz et al., 2009; Stoll et al. and NICHD Neonatal Research Network, 2010).

## REFERENCES

Adamkin, D.H., Radmacher, P.G. and Lewis S. Nutrition and selected disorders of the gastrointestinal tract. In A.A. Fanaroff and J.M. Fanaroff (Eds.): *Klaus & Fanaroff's care of the high risk neonate* (6th ed.). Philadelphia, 2013, Elsevier Saunders, pp. 151–200.

American Academy of Pediatrics, Section on Breastfeeding: Breastfeeding and the use of human milk. *Pediatrics*, 129(3):e827–e841, 2012.

Arslanoglu, S., Bertino, E.Coscia, A., et al.: Update of adjustable fortification regimen for preterm infants: A new protocol. *Journal of Biological Regulators & Homeostatic Agents*, 26(3):65–67, 2012.

Arslanoglu, S., Ziegler, E.E. and Moro, G.E.: WAPM Working Group on Nutrition: Donor human milk in preterm infant feeding: Evidence and recommendations. *Journal of Perinatal Medicine*, 38(4):347–351, 2010.

Atkinson, S.: Nutrition for premature infants with bronchopulmnary dysplasia. In P. Thureen, and W. Hay (Eds.): *Neonatal nutrition and metabolism* (2nd ed.). New York, 2006, Cambridge University Press, pp. 522–532.

Auron, A. and Mhanna, M.J.: Serum creatinine in very low birth weight infants during their first days of life. *Journal of Perinatology*, 26(12):755–760, 2006.

Barry, J.S. and Thureen, P.J.: Nutrition in infants with congenital heart disease. In P. Thureen and W. Hay (Eds.): *Neonatal nutrition and metabolism* (2nd ed.). New York, 2006, Cambridge University Press, pp. 533–543.

Belfort, M.B., Rifas-Shiman, S.L.Sullivan, T., et al.: Infant growth before and after term: Effects on neurodevelopment in preterm infants. *Pediatrics*, 128(4): e899–e906, 2011.

Berseth, C.L.: Development and physiology of the gastrointestinal tract. In P. Thureen and W. Hay (Eds.): *Neonatal nutrition and metabolism* (2nd ed.). New York, 2006, Cambridge University Press, pp. 1071–1085.

Bertino, E., Giuliani, F.Occhi, L., et al.: Benefits of donor human milk for preterm infants: Current evidence. *Early Human Development*, 85(10, Suppl.):S9–S10, 2009.

Bhatia, J.: Growth curves: How to best measure growth of the preterm infant. *Journal of Pediatrics*, 162(3, Suppl.):S2–S6, 2013.

Bhatia, J. and Greer, F.: Use of soy protein-based formulas in infant feeding. *Pediatrics*, 121(5):1062–1068, 2008.

Bhatia, J., Griffin, I.Anderson, D., et al.: Selected macro/micronutrient needs of the routine preterm infant. *Journal of Pediatrics*, 162(3, Suppl.):S48–S55, 2013.

Biasini, A., Marvulli, L.Neri, E., et al.: Growth and neurological outcome in ELBW preterms fed with human milk and extra-protein supplementation as routine practice: Do we need further evidence? *Journal of Maternal-Fetal and Neonatal Medicine*, 25(Suppl. 4): 64–66, 2012.

Blackburn, S.T.: *Maternal, fetal, and neonatal physiology: A clinical perspective* (4th ed.). St. Louis, 2013, Elsevier Saunders.

Boiron, M., DaNobrega, L.Roux, S., et al.: Effects of oral stimulaton and oral support on non-nutritive sucking and feeding performance in preterm infants. *Developmental Medicine and Child Neurology*, 49: 439–444, 2007.

Botet, F., Figueras-Aloy, J.Miracle-Echegoyen, X., et al.: Trends in survival among extremely-low-birthweight infants (less than 1000 g) without significant bronchopulmonary dysplasia. *BMC Pediatrics*, 12(63):1–7, 2012.

Cirgin-Ellett, M.L., Cohen, M.D.Perkins, S.M., et al.: Predicting the insertion length for gastric tube placement for neonates. *Journal of Obstetrical, Gynecologic and Neonatal Nurses*, 40:412–421, 2011.

Corvaglia, L., Rotatori, R.Ferlini, M., et al.: The effect of body positioning on gastroesophageal reflux in premature infants: Evaluation by combined impedance and pH monitoring. *Journal of Pediatrics*, 151: 591–596, 2007.

Dani, C. and Poggi, C.: Nutrition and bronchopulmonary dysplasia. *Journal of Maternal-Fetal and Neonatal Medicine*, 25(Suppl. 3):37–40, 2012.

Davis, M.K. and Andres, J.M.: Cholestasis in neonates and infants. In J. Neu (Ed.): *Gastroenterology and nutrition: Neonatology questions and controversies.* Philadelphia, 2008, Elsevier Saunders.

Decaro, M.H. and Vain, N.E.: Hyperglycaemia in preterm neonates: What to know, what to do. *Early Human Development*, 87(Suppl.):S19–S22, 2011.

Dell, K.M.: Fluid, electrolytes, and acid-base homeostasis. In R.J. Martin, A.A. Fanaroff, and M.C. Walsh (Eds.): *Neonatal-perinatal medicine: Diseases of the fetus and infant*, (9th ed., Vol. 1). St. Louis, 2011, Elsevier Saunders.

deRegnier, R.A.O. and Georgieff, M.K.: Fetal and neonatal iron metabolism. In R.A. Polin, W.W. Fox, and S.H. Abman (Eds.): *Fetal and neonatal physiology*, (4th ed., Vol. 1). Philadelphia, 2011, Elsevier Saunders.

Dimmitt, R.A. and Sibley, E.: Developmental anatomy and physiology of the gastrointestinal tract. In C.A. Gleason and S.U. Devaskar (Eds.): *Avery's diseases of the newborn* (9th ed.). Philadelphia, 2012, Elsevier Saunders.

Ditzenberger, G.R., Collins, S.D. and Binder, N.: Continuous insulin intravenous infusion therapy for VLBW infants. *Journal of Perinatal & Neonatal Nursing*, 13 (3):70–82, 1999.

Elser, H.E.: Positioning after feedings: What is the evidence to reduce feeding intolerances? *Advances in Neonatal Care*, 12(3):172–175, 2012.

Fanaro, S.: Strategies to improve feeding tolerance in preterm infants. *Journal of Maternal-Fetal and Neonatal Medicine*, 25(Suppl. 4):46–48, 2012.

Franz, A.R., Pohlandt, F.Bode, H., et al.: Intrauterine, early neonatal, and postdischarge growth and neurodevelopmental outcome at 5.4 years in extremely preterm infants after intensive neonatal nutritional support. *Pediatrics*, 123(1):e101–e109, 2009.

Gomella, T.L.: *Neonatology: Management, procedures, on-call problems, diseases, and drugs* (7th ed.). New York, 2013, Lange Medical Books/McGraw-Hill.

Greer, F.: Macro and micronutrients. In J. Neu (Ed.): *Gastroenterology and nutrition: Neonatology questions and controversies.* Philadelphia, 2008, Elsevier Saunders.

Greer, F.: Vitamins. In P.J. Thureen and W.W. Hay (Eds.): *Neonatal nutrition and metabolism* (2nd ed.). New York, 2006, Cambridge University Press, pp. 161–184.

Groothuis, J. and Makari, D.: Definition and outpatient management of the very low-birth-weight infant with bronchopulmonary dysplasia. *Advances in Therapy*, 29 (4):297–311, 2012.

Gutierrez, I.M., Kang, K.H. and Jaksic, T.: Neonatal short bowel syndrome. *Seminars in Fetal and Neonatal Medicine*, 16(3):157–163, 2011.

Hambidge, K.M.: Trace minerals. In P.J. Thureen and W.W. Hay (Eds.): *Neonatal nutrition and metabolism* (2nd ed.). New York, 2006, Cambridge University Press, pp. 273–290.

Hambidge, S.J. and Krebs, N.F.: Zinc in the fetus and neonate. In R.A. Polin, W.W. Fox, and S.H. Abman (Eds.): *Fetal and neonatal physiology* (Vol. 1). Philadelphia. 2011, Elsevier Saunders, pp. 403–408.

Hartman, D.M. and Medoff-Cooper, B.: Transition to home after neonatal surgery for congenital heart disease. *MCN: American Journal of Maternal and Child Nursing*, 37(2):95–100, 2012.

Haumont, D., Deckelbaum, R.J.Richelle, M., et al.: Plasma lipid and plasma lipoprotein concentrations in low birth weight infants given parenteral nutrition with twenty or ten percent lipid emulsion. *Journal of Pediatrics*, 115(5):787–793, 1989.

Hay, W.W., Regnault, T.R.H. and Brown, L.D.: Fetal requirements and placental transfer of nitrogenous compounds. In R.A. Polin, W.W. Fox, and S.H. Abman (Eds.): 4th ed.). *Fetal and neonatal physiology*, Vol. 1. Philadelphia, 2011, Elsevier Saunders.

Heird, W.C.: Intravenous feeding. In P.J. Thureen and W.W. Hay (Eds.): *Neonatal nutrition and metabolism* (2nd ed.). New York, 2006, Cambridge University Press.

Horvath, A., Dziechciarz, P. and Szajewska, H.: The effect of thickened-feed interventions on gastroesophageal reflux in infants: Systematic review and meta-analysis of randomized, controlled trials. *Pediatrics*, 122(6):e1268–e1277, 2008.

Husain, S.M., Mughal, M.Z. and Tsang, R.C.: Calcium, phosphorus, and magnesium transport across the placenta. In R.A. Polin, W.W. Fox, and S.H. Abman (Eds.): *Fetal and neonatal physiology* (Vol. 1). Philadelphia, 2011, Elsevier Saunders.

Itani, O. and Tsang, R.C.: Normal bone and mineral physiology and metabolism. In P.J. Thureen, and W.W. Hay (Eds.): *Neonatal nutrition and metabolism* (2nd ed.). New York, 2006, Cambridge University Press, pp. 185–228.

Jacobi, S.K. and Odle, J.: Nutritional factors influencing intestinal health of the neonate. *Advances in Nutrition: An International Review Journal*, 3(5):687–696, 2012.

Jadcherla, S.R.: Gastrointestinal reflux. In P.J. Thureen, and W.W. Hay (Eds.): *Neonatal nutrition and metabolism* (2nd ed.). New York, 2006, Cambridge University Press, pp. 445–453.

Jobe, A.H.: The new bronchopulmonary dysplasia. *Current Opinion in Pediatrics*, 23(2):167–172, 2011.

Johnson, L.H. and Bhutani, V.K.: Vitamin E metabolism in the fetus and newborn. In R.A. Polin, W.W. Fox, and S.H. Abman (Eds.): 4th ed.). *Fetal and neonatal physiology*, Vol. 1. Philadelphia, 2011, Elsevier Saunders.

Jones, E.: Transition from tube to breast. In E. Jones and C. King (Eds.): *Feeding and nutrition in the preterm infant*. Edinburgh, 2005, Churchill Livingstone, pp. 151–163.

Jones, L.: Oral feeding readiness in the neonatal intensive care unit. *Neonatal Network: The Journal of Neonatal Nursing*, 31(3):148–155, 2012.

Kashyap, S.: Enteral intake for very low birth weight infants: What should the composition be? *Seminars in Perinatology*, 31:74–82, 2007.

Kashyap, S. and Heird, W.C.: Protein and amino acid metabolism and requirements. In R.A. Polin, W.W. Fox, and S.H. Abman (Eds.): *Fetal and neonatal physiology*, (4th ed., Vol. 1). Philadelphia, 2011, Elsevier Saunders.

Kashyap, S. and Putet, G.: Lipids as an energy source for the premature and full-term neonate. In R.A. Polin, W.W. Fox, and S.H. Abman (Eds.): *Fetal and neonatal physiology* (Vol. 1). Philadelphia, 2011, Elsevier Saunders.

Kirk, A.T., Alder, S.C. and King, J.D.: Cue-based oral feeding clinical pathway results in earlier attainment of full oral feeding in premature infants. *Journal of Perinatology*, 27:572–578, 2007.

Kleinman, R.E. American Academy of Pediatrics, Committee on Nutrition: *Pediatric nutrition handbook* (6th ed.). Elk Grove Village, IL, 2009, American Academy of Pediatrics.

Lapillonne, A. and Griffin, I.J.: Feeding preterm infants today for later metabolic and cardiovascular outcomes. *Journal of Pediatrics*, 162(3, Suppl.):S7–S16, 2013.

Lapillonne, A., O'Connor, D.L., Wang, D. and Rigo, J.: Nutritional recommendations for the late-preterm infant and the preterm infant after hospital discharge. *Journal of Pediatrics*, 162(3, Suppl.):S90–S100, 2013.

Limperopoulos, C., Soul, J.S.Gauvreau, K., et al.: Late gestation cerebellar growth is rapid and impeded by premature birth. *Pediatrics*, 115:688–695, 2005.

Lucchini, R., Bizzarri, B., Giampietro, S. and De Curtis, M.: Feeding intolerance in preterm infants: How to understand the warning signs. *Journal of Maternal-Fetal and Neonatal Medicine*, 24(Suppl. 1): 72–74, 2011.

McCain, G.C., Del Moral, T.Duncan, R.C., et al.: Transition from gavage to nipple feeding for preterm infants with bronchopulmonary dysplasia. *Nursing Research*, 61(6):380–387, 2012.

Moore, K.L., Persaud, T.V.N. and Torchia, M.G.: *The developing human: clinically oriented embryology* (9th ed.). Philadelphia, 2013, Elsevier Saunders.

Moore, T.A.: Feeding intolerance. *Advances in Neonatal Care*, 11(3):149–152, 2011.

Moya, F., Sisk, P.M., Walsh, K.R. and Berseth, C.L.: A new liquid human milk fortifier and linear growth in preterm infants. *Pediatrics*, 130(4): e928–e935, 2012.

Moyer-Mileur, L.J.: Anthropometric and laboratory assessment of very low birth weight infants: The most helpful measurements and why. *Seminars in Perinatology*, 31(2):96–103, 2007.

Natarajan, G., Johnson, Y.R.Brozanski, B., et al.: Postnatal weight gain in preterm infants with severe bronchopulmonary dysplasia. *American Journal of Perinatology*, 31(3):223–230, 2014.

Nedergaard, J. and Cannon, B.: Brown adipose tissue: Develpment. In R.A. Polin, W.W. Fox, and S.H. Abman (Eds.): *Fetal and neonatal physiology* (Vol. 1). Philadelphia, 2011, Elsevier Saunders.

Neu, J., Mihatsch, W.A.Zegarra, J., et al.: Intestinal mucosal defense system, part 1. Consensus recommendations for immunonutrients. *Journal of Pediatrics*, 162(3, Suppl.):S56–S63, 2013.

Neville, M.C. and McManaman, J.L.: Milk secretion and composition. In P.J. Thureen, and W.W. Hay (Eds.): *Neonatal nutrition and metabolism* (2nd ed.). New York, 2006, Cambridge University Press, pp. 377–389.

Nye, C.: Transitioning premature infants from gavage to breast. *Neonatal Network: The Journal of Neonatal Nursing*, 27(1):7–13, 2008.

Ogilvy-Stuart, A.L. and Beardsall, K.: Management of hyperglycaemia in the preterm infant. *Archives of Disease in Childhood: Fetal and Neonatal Edition*, 95(2): F126–F131, 2010.

Olsen, I.E., Groveman, S.A.Lawson, M.L., et al.: New intrauterine growth curves based on United States data. *Pediatrics*, 125(2):e214–e224, 2010.

Pieltain, C., de Halleux, V., Senterre, T. and Rigo, J.: Prematurity and bone health. *World Review of Nutrition and Dietetics*, 106:181–188, 2013.

Poindexter, B.B. and Dunne, S.C.: Parenteral nutrition. In C.A. Gleason and S.U. Devaskar (Eds.): *Avery's diseases of the newborn* (9th ed.). Philadelphia, 2012, Elsevier Saunders.

Puckett, B., Grover, V.K., Holt, T. and Sankaran, K.: Cue-based feeding for preterm infants: A prospective trial. *American Journal of Perinatology*, 25(EFirst):623–628, 2008.

Pye, S. and Green, A.: Parent education after newborn congenital heart surgery. *Advances in Neonatal Care*, 3(3):147–156, 2004.

Ramírez-Santana, C., Pérez-Cano, F.J.Audí, C., et al.: Effects of cooling and freezing storage on the stability of bioactive factors in human colostrum. *Journal of Dairy Science*, 95(5):2319–2325, 2012.

Roggero, P., Giannì, M.L.Morlacchi, L., et al.: Blood urea nitrogen concentrations in low-birth-weight preterm infants during parenteral and enteral nutrition. *Journal of Pediatric Gastroenterology and Nutrition*, 51 (2):213–215, 2010.

Shenai, J.P.: Vitamin A metabolism in the fetus and neonate. In R.A. Polin, W.W. Fox, and S.H. Abman (Eds.): 4th ed.). *Fetal and neonatal physiology*, Vol. 1. Philadelphia, 2011, Elsevier Saunders.

Sinclair, J.C., Bottino, M. and Cowett, R.M.: Interventions for prevention of neonatal hyperglycemia in very low birth weight infants. *Cochrane Database of Systematic Reviews*, (3):CD0007615, 2009.

Slutzah, M., Codipilly, C.N.Potak, D., et al.: Refrigerator storage of expressed human milk in the neonatal intensive care unit. *Journal of Pediatrics*, 156(1):26–28, 2010.

Soundheimer, J.: Neonatal short bowel syndrome. In P.J. Thureen and W.W. Hay (Eds.): *Neonatal nutrition and metabolism*. New York, 2006, Cambridge University Press, pp. 492–507.

Stoll, B.J., Hansen, N.I., Bell, E.F., et al., and NICHD Neonatal Research Network: Neonatal outcomes of extremely preterm infants from the NICHD Neonatal Research Network. *Pediatrics*, 126(3):443–456, 2010.

Thomas, J.A., Tsai, A. and Bernstein, L.: Nutrition therapies for inborn errors of metabolism. In P.J. Thureen, and W.W. Hay (Eds.): *Neonatal nutrition and metabolism*. New York, 2006, Cambridge University Press, pp. 544–568.

Thureen, P.J. and Hay, W.W.: Nutritional requirements of the very low birth weight infant. In J. Neu (Ed.): *Gastroenterology and nutrition: Neonatology questions and controversies* Philadelphia, 2009, Elsevier Saunders.

Torowicz, D., Lisanti, A.J., Rim, J.-S. and Medoff-Cooper, B.: A developmental care framework for a cardiac intensive care unit. *Advances in Neonatal Care*, 12(5, Suppl.):S28–S32, 2012.

Tudehope, D., Fewtrell, M., Kashyap, S. and Udaeta, E.: Nutritional needs of the micropreterm infant. *Journal of Pediatrics*, 162(3, Suppl.):S72–S80, 2013.

Tudehope, D.I.: Human milk and the nutritional needs of preterm infants. *Journal of Pediatrics*, 162(3, Suppl.): S17–S25, 2013.

Underwood, M.A.: Human milk for the premature infant. *Pediatric Clinics of North America*, 60 (1):189–207, 2013.

Vieira, A.A., Soares, F.V.M.Pimenta, H.P., et al.: Analysis of the influence of pasteurization, freezing/thawing, and offer processes on human milk's macronutrient concentrations. *Early Human Development*, 87(8):577–580, 2011.

Williford, A., Pare, L. and Carlson, G.: Bone mineral metabolism in the neonate: Calcium, phosphorus, magnesium, and alkaline phosphatase. *Neonatal Network: The Journal of Neonatal Nursing*, 27(1):57–63, 2008.

Wojcik, K.Y., Rechtman, D.J.Lee, M.L., et al.: Macronutrient analysis of a nationwide sample of donor breast milk. *Journal of the American Dietetic Association*, 109 (1):137–140, 2009.

Young, L., Morgan, J., McCormick, F.M. and McGuire, W.: Nutrient-enriched formula versus standard term formula for preterm infants following hospital discharge. *Cochrane Database of Systematic Reviews*, 0:CD0004696, 2012.

CHAPTER

# 11 Developmental Support

CAROL TURNAGE SPRUILL

**OBJECTIVES**

1. Assess physiologic and behavioral organization of preterm and ill newborn infants using the neurobehavioral subsystems from Als' Synactive Framework.
2. Design a developmental care plan that respects and supports each infant's unique needs as related to the environment, direct caregiving, parent support, and consistency of care.
3. Engage parents in active participation in their infant's plan of care.

Individualized developmentally supportive care (IDSC) is based on a philosophy of respect for the unique needs of preterm and high-risk infants susceptible to neurodevelopmental disadvantage in part due to the complex, atypical environment of the neonatal intensive care unit (NICU) and separation from the nurturing of parents (Fig. 11-1). Family-centered IDSC promotes a culture that supports family adaptation and involvement so that parents can be parents to their recovering infant.

Preterm infants are especially vulnerable to cognitive, neuromotor, and neurosensory problems after discharge from the NICU. Fluctuations in cerebral circulation have been demonstrated in routine care procedures, and smaller than expected brain volumes at 36 to 40 weeks may play a significant role in increased morbidity in these infants. Altered cerebral oxygenation and blood volume measured with near-infrared spectroscopy have been exhibited during diaper changes, endotracheal tube suctioning, repositioning, physical exam, and nasogastric tube insertion (Limperopoulos et al., 2008). These brain changes are associated with early parenchymal abnormalities.

## EARLY EXPERIENCE

A. **The influence of early environmental, medical, and other perinatal atypical exposures is not clear even though developmental problems are more frequent in preterm infants after their NICU stay.** Preterm infants display a different pattern of behavior on the NICU Network Behavioral Scale at term equivalent as compared with full-term infants (Pineda, et al., 2013).
   1. Weaker orientation ($P < 0.001$).
   2. Less ability to tolerate handling ($P < 0.001$).
   3. Poorer self-regulation ($P < 0.001$).
   4. Weaker reflexes ($P < 0.001$).
   5. Higher stress response ($P < 0.001$).
   6. More hypertonicity or hypotonia ($P < 0.001$).
   7. Increased tendency toward excitability ($P < 0.007$).

B. **Important changes were observed in behaviors of preterm infants at 34 weeks postconceptional age compared to term equivalent.**
   1. Increasing arousal and excitability ($P < 0.001$).
   2. Decreasing quality of movement ($P = 0.006$).
   3. Increasing levels of hypertonia ($P < 0.001$) and decreasing hypotonia ($P = 0.001$).
   4. Less lethargy ($P < 0.001$).

C. **Infants with brain injury demonstrated more excitability ($P = 0.002$).** These neurobehavioral changes highlight the importance of interventions beginning immediately in the delivery room and throughout the NICU stay.

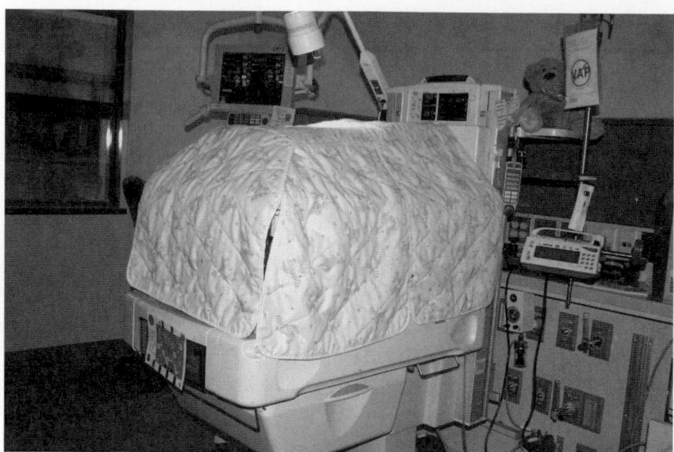

FIGURE 11-1 ■ High-risk infant in NICU environment. (Courtesy of Texas Children's Hospital, Houston, Tex.; photographer Carol Turnage Spruill.)

1. Developmental support during care is a strategy to reduce the influence of environment, care practices, handling, and other disruptions stressful to the NICU infant to optimize outcomes.

## WHAT IS DEVELOPMENTAL CARE?

A. **Developmental care is more about the caregiver who:**
   1. Acknowledges the environmental risks of the NICU on the developing brain and body of the high-risk newborn.
   2. Recognizes that health and neurodevelopmental problems occur at much higher frequency in preterm infants.
   3. Realizes infants need early developmental support to reach optimal cognitive, physical, and social/emotional potential.
   4. Commits to providing developmental support during all care and procedures; adapts the environment to better suit the individual infants.
   5. Supports parents as essential to their infant's physical and developmental progress from the moment of birth.

B. **The Universe of Developmental Care (UDC):** expands Als' Synactive Theory (Lawhon and Als, 2010) to accentuate the neurodevelopmental interface of the infant's skin that links the baby to the environment of care and caregivers (Fig. 11-2). Aside from tactile opportunities, this shared surface is integrated with the entire sensory system (visual, auditory, vestibular, etc.) and affords the caregiver a practical approach to care through an interactive link to the actual body surface within the NICU context (Gibbins et al., 2008).
   1. The model is based on a solar system concept where the inner circle or sun is the core that explains the planetary movement and purpose while also keeping the entire system together. In the UDC, the infant's position is equivalent to the sun so the model is focused on the patient. The family is closest to the infant so they can be involved in care and parenting. The ring closest around the infant is composed of physiologic systems needed for optimal functioning and is where medical and nursing care is necessary should there be a disruption in one or more systems. These physiologic systems are also influenced by the infant's sleep–wake behavioral states surrounding the physiologic ring.
   2. The planets represent aspects of care practices based on systematic reviews and meta-analyses of literature on developmental care and infant outcomes. Staff orbit protectively around the infant and family, accessing the shared care surface during nursing care customized to the infant's individual requirements from knowledge of the available evidence-based practice symbolized by the planets that circumnavigate around the core (sun–infant).

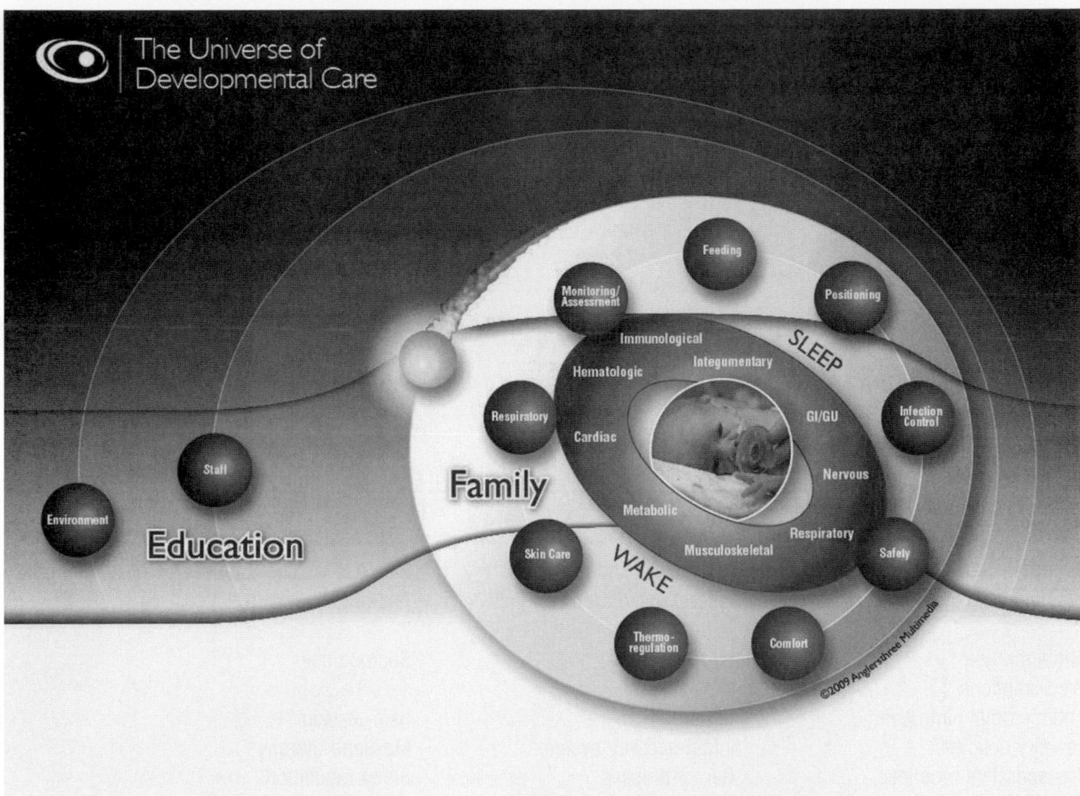


FIGURE 11-2 ■ The Universe of Developmental Care. (Copyright 2009, Koninklijke Philips N.V. Used with permission.)

3. The context for all interaction is the physical, human, and operations of the health care setting or NICU. The Milky Way exemplifies education as a persistent theme encompassing all orbital planes. Learning needs extend across staff, physicians, leaders, and families committed to safe, quality care and optimal outcomes.
4. The skin as the shared surface for interaction makes sense especially since it originates from the ectodermal layer during embryology, as does the brain. As the neurodevelopmental interface for care, the outer layer of the skin may be viewed as the brain's surface. Obviously the brain cannot be observed directly in the NICU, therefore, caregivers use the skin or shared surface to operationalize or translate this model into bedside application of developmental care practices (Table 11-1).

## OPERATIONALIZING DEVELOPMENTAL CARE

A. **Physical and behavioral assessment.**
   1. Assessment of stable or self-regulating behavior, as well as stress responses (Fig. 11-3), is ongoing during care and periods of rest and provides the information necessary for developmentally supportive care individual to each infant (Table 11-2). The framework for understanding preterm infant behavior is based on the work of Dr. Heidelise Als (1998). An infant's observable channels of communication are used in a systematic assessment by caregivers to provide individualized, developmentally appropriate care. Als' Synactive Theory proposes the hierarchical integration of subsystem development, integration with the other developing subsystems to eventual competent functioning without physiologic or autonomic stress and destabilization.
      a. Autonomic/visceral cues—changes in infant color, heart rate, respiratory patterns.
      b. Motor system—quality of tone and movement, posture.
      c. State system—quality and range of states, transitions between states.

■ TABLE 11-1
■ ■ **Expanded Developmental Care Practices Within the Universe of Developmental Care Model**

| **Monitoring/Assessment** | **Feeding** | **Positioning** |
|---|---|---|
| Vital sign assessment | Early feeds | Supine |
| Behavioral assessment | Trophic | Prone |
| Electrodes | Donor milk | Side-lying |
| Invasive catheters | Cue-based feeds | Flexion |
| Invasive/noninvasive monitoring | Nonnutritive sucking | Containment |
| $CO_2$ monitor | Breast milk mouth care | Midline orientation (proper body alignment) |
| Saturation monitor | Enteral feedings | Boundaries |
| Cerebral monitor | Breast shields | Hand-to-mouth opportunity |
| | Bottlefeed | Safety |
| | Breastfeed | |
| | NGT feeds | |
| **Infection Control** | **Safety** | **Comfort** |
| Occlusive dressings | Patient ID bands | Pain assessment practices |
| Handwashing | Enteral only/Parenteral only tubings | Pharmacological practices |
| Antibiotic use | | Sucrose use |
| Prep solutions | | |
| Antimicrobial ointments | Gentle touch | Skin-to-skin |
| Jewelry policies | Infant security systems | Massage therapy |
| Postoperative practices | Gel mattresses | Sleep regulation |
| Environmental issues (ventilation, garbage disposal) | Environmental issues (flooring, equipment) | Environmental factors |
| **Thermoregulation** | **Skin Care** | **Respiratory Care** |
| Humidity control | Touch | Intubation practices |
| Temperature control | Soaps and emollients | CPAP interface |
| Swaddling | Bathing practices | Oxygen delivery systems |
| Plastic wrap | Cleansers and solutions | Instillations (surfactant, saline, nebulizers) |
| Room temperature | Adhesive removal | Suctioning practices |
| Solution temperature | Transdermal drug interface | |
| Clothing | Topical anesthetics | |
| Bedding | Wound care | |
| **Family** | **Staff** | **Environment** |
| Satisfaction | Satisfaction | Light levels |
| Level of involvement | Knowledge | Noise levels |
| Knowledge | Autonomy | Cultural, racial, religious sensitivity |
| Autonomy | | Leadership quality |

From Gibbins, S., Hoath, S., and Coughlin, M.: The Universe of Developmental Care: A new conceptual model for application in the neonatal intensive care unit. *Advances in Neonatal Care*, 8(3):145, 2008. Reprinted with permission of Walter Kluwer Health.
*CPAP*, continuous positive airway pressure; *NGT*, nasogastric tube.

(1) Attention and interaction.
(2) Self-regulation.

2. For example, competent functioning is demonstrated when Misha, now 35 weeks, is able to focus on suck, swallow, and breathing during an oral examination while maintaining physiologic and motor stability in a quiet, alert state.

**B. Individualized developmental care relies on both the moment-to-moment caregiver adaptations while in interaction with an infant and the formal plans based on infant assessment**

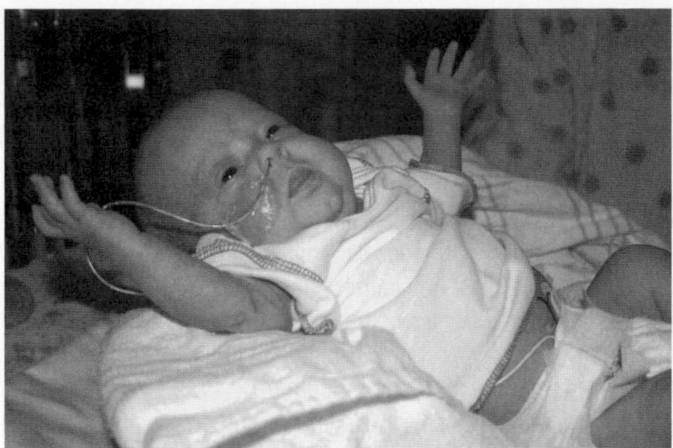

FIGURE 11-3 ■ NICU infant demonstrating stress cues. (Courtesy of Texas Children's Hospital, Houston, Tex.; photography by Carol Turnage Spruill.)

■ TABLE 11-2
### ■ ■ Neurobehavioral Organization and Facilitation

| Subsystem | Signs of Stress | Signs of Stability | Interventions |
|---|---|---|---|
| **AUTONOMIC** | | | |
| Respiratory | Tachypnea, pauses, irregular breathing pattern, slow respirations, sighing, or gasping | Smooth, unlabored breathing; regular rate and pattern | Reduce light, noise and activity at bedside (place pagers/phone on vibrate, lower conversation levels at bedside) |
| Color | Pale, mottled, red, dusky, or cyanotic | Stable, overall pink color | Use hand containment and pacifier during exams, procedures, care<br>Slowly awaken with soft voice before touch including all procedures, exams, and care unless hearing impaired, use slow movement transitions |
| Visceral | Several coughs, sneezes, yawns; hiccups, gagging, grunting and straining associated with defecation, spitting up | Visceral stability, smooth digestion, tolerates feeding | Pace feedings by infant's ability and cues |
| Autonomic-related motor patterns | Tremors, startles, twitches of face and/or body, extremities | Tremors, startles, twitching not observed | Gently reposition while containing extremities close to body if premature<br>Minimize sleep disruption<br>Position appropriately for neuromotor development and comfort; use nesting/boundaries or swaddling as needed to reduce tremors, startles<br>Manage pain appropriately |
| **MOTOR** | | | |
| Tone | Either hypertonia or hypotonia; limp/flaccid body, extremities and/or face; hyperflexion | Consistent, reliable tone for postmenstrual age (PMA); controlled or more control of movement, activity, and posture | Support rest periods/reduce sleep disruption; minimize stress; contain or swaddle |
| Posture | Unable to maintain flexed, aligned, comfortable posture | Improved or well-maintained posture; with maturation posture sustainable without supportive aids | Provide boundaries, positioning aids, or swaddling for flexion, containment, alignment, and comfort as appropriate |

*Continued*

■ TABLE 11-2
■ ■ **Neurobehavioral Organization and Facilitation—cont'd**

| Subsystem | Signs of Stress | Signs of Stability | Interventions |
|---|---|---|---|
| **MOTOR—cont'd** | | | |
| Movement | Stiff extension of arms and/or legs, fingers stiffly outstretched (salute), arching, neck hyperextension; jerky, flailing movements | Less self-stimulating motor arousals; control of movement improving; smoother, less awkward; may get hands together or to face/mouth | Use swaddling, boundaries, nesting, or hand containment to minimize motor arousal and support overall calming, assist hands to face/mouth |
| Level of activity | Frequent squirming, frantic flailing activity or little to no movement | Activity consistent with environment, situation and PMA | Intervene as needed for pain management, environmental modification, less stimulation; encourage skin to skin holding |
| **STATE** | | | |
| Sleep | Restless, facial twitching, movement, irregular respirations, fussing, grimacing, whimpers or makes sounds; responsive to environment | Quiet, restful sleep periods, less body/facial movement, little response to environment | Comfortable and age appropriate positioning for sleep with a quiet, dim environment and no interruptions except medical necessity<br>Position with hands to face or mouth or so they can learn to achieve this on their own. |
| Awake Attention/ Interaction | Low level arousal with unfocused eyes; hyperalert expression of worry/panic; cry face or crying; actively avoids eye contact by averting gaze or closing eyes; irritability, prolonged awake periods; difficult to console or inconsolable | Alert, bright, shiny eyes with focused attention on an object or person; robust crying; calms quickly with intervention, consolable in 2 to 5 minutes | Encourage parent holding as desired either traditional or skin-to-skin<br>May be ready for brief eye contact around 30 to 32 weeks without displaying stress cues<br>Support awake moments with postmenstrual age (PMA) appropriate activity based on stress and stability data for individual infant |
| Self-regulation | Little attempt to flex or tuck body, few attempts to push feet against boundaries, unable to maintain hands to face or mouth, sucking a pacifier may be more stressful than soothing | Strategies for self-regulation include: Foot bracing against boundaries or own feet/leg; hands grasped together; hand to mouth or face, grasping blanket or tubes, tucking body/trunk; sucking; position changes | Examine using blanket swaddle or nest to support infant regulation by removing only a small part of the body at a time while keeping most of body contained<br>Ask a parent or nurse to provide support during exams, tests, procedures<br>Swaddle or contain as needed to keep limbs close to body during care or exams and to provide boundaries for grasping or foot bracing<br>Position for sleep with hands to face or mouth<br>Provide pacifier intermittently when awake and at times other than exams, care or procedures |
| State transitions | Rapid state transitions, unable to move to drowsy or sleep state when stressed, states are not clear to observers | Transitions smoothly from high arousal states to quiet alert or sleep state; focused attention on an object, person; maintains quiet alert state without stress or with some facilitation | Give older infants something to hold (maybe a finger or blanket)<br>Encourage parenting to support parenting skill; teach parents communication cues and behaviors; model appropriate responses to cues |

■ TABLE 11-2
■ ■ **Neurobehavioral Organization and Facilitation—cont'd**

| Subsystem | Signs of Stress | Signs of Stability | Interventions |
|---|---|---|---|
| **STATE—cont'd** | | | |
| | | | Consistently avoid rapid disruption of state behavior (e.g., starting an exam without preparing the baby for the intrusion) by: awakening slowly with soft speech or touch, use indirect lighting or shield eyes depending on PMA during exams, care |
| | | | Assist return to sleep or quiet alert state after handling |
| | | | Provide auditory and facial visual stimulation for quietly alert infants based on cues; premature infants may need to start with only one mode of stimulation initially, adding others based on cues |
| | | | Swaddling or containment to facilitate state control or maintenance |

From Spruill-Turnage, C., and Papile, L.A.: Developmentally supportive care. In J.P. Cloherty, E.C. Eichenwald, A.R. Hansen, and A.R. Stark (Eds.): *Manual of neonatal care* (7th ed.). Philadelphia, 2012, Lippincott, Williams, & Wilkins; reprinted with permission. Modified from Als, H.: Toward a synactive theory of development: Promise for the assessment and support of infant individuality. *Infant Mental Health Journal*, 3:229-243, 1982; Als, H. A synactive model of neonatal behavior organization: Framework for the assessment of neurobehavioral development in the premature infant and for support of infants and parents in the neonatal intensive care environment. *Physical and Occupational Therapy in Pediatrics*, 6:3-55, 1986; Hunter, J.G.: The neonatal intensive care unit. In J. Case-Smith, A.S. Allen, and P.N. Pratt (Eds.): *Occupational therapy for children*. St. Louis, 2001, C.V. Mosby, p. 593; and Carrier, C.T., Walden, M., and Wilson, D.: The high-risk newborn and family. In M.J. Hockenberry (Ed.): *Wong's nursing care of infants and children* (7th ed.). St. Louis, 2003, C.V. Mosby.

**that provide overall guidance for care of that particular infant.** Both are flexible, in that changes may need to be made based on infant responses at any given moment.

1. Care is dynamic and responsive, although dependent on the caregiver being completely in tune and in interaction *with* the infant rather than performing care as tasks *on* the infant (Fig. 11-4). Cues without context or an experience make it difficult for caregivers to apply appropriate interventions during care and in the overall plan of care.
2. The Five Constructs of Developmental Care (Fig. 11-5) can be used as a learning tool to guide the caregiver through the whole experience of the infant by the process of using their assessment within the context of the environment and situation to initiate interventions in the moment or use patterns of responses for developing plans of care. Finally, continuity and consistency among caregivers require that this information is communicated to the infant's health care team and family to gather input on the developmental plan of care and link interventions to medical goals.
   a. The Five Constructs are a simple way to look at all the elements of operationalizing developmental principles into practical application (see Fig. 11-5).
      (1) Cues—observe infant cues and determine whether the behaviors indicate stability or stress.
      (2) Clues—check the situation and environment for clues to the observed behavior (Is the care stressful? Is the environment noisy?).
      (3) Consider—what is your best response given your knowledge of this infant and the cues/clues you identified within the best evidence available to the UDC. How is the shared interface useful in delivering care or interventions?
      (4) Connect—if you see a pattern of behavior, think about events that frequently trigger the infant's stress cues (weighing on scale elicits extended arms, stiffly outstretched fingers, and oxygen saturation decreases from 4% to 6%).

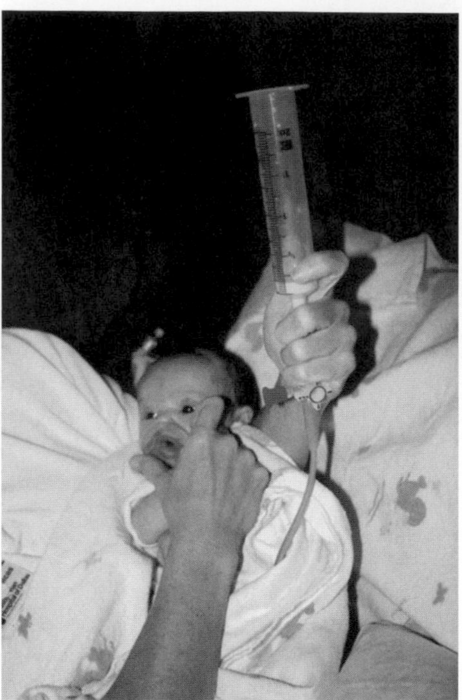

FIGURE 11-4 ■ Caregiver interacts with infant to promote enjoyment during a tube feeding. (Courtesy of Texas Children's Hospital, Houston, Tex.; photography by Carol Turnage Spruill.)

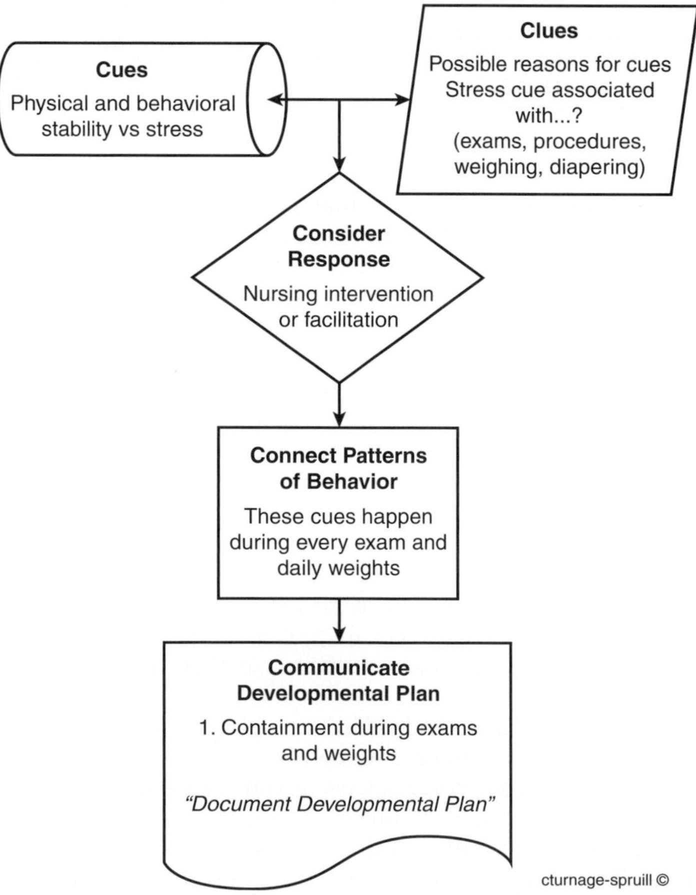


FIGURE 11-5 ■ The Developmental Care Experience: Five Constructs©. (Courtesy of Carol Spruill-Turnage.)

(5) Communicate—document and report the developmental plan based on your observation and analysis of individual behaviors and potential triggers to ensure consistent responses among caregivers.

C. **Evaluate developmental care practices in NICU**
   1. Core measures for developmentally supportive care (Table 11-3) are based on five repetitive themes from the evidence base of developmental and quality care practices for NICU patients (Coughlin et al., 2009). Each measure includes attributes with corresponding criteria that set the minimum requirements for successful attainment. These criteria can be translated into measurable indicators to monitor, benchmark, and analyze the current quality of developmental care practices in the NICU (Table 11-4). The ability to substantiate and quantify developmentally supportive nursing care using metrics based on the core measures may provide data on the impact of this care model on family/staff satisfaction and clinical and economic outcomes.
   2. Core measures of developmental care:
      a. Protected sleep—behavioral state guides caregiving activities, interventions to promote sleep, and parents' education about sleep protection in NICU and at home.
      b. Assessment and management of stress and pain—defined intervals of stress/pain assessment with validated pain scoring tool and infant cues, interventions for stress/pain documented and reassessed at appropriate intervals, nonpharmacologic and/or pharmacologic interventions for stress/pain utilized and documented.
      c. Developmentally supportive daily living activities—positioning, infant-driven feeding, and skin care.
      d. Family-centered care—opportunities to participate in care, daily rounds, and change-of-shift report, receive education on their infant's cues and care, input on plan of care; culturally sensitive interactions; access to social, spiritual and financial support.
      e. Healing environment—human, physical, and organizational environment that includes evidence-based policies, procedures, and appropriate resources. A bloodstream infection bundle is part of a healing environment of care.

## DEVELOPMENTALLY SUPPORTIVE ENVIRONMENT

A. **Many NICUs are building single-family rooms to improve the environment of care for both infant and family.** Just because a room is "private," that does not mean it is necessarily designed to reduce or minimize the effects of light and sound. Healthy environments without toxic products containing volatile compounds or formaldehyde are still being used for building materials and furniture in hospital facilities. There are also areas where building or renovating is not an immediate option. Resources and professionals exist to help leaders and administrators improve the NICU environment (White et al. and Committee to Establish Recommended Standards for Newborn ICU Design, 2013). Environmental modifications are intended to reduce stress, protect sleep, and allow parent–infant interaction with less distraction.
   1. Sound environment: the money spent on a professional acoustic engineer is well spent when deciding to renovate or build an NICU for sound abatement. The sound "floor" or baseline for sound levels prior to adding equipment, patients, and staff has to be much lower than the 45-dB level for ambient sound, and an acoustical engineer can make that happen. Standards for the neonatal hospital environment can be found in the American Academy of Pediatrics and American College of Obstetricians and Gynecologists *Guidelines for Perinatal Care* (2012) and Recommended Standards for Newly Designed NICUs (White et al. and Committee to Establish Recommended Standards for Newborn ICU Design, 2013). It is not recommended that infants wear eye goggles or earmuffs for protection against NICU noise and light due to increased stress responses of premature infants while such devices are in place (Aita et al., 2012).
      a. Ototoxic medications coupled with a noisy NICU environment may contribute to hearing loss in preterm infants (Zimmerman and Lahav, 2013).
      b. Most hearing loss in preterm infants has no known etiology.
      c. Potential for atypical development of auditory pathways from NICU noise experience.

■ TABLE 11-3
■ ■ **Core Measures of Developmental Care**

| Attribute | Criteria |
|---|---|
| **1. PROTECTED SLEEP** | |
| Infant sleep-wake states assessed and documented and guide all infant interactions | ■ All non-emergent caregiving is provided during wakeful states<br>■ Support integration of hunger cues with sleep cycles<br>■ Scheduled caregiving contingent on infant's sleep-wake states and adapted accordingly |
| Care strategies that support sleep are individualized for each infant and documented | ■ Provide caregiving activities that promote sleep, i.e., facilitative tuck, swaddled bathing and kangaroo care<br>■ All caregiving activities are modified according to infant's state<br>■ Maintain light and sound levels within recommended range and implement cycled lighting to support nocturnal sleep |
| Families are educated on importance of sleep safety in the hospital and the home; this education is documented | ■ Family education on caregiving activities that promote safe sleep is provided<br>■ Parenting opportunities are provided to promote infant sleep<br>■ Staff role model "Back to Sleep" practices for families once the infant has demonstrated physiologic flexion of the upper body in supine and discharge home is anticipated |
| **2. PAIN AND STRESS: ASSESSMENT AND MANAGEMENT** | |
| Assessments of pain and/or stress are performed routinely and documented | ■ Each infant is assessed for pain/stress at a minimum every four hours or with each infant interaction<br>■ Each infant is assessed for pain/stress during all procedures and caregiving activities<br>■ A valid pain assessment tool is utilized |
| Pain and/or stress is managed before, during and after all procedures until infant reaches baseline; interventions and infant responses are documented | ■ Utilize non-pharmacologic and/or pharmacologic measures prior to anticipated stressful/painful procedures.<br>■ Adapt caregiving activities to minimize pain and stress.<br>■ Document infant's response to pain/stress relieving interventions. |
| Family is involved and informed of pain and stress management plan for their infant(s); involvement and information sharing is documented | ■ Family is offered choice to be present during invasive procedures<br>■ Family education regarding infant pain and stress cues is provided<br>■ Family is encouraged to provide comfort to their infant |
| **3. DEVELOPMENTALLY SUPPORTIVE ACTIVITIES OF DAILY LIVING** | |
| Positioning: Infant positioning will provide comfort, safety, physiologic stability and optimal neuromotor development and is documented | ■ Each infant is positioned and handled in flexion, containment and alignment during all caregiving activities<br>■ Infant position is evaluated with every infant interaction and modified to support symmetric development<br>■ Positioning aides are gradually removed and Back to Sleep and Tummy to Play Practices are implemented as the infant demonstrates physiologic flexion |
| Feeding: Feeding will be infant-driven, individualized, nurturing, functional and developmentally appropriate to ensure safety | ■ Offer NNS with each non-oral feeding contingent on infant's state<br>■ Feeding readiness and quality of nippling and appropriate caregiver techniques are utilized<br>■ Education regarding benefits of breastmilk is provided and family choice is supported |
| Skin care: Infant skin integrity is assessed and protected and care is documented | ■ Infants are bathed no more frequently than every three days or as indicated on individualized assessment |

■ TABLE 11-3
■ ■ **Core Measures of Developmental Care—cont'd**

| Attribute | Criteria |
|---|---|
| **3. DEVELOPMENTALLY SUPPORTIVE ACTIVITIES OF DAILY LIVING—cont'd** | |
| | ■ Skin integrity is assessed using a reliable assessment tool once per shift and documented (Braden Q Scale or similar neonatal tool)<br>■ Skin surface interface is protected during application, utilization and removal of adhesive products |
| **4. FAMILY-CENTERED CARE** | |
| Family (defined by infant's parents and/or guardians) has 24 hour unrestricted access to their infant and is provided opportunity to parent; family definition and participation is documented | ■ Family is offered opportunity to be present and/or participate in medical rounds and change of shift report<br>■ Family is offered opportunity to be present during invasive procedures and/or resuscitative interventions to provide comfort and reassurance<br>■ Family is supported in parenting activities to include kangaroo care, holding, feeding activities, dressing, bathing, diapering, singing and bonding interactions |
| Family's level of emotional well-being and parental confidence and competence is assessed and documented weekly | ■ Mental health professionals (social/spiritual) resource families accessible to family weekly<br>■ Family observations and input regarding infant are sought by direct care provider and documented in the medical record<br>■ Health care providers share unbiased infant information weekly with family |
| Family has access to resources and support that assist in short- and long-term parenting, decision making and parental well being | ■ Families are invited to participate in a support group<br>■ Culturally sensitive family education on infant safety and infant care is available in various formats<br>■ Resources for the social, spiritual and financial needs of families are provided |
| **5. THE HEALING ENVIRONMENT** | |
| A quiet, dimly lit, private environment that promotes safety and sleep | ■ Continuous background sound and transient sound in the NICU shall not exceed an hourly Leg of 45 dB and an hourly L10 of 50 dB; transient sounds or Lmax shall not exceed 65 dB<br>■ Ambient light levels ranging between 10-600 lux or 1-60 ftc shall be adjustable and measured at each infant bedspace<br>■ Physical and auditory privacy is offered at each patient bedspace |
| A collaborative healthcare team that emanates teamwork, mindfulness and caring | ■ Interdisciplinary care rounds occur at least weekly<br>■ Direct care providers demonstrate caring behaviors which include adherence to hand hygiene protocols, cultural sensitivity, open listening skills, and a sensitive relationship orientation<br>■ RN-MD collaboration is defined, practiced and reinforced on a daily basis |
| Evidence-based policies, procedures and resources are available to sustain the healing environment over time | ■ Core measures of developmental care provide the standard of care for all patient care providers<br>■ Resources are available 24/7 to support implementation of developmental care<br>■ A system is present to ensure staff accountability for the practice of core measures of developmental care |

From Coughlin, M., Gibbins, S., and Hoath, S.: Core measures for developmentally supportive care in neonatal intensive care units: Theory, precedence and practice. *Journal of Advanced Nursing*, 65(10):2243-2245, 2009, with permission of John Wiley and Sons.

■ TABLE 11-4
■ ■ **Example of Protected Sleep Core Measure with Attribute and Criteria with Potential Quality Measurement**

| Core Measure | Attribute | Criteria | Quality Indicator |
|---|---|---|---|
| **Protected Sleep** | Nursing care that is individualized to promote sleep for each infant is documented and reported | 1. Care is adapted based on infant state<br>2. Sleep is promoted with care such as hand containment, swaddled bathing, skin-to-skin holding<br>3. Light and sound levels are within recommended range (White et al. and Committee to Establish Recommended Standards for Newborn ICU Design, 2013) | 1. Sleep–wake states are assessed and documented correctly with vital signs and care activities in 95% of audited records<br>2. Skin-to-skin holding by parent choice is documented in 100% of records audited<br>3. Random light and sound levels of monthly audits do not exceed 45 dB for continuous background sound or 65 dB for transient loud sounds |

2. Noise abatement.
   a. Monitor noise levels either continuously or intermittently.
   b. Heighten awareness of physicians, staff, and parents regarding the effects of noise and their responsibility in decreasing it at the individual level.
   c. Communication devices such as phones and pagers can be used on the vibration setting.
   d. Locate sources of loud sounds and request the facilities or building department to assist in reducing or eliminating those sounds whenever possible.
   e. Eliminate overhead paging.
   f. Intense noise levels (>55 to 60 dBA) disrupt sleep states and interfere with brain development and organization (White et al. and Committee to Establish Recommended Standards for Newborn ICU Design, 2013).
   g. Ambient noise must be low enough for an infant to distinguish the maternal voice to optimize auditory development.
3. Lighting
   a. While sound must be managed overall, lighting needs to be individualized to the patient (Lasky and Williams, 2009).
   b. Quilted incubator covers that are dark on the infant's side will reduce both light and sound.
   c. Sudden increase in light poses a stressor to premature infants and can influence physiologic stability; gradual increases are better tolerated (Ozawa et al., 2010).
   d. Visual stimulation around 30 to 32 weeks frequently results in observable stress responses.
   e. Protection from light during procedures is especially important as procedure lights are more intense than ambient light levels.
   f. Stiff stand-alone tents made from several blankets can shade the eyes without touching the skin during care/procedures.
4. Healthy environment (White et al. and Committee to Establish Recommended Standards for Newborn ICU Design, 2013).
   a. Ceilings, wall, flooring surfaces, furnishings, countertops, and other facility structures should not contain substances that are teratogenic, mutagenic, carcinogenic, or known to cause harm to humans.
   b. Cleaning of surfaces and furniture should be simple and require no toxic chemicals; soap and water preferred.
   c. Polyvinyl chlorides (PVCs) such as in vinyl flooring can affect air quality and should not be used.

d. Volatile organic compounds (VOCs) and persistent bioaccumulative toxins (PBTs) such as found in some paints and ceiling tiles are not recommended.
e. Rubber flooring (latex) must be certified as nonallergenic.
f. A minimum of 2 weeks is needed for adhesives and flooring material to be ready for infants to move into any new space.
g. The benchmark organization for green buildings is Leadership in Energy and Environmental Design (LEED), which has standards to help hospitals choose smart designs that are environmentally responsible and healthy for humans (http://www.leed.net).

B. **Nurses and other health team members can learn more about environments that can compromise patient care and safety.** Websites such as http://www.noharm.org, http://www.greennicu.com, and http://www.ewg.org, to name a few, are educational for staff interested in learning more about environmental safety. A pregnant woman passes chemicals to the fetus through the placenta. The Environmental Working Group reported 287 chemicals found in neonatal cord blood were linked to cancer, neurotoxins, and birth defects (Environmental Working Group, 2009; Houlihan et al., 2005). Neurotoxins transmitted to the developing fetus may interfere with processes required for normal brain development and function. By improving knowledge about healthy environments and keeping up-to-date, nurses can be prepared to advocate for better hospital environments for mothers and babies.

## DEVELOPMENTAL CARE PRACTICES

A. **Developmental care of infants within a medical context necessitates a collaborative team with family participation.** Various models of care delivery attempt to make this happen with a primary team that stays with the baby and family, building trust and learning the infant's cues and support needs. Essential to the continuity and consistency of care is sharing the infant's cues and needs with parents, other staff, therapists, consultants, and the health care team. Documentation in the medical record, plan of care, shift huddle, and report are ways to communicate important developmental support information.
   1. Examinations, nursing care, therapy, and procedures are carried out as often as possible around infant state while attentive and responsive to the infant's communication cues.
      a. Care is provided when infant is in the alert state.
      b. Care providers prepare infant for touch by speaking softly as they approach the bed.
      c. Infants are further prepared for care or touch with hand containment prior to moving hands for care/procedures so an infant can adjust to touch.
      d. Sleep cycles are protected with the understanding that synaptic connections around learning and memory are being wired.
      e. Behavioral cues are respected and responses prompt to avoid escalation of stress when stress cues are identified.

B. **Interventions that support positioning depend on the individual infant's needs.** For infants who are immobile or cannot maintain their own posture, supportive positioning will be essential to avoid acquired deformities. Positioning support devices should not cause restraint so infants have enough room to push against boundaries and develop their neuromuscular and skeletal systems (Fig. 11-6). Positioning interventions include (Hunter, 2010):
   1. Flexion, containment, midline alignment regardless of position (Fig. 11-7).
   2. Assessment of comfort (physiologic and behavioral) after positioning.
   3. Use of aids to support and maintain positions without restriction so an infant can move and push against boundaries without loss of motor stability (materials for "nest" or boundaries are blanket rolls, commercially available positioning aids; Fig. 11-8).
   4. Repositioning is often every 3 to 4 hours depending on the infant age and condition; however, an infant may become uncomfortable before time to reposition. Signs of discomfort such as squirming, irritability, frowning, or grimacing may indicate a need to reposition before schedule.

C. **Handling preterm infants using developmental principles minimizes the stress of movement by combining flexion and containment with a slow transfer.** Smaller infants can be transferred by gently containing the extremities and lifting in prone or side-lying with less disruption and stress (Fig. 11-9). Diaper changes can be made with an infant in side-lying position

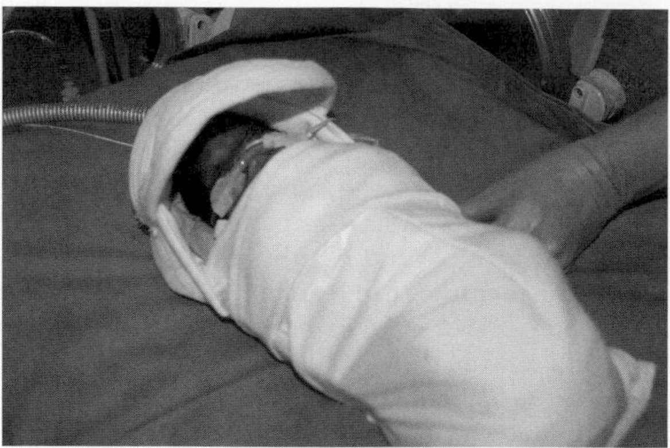

FIGURE 11-6 ■ Positional support that allows movement against boundaries and eye shielding. (Courtesy of DandleLION, Inc.)

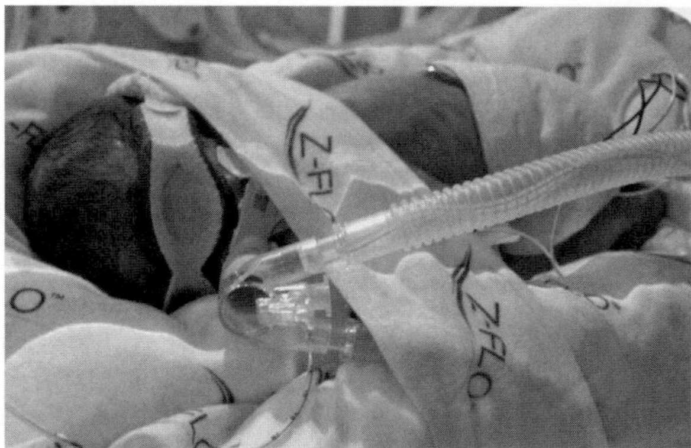

FIGURE 11-7 ■ Positioning principles applied for flexion, containment, alignment, and comfort. (Courtesy of Texas Children's Hospital, Houston, Tex.; photographer Carol Turnage Spruill.)

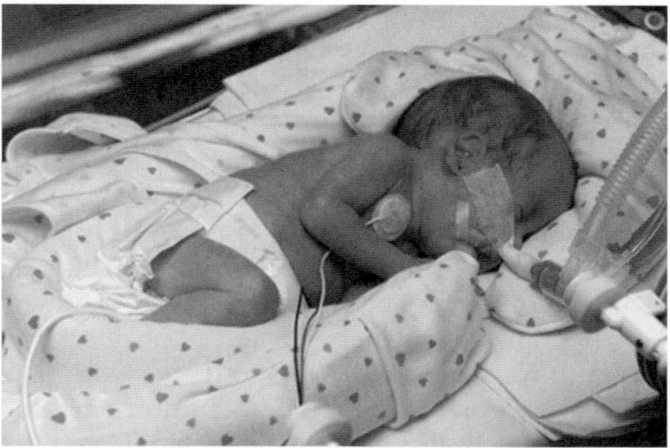

FIGURE 11-8 ■ Positioning can be accomplished using commercially available positioning supports or carefully rolled towels. Consider the external forces against the baby and select an appropriate mattress to reduce the risk of pressure ulcers. (Photograph provided courtesy Philips Healthcare.)

with less handling and without lifting lower body above the head (Comaru and Miura, 2009). Every opportunity to rethink care in a more supportive manner impacts the neurodevelopmental interface and the information received repeatedly by the evolving brain.

D. **Feeding is frequently viewed as a routine task.** The preterm infant's transition to breast or bottle requires thoughtful planning for developmental support as he or she learns to feed. Developmental support during feeding requires consideration of (McGrath et al., 2010):

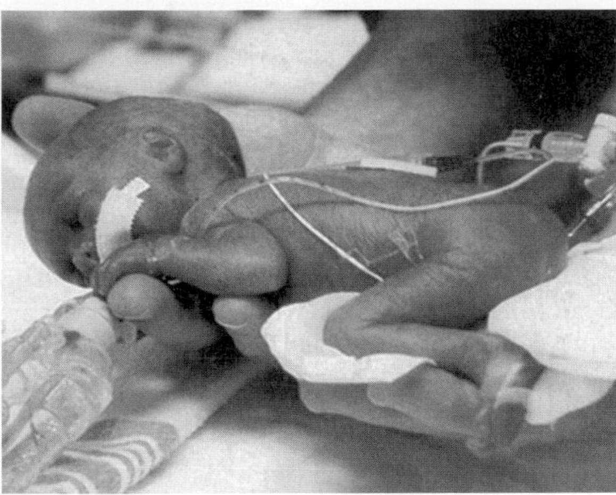

FIGURE 11-9 ■ Transfer small preterm infants with extremities contained and slowly transition to parent for skin-to-skin holding or for repositioning. (Courtesy of Texas Children's Hospital, Houston, Tex.; photography by Carol Turnage Spruill.)

1. Preparing the environment to minimize distraction and stressors (bright light, noise, swaddling).
2. Infant feeding readiness cues to start feedings without the confines of specific time intervals and duration.
3. Removing gavage tubes to enhance the experience.
4. Trying feedings when infant displays more energy.
5. Providing opportunities often for parents to feed their infant.

E. **The tactile sensation is the first sensory system to begin functioning, at about 7 weeks, in the fetus and through the skin becomes the neurodevelopmental interface between the infant and the world upon arrival at birth.** Tactile stimulation using various methods can be pleasant or unpleasant to an infant, especially if high-risk or premature. Touch is fundamental for newborn development; however, there continues to be reluctance in supporting parents in the early days of their newborn's critical illness or prematurity even though stressful and/or painful procedures/test are often performed. Touch by parents can begin on admission with sensitive nurses guiding them on techniques (Livingston et al., 2009) that are nurturing and less likely to elicit a stress response.

1. Hand containment or facilitated tuck can be taught to parents on the first day. This approach of low-stress touch has been associated with a decreased stress and pain response (Fig. 11-10).

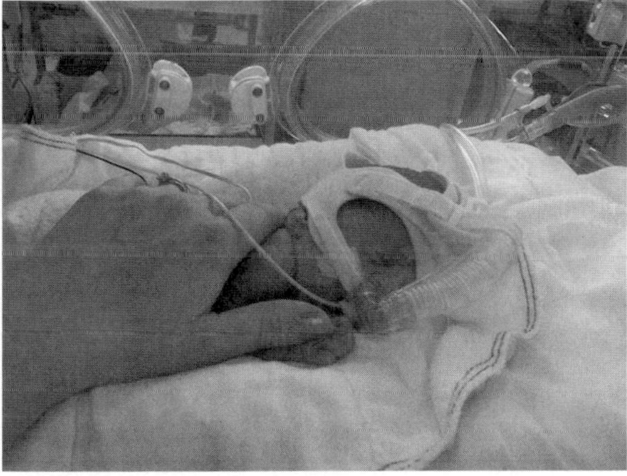

FIGURE 11-10 ■ Hand containment supports neurobehavioral organization and modifies pain response. (Courtesy DandleLION, Inc.)

2. Kangaroo care (KC) or skin-to-skin holding is associated with improved outcomes in both infant (i.e., fewer respiratory complications, better weight gain, temperature stability, decreased mortality in developing countries, duration of quiet sleep, modulation of pain, etc.) and mother (i.e., increased breast milk volume, increased parenting confidence, more positive and adaptive to infant cues, longer breastfeeding duration, etc.) (Jeffries and the Canadian Paediatric Society, Fetus and Newborn Committee, 2012; Spruill-Turnage and Papile, 2012).
   a. KC has positive benefits for both infants and mothers even after discharge from the NICU (Fig. 11-11). No adverse effects of KC on physiologic stability in preterm infants as young as 26 weeks' gestational age, even those on mechanical ventilation, have been reported. Fathers should be given opportunities for holding their infant KC style (Fig. 11-12). Resources for practice guidelines are available for developing specific unit KC guidelines (Jeffries and the Canadian Paediatric Society, Fetus and Newborn Committee, 2012; Nyqvist et al. and an Expert Group of the International Network on Kangaroo Mother Care, 2010a; Nyqvist et al., 2010b). When there is a question whether KC is an appropriate intervention, the health care team and family can evaluate the situation and decide on timing.
3. Massage is another intervention for preterm and term infants who are stable and might gain from a variation in tactile stimulation (Galicia-Connolly et al., 2012). Often infants are around 32 weeks when massage is considered, but there may be individual differences as to when it is beneficial.
   a. Benefits for caregivers (Richman and Caple, 2010):
      (1) Improved mood, confidence, and caregiver–infant attachment.
      (2) Decrease in maternal postnatal depression symptoms following massage classes compared with mothers in a support group.
   b. Benefits for infants (Richman and Caple, 2010):
      (1) Enhanced growth and development when massaged with moderate pressure.
      (2) Infants receiving moderate pressure massage gain more weight, sleep better, and cry/fuss less than those getting light pressure.
      (3) Decreased length of stay.
      (4) Less late-onset sepsis in the less than 32-week infant.
   c. The technique is taught to parents who provide the massage to their infant with support from a certified infant massage therapist trained to perform this skill on hospitalized preterm and term infants in the NICU. Parents often attend a class on infant massage to learn

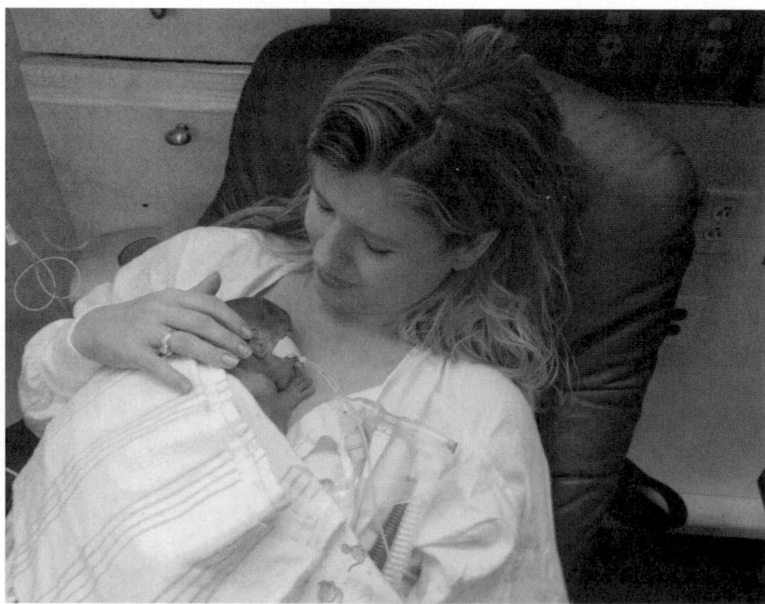

FIGURE 11-11 ■ Kangaroo or skin-to-skin holding in the NICU. (Courtesy of the Salinas Family, Houston, Tex.)

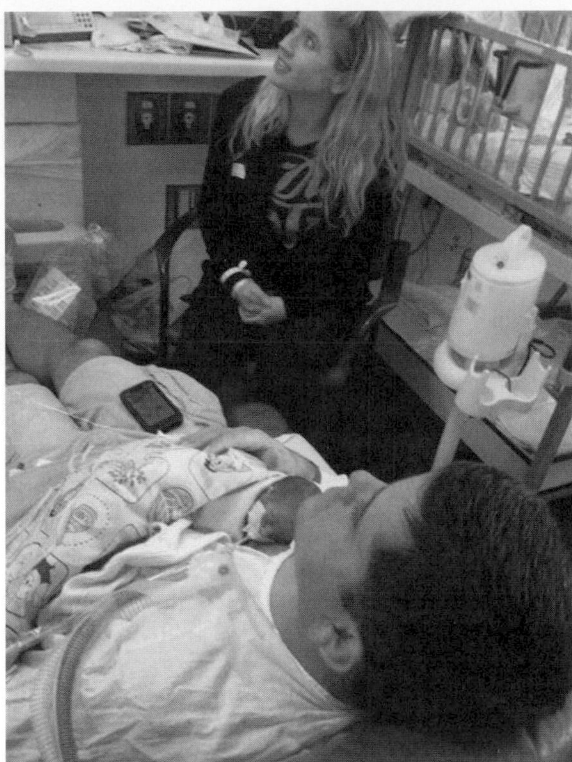

FIGURE 11-12 ■ Not for mothers only; fathers enjoy kangarooing their infant too. (Courtesy of the Salinas Family, Houston, Tex.)

and practice before attempting on their infant. Abdominal massage should be limited to trained providers since intestinal volvulus has been reported in preterm infants following massage therapy (Galicia-Connolly et al., 2012). Massage is considered a safe, effective opportunity to bring infant and parents together for a nurturing experience.

**d.** Adverse physiologic effects of massage are more likely when an infant cannot tolerate additional stimulation, is clinically unstable, has skin problems or wounds, is easily overstimulated, or has a reaction to massage oil after a skin test.

## PARENT SUPPORT AND INVOLVEMENT

Parents have expressed a variety of emotions about having to wait to touch or hold their baby in the NICU. They sometimes convey feelings of fear due to the NICU environment, their fragile baby, and all the medical devices on or around their infant. On the first day of admission, parents need assistance in understanding ways to touch their premature or sick infant that are nurturing and will not provoke stress responses. Helping parents recognize their own baby's specific behaviors will lead them to respond more appropriately. This time is an incredible opportunity to model nurturing, behaviorally supportive care that may be sustained after discharge. Encouraging parents to attend rounds, ask questions, and provide suggestions on supportive care directly influences their team involvement.

Becoming a parent in the NICU is a challenge since the environment is so foreign and providing care so publicly may impact the ability to achieve one's role as a parent. The more parents have an understanding of their infant's communication, the better they can participate in everyday care. Getting to know their baby as a unique individual who can convey needs and emotions is essential for attachment.

**A. Parental support strategies.** The key to supporting mutually satisfying parent–infant interaction is to establish a family-centered approach on admission that will empower the parents to assume the natural parental role of advocating for their child's needs and desires and become the primary nurturer to their infant. Supporting the parents' ability to understand their infant's level of communication through the infant's behavior will place the parents in a better position to respond to and interact with their infant in a developmentally supportive manner. Positive outcomes are associated with more parent visitation (Reynolds et al., 2013), such as increased holding ($P<0.001$) while infants had better movement quality ($P<0.02$), were less aroused ($P=0.01$), and were less excitable ($P=0.03$). The increased infant holding was also associated with better movement quality ($P<0.01$), lower stress ($P<0.01$), and fewer episodes of arousal ($P=0.04$) and excitability ($P<0.01$).

1. Establish an atmosphere in the NICU that is welcoming to parents and does not treat them as "visitors," but as parents who deserve respect as important members of their infant's care team (invite parents to join daily team rounds).
2. Help parents identify the most effective techniques for interacting with their infant (e.g., recognizing stress and time-out signs). Place parents in situations in which they will succeed in interacting positively with their infant.
3. Help parents identify both the consoling measures unique to their infant and how their child is providing feedback concerning the consoling measures. Parents can add to the developmental plan of care after they discover the likes/dislikes and learn the supportive techniques their baby responds to in certain situations.
4. Recommend the caregiving team work with parents to plan specific activities (i.e., KC or skin-to-skin holding, biologically meaningful smells and tastes, verbal interaction, eye contact, use of toys, therapeutic touch) for parental interaction when appropriate.
5. Encourage parents to assume caregiving responsibilities as soon and as much as possible.
6. Discuss parents' expectations and goals for themselves and their infant. Encourage families to write down these expectations and goals. Writing down these dreams and goals or journaling will be the beginning of a lifelong care plan.
7. Encourage the parents to use their child's medical record as a communication tool.

B. **Be aware of and involve the family's support system.** Encourage parent-to-parent support if possible, either in a formal or an informal manner. Recognize that the parents are the constant in the child's life and that health professionals will come and go. Parents and families will have the most effect on their infants' outcomes in the long term. NICU professionals must be ready to engage, interact, teach, respect, and build a relationship with them that supports the assimilation of the knowledge, skills, and attitudes they need to succeed as parents long after their infant is discharged from the NICU.

## TEAMWORK AND CONTINUITY OF CARE

A. **Collaboration fosters care that is consistent among caregivers.** Consistency and collaboration by caregivers who establish familiarity and predictable routine inspire trust from both infant and family. Consistency of caregivers is not only important for developmental planning and intervention but provides a measure of safety toward the recognition of clinical and behavioral changes requiring prompt intervention. The evolution of larger and larger NICUs requires critical appraisal of ways to maintain continuity, consistency, and communication to sustain safe clinical and developmental care (Goldschmidt and Gordin, 2006).

1. Consistency of care is a continuum that requires documentation of individual stress and stability cues, written plans of care based on individual assessment of each infant's response to the environment, care, procedures, and medical treatments.
2. Communication through the medical record, easily accessible assessment and care plans, and direct communication between and among caregivers at shift report and/or daily medical/nursing rounds foster collaborative practice and enhance consistent care.
3. A familiar group of people who care for individual infants provides reassurance that establishes trust and builds a partnership that is rewarding to the entire team, especially the family.

B. **Safe, quality care happens by design and not by accident.** Communication among caregivers who know the infant and family through repeated interactions enables them to deliver quality developmental care safely and effectively.

## REFERENCES


Aita, M., Johnston, C., Goulet, C., et al.: Intervention minimizing preterm infants' exposure to NICU light and noise. *Clinical Nursing Research*, 20(10):1–22, 2012.

American Academy of Pediatrics and American College of Obstetricians and Gynecologists: *Guidelines of perinatal care:* (7th ed.). Elk Grove Village, IL, and Washington, DC, 2012, American Academy of Pediatrics and American College of Obstetricians and Gynecologists.

Als, H.: Developmental care in the newborn intensive care unit. *Current Opinion in Pediatrics*, 10 (2):138–142, 1998.

Comaru, T. and Miura, E.: Postural support improves distress and pain during diaper change in preterm infants. *Journal of Perinatology*, 29(7):504–507, 2009.

Coughlin, M., Gibbins, S. and Hoath, S.: Core measures for developmentally supportive care in neonatal intensive care units: Theory, precedence and practice. *Journal of Advanced Nursing*, 65(10):2239–2248, 2009.

Environmental Working Group: Pollution in minority newborns. 2009: Retrieved May 4, 2013, from http://www.ewg.org/research/minority-cord-blood-report/executive-summary.

Galicia-Connolly, E., Shamseer, L. and Vohra, S.: Complementary, holistic, and integrative medicine: Therapies for neurodevelopment in preterm infants. *Pediatrics in Review*, 33(6):276–278, 2012.

Gibbins, S., Hoath, S.B., Coughlin, M., et al.: The universe of developmental care: A new conceptual model for application in the neonatal intensive care unit. *Advances in Neonatal Care*, 8(3):131–147, 2008.

Goldschmidt, K. and Gordin, P.: A model of nursing care microsystems for a large neonatal intensive care unit. *Advances in Neonatal Care*, 6(2):81–88, 2006.

Houlihan, J., Kropp, T., Wiles, R., et al.: Body burden: The pollution in newborns. 2005: Retrieved May 4, 2013, from http://www.ewg.org/research/body-burden-pollution-newborns/about-report.

Hunter, J.: Therapeutic positioning: Neuromotor, physiologic, and sleep implications. In C. Kenner, and J.M. McGrath (Eds.): *Developmental care of newborns and infants: A guide for health professionals* Glenview, IL, 2010, National Association of Neonatal Nurses, pp. 285–312.

Jeffries, A.L. and the Canadian Paediatric Society, Fetus and Newborn Committee: Kangaroo care for the preterm infant and family. *Paediatric and Child Health*, 17 (3):141–143, 2012.

Lasky, R.E. and Williams, A.L.: Noise and light exposures for extremely low birthweight newborns during their stay in the neonatal intensive care unit. *Pediatrics*, 123:540–546, 2009.

Lawhon, G. and Als, H.: Theoretical perspective for developmentally supportive care. In C. Kenner, and J.M. McGrath (Eds.): *Developmental care of newborns and infants: A guide for health professionals* Glenview, IL, 2010, National Association of Neonatal Nurses, pp. 20–24.

Limperopoulos, C., Gauvreau, K.K., O'Leary, H., et al.: Cerebral hemodynamic changes during intensive care of preterm infants. *Pediatrics*, 122(5): e1006–e1013, 2008.

Livingston, K., Beider, S. and Kant, A.J.: Touch and massage for medically fragile infants. *Evidence-Based Complementary and Alternative Medicine*, 6(4):473–482, 2009.

McGrath, J.M., Medoff-Cooper, B., Hardy, W. and Darcy, A.M.: Oral feeding and the high-risk infant. In C. Kenner, and J.M. McGrath (Eds.): *Developmental care of newborns and infants: A guide for health professionals* Glenview, IL, 2010, National Association of Neonatal Nurses, pp. 313–340.

Nyqvist, K.H., Anderson, G.C. and Bergman, N.: an Expert Group of the International Network on Kangaroo Mother Care: State of the art and recommendations. Kangaroo mother care: Application in a high-tech environment. *Acta Paediatrica*, 99:812–819, 2010a.

Nyqvist, K.H., Anderson, G.C., Bergman, N., et al.: Towards universal Kangaroo Mother Care: Recommendations and report from the First European conference and Seventh International Workshop on Kangaroo Mother Care. *Acta Paediatrica*, 99:820–826, 2010b.

Ozawa, M., Sasaki, M. and Kanda, K.: Effect of procedure light on physiological responses of premature infants. *Japan Journal of Nursing Science*, 7:76–83, 2010.

Pineda, R.G., Tjoeng, T.H., Vavasseur, C., et al.: Patterns of altered neurobehavior in preterm infants within the neonatal intensive care unit. *Journal of Pediatrics*, 162(3):470–476, 2013.

Reynolds, L.C., Duncan, M.M., Smith, G.C., et al.: Parental presence and holding in the neonatal intensive care unit and associations with early neurobehaviour. *Journal of Perinatology*, 33(8):636–641, 2013.

Richman, S. and Caple, C.: Evidence-based care sheet: Infant massage. Glendale, CA, 2010, Cinahl Information Systems.

Spruill-Turnage, C. and Papile, L.A.: Developmentally supportive care. In J.P. Cloherty, E.C. Eichenwald, A.R. Hansen, and A.R. Stark (Eds.): *Manual of neonatal care* (7th ed.). Philadelphia, 2012, Lippincott Williams & Wilkins, pp. 174–175.

White, R.D., Smith, J.A. and Shepley, M.M.: Committee to Establish Recommended Standards for Newborn ICU Design: Recommended standards for newborn ICU design, eighth edition. *Journal of Perinatology*, 33:S2–S16, 2013.

Zimmerman, E. and Lahav, A.: Ototoxicity in preterm infants: Effects of genetics, aminoglycosides, and loud environmental noise. *Journal of Perinatology*, 33:3–8, 2013.

CHAPTER

# 12 Pharmacology

CHRISTINE D. DOMONOSKE

**OBJECTIVES**

1. Define the concepts of (a) pharmacology, (b) pharmacodynamics, and (c) pharmacokinetics.
2. Describe the developmental changes that affect medication absorption, distribution, metabolism, and elimination.
3. Identify specific considerations when one is administering medications of the following types to a neonate: (a) antimicrobial agents, (b) cardiovascular agents, (c) central nervous system agents, (d) diuretics, and (e) immunizations.
4. Describe nursing responsibilities and interventions when administering medication to the neonate.

The study and clinical application of neonatal pharmacology can facilitate safe medication administration in the neonate. The application of pharmacologic principles involves evaluating existing knowledge related to the pharmacodynamic and pharmacokinetic responses of the neonate to specific medications. Unfortunately, this body of knowledge is extremely limited in the neonatal population owing to a lack of controlled clinical trials with these patients. Confounding factors relative to gestational and chronologic age, weight, fluid status, and the health–illness state of individual organ systems make dosing medications in this population a challenging and perpetual learning process. The decision to administer a medication should be evaluated for the desired response and the potential for an undesirable reaction. The nurse is in the ideal position to observe and evaluate both response and reaction and to intervene if necessary.

This chapter provides pharmacologic information specific to the neonate. Information on medication dosages and implications for medication administration is provided in individual clinical chapters. Additional current reference materials should also be available in the neonatal intensive care unit (NICU).

## PRINCIPLES OF PHARMACOLOGY

### Terminology

A. **Pharmacology:** the science of the properties of medications and their effects in the body.
   1. **Pharmacotherapy:** the administration of a medication to a patient with the intent of preventing, diagnosing, or treating disease.
   2. **Medication:** any substance or mixture of substances intended to be used for the cure, mitigation, or prevention of disease in human beings or animals.
   3. **Pharmacodynamics:** the relationship between medication concentrations at the site of action and the pharmacologic response (intensity and time course of therapeutic and adverse effects). This is what the drug does to the body.
   4. **Pharmacokinetics:** the fate of a medication in the body from the time it enters until it and all of its metabolites are removed. This includes medication absorption, distribution, metabolism, and excretion. It is also the specialized study of the mathematical relationship between a medication dosage regimen and the resulting serum concentration. This is what the body does to the drug.
   5. **Bioavailability:** the portion of the administered dose that reaches the site of action in the body. This is usually the amount entering the circulation and may be reduced when medications are given by mouth versus when given intravenously.
   6. **Therapeutic range:** a range of medication concentrations within which the probability of the desired clinical response is relatively high and the probability of unacceptable toxicity or subtherapeutic response is relatively low.

7. **Therapeutic drug monitoring (TDM):** determinations of plasma medication concentrations to optimize medication therapy. TDM is valuable when:
    a. A good correlation exists between the pharmacologic response and plasma concentration.
    b. Wide intersubject variation in drug plasma levels results from a given dose.
    c. The medication has a narrow therapeutic range.
    d. The medication's desired pharmacologic effects cannot be readily assessed by other simple means.
8. **Steady state:** a term used to refer to a situation in which the amount of medication administered is equal to the amount of medication eliminated. When steady state is reached in a patient, the blood concentrations remain "steady." Therefore, at steady state, all peak drug levels and all trough drug levels should be the same.
9. **Half-life:** the time necessary for a measured medication concentration to fall to half its original value. A medication's duration of action is often related to its half-life, and the half-life may also indicate when another dose should be given. It takes approximately five half-lives to reach steady state.
10. **Types of medication levels:**
    a. *Peak level:* a drug level that is drawn after the dose is given and after adequate time is allowed for the drug to distribute throughout the body. The time for the drug to distribute varies with each medication and the route of administration.
    b. *Trough level:* a drug level that is drawn just prior to the dose.
    c. *Random level:* a drug level that is drawn at any time after a dose is given. These levels are often used to follow drug levels in patients with changing renal function or changing volume status.

## PHARMACODYNAMICS

A. **Receptor concept:** The principle that medications act by forming a complex with a specific macromolecule in a way that produces a given response. This response may include inhibition or potentiation of the macromolecule's activity to create the desired medication effect. Receptor effects are as follows:
    1. The medication's affinity for binding to the receptor plays a large part in the determination of the concentration of the medication required to achieve the desired response.
    2. The individual characteristics of the receptor are responsible for the selective nature of medication response.
    3. Receptor theory of medication action allows an explanation of medication antagonists. The antagonist medication may alter the characteristics of the receptor molecule in a way that limits or inhibits the response to the original medication (e.g., naloxone and morphine) or stimulus (e.g., a β-blocker such as propranolol).
    4. Some medications do not appear to act through receptors. Their action is related to a direct response in the recipient.

B. **General mechanisms of medication action.**
    1. Based on the nature of the receptor medication complex.
    2. Types of receptor–medication complexes.
        a. Receptor–medication complexes that regulate gene expression.
            (1) One common class of medications acts by mediating a response that ultimately involves gene expression and new protein synthesis.
            (2) These medications generally do not have a rapid effect after initial administration (e.g., epoetin alfa).
        b. Receptor–medication complexes that change cell membrane permeability.
            (1) Many clinically useful medications act by changing the cell membrane permeability and therefore altering membrane characteristics.
            (2) These medications may have a relatively short lag time between administration and response (e.g., penicillin).
        c. Receptor–medication complexes that increase the intracellular concentration of a second messenger molecule.

(1) These medications increase production and activity of enzyme systems within the cell.
(2) These medications may stimulate a rapid response in changing cell characteristics (e.g., dopamine).

**C. Relationship between medication dose and clinical response.**

1. Individuals in a population receiving a medication may have a wide range of responses to a medication dose. An idiosyncratic medication response is an abnormal response to a medication that is not usually observed. These unpredictable responses include the following:
   a. Low sensitivity: a patient who, on receiving the usual medication dose, exhibits a clinical or biological response that is less intense than expected (e.g., inadequate pain relief with usual doses of analgesic medications).
   b. Extreme sensitivity: a patient whose response to a medication is more intense than is expected (e.g., severe hypotension from an antihypertensive agent).
   c. Unpredictable adverse reaction: a patient whose medication reaction is substantially different from what would have been predicted and may differ from the usual response in most patients (e.g., an anaphylactic reaction).
   d. Tolerance: a diminished response to a given medication dose that is related to long-term administration of a medication (e.g., fentanyl doses must be increased as the length of therapy increases to achieve the same effects).
   e. Tachyphylaxis: a rapidly diminished medication response without a medication dosage change. This may be caused by any of a number of factors, including a limited number of receptor sites or limited numbers of transmitter chemicals (e.g., response to albuterol may diminish if given frequently).
2. Factors that may affect individual medication response are as follows:
   a. Alterations in medication concentration: a change from the expected norm in the amount of medication that reaches the receptor molecule.
   b. Variation in amounts of antagonistic substances: an unusually large or limited amount of antagonistic substances that alter receptor molecule response.
   c. Alterations in numbers or function of receptor molecules: an increased or diminished number of receptor molecules changes the number of potential medication–receptor complexes.
   d. Changes in concentration of molecules other than receptor molecules: if medication response is ultimately dependent on an effect on molecules other than those of the medication–receptor complex, medication response may be limited by the amount of the third molecule type (e.g., prodrugs such as fosphenytoin).

**D. Desired versus undesired effects of medications.**

1. No medication causes only one effect; all medications have several effects, which can be divided into four groups:
   a. Desired, or therapeutic, effects: those effects that are the desired outcome of the medication administration (e.g., reduction in apnea episodes with theophylline treatment).
   b. Subtherapeutic effect: those effects that are less than the desired outcome of the medication administration (e.g., continued apnea episodes with low theophylline levels).
   c. Side effects: those medication effects that result from medication administration and that are in addition to the desired effects. All medications have some side effects, varying from minor and clinically insignificant to major side effects that are sufficiently adverse to require discontinuation of the medication therapy (e.g., tachycardia with theophylline treatment).
   d. Toxic effects: medication response that results from a medication overdose or unexpected high serum medication concentrations (e.g., seizures from a high theophylline level).
2. It is the responsibility of the health care provider to weigh the benefits of the therapeutic effect against the risk of undesirable side effects and toxic effects or subtherapeutic responses and make adjustments accordingly.

## PHARMACOKINETICS

**A. Principles of medication absorption (Fig. 12-1).**

1. General principles of medication absorption.
   a. The movement of a medication from the site of administration to the bloodstream.

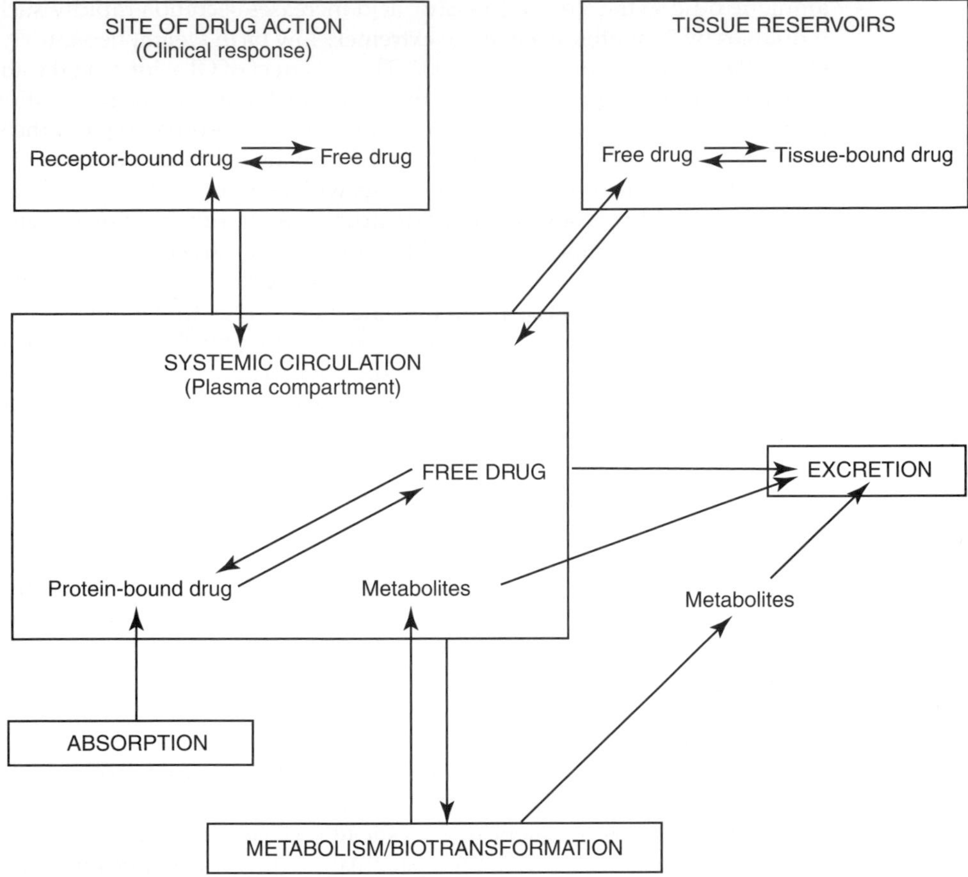


FIGURE 12-1 ■ Principles of medication absorption. (Adapted from McClary, J., Blumer, J.L., and Aranda, J.V.: Developmental pharmacology. In R.J. Martin, A.A. Fanaroff, and M.C. Walsh [Eds.]: *Fanaroff and Martin's neonatal-perinatal medicine: Diseases of the fetus and infant* [9th ed.]. Philadelphia, 2011, Elsevier Mosby.)

**b.** Regardless of the route of administration, most medications must cross cell membranes to reach their site of action.
   (1) Most medications cross cell membranes by passive diffusion. Physiochemical properties of the medication molecule have a major impact on the ease of diffusion.
   (2) Medications can enter the cell through other mechanisms also, such as active transport or facilitated diffusion.

**c.** The absorption of a medication is dependent, in large part, on the route of administration. The common sites of administration are as follows:
   (1) **Gastrointestinal (GI):** commonly used because of minimal infection risk, decreased cost, and convenience.
      (a) Gastric emptying and intestinal transit times: prolonged and irregular; approaches adult values at 6 to 8 months of age. Gastric and intestinal motility are reduced with prematurity, asphyxia, gastroesophageal reflux, and respiratory distress syndrome. Administration of hypocaloric feeds, human milk, or prokinetic agents (e.g., metoclopramide, erythromycin) can increase motility. Prolonged transit times and enterohepatic recirculation may also increase the bioavailability and pharmacologic effect of some substances (Chemtob, 2011; van den Anker et al., 2011). However, the bioavailability of the medication may decrease because of increased first-pass loss, increased GI destruction of medication or shortened transit times from diarrhea or emesis.
      (b) GI tract acidity: the presence of marked changes in pH from the stomach through the distal portion of the GI tract may affect absorption. The pH of the GI tract is nearly neutral or slightly alkaline at birth owing to the presence of

amniotic fluid in the stomach. Gastric acid increases secretion rapidly such that it doubles by 2 months, even in the extremely low birth weight neonate (Kearns et al., 2003; van den Anker et al., 2011). The net effect of GI acidity on the absorption of medications is dependent on the pH characteristics of the medication and preparation. Medications that normally may not be absorbed well in the stomach may be absorbed at a higher rate in the neonate because of decreased stomach acidity. The absorption of acidic drugs will be reduced (e.g., phenobarbital, phenytoin) and the absorption of basic drugs will be enhanced (e.g., penicillin, erythromycin) as compared with adults (Funk et al., 2012).

(c) GI enzyme activity: neonates are deficient in pancreatic enzymes at birth. This deficiency may inhibit absorption of some medications that require pancreatic enzymes for efficient absorption. One compensating mechanism that neonates have is an increased β-glucuronidase secretion. This is an enzyme produced by organisms normally present in the small intestine that are capable of metabolizing some medications. It is present in neonates at up to seven times the adult amounts (Kearns et al., 2003; van den Anker et al., 2011).

(d) Bacterial flora: composition and rate of colonization of the GI tract by the normal bacterial flora may affect both GI tract motility and the metabolism of some medications. Colonization is dependent on oral intake, antibiotic administration, or disease states such as necrotizing enterocolitis or infectious gastroenteritis. Normal colonization in vaginally born term neonates occurs by 4 to 6 days of age. Intestinal flora are required for the production of vitamin K (Chemtob, 2011).

(e) GI tract perfusion: in very ill neonates, hypoperfusion of the gut may decrease medication absorption.

(f) Underlying disease states: underlying disease states such as diarrhea, emesis, or the presence of nasogastric suction may reduce the time available for medication absorption. Diseases of genetic (e.g., cystic fibrosis) or circulatory (e.g., necrotizing enterocolitis) origin will alter pancreatic enzymes or intestinal mucosa, decreasing GI absorption.

(2) **Rectal:** may be a very rapid and efficient means of medication absorption.

(a) Useful when rapid intravenous (IV) access is not available (e.g., patients in status epilepticus in need of anticonvulsant agents).

(b) Serum levels of some medications may be as high as levels obtained through the IV route of administration (Kearns et al., 2003).

(c) Routine administration by rectal route is discouraged. Relative volume and fragility of the neonatal rectum must be considered.

(d) The retention time is the rate-limiting step.

(3) **Inhalation:** useful for gaseous or easily vaporized medications.

(a) Absorption is favored owing to the large surface area of the alveolar membranes and the generous blood flow. Medication response may be very rapid.

(b) Medications administered by this route have a particular advantage when the site of desired action is the tracheobronchial tree (e.g., albuterol).

(c) There is a potential for fewer side effects when medications are administered this way, because much of the medication may not be systemically absorbed (e.g., inhaled corticosteroids).

(d) Most frequently used in neonatal intensive care for the administration of various surfactant preparations.

(e) Certain medications (e.g., epinephrine and lidocaine) can be given through the endotracheal tube in emergency situations when IV access is not readily available.

(f) This route may be less effective in a neonate with pulmonary hypertension and poor or abnormally distributed pulmonary blood flow.

(4) **Topical/percutaneous:** utility is limited to medications whose absorptive characteristics allow permeation through the skin or mucous membranes. Percutaneous absorption has particular advantages as well as risks in the neonate.

(a) The rate of absorption is inversely related to skin thickness and directly related to skin hydration. With increasing gestational age, skin thickness increases and water content decreases, thus reducing the amount of absorption from this route. Maturation of the epidermis occurs between 23 and 33 weeks of gestation. The stratum corneum forms after 23 to 24 weeks of gestation. Formation of this layer of the skin greatly decreases the permeability of the skin to water and infection (Hoath, 2011). This allows much more efficient percutaneous absorption of medications in neonates of lower birth weight and younger gestational age. However, this poses a particular hazard in care, because substances that may be safely applied to the skin of a more mature patient may be absorbed in dangerous amounts in the immature neonate (van den Anker et al., 2011).

(b) The ratio of body surface area to body weight is higher in neonates than adults, providing a relatively larger absorptive surface in comparison with body mass.

(c) The absorptive response time is variable and may be limited to the local area of application; however, some topically applied medications (e.g., nitroglycerin) can have a systemic effect. As a result, products that contain alcohol and hexachlorophene skin washes should be avoided. Any treatment with topical steroids should be limited to less than 2 weeks to prevent adrenal suppression. On the other hand, antibiotic ointments will be more readily absorbed to treat infections, povidone–iodine (Betadine) absorption can prevent iodine deficiency, and topical safflower oil may prevent essential fatty acid deficiency.

(d) Occlusive dressings will increase the extent of absorption.

(5) **Intramuscular/subcutaneous:** administration into muscle or subcutaneous tissue.

(a) Minimal subcutaneous tissue and muscle mass significantly limit these two routes of administration, particularly in the low birth weight neonate.

(b) These routes are limited to medications that do not cause tissue damage at the administration site and are soluble at physiologic pH.

(c) These routes will achieve slower responses as compared with the IV route because of the lag time between administration and achievement of blood concentration.

(d) Response time is dependent on blood flow to muscle and may be greatly delayed in hypoperfused tissue. Poor peripheral blood flow and low blood pressure are common in neonates. These problems become less common with increasing gestational age but can occur in the presence of many neonatal disease states. Poor cardiac output frequently occurs with many illness states in the neonatal period. Subsequent increases in the peripheral perfusion after resolution of the primary illness states may put the neonate at risk of having an increase in the rate and amount of medication absorption.

(e) Diminished muscle activity in the ill neonate decreases muscle perfusion and consequently may limit absorption of medications administered by this route.

(6) **Intravenous:** direct administration into the bloodstream.

(a) Bypasses all absorptive barriers.

(b) Most effective and reliable method of medication administration because the medication is delivered directly to the circulating plasma volume.

(c) Significant medication serum concentrations are reached rapidly, allowing for immediate medication response. This includes both desired and undesired or toxic reactions.

(d) Adequate and equal distribution to all organs or compartments is not guaranteed. Characteristics of some biological membranes may limit medication distribution to body compartments (e.g., blood–brain barrier).

(e) Rapid achievement of potentially dangerous serum medication concentrations may require administration of the IV medication over a prolonged period rather than by IV push (e.g., vancomycin, amphotericin, and aminoglycosides).

**B. Principles of medication distribution.**

1. **Distribution:** movement of the medication to and through various body compartments. The extent of this movement, the "size" of the compartment, the number and character of the binding sites, and the amount of the medication administered determine the amount

of medication at the desired site of action. When medication movement reaches a steady state, the volume of distribution is defined as the hypothetical volume of body fluid that would be required to dissolve the total amount of medication as found in the serum. This volume is sometimes described as apparent volume of distribution. This volume may be larger than the total body volume if the medication is highly protein- or tissue-bound.

2. **Body compartments.**
   a. *Total body water:* as age increases, total body water, as a percentage of total body mass, decreases. Total body water in adults comprises approximately 55% of total body weight; in term infants it is 75%, and in preterm infants it is 85% (Funk et al., 2012).
      (1) As body water increases, as a percentage of body mass, water-soluble medications have a larger volume of distribution.
      (2) Because of increased total body water, a less mature neonate may require a larger per-kilogram dose to achieve the same peak medication concentration and effect as an older patient (e.g., aminoglycosides).
      (3) In the first several days after birth, total body water decreases, causing the volume of intracellular fluid to be increased relative to the amount of extracellular water (van den Anker et al., 2011). This leads to rapid changes in the volume of distribution for water-soluble medications, in relation to normal physiology and illness states.
      (4) Body water loss is divided into two main categories: sensible and insensible. Sensible losses can be measured and quantified. In term neonates, insensible losses occur in a strong relationship to metabolism. In extremely premature neonates, insensible losses occur primarily through evaporative loss, independent of metabolic rate. Insensible losses are difficult to quantify (Chemtob, 2011).
      (5) Medications frequently administered to the neonate (e.g., diuretics, indomethacin) may have a major impact on body water volume and, as a side effect, may alter the volume of distribution (Chemtob, 2011).
      (6) Neonates with disease states that alter water excretion (e.g., primary renal disease, syndrome of inappropriate antidiuretic hormone [SIADH], congestive heart failure, capillary leak syndromes) may have expansion of body water as a result of this dysfunction.
      (7) The preceding alterations make dosing medications that are primarily distributed in body water (e.g., aminoglycosides) difficult.
      (8) Frequent monitoring of medication levels may be required as the mentioned changes in body compartment volumes occur.
   b. *Fat:* wide variability of neonatal values, based on gestational age and intrauterine and postnatal growth patterns. This percentage increases from 1% of body weight at 28 weeks of gestation to approximately 15% in a term neonate (Stewart and Hampton, 1987).
      (1) Medications with more lipid solubility have affinity for this tissue.
      (2) Reduced amounts of the percentage of body fat may make the volume of distribution smaller for medications distributed primarily in fatty tissue. Hence the plasma levels of these medications will be higher because less drug will be bound in the fat tissue, resulting in a greater potential for side effects and toxicity (e.g., morphine, lorazepam).
   c. *Blood components:* potential sites for medication binding.
      (1) Erythrocytes: neonates have 2.5 times more binding sites for digoxin as compared with the erythrocytes in adults. This results in the need for much higher doses per total body weight in neonates than adults (Stewart and Hampton, 1987).
      (2) Plasma protein concentrations: medications may form a complex with large circulating molecules (usually proteins).
         (a) The amount of medication that binds to these sites has a direct effect on the amount of medication available for the desired pharmacologic effect. This binding may result in a limited medication response because only the unbound medication can be distributed to active receptor sites. When more of the medication is protein-bound, less is available for the desired medication effect: serum concentration = protein-bound medication + unbound medication.

(b) The primary binding protein for acidic medications (e.g., phenytoin, indomethacin, and furosemide) in the serum is albumin (Chemtob, 2011).
(c) Serum albumin levels may be markedly decreased in the ill, extremely low birth weight neonate.
(d) The primary binding proteins for basic molecules (e.g., lidocaine, propranolol) are lipoproteins, glycoproteins, and β-globulins (Chemtob, 2011).
(e) *Unconjugated bilirubin:* many neonates have increased plasma unconjugated bilirubin levels. Fetal albumin has an increased affinity for bilirubin and a decreased affinity for medications. This causes the unconjugated bilirubin to displace some medications from the albumin-binding sites, making more free medication available for action. In contrast, some medications (e.g., ceftriaxone, sulfonamides) may displace unconjugated bilirubin from albumin-binding sites. This may lead to the deposition of unconjugated bilirubin in the neonatal brain, causing kernicterus (Kearns et al., 2003). These medications should be avoided if possible in patients younger than 2 months of age or in patients with high unconjugated bilirubin levels.
(f) *Free fatty acids:* increased serum free fatty acid concentrations have been shown to displace some medications from plasma albumin-binding sites (Chemtob, 2011).
(g) *Blood pH:* acidosis is a common finding associated with many neonatal disorders. Changes in blood pH have been shown to change albumin-binding characteristics. This may cause medication displacement from albumin. Changes in blood pH may also cause medications to displace unconjugated bilirubin (see above).

**d.** *Blood–brain barrier:* incomplete in the neonate, causing a greater permeability to lipophilic medications (e.g., phenytoin, benzodiazepines). This incomplete barrier may be beneficial when treating neonatal meningitis because the antibiotics penetrate the cerebrospinal fluid more readily (Stewart and Hampton, 1987).

**3. Medication movement:** an important part of medication distribution involves medication movement from the site of administration to sites throughout the body. It is dependent on the blood flow and medication solubility.

**a.** *Blood flow:* amount and distribution of blood flow to the target organ or cell affect the delivery of a medication absorbed into the bloodstream. Continued adequate blood flow and serum medication concentration are required to maintain an adequate concentration of the medication at the target organ. Several neonatal conditions affect blood flow:
(1) Hypotension: may affect peripheral medication absorption and/or distribution.
(2) Distributive shock: caused by inappropriate vasodilation; seen with sepsis. Medication distribution to specific organs may be limited by local hypoperfusion.
(3) Pulmonary hypertension: may impede medication delivery to the pulmonary vascular bed.
(4) Patent ductus arteriosus: blood flow may be distributed preferentially to either the pulmonary or systemic circulation, depending on the pressure differential.
(5) Congestive heart failure: may affect peripheral medication absorption or distribution.

**b.** *Medication solubility:* in biological tissues, the relative ability of the medication to dissolve in biological fluids.
(1) Medications with low lipid solubility do not distribute well through lipid membranes, though they may be distributed well through the body water spaces. Highly lipid-soluble medications are distributed readily through most lipid membranes but are not distributed well through body water spaces.
(2) The relative medication solubility may make some medication use inappropriate. A medication with low lipid solubility may not reach therapeutic concentrations in an organ that is primarily fat tissue (e.g., aminoglycosides do not readily cross the blood–brain barrier).

**C. Principles of medication metabolism.**

**1. General principles of medication metabolism.** Many medications must be converted into more water-soluble compounds before they can be removed from the body. Metabolism (biotransformation) is the *chemical change* of a medication into another form. This transformed medication may be pharmacologically active or inactive. The liver, kidney, GI tract, lung, adrenal gland, blood, and skin are tissues capable of biotransforming certain compounds. Of these sites, the liver is the principal organ for medication metabolism.

a. Liver.
   (1) Metabolic activity is divided into two main types.
      (a) Phase I (nonsynthetic) metabolism of medications: primarily oxidation, reduction, hydrolysis, or demethylation reactions, which generally occur in the smooth endoplasmic reticulum of the hepatocyte. The function of these enzymes in the full- and preterm neonate is approximately 50% to 70% of adult values. Maturation occurs as a function of chronologic rather than postconceptional age, with a wide range of variability. Maturation of nonsynthetic enzyme systems during the first several days of life requires careful monitoring of serum levels of some classes of medications (e.g., anticonvulsants). For instance, at term gestation, neonates have approximately 30% of adult ability to metabolize phenytoin, hence the half-life is significantly prolonged. Within several weeks of medication exposure, metabolic enzyme activity for phenytoin surpasses adult activity (Funk et al., 2012; van den Anker et al., 2011).
      (b) Phase II (synthetic) metabolism of medications: primarily involves the acetylation, methylation, or conjugation of the medication with another substance. The function of these enzymes is also immature, and they may not reach adult levels in concentration and function until well after the neonatal period.
   (2) Hepatic uptake of the medication is dependent on the concentration of the medication in the liver (dependent on hepatic blood flow) and the hepatocyte concentration of ligandin (Y-protein). This protein is responsible for substrate uptake by hepatic cells.
   (3) In the first-pass effect, hepatic biotransformation may markedly alter medication availability by directly metabolizing medications absorbed from the GI tract, before those medications reach other organs. Slow GI motility may increase the potential for first-pass effect. Prolonged GI transit times may increase potential for hepatic metabolism and eventual excretion of orally administered medications.
   (4) Certain medications (e.g., phenobarbital) are thought to induce enzyme maturity in the fetus and neonate, resulting in increased rates of medication elimination.
   (5) Both hepatic enzyme systems may be vulnerable to hypoxic–ischemic insult.
   (6) Maturational changes in medication metabolism can have a major clinical significance. Careful monitoring of serum levels of some medication classes (e.g., anticonvulsants) is necessary in the first weeks of life.

**D. Principles of medication excretion.**

1. **General principles of medication excretion.** Excretion is the final elimination of medication from the body. The process of excretion begins with administration of the medication and ends when the medication is completely eliminated from the body. There are several important organs of excretion:
   a. **Salivary, sweat, and mammary glands:** small amounts of medication may be excreted through these minor organs. Very limited sweat production makes excretion by this mode insignificant in the neonate.
   b. **Lungs:** the lungs are an important route of excretion of gaseous anesthetics but are relatively less important for other medications. Excretion by the lungs is not well studied in the neonatal population. Because lung disease is common in newborn infants, adult data indicate that this may affect or limit the ability to excrete medications by this method.
   c. **GI tract:** the large, lipid-soluble surface of the GI tract allows diffusion of medications into the bloodstream. The limited motility in neonates affects excretion and increases the potential for reabsorption of medications or metabolites back into the circulation.
   d. **Liver:** the most important site of medication biotransformation also serves as an important site of medication excretion. The excretion of bile is an important means of medication elimination.

(1) Limited oral intake, long-term parenteral nutrition, or intrinsic hepatic disease may reduce bile flow. This may reduce the efficacy of this route of elimination.
(2) Metabolite or medication elimination in bile is dependent on the solubility characteristics of that substance in bile.

e. **Kidneys:** the most important site for medication excretion.
(1) *Renal blood flow*:
(a) Clamping of the umbilical cord is a significant event that signals a major increase in renal blood flow.
(b) As a percentage of cardiac output, renal blood flow is limited in neonates in comparison with older children and adults. Limited renal blood flow as an absolute value and as a percentage of cardiac output restricts medication or metabolite delivery to the kidney for excretion.
(c) Renal blood flow increases with increasing gestational and postnatal age.
(d) High umbilical artery catheter placement may reduce the renal blood flow.
(2) *Glomerular filtration rate (GFR)*: the removal, by passive filtration, of small unbound medication molecules at the glomerulus. Glomerular filtration is dependent on renal blood flow, the characteristics of the glomerular membranes, and the water solubility of the medication.
(a) The GFR function is extremely limited in neonates (full-term neonates have 30% of adult values, per unit of body surface area; adult values are reached by 8 to 12 months of age) (Stewart and Hampton, 1987; van den Anker et al., 2011).
(b) GFR is related to gestational age; the lower the gestational age, the lower the GFR. Neonates born at less than 34 weeks of gestation have fewer glomeruli, with total glomerular mass proportional to gestational age (Stewart and Hampton, 1987). Glomerular filtration has been shown to mature rapidly the first 2 weeks of life, although GFR in premature neonates remains significantly suppressed as compared to full-term neonates (Funk et al., 2012).
(c) GFR can be further compromised with asphyxia, hypoxia, or indomethacin treatment. Limited glomerular filtration reduces removal of medications or metabolites at the glomerulus.
(d) Medication excretion dependent on glomerular filtration includes indomethacin, digoxin, aminoglycosides, and vancomycin.
(3) *Tubular secretion*: the active secretion of molecules into the tubular urine. Tubular secretion is dependent on the efficiency of tubular function.
(a) Neonates have a relatively small mass of functional tubular cells, as well as an immaturity of tubular function. This functional limitation is thought to be caused in part by a decrease of renal blood flow to the renal tubular region and by shortened renal tubules (Stewart and Hampton, 1987).
(b) The limitation in tubular mass and function causes poor excretion of medications and metabolites removed by this method.
(c) Tubular secretion matures much more slowly than glomerular filtration.
(d) Tubular secretion is also vulnerable to hypoxic–ischemic insult.
(e) Medications dependent on tubular secretion for excretion include penicillins, morphine, and thiazide diuretics.
(4) *Tubular reabsorption*: reabsorption, for some medications, back into the circulating plasma.
(a) May occur through either passive diffusion or active transport.
(b) Passive diffusion appears to be the most important process.
(c) Tubular reabsorption matures much more slowly than glomerular filtration.
(d) Substances dependent on tubular reabsorption include caffeine, glucose, phosphate, and sodium.
(5) *Urinary output*:
(a) Because of changes in renal blood flow, glomerular filtration, and tubular secretion in the neonate, urinary output is not a reliable sign of renal excretion of medications.

(b) Blood level monitoring is required to ensure safe serum levels of renally excreted medications.

# MEDICATION CATEGORIES

## Antimicrobial Agents

A. **Introduction.** The use of a larger variety of antimicrobial agents in the neonatal population has occurred in the past several years for several reasons. As the threshold of viability is pushed, the length of stay of NICU infants is increasing. The additional numbers of antibiotic courses, coupled with increasing antibiotic resistance patterns, necessitate more broad-spectrum antibiotic usage as well as increased use of antifungal agents.

B. **Definitions.**

1. **Antimicrobial medications:** medications that inhibit the growth of or kill microorganisms such as bacteria, fungi, viruses, protozoa, and amebae.
   a. Bacteriostatic medications: agents that inhibit the growth of microorganisms, thereby allowing normal body defense mechanisms to control spread of the organism (e.g., clindamycin, fluconazole).
   b. Bactericidal medications: agents that kill microorganisms. At lower concentrations they may be bacteriostatic (e.g., aminoglycosides, penicillin, cephalosporins).
2. **Minimal inhibitory concentration (MIC):** the lowest concentration of a medication that stops visible organism growth in a laboratory setting. In the body, this cannot be directly measured and is dependent on achieved tissue concentration and bacterial count. This is easily measured in the microbiology laboratory and is used to measure the susceptibility of the microorganism to antimicrobial agents.
3. **Minimal bactericidal concentration (MBC):** the lowest concentration of a medication that results in a $\geq$99.9% decline in microbial number, measured in the laboratory setting. It is useful when compared with known potential toxic concentration levels to choose the antimicrobial regimen that does the greatest good with the fewest adverse or toxic effects.
4. **Resistance:** the ability of microorganisms to counteract the bacteriostatic or bactericidal effects of an antimicrobial agent.
   a. Resistance interferes with the medication's action either through changes in the microorganism's cellular structure or through production of enzymes that reduce antimicrobial activity.
   b. Microorganisms develop resistance by:
      (1) Enzymes: microorganisms produce various enzymes to inactivate antimicrobial agents (e.g., β-lactamase inactivates penicillins and cephalosporins).
      (2) Decreased cellular penetration: microorganisms alter their cell wall permeability to prevent penetration of antimicrobial agents into the cell (e.g., *Pseudomonas aeruginosa* alters porin channels to limit the entry of ceftazidime, imipenem–cilastatin).
      (3) Altered target proteins: microorganisms change target proteins so that antimicrobial agents cannot bind and elicit antimicrobial activity (e.g., *Streptococcus pneumoniae*'s resistance to penicillin).
      (4) Efflux pump: microorganisms pump the antimicrobial agent out of the cell before the antimicrobial agent can kill the microorganism (e.g., *Streptococcus pneumoniae*'s resistance to erythromycin).

C. **Basic principles of antimicrobial use.**

1. Antibiotics must reach the target tissue in a concentration adequate to inhibit the growth of or to kill the desired microorganism. This concentration:
   a. Ideally would be such that it would have limited side effects or toxic effects on target tissues or the patient as a whole.
   b. Must be readily achievable and sustainable for the desired duration of antimicrobial therapy.
2. The choice of antimicrobial agent(s) must be taken into account:
   a. Microorganism susceptibility to available antimicrobial agents.
   b. Relative permeability of the target tissue to agent of choice (e.g., blood–brain barrier).

c. Bioactivity of chosen antimicrobial agent in target tissue (e.g., bactericidal or bacteriostatic).
d. Known MIC/MBC in relation to existing body of knowledge concerning side effects and toxic effects in the specific population.
e. Specific characteristics of the individual patient in relation to the chosen antimicrobial's toxicities (e.g., the blood levels of a nephrotoxic antimicrobial such as gentamicin should be closely monitored in patients with impaired renal function).

**D. Specific considerations in the neonatal population.**
1. Pharmacodynamics.
   a. Tissue concentration of medication may be altered by clinical and physiologic conditions that may increase or decrease bioavailability of the medication in the target tissue (e.g., cerebrospinal fluid penetration by antibiotics may be excellent early in meningitis. As meningeal inflammatory response subsides, penetration into the cerebrospinal fluid diminishes).
   b. Differences in response or potential for toxic effects may result from immaturity and/or illness state.
2. Pharmacokinetics.
   a. To optimize the probability of response to antibiotics, the unpredictable pharmacokinetic influences should be minimized; hence, the IV route is preferred for septic patients.
   b. Absorption.
      (1) Changes in GI tract pH affect absorption of oral medication: may be increased or decreased (e.g., oral penicillin G is absorbed better in neonates than in older infants and children because of increased gastric pH).
      (2) Changes in skin permeability in the extremely immature neonate may allow topically applied antimicrobial agents to be absorbed systemically.
      (3) Blood flow changes may affect absorption and distribution of antimicrobials administered intramuscularly or subcutaneously (e.g., repeated intramuscular administration of aminoglycosides to premature neonates may result in local tissue damage and unacceptably variable rates of absorption).
   c. Distribution: Decreasing body water and increasing body fat concentration in more mature neonates affect the volume through which the antimicrobial agent is distributed. This may make dosage adjustments necessary in the first days of life.
   d. Metabolism: Limited hepatic function, because of immaturity or illness state, may affect dosage regimen of some antibiotics, requiring smaller or less frequent doses of some antibiotics (e.g., nafcillin, erythromycin).
   e. Excretion:
      (1) Limited renal function with lower gestational age may prolong the half-life of antimicrobials excreted by the kidneys (e.g., aminoglycosides, cephalosporins, penicillins, vancomycin). This limited renal function (GFR and tubular secretion) commonly improves significantly in the first few days of life and with advancing chronologic age. For this reason, serum antibiotic levels must be monitored closely and dosage adjustments made accordingly.
      (2) Limited renal function or failure may cause toxic effects as a result of accumulation of medication or metabolites (e.g., nephrotoxicity from aminoglycosides).
      (3) Medication may have a direct effect on renal function.
         (a) Blood flow to kidney may be diminished (e.g., amphotericin can cause renal artery vasospasms).

## Cardiovascular Agents

**A. Introduction.**
1. A broad group of medications that affect the regulation, inhibition, or stimulation of the cardiovascular system.
2. The use of cardiovascular agents is increasing in the care of neonates.

**B. Basic principles of cardiovascular medication use.**

1. The wide range of pharmacologic actions of this class of medications requires specific in-depth knowledge about each medication and about concurrent medication therapy.
2. Knowledge of the pathophysiologic basis of neonatal cardiovascular disease is necessary to ensure proper application of this class of medications.
3. Many of these medications have overlapping or synergistic effects. This overlap in clinical response makes the optimal choice of a medication and dose difficult.
4. Extensive knowledge and application of invasive and noninvasive cardiovascular monitoring techniques in the neonatal population are necessary to allow titration of the medication dose to the clinical response.

C. **Types of cardiovascular medications.**
1. Inotropic/vasopressive agents.
   a. Includes a broad range of medications that act to improve cardiac output by increasing the heart rate (chronotropic effect), the force of myocardial contraction (inotropic effect), and the vascular tone.
   b. Used both for cardiovascular resuscitation and long-term support of the myocardium.
   c. Specific inotropic agents:
      (1) Digitalis glycosides (e.g., digoxin). Inhibit the sodium–potassium pump to increase intracellular calcium, thus increasing myocardial contractility. They also decrease conduction through the sinoatrial and atrioventricular nodes to slow the ventricular rate in tachyarrhythmias.
      (2) Sympathomimetic amines (e.g., epinephrine, dopamine, dobutamine, isoproterenol).
         (a) Clinical responses stimulated by this group of medications are classified according to their effects on the "receptors" in the body. These receptors are categorized as either $\alpha$-, $\beta$-, or dopamine types.
            i. $\alpha_1$-adrenergic receptor response: contractions of vascular smooth muscle and constriction of blood vessels.
            ii. $\alpha_2$-adrenergic receptor response: activation of central nervous system (CNS) receptors in the brain to suppress outflow of the sympathetic nervous system activity from the brain. Results in decreased motility and tone of intestine and stomach.
            iii. $\beta_1$-adrenergic receptor response: increased strength and rate of myocardial contraction.
            iv. $\beta_2$-adrenergic receptor response: vascular smooth muscle dilation and bronchial muscle relaxation.
            v. Five different dopamine receptors are located in multiple organs and have mixed actions involving motor function, cardiovascular (e.g., vasodilating properties), renal (e.g., intrarenal vasodilator), behavioral, and hormonal (e.g., prolactin secretion) systems.

            For example, epinephrine increases blood pressure by stimulating the $\alpha_1$- and $\beta_1$- receptors. Dobutamine increases cardiac output by stimulating the $\beta_1$-receptors.
         (b) Response to each of these medications depends on relative amounts of $\alpha$-, $\beta$-, and dopamine receptor effects.
         (c) Prolonged administration of sympathomimetic amines may result in diminished clinical efficacy secondary to diminished responses of $\alpha$- and $\beta$-receptors, referred to as tachyphylaxis.
2. Antihypertensives/vasodilators.
   a. Used to normalize blood pressure in patients with hypertension, reduce vascular resistance in patients with poor myocardial function, and reduce pulmonary vascular resistance in conditions associated with pulmonary hypertension.
   b. May be used to inhibit pathophysiologic changes that cause increased blood pressure (e.g., captopril, propranolol) or directly reduce blood pressure through changes in intravascular volume (e.g., diuretics) or vascular resistance (e.g., hydralazine).
3. Antiarrhythmics.
   a. Used to treat cardiac dysrhythmias causing adverse effects on cardiovascular stability.
   b. Include adenosine, digoxin, esmolol, and lidocaine.

**D. Specific considerations in the neonatal population.**

1. Pharmacodynamics.
   a. Specific in-depth knowledge about neonatal cardiovascular physiology and pathophysiology is required to determine the need for these medications.
   b. Cardiovascular medications are commonly used in conjunction with other medications that may affect the neonate's response to the medication regimen (e.g., the digoxin–furosemide combination may result in electrolyte loss with the diuretic, which in turn may potentiate a toxic response to the digoxin).
2. Pharmacokinetics.
   a. Absorption: Many cardiovascular medications cannot be given effectively through any significant absorptive barrier. For this reason, IV administration is necessary in many cases (e.g., pressors, inotropes).
   b. Distribution.
      (1) Poor cardiac output/shock states may affect the distribution of medication to all tissues.
      (2) Medication administered for a desired response to one target organ may cause an undesirable systemic response (e.g., dobutamine increases cardiac output but may cause decreased blood pressure, furosemide reduces pulmonary edema but may decrease blood pressure).
      (3) Some cardiovascular medications are highly albumin-bound; this raises the possibility of unconjugated bilirubin displacement from albumin.
   c. Metabolism.
      (1) Hepatic metabolic activity may markedly affect the bioavailability of the medication (e.g., the high rate of first-pass metabolism of oral propranolol causes the IV and oral dosing to be significantly different).
      (2) Medication metabolites may cause a toxic response (e.g., cyanide liberation as a result of nitroprusside metabolism).
      (3) Rapid metabolism and serum clearance may require continuous IV infusion (e.g., dopamine, dobutamine).
   d. Excretion:
      (1) Impaired renal function will markedly affect the excretion of some medications (e.g., captopril, furosemide). This requires careful monitoring of the clinical response and serum medication levels.
      (2) Medication may have a direct effect on renal function.
         (a) Urinary output may be diminished (e.g., indomethacin reduces the glomerular filtration rate).

## Central Nervous System Medications

**A. Introduction.**

1. In adult patients, these are the most widely used group of medications.
2. The value of pain control and mood alteration in the neonatal population has only recently been recognized.
3. Recent increased interest in the use of CNS medications in the neonatal population has caused a recognition that the body of knowledge about these medications is limited.
4. The use of these medications is increasing as neurobehavioral assessment skills increase among neonatal caregivers.

**B. Definitions.**

1. Analgesic medication: a medication (e.g., morphine, acetaminophen) that provides diminished sensation of pain. These help to promote control of undesirable responses to a painful event.
2. Anesthetic medication: a medication that removes pain sensation either through peripheral nerve block (e.g., lidocaine) or through CNS effects (e.g., high-dose fentanyl). Not all anesthetic medications provide pain relief (e.g., inhalation gases, propofol).

3. Sedative–hypnotic medications: medications that provide mood alteration in patients with anxiety. These are divided into two groups: barbiturates (e.g., phenobarbital) and nonbarbiturates (e.g., chloral hydrate, lorazepam). These medications do not provide relief from pain.
4. Addiction: a lifestyle change that occurs in a medication-dependent person. This lifestyle change involves a focus on medication use. This behavior cannot occur in a neonate.
5. Tolerance: a condition that may occur with many types of medications. Tolerance exists when larger doses and higher serum concentrations of the medication are required to achieve the desired response, and commonly occurs in conjunction with physical dependence.
6. Dependence: a physiologic state in which the individual requires regular medication administration for continued physiologic well-being. Patients who develop dependence on a medication may need a dosage-tapering regimen rather than abruptly discontinuing the medication in order to prevent withdrawal symptoms. In neonates, dependence can develop from either placental transfer of medications or iatrogenically due to long-term infusions of sedatives and/or narcotics.

**C. Basic principles of CNS medication use.**

1. Mechanism of action of most CNS medications is not clearly understood.
2. Assessment of need for these medications must be carefully performed as an ongoing process.
   a. Close attention must be paid to differentiation of need for sedation, pain relief, or both.
   b. These medications may cause the development of medication tolerance and/or dependence.
3. Consideration must be made for the risks and benefits of the medication in relation to potential side effects or toxicities.
4. The science of the study of neonatal neurologic development is still emerging, and much is yet to be learned. The effect that CNS medications may have on that development is largely unknown.

**D. Specific considerations in the neonatal population.**

1. Pharmacodynamics.
   a. Limited knowledge of CNS development in premature and term neonates mandates a special need for caution in the use of CNS-active medications.
   b. Specific physiologic characteristics in the neonatal population require careful observation for harmful side effects or toxicities (e.g., reduction in blood pressure with IV bolus doses of morphine, chest wall rigidity with fentanyl).
   c. Narcotic analgesics may cause respiratory depression and may precipitate respiratory failure in neonates. Therefore, the lowest possible dose that relieves the patient's pain should be used.
   d. Careful assessment of clinical response is necessary to determine the most safe and effective dose and interval.
2. Pharmacokinetics.
   a. Absorption.
      (1) Poor GI motility and high first-pass clearance may make oral administration highly unpredictable for many medications (e.g., morphine).
      (2) Oral or rectal absorption of mild analgesics and sedatives is often adequate (e.g., acetaminophen).
   b. Distribution.
      (1) Because these agents work in the CNS, they must be lipid soluble in order to cross the blood–brain barrier.
      (2) As neonates increase their proportion of body fat, the doses required will increase.
      (3) Because these agents are stored in the body fat, patients must be monitored for the accumulation of these agents and hence prolonged effects.
   c. Metabolism.
      (1) Slower hepatic metabolism may cause a prolonged half-life.
      (2) Hepatic disease may markedly increase the risk of toxic effects (e.g., chloral hydrate).
      (3) Hepatic metabolism may convert medications to either toxic metabolites or active metabolites (e.g., theophylline converts to caffeine).

d. Excretion.
(1) Limited renal function or failure may cause toxic effects as a result of accumulation of medication or metabolites (e.g., seizures from penicillin).

## Diuretics

A. **Introduction.**
1. Commonly used in neonatal patients to promote the removal of excessive extracellular fluid.
2. Site of action of nearly all diuretic agents is the luminal surface of the renal tubular cell.

B. **Basic principles of diuretic use.**
1. Use must be based on a thorough understanding of the functions of the various segments of the nephron in the neonatal population.
2. Diuretic medications whose primary purpose is to cause the excretion of excess extracellular fluid commonly cause a secondary or side effect of loss of electrolytes, along with the desired water loss. Knowledge of the specific action of each diuretic medication will assist the clinician in monitoring electrolytes for undesirable losses.
3. The pharmacologic response is dependent on the existing level of renal function and the medication's ability to reach the target tissue in amounts adequate to produce the desired diuretic effect.
4. Any medication or therapy that increases the GFR may have an indirect diuretic effect. Some medications that act on the cardiovascular system to increase cardiac output or increase renal blood flow through vasodilation may cause diuresis (e.g., dopamine). Maximal water and electrolyte excretion usually occurs in the first days of use. Later, decreased GFR and hyperaldosteronism resulting from diuretic-induced hypovolemia limit these losses.

C. **Specific considerations in the neonatal population.**
1. Pharmacodynamics.
a. Many diuretic medications are dependent on reaching the lumen of the proximal tubule to achieve diuresis.
b. The renal tubular function is limited in all neonates and is more limited in less mature neonates.
c. The clinical response to diuretic agents is commonly decreased because of existing poor renal tubular absorption. Therefore, a larger dose is needed to achieve the response.
d. Limited tubular function potentiates electrolyte loss with many diuretic agents (e.g., furosemide, hydrochlorothiazide).
2. Pharmacokinetics.
a. Absorption. Oral absorption may be limited, requiring a larger per-kilogram dose as compared with the IV dose to achieve the desired effect (e.g., furosemide). Other diuretics (e.g., hydrochlorothiazide, spironolactone) are well absorbed orally.
b. Distribution. Some diuretic medications are strongly protein-bound. Some concern has been raised over the displacement of bilirubin from albumin-binding sites (e.g., furosemide, spironolactone).
c. Metabolism. Some diuretics are primarily metabolized by the liver (e.g., spironolactone).
d. Excretion.
(1) Low renal blood flow and low GFR, along with limited renal tubular function, may delay excretion and limit the effectiveness of the medication (e.g., the plasma clearance of furosemide is prolonged in extremely premature neonates and in neonates with renal failure).
(2) Some diuretics are primarily eliminated unchanged in the urine (e.g., furosemide, hydrochlorothiazide).

## Immunizations

A. **Introduction.**
1. Vaccines are commonly given to the hospitalized neonatal patient.
2. Each year in January, the Centers for Disease Control and Prevention (CDC) Advisory Committee on Immunization Practices publishes an updated version of the recommended immunization guidelines. Each nurse should be familiar with these guidelines.

3. The following documentation is required when vaccines are given:
   a. Name, title, and business address of person administering the vaccine.
   b. Vaccine administered.
   c. Manufacturer of the vaccine.
   d. Lot number of the vaccine.
   e. Expiration date of vaccine.
   f. Date of administration.
   g. Site of administration.
   h. Route of administration.
   i. Documentation that the vaccine information statement (VIS) has been given to the parents/guardians.
   j. Documentation of the VIS publication date (the most current version must be used).

**B. Basic principles of immunization use.**
1. The goal of immunization is to prevent many viral and bacterial diseases and their sequelae.
2. For maximum effectiveness, the immunizations must be given at specific ages before the recipients have been exposed to the diseases.
3. Live-virus vaccines (e.g., measles-mumps-rubella [MMR], rotavirus, varicella) should NOT be administered in the NICU.
4. All adverse events associated with immunization should be reported in detail in the patient's medical record and also on the Vaccine Adverse Event Reporting System (VAERS) form found on the U.S. Food and Drug Administration (FDA) website.

**C. Types of immunizations.**
1. Active immunization.
   a. Involves the administration of all or part of a microorganism or a modified product of that microorganism to evoke an immunologic response mimicking that of natural infection. This usually presents little or no risk to the recipient.
   b. Some immunizing agents provide complete protection against disease for life (e.g., polio vaccine), some provide partial protection (e.g., influenza vaccine), and some must be readministered at intervals (booster doses) (e.g., tetanus vaccine).
   c. Vaccines may be either live (attenuated) or killed (inactivated). Inactivated vaccines may not elicit the range of immunologic response provided by attenuated agents.
2. Passive immunization.
   a. Involves the administration of preformed antibody to a recipient.
   b. Most often used when a person exposed to a disease has a high likelihood of complications from that disease and time does not permit adequate protection by active immunization alone.
   c. Can be used when a disease is already present with the hope of reducing the reaction to the disease.
   d. Accomplished through the use of immune globulin preparations (e.g., hepatitis B immune globulin, palivizumab).
   e. There are strict indications for the use of these products (American Academy of Pediatrics [AAP], 2012).

**D. Specific considerations in the neonatal population.**
1. Pharmacodynamics.
   a. Most immunizations are usually given starting at 2 months of age; the immune response to the vaccines may be limited if given before this age. Resistance to certain diseases before this time may be provided from the mother's antibodies that are transferred across the placenta.
   b. Preterm infants who are medically stable should receive the immunizations at the recommended chronologic age as long as the following criteria are met:
      (1) The infant does not require ongoing treatment for serious infections or metabolic disease.
      (2) The infant does not have acute renal, cardiovascular, or respiratory illness.
      (3) The infant demonstrates a clinical course of sustained recovery and pattern of steady growth (AAP, 2012).

c. The dose should NOT be decreased in preterm infants.
d. Antibody titers may be measured to prove adequate immune responses.

2. Pharmacokinetics.
   a. Absorption.
      (1) Injectable vaccines should be administered in sites that limit the risk of neural, vascular, or tissue injury.
      (2) The preferred site for administration is the anterolateral aspect of the upper thigh.
      (3) The deltoid area of the upper arm can be used in older infants (>1 year).
      (4) The upper, outer aspect of the buttocks should not be routinely used because of the possibility of damaging the sciatic nerve and reduced immunogenicity.
      (5) When necessary, two vaccines can be given in the same limb but should be separated by at least 1 inch if possible so that local reactions are not likely to overlap.
      (6) The recommended routes of administration are included in the package inserts of the vaccines (e.g., intramuscular, subcutaneous).
   b. Distribution. Vaccines should be held when the neonate is on pressor agents because the blood flow to the muscle and subcutaneous tissues may be limited.
   c. Metabolism/Excretion: Kidney and/or liver failure should not prevent the administration of vaccines.

E. **Misconceptions about vaccine contraindications:** The nurse should be familiar with the specific contraindications listed in the package inserts of the vaccines so that immunizations are not withheld unnecessarily (AAP, 2012).

## NURSING IMPLICATIONS FOR MEDICATION ADMINISTRATION IN THE NEONATE

There are several areas in which the nursing staff are an invaluable resource for the patient in helping to prevent errors in this fragile patient population.

A. **Correct order-writing policies** should be followed to reduce the potential for error. Unapproved abbreviations should be avoided, trailing zeros should be avoided (e.g., 1.0), leading decimals should be used (e.g., 0.1), and all verbal orders should be read back to the physician for clarification.
B. **Standard concentrations** for IV continuous infusions should be used rather than relying on concentrations based on weight.
C. **Double check of medication doses** involves recalculating the weight-based doses and comparing prescribed doses with current medication dosing reference books to prevent potential medication dosing errors. In addition, smart pump technology that includes dosing ranges for both intermittent and continuous infusions for IV medications should be used with IV pumps to avoid programmable errors.
D. **Cross-checking** on a regular basis is a nursing responsibility. Because of the very small volumes of medications commonly given to the NICU patient, a system for regular cross-checking of medications' volume accuracy with medication concentration before administration should be established for all medications and especially with high-risk medications.
E. **Monitoring renal function through intake and output measurements** may alert the care team to potential changes in medication metabolism and/or excretion.
F. **Meticulous medication administration and documentation** involves administering the medication at the correct time and at the correct time interval. In addition, documenting the medication administration date, time, dose, route, and interval and the time medication levels are obtained is important in interpreting patient response to therapy.
G. **Facilitation of medication serum level monitoring with absolute accuracy** makes safe administration of medications—with a narrow margin between effective and toxic levels—possible.
H. **Careful assessment of vital sign parameters and clinical responses** may assist in the evaluation of desirable or undesirable medication responses.
I. **Careful observation of the neonate for therapeutic and toxic medication effects** will allow medication administration to achieve the maximal desired response while minimizing toxic responses.

J. **Medication precautions** must be observed. Any medication or medication preparation known to have a high risk of adverse effects in the neonate should be removed from the patient care area (e.g., concentrated potassium vials) or should be specifically labeled to avoid inadvertent administration.

K. **Facilitation of or participation in clinical trials** designed to evaluate a medication's efficacy does much to advance the body of knowledge related to neonatal pharmacology.

L. **Recognition of established clinical experience with individual medications in the neonatal population is essential.** Because some medications are introduced into the clinical area after only minimal study of specific medication response in the neonate, early observation of potential toxic effects may avert a later disaster.

## REFERENCES


American Academy of Pediatrics: Active and passive immunization. In L.K. Pickering (Ed.): *2012 Red Book: Report of the Committee on Infectious Diseases* (29th ed.). Elk Grove Village, IL, 2012, American Academy of Pediatrics, pp. 1–109.

Chemtob, S.: Basic pharmacologic principles. In R.A. Polin, W.W. Fox, and S.H. Abman (Eds.): *Fetal and neonatal physiology* (4th ed.). Philadelphia, 2011, Elsevier Saunders, pp. 211–223.

Funk, R.S., Brown, J.T. and Abdel-Rahman, S.M.: Pediatric pharmacokinetics: Human development and drug disposition. *Pediatric Clinics of North America*, 59:1001–1016, 2012.

Hoath, S.B.: Physiologic development of the skin. In R.A. Polin, W.W. Fox, and S.H. Abman (Eds.): *Fetal and neonatal physiology* (4th ed.). Philadelphia, 2011, Elsevier Saunders, pp. 679–695.

Kearns, G.L., Abdel-Rahman, S.M., Alander, S.W., et al.: Developmental pharmacology—drug disposition, action, and therapy in infants and children. *New England Journal of Medicine*, 349(12):1157–1167, 2003.

Stewart, C.F. and Hampton, E.M.: Effect of maturation on drug disposition in pediatric patients. *Clinical Pharmacy*, 6(7):548–564, 1987.

van den Anker, J.N., Schwab, M. and Kearns, G.L.: Developmental pharmacokinetics. *Handbook of Experimental Pharmacology*, 205:51–75, 2011.

CHAPTER 13

# Laboratory and Diagnostic Test Interpretation

DIANE M. SZLACHETKA

**OBJECTIVES**

1. Identify the types of laboratory testing in the neonatal intensive care unit.
2. Discuss the purpose of laboratory testing and diagnostics.
3. Review the process of specimen collection and the principles of test utilization.
4. Review the principles of laboratory interpretation.
5. Describe iatrogenic sequelae associated with laboratory testing and diagnostic procedures.
6. Discuss strategies to minimize iatrogenic sequelae associated with laboratory testing and diagnostic procedures.
7. Discuss the decision-making process of ordering and interpreting laboratory values—a decision tree.

Newborns delivered in the United States receive an average of one or two laboratory tests, typically in the form of screening for jaundice, genetic disorders, and birth defects. In addition, all infants admitted to the neonatal intensive care unit (NICU) require laboratory testing to assess their clinical status. Given the U.S. birth rate of 3.95 million infants (Centers for Disease Control and Prevention [CDC], 2013) and average NICU admission rates of 7% of live births (CDC, 2011), this translates to a minimum of 7.9 million screening/laboratory tests per year.

It has been estimated that approximately 3% (Rusckowski, 2012) of the U.S. national health budget is spent on laboratory testing, constituting 15% to 20% of each patient's hospital bill (Sacher et al., 2000d). The impact of laboratory testing on the patient, health care, and its cost is significant.

Because all health care workers in the NICU are in some way involved in obtaining laboratory samples, understanding the principles of laboratory testing and the contribution of laboratory tests to patient care and cost is essential. Developing skills in laboratory interpretation at the NICU bedside provides a key element in comprehensive patient care.

This chapter features a review of the types and purposes of laboratory testing in the NICU, describes principles of laboratory testing and interpretation, and discusses potential iatrogenic sequelae. Included is a discussion of strategies to avoid sequelae, when to obtain laboratory testing, and a strategy to interpret results for patient care. A decision-making process for laboratory testing and interpretation is presented.

## LABORATORY TESTS IN THE NICU

A. **Laboratory testing occurs daily in the NICU.** Why and when laboratory testing is performed is driven by patient history and presenting symptoms. By one estimate, 70% of all medical decisions are based on laboratory results (Kurec and Lifshitz, 2011; Rusckowski, 2012). Data obtained from laboratory analyses assist clinicians in determining diagnosis, measuring success of treatment, and monitoring trends in an infant's clinical course. The common laboratory tests performed in the NICU include the following (Table 13-1):

TABLE 13-1

**Common Laboratory Tests in the NICU by System**

| Fluids Electrolytes Nutrition | Respiratory | Cardiac | Gastrointestinal | Renal | Endocrine/Metabolic | Neurologic | Hematologic | Other |
|---|---|---|---|---|---|---|---|---|
| Electrolytes (serum) | Blood gas | Isoenzymes | Alkaline phosphatase | BUN (serum) | Thyroxine level | Phenobarbital level | CBC w/differential | Chromosome levels |
| Calcium (serum) | pH | | Triglyceride levels | Creatinine (serum) | Thyroid-stimulating hormone level | Dilantin level | Hct | Buccal smear |
| Magnesium (serum) | $Paco_2$ | | AST (SGOT) | Specific gravity | Cortisol level | Ammonia (serum) | Plt<br>Plt antibody | CRP |
| Phosphorus (serum) | $Pao_2$ | | ALT (SGPT) | Urine sodium | Insulin level | Amino acid (serum) | Reticulocyte count | Drug levels |
| Alkaline phosphorus | Bicarbonate ($HCO_3^-$) | | GGT (GGTP) | Urine potassium | Growth hormone level | Amino acid (urine) | Direct Coombs' test/DAT | Urine toxicology screen |
| Glucose (serum) level | Base excess | | Bilirubin (total and direct) | Urine osmolality | Testosterone level | Organic acids (urine) | Blood type | Cultures (all sources) |
| Vitamin levels | Theophylline level | | Ammonia (serum) | Drug levels | Aldosterone (serum and urine) level | Glycine (serum and CSF) | G6PD | RPR |
| Serum osmolality | Caffeine level | | $\alpha_1$-antitrypsin | Uric acid (serum) | 17-hydroxy corticosteroids | Pyridoxine level | Sedimentation rate | Occult blood (fecal) |
| Albumin (serum) | | | Trypsin (stool) | Urinalysis | Parathyroid hormone level | Lactic acid | Folic acid | PCR (serum) |
| Total protein | | | Pyridoxine level | | State metabolic screening | | Fibrinogen<br>PT<br>PTT<br>Immunoglobulins<br>Methemoglobin | State Screening<br>Kleihauer-Betke test (maternal) |

*ALT (SGPT)*, Alanine aminotransferase (serum glutamic-pyruvic transaminase); *AST (SGOT)*, aspartate aminotransferase (serum glutamic-oxaloacetic transaminase); *BUN*, blood urea nitrogen; *CBC*, complete blood count; *CRP*, C-reactive protein; *CSF*, cerebrospinal fluid; *DAT*, direct antiglobulin test; *GGT (GGTP)*, $\gamma$-glutamyltransferase ($\gamma$-glutamyl transpeptidase); *G6PD*, glucose-6-phosphate dehydrogenase; *Hct*, hematocrit; *PCR*, polymerase chain reaction; *Plt*, platelet; *PT*, prothrombin time; *PTT*, partial thromboplastin time; *RPR*, rapid plasma reagin.

1. Chemistry analysis: serum tests that measure the chemical activity or state of the body. Serum is the by-product of clotted blood that is centrifuged to remove the clot and any other cells (Laposata, 2002). Chemical substances reflect metabolic processes and disease states in the body. Measuring changes in chemical concentrations (chemical substances) is useful in diagnosis, planning care, monitoring of therapy, screening, and determining the severity of disease and response to treatment (Sacher et al., 2000a).
   a. Four categories of chemical analyses include:
      (1) Chemical substances normally present with function in the circulation. Laboratory examples: sodium, potassium, calcium, magnesium, phosphorus, total proteins, albumin, hormones, and vitamins.
      (2) Metabolites: nonfunctioning waste products in process of being cleared. Laboratory examples: bilirubin, ammonia, blood urea nitrogen (BUN), creatinine, and uric acid.
      (3) Substances released from cells as a result of cell damage and abnormal permeability or abnormal cellular proliferation. Laboratory examples: alkaline phosphatase, alanine aminotransferase (ALT), aspartate aminotransferase (AST), and creatinine kinase.
      (4) Drug and toxic substances. Laboratory examples: antibiotics, theophylline, caffeine, digoxin, phenobarbital, and substances of abuse.
2. Hematologic tests: study of the blood and blood-forming tissues of the body such as the bone marrow and reticuloendothelial system (Sacher et al., 2000b). This area of testing also includes the study of hemoglobin (Hgb) structure, red cell membrane, and red cell enzyme activity. Whole blood is composed of blood cells suspended in plasma fluid (see also Chapter 31). Plasma is unclotted blood that has been centrifuged to remove any cells (Laposata, 2002). Plasma contains the protein fibrinogen, which is converted to the substance composing the fibrin clot (Kee, 2010).
   a. Blood cells: erythrocytes (red blood cells), leukocytes (white blood cells), and thrombocytes (platelets). Laboratory examples: hematocrit (Hct), reticulocyte (Retic) count, platelet (Plt) count, peripheral blood smear, complete blood count (CBC), Kleihauer-Betke test, white blood cell (WBC) count, and WBC differential count.
   b. Plasma: plasma proteins, coagulation factors I through XIII, immunoglobulins. Laboratory examples: total protein, albumin, fibrinogen (factor I), prothrombin (factor II), thromboplastin (factor III), factors IV through XIII assays, immunoglobulin G (IgG), immunoglobulin A (IgA), and immunoglobulin M (IgM).
3. Microbiology tests: identification of infectious microorganisms causing disease. Tests include diagnostic bacteriology, mycology, virology, parasitology, and serology. Laboratory examples: culture of any body fluid, bacterial stain, and bacteria antigen detection.
4. Microscopy tests: examination of body fluids and tissues under a microscope. Laboratory examples: cell counts, fecal blood, fecal fat, Apt test, and urinalysis.
5. Blood bank tests (transfusion medicine): area of blood component preparation, blood donor screening and testing, blood compatibility testing, and blood and stem cell banking.
   a. Common blood bank tests:
      (1) Blood typing and cross-match.
      (2) Direct antiglobulin test (DAT)/Coombs' test.
      (3) Indirect antiglobulin test (IAT)/indirect Coombs' test.
      (4) Erythrocyte rosette test, Kleihauer-Betke test for fetomaternal hemorrhage.
6. Immunoassays: laboratory method based on antigen–antibody reactions employed in therapeutic drug monitoring, toxicology screening, detection of plasma proteins, and certain endocrine testing. Laboratory examples: urine and meconium toxicology test for "street drugs," latex agglutination test, and drug levels.
7. Cytogenetic tests: testing used to determine genetic composition by chromosome analysis. Laboratory examples: simple karyotype (blood, amniotic fluid, tissue, bone marrow, buccal swab), chromosome-specific probes, and fluorescent in-situ hybridization (FISH).
8. Immunology tests: laboratory evaluation measuring immune system activity (Sacher et al., 2000c). This consists of complement activity and its cascade of activation, humoral, and cell-mediated immunity. Tests are used to diagnose inflammatory responses, immunodeficiency, and autoimmune disorders. Laboratory examples: C-reactive protein, cytokine measurement, complement C3 and C4, IgG, IgM, and IgA.

## PURPOSE OF LABORATORY TESTING

A. **Laboratory testing in the NICU is multidimensional.** The rationale for selecting, ordering, and interpreting laboratory tests needs to be scrutinized (considered) in order to maximize patient care, minimize patient risk, and contain health care costs. The purpose of laboratory testing is to:
1. Determine the health state of the patient.
2. Monitor the clinical status, trends, and disease severity.
3. Assist in a differential diagnosis.
4. Confirm a diagnosis or cure.
5. Screen for common disorders and disease prevention.
6. Measure the effect of therapy.
7. Assist in the management of disease.
8. Establish a prognosis.
9. Assist in genetic counseling.
10. Evaluate specific events—example: medication errors, sudden clinical decompensation, medical–legal problems, and postmortem evaluation.

## PROCESS OF LABORATORY COLLECTION

A. **Collection of laboratory specimens requires meticulous technique to ensure the best possible results.** Proper technique, source of laboratory sample, use of collection tubes, labeling, and laboratory processing combine to play a key role in patient treatment, in minimizing blood loss and painful stimuli, and in reducing the costs of NICU care. Anticipatory pain management is needed prior to heel sticks, venipuncture, and arterial puncture (American Academy of Pediatrics [AAP] and Canadian Paediatric Society [CPS], 2007; Folk, 2007; see also Chapter 16) as well as other specimen collection procedures such as lumbar puncture and suprapubic bladder tap.
1. **Types of laboratory collection (see also Chapter 15).**
   a. *Capillary blood sampling*: admixture of arterial, venous, and capillary blood and tissue fluid obtained from a well-perfused heel. Heel sticks should not be performed on infants whose feet are edematous, injured, bruised, infected, or anomalous (Folk, 2007). NOTE: Fingerstick sampling is contraindicated in infants, because distance from skin surface to bone is less than 1.5 mm (Olsowka and Garg, 2001). NOTE: The Cochrane Database of Systematic Reviews concludes that venipuncture, performed by skilled phlebotomists, appears to be the method of choice for blood sampling in term neonates (Shah and Ohlsson, 2011).
      (1) Most common route for obtaining small blood samples in the infant.
      (2) Heel stick less than 2 mm (Garza and Becan-McBride, 2010c, 2010d) and with heel-stick devices ranging from 0.65 to 1 mm depending on infant size (Vedder and Sawyer, 2011).
      (3) Avoid squeezing or milking site to obtain blood (Folk, 2007; Garza and Becan-McBride, 2010c). NOTE: Excessive scooping of blood from nearby skin with the lip of collection tube can interfere with the laboratory result (Vedder and Sawyer, 2011).
      (4) Cell counts such as WBC, platelet count, or blood gas $Po_2$ may not be accurate.
      (5) Anticipatory pain management should be considered (see also Chapter 16).
   b. *Venipuncture*: venous blood typically obtained from the hand, arm, foot, leg, or scalp. Venous blood can also be obtained from an umbilical vein catheter, tunneled central venous catheter, or peripherally inserted central catheter (PICC) (Folk, 2007). In term infants, venipuncture has been shown to be a less painful procedure than heel stick when performed by skilled phlebotomists (Shah and Ohlsson, 2011).
      (1) May need use of tourniquet to distend peripheral veins. Recommended time for tourniquet application is $\leq$1 minute. Tourniquet application $\geq$3 minutes may alter laboratory test results (Garza and Becan-McBride, 2010b, 2010f; Kee, 2010).
      (2) Venipuncture may be difficult to obtain in small infants.
      (3) May wish to ration available veins for future intravenous (IV) sites versus use for laboratory drawing (Folk, 2007; Vedder and Sawyer, 2011).
      (4) Anticipatory pain management should be considered (see also Chapter 16).

c. *Arterial puncture* (see also Chapter 15): arterial blood typically obtained from an artery stick of the radial, tibial, or temporal arteries. Brachial artery stick is performed less often due to potential for arteriospasm of brachial artery supplying the lower arm. Femoral artery stick is rarely performed in the NICU population. Arterial blood can also be obtained from an umbilical artery catheter or percutaneous arterial line.
   (1) Allen test (modified) should be done prior to radial artery stick (Garza and Becan-McBride, 2010a).
   (2) Anticipatory pain management should be considered (see also Chapter 16).

d. *Point-of-care testing* (POCT), alternate-site testing, near-patient testing, patient-focused testing: tests done in a variety of settings, often at the bedside (Threatte and Schexneider, 2011).
   (1) Uses whole blood obtained from capillary stick, arterial, or venous sources.
   (2) Provides "real-time," rapid testing.
   (3) Uses small blood volumes (<0.5 mL).
   (4) Common POCT assays obtained in the NICU include levels of electrolytes, ionized calcium, BUN, creatinine, Hct, Hgb, blood gases, and glucose.
   (5) Anticipatory pain management should be considered (see also Chapter 16).

e. *Lumbar puncture* (see Chapter 15): procedure done to remove cerebrospinal fluid (CSF) from the spinal canal.
   (1) CSF evaluated in the laboratory for:
      (a) Infection.
      (b) Hemorrhage.
      (c) Demyelinating diseases.
      (d) Malignancy.

f. *Urine sampling* (see also Chapter 15): urine obtained for chemical analysis, bacterial cultures, or microscopic examination.
   (1) Techniques for obtaining samples include:
      (a) Bag collection.
      (b) Straight catheterization.

g. *Thoracentesis* (see also Chapter 15): procedure using a needle tap or chest tube to remove abnormal collection of fluid (effusion) from the thoracic cavity.
   (1) Thoracic cavity fluid evaluated in laboratory for:
      (a) Microorganisms: cultures, Gram stains.
      (b) Chemistries: levels of electrolytes, total protein, albumin, glucose, and triglycerides.
      (c) Hematology: WBC count and WBC differential count.

h. *Peritoneal tap*: procedure using a needle tap to remove an abnormal collection of fluid (ascites) from the abdomen.
   (1) Peritoneal cavity fluid evaluated in laboratory for:
      (a) Microorganisms: cultures, Gram stains.
      (b) Chemistries: levels of electrolytes, total protein, albumin, glucose, and triglycerides.
      (c) Hematology: WBC count and WBC differential count.

2. **Process of laboratory collection.**
   a. Order request for test.
   b. Check for appropriateness of order.
   c. Cluster laboratory drawing as much as possible.
   d. Check patient identification prior to laboratory sampling per hospital protocol.
   e. Prepare infant for laboratory test, for example:
      (1) Wrap foot with a heel warming device for capillary specimen—a warmed foot arterializes specimen and helps promote blood flow (Garza and Becan-McBride, 2010c; Kaplan and Tange, 1998; Olsowka and Garg, 2001). Some studies suggest that heel warming has not resulted in greater blood volume yield (Folk, 2007).
      (2) Provide pain management.
   f. Observe strict aseptic technique per institution guidelines.
   g. Observe Standard Precautions per institution guidelines.

h. Obtain laboratory test using an appropriate route, for example:
   (1) Capillary versus arterial versus venous.
i. Discard the initial few drops of blood after lancing the heel—along with prewarming the heel, this reduces the magnitude of capillary and venous laboratory value differences (Blackburn, 2013; Kee, 2010).
j. Obtain blood cultures first, hematology specimens next to minimize platelet clumping, then chemistry and blood bank samples (Folk, 2007; Garza and Becan-McBride, 2010e; Sanford and McPherson, 2011) or per institution protocol. Note: Blood cultures cannot be obtained via capillary source.
k. Insert proper amount of specimen into proper specimen container.
l. Label specimen.
m. Place specimen in biohazard container or bag per institutional guidelines.
n. Promptly send specimen to laboratory.

3. **Specimen tubes:** standardized, color-coded containers indicating whether they contain whole blood, plasma (which contains fibrinogen), or serum (Kee, 2010). Specimen tubes can be glass or plastic, with many labs converting to plastic collection tubes to increase occupational safety (Sanford and McPherson, 2011). Tube colors in the NICU typically come in red, blue, green, lavender, and yellow. Plastic microtainers are the most common types of specimen collection tubes in the NICU. Microtainers allow use of smaller blood volumes to obtain laboratory results. Blood culture tubes, sterile swabs, and glass slides are also used in the NICU for specimen collection. Tubes with anticoagulant coating should be gently inverted, end over end, 7 to 10 times for proper anticoagulant–blood mixing (Fischbach, 2009; Garza and Becan-McBride, 2010a). Tubes with anticoagulant must be filled to the indicated fill line to properly dilute anticoagulant and avoid potential erroneous results.
   a. *Red tube (plain)*: no additives or anticoagulant. Clotted blood for *serum* testing. Hemolysis should be avoided. Laboratory examples: electrolytes, serology, blood bank, proteins, hormones, and drug monitoring.
   b. *Blue tube (light)*: contains sodium citrate, an anticoagulant that removes calcium to prevent clotting (Fischbach, 2009). Use for unclotted blood–*plasma* specimens. Laboratory specimens: prothrombin time (PT), partial thromboplastin time (PTT), factor assays. Another light-blue tube containing thrombin and soybean trypsin inhibitor is useful for measurement of fibrin degradation products (Sanford and McPherson, 2011).
   c. *Green tube*: contains anticoagulant heparin (sodium, lithium, ammonium) that inhibits thrombin activation to prevent clotting. Used for unclotted blood–*plasma* specimens. Laboratory examples: chromosome analysis (use sodium heparin tube), ammonia levels, and hormone levels.
   d. *Lavender tube*: contains ethylenediaminetetraacetic acid (EDTA) that removes calcium to prevent clotting. Tube used for whole blood and *plasma* specimens. Laboratory examples: CBC, Retic count, platelet count, Hct.
   e. *Yellow tube/bottle cap* (SPS)—sterile, contains sodium polyanethol sulfonate (SPS) that aids in bacterial recovery by inhibiting complement, phagocytes, and certain antibiotics (Sanford and McPherson, 2011). Whole blood used for blood cultures. These cultures should be processed quickly to minimize the potential for decreased yield owing to storage or prolonged exposure to SPS (Olsowka and Garg, 2001). A yellow, acid citrate dextrose (ACD) tube is not typically used in the NICU; however, it is used for human leukocyte antigen (HLA) phenotyping and paternity testing (Sanford and McPherson, 2011).

## CONCEPTS OF LABORATORY TEST INTERPRETATION

A. **It is important to be familiar with the limitations and applications of the laboratory data as they apply to patient care.** Many factors influence blood values and their interpretation in the newborn, including timing, site and amount of blood sample, placental transfusion, and infant growth rate (Blackburn, 2013; Letterio et al., 2013). A laboratory test has certain characteristics that influence how it is interpreted and used in the clinical setting. The following concepts are integral in the process of laboratory interpretation:

1. **Accuracy:** synonymous with "correctness," this term refers to how close a test result is to the true value (Laposata, 2002; Oxley et al., 2001).
   a. Point-to-point variability in test results exists.
   b. Variation in value may be more reflective of an analytic variation of automated chemistry systems than actual patient status.
2. **Precision:** synonymous with "reproducibility," this term describes the distribution of results when a sample is analyzed repeatedly.
   a. Imprecision is known as random error.
   b. Test precision is a more desirable test characteristic than accuracy in measuring treatment response or clinical changes.
3. **Sensitivity:** the ability of a test to correctly identify an individual with disease and not miss anyone by falsely testing "healthy." It refers to a test's ability to generate more true-positive results and fewer false-negative results.
   a. Sensitive tests have a low threshold for abnormality.
   b. Sensitive tests usually have a low specificity.
   c. Certain testing requires sensitivity over specificity—example: blood bank donors screened for infectious diseases, when it is better to err in excluding donors who are falsely positive than include donors who are falsely negative.
4. **Specificity:** the ability of a test to identify only those individuals with disease as opposed to individuals testing positive when there is no disease. It refers to a test's ability to generate more true-negative results and fewer false-positive results.
   a. Specific test has a high threshold for "normal" or negative test results.
   b. Specific test usually has low sensitivity.
   c. Certain testing requires specificity over sensitivity—examples: urine toxicology screen to detect presence of cocaine, cardiac isoenzymes to rule out a myocardial infarct.
   d. Positive predictive value (yield): the probability that an individual with a positive screening test really *has* the disease. It is dependent on the prevalence of the disease in the population being tested (LaMorte, 2013).
      (1) Probability ratio is a percentage based on the population screened.
      (2) Computation based on a 2 × 2 contingency table.
         (a) Compare all who test positive with those who actually *have* the disease to obtain the percentage of probability that the individual who tested positive *has* the disease.
         (b) Certain testing, such as state screening programs, considers this probability.
   e. Negative predictive value: the probability that an individual with a negative screening test really *does not have* the disease.
      (1) Probability ratio is a percentage based on the population screened.
      (2) Computation based on a 2 × 2 contingency table.
         (a) Compare all who test negative with those who actually *do not* have the disease to obtain the percentage of probability that the individual who tested negative *does not have* the disease.
5. **Reference range:** established upper and lower boundary levels of a laboratory value by which a patient's result will be measured for presence of disease. The range of normality (mathematical) is dependent on population subsets such as age, gender, pregnancy, and other patient attributes.
   a. Often referred to as "normal" range.
   b. Term *normal* is misleading—reference range determined based on specific attributes of a population subset, not due to "normalcy" (Oxley et al., 2001).
   c. Approximately 5% of "healthy" laboratory results fall outside the reference range.
   d. Reference range can vary from laboratory to laboratory.

## PRINCIPLES OF TEST UTILIZATION

A. **Patient management depends on good clinical skills, judicious use of laboratory testing, and careful interpretation of laboratory data.** Once a laboratory value is determined and the patient's clinical status evaluated, the combined information is used to direct treatment. In an effort to optimize care, minimize patient discomfort, and contain health care costs, Wallach (2007) identifies key principles of test utilization:

1. Even under the best of circumstances, no test is perfect.
   a. Results can be misleading.
   b. Specificity or sensitivity of a test is never 100%.
2. Choice of tests should be based on the prior probability of the diagnosis being sought, which affects the predictive value of the test.
   a. History, physical examination, and prevalence of a disease determine the probability of diagnosis.
   b. Patient history and examination should precede choice of laboratory tests.
3. The combination of short-term physiologic variation and analytic error is sufficient to render the interpretation of single determinations difficult when the concentrations are in the borderline range.
   a. Despite the high quality of a laboratory, any laboratory result may be incorrect.
   b. Laboratory tests may need to be rechecked or redrawn, at times in another laboratory.
4. Reference ranges vary from one laboratory to another.
   a. Age, gender, race, size, and physiologic status must be considered.
   b. 5% of test results will be outside the reference range in the absence of disease.
5. Tables of reference values represent statistical data for 95% of the population; values outside these ranges do not necessarily represent disease.
   a. Test results falling within the reference range may be abnormal from the patient's baseline range.
   b. Certain conditions warrant serial testing.
6. An individual's test values when performed in a good laboratory tend to remain fairly constant over a period of years.
   a. Comparing patient laboratory values obtained when not ill often provides a better reference value than "normal" ranges.
7. Multiple test abnormalities are more likely to be significant than single test abnormalities.
   a. Two or more positive tests for a given disease reinforce diagnosis.
8. The greater the degree of abnormality of a test result, the more likely that a confirmed value is clinically significant or represents a real disorder.
9. Characteristic laboratory test profiles representing full-blown or advanced disease may all be present in only one third of patients with said condition.
   a. Other disorders or conditions may produce exactly the same combination of laboratory test changes.
10. Excessive repetition of tests is wasteful, and the excess burden increases the possibility of laboratory errors.
    a. Patient's acuity should dictate testing interval.
11. Tests should be performed only if they will alter the patient's diagnosis, prognosis, treatment, or management.
12. Clerical errors are far more likely than technical errors to cause incorrect results.
13. The effect of drugs on laboratory test values must never be overlooked.
    a. Certain drugs can produce false-negative and false-positive results; examples: anticonvulsants, antihypertensives, and antiinfectives.
14. The effect of artifacts can cause spurious values and factitious disorders, especially in the face of discrepant laboratory results.
15. Negative laboratory tests (or any other type of tests) do not necessarily rule out a clinical disease.

## IATROGENIC SEQUELAE OF LABORATORY TESTING—PREVENTIVE STRATEGIES

A. **The goal of laboratory testing is to help diagnose and guide management of disease.** Estimates suggest an average of 61 invasive procedures are performed on NICU patients during their stay, with the smallest of infants experiencing the largest amount of painful procedures (Walden, 2007). Inadvertently, the pain of laboratory testing can complicate patient care by creating additional illness, stress, injury, and/or cost. An understanding of the potential sequelae associated with laboratory sampling and strategies that can be used to minimize sequelae is integral to patient care.

1. **Physiologic stress.**
   - **a.** Adverse physical symptoms triggered by pain stimuli, sensory stimuli, and/or disease state.
   - **b.** Laboratory sampling via skin puncture elicits a painful stimulus creating physiologic stress.
   - **c.** Common physiologic stress symptoms include the following (AAP and CPS, 2007) (see also Chapter 11):
     - (1) Tachycardia or bradycardia.
     - (2) Hypertension or hypotension.
     - (3) Apnea or crying.
     - (4) Cyanosis or respiratory distress.
     - (5) Changes in skin color and temperature.
   - **d.** An event creating physiologic stress can potentially alter a laboratory sample result; for example:
     - (1) Change in $Pco_2$ and $Po_2$ reading when infant cries (Kaplan and Tange, 1998).
     - (2) Altered blood pH if infant becomes hypothermic.
   - **e.** Strategies to minimize sampling-induced physiologic stress include the following:
     - (1) Minimize skin punctures for laboratory sampling by minimizing or combining lab work.
     - (2) Utilize existing indwelling catheters (when available) to obtain laboratory samples.
     - (3) Use noninvasive pain management techniques to assist infant in coping with painful stimuli (AAP and CPS, 2007; see also Chapter 16).
     - (4) Use spring-loaded lancets for heel-stick sampling (Folk, 2007; Walden, 2007).
     - (5) Ensure quick, efficient execution of laboratory sampling.
     - (6) Apply warm compress to the heel, which might promote blood flow and improve testing accuracy, thus avoiding repeat laboratory sampling.
     - (7) Venipuncture may be preferable to the heel-stick procedure in minimizing procedure-related pain in term neonates (Shah and Ohlsson, 2011).
     - (8) Careful specimen collection, handling, and labeling can decrease repeat laboratory draws.
2. **Pain** (see also Chapter 16).
   - **a.** An unpleasant sensory and emotional experience associated with actual or potential tissue invasion (Walden, 2007).
   - **b.** Laboratory sampling by skin puncture evokes pain.
   - **c.** Pain causes adverse physiologic stress (see 1. c., this section), including potential central nervous system (CNS) alterations (AAP and CPS, 2007).
   - **d.** It is difficult to differentiate between acute and chronic pain in the infant (AAP and CPS, 2007).
   - **e.** Strategies to minimize sampling-induced pain include the following:
     - (1) Strategies that minimize physiologic stress (see 1. e., this section).
     - (2) Nonpharmacologic pain management strategies; examples: swaddling, facilitated tucking, nonnutritive sucking, skin-to-skin contact (AAP and CPS, 2007; Folk, 2007).
     - (3) Pharmacologic pain management strategies; examples: 24% sucrose, local anesthetic, and opioid and nonopioid analgesics.
     - (4) Usefulness of topical local anesthesia for pain control in infants can be helpful for procedures such as venipuncture, lumbar puncture, and IV catheter insertion. It is not effective for heel sticks (AAP and CPS, 2007).
     - (5) Using venipuncture when obtaining blood samples may be less painful and have less potential sequelae (i.e., nerve damage, arterial spasm) compared with arterial puncture.
     - (6) In term infants, venipuncture has been shown to be less painful a procedure than heel stick when performed by skilled personnel (Shah and Ohlsson, 2011).
3. **Skin injury.**
   - **a.** Alteration in normal barrier function of skin as a result of invasive procedures, adhesives to skin, reaction to skin antiseptics, and/or disease states (Lund and Kuller, 2007).

b. Arterial punctures, venipunctures, and capillary heel sticks used to obtain laboratory samples may potentially create skin injury (LeFrak and Lund, 2013).
c. Potential skin injury from peripheral laboratory samples includes:
   (1) Bruising.
   (2) Hematoma.
   (3) Abrasion from antiseptic solutions, friction, or tape application.
   (4) Dermal stripping from friction or tape application.
   (5) Scarring from multiple punctures.
   (6) Calcifications.
   (7) Burns secondary to prewarming heel with a soak that is too hot; warm soak should not exceed 44° F.
   (8) Chemical burns secondary to antiseptic skin-cleansing agents.
d. Strategies to minimize sampling-induced skin injury from skin puncture include:
   (1) Minimize lab work.
   (2) Avoid excessive "squeeze" when obtaining capillary blood sample.
   (3) Apply adequate pressure to puncture sites to minimize bleeding and formation of hematoma.
   (4) Use nonadhering products to apply as a dressing to puncture site; example:
      (a) Loose elastic wrap (Coban™) around extremity holding gauze in place.
   (5) Thoroughly wash skin of antiseptic solutions.
   (6) Use proper skin puncture devices when obtaining blood; example:
      (a) Spring-loaded lancet of proper length (<2 mm) (Garza and Beacon-McBride, 2010b) and with heel-stick devices ranging from 0.65 to 2 mm depending on infant size (Folk, 2007).
      (b) Butterfly needle of proper gauge and length for site.

**4. Infection.**
a. An important skin function is to provide a barrier to infection.
b. Any break in skin barrier creates potential for infection.
c. Common infections associated with altered skin barrier include:
   (1) Bacterial/candidal skin surface infection.
   (2) Cellulitis.
   (3) Abscess formation at puncture site.
   (4) Septicemia.
   (5) Osteomyelitis.
   (6) Urinary tract/bladder infection.
   (7) Meningitis.
d. Strategies to minimize sampling-induced infection include:
   (1) Minimize laboratory sampling.
   (2) Avoid sampling in area of existing skin injury.
   (3) Avoid repeated sampling from dedicated central lines (Folk, 2007); example: routine laboratory sampling via PICC or Broviac® catheter.
   (4) Meticulous aseptic technique when obtaining a laboratory sample.
   (5) Use of nursing strategies to maintain optimal skin integrity (see Chapter 36).

**5. Organ/nerve injury.**
a. Needle puncture for laboratory sampling can potentially contribute to organ injury.
b. Potential organ injury associated with needle puncture includes:
   (1) Damage to nerve and/or tissues in wrist or brachial area from arterial puncture.
   (2) Damage to lung and/or breast tissue from thoracentesis.
   (3) Damage to abdominal organs from peritoneal tap.
   (4) Damage to nerves or tissue of spine from lumbar puncture.
   (5) Damage to skin as mentioned in 3., this section.
   (6) Tissue ischemia from arterial vasospasm secondary to arterial puncture.
c. Strategies to minimize sampling-induced organ/nerve injury include the following:
   (1) Prudent use of laboratory sampling.
   (2) Proper technique for needle-stick sampling (see also Chapter 15).
   (3) Ultrasound guidance as needed for pleural and peritoneal aspiration.

6. **Anemia.**
   a. Iatrogenic anemia owing to blood loss from laboratory sampling (Bagwell, 2007; Kaplan and Tange, 1998).
   b. Iatrogenic anemia, along with physiologic anemia, constitute the most common causes of chronic anemia in infants (Bagwell, 2007).
   c. Despite microsampling and conservative laboratory sampling, sick infants can lose more than 5 mL of blood per day (Letterio et al., 2013).
   d. Removal of 1 mL of blood from a 1-kg infant equals removal of 70 mL of blood from an adult (Blackburn, 2013).
   e. Iatrogenic blood loss correlates with degree of illness.
   f. Laboratory sample overdraws (19% ± 1.8% more than needed) are common in the NICU (Blackburn, 2013).
   g. Strategies to minimize sampling-induced anemia include:
      (1) Judicious use of laboratory sampling.
      (2) Microsampling when possible.
      (3) Accurate documentation of blood loss.
      (4) Avoiding overdrawing of blood samples.
7. **False diagnosis.**
   a. Even under the best circumstances, no test is perfect.
   b. Excess repetition of a test increases the possibility of laboratory error.
   c. The more laboratory samples drawn, the more likely one or more results will be outside the reference range.
   d. Clinical decision making should be based on trends or multiple laboratory values pointing to disease versus spurious results.
   e. Strategies to minimize sampling-related false diagnosis include:
      (1) Obtain laboratory samples only when necessary to assist in diagnosis, prognosis, treatment, or management.
      (2) Verify spurious laboratory values.
      (3) Draw laboratory samples using proper technique and conditions.
8. **Cost factor.**
   a. 2.3% to 3% of a patient's hospital bill results from laboratory sampling (Rusckowski, 2012).
   b. If the average daily cost of a NICU stay is $3000 (Kornhauser and Schneiderman, 2010), a patient minimally spends $90 per day for laboratory testing.
   c. Cost of hospitalization in the NICU is inversely related to gestational age. The average cost of healthy, term newborn is $2830, while premature infant costs range from $41,610 to greater than $250,000 (Kornhauser and Schneiderman, 2010).
   d. Rising cost of medical care is complicating delivery of care.
   e. Strategies to minimize sampling-related laboratory costs include:
      (1) Minimize laboratory sampling.
      (2) Prudent medical and nursing decision making regarding laboratory sampling.
      (3) Minimizing laboratory errors precipitating repeat sampling.

## DECISION—QUESTIONS TO ASK PRIOR TO OBTAINING A LABORATORY TEST

A. **Judicious use of laboratory testing is critical in any setting, particularly in the NICU, where acuity is high.** Below are questions to consider prior to ordering and/or obtaining a laboratory sample. Asking oneself these questions will assist in refining critical thinking skills and aid in selective use of lab work (Box 13-1). To simplify the discussion process, one presenting symptom—*jittery infant*—will be used and applied to all phases of critical thinking.
   1. **Does the patient require the laboratory test?**
      a. Are the patient examination results abnormal, whereby a laboratory test will help in diagnosis?
         (1) Example:
            (a) Abnormal finding: *model–jittery infant*.
            (b) Possible laboratory tests: glucose, calcium, and urine toxicology screen.

**BOX 13-1**
**QUESTIONS TO ASK *BEFORE* OBTAINING A LABORATORY TEST**

- Does the patient require the laboratory test?
  - Are the patient examination results abnormal, whereby a laboratory test will help in diagnosis?
  - Is the medical history helpful in directing which laboratory test to order?
- Will the laboratory test requested answer the "so what" question?
  - Is the laboratory result integral to the immediate clinical management of the infant?
  - Is the laboratory result contributory to a patient's diagnosis?
- Is the laboratory test requested still applicable to the current clinical status?
  - Has the outcome of the infant's clinical examination changed?
  - Has the infant recovered?
- Is the timing of the laboratory test appropriate?
  - When should the labwork be obtained?
- Is the laboratory test ordered the "best" test to answer the clinical question?
- Does the laboratory test require too much blood volume?
- Does the potential benefit of the laboratory test outweigh the risk of sequelae in the patient?
- If the laboratory sample is inadequate, faulty, or "lost," is it necessary to redraw?
  - Has the clinical status changed?
  - Has the infant recovered?

**b.** Is the medical history helpful in directing which laboratory test to order?
(1) *Example: model–jittery infant.*
(a) Infant of a gestational, class A1, diabetic mother (IDM-A1)? Might choose to obtain a serum glucose and/or serum calcium level versus a urine toxicology screen.
(b) Infant with delayed drying of skin after birth and axilla/skin temperature of 96° F? Might choose to place infant under heat source and not obtain lab work.
(c) Infant 1800 g, IDM-A1, and mother with minimal prenatal care? Might choose to obtain all possible laboratory tests.

**2. Will the laboratory test requested answer the "so what" question?** *Model–jittery infant.*
**a.** Is the laboratory result integral to the immediate clinical management of the infant?
(1) Hypoglycemia in an IDM-A1 will mandate increasing the carbohydrate intake to treat the problem.
(2) Mild hypothermia in an otherwise healthy infant will not require a change in management directed by lab work.
**b.** Is the laboratory result contributory to the infant's diagnosis?
(1) Serum glucose test result will help diagnose hypoglycemia as a cause of jitteriness.
(2) Serum glucose test result will not help diagnose respiratory distress syndrome.

**3. Is the laboratory test requested still applicable to current clinical status?**
**a.** *Example: model–jittery infant.*
(1) **Has the infant's clinical status changed?**
(a) An hour-old IDM-A1 whose jitteriness has changed to tonic–clonic movements of extremities—in addition to serum glucose and calcium levels—will need consideration of a urine toxicology screen and electrolytes.
(b) An hour-old IDM-A1 who breastfed for 20 minutes and is no longer jittery may not require further testing, particularly if the original serum glucose level was normal.
(c) The hypothermic infant who continues to remain hypothermic after 2 hours under heat source may need serum glucose test and sepsis evaluation.
**b.** *Example: model–jittery infant.*
(1) **Has the infant recovered?**
(a) Infant with multiple normal glucose test results may no longer require frequent glucose testing.
(b) Infant no longer jittery after acquiring a normal body temperature—may need to cancel lab work ordered to evaluate jitteriness.

4. **Is the timing of the laboratory test appropriate?**
   a. *Example: model–jittery infant.*
      (1) **When should the lab work be obtained?**
         (a) IDM-A1 at birth—might wait to check serum glucose level at 30 minutes of age when the result would reflect infant's status versus that of the maternal environment.
         (b) Jittery infant with normal serum glucose and calcium levels—might obtain first voided specimen for a urine toxicology screen.
5. **Is the laboratory test ordered the "best" test to answer the clinical question?**
   a. *Example: model–jittery infant.*
      (1) Should the jittery infant have a serum glucose sample sent to the laboratory or should a whole-blood glucose level be obtained at the bedside by POCT or near-patient testing? A POCT glucose result is available in seconds, allowing for rapid clinical intervention.
      (2) Should the jittery infant with polycythemia have a POCT whole-blood glucose test or should a serum glucose sample be sent to the laboratory? A POCT glucose result may not be accurate in the face of polycythemia.
6. **Does the laboratory test require too much blood volume?**
   a. *Example: model–jittery infant.*
      (1) A 500-g infant with every-2-hour serum glucose—POCT whole-blood glucose testing requires average sample size of one drop to 0.1 mL of blood, whereas serum glucose test requires an average sample size of 0.5 mL.
      (2) A 5-mL sample of blood is required for metabolic screening in a 500-g infant—10% blood volume loss may not be tolerated; need to prioritize lab work and draw in stages based on most common to least common disorders.
7. **Does the potential benefit of the laboratory test outweigh the risk of sequelae in the patient?**
   a. *Example: model–jittery infant.*
      (1) A 500-g infant with hypoglycemia—frequent glucose testing needed to monitor treatment; benefit outweighs potential harm of blood loss. Also, POCT use can minimize blood loss.
      (2) A 5-mL blood sample for metabolic screening in a 500-g, symptomatic infant—potential harm of an acute 10% blood loss outweighs the need to simultaneously obtain all the ordered metabolic screening laboratories.
8. **If the laboratory sample is inadequate, faulty, or "lost," is it necessary to redraw?**
   a. *Example: model–jittery infant.*
      (1) **Has the clinical status changed?**
      (2) **Has the infant recovered?** (See 3., this section.) If the status improves or the infant recovers while waiting for sample, repeat sampling may not be indicated.

## LABORATORY INTERPRETATION—DECISION TREE

A. **Careful laboratory data interpretation is essential in providing accurate therapeutic interventions.** Asking focused questions will assist in refining critical thinking skills related to utilization of laboratory values in patient management. Below are questions to consider when using laboratory results to direct patient care.
   1. **Laboratory test result. Is it reliable? Is it believable? (Box 13-2) A question tree *if result too low.***
      a. Is the sample diluted? Examples:
         (1) A laboratory specimen can be contaminated with or diluted by fluids infusing through indwelling arterial and/or venous lines if the line is not properly cleared.
         (2) A laboratory specimen can be diluted by interstitial fluid from the skin tissues if heelstick puncture is not fresh, the puncture site is not prewarmed, or the infant is exceedingly edematous.
      b. Was the sample handled correctly? Examples:
         (1) A serum bilirubin count can be falsely low if obtained while the infant is under phototherapy or if exposed to the daylight or fluorescent light too long before analysis.

**BOX 13-2**

**LABORATORY INTERPRETATION: IS IT RELIABLE? IS IT BELIEVABLE?**

**Laboratory test result. Is it *reliable?* Is it *believable*?**

**Yes**
- Implement an appropriate clinical intervention, if needed.

**No**
- Consider repeating the laboratory test when the appropriate correction is made.
- Consider repeating the laboratory test if the clinical status continues to warrant a laboratory test.

**Laboratory test result. Is it *reliable*? Is it *believable*?**

**If Result too Low**
- Is the sample diluted?
- Was the sample handled correctly?
- Was the timing of the test an issue?
- Was medical therapy not implemented or inadequate?
- Was the specimen site condition a factor?
- Was the POCT device calibrated?
- Was there interference from a past medical therapy?

**If Result too High**
- Was the laboratory specimen drawn too early?
- Was the sample handled correctly?
- Was medical therapy not implemented or inadequate?
- Was the source of the laboratory sample not appropriate?
- Was the POCT device calibrated?

*POCT*, Point-of-care testing.

(2) A serum glucose level can be falsely low if left in a microtainer and not processed and analyzed promptly.
(3) An overfilled or underfilled hematology sample can precipitate clotting and falsely decrease platelet count.

**c.** Was the timing of the test an issue? Examples:
(1) A serum gentamicin, vancomycin, or theophylline level will be too low if drawn too early in the drug treatment.
(2) A serum glucose or POCT glucose level obtained too soon after feeding the infant may remain falsely low due to lack of digestion time.
(3) Electrolyte levels may remain falsely low if obtained too soon after electrolyte replacement.

**d.** Was medical therapy not implemented or inadequate? Examples:
(1) A blood gas level obtained prior to weaning the ventilator for a $P_{CO_2}$ of 25.
(2) A serum glucose or POCT glucose level obtained prior to medical intervention for hypoglycemia.
(3) A serum gentamicin, vancomycin, or theophylline level will be too low if the dose is inadequate or dosing interval too long.
(4) A theophylline level may be low because intermittent doses are held as a result of tachycardia in the infant.

**e.** Was the specimen site condition a factor? Examples:
(1) A capillary blood sample from an edematous infant can be falsely low due to excessive tissue fluids.
(2) A nonwarmed heel can falsely lower a capillary blood gas pH, $P_{O_2}$.

**f.** Was the POCT device calibrated? Examples:
(1) Laboratory test results may be unreliable if the:
(a) POCT device was not calibrated recently.
(b) POCT device was calibrated improperly.
(c) Reagent used for calibration had expired.
(d) Sample cartridge expired or was not kept at room temperature.

**g.** Was there interference from past medical therapy? Examples:
(1) An infant's blood culture result may be falsely negative if a mother was treated with antibiotics during labor.
(2) Phenobarbital use may decrease theophylline concentrations.

2. **Laboratory test result. Is it *reliable?* Is it *believable*? A question tree *if result too high.***
   a. Was the laboratory specimen drawn too early? Examples:
      (1) A triglyceride level may be falsely elevated if drawn too soon after lipid infusion.
      (2) A serum calcium level may be falsely increased if drawn soon after a calcium gluconate bolus.
      (3) Electrolytes can remain abnormal if drawn too soon after corrective action.
   b. Was the sample handled correctly? Examples:
      (1) A serum potassium level may be falsely elevated due to hemolysis from squeezing the heel for capillary laboratory sampling.
      (2) A serum protein or potassium level may be falsely elevated if a tourniquet is applied too tightly or too long ($\geq$3 minutes).
      (3) An Hct count can be falsely elevated if drawn from a poorly perfused heel.
   c. Was medical therapy not implemented or inadequate? Examples:
      (1) A serum bilirubin count can remain elevated if phototherapy is not instituted long enough to measure change.
      (2) A $Pco_2$ can remain elevated if ventilator setting changes are not sufficient to correct for the respiratory ailment or the sample is drawn too soon after corrective intervention.
   d. Was the source of the laboratory sample not appropriate? Examples:
      (1) An Hct can be falsely elevated from a capillary sample versus an arterial or venous sample.
      (2) An ammonia level can be falsely elevated if hemolyzed, so needs to be drawn via an artery or vein.
   e. Was the POCT device calibrated? Examples:
      (1) Laboratory result may be unreliable if the POCT device was not recently calibrated or was calibrated improperly, if the reagent for calibration had expired, or the sample cartridge either expired or was not stored properly.
3. **Laboratory test result. Is it *reliable*? Is it *believable*? YES.**
   a. Implement appropriate clinical intervention, if needed. Examples:
      (1) Alert the primary care provider of laboratory result and implement appropriate medical or nursing corrective intervention as needed:
         (a) Medication dosage change for inadequate drug level.
         (b) Ventilator setting change for under- or overventilation.
         (c) Blood product transfusion for anemia, thrombocytopenia.
         (d) Change in IV fluid concentration or rate for electrolyte imbalance or dehydration.
         (e) Change feeding interval for hypoglycemia.
4. **Laboratory test result. Is it *reliable*? Is it *believable*? NO.**
   a. Consider repeating laboratory test when the appropriate correction is made. Examples:
      (1) Repeat laboratory test at an appropriate time for drug level measurement.
      (2) Warm heel prior to obtaining capillary sample.
      (3) Wait 30 minutes to 1 hour after a milk feeding to test a postfeed serum glucose level.
   b. Consider repeating laboratory test if clinical status continues to warrant laboratory test. Examples:
      (1) A clotted CBC sample after red blood cell transfusion or after antibiotic therapy: may not require a repeat sample or might wait for redraw until another blood sample is needed.
      (2) A high Hct value taken from an acrocyanotic heel in a hypoglycemic infant would need a central Hct to determine if polycythemia is a cause of hypoglycemia.
5. **Laboratory test result. Is it *normal*? YES (Box 13-3)**
   a. Consider a change in medical management. Examples:
      (1) Normal electrolyte results in the face of electrolyte replacement may signal a need to decrease or stop the electrolyte supplementation.
      (2) A normal Hct may warrant cancellation of a projected red blood cell transfusion.
   b. Consider implementing surveillance plans. Examples:
      (1) Normal serum calcium, phosphorus, and alkaline phosphatase may need weekly surveillance in very low birth weight infants to monitor for potential rickets.
      (2) Normal electrolytes may need frequent monitoring when initiating diuretic therapy.

BOX 13-3
**LABORATORY INTERPRETATION: IS IT NORMAL?**

**Laboratory Test Result. Is it *normal*?**

**Yes**
- Consider a change in medical management.
- Consider implementing surveillance plans.

**No**
- Consider calling the laboratory to verify the specimen.
- Is the laboratory result in the appropriate reference range?
- Review patient care practice at the time of laboratory specimen sampling.
- Consider medication interactions as etiology.
- Institute corrective medical and/or nursing action.

BOX 13-4
**LABORATORY INTERPRETATION: TEST FOLLOW-UP**

**Laboratory Test *Follow-up***

**Normal Test Result**
Continue to watch for potential sequelae of treatment.
Consider a plan for implementing maintenance laboratory surveillance.

**Abnormal Test Result**
Consider a change in clinical practice.
Allow time for corrective action, then repeat laboratory test to measure effective therapy.

6. **Laboratory test result. Is it *normal*? NO (see Box 13-3).**
   a. Consider calling the laboratory to verify specimen. Examples:
      (1) See 1., 2., and 4., this section.
      (2) Call laboratory to verify that the result is indeed that of the patient in question.
      (3) Ascertain that the abnormal laboratory value was taken from the patient in question.
   b. Is the laboratory result in the appropriate reference range? Examples:
      (1) A critical Hct value differs with age. An Hct of 55% in a newborn is normal as compared with an adult.
      (2) Laboratory methods and equipment vary among different laboratories; need to confirm laboratory result with the laboratory that analyzed the sample.
   c. Review patient care practice at time of laboratory specimen sampling. Examples:
      (1) See 1., 2., and 4., this section.
   d. Consider medication interactions as etiology. Examples:
      (1) Heparin in a blood sample will prolong PT and PTT.
      (2) Narcotic sedation may depress respirations and increase $P_{CO_2}$ level.
      (3) Sulfonamides can increase serum bilirubin.
      (4) Stool Hematest can be falsely positive when patient is on iron supplement, indomethacin, potassium preparations, or steroids.
   e. Institute corrective medical and/or nursing action. Example:
      (1) See 3., this section.
7. **Laboratory test *follow-up*—normal test result (Box 13-4).**
   a. Continue to watch for potential sequelae of treatment. Examples:
      (1) Periodic monitoring of electrolytes is needed when the patient is on diuretic therapy.
      (2) Periodic monitoring of renal function and electrolytes is needed when the patient is on antifungal therapy.
   b. Consider a plan for implementing maintenance laboratory surveillance. Examples:
      (1) Routine weekly monitoring of electrolytes, liver function, and renal function when the infant is on prolonged hyperalimentation.
      (2) Routine monitoring of skeletal integrity of the premature infant susceptible for rickets.

8. **Laboratory test *follow-up*—abnormal test result (see Box 13-4).**
   a. Consider a change in clinical practice. Examples:
      (1) See 3., this section.
   b. Allow time for corrective action, then repeat laboratory test to measure effective therapy. Examples:
      (1) Weaning from ventilatory support may warrant blood gas analyses every half hour to every 4 hours for an overventilated infant recovering from primary atelectasis.
      (2) Repeated serum glucose level checks every half hour to every hour may be necessary after a hypoglycemic infant receives an IV glucose bolus.
      (3) Weekly or biweekly serum electrolyte tests may be necessary when adjusting oral electrolyte supplementation for borderline low serum electrolyte levels in infants on diuretics for chronic lung disease.

## REFERENCES


American Academy of Pediatrics and Canadian Paediatric Society: Prevention and management of pain in the neonate: An update. *Advances in Neonatal Care*, 7 (3):151–160, 2007.

Bagwell, G.A.: Hematologic system. In C. Kenner, and J.W. Lott (Eds.): *Comprehensive neonatal nursing: An interdisciplinary approach* (4th ed.). St. Louis, 2007, Elsevier Saunders, pp. 221–253.

Blackburn, S.T.: Hematologic and hemostatic systems. In S.T. Blackburn (Ed.): *Maternal, fetal and neonatal physiology: A clinical perspective* (4th ed.). St. Louis, 2013, Elsevier Saunders, pp. 238–239.

Centers for Disease Control, Prevention: Births: Final data for 2011. *National Vital Statistics Reports*, 62 (1), 2013. Retrieved September 22, 2013, from www.cdc.gov/nchs/data/nvsr/nvsr62/nvsr62_01.pdf.

Centers for Disease Control, Prevention: Births: Preliminary data for 2011. *National Vital Statistics Reports*, 57 (7), 2011. Retrieved March 21, 2013, from www.cdc.gov/nchs/data/nvsr/nvsr59/nvsr59_07.pdf.

Fischbach, F.: Diagnostic testing. Intratest phase: Elements of safe, effective, informed care. In F. Fischbach (Ed.): *A manual of laboratory & diagnostic tests* (8th ed.). Philadelphia, 2009, Lippincott Williams & Wilkins, pp. 25–41.

Folk, L.A.: Guide to capillary heelstick blood sampling in infants. *Advances in Neonatal Care*, 7(4):171–178, 2007.

Garza, D. and Becan-McBride, K.: Arterial, intravenous (IV), and special collection procedures. In D. Garza, and K. Becan-McBride (Eds.): *Phlebotomy handbook: Blood specimen collection from basic to advanced* (8th ed.). Upper Saddle River, NJ, 2010a, Pearson Education, pp. 465–498.

Garza, D. and Becan-McBride, K.: Blood collection equipment. In D. Garza, and K. Becan-McBride (Eds.): *Phlebotomy handbook: Blood specimen collection from basic to advanced* (8th ed.). Upper Saddle River, NJ, 2010b, Pearson Education, pp. 248–279.

Garza, D. and Becan-McBride, K.: Capillary blood specimens. In D. Garza, and K. Becan-McBride (Eds.): *Phlebotomy handbook: Blood specimen collection from basic to advanced* (8th ed.). Upper Saddle River, NJ, 2010c, Pearson Education, pp. 363–381.

Garza, D. and Becan-McBride, K.: Pediatric and geriatric procedures. In D. Garza, and K. Becan-McBride (Eds.): *Phlebotomy handbook: Blood specimen collection from basic to advanced* (8th ed.). Upper Saddle River, NJ, 2010d, Pearson Education, pp. 405–442.

Garza, D. and Becan-McBride, K.: Preanalytical complications causing medical errors in blood collection. In D. Garza, and K. Becan-McBride (Eds.): *Phlebotomy handbook: Blood specimen collection from basic to advanced* (8th ed.). Upper Saddle River, NJ, 2010e, Pearson Education, pp. 281–299.

Garza, D. and Becan-McBride, K.: Venipuncture procedures. In D. Garza, and K. Becan-McBride (Eds.): *Phlebotomy handbook: Blood specimen collection from basic to advanced* (8th ed.). Upper Saddle River, NJ, 2010f, Pearson Education, pp. 301–361.

Kaplan, L.A. and Tange, S.M. (Eds.): *Standards of laboratory practice* Washington, DC, 1998, National Academy of Clinical Biochemistry.

Kee, J.L.: The importance of specimen collection. In J.L. Kee (Ed.): *Laboratory and diagnostic tests with nursing implication* (8th ed.). Upper Saddle River, NJ, 2010, Prentice Hall, pp. xiii–xviii.

Kornhauser, M. and Schneiderman, R.: How plans can improve outcomes and cut costs for preterm infant care. Managed Care January:1-6, 2010. Retrieved March 3, 2013, from www.managedcaremag.com/print/archives/1001/1001.preterm.html.

Kurec, A.S. and Lifshitz, M.S.: General concepts and administrative issues. In R.A. McPherson and M.R. Pincus (Eds.): *Henry's clinical diagnosis and management by laboratory methods* (22nd ed.). Philadelphia, 2011, Elsevier Saunders, pp. 3–12.

LaMorte, W.W.: Screening for disease. Boston University MPH Module. 2013: Retrieved March 21, 2013, from http://sph.bu.edu/otlt/MPH-Modules/EP/EP713-Screening/EP713-Screening-print.html.

Laposata, M.: *Laboratory medicine: Clinical pathology in the practice of medicine.* Chicago, 2002, American Society for Clinical Pathology, p. 14.

LeFrak, L. and Lund, C.H.: Nursing practice in the neonatal intensive care unit. In M.H. Klaus, and A.A. Fanaroff (Eds.): *Care of the high-risk neonate* (6th ed.). Philadelphia, 2013, Elsevier Saunders, pp. 225–243.

Letterio, J., Ahuja, S.P. and Petrosiute, A.: Hematologic problems. In M.H. Klaus, and A.A. Fanaroff (Eds.):

*Care of the high-risk neonate* (6th ed.). Philadelphia, 2013, Elsevier Saunders, pp. 432–444.

Lund, C.H. and Kuller, J.M.: Integumentary system. In J. Kenner, and J.W. Lott (Eds.): *Comprehensive neonatal nursing: An interdisciplinary approach* (4th ed.). St. Louis, 2007, Elsevier Saunders, pp. 65–91.

Olsowka, E.S. and Garg, U.: Specimen collection and point-of-care testing. In D.S. Jacobs, D.K. Oxley, and W.R. DeMott (Eds.): *Jacobs & DeMott laboratory test handbook* (5th ed.). Hudson, OH, 2001, Lexi-Comp, pp. 35–48.

Oxley, D.K., Garg, U. and Olsowka, E.S.: Maximizing the information from laboratory tests—the Ulysses syndrome. In D.S. Jacobs, D.K. Oxley, and W.R. DeMott (Eds.): *Jacobs & DeMott laboratory test handbook* (5th ed.). Hudson, OH, 2001, Lexi-Comp, pp. 15–23.

Rusckowski, S.: The growing role of diagnostics in health care. In *American Medical Technologists: G-2 Lab Institute report*, 2012. Retrieved March 13, 2013, from www.americanmedtech.org/NewsAdvocacy/View/tabid/95/Articled/12/G-2-Lab-Institute-Report-2012.aspx.

Sacher, R.A., McPherson, R.A. and Campos, J.M.: General chemistry. In R.A. Sacher, R.A. McPherson, and J.M. Campos (Eds.): *Widmann's clinical interpretation of laboratory tests* (11th ed.). Philadelphia, 2000a, F.A. Davis, pp. 445–446.

Sacher, R.A., McPherson, R.A. and Campos, J.M.: Hematological methods. In R.A. Sacher, R.A. McPherson, and J.M. Campos (Eds.): *Widmann's clinical interpretation of laboratory tests* (11th ed.). Philadelphia, 2000b, F.A. Davis, pp. 31–32.

Sacher, R.A., McPherson, R.A. and Campos, J.M.: Principles of immunology and immunology testing. In R.A. Sacher, R.A. McPherson, and J.M. Campos (Eds.): *Widmann's clinical interpretation of laboratory tests* (11th ed.). Philadelphia, 2000c, F.A. Davis, p. 325.

Sacher, R.A., McPherson, R.A. and Campos, J.M.: Principles of interpretation of laboratory tests. In R.A. Sacher, R.A. McPherson, and J.M. Campos (Eds.): *Widmann's clinical interpretation of laboratory tests* (11th ed.). Philadelphia, 2000d, F.A. Davis, pp. 3–27.

Sanford, K.W. and McPherson, R.A.: Preanalysis. In R.A. McPherson, and M.R. Pincus (Eds.): *Henry's clinical diagnosis and management by laboratory methods* (22nd ed.). Philadelphia, 2011, Saunders, pp. 24–36.

Shah, V. and Ohlsson, A.: Venipuncture versus heel lance for blood sampling in term neonates. *Cochrane Database of Systematic Reviews,* (4):CD001452, 2011.

Threatte, G.A. and Schexneider, K.I.: Point of care and physician office laboratories. In R.A. McPherson, and M.R. Pincus (Eds.): *Henry's clinical diagnosis and management by laboratory methods* (22nd ed.). Philadelphia, 2011, Elsevier Saunders, pp. 73–79.

Vedder, T. and Sawyer, T.L.: Heel sticks. In T. Rosenkrantz (Ed.): Medscape Reference Drugs, Diseases, & Procedures. emedicine, November 2:1-6, 2011. Retrieved March 21, 2013, from http://emedicine.medscape.com/article/1413486-0verview#a01.

Walden, M.: Pain in the newborn and infant. In C. Kenner, and J.W. Lott (Eds.): *Comprehensive neonatal nursing: An interdisciplinary approach* (4th ed.). St. Louis, 2007, Elsevier Saunders, pp. 360–371.

Wallach, J.: Introduction to normal values (reference range). In J. Wallach (Ed.): *Interpretation of diagnostic tests* (8th ed.). Philadelphia, 2007, Wolters Kluwer/Lippincott Williams & Wilkins, pp. 3–7.

CHAPTER

# 14 Radiologic Evaluation

LINDA LANE EHRET

**OBJECTIVES**

1. Define common radiologic terms used to describe an x-ray.
2. Differentiate various densities that are evident on an x-ray.
3. Describe radiologic findings that are commonly seen in neonatal disease states.
4. Differentiate normal from abnormal findings on a chest x-ray.
5. Recognize findings on an x-ray that are consistent with congenital heart disease.
6. Describe an x-ray consistent with necrotizing enterocolitis.
7. Review correct indwelling line and tube placement on an x-ray.

Radiographic medical imaging of abnormalities in a sick newborn infant is an established part of diagnostic evaluation. This evaluation assists the clinician in determining a diagnosis or formulating a differential diagnosis for treatment of the patient. Rarely is a newborn infant admitted to the neonatal intensive care unit (NICU) without having at least one x-ray taken, and frequently several additional films are needed during the course of treatment. Nurses need to become familiar with common radiographic findings to add to the knowledge base on which patient care is founded. This chapter reviews essentials of radiologic interpretation, discusses pathologic findings, and presents x-rays with common findings.

## BASIC CONCEPTS

A. **Radiographs are images produced on a radiosensitive surface, such as film, when x-ray beams are passed through an object to the surface below (Stedman's Medical Dictionary, 2013).**

B. **By comparing densities and shapes from the image produced on the film, information can be deduced or inferred regarding anatomy, pathology, and function.**

## TERMINOLOGY

A. **Air bronchogram:** air in the bronchial tree visualized against a background of generalized alveolar atelectasis (Stedman's Medical Dictionary, 2013).

B. **Artifact:** an unnaturally occurring silhouette that is artificially reproduced on an x-ray and is not a part of the patient (e.g., electrocardiogram leads, temperature probes).

C. **Cardiothoracic ratio:** computed by dividing the maximum cardiac width by the maximum thoracic width to determine the heart size.

D. **Carina:** bifurcation of the trachea, usually about the level of the third and fourth thoracic vertebrae (Stedman's Medical Dictionary, 2013). Used in determining location of endotracheal tube.

E. **Expiratory film:** obtained when the infant is in expiration; appears to increase cardiac size, accentuate lung markings, and decrease normal lung expansion.

F. **Exposure:** amount of radiation used, producing a film ranging from light to dark. An underpenetrated (underexposed) film causes images to appear light and hazy. Overpenetration (overexposure) causes the film to be dark and to lack contrast, in comparison with an appropriately penetrated and exposed film.

G. **Hyperexpanded lungs:** lungs expanded to greater than the ninth rib.

H. **Hypoexpanded lungs:** lungs expanded to less than the seventh rib.

I. **Inspiratory film:** obtained when infant is in full inspiration and the lungs project to the eighth rib above the right diaphragmatic dome, with the trachea shown in a straight projection. This is the optimal for chest film interpretation.
J. **Interlobar fissure:** accumulation of fluid in the pleural space between the lung lobes. The fissure may be fluid filled and may appear as a distinctive line.
K. **Perihilar:** pertaining to radiographic area bordering mediastinal structures.
L. **Pleural effusion:** abnormal collection of fluid in the pleural space (Stedman's Medical Dictionary, 2013).
M. **Radiolucent:** pertaining to substances with varying degrees of transparency (Stedman's Medical Dictionary, 2013).
N. **Radiopaque:** pertaining to substances that are dense and nonpenetrable to x-rays (Stedman's Medical Dictionary, 2013).
O. **Rad:** fundamental unit of radiation measurement (Stedman's Medical Dictionary, 2013).
P. **Roentgen:** unit of exposure (Stedman's Medical Dictionary, 2013).
Q. **Rotation:** turned from the midline. Chest structures closest to the beam are magnified, making their shadows appear enlarged and distorted.
R. **Skinfold:** the most common artifact seen in the neonate. Manifests as a straight line of variable length that can travel across or outside the chest or across the diaphragm and into the abdomen. Results from folding of excessive skin; may mimic a pneumothorax. However, the obliquity of the line produced by a skinfold is opposite to that produced by the edge of the lung in pneumothorax.
S. **Proper technique:** signifies correct exposure, positioning, and timing in relation to inspiration and proper labeling of a film.
T. **X-ray:** a form of electromagnetic radiation with shorter wavelengths than normal light. X-rays can penetrate most structures (Stedman's Medical Dictionary, 2013).

## X-RAY VIEWS COMMONLY USED IN THE NEWBORN INFANT (FIG. 14-1)

A. **Anteroposterior view.** X-ray tube is positioned above the infant's chest, with the x-ray beam passing through from front to back. Most common view used in the neonate for general assessment.

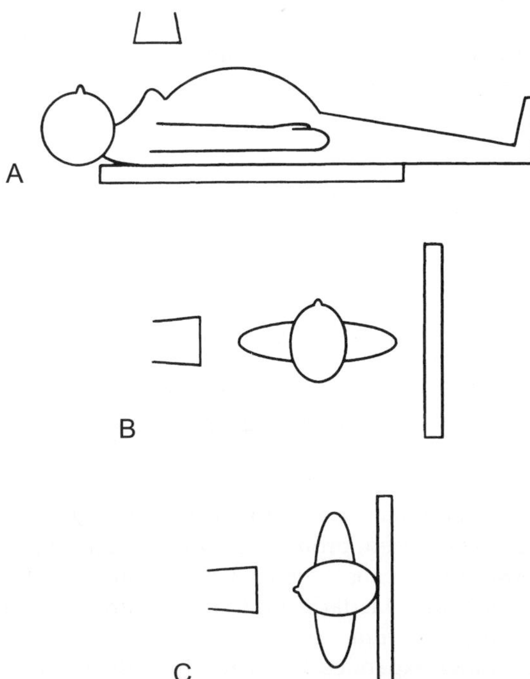


FIGURE 14-1 ■ X-ray views commonly used for the newborn infant. **A,** Anteroposterior view. **B,** Cross-table lateral view. **C,** Lateral decubitus view. (Courtesy Peter Honeyfield, M.D.)

B. **Cross-table lateral view.** X-ray beam passes horizontally through infant in the supine position. Used for general assessment, assessment of free air in the chest, and to verify line placement.
C. **Lateral decubitus view.** X-ray beam passes horizontally through the infant, who is positioned with suspect side uppermost. The film is placed on the infant's back, and the infant is placed perpendicular to the bed, facing the x-ray tube. The infant is usually elevated on foam pads or blankets, with the arm positioned above the head and out of the field of view. Free air will rise to the highest portion of the thorax if a pneumothorax is present. If an abdominal perforation is present, free air will also rise above the liver when the infant is positioned with the left side down.

## RADIOGRAPHIC DENSITIES

A. **Radiodensities of various substances and tissues differ according to their composition.**
   1. The least dense (radiolucent) substance will radiograph black or dark gray because the sparse molecules offer no obstacle to the rays.
   2. A very dense (radiopaque) object such as lead will radiograph gray or white because no rays or few rays will penetrate it, so the film underneath will remain unchanged.
   3. Subcutaneous fat is very radiolucent and produces a dark gray shadow on x-ray film.
   4. Blood, muscle, and liver are of similar densities and will be seen as white and medium gray. Moist solid or fluid-filled organs and tissue masses have about the same radiodensity—greater than air but less than bone or metal.
   5. Bone is composed of an organic matrix into which the complex bone mineral (primarily calcium) is precipitated. Organic substances will reduce the radiodensity of bone and will be seen as white with a tinge of gray.
   6. Metal such as the surgical clip used for patent ductus arteriosus ligation is very dense and radiopaque. All the x-rays are absorbed by the metal, producing a white image on the film.
B. **Differentiation of densities is the basis for interpretation of an x-ray film.** For example, because of the contrast in densities between the fluid-filled heart, which radiographs white, and the air-filled lungs, which radiograph black, the heart can be seen against the lungs. Organs of the same density that are located side by side, such as the heart and the thymus, may be difficult to distinguish from each other. Changes in normal density can indicate a pathologic process, such as severe respiratory distress syndrome. Surfactant-deficient lungs will appear on the film completely white instead of black, indicating areas of alveolar collapse.

## RISKS ASSOCIATED WITH RADIOGRAPHIC EXAMINATION IN THE NEONATE

A. **Radiation effects and risks (Daldrup-Link and Gooding, 2010).**
   1. Adverse effects of x-rays do not occur unless a threshold amount of radiation is delivered.
   2. Virtually all radiation doses for diagnostic imaging fall below the threshold for adverse effects.
B. **Risks to personnel.**
   1. Risks to personnel in the area, when studies and technique are properly done, are low.

## APPROACH TO INTERPRETING AN X-RAY

A. **Develop a systematic approach and a definite order for assessing a film to ensure that no pathology is missed.**
B. **Labeling.** Note name or identification of the patient, date and time of the film, and radiographic labeling on right or left side of the film.
C. **Assess for correct exposure of the film.**
D. **Note positioning.** Clavicles and ribs should be even on both sides of the chest. Rotation distorts structures.

**E. Individually assess all anatomic and pathologic changes on each film.**

1. Lung fields.
   a. Normal lung expansion: eight ribs projecting above the right diaphragmatic dome, with the trachea in a slightly curved, near-midline position. Consider areas of density and areas of lucency (Daldrup-Link and Gooding, 2010).
   b. Lung volume, determined by noting the number of ribs expanded on an inspiratory film.
   c. Pulmonary vascularity: vessels branching from the lung root (hilum) and decreasing in size, with extension into the lung fields. Vascularity will be increased or diminished depending on pathologic state.
   d. Presence of free air: pneumothorax, pneumoperitoneum, pneumopericardium, and pneumomediastinum.
2. Mediastinum.
   a. Heart.
      (1) Size.
      (2) Malposition: any inappropriate position of the heart—that is, any position other than the usual position in the hemithorax.
      (3) Contour: variable because of the influence of patient position and angulation of the x-ray beam.
      (4) Shape: may indicate pathologic change—for example, boot-shaped heart in tetralogy of Fallot and egg-shaped heart in transposition of the great vessels (Daldrup-Link and Gooding, 2010).
      (5) Pulmonary vascular markings: may be significantly diminished, as in pulmonary atresia, or increased, as in congestive heart failure [CHF] (Daldrup-Link and Gooding, 2010).
   b. Trachea.
      (1) Normally located within the mediastinum.
      (2) Assessment on x-ray film for presence and position of endotracheal tube.
   c. Thymus.
      (1) Size.
      (2) Presence or absence.
      (3) Presense of "sail sign" when mediastinal air lifts the thymus upward.
   d. Diaphragm.
      (1) General pattern: two smooth, curved shadows on either side of the heart, taking off from the midline at the origin of the 10th and 11th ribs (Daldrup-Link and Gooding, 2010).
      (2) Contour: possibly flattened with lung overdistention or elevated if there is abdominal distention.
      (3) Diaphragmatic hernia: abdominal contents passing through a hole in the diaphragm.
      (4) Eventration: herniation of bowel and liver against a weakened hemidiaphragm. The diaphragm remains intact but is abnormally elevated.
   e. Gastrointestinal (GI) tract.
      (1) Esophagus is typically air filled and linear. Distended, air-filled esophageal pouch may be visible in esophageal atresia.
      (2) Tracheoesophageal fistula. Fistula is present if an esophageal atresia exists and if air is visible in the stomach and intestine.
      (3) Passage of air through stomach and intestines.
      (4) Location of stomach bubble.
      (5) Bowel gas pattern.
      (6) Presence of pneumatosis intestinalis.
      (7) Presence of calcifications as a result of bowel perforation in utero.
      (8) Fluid, seen as a gasless abdomen. It is necessary to distinguish fluid from masses.
      (9) Pneumoperitoneum. Free air is seen within the peritoneal cavity.
      (10) Obstructions. Gaseous distention of the bowel is seen at various levels, depending on the location of the obstruction.

f. Skeletal system.
   (1) General skeletal assessment. Assess for symmetry, size, continuity, intactness, and abnormalities.
   (2) Fractures of long bones, clavicles, ribs, and skull. A dark line is seen along any portion of a fractured bone because of the air or tissue that settles between the bone fragments (Stedman's Medical Dictionary, 2013).
g. Tubes and catheters.
   (1) Position of endotracheal tube, gastric tube, or chest tube.
   (2) Umbilical catheter placement.
   (3) Central venous line placement.

## RESPIRATORY SYSTEM

**A. The normal chest (Fig. 14-2).**
1. Complete aeration of the chest occurs within a few breaths after onset of respirations at delivery (Kenner and Lott, 2007).
2. Residual fluid may be present in the alveoli after delivery. Early films (<6 hours after delivery) may show increased bronchovascular markings because of this fluid.
3. Normal lung pattern.
   a. Uniform radiolucent appearance.
   b. Hilar and perihilar regions show some increased density because of vascular, bronchial, and hilar structures, which produce some increase in density.
   c. Periphery shows few, if any, markings.
   d. Fluid in the various interlobar fissures represents a normal variation.

**B. Thymus.**
1. Occupies the anterior part of the superior portion of the mediastinum and consists of right and left lobes (Daldrup-Link and Gooding, 2010).
2. Appears as a smoothly rounded outline superior to the cardiac shadow and blending imperceptibly with the cardiac silhouette.
3. Definite notch visible in some cases at the junction of the cardiac silhouette and the thymus.
4. Generally more prominent on the right.
5. Shape may alter markedly with degree of inspiration.
6. Rapid involution during times of stress.
7. Aplasia of the thymus (DiGeorge syndrome).
8. Creation of "sail sign" when mediastinal air lifts the thymus upward.

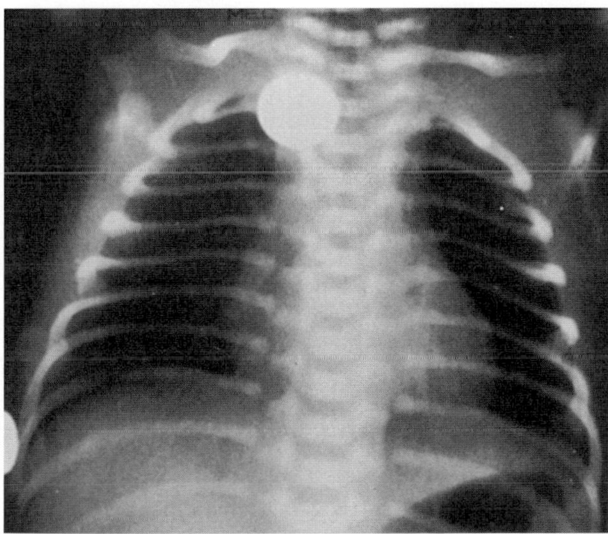

FIGURE 14-2 ■ Normal appearance of chest on x-ray film.

C. **Trachea.**
1. Trachea is normally displaced slightly to the right by the left aortic arch.
2. Deviated trachea supports a mediastinal shift.
3. On inspiration, the trachea dilates and lengthens.
4. On expiration, the trachea constricts and shortens.
5. On deep inspiration, the trachea and major bronchi are well distended and are easily identifiable.

## PULMONARY PARENCHYMAL DISEASE

A. **Respiratory distress syndrome (hyaline membrane disease) (Fig. 14-3, *A*).**
1. Pronounced under aeration. Fewer than eight ribs expand on inspiration on anteroposterior film with doming of the hemidiaphragms on lateral view.
2. Bilateral diffuse alveolar infiltrates. Reticulogranular (ground-glass) appearance is due to microatelectasis of the alveoli (Kenner and Lott, 2007).
3. Homogeneous pattern throughout both lung fields.
4. Air bronchograms. Air-filled bronchi (black) are contrasted against the more radiopaque (whiter) lung fields (Daldrup-Link and Gooding, 2010).
5. With severe disease, a generalized opacity or frank "white-out" appearance (see Fig. 14-3, *B*).
6. Reticulogranular pattern and air bronchograms. May resemble those seen in group B streptococcal pneumonia and may be impossible to distinguish from respiratory distress syndrome.
7. X-ray findings after surfactant administration (Fig. 14-4).
   a. Improvement in pulmonary aeration on x-ray.
   b. Asymmetrical distribution of surfactant, showing areas of improved lung alternating with areas of unchanged respiratory distress syndrome (RDS).
   c. Poor prognosis with pulmonary interstitial emphysema after surfactant therapy.

B. **Transient tachypnea of the newborn (retained fetal lung fluid, wet lung disease) (Fig. 14-5).**
1. Bilateral, symmetrical perihilar streakiness due to increased interstitial and alveolar fluid (Fanaroff and Martin, 2010).
2. Mild to moderate overaeration of the lungs and streaky appearing densities (Daldrup-Link and Gooding, 2010).

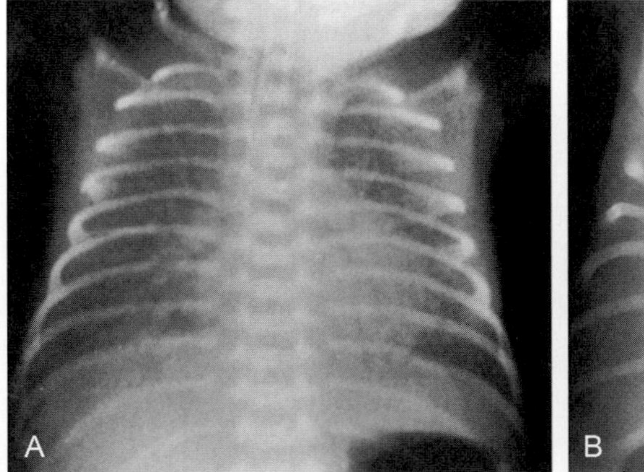

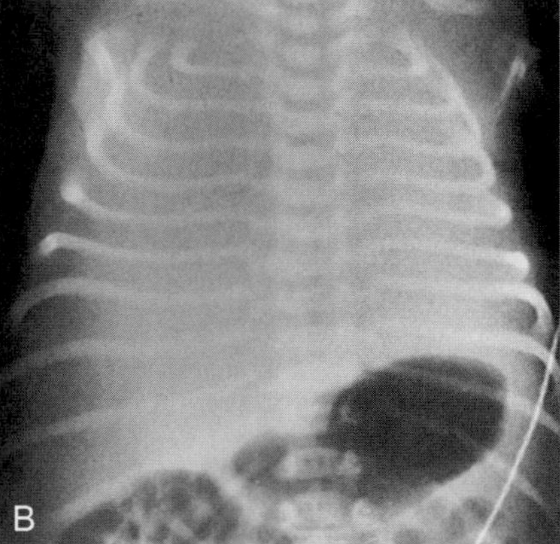


FIGURE 14-3 ■ **A,** Hyaline membrane disease. Note reticulogranular lung pattern and air bronchograms. **B,** Severe hyaline membrane disease. Note "white-out" appearance bilaterally with faint air bronchograms visible.

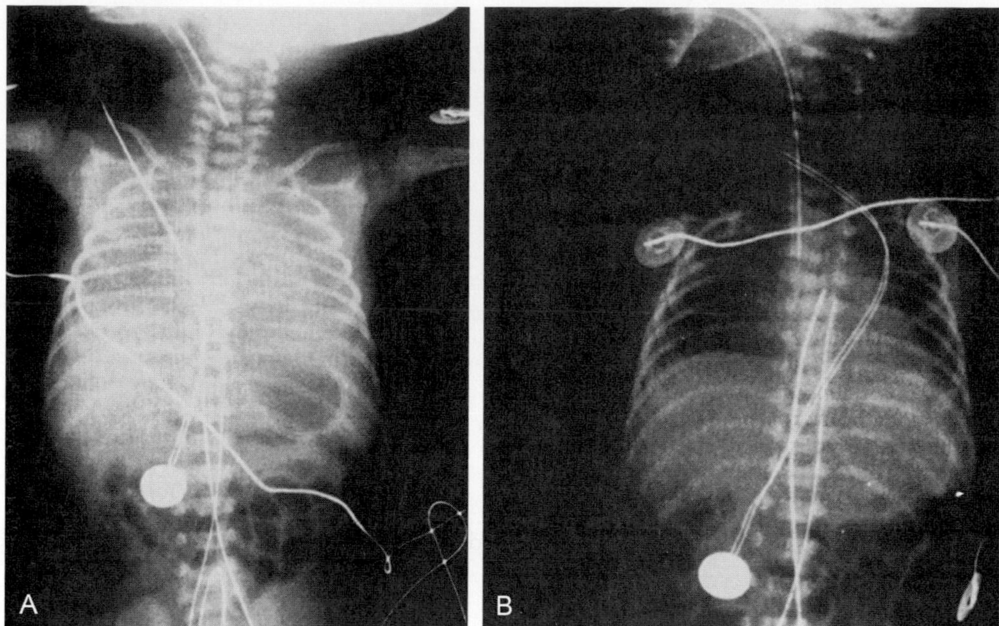


FIGURE 14-4 ■ Hyaline membrane disease before administration of surfactant **(A)** and significant clearing after administration **(B)**.

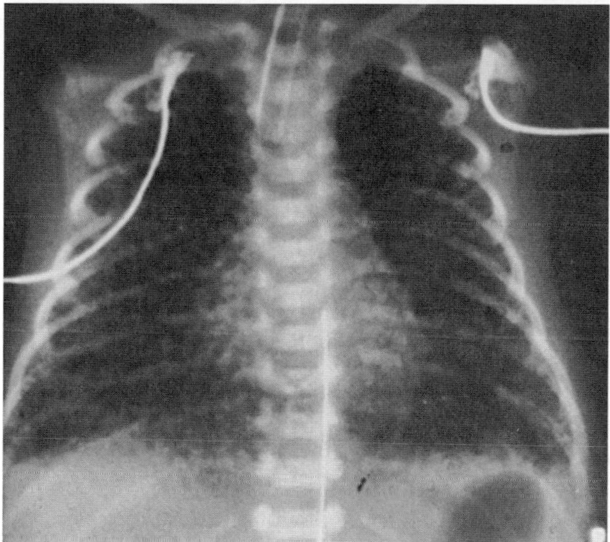

FIGURE 14-5 ■ Transient tachypnea of the newborn. Note mild hyperexpansion and perihilar streakiness. A small pleural effusion is also present on right side.

3. Possible fluid in minor (or horizontal) fissure and major (or oblique) lobar fissure.
4. Mildly enlarged cardiothymic silhouette.
5. Lung fields begin to clear in 24 to 48 hours.

C. **Bronchopulmonary dysplasia (BPD) (Fig. 14-6).**
   1. Initial x-ray picture shows lung disease (e.g., RDS, meconium aspiration syndrome).
   2. Radiologic appearance and course of BPD have changed since Northway and Rosan (1968) described their four stages.

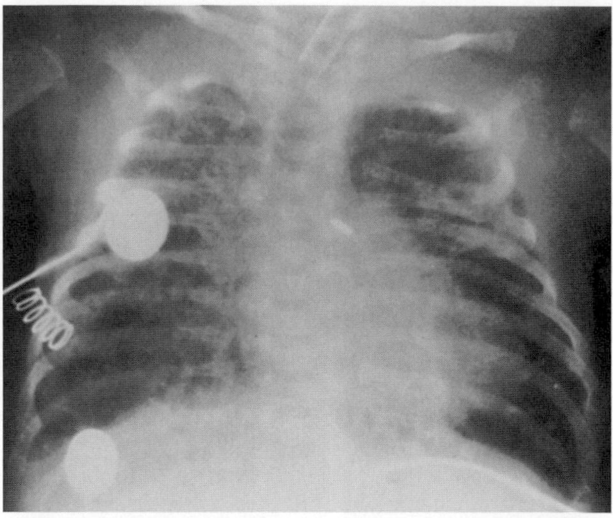

FIGURE 14-6 ■ Bronchopulmonary dysplasia. Note ill-defined densities bilaterally. Also note fractured rib in upper left portion of chest and pale-appearing ribs.

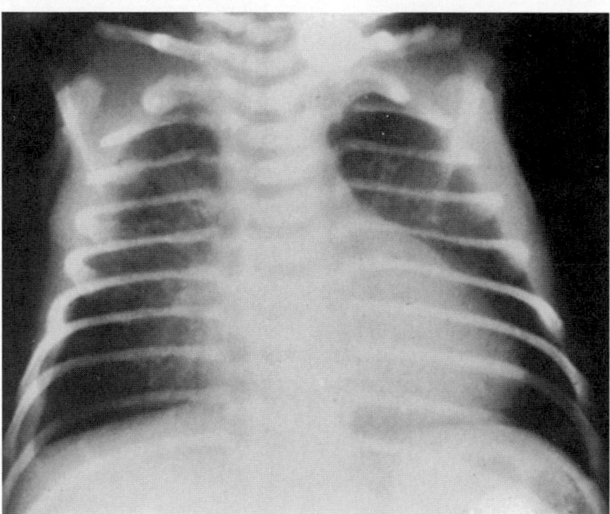

FIGURE 14-7 ■ Pulmonary interstitial emphysema. Note hyperexpansion bilaterally and pinpoint dark bubbles throughout both lung fields.

a. By the end of the first or second week, there is a persistent haziness of vessel margins progressing to linear densities that persist into the third or fourth week of life.
b. Subsequently there is gradual development of a bubbly appearance of the lungs in association with hyperaeration, which is more pronounced at the lung bases. This persists after 1 month of age and represents a modified form of BPD (Fanaroff and Martin, 2010).

D. **Pulmonary interstitial emphysema (Fig. 14-7).**
1. Alveolar overdistention is due to assisted ventilation, visualized as multiple small, cystlike radiolucencies that are bilateral, unilateral, localized, or in a diffuse pattern (Kenner and Lott, 2007).
2. Condition may lead to a pneumothorax or other air leak.

E. **Meconium aspiration syndrome (Fig. 14-8).**
1. Mild cases may show a normal lung pattern to mild infiltrates with overexpanded lungs.
2. Bilateral asymmetrical areas of atelectasis; hyperaeration and air trapping due to debris, with flattened hemidiaphragms (Daldrup-Link and Gooding, 2010).
3. Possible air leaks (pneumothorax or pneumomediastinum) resulting from overdistention and rupture of the alveoli.

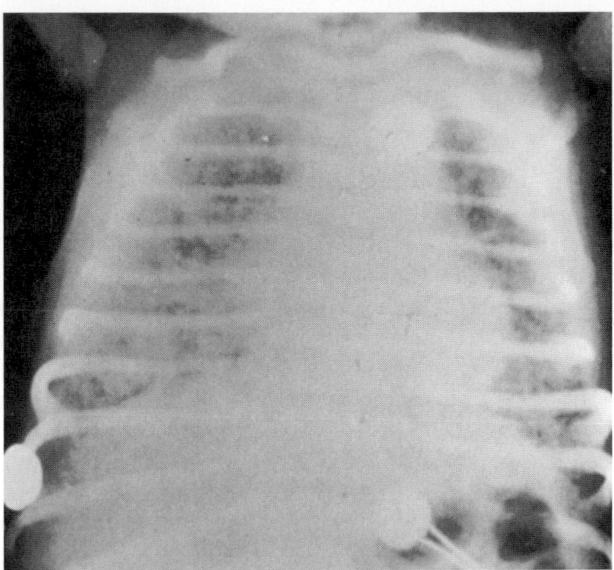

FIGURE 14-8 ■ Meconium aspiration syndrome. Note coarse, patchy infiltrates bilaterally.

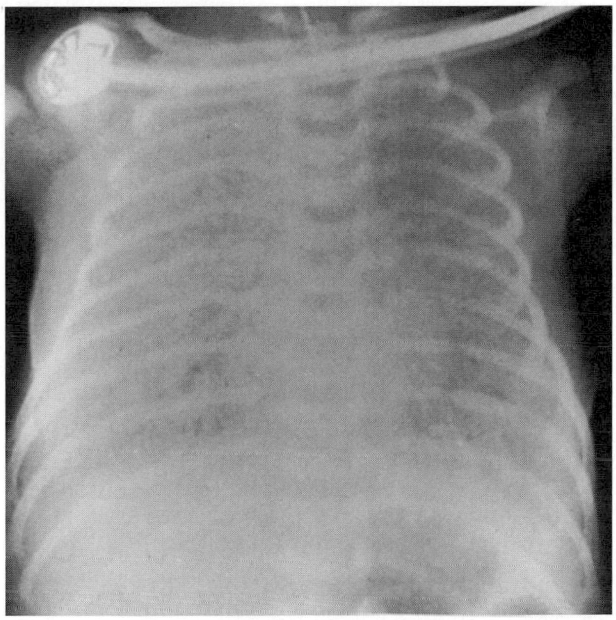

FIGURE 14-9 ■ Group B streptococcal pneumonia. Note reticulogranular appearance seen with hyaline membrane disease.

F. **Pneumonia.**

1. Occasionally asymmetrical, patchy, or streaky bilateral interstitial infiltrate. A nodular pattern may predominate in hazy lungs, and an effusion is a common occurrence (Daldrup-Link and Gooding, 2010).
2. Reticulogranular pattern similar to that of RDS. Some alveoli contain inflammatory exudate, which will appear more opaque on x-ray than those filled with air (Daldrup-Link and Gooding, 2010).
3. Group B streptococcal pneumonia is often difficult to diagnose on x-ray due to variable lung volumes and variable densities. May be indistinguishable from RDS (Kenner and Lott, 2007) (Fig. 14-9).

## PULMONARY AIR LEAKS

A. **Pneumothorax (Fig. 14-10, *A*).**
  1. Accumulation of air in the pleural space. Air can outline the lung circumferentially or can accumulate.
  2. Mediastinal shift of structures away from the affected side as air accumulates (tension pneumothorax) (Daldrup-Link and Gooding, 2010).
  3. Outline of the collapsed lung, with a band of hyperlucency between the chest wall and the underlying lung (Daldrup-Link and Gooding, 2010).
  4. Other findings related to pneumothorax.
    a. Pneumothorax not under tension may not exhibit a mediastinal shift.
    b. Diaphragm on affected side of a pneumothorax under tension will be flattened because of tension placed on it by air accumulation superior to it (Kenner and Lott, 2007).
    c. Skinfold may mimic a pneumothorax (Kenner and Lott, 2007) (see Fig. 14-10, *B*).

B. **Pneumomediastinum (Fig. 14-11).**
  1. Mediastinal air collection, which produces irregular gas collections within the soft tissues of the superior mediastinum, with air frequently outlining the undersurface of the thymus gland and thus creating a "sail sign" (Daldrup-Link and Gooding, 2010).
  2. Can accompany a pneumothorax.
  3. On cross-table lateral film, a radiolucent area of hyperlucency in the superior retrosternal space.

C. **Pneumopericardium (Fig. 14-12).**
  1. Radiolucent halo of free air surrounds the heart as air accumulates within the pericardial space (Daldrup-Link and Gooding, 2010).
  2. Width of air around the heart is proportional to the amount of air present. Air is limited to the pericardium and cannot extend beyond the origins of the aorta and pulmonary artery.
  3. Decreased cardiac size may indicate cardiac tamponade.
  4. Other pulmonary air leaks and/or pulmonary interstitial emphysema are generally present.
  5. Pneumopericardium is rare in the absence of assisted ventilation.

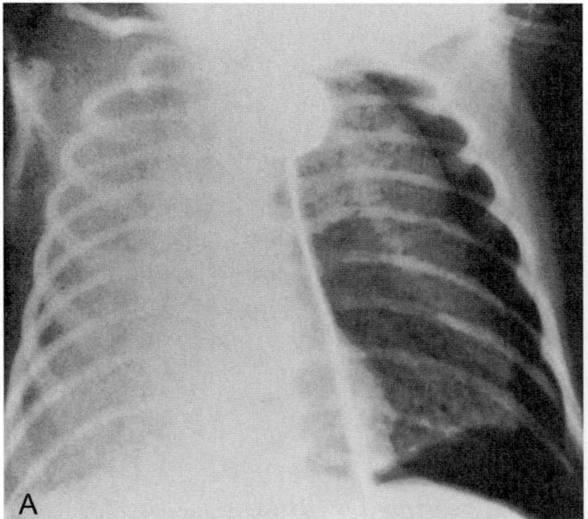


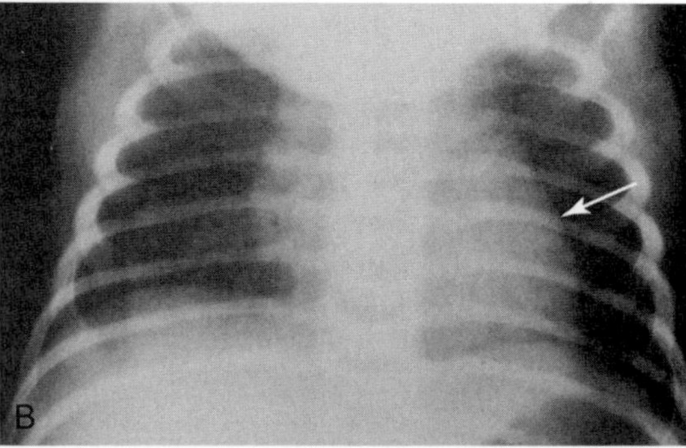


FIGURE 14-10 ■ **A,** Left tension pneumothorax. Note mediastinal shift toward right side. **B,** Note skinfold on right (*arrow*). It can be mistaken for a pneumothorax. It extends beyond chest and crosses over diaphragm.

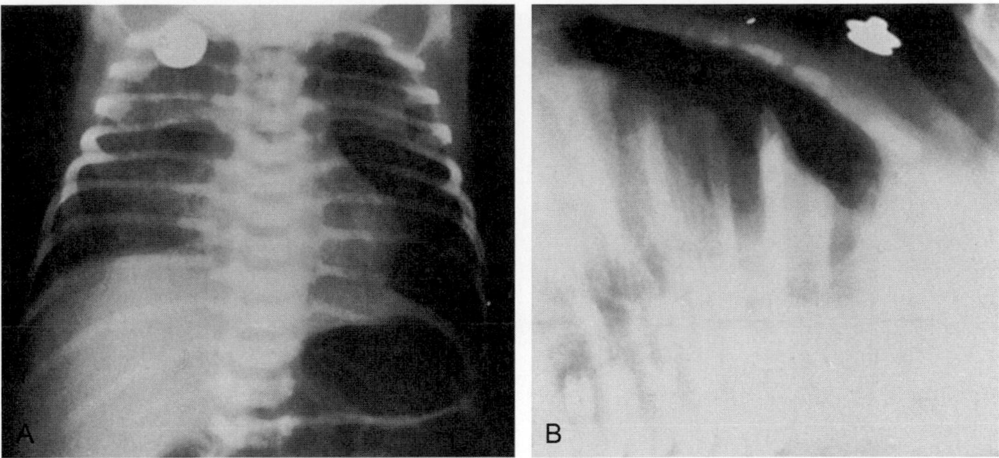


FIGURE 14-11 ■ **A,** Pneumomediastinum with thymus lifted, demonstrating the "sail sign." **B,** Pneumomediastinum on lateral view. Note air in anterior chest outlines thymus.

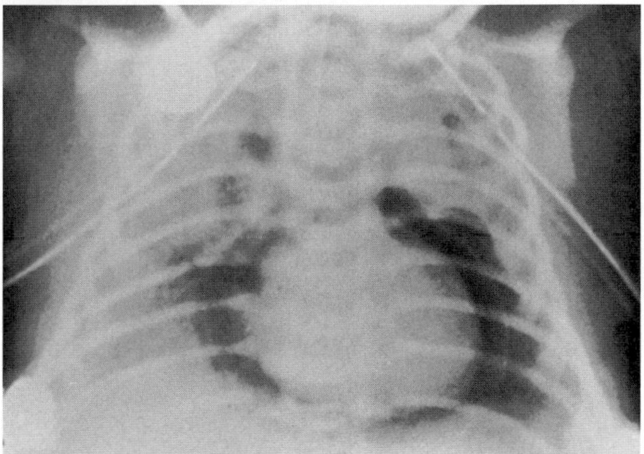

FIGURE 14-12 ■ Pneumopericardium. Note air completely encircles heart. Bilateral chest tubes are also in place.

## MISCELLANEOUS CAUSES OF RESPIRATORY DISTRESS

A. **Diaphragmatic paralysis (phrenic nerve injury) (Fig. 14-13).**
   1. Elevation and fixation of a diaphragmatic leaflet (Daldrup-Link and Gooding, 2010).
   2. More common on the right than the left side and usually unilateral.
   3. Mediastinum may be shifted away from the affected side.
   4. Most often results from obstetric injury to the brachial plexus (Erb's palsy), an associated finding.

B. **Eventration of the diaphragm (Fig. 14-14).**
   1. Weakness of the hemidiaphragm, with abdominal organs pushing up against it but not entering the chest because no opening exists.
   2. Either partial or complete; usually right-sided (Daldrup-Link and Gooding, 2010).

C. **Pulmonary edema (Fig. 14-15).**
   1. Increased pulmonary permeability is common in premature infants with lung injury that can manifest as diffuse haziness of the lungs to a white-out appearance (Daldrup-Link and Gooding, 2010).
   2. Association between high fluid intake and subsequent occurrence of a clinically significant patent ductus arteriosus and BPD (Kenner and Lott, 2007).
   3. Common with certain congenital heart defects due to increased pulmonary blood flow (coarctation of the aorta, hypoplastic left heart syndrome).

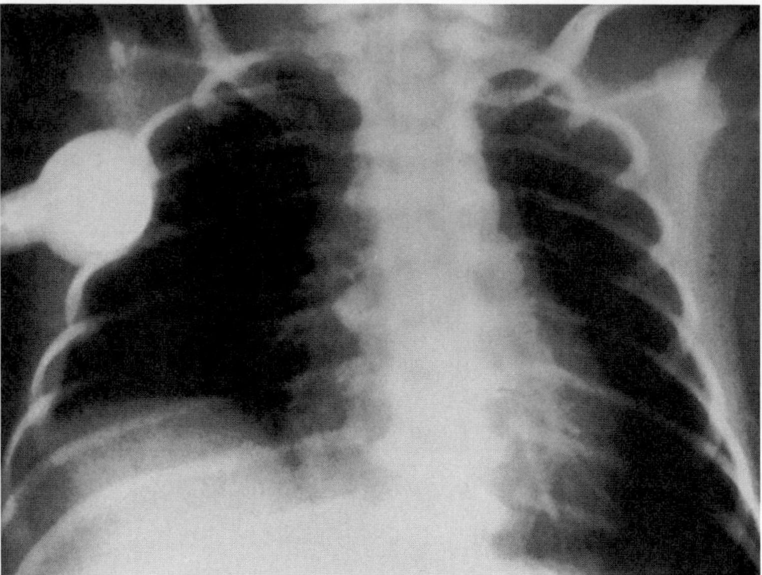

FIGURE 14-13 ■ Paralysis of right side of diaphragm. Note right side of diaphragm is markedly elevated in comparison with left side of diaphragm.

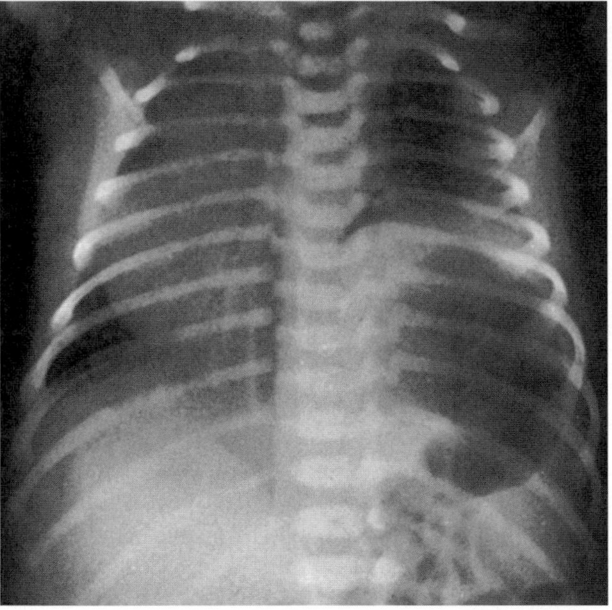

FIGURE 14-14 ■ Eventration of diaphragm. Note left side of diaphragm bulging upward, with stomach pushing upward against it.

# THORACIC SURGICAL PROBLEMS

**A. Congenital diaphragmatic hernia (Fig. 14-16, *A*).**

1. Herniation of abdominal contents through various portions of the diaphragm into the thoracic cavity, most commonly through the foramen of Bochdalek (Daldrup-Link and Gooding, 2010).
2. The majority occur on the left side.
3. Hemithorax filled with loops of bowel, stomach, and often liver; displaces the mediastinal structures away from the affected side.
4. Abdomen relatively gasless and may be scaphoid.

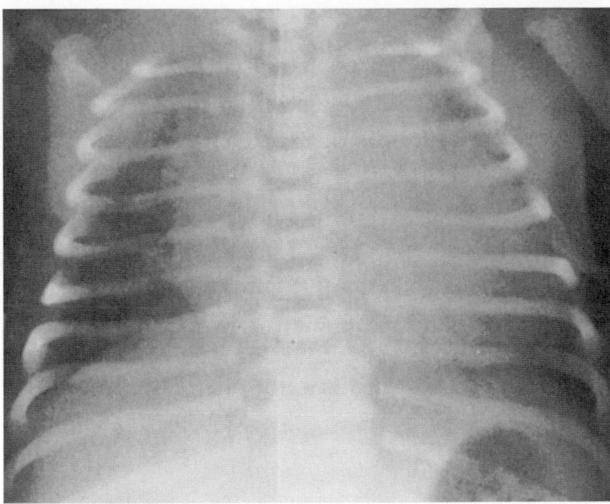

FIGURE 14-15 ■ Pulmonary edema. Note congested lung fields and cardiomegaly.

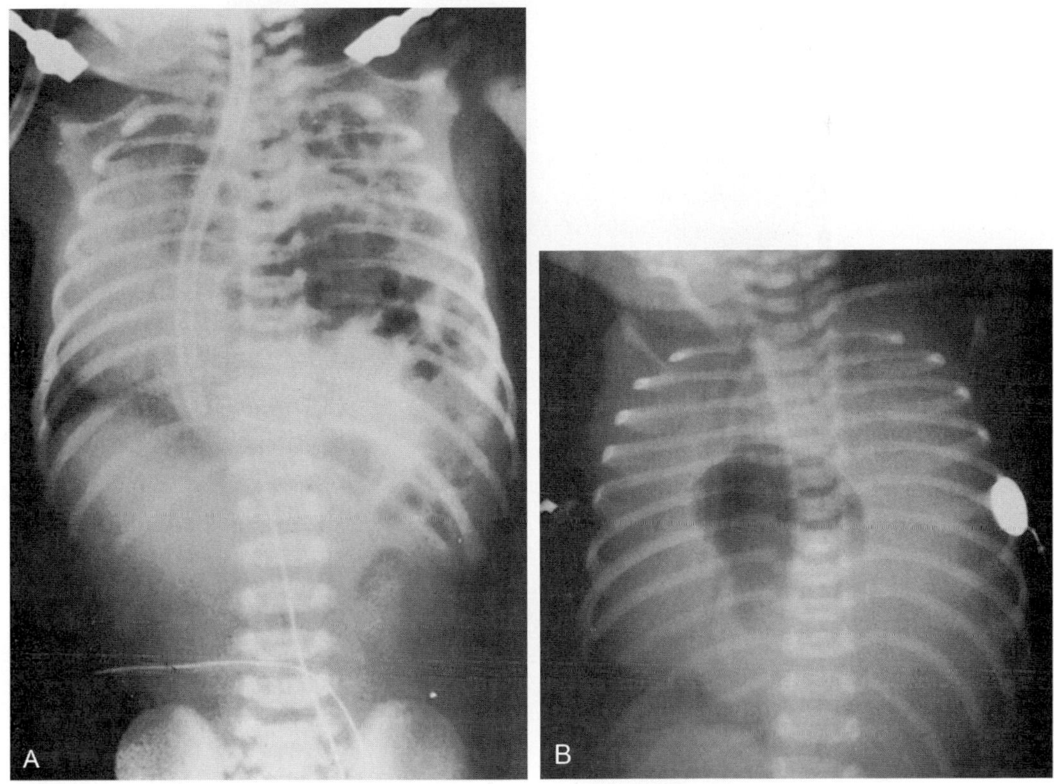


FIGURE 14-16 ■ **A,** Left diaphragmatic hernia. Note presence of bowel in left side of chest, a mediastinal shift to right, and lack of bowel in abdomen. **B,** Left diaphragmatic hernia before much air has expanded bowel. Note that trachea and heart have shifted to right.

5. Contralateral pneumothorax possible with assisted ventilation or as a result of pulmonary hypoplasia on the unaffected side.
6. If the x-ray is obtained before the bowel is expanded with air, the affected hemithorax may appear entirely opacified with the mediastinal structures shifted to the opposite side (Daldrup-Link and Gooding, 2010) (see Fig. 14-16, *B*).

B. **Congenital lobar emphysema (Fig. 14-17).**
   1. Most common cause of cystic malformation of the lung.
   2. Air trapped within one or more lung lobes at birth, resulting in obstructive emphysema.
   3. Overdistended affected lobe, with mediastinum shifted to contralateral side.
   4. Possibly hyperlucent but may also be opaque because of fluid accumulation distal to the obstruction (Fanaroff and Martin, 2010).
   5. Generally limited to the upper lobes.

C. **Cystic adenomatoid malformation (Fig. 14-18).**
   1. Overdistention of affected lobe, with mediastinal shift to contralateral side.
   2. Lobar overdistention, caused by air and fluid.
   3. Upper lobes most frequently affected (Fanaroff and Martin, 2010).
   4. X-ray findings: multiple air-filled cysts, mediastinal shift, and compression of opposite lung. Diaphragmatic hernia must be ruled out.

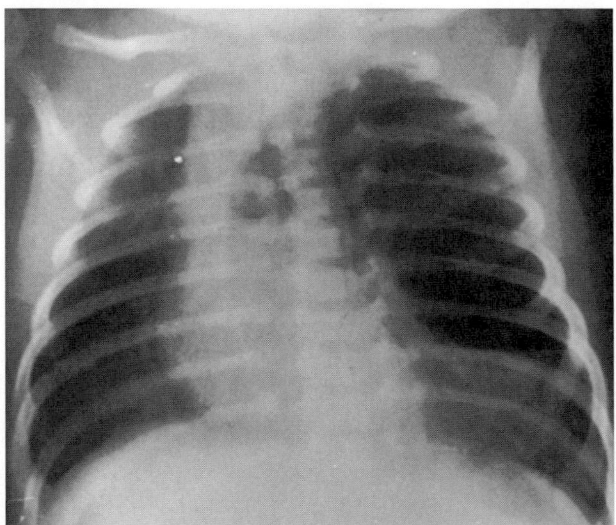

FIGURE 14-17 ■ Congenital lobar emphysema. Note hyperlucency of left upper lung lobe, with mediastinal shift toward right.

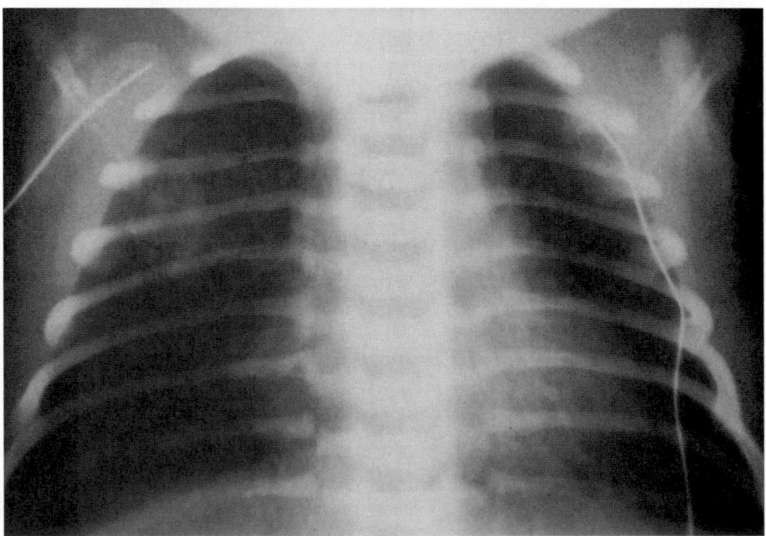

FIGURE 14-18 ■ Cystic adenomatoid malformation in right lung.

## CARDIOVASCULAR SYSTEM

**A. Size of the heart.**

1. Difficult to assess on anteroposterior film because of a large thymus. Lateral film assessing a specific chamber enlargement may be more useful.
2. Enlargement suggested by cardiothoracic ratio greater than 65% (Daldrup-Link and Gooding, 2010) (Fig. 14-19).
3. Malpositioning: may represent cardiac displacement, developmentally abnormal cardiac position, or ambiguous rotation or site.
4. Possible transient enlargement as a result of polycythemia, perinatal anoxia, or normally increased fluid present at birth (Kenner and Lott, 2007).

**B. Pulmonary vascularity.**

1. Normal vascular markings are seen in the middle one third of the lung fields (Fig. 14-20).
2. Decreased vascular markings occur with obstruction along the right ventricular outflow tract of the heart and are manifested as hyperlucency in both lung fields (Fig. 14-21).
3. Increased pulmonary vascularity occurs when excess blood flow causes congestion in the blood vessels and is manifested as increased streakiness, hazy lung fields, and increased densities as the condition worsens.

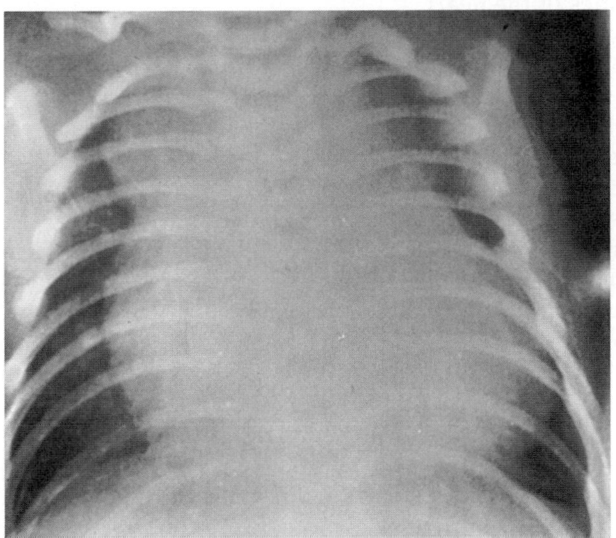

FIGURE 14-19 ■ Cardiomegaly. Note enlarged heart occupies majority of thorax.

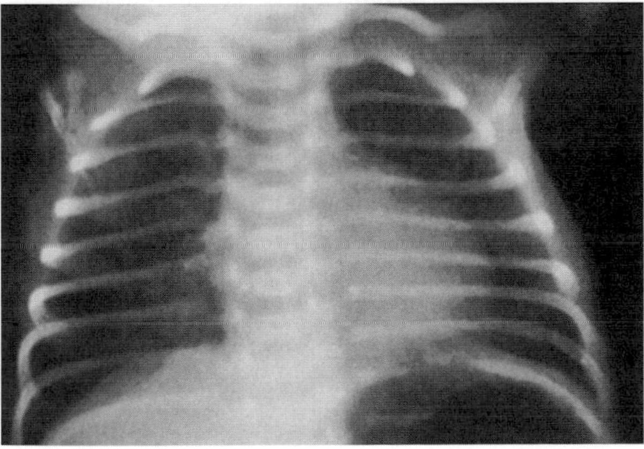

FIGURE 14-20 ■ Normal pulmonary vascularity. Note presence of vascularity radiating from perihilar region.

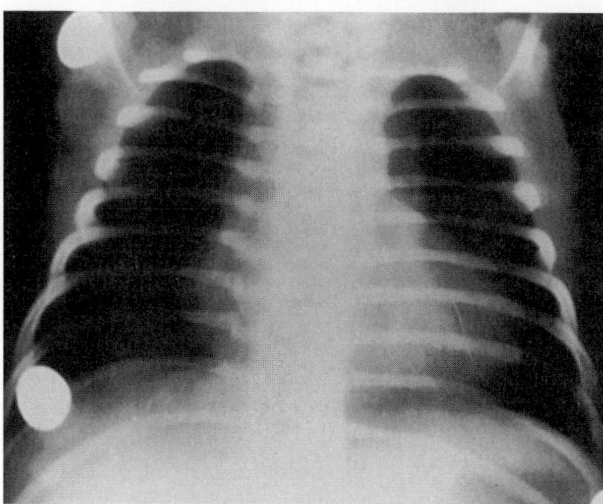

FIGURE 14-21 ■ Hyperlucent lung fields because of decreased blood flow to lungs.

**C. Positional anomalies of the heart.**

1. Types of malposition are as follows (Falkensammer et al., 2008):
   a. Dextrocardia: mirror image of its normal position with apex pointed to the right.
   b. Mesocardia: midline heart.
   c. Extrathoracic: heart develops outside the thoracic cavity, as in ectopia cordis.
2. Position of other organs in relation to the heart is also incorporated into the definition of cardiac malposition. Positions of the abdominal organs are as follows:
   a. Situs solitus: normal abdominal organ position.
   b. Situs inversus: stomach and spleen on right, liver on left, and left atrium on right.
   c. Situs ambiguus: abdominal organs and atrial position are anatomically uncertain. The liver may be symmetrical and at midline, and the stomach may be central. There may be duplication or absence of unilateral structures such as the spleen (asplenia or polysplenia).
3. "Mirror image" dextrocardia with situs inversus is the most common type of malposition (Falkensammer et al., 2008) (Fig. 14-22).
4. Concomitant congenital heart disease occurrs in approximately 50% of patients with cardiac malposition (Falkensammer et al., 2008).
5. Cardiac malposition caused by shift of the heart within the thorax must be differentiated from extracardiac causes, such as pneumothorax, hypoplastic lung, diaphragmatic hernia, decreased lung volume, and lung mass.

**D. Lesions with increased pulmonary vascularity.**

1. Left-to-right shunt or intracardiac mixing.
   a. Transposition of the great vessels. Plain film shows "egg on a string" appearance. Cardiac silhouette of normal size or mild cardiomegaly may be seen (Daldrup-Link and Gooding, 2010). Pulmonary vascularity is variable, depending on the presence or absence of a ventricular septal defect or a patent ductus arteriosus.
   b. Total anomalous pulmonary venous return. X-ray film shows cardiomegaly; increased pulmonary vascularity; and enlargement of the right atrium, right ventricle, and pulmonary artery. The "snowman" appearance of the heart, caused by a characteristic widening of the superior mediastinum due to the connecting blood vessels, is rarely seen in the neonate because of the slow development of excessive pulmonary blood flow (Daldrup-Link and Gooding, 2010).
   c. Atrioventricular canal defect (endocardial cushion defect). Pulmonary vascular resistance usually remains high enough to delay the onset of CHF until after the first 1 to 2 weeks, after which marked cardiomegaly and vascular congestion are evident.
   d. Truncus arteriosus. Right and left ventricles are prominent, with left atrial dilation. As CHF develops, pulmonary vessels become indistinct and obscured by pulmonary edema.

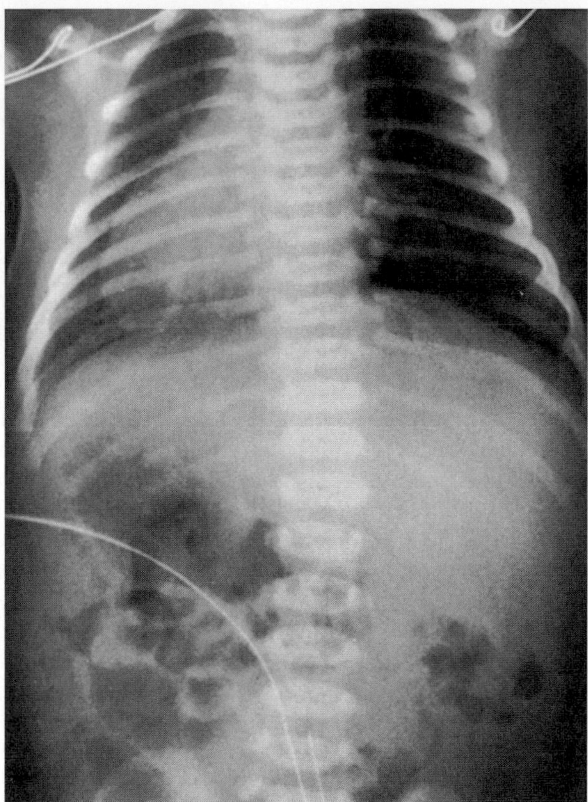

FIGURE 14-22 ■ "Mirror image" dextrocardia. Note apex of heart pointing to right, with stomach located on right and liver on left.

e. Atrial septal defect. Chest x-ray may be normal, with small defects. With large left-to-right shunts, there are moderate cardiac enlargement and increased pulmonary vascularity. The right atrium and right ventricle are enlarged.

f. Ventricular septal defect. With small defects the heart size and vascularity may be normal. With moderate-sized defects, heart size may be enlarged, with increased pulmonary vascular markings. With large defects and increased blood flow, cardiomegaly is evident because of right and left ventricular enlargement. Pulmonary vascularity is markedly increased. CHF, interstitial edema, and alveolar fluid may be present.

g. Patent ductus arteriosus. Pulmonary vasculature and cardiac silhouette may be obscured by underlying lung disease of RDS. Lung fields may show pulmonary edema and increasing heart size compared with heart size on previous x-ray films (Daldrup-Link and Gooding, 2010).

2. Left-sided obstruction. Outflow of blood from the left side of the heart or return of blood from the lungs is obstructed, which will eventually cause CHF (Kenner and Lott, 2007).

a. Hypoplastic left heart syndrome (aortic atresia, mitral atresia). Pulmonary vascularity may appear normal until significant cardiac decompensation is present, and then cardiomegaly and CHF become evident. Right atrial enlargement may also be seen (Daldrup-Link and Gooding, 2010).

b. Coarctation of the aorta. Heart size is normal, but left ventricular enlargement may subsequently be seen on lateral views (Kenner and Lott, 2007). X-ray findings vary according to the degree of patency of the patent ductus arteriosus and the severity of the obstruction at the coarctation site. CHF occurs, with ductal closure resulting in cardiomegaly and pulmonary venous congestion.

c. Aortic stenosis. Normal cardiac size and vasculature may be seen, with mild stenosis of the aortic valve. Left ventricular enlargement occurs, with cardiac decompensation or associated aortic regurgitation resulting in cardiomegaly and venous congestion.

3. Lesions with decreased pulmonary vascularity. All these lesions involve some form of obstruction to the normal flow of blood through the right outflow tract. They can be located anywhere from the tricuspid valve to the pulmonary artery.
   a. Pulmonary valve atresia with intact ventricular septum. Pulmonary vascularity is reduced or normal, depending on alternative sources of pulmonary blood flow, such as a patent ductus arteriosus. A shallow or concave pulmonary artery is evident. Closure of the ductus arteriosus and obstruction of the right ventricular outflow tract cause decreased pulmonary blood flow. Pulmonary vessels are underfilled and appear small and thin, which results in dark, hyperlucent lung fields. Heart size is variable, but cardiomegaly is usually present because of right atrial and left ventricular enlargement.
   b. Tricuspid atresia. Tricuspid valve has complete atresia, and the right ventricle and right outflow tract are underdeveloped. Chest x-ray shows a normal or small heart and diminished pulmonary blood flow.
   c. Tetralogy of Fallot. Cardiac size and shape are frequently normal. Pulmonary vascular markings are decreased. A "boot-shaped" contour may occur from a small, concave pulmonary artery and a prominent cardiac apex as a result of right ventricular hypertrophy.
   d. Pulmonary stenosis. Severe valvular obstruction is associated with hypoxemia because of a right-to-left shunt at the foramen ovale. This is referred to as critical pulmonary stenosis. Neonate's chest x-ray is normal, but cardiomegaly with predominant right atrium and right ventricle, decreased pulmonary vascularity, and dilation of the pulmonary artery eventually occur.

## GASTROINTESTINAL SYSTEM

**A. Characteristics of the normal abdomen (Fig. 14-23).**

1. Air is present in the stomach immediately after birth because of respiratory movement of the thorax and swallowing of air. By 24 hours of life, air should appear in the rectum (Kenner and Lott, 2007).
2. A gasless abdomen may be seen in infants with decreased swallowing or obstruction, decreased GI motility (i.e., with intubation or chemical paralysis), vomiting, or gastric decompression from suctioning.
3. Resuscitation may increase the amount of bowel gas seen on an x-ray.

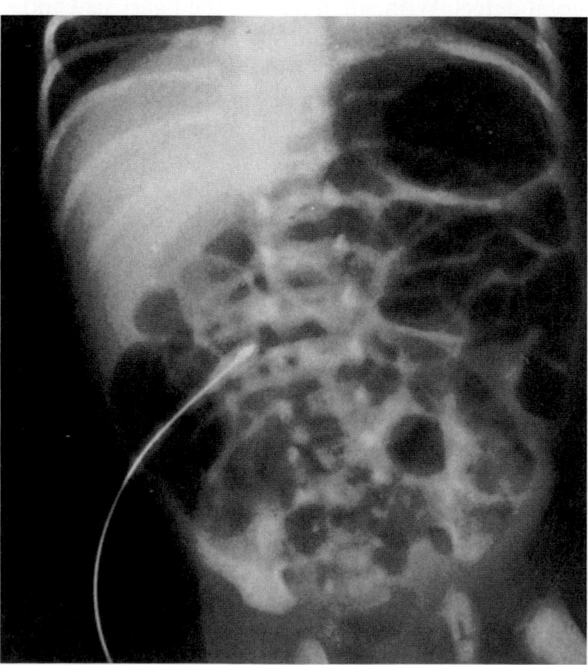

FIGURE 14-23 ■ Normal bowel gas pattern. Note presence of stomach bubble and air through entire abdomen to rectum.

**B. The esophagus.**

1. May show indentations near the aortic arch and left mainstem bronchus.
2. May assume peculiar configurations because of flexibility during the respiratory cycle.
3. Air in the esophagus is a normal finding on regular chest films.

**C. Esophageal abnormalities.**

1. Esophageal atresia (Fig. 14-24, *A*). A portion of the esophagus is atretic, and both distal and proximal portions of the esophagus end in blind pouches.
   a. On x-ray a radiolucent, air-filled, distended proximal esophageal pouch is present. The abdomen is gasless because no air can enter. The proximal pouch can be identified by passing a radiopaque tube and obtaining a chest film. The tube will not advance beyond 9 to 11 cm (Kenner and Lott, 2007).
   b. Aspiration pneumonitis of the upper lobes, especially the right upper lobe, is a common finding.

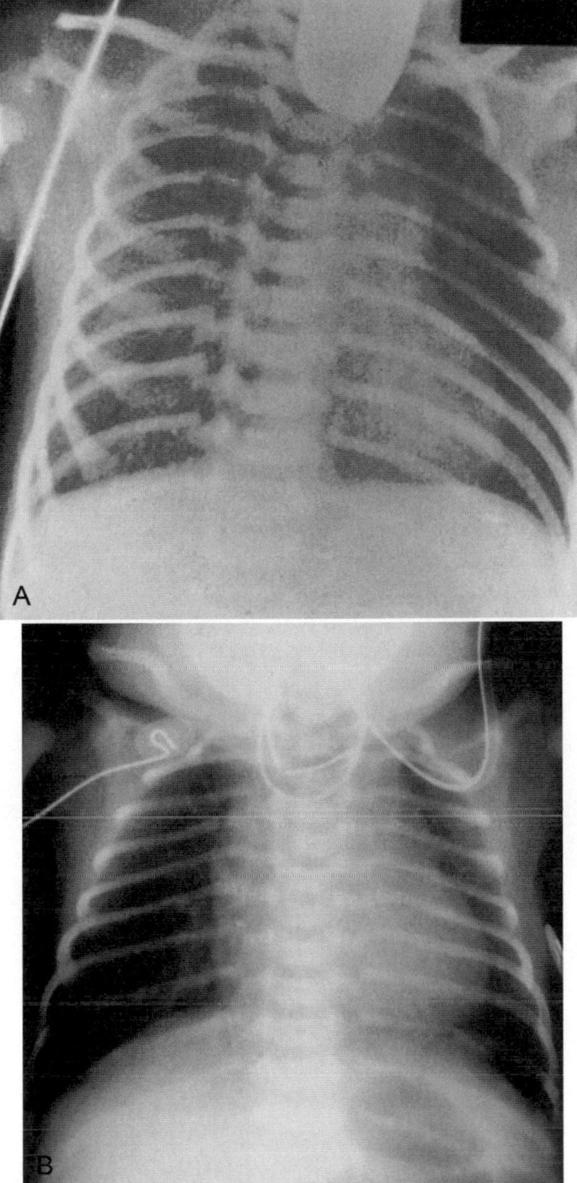


FIGURE 14-24 ■ **A,** Esophageal atresia. Contrast medium outlines esophagus, which ends in blind pouch. **B,** Esophageal atresia with tracheoesophageal fistula. Gastric tube cannot be advanced because of esophageal atresia. Air is in abdomen, confirming presence of tracheoesophageal fistula.

2. Esophageal atresia with tracheoesophageal fistula (see Fig. 14-24, *B*).
   a. Esophageal atresia with fistulous connection to the distal esophageal pouch is the most common esophageal anomaly.
   b. Excessive dilation of the stomach and/or small bowel, resulting from distal fistula communication between the lungs and the stomach, may occur.
   c. Chest film should be obtained with a radiopaque tube in place. The tube will not advance into the stomach, and air will be present in the GI tract.
3. Tracheoesophageal fistula with no esophageal atresia (H type of fistula).
   a. Difficult to identify without a contrast study.
   b. Fistula characteristically assumes an upwardly oblique configuration on contrast study.
   c. Widespread pulmonary infiltrates are commonly present because of constant aspiration through the fistula into the lungs.

**D. The stomach.**
1. Visible directly beneath the left diaphragm.
2. Often appears large in the neonate as a result of dilation with air.
3. Mucosal folds are absent. Stomach wall appears smooth.
4. Begins to empty moments after being filled.

**E. Abnormalities of the stomach.**
1. Pyloric stenosis.
   a. Symptoms develop 2 to 8 weeks after birth (Kenner and Lott, 2007).
   b. Plain films demonstrate a distended stomach and duodenum, with disproportionately less gas in the small bowel.
   c. Ultrasonography is the study of choice for the diagnosis.
2. Gastric perforation.
   a. Uncommon, but may result from gastric ulcers, hypoxia-induced focal necrosis, gastric tubes, or indomethacin therapy for closure of ductus arteriosus.
   b. Possible overinflation due to distal obstruction, as with mechanical ventilation.
   c. Common finding of free air (pneumoperitoneum) with absence of gastric gas.

**F. Duodenal abnormalities (Fig. 14-25).**
1. Duodenal atresia and stenosis.
   a. Infants with duodenal atresia present with vomiting in the first few hours of life. Those with stenosis present at variable times, depending on the degree of stenosis.
   b. Duodenal atresia and stenosis are present in approximately 25% to 40% of infants with Down syndrome (trisomy 21) (Karrer et al., 2012).
   c. X-ray demonstrates dilation of the stomach and proximal duodenum, producing the characteristic "double bubble" pattern. No air is present distal to the duodenum.

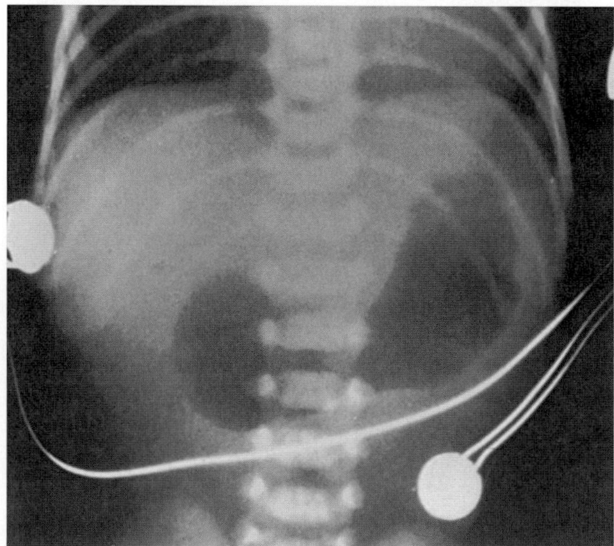

FIGURE 14-25 ■ Duodenal atresia with characteristic "double bubble" pattern.

2. Annular pancreas.
   a. Pancreas grows in the form of an encircling ring around the duodenum (Kenner and Lott, 2007).
   b. Presentation is similar to that of duodenal atresia or stenosis.
   c. X-ray findings are generally indistinguishable from duodenal atresia or stenosis. Identification is made with ultrasonography.

G. **Abnormalities of the small bowel.**
   1. Small-bowel atresia and stenosis.
      a. Single or multiple areas of atresia or stenosis may exist.
      b. Clinically, abdominal distention and bile-stained vomiting are apparent early on.
      c. Types of small-bowel atresia.
         (1) High jejunal obstruction: one or two loops of bowel are visible on x-ray.
         (2) Midjejunal obstruction: more dilated loops are visible on x-ray.
         (3) Distal ileal atresia: many dilated loops are visible on x-ray.
   2. Meconium ileus (Fig. 14-26).
      a. Approximately 13% to 17% of infants with cystic fibrosis present with meconium ileus at birth (van der Doef et al., 2011).
      b. Obstruction results from impaction of thick, tenacious meconium in the distal portion of the small bowel. Ileal atresia or stenosis, ileal perforation, meconium peritonitis, and volvulus are common complications.
      c. Clinical presentation includes bile-stained vomiting, abdominal distention, and failure to pass meconium.
      d. X-ray shows a low small-bowel obstruction with numerous, variably sized air-filled loops of bowel. There is a "soap bubble" appearance in the right lower quadrant as a result of trapping of air in meconium.
      e. A contrast-enema study will demonstrate a microcolon. A water-soluble contrast agent draws large amounts of fluid into the intestine and lubricates the meconium, allowing it to pass without surgical intervention. This technique along with medical laxative treatment can decrease the need for surgical interventions.
   3. Midgut volvulus.
      a. Most common form of small-bowel volvulus.
      b. Twisting and spiraling of entire gut around the superior mesenteric artery, resulting in vascular compromise, necrosis, perforation, and gangrene.
      c. May present with bilious vomiting.

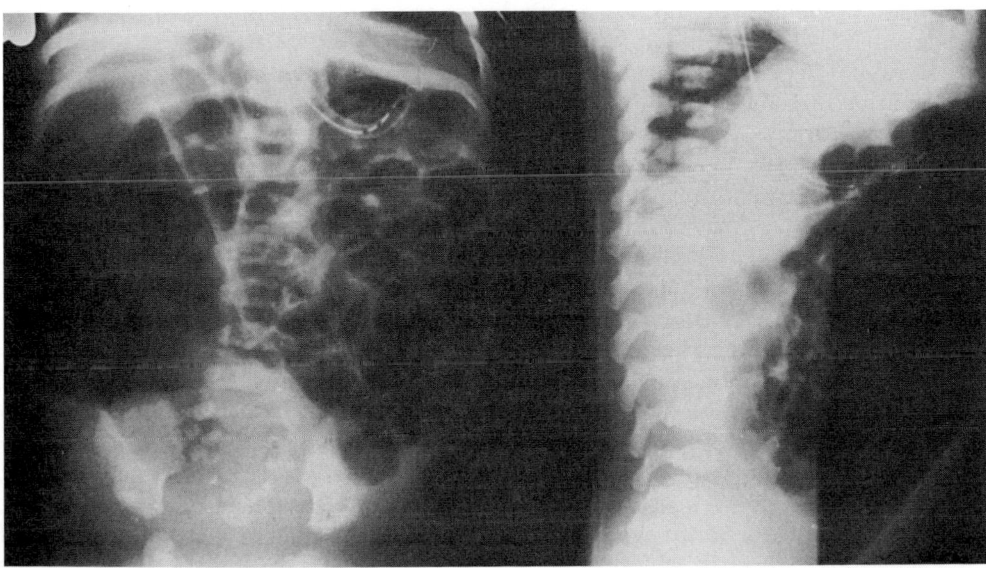

FIGURE 14-26 ■ Meconium ileus with perforation and free air visible on lateral film.

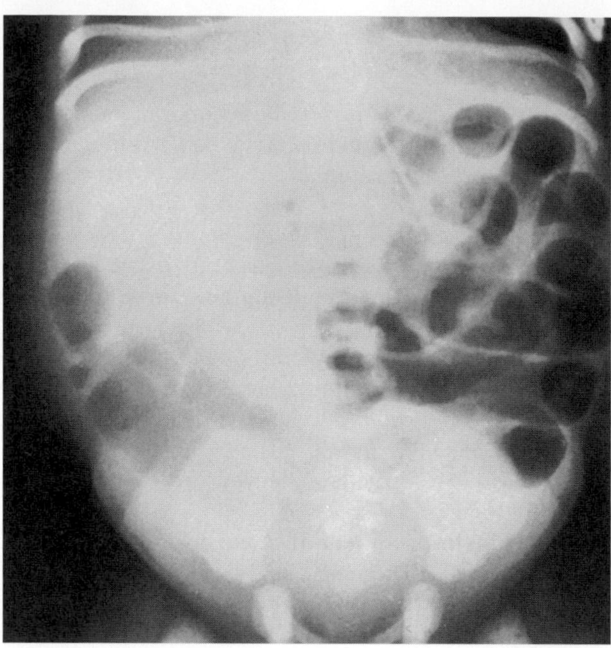

FIGURE 14-27 ■ Hirschsprung's disease. Note abdominal distention with dilated loops of bowel and lack of air present in distal portion of bowel.

d. May be difficult to determine on x-ray because findings are variable, from a normal abdomen to one suggesting a gastric outlet obstruction, partial obstruction of the duodenum, or small-bowel obstruction.
e. Ultrasonography, barium enema, or x-ray of upper GI tract may be needed for diagnostic purposes or to demonstrate complete obstruction of third portion of duodenum.

**H. Abnormalities of the colon.**

1. Hirschsprung's disease (aganglionosis of the colon) (Fig. 14-27).
   a. Typical presentation is vomiting, obstruction, and failure to pass meconium within the first 24 to 36 hours of life.
   b. Commonly involves the distal colonic segment—rectal and rectosigmoid areas.
   c. Plain films show some degree of low small-bowel or colonic obstruction, air–fluid levels, and distention of the bowel (Kenner and Lott, 2007). Rectal gas may be absent or sparse.
   d. Barium enema will support the findings, and a rectal biopsy will show absence of ganglion cells.
2. Meconium plug syndrome/small left colon syndrome.
   a. Normal meconium becomes impacted in the distal portion of the colon. In meconium plug syndrome, the obstruction is generally in the sigmoid colon. In small left colon, the site of obstruction is the splenic flexure.
   b. Functional immaturity of the colon is thought to be the cause of the initial inability to pass meconium.
   c. Condition is manifested within the first 23 to 36 hours of life with abdominal distention, bilious vomiting, and failure to pass meconium.
   d. Diagnosis is by contrast-enema examination. The examination may also be therapeutic by dislodgment of the meconium.
   e. Plain films are nonspecific and usually show a low small bowel with distention of the bowel obstruction.
3. Necrotizing enterocolitis (Fig. 14-28).
   a. X-ray findings include generalized distention caused by paralytic ileus, asymmetrical distribution of bowel gas, and localized distention of bowel loops.
   b. X-ray films are obtained every 6 to 8 hours to follow the progression of the disease in the acute phase. A cross-table lateral view, along with plain film, should be obtained to detect free air.

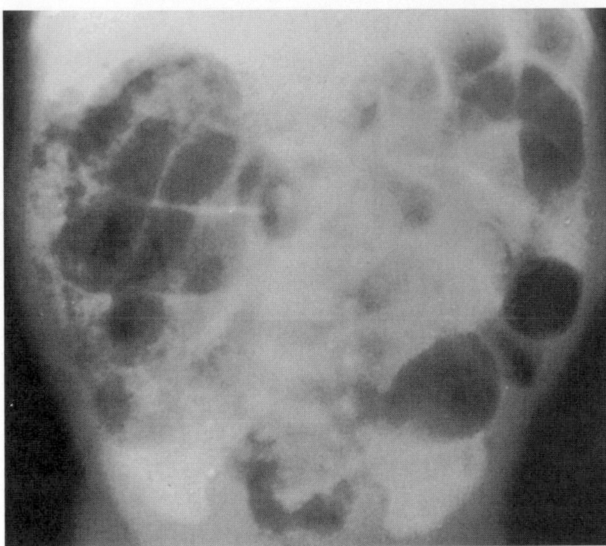

FIGURE 14-28 ■ Necrotizing enterocolitis. Note presence of distended bowel loops and pneumatosis intestinalis.

c. Subsequently, individual loops may become tubular, with thickened bowel walls.
d. Persistently dilated loops may be evident on consecutive films.
e. At any point, pneumatosis cystoides intestinalis can be seen. This represents gas formed in the intestinal wall by bacteria. The typical picture is linear or of a bubbly or foamy appearance. Air may be located in the submucosal or subserosal layer and can enter the GI tract or portal venous system (Kenner and Lott, 2007).
f. Right segment of colon and terminal ileum are most likely to be affected, although the entire colon may be affected.
g. The most common cause of intestinal perforation, seen as free abdominal gas on plain film or in left lateral decubitus view.

**I. Pneumoperitoneum (see Fig. 14-26).**

1. Most commonly a result of perforation of the GI tract because of perinatal asphyxia, indomethacin therapy, gastric overdistention, iatrogenic perforation with a thermometer, and as a complication of necrotizing enterocolitis and GI obstruction (Kenner and Lott, 2007).
2. Air may dissect from the neonate's chest during positive pressure ventilation.
3. Presents with abdominal distention and respiratory distress, or abdominal wall erythema.
4. Supine x-ray may not reveal free air (Kenner and Lott, 2007), necessitating lateral decubitus or cross-table view.
5. Abdomen is distended and radiolucent on x-ray (Kenner and Lott, 2007). Individual loops of bowel are visible because of air inside and outside the bowel wall. Falciform ligament (an opaque stripe) may be visualized in the right upper quadrant or upper midportion of the abdomen.

**J. Meconium peritonitis.**

1. Results from intrauterine GI perforation due to obstruction (atresia, stenosis, imperforate anus) and/or volvulus associated with meconium ileus (van der Doef et al., 2011).
2. Calcifications, which are easily identifiable on x-ray, assume a focal or diffuse, patchy, irregular pattern. Multiple white-speckled areas are seen in one area or throughout the abdomen and may be present in the scrotum.
3. Calcifications will slowly disappear.

**K. Abdominal ascites (Fig. 14-29).**

1. Cases include infants with fetal hydrops, GI obstruction with perforation, and peritonitis.
2. Uniform density to the distended abdomen is noted with a gasless or centralized bowel gas pattern. Body wall edema may also be present in infants with fetal hydrops.

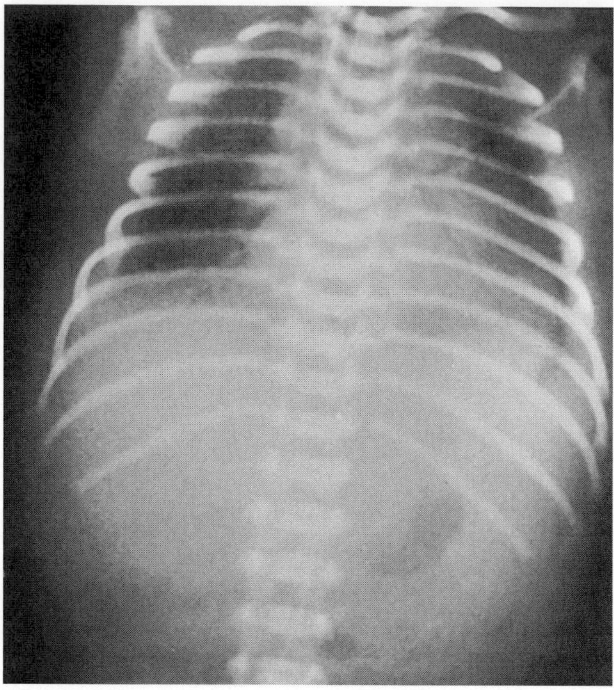

FIGURE 14-29 ■ Abdominal ascites with bilateral pleural effusions.

## SKELETAL SYSTEM

A. **Fractures:** occur most often during delivery, with an increased incidence during breech deliveries. In breech deliveries, fractures can occur in both upper and lower extremities.
   1. Clavicle: fractured during delivery (Fig. 14-30). Fractures occur at the midclavicle most commonly. Fractured clavicle is common in large infants during difficult vaginal delivery (Kenner and Lott, 2007).
   2. Rib fractures: may occur at delivery or related to performance of compressions and be asymptomatic. With multiple fractures, the infant may show signs of respiratory distress and pain. Premature infants may have rib fractures as a result of osteopenia of prematurity 8 to 16 weeks after birth (Fig. 14-31) (Fanaroff and Martin, 2010). These bones are fragile and will fracture with handling and chest physiotherapy. Fractures may be preceded by a thin, "washed out" appearance to the ribs or extremities.
   3. Skull fractures.
      a. Can be linear, buckled, or frankly depressed.
      b. Linear and buckling fractures most often occur in the parietal bone and may be suspected in the presence of cephalhematoma or other skull trauma.

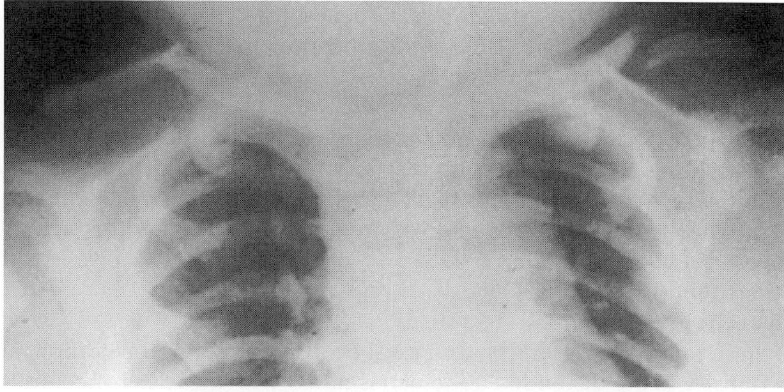

FIGURE 14-30 ■ Fractured left clavicle.

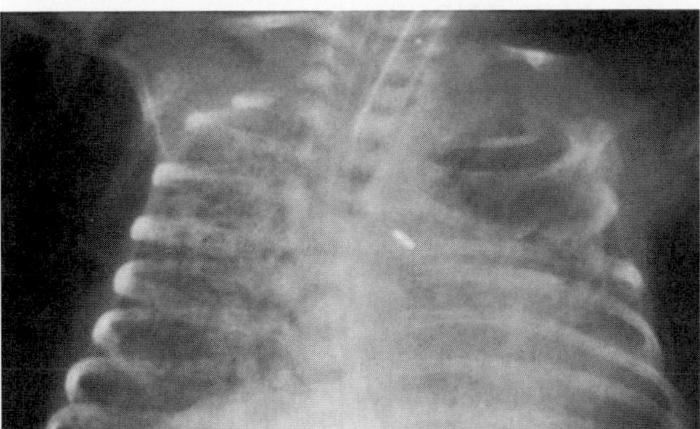

FIGURE 14-31 ■ Fractured rib on left, with pale, "washed out" ribs.

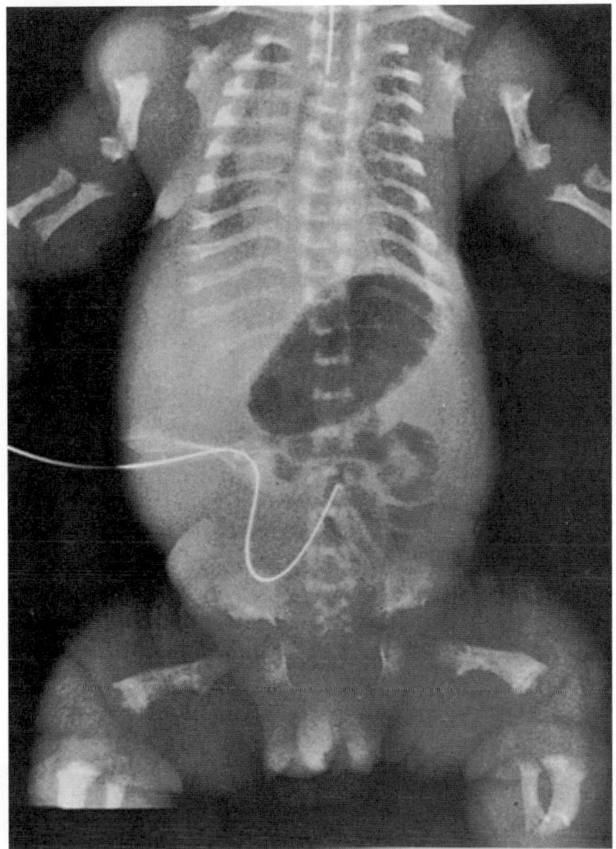

FIGURE 14-32 ■ Thanatophoric dwarf. Note small, narrow thorax and shortness of long bones.

c. Computed tomography (CT) scan is more helpful than plain films for evaluation of skull fractures.

B. **Bony dysplasias.**
1. Osteogenesis imperfecta (see Chapter 35).
2. Dwarfism (common types).
a. Achondroplasia: short extremities and marked flaring of the metaphyses. Classic signs include spinal curvature and narrowed spinal canal; short, squared-off iliac wings; deep-set sacrum; flat acetabular roofs; and bulky proximal femurs.
b. Thanatophoric dwarfism (type I) (Fig. 14-32): marked underdevelopment of the skeleton; extremely short, bent, or curved long bones; and flaring of the metaphyses. Vertebral bodies are very flat and underdeveloped. Thorax is small and narrow, with pulmonary hypoplasia. Condition is uniformly fatal in the perinatal period.

## INDWELLING LINES AND TUBES

A. **Endotracheal tube.**
   1. Placement is approximately 1 cm below the vocal cords and 2 cm above the carina, with the neonate's head in neutral position (Carlo and Ambalavanan, 2013).
   2. Placement beyond the carina results in occlusion of a bronchus (usually the right mainstem bronchus), with subsequent atelectasis and clinical deterioration (Fig. 14-33).

B. **Umbilical artery catheter (Fig. 14-34, *A*).** Proceeds from the umbilicus down toward the pelvis, making an acute turn into the internal iliac artery and common iliac artery and advancing into the aorta (Gomella, 2009).
   1. Low placement: at third and fourth lumbar vertebrae.
   2. High placement: at sixth through ninth thoracic vertebrae.

C. **Umbilical venous catheter (see Fig. 14-34, *B*).** Proceeds from the umbilicus cephalad to join the left portal vein.
   1. On lateral view, the catheter is directly distal to the abdominal wall until it passes through the ductus venosus.
   2. Correct placement is 1 to 2 cm above the diaphragm, with the catheter tip at thoracic vertebrae eight to nine (Gomella, 2009).

D. **Chest tube (see Fig. 14-12).**
   1. X-rays are obtained to determine placement and effectiveness in reinflating the lung.
   2. Lateral chest x-ray film will determine anterior or posterior placement. For air evacuation, anterior placement is desirable. For fluid evacuation, posterior placement is most effective.

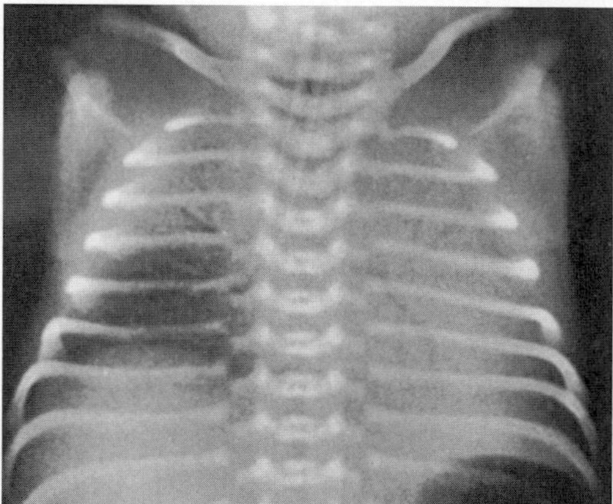

FIGURE 14-33 ■ Endotracheal tube is down right mainstem bronchus, causing atelectasis of right upper lobe and entire left lung.

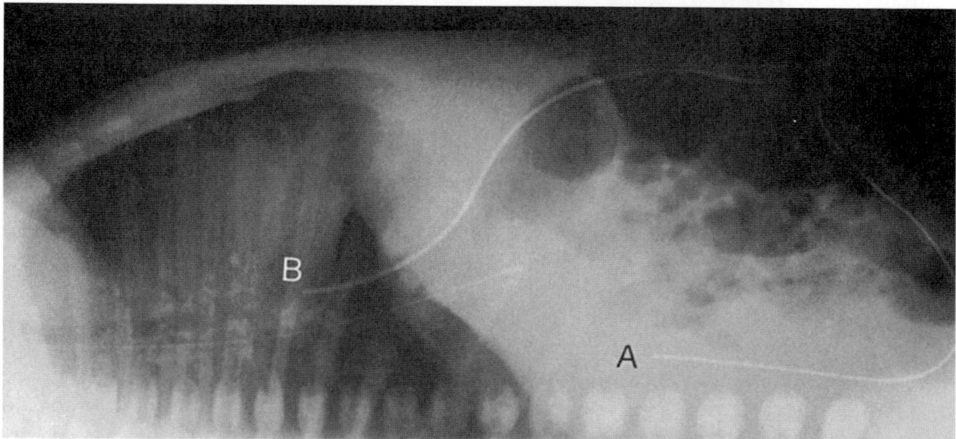


FIGURE 14-34 ■ Umbilical artery catheter **(A)** enters abdomen and proceeds distally as it enters aorta. Umbilical venous catheter **(B)** proceeds toward head, passes through ductus venosus, and lies in inferior vena cava.

3. Correct placement will show the tube in the midclavicular line with the distal chest tube hole inside the thoracic space (Gomella, 2009).

E. **Percutaneous central venous line.** If placed in an upper extremity, the tip of the catheter should be located in the superior vena cava and is considered central once it crosses the midclavicular line and is above the right atrium of the heart (Gomella, 2009). If placed in a lower extremity, the line should be positioned in the inferior vena cava and is considered central once it crosses to the pelvic cavity and rests below the right atrium of the heart (Gomella, 2009).
   1. A chest x-ray is obtained to confirm placement of a catheter placed in an upper extremity. Arm placement will affect the position of the line. The arm should be extended and at a 45-degree angle from the body to best represent normal arm position.
   2. An abdominal x-ray is obtained to confirm placement of a catheter placed in a lower extremity. Lower extremities should be extended and held in place for the abdominal x-ray.

## DIAGNOSTIC IMAGING

A. **Ultrasound.**
   1. Uses sound waves to depict anatomic and functional motion of tissue. The sound waves evaluate varying density of tissues, the movement of tissue, and blood flow. The sound waves can be directed in a variety of planes and angles to enhance imaging (Kenner and Lott, 2007).
   2. Utilized to evaluate internal anatomic structures and some function. Unlike conventional radiography, ultrasound does not emit radiation. The images are typically recorded digitally.
   3. Ultrasound is less expensive than CT or magnetic resonance imaging (MRI), is portable, and therefore more convenient for the evaluation of the unstable patient.
   4. Ultrasound is painless and generally does not require sedation. The procedure is performed at the bedside and the infant's environment is minimally disrupted. Peripheral intravenous lines placed in the area of the anterior fontanelle may need to be relocated if brain imaging is required.
   5. Poor imaging technique, presence of bone and air in the imaging area, and patient position adversely affect quality of the examination. Infant should be supine for cranial imaging and the head should be in midline position.
   6. The nurse's role during an ultrasound examination is to correctly position the infant, offer comfort measures if necessary, and monitor vital signs and the infant's tolerance of the procedure.
   7. Ultrasound is commonly used to evaluate brain parenchyma and ventricular size, myocardial function and structure, urinary tract anatomy and pathology, pelvic masses, liver anatomy, and blood flow in major vessels.

B. **Computed Tomography.**
   1. Obtains cross-sectional images of structures by emitting multiple x-ray beams through tissue. CT passes multiple fan x-ray beams through the same cross-sectional slice of tissue at different angles during different time intervals. The beams rotate about the infant, pass through the body, and the exit transmission of x-ray beam is monitored by a series of detectors (Kenner and Lott, 2007).
   2. CT provides a two-dimensional visualization of anatomy and can be further enhanced by the use of a radiographic contrast agent. Contrast enhancement can assist in the evaluation of blood flow and help define pathologic abnormalities.
   3. CT can distinguish changes in density in very small areas of tissue and allows identification of a variety of soft tissues. This allows for superior anatomic detail and precise clarity of tissue structure.
   4. CT requires the infant to be transported to the radiology department, so the infant's environment is disrupted. CT is painless but may require sedation depending on the infant's state.

5. Utilized to evaluate structure, function, malformation, and extent of disease process. Used commonly in the NICU to evaluate brain anatomy; intraventricular hemorrhage and extent of parenchymal disease; and subgaleal, subarachnoid, and subdural bleeds (Kenner and Lott, 2007).
6. The nurse's role in caring for an infant undergoing a CT examination is to swaddle the infant to decrease movement while in the scanner, thus diminishing artifacts from scan. The nurse must also provide comfort measures, evaluate the need for sedation, and monitor vital signs and infant's tolerance of procedure.

**C. Magnetic Resonance Imaging.**

1. Utilizes radio waves to image protons and hydrogen ions within the body (Kenner and Lott, 2007). The image quality is excellent and the increased sensitivity allows for more precise imaging of even the smallest structures.
2. Does not use ionizing radiation and has less artifact to obscure visualization.
3. Is costly and has limited availability. The magnetic field can interfere with monitoring devices and may restrict the availability to unstable infants.
4. Requires that the infant be transported to the MRI department, so the infant's environment is disrupted. MRI is painless, but heavy sedation may be required for an optimal study, which may require mechanical ventilation.
5. May be useful in the early diagnosis of periventricular leukomalacia, or when more accurate definition of tissue structures is needed for evaluation and diagnosis (Kenner and Lott, 2007).
6. The nurse's role in MRI includes swaddling the infant and positioning in the scanner. The infant must be placed on a monitor designed to function within a magnetic field; specialty ventilators are also available for use with MRI. The nurse provides comfort measures and sedation as ordered, as well as monitoring vital signs and infant's tolerance of procedure.

**D. Echocardiogram (ECHO).**

1. Noninvasive diagnostic tool to evaluate cardiac structure and function.
2. High-frequency sound waves send vibrations through the heart, which reflect energy, which is transmitted into a visual image.
3. Poor imaging technique and infant movement adversely affect ECHO quality. It is portable and therefore available for even the unstable infant.

**E. Barium enema.**

1. Used to evaluate the structure and function of the large intestine and diagnose disorders such as Hirschsprung's disease, malrotation, and meconium plug syndrome.
2. A water-soluble contrast solution is instilled and a series of x-rays are taken under fluoroscopy. A series of follow-up x-rays may be taken at timed intervals to evaluate the evacuation of the solution from the bowel.

**F. Upper GI series with small bowel follow-through.**

1. Used to evaluate the structure and function of the upper GI tract. The three main areas examined are (1) the esophagus (for size, patency, reflux, and presence of fistula or swallowing abnormalities); (2) the stomach (abnormalities and motility); and (3) the small intestine (for strictures, patency, and function).
2. A water-soluble contrast solution is swallowed and a series of x-rays are taken under fluoroscopy. A series of follow-up x-rays are obtained to evaluate emptying ability of the stomach, intestinal motility, and for potential obstruction (van der Doef et al, 2011). Complications include reflux of the contrast solution, vomiting, and potential for aspiration.

**G. Voiding cystourethrogram (VCUG).**

1. Used to evaluate the structure and function of the kidneys, bladder, and lower urinary tract.
2. The infant's bladder is emptied by catheterization and then filled with a contrast solution. A series of x-rays are taken under fluoroscopy in a variety of positions during voiding. After voiding, follow-up x-rays are taken to evaluate residuals in the bladder and any reflux into the kidneys (Kenner and Lott, 2007).
3. The infant should be monitored for hematuria and signs of infection related to a contaminated catheterization.

## REFERENCES

Carlo, W.A. and Ambalavanan, N.: Assisted ventilation. In A.A. Fanaroff and J.M. Fanaroff (Eds.): *Klaus & Fanaroff's Care of the High Risk Neonate*. Philadelphia, 2013, Elsevier Saunders, p. 270–288.

Daldrup-Link, H. and Gooding, C.: *Essentials of pediatric radiology*. New York, 2010, Cambridge University Press.

Falkensammer, C., Ayres, N., Altima, C., et al.: Fetal cardiac malposition: Incidence and outcomes of associated cardiac and extra cardiac malformations. *American Journal of Perinatology*, 25 (5):277–281, 2008.

Fanaroff, A.A. and Martin, R.J. (Eds.): *Neonatal perinatal medicine: Diseases of the fetus and infant* (9th ed.). St. Louis, 2010, Elsevier Mosby.

Gomella, T.L.: *Neonatology: Management, procedures, on-call problems, diseases, and drugs* (6th ed.). New York, 2009, Lange Medical Books/McGraw-Hill.

Karrer, F., Potter, D., and Calkins, C.: Pediatric duodenal atresia. 2012. Retrieved from Medscape at http://emedicine.medscape.com/article/932917.

Kenner, C. and Lott, J.W.: *Comprehensive neonatal care: An interdisciplinary approach* (4th ed.). St. Louis, 2007, Elsevier Saunders.

Northway, W.H., Jr. and Rosan, R.C.: Radiographic features of pulmonary oxygen toxicity in the newborn: Bronchopulmonary dysplasia. *Radiology*, 91 (1):49–58, 1968.

*Stedman's Medical Dictionary* (28th ed.). Baltimore, 2013, Lippincott Williams & Wilkins. Retreived May 1, 2013, from http://dictionary.reference.com.

Van der Doef, H., Kokke, F., van der Ent, C., and Houwen, R.: Intestinal obstruction syndromes in cystic fibrosis: Meconium ileus, distal intestinal obstruction syndrome, and constipation. *Current Gastroenterology Report*, 13(3):265–270, 2011.

CHAPTER

# 15 Common Invasive Procedures

TERESA BAILEY

**OBJECTIVES**

1. Understand the indications for common procedures performed in the neonatal intensive care unit (NICU), such as endotracheal tube (ETT) intubation and suctioning, vascular access methods, blood sampling methods, bladder catheterization, bladder aspiration, thoracentesis, and lumbar puncture.
2. Know the equipment and supplies needed to perform common fundamental and advanced invasive procedures in the neonate.
3. Identify pertinent anatomic landmarks for commonly performed invasive procedures in the NICU.
4. Describe the precautions and contraindications for each invasive procedure.
5. Describe potential complications associated with each invasive procedure.

Approximately 250,000 to 350,000 newborn infants are admitted into the NICU in the United States annually and undergo hundreds of diagnostic and/or therapeutic procedures during their hospitalization. This chapter incorporates many of the diagnostic and therapeutic interventions that are commonly performed in the NICU. These procedures are crucial to the infant's survival; however, they expose the infant to pain and stress that can result in harmful long-term consequences. Therefore, pain management is essential when performing interventions in the NICU.

In many NICUs today, qualified registered nurses or advanced practice nurses, rather than physicians, perform many invasive procedures. Prior to performing any procedure, it is essential that one have knowledge of the indications, precautions, and complications associated with each procedure. Infants are extremely vulnerable; therefore, the ability to perform the procedure proficiently is a major requirement to prevent harm.

The details pertaining to each of the covered procedures comprise this chapter. Aspects that are common to each include the crucial issues listed below.

- Know your institution's protocols about the qualifications needed to perform any procedure.
- Know your institution's protocols about any specific ways in which procedures differ from the descriptions included here.
- Obtain informed consent whenever required for an invasive procedure. Discussion with family is key, even if signed informed consent is not required.
- Always use standard infection control precautions and implement aseptic technique whenever indicated.
- Provide for pain and comfort control before, during, and after the procedure.
- Monitor the patient's clinical status during the procedure. Minimally, monitoring will include oxygenation, ventilation, temperature, and reaction to the procedure, including pertinent vital signs.
- Make written documentation about pertinent aspects of the procedure and enter this into the medical record.
- Perform time out before procedure to ensure patient safety.

## AIRWAY PROCEDURES

### Endotracheal Tube Suctioning: Fundamental Procedure

**A. Indications.**

1. Facilitate oxygenation and ventilation.
2. Maintain patent airway.

3. Clearance of tracheobronchial secretions.
4. Obtain tracheal aspirate specimens.

B. **Contraindications.**
1. Recent surgical procedure to area.
2. Recent surfactant administration.
3. Pulmonary hemorrhage—suction only if needed to maintain tube patency.

C. **Precautions.**
1. Suctioning should be done only when the infant needs it and not on a routine schedule.
2. Maintain aseptic technique.
3. Monitor vital signs and for adverse responses to procedure, such as bradycardia and oxygen desaturations.
4. Avoid hyperoxygenation, hyperinflation, and hyperventilation techniques if possible. Hyperoxygenation in preterm neonates is discouraged owing to risk of retinopathy of prematurity (ROP). If the infant easily becomes hypoxic or oxygenation status is critical, oxygen can be increased by 10% to 20% above baseline to maintain adequate oxygenation. Hyperinflation should be avoided as this places the neonate at risk for air leaks. The effect of hyperventilation alone in neonates is unclear and therefore discouraged (Davis and Rosenfeld, 2005).
5. Loss of lung volume can occur with suctioning. Increased loss of lung volume and hypoxia are associated with open catheters versus closed "in-line" catheters (Tingay et al., 2007).
6. Keep infant's head midline during suctioning to prevent jugular vein distention, which can increase intracranial pressure (ICP).
7. Pulmonary hemorrhage may be exacerbated by suctioning. However, suctioning may be needed to clear the blood from the airway or tube.
8. Always suction ETT before suctioning mouth.
9. When feasible, use two caregivers to perform endotracheal suctioning if the closed (in-line) system is not in use. This may minimize adverse responses and shorten procedure time.

D. **Equipment and supplies.**
1. Sterile gloves.
2. Choose the appropriate-sized catheter. Catheter should be no larger than half the inside diameter of the ETT.
   a. Use 8 F for ETT $\geq$3.5 mm.
   b. Use 6 F for ETT less than 3.5 mm.
3. Resuscitation bag with 100% oxygen source and oxygen blender.
4. Suction source with vacuum control setting.
5. Manometer.
6. Stethoscope.
7. Specimen trap (if applicable).

E. **Procedure.**
1. Determine the need to suction and suction only when indicated. Suctioning should be individualized based on changes in the patient's physical assessment and not on a routine schedule (Gardner et al., 2011). The following situations may warrant suctioning:
   a. Falling oxygen saturations.
   b. Increasing oxygen requirements.
   c. Diminished breath sounds.
   d. Changes in vital signs.
   e. Changes in blood gases.
   f. Changes in respiratory rate and pattern.
   g. Agitation.
   h. Visible secretions in ETT.
   i. Pattern change in ventilator graphics.
   j. Loss of or poor chest wall excursion with ventilator breaths.
2. Wash hands and ensure that equipment is in working order.
3. Shallow suctioning technique is the preferred method. Deep suctioning should be avoided as this has been shown to cause tissue damage and inflammation.

   a. Determine suction catheter insertion depth by summing the length of the ETT and its adapter. The catheter should not be inserted more than 1 cm beyond the total distance determined (Hagler and Traver, 1994).
4. Gather supplies.
   a. Commercially prepared suction catheter kit or sterile suction catheter and sterile gloves. Closed-system (in-line) suction catheter kits are available that remain attached to the ETT adapter and should be used per manufacturer's recommendations. The closed-system suction technique is preferred as it allows the infant to be suctioned without being removed from the ventilator. Closed-system suction devices may decrease respiratory contamination and pulmonary infections and have been shown to have decreased physiologic consequences such as bradycardia and desaturation (Choong et al., 2003; Kalyn et al., 2003; Tan et al., 2005).
   b. Appropriate-sized suction catheter with measurement markings.
   c. If using a commercially prepared suction kit, open package and maintain sterility of contents. Remove and don sterile gloves, then remove catheter. If using separate gloves and catheter supplies, open suction catheter package, maintaining sterility of catheter, then open and don gloves. Continue to maintain aseptic technique and remove catheter from package.
5. While maintaining aseptic procedure, attach suction catheter to suction tubing with nondominant hand (now considered contaminated). With sterile dominant hand, hold suction catheter and maintain sterility of catheter.
6. Release suction tubing from nondominant hand and remove infant from ventilator. Provide oxygen and ventilation at necessary levels to maintain the heart rate and provide adequate oxygen saturation. Infant may be ventilated by hand or by providing manual breaths from ventilator. If manual breaths are provided by the ventilator, use caution to avoid hyperinflation and to allow adequate exhalation times.
7. Suction at 60 to 100 mm Hg or with just enough suction to extract secretions through catheter.
8. Advance catheter only to a predetermined distance. If a cough reflex is initiated, catheter distance is too far.
9. Apply suction only when withdrawing catheter and limit suction duration to 5 to 10 seconds. Allow patient to recover between suction passes while monitoring vital signs, oxygen saturation, and chest wall movement.
10. Routine normal saline (NS) irrigation is not recommended as this may dislodge viable bacteria from colonized ETT into the lower airway (Gardner et al., 2011).
11. Limit the number of suction passes. Suction until secretions are removed or infant shows signs of intolerance. Clear suction catheter with NS between suction passes. Most secretions can be cleared in one or two passes.
12. If obtaining tracheal specimen, attach sterile specimen trap to suction catheter and suction tubing for specimen prior to general suctioning.
13. Return infant to previous oxygen requirement as tolerated, if applicable.
14. Label and send tracheal specimen to laboratory, if applicable.
15. Document patient's tolerance, character of secretions (amount, color, and consistency), and breath sounds.
16. If using a closed-system (in-line) catheter device, change per manufacturer's recommendation or per institution's policy if sooner.

F. **Complications.**
1. Hypoxia.
2. Bradycardia.
3. Apnea.
4. Accidental extubation or malpositioning of tube.
5. Trauma to trachea or bronchi.
6. Hemorrhage.
7. Loss of lung volume.
8. Atelectasis.
9. Infection/pneumonia.
10. Pneumothorax.

11. Increased ICP.
12. Granular tissue formation.
13. Bronchial stenosis.
14. Tracheal laceration.

## Oral Endotracheal Intubation: Advanced Practice Procedure

A. **Indications.**
   1. To perform resuscitation.
   2. Bag-and-mask ventilation is ineffective or undesirable.
   3. Need for mechanical ventilation.
   4. Tracheal suctioning or lavage is required, such as to remove meconium from the trachea.
   5. To obtain sterile tracheal aspirate specimen.
   6. Protection of the airway is required.
   7. Diaphragmatic hernia is present.
   8. Administration of exogenous surfactant.
   9. To relieve critical upper airway obstruction.

B. **Precautions.**
   1. Patient's heart rate and oxygen saturation should be monitored continuously during the procedure and stabilized with bag-and-mask ventilation if possible prior to intubation.
   2. Hypoxia during the procedure should be minimized.
   3. Use free-flow oxygen held near the mouth and nose of any infant with respiratory effort, to maximize oxygenation during the procedure.
   4. Limit intubation attempts to 20 seconds. The infant's condition should be stabilized with bag-and-mask ventilation between attempts.
   5. Have all equipment necessary for intubation prepared and in working order prior to initiating procedure.
   6. For nonemergent intubations, infant pain management is recommended prior to procedure using institutional protocol (Allen, 2012).
   7. Maintain thermal homeostasis and developmental care.

C. **Equipment and supplies.**
   1. Pediatric laryngoscope handle.
   2. Laryngoscope blade with functioning secure bulb.
      a. Size 00 blade for preterm infants weighing less than 1000 g.
      b. Size 0 blade for infants weighing 1000 to 3000 g. Most infants weighing 3000 to 4000 g can be successfully intubated with a size 0 blade. However, if unable to visualize landmarks, a size 1 blade may be necessary.
      c. Size 1 blade for infants weighing more than 4000 to 5000 g.
      d. Types of blades:
         (1) Miller straight blade.
         (2) Macintosh curved blade.
   3. ETT size:
      a. Internal diameter (ID) 2.5 mm for infants weighing less than 1000 g or less than 28 weeks of gestation.
      b. ID 3 mm for 1000- to 2000-g infants or infants with a gestational age of 28 to 34 weeks.
      c. ID 3.5 mm for 2000- to 3000-g infants or infants with a gestational age of 34 to 38 weeks.
      d. ID 3.5 to 4 mm for infants weighing more than 3000 g or greater than 38 weeks of gestation.
   4. Stylet (though use is optional, it should be available).
   5. Suction catheters (size 5 F to 10 F) and suction source set at 60 to 100 mm Hg of negative pressure.
   6. Resuscitation bag and mask of appropriate sizes. Alternatively, availability of infant ventilation device, such as a T-piece resuscitator (i.e., NeoPuff).
   7. 100% oxygen source with blender providing an appropriate $FiO_2$ for the patient, minimally at a flow rate of 5 to 10 L/min, with attached manometer.
   8. Tape and other supplies to secure ETT according to hospital policy.

9. Cardiorespiratory monitor and oxygen saturation monitor.
10. Stethoscope.
11. Meconium aspirator, if applicable.
12. End-tidal $CO_2$ ($EtCO_2$) detector, colorimetric device such as the Pedi-Cap to confirm intubation.
    a. Limitations of neonatal colorimetric $EtCO_2$ detection devices (DeBoer and Seaver, 2004).
        (1) Decreased peripheral perfusion—adapter may not change color quickly, if at all, when the neonate has little to no perfusion.
        (2) False-positive readings—verify ETT placement after at least 6 breaths have been given via ETT with attached $EtCO_2$ device.
        (3) Detector contamination—detector may be contaminated with bodily fluids or medication and limit ability to display color change. False-positive color change has been reported with atropine, epinephrine, calfactant (Infasurf), and naloxone (Narcan) (Hughes et al., 2007).
        (4) Limited time accuracy—sufficient exhalation time must be allowed for device to detect $CO_2$ and display color change (may take up to six ventilations with a resuscitation bag), device is good for up to 24 hours of intermittent use or 2 hours of continuous use.
13. Devices for difficult intubation—ideally, a difficult airway should be identified prior to intubation. The following devices should only be used by personnel with extensive training and experience, such as a neonatologist, otolaryngologist, or anesthesiologist. If this is not possible, arrangements should be made for transfer to a center where personnel and equipment are available (Kumar et al. and Committee on Fetus and Newborn, Section on Anesthesiology and Pain Medicine, 2010).
    a. Laryngeal mask airway (LMA) should be available at all intubations in the event intubation is unsuccessful (Kumar et al. and Committee on Fetus and Newborn, Section on Anesthesiology and Pain Medicine, 2010).
        (1) All personnel who are trained in neonatal intubation should also be trained in the use of LMA.
        (2) This is not an acceptable long-term airway; however, it may be used while preparations are made for a secure airway.
    b. Specialized stylets such as lighted and fiberoptic stylets, intubating introducers such as the gum elastic bougie, and fiberoptic flexible bronchoscopes.
    c. Indirect rigid laryngoscopes.
    d. Video laryngoscopes.

**D. Procedure.**

1. Gather ancillary personnel and ensure that all equipment is in working order (i.e., stethoscope, bag, and mask at bedside; suction on and functioning; laryngoscope with secured working light source; etc.).
2. Wash hands and verify patient and procedure to be performed.
3. It is recommended that an analgesic be given prior to all nonemergent intubation, and use of a vagolytic be considered. Premedication can decrease adverse effects of intubation, such as bradycardia, hypoxia, and increased intracranial pressure, by treating pain and calming a patient during an uncomfortable procedure (Kumar et al. and Committee on Fetus and Newborn, Section on Anesthesiology and Pain Medicine, 2010). When writing a unit policy for preintubation medications, consider use of agents that are rapid onset with the shortest possible duration of action. See Table 15-1 for common medications used in intubation (adapted from Allen, 2012; Kumar et al. and Committee on Fetus and Newborn, Section on Anesthesiology and Pain Medicine, 2010):
    a. Analgesics: Preferred American Academy of Pediatrics (AAP) analgesic is fentanyl, with morphine and remifentanil listed as acceptable.
    b. Sedative–hypnotic (optional): Due to limited data and side effect profile, there are no AAP-preferred sedative–hypnotic agents. Acceptable agents are thiopental and propofol in preterm and term infants, and midazolam is acceptable in term infants. A sedative alone without analgesia should not be used (Kumar et al. and Committee on Fetus and Newborn, Section on Anesthesiology and Pain Medicine, 2010).

■ TABLE 15-1
■ ■ **Medications for Use With Intubation**

| Medication | Onset of Action | Duration of Action | Dose | Considerations |
|---|---|---|---|---|
| **ANALGESICS** | | | | |
| Fentanyl (preferred) | Almost immediate IV, 7 to 15 minutes IM | 30 to 60 minutes IV, 1 to 2 hours IM | 1 to 4 mcg/kg IV or IM | Give slowly (over 1 to 2 minutes minimally) as rapid infusion may cause thoracic and skeletal muscle rigidity. May cause apnea, hypotension, and CNS depression; reversed with naloxone. |
| Remifentanil | Almost immediate | 3 to 10 minutes | 1 to 3 mcg/kg IV | Give slowly (over 1 to 2 minutes minimally) as rapid infusion may cause thoracic and skeletal muscle rigidity. May cause apnea, hypotension, and CNS depression. |
| Morphine | 5 to 15 minutes IV, 10 to 30 minutes IM | 3 to 5 hours IV or IM | 0.1 to 0.3 mg/kg IV or IM | May cause apnea, hypotension, and CNS depression; reversed with naloxone. |
| **SEDATIVE–HYPNOTIC** | | | | |
| Thiopental | 30 to 60 seconds | 5 to 30 minutes | 2 to 6 mg/kg IV | May cause apnea, hypotension, and bronchospasm. |
| Propofol | Within 30 seconds | 3 to 10 minutes | 1 to 2.5 mg/kg | May cause apnea, hypotension, bronchospasm, bradycardia, and pain at injection site. |
| Midazolam | 1 to 5 minutes IV, 5 to 15 minutes IM | 20 to 30 minutes IV, 1 to 6 hours IM | 0.05 to 0.1 mg/kg IV or IM | Has not been established as safe for use in very preterm infants due to risk of benzyl alcohol toxicity. May cause apnea, hypotension, and CNS depression. Effects reversed with flumazenil. |
| **NEUROMUSCULAR BLOCKING AGENTS** | | | | |
| Succinylcholine | 30 to 60 seconds IV, 2 to 3 minutes IM | 4 to 6 minutes IV, 10 to 30 minutes IM | 1 to 2 mg/kg IV, 2 mg/kg IM | Do not use in neonates with hyperkalemia, suspicion of muscular dystrophy, increased ICP, or a family history of malignant hyperthermia; monitor for bradycardia (pretreatment with atropine minimizes bradycardia). |
| Vecuronium | 2 to 3 minutes | 30 to 40 minutes | 0.05 to 0.10 mg/kg IV | Minimal cardiovascular side effects; however, decrease in heart rate and blood pressure has been observed when used concurrently with narcotics. Reversed with neostigmine and atropine. |
| Rocuronium | 1 to 2 minutes | 20 to 30 minutes | 0.5 mg/kg IV | May cause hyper- or hypotension, tachycardia, arrhythmias, and bronchospasm. |
| Pancuronium | 1 to 3 minutes | 40 to 60 minutes | 0.05 to 0.10 mg/kg IV | May cause hypertension, tachycardia, bronchospasm, and excessive salivation; reversible with atropine and neostigmine. |
| **VAGOLYTICS** | | | | |
| Atropine | 1 to 2 minutes | 0.5 to 2 hours | 10 to 20 mcg/kg IV or IM | May cause tachycardia and dry skin. |
| Glycopyrrolate | 1 to 10 minutes | ~6 hours | 5 mcg/kg IM | May cause tachycardia, arrhythmias, and bronchospasm. |

*CNS*, Central nervous system; *ICP*, intracranial pressure; *IM*, intramuscularly; *IV*, intravenously.

   c. Neuromuscular blocking agents (optional): Muscle relaxants are contraindicated in situations where intubation may be difficult, such as micrognathia and cleft lip/palate or with health care providers with limited neonatal intubations. Sensation remains intact with neuromuscular blockade, and thus, analgesia must be used in combination.
   d. Vagolytics: These drugs may help prevent reflex bradycardia during intubation. Atropine is the AAP-preferred vagolytic, but glycopyrrolate may be used as a second option.
4. Select ETT of the appropriate size.
5. Insert stylet (optional) and shape the ETT as desired. The stylet must be secured so that its tip does not extend below the tip of the ETT and also so the stylet cannot advance during the procedure. Keep the tube and stylet as clean as possible.
6. Determine ETT insertion depth. A variety of methods has been reported for predicting insertional length such as nasal–tragus length, sternal length, foot length, and weight. The American Heart Association (AHA) Neonatal Resuscitation Program use the 7-8-9 Rule (AAP and AHA, 2011).
   a. 6 plus the weight in kilograms (e.g., in a 2-kg neonate, the ETT should be inserted to the 8-cm marking: 2 kg + 6 = 8 cm)
      (1) The 7-8-9 Rule has been associated with overestimated depth insertion in infants weighing less than 750 g (Peterson et al., 2006).
7. Aspirate gastric contents and suction the oropharynx.
8. Position the patient supine on a flat surface, with the head midline and the neck slightly extended (optional: place a soft flat roll under neck) in a "sniffing" position. The person performing intubation must have easy access to the airway and equipment while positioned at the patient's head.
9. Hold the laryngoscope in the left hand between the thumb and first finger, with the blade pointing away. The laryngoscope is designed to be held with the left hand only.
10. Open the patient's mouth with the fingers of the right hand and gently slide the blade into the right side of the mouth.
11. Stabilize the left hand against the left side of the patient's face, advance the blade tip to the base of the tongue, and move the blade to the midline, pushing the tongue to the left.
12. Expose the pharynx by lifting the entire blade upward in the direction in which the handle is pointing. Do not rock the tip of the blade upward or use the upper gum as a fulcrum.
13. If unable to see the glottis, apply gentle external tracheal pressure (cricoid pressure) with the fifth finger of the left hand or have an assistant perform this and withdraw the blade slowly until the glottis is visible.
14. Remove any secretions that interfere with visualization by suctioning. Direct suctioning under laryngoscopy is ideal.
15. Identify anatomic landmarks.
   a. Epiglottis is uppermost.
   b. Glottis is anterior, with vocal cords closing side to side.
   c. Esophagus is posterior.
16. After identifying the vocal cords, and with the cords in clear view, place the ETT into the right side of the patient's mouth with the right hand.
17. Keeping the cords in view, pass the ETT between the cords 1 to 2 cm into the trachea on inhalation (level of the vocal cord guide mark on the ETT). This should position the tip of the tube midway between the thoracic inlet and the carina, approximately at the second and third thoracic vertebrae. If the vocal cords are closed or will not open, wait for spontaneous breath, or stimulate a breath by stroking the soles of the feet.
18. With the right index finger, firmly hold the ETT against the roof of the mouth, stabilize the right hand against the patient's face, and carefully remove the laryngoscope with the left hand.
19. Carefully remove the stylet, if used, from the ETT.
20. Attach the resuscitation bag and $EtCO_2$ detector if applicable and assess tube placement.
   a. Auscultate both sides of the chest for the presence and intensity of breath sounds.
   b. Assess chest movement with inflationary breaths.
   c. Auscultate over the epigastrium and visually assess for distention.

d. Check for condensation in tube during exhalation.
e. Check for color change on $CO_2$ detector, if available.

21. Following confirmation of successful intubation, attach ETT to bag or special ventilation device such as a T-piece resuscitator and deliver breaths.
22. If the tube is in too far and placed in a right or left mainstem bronchus, auscultation may reveal unilateral or unequal breath sounds. The tube should be withdrawn very gradually and assessed until equal bilateral breath sounds are auscultated. If the tube is in the esophagus:
    a. Air may be heard entering the stomach with inflationary breaths.
    b. The stomach may become distended.
    c. A strong cry or cough may be noted.
    d. No breath sounds will be heard on auscultation of the chest during inflationary breaths, though air movement may be heard, especially over the lower portion of the chest.
    e. No color change with $EtCO_2$ detector.
    f. Remove the ETT and discard it and hand ventilate with bag and appropriate-sized mask.
23. In very small infants, breath sounds may seem audible even with an ETT in the esophagus.
24. When the tube is assessed to be in good position, note the markings and secure the tube according to hospital policy.
25. Position of the tube must be confirmed by chest radiograph.
    a. Obtain chest x-ray in anterior–posterior (AP) view with head midline and not in a flexed position.
    b. Tip of ETT should lie approximately 0.5 to 1 cm above the carina.
26. After confirming tube placement by chest radiograph, any length of tube that extends more than 4 cm beyond the lip should be cut off to limit dead space and to prevent kinking.
27. Document according to hospital policy: date, time, ETT size, centimeter marking at lip, $EtCO_2$ results, chest radiograph, and patient's tolerance of procedure. Medications given, if any, should also be documented.

**E. Complications.**

1. Hypoxia.
    a. During the procedure.
    b. Due to misplacement of tube.
2. Bradycardia.
    a. Due to hypoxia.
    b. Due to vagal stimulation from the laryngoscope, ETT, or suction catheter.
3. Infection.
4. Perforation of esophagus or trachea.
5. Trauma/edema to oropharyngeal and laryngeal tissues.
6. Vocal cord injury.
7. Subglottic stenosis associated with long-term (>3 to 4 weeks) intubation.
8. Palatal grooves from prolonged intubation.
9. Misplacement of tube into esophagus or bronchus.
10. Interference of oral development caused by oral ETT.
11. Abnormal dentition.
12. Ingestion/aspiration of laryngoscope bulb.
13. Tube obstruction or kinking.
14. Pain, agitation, or discomfort.

## Thoracentesis: Advanced Practice Procedure

**A. Indications.**

1. Emergency evacuation of pneumothorax.
2. Emergency evacuation of pleural fluid.

**B. Equipment and supplies.**

1. Skin antiseptics according to hospital policy.
2. Large-bore over-the-needle intravenous (IV) catheter (14 to 22 gauge).
3. Three-way stopcock.

4. Syringe, 20 to 35 mL.
5. Local anesthetic, tuberculin (TB) syringe with small-bore needle, if medical condition permits.

C. **Procedure.**
1. Position the infant supine and restrain limbs if necessary.
2. Provide pharmacologic pain management if medical condition permits.
3. Identify entry site. Use second or third intercostal space along the midclavicular line.
4. Prepare skin with antiseptic as per hospital policy.
5. Infiltrate the area with 1 mL of local anesthetic using a TB syringe and 25- to 27-gauge needle.
6. Puncture skin at 45-degree angle, angling over third or fourth rib, and advance needle/catheter at a 90-degree angle. Inserting the catheter over the top of the rib will avoid blood vessels and nerves that run along the bottom of the rib. If thoracentesis is being done because of pleural fluid or effusion, the thorax should be punctured between the fifth and sixth intercostal spaces, midaxilla.
7. Remove needle from IV catheter while sliding the catheter into the pleural space.
8. Attach catheter hub to stopcock and syringe. The stopcock allows for aspiration of free air or fluid into the syringe and emptying of the syringe while maintaining a closed system.
9. When free air or fluid is obtained, stabilize the catheter and continue to aspirate until preparation for chest tube insertion is complete, or until the air leak or fluid accumulation is evacuated.
10. Document according to hospital policy: date, time, catheter size, location, amount of air/fluid evacuated, patient's tolerance of procedure. Pharmacologic interventions performed should also be documented.

D. **Complications.**
1. Hemorrhage.
2. Infection.
3. Needle injury to lung or adjacent structures.
4. Damage to breast tissue.
5. Pain.

# CIRCULATORY ACCESS PROCEDURES

## Peripheral Intravenous Line Placement: Fundamental Procedure

A. **Indications.**
1. Administration of medications.
2. Administration of fluids, volume expanders, or blood products.
3. Administration of parenteral nutrition.

B. **Precautions.**
1. Avoid areas of infection or loss of skin integrity near selected puncture site.
2. Use caution in infants with coagulation disorders, which may result in bleeding into surrounding tissues.
3. Padded armboard is to be used only if necessary to maintain line placement and must be of an appropriate size for gestational age.
4. Choose an access site based on patient's condition, prescribed therapy, and inserter's experience (Alexander and Infusion Nurses Society (INS), 2011).
   a. Consider conserving areas that may later be needed for central line placement, such as the basilic, cubital, cephalic, and saphenous veins.
   b. The inserter should be familiar with anatomic characteristics and acceptable venipuncture sites.
   c. Recommended for short-term IV therapy (<1 week).
   d. Avoid infusion of hyperosmolar fluids (<600 mOsm/L) and acidotic (pH <5) or alkalotic (pH >9) fluids because of the risk of injury.

C. **Equipment and supplies.**
1. 22- to 24-gauge over-the-needle safety catheter.
2. Tape and dressing supplies as per hospital policy.
   a. Catheter stabilization device if available.
   b. Transparent semipermeable membrane to allow visualization of insertion site.

3. Skin antiseptics as per hospital policy.
4. Tourniquet (a sanitized rubber band will suffice).
5. NS flush solution in a 3-mL syringe.
6. Transilluminator, if necessary to visualize vessels.
7. Small scissors or safety razor, if necessary.
8. Appropriately sized padded armboard, if necessary.
9. Nonsterile gloves.
10. Additional tubing and infusate as indicated per hospital policy.
11. Pain/developmental management: pacifier, sucrose pacifier, blankets for developmental swaddling, eye protection from bright lights.

D. **Procedure.**
1. Verify order from licensed health care provider for placement of a vascular access device.
2. Gather supplies, use hand hygiene as indicated by hospital policy, and don gloves.
3. Provide pain management such as pacifier for nonnutritive sucking, sucrose pacifier, and/or developmental care with facilitated tucking or swaddling. Shield eyes from bright lights.
4. Flush connecting tubing with NS flush solution.
5. Determine vein for cannulation (Fig. 15-1). Accomplish distention of the vessel by applying a gentle tourniquet proximal to the selected insertion site. Alternatively, an assistant may encircle the proximal extremity with hand/fingers and apply direct pressure for the same effect.
   a. Transilluminate to locate vein, if necessary (use caution to avoid skin burns from heated device).
   b. Apply warm compress for 5 minutes if needed to help dilate veins and make them more visible.
   c. If a scalp vein will be cannulated, trim hair with scissors rather than shaving to help visualize and secure IV tubing.
6. Choose appropriate-sized catheter for patient's size and vein.
7. Prepare skin at selected puncture site with antiseptic as per hospital policy, using aseptic technique.
8. Position and stabilize puncture site, keeping skin taut.
9. Beginning a few millimeters distal to the anticipated site of the vessel puncture, insert the needle bevel-up, at a 10- to 20-degree angle, depending on location of vein. Puncture skin in the direction of blood flow and advance needle in 1- to 2-mm increments.
10. If resistance is met or vein is not punctured, withdraw needle slowly to just below the level of the skin, relocate vein, and advance the needle again.

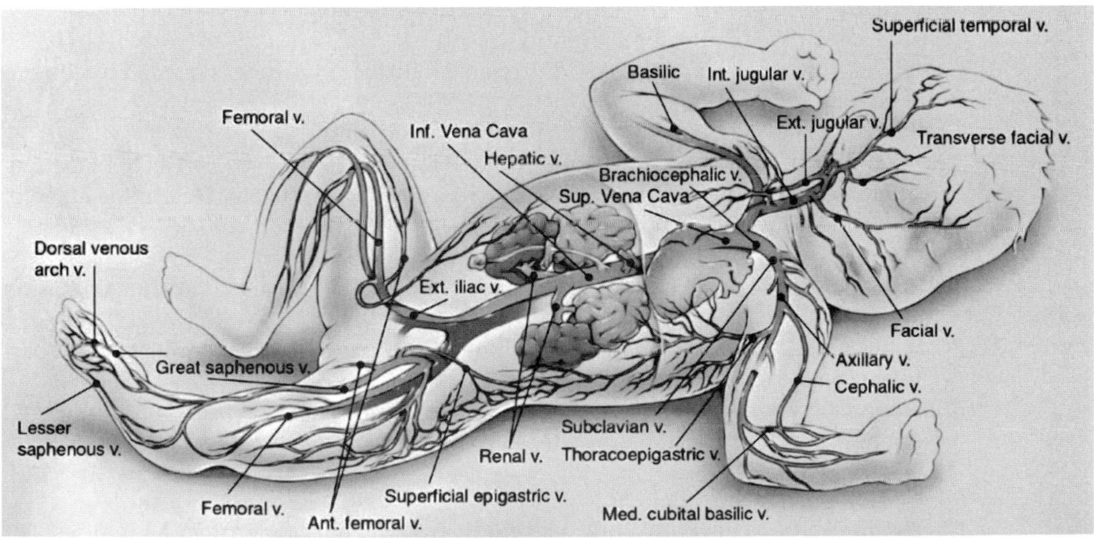


FIGURE 15-1 ■ The major veins that may be used for peripheral intravenous line placement in young infants. (Courtesy and copyright Becton Dickinson and Company.)

11. If a hematoma develops or bleeding occurs, occlude the vessel with pressure just proximal to the puncture site, remove tourniquet, withdraw the needle or catheter, and apply pressure until hemostasis has occurred.
12. If cannulation appears to be successful (i.e., flashback of blood in hub), remove the tourniquet and catheter needle (if using over-the-needle catheter), connect the tubing to the catheter hub, and inject some of the flush solution gently to evaluate patency of the catheter. If flush solution infiltrates the tissues surrounding the catheter tip, occlude the vessel with pressure just proximal to the puncture site, withdraw the needle or catheter, and apply pressure until hemostasis has occurred.
13. Each inserter should attempt access no more than two times to limit damage to future access sites and patient pain (Alexander and INS, 2011). Access attempts should be limited with considerable thought given to alternative treatments or access should attempts continue to be unsuccessful.
14. If cannulation was successful and flush solution infuses without complications, connect T-connector and IV tubing with appropriate fluid to catheter, if applicable.
15. Tape catheter in position that is developmentally appropriate and per hospital policy. Tape, dressing, and restraint must allow for easy inspection of insertion site, circulation of the distal extremity, and patency of the IV tubing. Avoid occlusion of the IV tubing with the tape or dressing.
16. Activate safety device upon removal of needle and dispose of needle(s) in appropriate sharps container.
17. Document date, time, catheter size, site location, and patient's tolerance of procedure, according to hospital guidelines. Pain management interventions should also be documented.
18. Monitor for tissue infiltration or device dislodgment. If signs of infiltration are present, stop infusion immediately. Adverse signs may include the following:
    - **a.** Redness, blanching, or discoloration at or near IV insertion site.
    - **b.** Edema or swelling of extremity.
    - **c.** Blistering at site.
    - **d.** Pain with flushing.
    - **e.** Resistance with flushing.
    - **f.** Leaking at site.
    - **g.** Coolness of skin around insertion site/extremity.
19. Treatment for infiltration/extravasation (Fox, 2011; Sawatzky-Dickson and Bodnaryk, 2006; Thigpen, 2007):
    - **a.** Immediately stop all infusion of fluids and/or medications.
    - **b.** Remove any constricting bands that may interfere with blood flow.
    - **c.** Consider elevation of affected extremity.
    - **d.** Use of cold or warm compresses is controversial; further evidence is needed to demonstrate benefit.
    - **e.** Notify physician or advanced practice nurse immediately.
    - **f.** Assess and document appearance of infiltrated area, including size, areas of blanching or erythema, pulses, perfusion, and estimated amount of infusate. Determine stage of extravasation (Sawatzky-Dickson and Bodnaryk, 2006; Thigpen, 2007):
        - (1) Stage 1: IV difficult to flush, pain at site without redness or swelling.
        - (2) Stage 2: Slight swelling and redness at site, pain, good pulse and normal perfusion below site.
        - (3) Stage 3: Moderate swelling and blanching at site, pain, good pulse and normal perfusion below site, skin cool to touch.
        - (4) Stage 4: Severe swelling and blanching at site, pain, decreased pulse and prolonged or absent capillary refill below site, skin cool to touch with evidence of breakdown or necrosis.
    - **g.** Pharmacologic intervention:
        - (1) Hyaluronidase (Vitrase)—indicated for the treatment of Stage 3 and 4 injuries. For best results, use hyaluronidase within 1 hour of infiltration but may be given up to 3 hours after infiltration. Reconstitute product with NS. The recommended dose is

15 units/mL. After cleaning the area with an antimicrobial agent, inject five 0.2-mL injections subcutaneously around the periphery of the infiltration (do not inject directly into affected area), using a different 25- to 27-gauge needle for each injection. Not recommended for IV use.

(2) Phentolamine (Regitine)—indicated for treatment of infiltration of α-adrenergic drugs such as dopamine, epinephrine, norepinephrine, and phenylephrine. For best results, use within 12 hours of infiltration. Dilute the available 5-mg/mL product to a concentration of 0.5 mg/mL. Inject subcutaneously into the area of infiltration using multiple small injections of 0.2 mL with a 25- to 27-gauge needle, changing the needle between each skin entry. Use cautiously in hemodynamically unstable infants. Monitor for hypotension.

(3) Nitroglycerin 2%—apply 4 mm/kg to affected area. Use with caution in neonates ≤34 weeks' postmenstrual age who are not greater than 21 days of age because of enhanced absorption through the thin immature skin, which may put them at risk for overdosage and toxicity. Apply only to intact skin. Monitor heart rate and blood pressure as it may cause tachycardia and hypotension.

**h.** Multiple puncture technique.

(1) To be used to express fluid in extreme infiltrations (stage 4) to reduce pressure and prevent skin necrosis.
(2) Prepare skin at site with antiseptic technique as per hospital policy.
(3) Provide pain management with swaddling, sucrose pacifier, and/or pain medication.
(4) Use a large-bore (18-gauge) sterile needle and make multiple perforations over the greatest area of swelling with strict aseptic technique.
(5) Allow for free flow of infiltrated fluid. May gently massage affected area.
(6) Cover skin with room-temperature saline-soaked dressing and elevate affected extremity.

**E. Complications.**

1. Hematoma.
2. Infection.
3. Air, clot, or particle embolus.
4. Tissue injury (phlebitis, infiltration) and possible necrosis after infiltration of infused solutions and/or medications.
5. Injury to extremity from restraint.
6. Compromised distal circulation.
7. Pressure necrosis over bony areas.
8. Limb deformity after prolonged immobilization.
9. Pressure injury of peripheral nerves.
10. Inadvertent arterial line placement.
11. Blood loss from inadvertent catheter or tubing dislodgment.
12. Pain from infiltration or ruptured blood vessel from unsuccessful cannulation.

## Peripherally Inserted Central Catheter and Midline Catheter: Advanced Practice Procedure

A midline catheter (MLC) is a peripherally inserted catheter that dwells deeper in the vein than those used for standard peripheral IV therapy but never enters the abdominal–thoracic cavity. Midline catheters are a form of intermediate IV therapy and should not be used in infants who require the use of a peripherally inserted central catheter (PICC). The Centers for Disease Control and Prevention (CDC) recommends insertion of an MLC or PICC if IV therapy is expected to exceed 6 days (CDC, 2011). Insertion of an MLC is the same as for a PICC (i.e., equipment, use of strict aseptic technique, need for continuous heparinized carrier fluid); however, their use is strictly that of a peripheral IV device. An MLC can remain in place for 2 to 4 weeks. MLC studies in neonates have reported MLC mean dwell times from 4 to 11 days (Leike-Rude and Haney, 2006; Pettit and Wyckoff, 2007; Wyckoff, 1999). The longer MLC dwell time therefore minimizes the frequent painful IV insertions associated with standard peripheral IV lines. It is important to note that, while MLCs have established safety, there are indications that catheters that dwell in near-central veins, past the head of the humerus or femur, have significantly higher rates of complications (Colacchio et al., 2012; Jain et al., 2013). These veins include the subclavian, internal jugular, axillary, and common iliac veins. The cephalic vein diameter may be too small to adequately accommodate an MLC (Alexander and INS, 2011). If a central placement is not possible, the catheter should be retracted and position confirmed outside the abdominal–thoracic cavity.

NOTE: Catheters with a stylet are available. A stylet may make advancing a catheter easier, and there is no evidence to support concerns that the stylet will damage or perforate vessels when used with care (Paulson and Miller, 2008). Hospital stock choice of catheter size, lumen, and manufacturer should be based on the evidence, patient population need, and cost-effectiveness. The stylet should not extend past the tip of the catheter, and should never be trimmed. Follow manufacturer's recommendations regarding trimming and flushing catheters with stylets prior to insertion.

**A. Indications.**

1. Intermediate or long-term IV therapy (>6 days).
2. Parenteral nutrition (strongly consider use of PICC, especially if anticipated dextrose or osmolarity requires central placement).
3. Antibiotic or other medicinal therapy.
4. Difficult venous access.
5. Irritating drug therapy (strongly consider central placement).
6. Strongly consider use of PICC in very low birth weight infant (<1500 g).

**B. Contraindications.**

1. Active bacteremia or sepsis; however, this is controversial. Consider deferring placement for at least 24 to 48 hours after antibiotic dosing is started.
2. Inadequate vessel for cannulation.
3. Anatomic irregularities in infant's extremities or chest that could interfere with proper insertion.
4. Avoid insertion in the right arm of infants with congenital heart defects resulting in decreased blood flow to the subclavian artery.
5. The infant can be adequately treated with a peripheral IV access.
6. Parental refusal.

**C. Precautions.**

1. Avoid areas of infection or loss of skin integrity near selected puncture site.
2. Avoid placement of a PICC in an extremity with inadequate or poor circulation.
3. Obtain parental informed consent for PICC insertion prior to the procedure per institutional policy.
4. Use caution in infants with coagulation disorders.
5. Use caution with high-frequency ventilation as pressure changes within the chest may lead to catheter migration, particularly with upper body insertions.
6. Do not measure blood pressure or perform venipuncture on the extremity containing the PICC/MLC.
7. Use aseptic technique during insertion and care of PICC/MLC.
8. Ensure attention to pain management, developmental care, and thermal homeostasis.
9. Infuse medication via medication infusion pump; avoid "pushes."
10. Use larger-bore syringes (>10 mL) that generate less pressure.
11. Avoid tension on catheter and tubing.
12. Never pull the catheter back through hollow needle introducer because of the risk of damage or shearing of catheter.
13. Monitor for bradycardia and hypoxia during procedure.
14. Follow manufacturer's recommendations regarding infusion of blood products or obtaining blood specimens from PICC or MLC.
15. When infusing fluids via MLC, follow the same precautions as with peripheral IV to avoid damage to noncentral vessels.

**D. Equipment and supplies.**

1. Commercially prepared catheter insertion kit, or the following:
   a. Antiseptic per hospital policy. Chlorhexidine gluconate is recommended by the CDC; however, it is only approved by the U.S. Food and Drug Administration for use in

infants over 2 months of age due to lack of evidence on absorption and safety. In infants under 2 months of age, use of povidone–iodine is still the best practice (Alexander and INS, 2011; Chapman et al., 2012). If institutional policy, use with care in premature infants or infants under 2 months of age as these products may cause irritation or chemical burns (U.S. Food and Drug Administration, 2012).

**b.** Nontoothed forceps.

**c.** Sterile measuring tape.

**d.** Sterile gown and gloves, mask, and surgical cap.

**e.** Sterile flush solution per institutional policy.

**f.** Sterile gauze pads.

**g.** Sterile drapes and towels.

**h.** Sterile tourniquet (optional with preterm infants).

(1) Sterile 5- to 10-mL syringes, as recommended by manufacturer.

**i.** Transparent, semipermeable dressing.

**j.** Sterile adhesive strips.

**k.** Extension set per hospital policy.

**l.** Select a neonatal percutaneous catheter of appropriate size. Catheter sizes include single-lumen 1.2 F and single- or double-lumen 1.9 F to 5 F (Alexander and INS, 2011). Usually lumens up to 3 Fr. are used in neonates.

**m.** Select an introducer of appropriate size to accommodate catheter.

(1) Different types of catheter introducers are available, depending on manufacturer:

(a) Breakaway needle—the vessel is cannulated and the catheter advanced through the needle to the premeasured distance. The needle is then retracted and broken along its longitudinal axis and discarded. These needles may be smaller in diameter than introducer-type devices, yet catheter shearing or damage may occur if the catheter is retracted through the needle.

(b) Peel-away plastic cannula—the vessel is punctured and the needle is removed, leaving the plastic cannula in the vessel for catheter insertion. Advance the catheter to the premeasured distance, then retract the plastic cannula from the vessel and pull the catheter apart along its longitudinal axis and discard.

(c) A device with a safety needle retractor should be used to avoid needle-stick injury.

**n.** Catheter trimming device per manufacturer's recommendation.

**E. Procedure.**

**1.** Verify order for PICC/MLC.

**2.** Check to ensure informed consent is obtained per institutional policy.

**3.** Gather equipment and supplies.

**4.** Provide pain management (Pettit and Wyckoff, 2007).

**a.** Developmentally supportive positioning, swaddling, and pacifier use.

**b.** Consider premedication with an analgesic and sedative.

**c.** Consider use of topical lidocaine cream if appropriate.

**5.** Maintain thermoregulation, provide environmental support by protecting infant's eyes from bright lights.

**6.** Select vein (see Fig. 15-1). Most common sites for neonates include the cephalic, basilic, and greater saphenous. A right-sided basilic or cephalic approach is preferred because of the shorter distance between the insertion site and the superior vena cava. Other sites include popliteal, temporal, and axillary veins.

**7.** Position infant so selected vein is accessible. Restrain infant if necessary to prevent contamination of sterile field.

**8.** Measure length of catheter to be inserted.

**a.** For PICC (central venous access) insertion (Pettit and Wyckoff, 2007):

(1) Upper body insertion: Tip should be in the superior vena cava.

(a) Measure from insertion site along the course of the vein to the third intercostal space, with the arm at a 90-degree angle for upper extremity placement.

(2) Lower body insertion: Tip should be in the inferior vena cava above the L4-L5 vertebrae or iliac crest and below the right atrium.
(a) Measure from insertion site to xiphoid process for lower extremity placement.

**b.** For MLC (peripheral venous access) insertion:
(1) Upper body insertion: Tip should end in the upper arm, distal to the head of the humerus.
(a) Measure from the insertion site to the desired site of catheter tip.
(2) Lower body insertion: Tip should end in the upper leg distal to the head of the femur.
(a) Measure from the insertion site to the desired site of catheter tip.

**9.** Don mask and cap and perform a 3-minute scrub.

**10.** Don sterile gown and gloves. Set up sterile field and open catheter kit, maintaining sterility of contents. Assemble equipment using an aseptic technique.

**11.** Trim catheter to predetermined length per manufacturer's recommendations and institution's policy.

**12.** Attach flush-syringe and prime catheter.

**13.** Prepare insertion site with antiseptic per hospital policy and allow to dry.

**14.** Change into new sterile gloves if contamination occurs.

**15.** Drape infant with sterile towels.

**16.** Apply sterile tourniquet (optional) and stabilize vein.

**17.** Take introducer and puncture vessel at an approximately 5- to 15-degree angle for shallow veins and approximately 15 to 30 degrees for deeper veins. After skin puncture, pause and let infant relax to prevent vasoconstriction. Entry into the vessel is signaled by blood leaking from puncture site or from the introducer needle/cannula.

**18.** Loosen tourniquet (if applicable) after advancing catheter a short distance. Remove needle, leaving peel-away plastic cannula in place if using this method.

**19.** Advance flushed catheter with forceps in 0.5- to 1-cm increments to predetermined distance. Catheter should advance smoothly and slowly to avoid vasospasm.

**20.** Once catheter is advanced 7 to 8 cm or to the predetermined distance, remove introducer. Catheter may be pulled out slightly during splitting technique and may need to be advanced slightly when complete. Gentle pressure with finger distal to puncture site may reduce blood loss.

**21.** Remove stylet (if present) slowly.

**22.** Aspirate on catheter to confirm blood return. If blood is obtained, flush catheter.

**23.** Temporarily secure catheter with sterile adhesive strips and obtain chest radiograph for catheter placement while maintaining sterile field and aseptic technique.

**24.** Radiographically confirming placement is central prior to any infusions. Pull back or advance catheter, if necessary, to appropriate distance. Check for blood return and obtain another chest radiograph to confirm satisfactory position.

**25.** If a lower extremity PICC is placed, consider performing a lateral abdominal radiograph in addition to AP view to verify that the catheter is in the inferior vena cava and not the ascending lumbar vein. As an alternative, 0.3 mL of contrast medium may be injected into the catheter with the AP view to verify central venous placement and avoid an additional radiograph (Sharpe et al., 2013; Trotter, 2009).

**26.** Remove antiseptic from surrounding skin with sterile water.

**27.** Secure and dress catheter per hospital policy.
**a.** Use of skin closure or Steri-Strips over the body of the catheter is contraindicated, due to risk of catheter shearing (Sharpe et al., 2013).
**b.** INS recommends a product-specific catheter securement device, if available (Alexander and INS, 2011).

**28.** Document procedure, including:
**a.** Indication for placement.
**b.** Parental education and consent.
**c.** Site preparation.
**d.** Catheter size, manufacturer, and lot number.
**e.** Catheter length if trimmed.

f. Presence of stylet.
g. Location and insertion distance.
h. Location of catheter tip on radiograph.
i. Pain management provided and patient tolerance.
j. Complications.
k. Type of dressing.
l. Name of clinician.

F. **Modified Seldinger technique**—this technique provides for central catheter placement using a peripheral IV catheter of smaller gauge than a standard PICC introducer (Fig. 15-2). Use of a smaller gauge may allow the inserter to access a smaller vessel, and minimizes vessel and surrounding nervous tissue trauma and hematoma formation. This procedure is now standard of practice in adult and pediatric patients, recommended by the INS to minimize damage to vessels (Alexander and INS, 2011; Pettit, 2007).

1. Supplies.
   a. All supplies previously described for PICC insertions.
   b. 24-gauge peripheral IV catheter.
   c. Guidewire:
      (1) 0.012 or 0.018 inch.
      (2) 15 to 20 cm.
   d. No. 11 scalpel blade or straight needle.

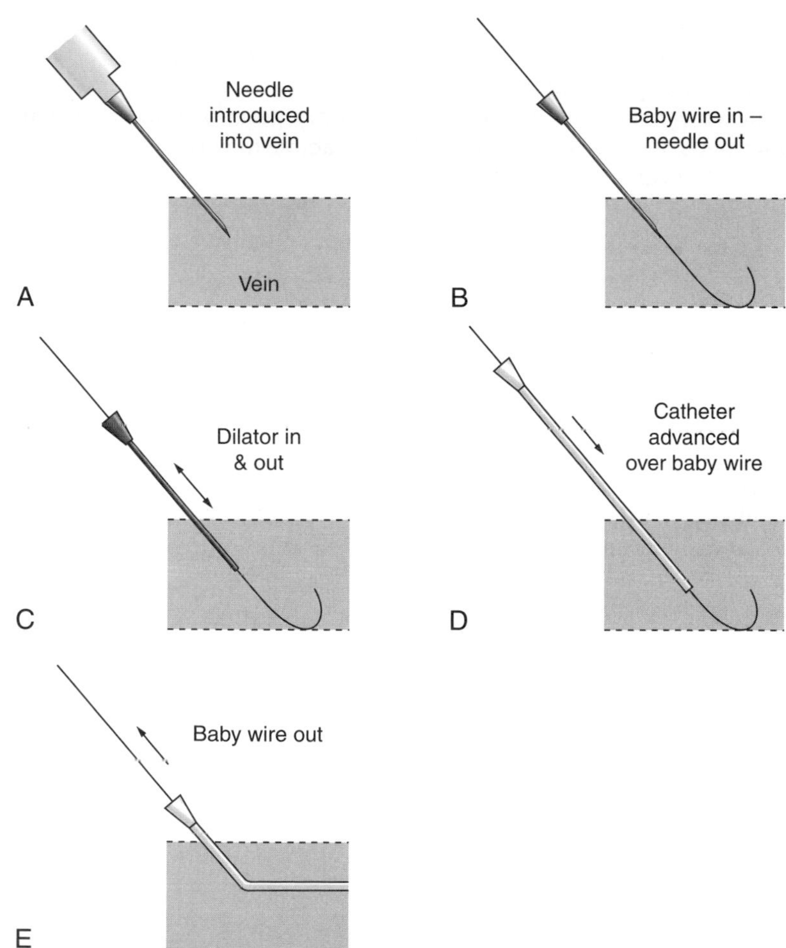


FIGURE 15-2 ■ The modified Seldinger technique for PICC insertion. (From Al-Shaikh, B. and Stacey, S.: *Essentials of anaesthetic equipment* [4th ed.]. London, 2013, Churchill Livingstone.)

2. Procedure.
   a. Identify vessel, trim catheter, and prepare the insertion site as previously described for PICC insertion.
   b. Apply tourniquet as needed.
   c. Perform venipuncture with 24-gauge peripheral IV catheter.
   d. When flashback of blood is noted, advance catheter into vein and remove inner needle.
   e. Thread guidewire through catheter into the vein, approximately 3 cm beyond the tip of the catheter.
      (1) Take caution to advance gently; do not apply force, as this may perforate the vessel.
      (2) Do not advance the guidewire past the infant's shoulder if placed in the arm.
   f. Remove the IV catheter while holding the guidewire in place. Take care to firmly stabilize the guidewire to prevent removal or embolization.
   g. Enlarge the insertion site by 1 to 2 mm.
      (1) Consider use of 1% lidocaine injected intradermally or topical lidocaine cream, or a systemic analgesic such as fentanyl.
      (2) Use forceps to gently dilate the insertion site, or
      (3) Thread a 20-gauge needle over the guidewire, and move side to side in the insertion site, or
      (4) Use a scalpel blade to make a dermatotomy, or small nick in the insertion site, taking care to avoid damaging the vessel.
   h. Slowly thread a plastic peel-away PICC introducer over the guidewire past the insertion site into the vessel. If the introducer cannot be advanced into the vein, the insertion site may need to be further dilated.
   i. Remove the guidewire, leaving the introducer in the vein.
   j. Remove tourniquet if applicable.
   k. Thread the catheter into the vein as previously described, to premeasured depth.
   l. Follow steps described for PICC placement above to verify blood return, assess proper placement of catheter, and apply dressing.
   m. Document procedure, including method of insertion, any additional steps taken, catheter length, patient tolerance, and any complications.

G. **Complications.**
   1. Cardiac arrhythmias.
   2. Pericardial effusion with cardiac tamponade.
   3. Atrial perforation with cardiac tamponade.
   4. Intravascular catheter shearing, followed by embolization of catheter fragment.
   5. Thrombus formation.
   6. Infection, local or systemic.
   7. Nerve damage.
   8. Air embolism.
   9. Rupture of catheter from using excessive infusion pressure (e.g., from using small-bore syringes).
   10. Infiltration/extravasation for MLC.
   11. Hemorrhage.
   12. Vascular perforation.

H. **Catheter maintenance.**
   1. INS recommends an evidence-based catheter care policy to include all aspects of insertion, care, and infusion (Alexander and INS, 2011). This may reduce infection rate and improve patient safety.
   2. Change dressing no more than weekly, or whenever damp, soiled, or nonocclusive.
      a. If gauze is used in the dressing, it must be changed every 48 hours.
   3. Monitor for infiltration or extravasation:
      a. Redness.
      b. Edema.
      c. Difficulty with flushing or fluid infusion.

## Removal of Peripherally Inserted Central Catheter: Fundamental Procedure

**A. Indications.**
1. No longer needed or indicated.
2. Septicemia, especially fungal.
3. Malfunctioning.

**B. Precautions.**
1. Avoid catheter disruption.
2. Venospasm (if resistance is met, do not force catheter; apply warm compress for 20 to 30 minutes and reattempt).

**C. Equipment and supplies.**
1. Sterile gauze.
2. Measuring tape.
3. Transparent dressing.
4. Nonsterile gloves.

**D. Procedure.**
1. Verify order for removal.
2. Wash hands and don gloves.
3. Remove securing tape and dressing carefully to avoid skin trauma.
4. Change gloves.
5. Cleanse site with povidone–iodine or antiseptic per hospital policy and allow to dry.
6. Slowly and carefully retract catheter 1 cm at a time, grasping the catheter near the insertion site until the catheter has been removed. Do not apply pressure over insertion site during catheter removal.
7. Apply sterile gauze over insertion site as withdrawal is complete.
8. Continue to apply pressure if needed with gauze until hemostasis is obtained. Once hemostasis is confirmed, cover site with transparent dressing. Dressing should remain in place for at least 24 hours.
9. Measure and inspect removed catheter and compare that distance with the recorded insertion depth.
   a. If any part has broken off during removal or the length of the catheter differs from the recorded insertion length, place a tourniquet on the affected extremity above the insertion site, such as upper arm or upper leg, to prevent advancement of the catheter piece into the right atrium. Check for pulses. If no pulse or the extremity is dusky, loosen the tourniquet. Immediately notify health care provider as catheter embolization is an emergency and may require removal via cardiac catheterization or via surgery.
10. Document date, time, site location, measurement of catheter removed in comparison to recorded insertion depth, patient's tolerance of procedure, and any complications according to hospital guidelines.

**E. Complications.**
1. Shearing of catheter inside patient, before complete removal.
2. Dislodgment of thrombus from tip.

## Umbilical Vessel Catheterization: Advanced Practice Procedure

**A. Indications.**
1. Arterial catheterization.
   a. Frequent arterial blood sampling.
   b. Continuous arterial blood gas monitoring.
   c. Continuous arterial blood pressure monitoring.
   d. Vascular access for IV fluids when other sites are not available or suitable.
   e. Exchange transfusion.
   f. Cardiac catheterization.

2. Venous catheterization.
   a. Emergency administration of drugs.
   b. Emergency measurement of $P_{CO_2}$ and pH.
   c. Fluid administration (hypertonic solutions or inadequate peripheral access).
   d. Exchange transfusion.
   e. Central venous pressure monitoring.
   f. Blood sampling.

**B. Contraindications.**
1. Abdominal wall defects.
2. Necrotizing enterocolitis (controversial).
3. Vascular compromise below level of umbilicus.
4. Omphalitis.
5. Peritonitis.

**C. Precautions.**
1. Maintain thermal homeostasis.
2. Monitor heart rate and oxygen saturation throughout the procedure.
3. Maintain aseptic technique.
4. Dilate artery before attempting vessel cannulation.
5. Do not force catheter past obstruction.

**D. Equipment and supplies.**
1. Commercially prepackaged sterile umbilical catheter tray or sterile instrument tray for umbilical catheterization to include the following:
   a. 4 × 4 gauze pads.
   b. Sterile drapes.
   c. Small container for antiseptic solution.
   d. Scissors.
   e. Umbilical tape.
   f. Measuring tape.
   g. Syringes, 10 mL.
   h. No. 11 scalpel with handle.
   i. Mosquito hemostats (2).
   j. Curved, nontoothed iris forceps (2).
   k. Toothed iris forceps (1).
   l. Needle holder.
   m. Umbilical catheter of either polyurethane or silicone material. Silicone catheters may be more difficult to insert owing to their lack of rigidity.
   n. Determine appropriate-sized catheter with either a single, double, or triple lumen or as desired by medical staff. Various sizes of catheters are available ranging from 2.5 F to 8 F. Generally, the following guidelines apply.
      (1) Size 3.5 F for infants weighing less than 1500 g.
      (2) Size 3.5 F, 4.0 F, or 5.0 F for infants weighing more than 1500 g.
      (3) A 2.5 F polyurethane catheter is available for use in the extremely premature infant.
   o. 3-0 silk suture.
   p. 4-0 silk suture with curved needle.
   q. Three-way Luer-Lok stopcock.
   r. Dressings for securing (clear occlusive dressing and a hydrocolloid skin barrier).
   s. Sterile heparin-flush solution (1 unit/mL).
2. Sterile antiseptic solution.
3. Mask, surgical cap, and sterile gown and gloves.
4. Standardized premeasurement graph or access to a formula to determine insertion depth.

**E. Procedure.**

**Umbilical Artery Catheterization.** NOTE: *Low position*, catheter tip placed between the third and fourth lumbar vertebrae (L3-L4). *High position*, catheter tip placed between the sixth and 10th thoracic vertebrae (T6-T10). Either position is accepted practice currently. Consult your institution's guidelines for desired positioning of umbilical artery catheters (UACs).

1. Inspect lower extremities for bruising and palpate pulses.

2. Assess umbilical cord to rule out umbilical anomaly, such as a small omphalocele.
3. Place infant supine and restrain limbs.
4. Calculate insertion depth.
   a. Measure shoulder-to-umbilical distance (adding length of umbilicus stump) and multiply by 0.66 to arrive at insertion depth for a "low" placement (L3-L4), or
   b. 2.5 times body weight in kilograms plus 9.7 cm ($2.5 \times$ weight$+9.7$) for a "high" placement (T6-T10).
5. Don mask and cap and perform a 3- to 5-minute scrub.
6. Don sterile gown and gloves.
7. Have assistant hold heparin-flush vial and draw up flush into sterile syringe.
8. Prepare catheter by attaching Luer-Lok stopcock to catheter and connect flush-filled syringe to stopcock and flush catheter.
9. Turn stopcock off to catheter.
10. Have assistant hold umbilical cord up and out of procedure area while cord is prepped with antiseptic solution. Scrub in a circular manner, moving from the cord to approximately 5 cm in radius on surrounding abdomen. Do not let antiseptic drip down infant's side or pool on abdomen because this may cause skin damage, especially in extremely premature infants.
11. Drape procedure area with sterile towels.
12. Tie umbilical tape using a single-hand knot tight enough to prevent bleeding at base of cord, not on the skin. Umbilical tape may have to be loosened to advance catheter or tightened to control bleeding.
13. Using a scalpel, cut through the umbilical cord 1 to 1.5 cm from skin.
14. Identify cord vessels.
    a. Arteries: two small, thick-walled, and white constricted vessels that may stick out slightly and are typically located at the 4 and 8 o'clock positions.
    b. Vein: single, large, thin-walled vessel, often open and typically located at the 12 o'clock position.
15. Stabilize cord stump.
    a. Grasp portion of cut edge of cord with hemostat and apply gentle traction.
    b. Apply hemostats to opposite sides of the cord and roll them away from each other, causing the arteries to protrude from the cut surface of the cord.
16. Dilate artery.
    a. Insert one tip of curved iris forceps into selected artery and probe gently to a depth of about 0.5 cm; withdraw forceps tip.
    b. With tips of forceps together again, gently probe artery to a depth of about 0.5 cm.
    c. Gently spread forceps apart, and then slowly withdraw forceps from artery, dilating lumen as forceps is withdrawn.
    d. Continue to dilate lumen (approximately 15 to 60 seconds) until forceps can easily be inserted to a depth of about 1 cm.
17. Insert catheter.
    a. Insert catheter into dilated artery.
    b. Thread catheter to predetermined depth.
    c. If resistance is met, do not force catheter. Apply gentle, steady pressure to catheter while applying gentle traction on cord.
    d. If catheter cannot be advanced to the desired distance, discontinue attempts and catheterize second artery.
    e. Observe for blanching of legs, toes, and/or buttocks.
18. Aspirate blood to ensure placement in vessel after catheter advanced approximately 5 cm. If blood is obtained, clear catheter by injecting 0.5 mL flush solution. If blood cannot be aspirated, remove catheter and attempt catheterization of second artery.
19. Obtain radiograph to confirm catheter position.
    a. If the catheter tip is too high, pull the catheter back to its proper position and obtain another radiograph.
    b. If the catheter tip is too low for "high position," pull back to "low position," if your institutional guidelines allow this.

c. If catheter tip is too low for "low position," it should be adjusted to an acceptable position. Keep in mind that a catheter that is no longer sterile should not be advanced.

20. Suture catheter in place.
    a. Place purse-string suture around cord. Avoid piercing the vessels and catheters. Secure to umbilical skin or cord depending on your institution's guidelines.
    b. Knot suture securely in cord close to catheter per manufacturer's recommendations.
    c. If suture is around catheter, it must be tight to prevent catheter from sliding, but not so tight that flow through catheter is obstructed.
21. Loosen umbilical tape.
22. Remove antiseptic as soon as possible from the skin to prevent irritation or breakdown.
23. Secure catheter per hospital policy. The following are various securing techniques used to secure catheters:
    a. Commercially manufactured securing devices.
    b. "Bridge" or "goalpost" taping technique.
    c. Hydrocolloid skin barrier applied to umbilical area with clear occlusive dressing.
24. Document procedure according to hospital policy, noting type of catheter, catheter size, distance catheter threaded, location of catheter tip on radiograph, adjustments made to catheter to correct malpositioned catheter, and assessment of color, pulses, and perfusion to lower extremities.

**Umbilical Vein Catheterization.** NOTE: Equipment for umbilical vein catheterization is the same as that for UAC insertion with the exception that an 8 F catheter may occasionally be used for infants weighing greater than 3500 g.

1. Maintain aseptic technique.
2. Prepare cord as for UAC and identify the thin-walled vein.
3. Grasp the base of the cord with curved hemostats or toothed forceps, hold upright, and dilate vessel with the tip of iris forceps.
4. Insert the catheter to predetermined distance.
    a. Emergency placement (temporary catheter, "low position"): Insert 2 to 3 cm into vessel until blood is obtained. Once emergency medications and fluids have been administered and the infant is stabilized, remove the catheter.
    b. Indwelling umbilical venous catheter:
        (1) Measure shoulder-to-umbilical distance and multiply by 0.75 to arrive at insertion depth, or
        (2) Calculate insertion depth with the formula 1.5 times body weight in kilograms plus 5.6 cm ($1.5 \times \text{weight} + 5.6$).
5. If resistance is met, withdraw the catheter 2 to 3 cm and attempt to reinsert. If cannulation remains unsuccessful, remove the catheter.
6. If cannulation is successful, connect and secure catheter and confirm position by radiograph. Correct radiographic position is 0.5 to 1 cm above the diaphragm.
7. Secure catheter per hospital policy.
8. Document procedure according to hospital policy, noting type of catheter, catheter size, distance catheter threaded, location of catheter tip on radiograph, and adjustments made to catheter to correct malpositioned catheter.

**F. Complications of using umbilical catheters.**

1. Vasospasm, embolism, thrombosis, and distal ischemia:
    a. Blanching, cyanosis, and mottling of skin.
    b. Sloughing of skin.
    c. Necrosis of extremities, possibly leading to loss of toes.
    d. Paraplegia.
    e. Intestinal necrosis and perforation.
2. Infection.
3. Mechanical complications:
    a. Perforation of vessels.
    b. Perforation of peritoneum.

c. False aneurysm.
d. Knot in catheter or breaking of catheter.
4. Malpositioned catheter:
a. Cardiac arrhythmias.
b. Pericardial effusion.
c. Cardiac tamponade.
d. Hydrothorax.
5. Necrotizing enterocolitis (controversial).
6. Perforation of colon.
7. Hepatic necrosis.
8. Skin burns from antiseptics.
9. Hemorrhage, exsanguination.
10. Portal hypertension.
11. Death.

## Radial Artery Catheterization: Advanced Practice Procedure

**A. Indications.**
1. Need for frequent blood sampling and umbilical artery catheterization cannot be done or UAC has been removed.
2. Need for continuous blood pressure monitoring.

**B. Precautions.**
1. Avoid areas of skin breakdown or infection.
2. Use caution in infants with coagulopathy, who may bleed excessively.
3. Inadequate ulnar artery blood flow.
4. Limb malformation.

**C. Equipment and supplies.**
1. 22- to 27-gauge over-the-needle IV catheter.
2. Antiseptic solution per institution policy.
3. 0.25 to 0.5 NS flush.
4. Occlusive dressing and tape per institution policy.
5. Transilluminator if needed.
6. Appropriately sized padded armboard.
7. Arterial pressure transducer and extension tubing per institution policy.
8. Nonsterile gloves.
9. 4-0 sutures if needed per institution policy.
10. T-connector as needed per institution policy.
11. Pain/developmental management: pacifier, sucrose pacifier, blankets for swaddling, and eye protection from bright lights.

**D. Procedure.**
1. Select site for catheterization:
a. Palpate radial artery pulse.
b. Transillumination may assist in identifying vessel.
2. Take care not to hyperextend wrist, as this will occlude arterial flow.
3. Perform modified Allen test to ensure adequate collateral circulation:
a. Elevate hand.
b. Occlude both radial and ulnar arteries.
c. Massage the palm toward wrist to blanch hand.
d. Release pressure on the ulnar artery.
e. Perfusion to hand should return in less than 10 seconds; if longer than 15 seconds, do not puncture artery.
4. Position and secure wrist as shown in Figure 15-3.
5. Provide pain management and developmental support.
6. Prepare site with antiseptic solution per institution policy.

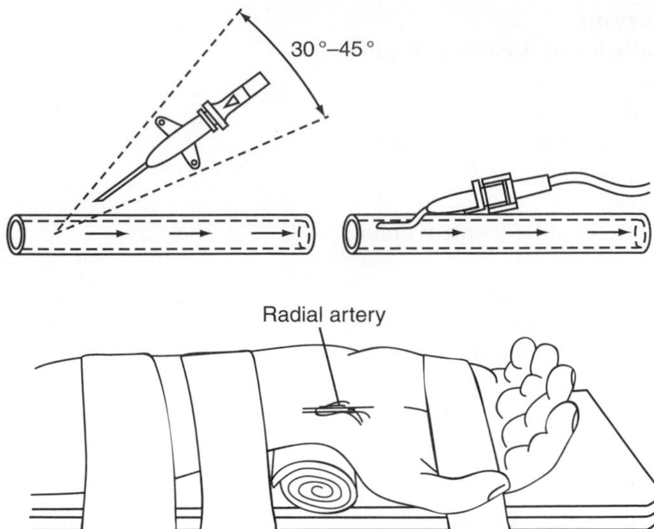


FIGURE 15-3 ■ Peripheral arterial line insertion. (From Gomella, T.L.: *Neonatology: Management, procedures, on-call problems, diseases and drugs* [6th ed.]. New York, 2009, Lange Medical Books/McGraw-Hill.)

7. Puncture the skin proximal to the wrist crease with the needle at a 30- to 45-degree angle (a deeper angle may be needed for larger babies).
8. Cannulate the artery using one of the following methods:
   a. Puncture both walls of the artery with the needle bevel up (blood return may be delayed). Remove the stylet and withdraw the catheter until blood return is noted. When blood return is seen, advance the catheter into the artery and flush. Flushing while advancing may stabilize the catheter and make advancing easier.
   b. Puncture the anterior wall of the artery until blood return is seen; at this point the catheter is in the artery. Advance the catheter while simultaneously withdrawing the stylet and flush.
9. Secure cannula with sutures or tape per institution policy.
10. Attach T-connector per institution policy and flush line. Luer-lock connections are preferred if they do not interfere with patency of the catheter.
11. Secure line with armboard and dressing per institution policy. Ensure visibility of insertion site and all fingers.
12. Attach pressure transducer and extension tubing per institution policy and ensure unobstructed flow of fluids by pump. Secure all connection sites to avoid backflow of blood into line.
13. Maintain patency of catheter with heparinized fluids.
14. Dispose of needle in designated sharps container.
15. Document date, time, location, catheter size, distal perfusion, and pain response to placement of catheter.
16. Monitor site for extravasation or leakage of fluids and/or blood.
17. Monitor fingers for adequate perfusion of all digits.

**E. Complications.**

1. Arteriospasm.
2. Infection.
3. Extravasation of fluids.
4. Hematoma or hemorrhage.
5. Embolism or thrombus formation leading to tissue ischemia or necrosis and possible loss of hand or digits.
6. Damage to surrounding tissues or structures.

# BLOOD SAMPLING PROCEDURES

## Choice of Method for Blood Sampling

A. **Amount of blood needed.**
   1. Capillary sampling is indicated for small amounts of blood, generally less than 1 mL.
   2. It may be easier to obtain large amounts of blood (>2 mL) from an arterial puncture.

B. **Type of testing indicated.**
   1. Newborn metabolic screens are primarily drawn via heel stick.
   2. Some laboratory results may be affected by hemolysis, clotting, or clumping of the blood, and a large-volume free-flowing specimen may be easier to obtain by venipuncture or arterial puncture (Folk 2007; Milcic, 2010).
      a. Chemistry levels.
      b. Platelet levels.
      c. Hematocrit.
      d. Coagulation studies.
   3. Collection of blood for cultures requires sterile technique and blood should be collected via venous or arterial puncture (Folk, 2007).
   4. Blood gas values will differ based on arterial, capillary, or venous sources. As exchange of oxygen for $CO_2$ occurs in peripheral tissues, $CO_2$ levels will be lowest in arterial blood, and highest in venous blood, and oxygen levels will be highest in arterial blood and lowest in venous blood. Blood pH will also vary, being lower in arterial and higher in venous sources. An arterial sample may be helpful to ascertain accurate pH, $Pao_2$, and $Paco_2$ levels.

C. **Pain of procedures.**
   1. Studies have shown venipuncture to be less painful than other sampling methods when drawn by a skilled phlebotomist (Folk, 2007). However, consideration should be given to preserving future IV sites in sick infants.
   2. Laboratory samples should be drawn with as few invasive procedures as possible to minimize pain. Consider the total volume of blood needed when choosing a sampling method, and try to cluster laboratory draws to avoid multiple punctures. For infants needing frequent blood draws, consider placement of an arterial catheter.

## Capillary Blood Sampling: Fundamental Procedure

A. **Indications.**
   1. Small amount of blood collection is needed (<1 mL) (Folk, 2007).
   2. Venous or arterial blood sample is not possible or necessary.
   3. Collection of blood specimen for blood gas sampling, routine laboratory sampling, state newborn metabolic screens.

B. **Contraindications.**
   1. Impaired circulation in selected limb or at puncture site.
   2. Infection near puncture site.

C. **Precautions.**
   1. Consider venipuncture if impaired skin integrity noted at selected puncture site (edema, bruising, multiple puncture marks).
   2. Consider venipuncture as an alternative to capillary sampling in term neonates, as it may be less painful (Shah and Ohlsson, 2007).
   3. Hyperviscous blood may render sampling difficult. Consider venipuncture in infants with polycythemia.
   4. Use caution in infants with coagulation disorders.
   5. Do not puncture the back of the heel; this may cause damage to the calcaneus bone.
   6. Avoid finger, great toe, and earlobe sticks.
   7. Avoid excessive squeezing that may cause hemolysis.

D. **Equipment and supplies.**
   1. Sterile alcohol swabs or other antiseptic, as per institutional guideline.
   2. Automated heel-lancing incision device based on infant size.
   3. Sterile gauze pad.

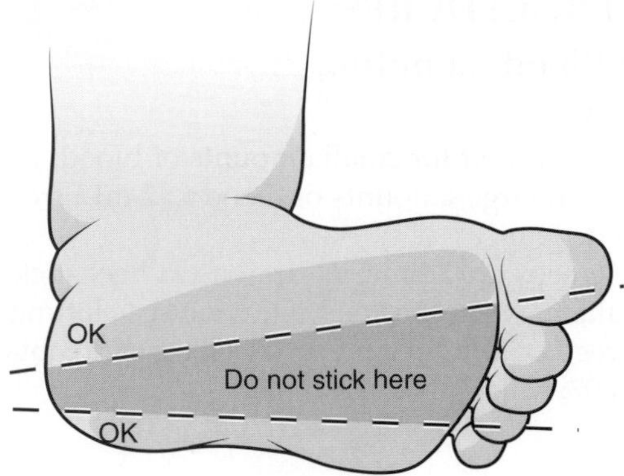


FIGURE 15-4 ■ Use shaded areas when performing heel stick in infant. (From Roberts, J.R.: *Roberts and Hedges' clinical procedures in emergency medicine* [6th ed.]. Philadelphia, 2014, Elsevier Saunders.)

4. Warm compress. Recent studies have shown that warming the heels may not be needed (Folk 2007). When warming heels, use a warm compress manufactured for use with infants, no warmer than 40° C.
5. Nonsterile gloves.
6. Appropriate specimen collection containers.
7. Pain management: pacifier, sucrose pacifier, and blankets for developmental swaddling.

**E. Procedure.**

1. Select puncture site on the lateral or medial aspect of the heel. Avoid other areas because of the possibility of nerve damage or osteomyelitis (Fig. 15-4).
2. Warm heel with compress for 5 to 10 minutes if desired.
3. Provide pain management:
   a. Pacifier for nonnutritive sucking.
   b. Consider 24% sucrose solution applied to pacifier or nipple 2 minutes prior to procedure, if patient age and status allow (Folk, 2007).
   c. Dim and quiet environment.
   d. Skin-to-skin holding, and/or blanket swaddling with selected extremity exposed.
4. Gather supplies, wash hands, and don gloves.
5. Prepare area selected for skin puncture with antiseptic or alcohol and allow to dry.
6. Puncture heel perpendicular to the skin.
7. Wipe away first drop of blood with sterile gauze pad.
8. Collect specimen from free-flowing drops at puncture site.
   a. Blood flow is increased if the puncture site is dependent relative to the extremity.
   b. Gentle "pumping" of the extremity above the puncture site may encourage blood flow.
9. After specimen is collected, elevate foot and apply pressure with sterile gauze pad until hemostasis has occurred.
10. Dispose of lancet in appropriate sharps container.
11. Label specimen per institutional policy.
12. Document the heel-stick procedure, specimen obtained, date and time, pain management, and patient's tolerance.

**F. Complications.**

1. Bruising or loss of skin integrity.
2. Infection.
3. Scarring.
4. Calcified nodules.
5. Cellulitis.
6. Osteomyelitis.
7. Nerve damage (Folk, 2007).
8. Pain.
9. Erroneous laboratory values may result from the following:
   a. Contamination of specimen with tissue fluid.

b. Contamination of specimen with alcohol.
c. Inadequate warming or poor circulation at puncture site.
d. Hemolysis of specimen.

## Venipuncture (Phlebotomy): Fundamental Procedure

A. **Indications.**
   1. Large quantity of blood required.
   2. Arterial sample not possible or necessary.
   3. Capillary sample not possible or sufficient.
   4. Sterile collection for blood culture.
   5. Specific laboratory tests requiring venous sampling.

B. **Contraindications.**
   1. Inadequate or impaired circulation in selected limb.
   2. Infection or loss of skin integrity near selected venipuncture site.

C. **Precautions.**
   1. Use caution in infants with coagulation disorders.
   2. Avoid sites that may be needed for possible central venous cannulation.
   3. Differentiate between arteries and veins.

D. **Equipment and supplies.**
   1. Antiseptic skin preparation per hospital policy.
   2. 23- to 25-gauge butterfly needle or hypodermic needle attached to syringe.
   3. Syringe(s) for specimen collection.
   4. Appropriate specimen collection tubes.
   5. Sterile gauze pad.
   6. Tourniquet or rubber band.
   7. Nonsterile gloves.
   8. Pain management: pacifier, sucrose pacifier, blankets for swaddling leaving venipuncture site accessible, and/or cloth to protect eyes from bright lights.

E. **Procedure.**
   1. Gather supplies, wash hands, and don gloves.
   2. Choose vein to be used. Accomplish distention of the vessel by applying a gentle tourniquet proximal to the selected insertion site. Alternatively, an assistant may encircle the proximal extremity with his or her hand or fingers and apply direct pressure for the same effect.
   3. Provide pain-relieving measures and developmentally position/swaddle infant with selected venipuncture site accessible.
   4. Stabilize and position the selected puncture site to allow puncture in direction of blood flow.
   5. Prepare skin at selected puncture site with antiseptic per hospital policy.
   6. Puncture skin at a 15- to 45-degree angle, with needle bevel up, just distal to anticipated vessel entry site, using shallow angle for smaller infants or superficial vessels.
   7. Advance needle until blood appears in the tubing.
      a. If resistance is met or vessel is not punctured, withdraw needle slowly to just below level of the skin, relocate vessel, and advance the needle again.
      b. If a hematoma develops or bleeding occurs, occlude the vessel with pressure just proximal to the puncture site, remove tourniquet, and withdraw needle. Apply pressure until hemostasis has occurred.
   8. On entrance of blood into tubing, attach syringe and gently aspirate to obtain specimen. If a hypodermic needle with an intact hub was used, blood specimen may drip into laboratory collection container.
   9. After specimen is obtained, using a gauze pad just proximal to puncture site, occlude vessel with pressure over entry site while removing tourniquet and withdrawing needle.
   10. Apply pressure to site until hemostasis has occurred.
   11. Dispose of needle in appropriate sharps container.
   12. Label specimens per institution policy.
   13. Document date, time, site location, specimen collected, amount of blood removed, nonpharmacologic interventions, patient's tolerance of the procedure, and any complications.

**F. Complications.**
1. Hematoma.
2. Infection.
3. Hemorrhage.
4. Needle injury to adjacent structures.
5. Pain.

## Radial Artery Puncture: Advanced Practice Procedure

**A. Indications.**
1. Venous and/or capillary sites are not satisfactory.
2. Other arterial line is unavailable for sampling.
3. Arterial blood gas sampling.
4. Need to sample large quantities of blood.

**B. Precautions.**
1. Avoid area of infection or loss of skin integrity near selected puncture site.
2. Use caution in infants with coagulation defects.
3. Avoid puncture in extremity with inadequate or impaired circulation.
4. Consider need to preserve arterial site for possible cannulation.
5. Avoid extremity with inadequate collateral circulation distal to the selected puncture site.
6. Use of small-gauge needle reduces potential complications.

**C. Equipment and supplies.**
1. Antiseptic supplies to prepare for arterial puncture per hospital policy.
2. 23- to 25-gauge butterfly needle or 23- to 25-gauge needle attached to a 3-mL syringe.
3. Extra syringes.
4. Sterile gauze pad.
5. Arterial blood gas syringe, other applicable laboratory specimen containers.
6. Transilluminator (optional).

**D. Procedure.**
1. Determine puncture site.
   a. Transillumination may assist in vessel location.
   b. Extend wrist; do not hyperextend, which may occlude vessel.
   c. Palpate artery at distal crease of wrist.
2. Perform modified Allen test to assess collateral circulation.
   a. Elevate hand.
   b. Apply pressure to occlude both radial and ulnar arteries.
   c. Massage the palm to blanch hand.
   d. Release pressure on ulnar artery.
   e. If color returns to hand in less than 10 seconds, adequate collateral circulation is suggested. If color returns in greater than 15 seconds, do not puncture artery because of poor collateral circulation.
   f. Doppler-flow evaluation of ulnar, radial, and palmar circulation can also help determine adequacy of collateral flow.
3. Provide pain management such as pacifier for nonnutritive sucking, sucrose pacifier, and/or developmental care with facilitated tucking or blanket swaddling.
4. Position and stabilize extended wrist to allow puncture against direction of arterial flow.
5. Prepare area with antiseptic for skin puncture (middle to outer third of wrist) per hospital policy.
6. Puncture skin with needle (bevel up) at a 15- to 45-degree angle, using shallower angle for smaller infants or more superficial arteries.
7. Advance needle slowly to puncture artery.
   a. If resistance is met or blood is not obtained, withdraw needle slowly to just below skin level, palpate artery, and advance needle again in the direction of the artery.
   b. If hematoma or bleeding develops, occlude artery with gauze and pressure just proximal to the puncture site, withdraw needle, and apply pressure until hemostasis has occurred (approximately 5 minutes of direct pressure).

8. If arterial cannulation is successful, when blood enters the butterfly tubing, attach syringe and aspirate gently to obtain sample.
9. Apply firm, but not occlusive, pressure to artery with gauze just proximal to puncture site and withdraw needle. Apply pressure to site for 5 minutes or until hemostasis has occurred.
10. Ensure distal circulation after puncture.
    a. Evaluate color and temperature.
    b. Check capillary refill time.
    c. Palpate arterial pulse.
11. Document the following: date, time, site location, Allen test result prior to procedure, pain management interventions, tolerance to procedure, specimen obtained, amount of blood drawn, hemostasis, distal circulation, and any complications if encountered.

E. **Complications.**
1. Hematoma.
2. Hemorrhage.
3. Infection.
4. Thrombosis, embolism.
5. Arteriospasm, tissue necrosis, possibly leading to loss of hand.
6. Needle injury to adjacent structures.
7. Pain.

# MISCELLANEOUS PROCEDURES

## Bladder Catheterization: Fundamental Procedure

A. **Indications.**
1. To obtain urine specimen/culture.
2. To monitor urinary output.
3. To monitor bladder residuals.
4. To relieve urinary retention.
5. To accomplish genitourinary testing such as cystogram or voiding cystourethrogram.

B. **Contraindications.**
1. Anatomic malformations.

C. **Precautions.**
1. Use caution in infants with coagulation disorders.
2. Maintain an aseptic technique.
3. Do not force the catheter, as this may lead to trauma to the urethra and bladder.
4. Remove catheter as soon as possible to minimize infection.
5. Use the smallest-diameter catheter to avoid trauma.

D. **Equipment and supplies.** Note: All equipment is sterile and is available in commercially prepared kits.
1. Urethral catheters.
    a. Size 3.5 F urinary catheter for infants weighing less than 1000 g may be used.
    b. Size 5 F urinary catheter for infants weighing greater than 1000 g may be used.
2. Urinary catheter tray.
    a. Sterile gloves.
    b. Povidone–iodine solution swabs.
    c. Sterile drapes.
    d. Lubricant.
    e. Sterile specimen container or closed urinary drainage system.

E. **Procedure.**

**Male Catheterization.**
1. Place infant supine and restrain legs or have assistant hold legs.
2. Don sterile gloves.
3. Clean penis:
    a. Hold the penis perpendicular to the body with the nondominant hand (which is now considered contaminated).

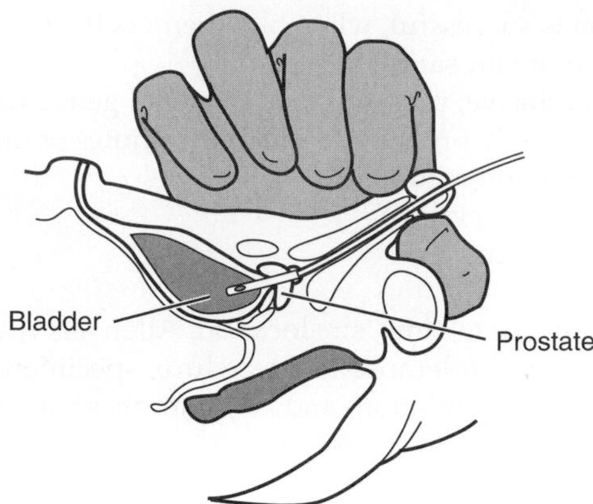


FIGURE 15-5 ■ Male bladder catheterization. (From Gomella, T.L.: *Neonatology: Management, procedures, on-call problems, diseases, and drugs* [6th ed.]. New York, 2009, Lange Medical Books/McGraw-Hill.)

b. Starting at the meatus and moving down the penis, clean with povidone–iodine solution swabs three times, using a new swab each time.

4. Drape sterile towels across infant's lower abdomen and across legs.
5. Apply sterile lubricant to appropriately sized catheter tip with the sterile dominant hand.
6. Place the catheter (held by the still-sterile dominant hand) into the meatus while maintaining perpendicular position of the penis with the nondominant hand. Advance catheter along the urethra until urine appears. Slight resistance may be felt as the catheter passes through the external bladder sphincter. Steady, gentle pressure is usually needed to pass beyond this area; however, never force the catheter (Fig. 15-5).
7. Advance catheter slightly past the point where urine flow began. Inflate the balloon per hospital policy and manufacturer's recommendations, if applicable. Usually the catheter will function satisfactorily if simply taped in place. Balloon inflation may injure the urethra if the catheter is not properly positioned in the bladder.
8. If catheter is to remain indwelling, tape it to lower abdomen or to penile shaft.
9. Collect urine specimen in the sterile container and send to the laboratory or attach to a closed urinary drainage system.
10. Document procedure, catheter type and size, patient's tolerance, quantity and characteristics of sample obtained, and any difficulties encountered.

**Female Catheterization.**

1. Place infant on back and secure legs in frog-leg position. You may secure with restraints or have an assistant hold the legs.
2. Don sterile gloves.
3. Separate the labia with the nondominant hand (which is no longer sterile). With the sterile dominant hand, clean the area around the meatus with the povidone–iodine solution swabs, using front-to-back strokes, repeating with three separate swabs.
4. Drape sterile towels across infant's lower abdomen and across legs.
5. Spread the labia and identify the meatus and urethra (Fig. 15-6).
6. Apply sterile lubricant to an appropriately sized catheter tip using the sterile dominant hand.
7. Insert the catheter into the urethra and advance until urine appears.
8. Advance catheter slightly past the point where urine flow began. Inflate balloon per hospital policy and manufacturer's recommendations, if applicable. Usually the catheter will function satisfactorily if simply taped in place. Balloon inflation may injure the urethra if the catheter is not properly positioned in the bladder.
9. If catheter is to remain indwelling, secure to inner thigh.
10. Collect urine specimen in the sterile container and send to the laboratory or attach to a closed urinary drainage system.
11. Document procedure, catheter type and size, patient's tolerance, quantity and characteristics of sample obtained, and any difficulties encountered.

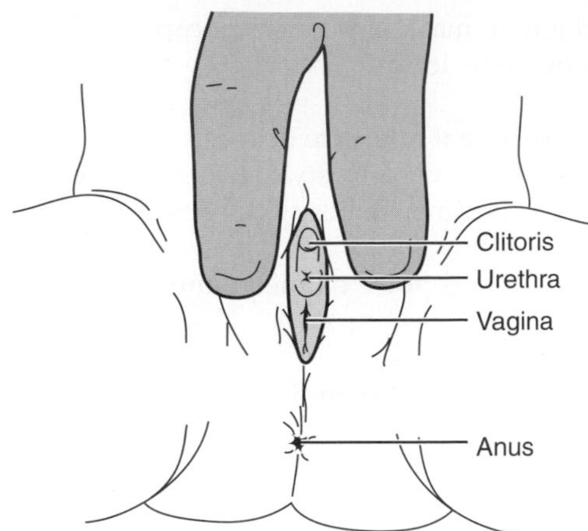


FIGURE 15-6 ■ Landmarks used in female bladder catheterization. (From Gomella, T.L.: *Neonatology: Management, procedures, on-call problems, diseases, and drugs* [6th ed.]. New York, 2009, Lange Medical Books/McGraw-Hill.)

**F. Complications.**
1. Infection.
2. Hematuria.
3. Trauma to urethra.
4. Stricture of urethra or at meatus.
5. Possible knotting of catheter.
6. Pain.

## Lumbar Puncture: Advanced Practice Procedure

**A. Indications.**
1. To obtain cerebrospinal fluid (CSF) to diagnose central nervous system (CNS) disorders such as infections or subarachnoid hemorrhage.
2. To monitor the efficacy of antibiotic therapy in the presence of CNS infection (rare).
3. To drain CSF in communicating hydrocephalus associated with intracranial hemorrhage.
4. To administer medication.
5. To assist in the diagnosis of certain metabolic disorders.

**B. Contraindications.**
1. Evidence of increased ICP. Performance of the procedure could cause herniation.
2. Lumbosacral anomalies.
3. Infants with uncorrected thrombocytopenia or coagulopathies.
4. Severe cardiorespiratory instability.

**C. Precautions.**
1. Avoid areas of infection or loss of skin integrity at puncture site.
2. Monitor for and be prepared to respond to cardiorespiratory instability.
3. Avoid flexion of the neck and ensure that a patent airway is maintained.
4. Always maintain aseptic technique.
5. Always use a needle with a stylet to avoid development of intraspinal epidermoid tumor.
6. To prevent traumatic tap caused by overpenetration, insert the needle slowly while removing the stylet at frequent intervals to detect CSF as soon as the subdural space is entered.
7. Never aspirate CSF with a syringe. Even a small amount of negative pressure can increase the risk of subdural hemorrhage or herniation.
8. Palpate landmarks accurately to prevent puncture above the L4 interspace.

**D. Equipment and supplies.**
1. Prepackaged lumbar puncture kit.
2. If a prepackaged kit is not available, gather the following supplies:

a. Sterile gloves and gown, mask, and surgical cap.
b. Sterile cup with povidone–iodine.
c. Sterile gauze pads.
d. Sterile towels or transparent aperture drape.
e. Spinal needle with short bevel and stylet (22-gauge needle).
f. Three or more sterile specimen tubes with caps.
g. Adhesive bandage.

3. Cardiorespiratory monitor and pulse oximeter and emergency equipment such as suction and oxygen source.
4. Analgesic agents and/or sedatives.
5. Pressure-monitoring equipment, if planning to obtain CSF pressures.

E. **Procedure.**

1. Obtain informed consent per institution's policy.
2. Gather equipment and supplies.
3. Provide anxiety/pain management by considering the following:
   a. Oral sucrose solution to minimize pain (Leef, 2006).
   b. Topical anesthetics such as EMLA, Ametop, or LMX4 over puncture site in term newborns per institution's policy and manufacturer's recommendations (Kaur et al., 2003; O'Brien et al., 2005). Use of topical local anesthetic has been shown to increase success rates (Baxter et al., 2006).
   c. Nonnarcotic relief such as acetaminophen.
   d. Local anesthesia: 1% lidocaine drawn up in a 1-mL syringe with a 27- to 25-gauge needle for injection.
   e. Opioid (fentanyl or morphine) or a benzodiazepine (Versed not recommended in premature infants).
4. Examine and determine puncture site:
   a. Grasp both iliac crests at their highest points and, following an imaginary line (that passes across the level of the fifth lumbar vertebra), palpate the interspace of the spinous process that falls immediately above or below the imaginary line drawn between the iliac crests (Fig. 15-7).
   b. The preferred puncture site is between L3-L4 and L4-L5 (MacDonald and Ramasethu, 2013).
   c. The puncture site can be marked by making a small nail print impression or using a surgical marker.
5. Don mask and cap and perform a 3-minute scrub, and then don gown and sterile gloves.

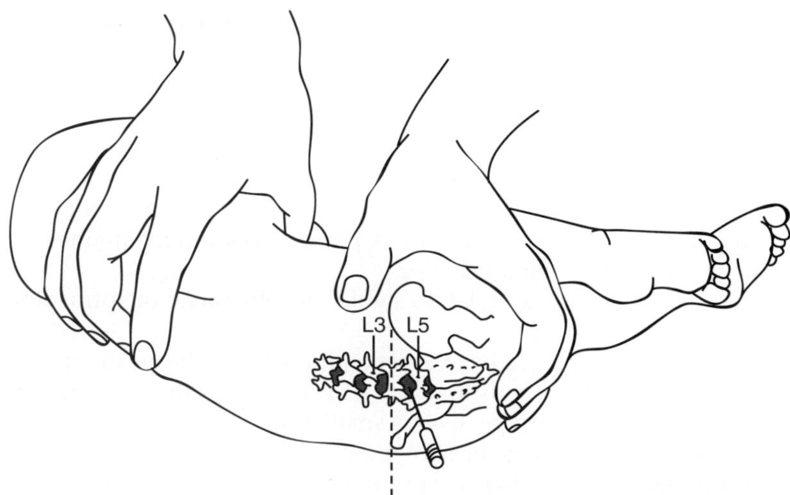


FIGURE 15-7 ■ Lumbar puncture positioning and landmarks. (From Gomella, T.L.: *Neonatology: Management, procedures, on-call problems, diseases, and drugs* [6th ed.]. New York, 2009, Lange Medical Books/McGraw-Hill.)

6. Have an assistant open tray while maintaining the sterility of its contents.
7. Have assistant restrain the infant with hips flexed and back arched in the lateral decubitus (knee–chest) or sitting position, with spine flexed. An intubated infant must be positioned in the lateral decubitus position. Avoid flexion of the neck and ensure that a patent airway is maintained.
8. Clean the lumbar area 3 times with antiseptic using a new swab each time.
   a. Begin at the desired interspace, using a circular motion from puncture site outward to up and over the iliac crests.
   b. Allow antiseptic to dry.
9. If used, inject a wheal of local anesthetic at the puncture site. After several minutes, infiltrate the deeper tissues also.
10. Place one sterile drape under the infant and another that covers the infant, with the exception of the puncture site and the infant's face. Transparent aperture drapes are available and recommended because they permit better observation of the infant.
11. Relocate the desired interspace and insert the needle in the midline.
    a. Angle slightly cephalad to avoid the vertebral bodies.
    b. If resistance is met, withdraw the needle slightly and redirect more cephalad.
    c. Hold a finger on the vertebral process above or below the interspace to aid in locating the puncture site if the infant moves.
12. Advance the needle slowly to a depth of approximately 1.0 to 1.5 cm depending on infant's size, in small increments (2 to 3 mm) to avoid puncture of posterior wall.
    a. Remove the stylet frequently to observe the needle hub for fluid. Always replace the stylet before readvancing the needle.
    b. A pop may be felt when the ligamentum flavum and dura are penetrated. Penetration of the dura may also be detected when a loss of resistance is met.
    c. Once fluid is noted in the needle hub, patiently wait for CSF, which may be slow.
13. Obtain pressure measurement reading, if desired.
    a. Opening pressure measurements are difficult and often unreliable, but possible in a quiet infant in the lateral decubitus position. If measuring pressure, attach the manometer and wait for the fluid oscillations to stabilize in the tube before recording the pressure. Normal mean lumbar CSF pressures in neonates and preterm infants are 100 and 95 mm $H_2O$, respectively (Marra et al., 2004).
14. Allow CSF to collect dropwise into the collection tubes; never aspirate with a syringe.
15. If no fluid is obtained, try gently rotating the needle. If no fluid is obtained after repositioning the needle, replace the stylet, remove the needle, and try one interspace above or below, using a new needle for each attempt.
16. Allow the CSF to drop from the needle hub to collect 0.5- to 1-mL aliquots of CSF in three or four of the specimen tubes for the following diagnostic studies:
    a. Tube 1: culture, Gram stain, and sensitivity studies.
    b. Tube 2: protein and glucose.
    c. Tube 3: cell count and differential.
    d. Tube 4: other diagnostic studies such as Venereal Disease Research Laboratory (VDRL) and/or viral studies.
    e. Note: If a traumatic (bloody) tap was performed, send the clearest specimen for cell count and differential. Bloody CSF can be differentiated from venous blood by dropping a sample onto filter paper. Bloody CSF will form a "water ring" around a central patch of erythrocytes.
17. Once specimens have been obtained, replace stylet and remove needle–stylet unit in a single outward motion to prevent injury to the spinal cord and nerves.
18. Apply local pressure to the puncture site for 3 to 5 minutes to minimize the risk of CSF leakage. Then place an adhesive bandage over the puncture site.
19. Remove the surrounding antiseptic with sterile water to avoid skin injury.
20. Document procedure according to hospital policy, noting position of the patient during procedure, needle size used, complications or difficulties encountered, CSF characteristics, pain management interventions, patient's tolerance, and specimens sent to laboratory for analysis.

**F. Complications.**

1. Infection from nonsterile conditions:
   a. Use of poor sterile technique.
   b. Bacteremia if blood vessel punctures during procedure, having passed through infected CSF.
2. Intraspinal epidermoid tumor from lack of stylet use.
3. Spinal cord and/or nerve damage if puncture performed above L4.
4. Cerebral herniation.
5. Apnea and/or bradycardia.
6. Hypoxia.
7. Spinal cord or epidural abscess.
8. Spinal or intracranial subdural hematoma.
9. Spinal or intracranial subarachnoid hematoma.
10. Spinal fluid leakage into epidural space.
11. Vertebral body osteomyelitis.
12. Persistent bleeding, especially in patients with an underlying coagulopathy.
13. Pain.

## SIMULATION

In the high-risk environment of the NICU, there are many delicate procedures that require proficiency, precision, and great skill. Opportunities for training in these skills are essential, as competence is critical to the survival of the tiny patients they serve (see Chapter 18).

---

## REFERENCES


Allen, K.A.: Premedication for neonatal intubation: Which medications are recommended and why. *Advances in Neonatal Care*, 12(2):107–111, 2012.

Alexander, M. (Ed.), and Infusion Nurses Society: Infusion Nursing Standards of Practice. *Journal of Infusion Nursing*, 34 (1S): S1–S110, 2011.

American Academy of Pediatrics and American Heart Association: *Textbook of neonatal resuscitation*, (6th ed.). Elk Grove Village, IL, 2011, American Academy of Pediatrics and American Heart Association.

Baxter, A.L., Fisher, R.G., Burke, B.L., et al.: Local anesthetic and stylet styles: Factors associated with resident lumbar puncture success. *Pediatrics*, 177 (3):876–881, 2006.

Centers for Disease Control and Prevention: *Guidelines for the prevention of intravascular-catheter related infections*, 2011. www.cdc.gov/hicpac/pdf/guidelines/bsi-guidelines-2011.pdf.

Chapman, A.K., Aucott, S.W. and Milstone, A.M.: Safety of chlorhexidine gluconate used for skin antisepsis in the preterm infant. *Journal of Perinatology*, 32:4–9, 2012.

Choong, K., Chatrkaw, P., Frndova, H., et al.: Comparison of loss in lung with open versus in-line catheter endotracheal suctioning. *Pediatric Critical Care Medicine*, 4(91):69–73, 2003.

Colacchio, K., Deng, Y., Northrup, V. and Bizzaro, M.J.: Complications associated with central and non-central venous catheters in a neonatal intensive care unit. *Journal of Perinatology*, 32:941–946, 2012.

Davis, J.M. and Rosenfeld, W.N.: Bronchopulmonary dysplasia. In M.G. MacDonald, M.D. Mullett, and M.M.K. Seshia (Eds.): *Avery's neonatology: Pathophysiology and management of the newborn* (6th ed.). Philadelphia, 2005, Lippincott Williams & Wilkins, pp. 578–599.

DeBoer, S. and Seaver, M.: End-tidal $CO_2$ verification of endotracheal tube placement in neonates. *Neonatal Network*, 23(3):29–38, 2004.

Folk, L.: Guide to capillary heelstick blood sampling in infants. *Advances in Neonatal Care*, 7(4):171–178, 2007.

Fox, M.: Wound care in the neonatal intensive care unit. *Neonatal Network*, 30(5):291–303, 2011.

Gardner, S.L., Enzman-Hines, M. and Dickey, L.A.: Respiratory diseases. In S.L. Gardner, B.S. Carter, M. Enzman-Hines, and J.A. Hernandez (Eds.): *Handbook of neonatal intensive care* (7th ed.). St. Louis, 2011, Elsevier Mosby, pp. 581–677.

Gomella, T.L.: *Neonatology: Management, procedures, on-call problems, diseases and drugs:* (6th ed.). New York, 2009, Lange Medical Books/McGraw-Hill.

Hagler, D.A. and Traver, G.A.: Endotracheal saline and suction catheters: Sources of lower airway contamination. *American Journal of Critical Care*, 3(6):444–447, 1994.

Hughes, S., Blake, B., Woods, S., et al.: False-positive results on a colorimetric carbon dioxide analysis in neonatal resuscitation: Potential for serious patient harm. *Journal of Perinatology*, 27(12):800–801, 2007.

Jain, A., Deshpande, P. and Shah, P.: Peripherally inserted central catheter tip position and risk of associated complications in neonates. *Journal of Perinatology*, 33:307–312, 2013.

Kalyn, A., Blatz, S., Feuerstake, S., et al.: Closed suctioning of intubated neonates maintains better physiologic stability: A randomized trial. *Journal of Perinatology*, 23(3):218–222, 2003.

Kaur, G., Gupta, P. and Kumar, A.: A randomized trial of eutectic mixture of local anesthetics during lumbar puncture in newborns. *Archives of Pediatric and Adolescent Medicine*, 157(11):1065–1070, 2003.

Kumar, P., Denson, S.E., Mancuso, T.J. and Committee on Fetus and Newborn, Section on Anesthesiology and Pain Medicine: Premedication for nonemergency endotracheal intubation in the neonate. *Pediatrics*, 125:608–615, 2010.

Leef, K.H.: Evidence-based review of oral sucrose administration to decrease the pain response in newborn infants. *Neonatal Network*, 25(4):275–284, 2006.

Leike-Rude, M.K. and Haney, B.: Midline catheter use in the intensive care nursery. *Neonatal Network*, 25 (3):189–199, 2006.

MacDonald, M.G. and Ramasethu, J.: *Atlas of procedures in neonatology:* (5th ed.). Philadelphia, 2013, Lippincott Williams & Wilkins.

Marra, C., Whitley, R. and Scheld, M.: Approach to the patient with central nervous system infection. In W.M. Scheld, R.J. Whitley, and C.M. Marra (Eds.): *Infections of the central nervous system* Philadelphia, 2004, J.B. Lippincott, p. 13.

Milcic, T.L.: The complete blood count. *Neonatal Network*, 29(2):109–115, 2010.

O'Brien, L., Taddio, A., Lyszkiewicz, D., et al.: A critical review of the topical anesthetic amethocaine (Ametop) for pediatric pain. *Paediatric Drugs*, 7(1):41–54, 2005.

Paulson, P.R. and Miller, K.M.: Neonatal peripherally inserted central catheters: Recommendations for prevention of insertion and postinsertion complications. *Neonatal Network*, 27(4):245–256, 2008.

Peterson, J., Johnson, N., Deakins, K., et al.: Accuracy of the 7-8-9 Rule for endotracheal tube placement in the neonate. *Journal of Perinatology*, 26(6):333–336, 2006.

Pettit, J.: Technological advances for PICC placement and management. *Advances in Neonatal Care*, 7 (3):122–131, 2007.

Pettit, J. and Wyckoff, M.M.: *Peripherally inserted central catheters: Guideline for practice:* (2nd ed.). Glenview, IL, 2007, National Association of Neonatal Nurses.

Sawatzky-Dickson, D. and Bodnaryk, K.: Neonatal intravenous extravasation injuries: Evaluation of a wound care protocol. *Neonatal Network*, 25(1):13–19, 2006.

Shah, V. and Ohlsson, A.: Venipuncture versus heel lance for blood sampling in term neonates. *Cochrane Database of Systematic Reviews*, (4)CD001452, 2007.

Sharpe, E., Pettit, J. and Ellsbury, D.L.: A national survey of neonatal peripherally inserted central catheter (PICC) practices. *Advances in Neonatal Care*, 13 (1):55–74, 2013.

Tan, A.M., Gomez, J.M., Mathews, J., et al.: Closed versus partially ventilated endotracheal suction in extremely preterm neonates: Physiologic consequences. *Intensive Critical Care Nurse*, 21(4):234–242, 2005.

Thigpen, J.L.: Peripheral intravenous extravasation: Nursing procedure for initial treatment. *Neonatal Network*, 26(6):379–384, 2007.

Tingay, D.G., Copnell, B., Mills, J.F., et al.: Effects of open endotracheal suction on lung volume in infants receiving HFOV. *Intensive Care Medicine*, 33:689–693, 2007.

Trotter, C.W.: Inadvertent catheterization of the ascending lumbar vein. *Neonatal Network*, 28(3):179–183, 2009.

U.S. Food and Drug Administration: *Safety Labeling Changes Approved By FDA Center for Drug Evaluation and Research*, 2012. www.fda.gov/Safety/MedWatch/SafetyInformation/Safety-RelatedDrugLabelingChanges/ucm307387.htm.

Wyckoff, M.M.: Midline catheter use in the premature and full-term infant. *Journal of Vascular Access Devices*, 4(3):26–29, 1999.

CHAPTER

# 16 Pain Assessment and Management

MARLENE WALDEN

**OBJECTIVES**

1. Review the physiology of acute pain in preterm neonates.
2. Discuss current standards for assessing and managing pain in neonates.
3. Identify behavioral and physiologic responses that are indicative of pain in the neonate.
4. Select a valid and reliable composite measure for assessment of pain in neonates.
5. Discuss the evidence base for nonpharmacologic and pharmacologic approaches to the management of pain in neonates.

Advances in neonatal care during the past several decades have led to the increased survival of extremely preterm and sick neonates who regularly are subjected to numerous diagnostic and therapeutic procedures that are painful but medically necessary to their care. The prevention of pain in these critically ill neonates not only is an ethical obligation but may also minimize the immediate and cumulative effects of repeated painful experiences on the developing brains of these vulnerable neonates. Despite impressive gains in the knowledge related to the assessment and management of pain in neonates over the last several decades, a large gap still exists between routine clinical practice and scientific evidence. This chapter will review pain pathways, identification of pain, and interventions to alleviate pain in the neonate.

## DEFINITION OF PAIN

**The International Association for the Study of Pain (IASP) defines pain as "unpleasant sensory and emotional experience associated with actual or potential tissue damage, or described in terms of such damage"** (IASP Subcommittee on Taxonomy, 1979, p. 250). The IASP definition implies that the meaning of pain must be learned through experience and articulated within the context of verbal language. This conceptualization of pain perpetuates the misconception that infants, who lack linguistic skills, do not experience pain (Anand and Craig, 1996). In neonates, physiologic, behavioral, and hormonal indicators provide objective and quantifiable information about the location, intensity, and duration of painful stimuli. These responses can be used in conjunction with other contextual indicators to infer the existence of pain.

## NEONATAL INTENSIVE CARE UNIT PROCEDURES THAT CAUSE PAIN

A. **Many activities and interventions in the neonatal intensive care unit (NICU) cause pain. The most frequently occurring painful procedures include nasal and endotracheal suctioning, heel stick, adhesive removal, and venous and arterial punctures (Carbajal et al., 2008).**
B. **Frequency of invasive procedures is inversely related to gestational age and severity of illness. Therefore, the smaller and sicker neonates are those subject to the greatest numbers of most painful procedures.**
   1. Carbajal and colleagues (2008) found that infants born between 24 and 42 weeks of gestation experienced on average a mean of 98 painful procedures during the first 14 days of admission, with one neonate having 364 painful procedures.
C. **The number of procedures encountered by infants in the NICU is partially due to a substantial number of failed attempts.**

1. In the study by Simons and colleagues (2003), the failure rates for placement of central venous catheters, peripheral arterial catheters, and intravenous (IV) cannulas were 45.6%, 37.5%, and 30.9%, respectively.
2. In the study by Carbajal et al. (2008), some of the most painful procedures needed as many as 10 to 15 attempts for completion.

**D. Despite safe, effective pharmacologic and nonpharmacologic interventions to prevent or minimize pain and distress, many painful procedures in the NICU are performed without analgesia.**

1. In the study by Simons et al. (2003), many of the procedures were rated by physicians and nurses to be painful (>4 on a 10-point scale); however, very few infants received any pharmacologic or nonpharmacologic procedural pain management.
2. Johnston and colleagues (2011) reported that 46% of tissue-damaging procedures (e.g., heel lance, venipuncture, lumbar puncture, endotracheal intubation, and ophthalmologic examination) and 57% of non–tissue-damaging procedures (e.g., endotracheal suctioning, tape removal, nasogastric tube insertion, catheter removal) were performed without analgesic interventions.
3. A descriptive survey of nurses and physicians noted that, rather than lack of knowledge, the most common reasons for withholding analgesia were related to fear of adverse drug reactions, absence of a unit pain policy, inadequate staffing, poor interdisciplinary communication about timing of procedures, forgetfulness, and taking advantage of the fact that "babies cannot protest" (Akuma and Jordan, 2012).
4. In a study by Johnston and colleagues (2011), parental presence predicted the use of sweet taste analgesia or nonpharmacologic interventions for tissue-damaging procedures.

**E. Procedural pain guidelines are available to help clinicians choose the most effective and safe pain control measures based on best evidence (Anand and International Evidence-Based Group for Neonatal Pain, 2001; Lago et al., 2009; Spence et al., 2010).**

1. Heel stick.
   a. Pain resulting from the heel-stick procedure is caused not only by the lancing procedure but also by the squeezing of the heel to obtain the blood sample.
   b. Spring-loaded mechanical lancets result in less bruising, less need for repeat punctures, and fewer behavioral and physiologic signs of pain.
   c. Heel warming has no effect on facilitating blood flow during the heel-stick procedure.
   d. Use of EMLA cream is not effective for management of pain associated with the heel-stick procedure.
   e. Evidence-based interventions include pacifier with sucrose, swaddling, containment, facilitated tucking, breastfeeding, and skin-to-skin contact with mother.
2. Venipuncture.
   a. May be preferable to heel stick in minimizing procedure-related pain in full-term infants. However, frequent venipuncture for blood sampling is not feasible for most infants in the NICU, necessitating the continued use of heel sticks.
   b. Use smallest-gauge trocar cannula, whenever possible.
   c. Evidence-based interventions include swaddling, facilitated tucking, pacifier with sucrose, and topical anesthetic cream in infants ≥37 weeks of gestation.
3. Lumbar puncture.
   a. Avoid extreme flexion of the neck and knees toward the chest as this may cause significant hypoxemia.
   b. Evidence-based interventions include sucrose, pacifier, and topical anesthetic cream in infants ≥37 weeks of gestation.
4. Chest tube insertion.
   a. If procedure is not urgent, apply topical anesthetic cream in infants ≥37 weeks of gestation. If urgent, infiltrate site with 1% subcutaneous lidocaine.
   b. If infant is intubated and ventilated, administer a slow IV opiate bolus such as fentanyl before the procedure.
5. Endotracheal intubation (Kumar et al. and Committee on Fetus and Newborn, Section on Anesthesiology and Pain Medicine, American Academy of Pediatrics, 2010).

a. Awake intubations should only be performed during resuscitation in the delivery room or after acute deterioration or critical illness.
b. Premedication with analgesic agents alone or in combination with vagolytic agents, muscle relaxants, or sedatives should be given.
c. Using appropriate analgesia and sedation reduces potentially harmful physiologic fluctuations and pain, decreases the time and number of attempts, and minimizes the potential for intubation-related airway trauma.

6. Ophthalmologic exam screening for retinopathy of prematurity.
a. Evidence-based interventions include the use of a pacifier, sucrose, containment, and local anesthetic eye drops.
b. Retinal surgery should be considered major surgery, and opiates should be provided.

F. **Technician expertise, such as the skill of the operator, influences pain responses in infants and should be monitored. Ensuring staff competence to perform required procedures may reduce the number of painful procedures to which an infant is exposed by reducing the number of failed attempts (Simons et al., 2003).**

## PHYSIOLOGY OF ACUTE PAIN IN PRETERM NEONATES

A. **An understanding of the physiology of acute pain in preterm neonates is essential for optimal pain management in the NICU. Pain responses exhibited by neonates are the result of a concurrent set of reactions within the peripheral nervous system, spinal cord, and higher centers involved at the supraspinal/integrative level, including the thalamus and cerebral cortex (Melzack, 1996).**

1. Peripheral nervous system (Evans, 2001).
a. Fully mature and functional by 20 weeks of gestation.
b. Consists of two types of neuronal afferent fibers.
(1) Delta fibers: thinly myelinated, rapid-conducting fibers associated with sharp pain or "first pain" (e.g., sharp, localized, pricking).
(2) C fibers: polymodal, unmyelinated, slow-conducting fibers associated with aching, burning, poorly localized, or "second pain."
c. Density of nociceptors is equal to or greater than that in adult skin.
d. Local tissue injury such as heel stick or venipuncture activates nociceptors of sensory afferent fibers to:
(1) Transmit pain impulses to spinal cord and central nervous system (CNS).
(2) Release biochemical mediators such as substance P and prostaglandins, which results in hyperalgesia (increased sensitivity to painful stimuli) or allodynia (pain caused by a stimulus that ordinarily does not cause pain). This decreased pain threshold may persist for days or weeks.
(3) Cause dendritic sprouting and hyperinnervation that result in hypersensitivity and lower pain threshold that may persist into adulthood.

2. Spinal cord (Evans, 2001).
a. During the first postnatal week, weak linkages exist between the peripheral nervous system and the dorsal horn, resulting in either prolonged pain responses or no reaction to the painful stimuli.
b. Receptive fields of the dorsal horn cells are larger than those of adults and begin to diminish 2 weeks after birth.
c. Local spinal cord response to pain impulses from peripheral afferent fibers stimulates efferent somatomotor neurons in the anterior horn and produce reflex withdrawal.
d. Afferent fiber neurotransmitters stimulate *N*-methyl-D-aspartate and tachykinin receptors in the dorsal horns, producing central sensitization (increased excitability of dorsal horn neurons that spreads to several adjacent segments of the spinal cord), "wind-up" phenomenon (perceived increase in intensity or duration of painful stimuli), or secondary hyperalgesia (hypersensitivity elicited by both painful and nonpainful stimuli that extends to areas beyond the site of injury).
e. Increases in autonomic responses such as heart rate and respiratory rate and facial responses such as brow bulge, eye squeeze, and nasolabial furrow in response to

heel-stick procedures provide evidence of maturity of ascending pathways by 20 weeks of gestation.

f. Preterm infants have a limited ability to modulate pain. Dopamine and norepinephrine are not available to modulate pain before 36 to 40 weeks of gestation. Serotonin is first released at approximately 6 to 8 weeks after birth.

3. Supraspinal/integrative level (Evans, 2001).
   a. Cerebral cortex has a full complement of neurons by 20 weeks of gestation.
   b. Cerebral cortex is functionally mature by 22 weeks of gestation and bilaterally synchronous by 27 weeks of gestation.
   c. Somatosensory evoked potentials are slow and simple before 29 weeks of gestation, but short and complex by 40 weeks of gestation.
   d. Cortical cell migration is complete at approximately 24 weeks of gestation. However, the support structure of the germinal matrix remains highly vascular until 28 weeks. Therefore, the neonate is vulnerable to intraventricular hemorrhage related to increases in blood pressure associated with pain.
   e. Maximum number of cortical neurons is reached at 28 weeks of gestation, and then approximately 70% of cortical neurons are lost before birth through apoptosis.
   f. Neonates as early as 27 weeks of gestation can differentiate touch (sham heel stick) from a noxious stimulus (heel stick) as evidenced by physiologic and facial response patterns.
   g. Neurologic connections are in place for the perception of, reaction to, and memory of pain on the cortical level as evidenced by mature visual and auditory response patterns on electroencephalogram in infants younger than 30 weeks of gestation and by measurements of in-vivo cerebral glucose in the sensory areas of the brain.

**B. Repetitive, unrelieved pain can lead to serious and adverse consequences for neonates.**

1. Short-term physiologic consequences of painful procedures include decreased oxygen saturations and increased heart rates that can place increased demands on the cardiorespiratory system.
2. Pain can cause elevation in intracranial pressure, thereby increasing risk of intraventricular hemorrhage in preterm neonates.
3. Pain and stress may also depress the immune system and contribute to increased susceptibility of neonates to infections.
4. The long-term effects of pain in animals are clear, with changes observed in pain thresholds, social behaviors, stress responses, and pain responses to nonpainful stimuli (Fitzgerald and Anand, 1993; Plotsky et al., 2000; Reynolds et al., 1997; Ruda et al., 2000). Preliminary human data suggest that early pain experiences may impair brain development and alter future pain responses (Bouza, 2009; Brummelte et al., 2012). Johnston and Stevens (1996) reported that neonates who were born at 28 weeks of gestation and were hospitalized in an NICU for 4 weeks (32 weeks of postconceptional age) had decreased behavioral response and significantly higher heart rate and lower oxygen saturation during a heel-stick procedure compared with newly born neonates at 32 weeks of gestation. In another study, Taddio and colleagues (1995) reported that males circumcised within 2 days of birth had significantly longer crying bouts and higher pain intensity scores at immunization at 4 or 6 months of age than males who were not circumcised.

## STANDARDS OF PRACTICE

**A. Recognition of the widespread inadequacy of pain management promoted various professional organizations to issue position statements and clinical recommendations in an effort to promote effective pain management in undertreated populations. Organizations that support the importance of optimal pain assessment and management in hospitalized neonates include the National Association of Neonatal Nurses (Walden and Gibbins, 2012) and the American Academy of Pediatrics and Canadian Paediatric Society (2000, 2006). There is considerable consistency in the recommendations set by these professional organizations. Core principles contained within these guidelines and standards that are applicable to pain assessment and management in the NICU include the following:**

1. Assess education and competency in pain assessment and management of new and current employees.
2. Regularly assess and reassess pain using a valid and reliable multidimensional pain assessment instrument.
3. Use both nonpharmacologic and pharmacologic approaches to prevent and/or manage pain.
4. Health care team members should collaborate together and with the infant's family in developing an approach to pain assessment and management.
5. Documentation should facilitate regular reassessment and follow-up intervention.
6. Policies and procedures should be established to provide consistency and quality of pain assessment and management practices.
7. Data should be collected to monitor the appropriateness and effectiveness of pain management practices.

B. **The clinical challenge remains on how to implement these standards in various institutional settings based on patient types, frequently occurring clinical procedures performed, and current staffing patterns.**

## PAIN ASSESSMENT

A. **Pain assessment has been advocated as the "fifth vital sign" and should be assessed routinely.**

B. **"The 'golden rule' of pain assessment must be: What is painful to an adult is painful to an infant until proven otherwise" (Franck, 1989). This rule, along with the use of valid and reliable tools, must be used for the assessment of and intervention for pain.**

C. **Because previous painful experiences may modify pain expression, further research is needed to develop and test an instrument to assess chronic pain in the infant requiring prolonged hospitalization who has been subjected to multiple painful clinical procedures.**

D. **Pain assessment is an essential prerequisite to optimal pain management.**

E. **Behavioral responses.**
1. Facial activity offers the most specificity as an indicator of pain, namely brow bulge, eye squeeze, and nasolabial furrow.
2. Acoustic and temporal characteristics of pain cries are different than other cry types in both preterm and full-term infants, including increases in peak fundamental frequency (pitch), peak spectral energy, cry duration, and intensity. However, differences in cry types are difficult to discriminate in the clinical setting.
3. Many preterm infants do not cry in response to a noxious stimulus. The absence of response may only indicate the depletion of response capability and not lack of pain perception.
4. Healthy full-term newborns use swiping motions by the unaffected leg to the lanced foot, as if trying to push away the noxious stimulus.
5. Preterm infants demonstrate an increase in motor extension patterns, including finger splay, "saluting," and "sitting on air" during painful clinical procedures. These hyperextension motor patterns are quickly replaced with flaccidity in infants at younger postconceptional ages.

F. **Physiologic responses.**
1. Preterm infants respond to noxious stimuli in patterns similar to those of full-term neonates, including increases in heart rate and decreases in oxygen saturation.
2. Although physiologic measures provide greater objectivity in the assessment of pain, they also reflect the body's nonspecific response to stress and thus are not specific to pain (Ranger et al., 2007). Therefore, physiologic measures should be converged with behavioral measures that have been demonstrated to be more consistent and specific to pain in neonates.
3. Physiologic measures should be used to assess pain in infants who are paralyzed for mechanical ventilation or who are severely neurologically impaired. Increases in heart rate and blood pressure during handling generally indicate the need for more analgesia and/or sedation in the pharmacologically paralyzed infant.

4. If the infant is sedated, variability in heart rate and blood pressure decreases. However, it is important to remember that, although sedatives may mask physiologic and behavioral signs of pain, sedatives do not provide pain relief.

G. **Contextual factors modifying pain responses.**

1. Developmental maturity, health status, and environmental factors may all contribute to an inconsistent, less robust pattern of pain responses between infants and even within the same infant over time and situations. Therefore, contextual factors that have been demonstrated to modify the pain experience must be considered when assessing for the presence of pain in neonates.
2. Infants in awake or alert states demonstrate a more robust reaction to painful stimuli than infants in sleep states.
3. Research examining facial as well as bodily activity has demonstrated that the magnitude of infant response has been observed to be less vigorous and robust with decreasing post-conceptional age. Craig and colleagues (1993) suggested that the less vigorous responses demonstrated by preterm infants "should be interpreted in the context of the energy resources available to respond and the relative immaturity of the musculoskeletal system" (p. 296).
4. Less mature behavioral responses to noxious stimuli are also noted with increased number of painful procedures to which the infant is exposed, increased postnatal age of the infant at time of observation, and shorter length of time since last painful procedure (Ranger et al., 2007).
5. When pain stimuli or pain persists for hours or days without intervention, the infant exhibits a decompensatory response. The sympathetic nervous system, or the "fight-or-flight" mechanism, can no longer compensate. As a result, the physiologic parameters return to baseline (Hummel and van Dijk, 2006). *Return to baseline* does not indicate that pain is no longer felt or is tolerated, but it does make the infant's pain more difficult to evaluate.

## PAIN ASSESSMENT INSTRUMENTS

A. **Select a composite or multidimensional instrument that incorporates both physiologic and behavioral measures of pain. Caregivers should select instruments with tested reliability, validity, and clinical utility. Infant population, setting, and type of pain experienced should also guide selection of a pain instrument (Duhn and Medves, 2004).**

B. **CRIES: a postoperative pain tool (Table 16-1) (Krechel and Bildner, 1995).**

1. Acronym for five behavioral and physiologic parameters: C = crying; R = requires oxygen to maintain saturation at greater than 95%; I = increased vital signs; E = expression; and S = sleeplessness.
2. Demonstrates validity and interrater reliability for use in infants born at 32 weeks of gestation and later. Initial establishment of clinical utility.
3. Tool scoring system, 0 to 10, is structured in the same fashion as the Apgar score and was designed to make the tool easy to use and remember.
4. Score was originally developed to assess postoperative pain, but has also been used in research related to procedural pain (Ahn, 2006; Belda et al., 2004).
5. A score of 4 or above indicates pain, and any assessment of 4 or above should receive pain intervention. The neonate should then be reevaluated 15 to 30 minutes after analgesia to assess for pain relief.

C. **The Premature Infant Pain Profile (Stevens et al., 1996).**

1. The Premature Infant Pain Profile (PIPP) is the most reliable and valid tool available to assess pain in the neonatal clinical setting and has been validated in over 62 studies (Stevens et al., 2010).
2. Seven-item, 4-point scale for assessment of pain in premature infants through term gestation.
3. PIPP score was originally developed to assess procedural pain, but has been used in research to assess postoperative pain in neonates (El Sayed et al., 2007; McNair et al., 2004; Suraseranivongse et al., 2006).

■ TABLE 16-1
■ ■ **CRIES: Neonatal Postoperative Pain Measurement Score***

| | Score | | | |
|---|---|---|---|---|
| | **0** | **1** | **2** | **Tips for Scoring CRIES** |
| Crying | No | High pitched | Inconsolable | Score 0: no cry or cry not high pitched<br>Score 1: high-pitched cry, but consolable<br>Score 2: high-pitched cry, inconsolable |
| Requires $O_2$ for saturation >95% | No | <30% | >30% | Score 0: no oxygen required from baseline<br>Score 1: oxygen requirement <30% from baseline<br>Score 2: oxygen requirement >30% from baseline |
| Increased vital signs | HR and BP ≤ preoperative values | HR or BP <20% of preoperative values | HR or BP ≥20% of preoperative values | Score 0: HR and BP are both unchanged or at less than baseline<br>Score 1: HR or BP is increased by <20%<br>Score 2: HR or BP is increased by >20%<br>*Note:* Measure BP last so as not to wake the infant. |
| Expression | None | Grimace | Grimace/grunt | Score 0: no grimace<br>Score 1: grimace only is present<br>Score 2: grimace and inaudible grunt present<br>*Note:* Grimace consists of lowered brow, eyes squeezed shut, deepening nasolabial furrow, and open lips and mouth. |
| Sleepless | No | Wakes at frequent intervals | Constantly awake | Score 0: continuously asleep<br>Score 1: awakens at frequent intervals<br>Score 2: awake constantly<br>*Note:* Based on infant's state during previous hour. |

From Krechel, S. and Bildner, J.: CRIES: A new neonatal post-operative pain measurement score: Initial testing of validity and reliability. *Paediatric Anaesthesia*, 5(1):53-61, 1995.
*BP*, Blood pressure; *HR*, heart rate.
*Neonatal pain assessment tool developed at the University of Missouri–Columbia.

4. Multidimensional: includes heart rate, oxygen saturation, brow bulge, eye squeeze, and nasolabial furrow.
5. Unique in that it includes two contextual modifiers (i.e., gestational age and behavioral state).
6. Total pain score of 7 to 12 indicates mild pain, and infant may benefit from use of nonpharmacologic comfort measures. Total pain score greater than 12 indicates moderate to severe pain and will most likely require pharmacologic intervention in conjunction with comfort measures.
7. The PIPP was revised in 2013 to enhance validity and feasibility (Stevens et al., 2013a). In the PIPP-R (Table 16-2), the decimal points in oxygen saturation were rounded to the nearest whole number and the scoring of facial features was changed from a percentage to the absolute duration of time the indicator was observed in the 30-second block. Instructions related to baseline behavioral state were clarified and made more specific.

■ TABLE 16-2
■ ■ **The Premature Infant Pain Profile: Revised**

| | Indicator Score | | | | |
|---|---|---|---|---|---|
| **Infant Indicator** | **0** | **+1** | **+2** | **+3** | **Infant Indicator Score** |
| Change in Heart Rate (bpm)<br>Baseline: ______ | 0 – 4 | 5 – 14 | 15 – 24 | >24 | |
| Decrease in Oxygen Saturation (%)<br>Baseline: ______ | 0 – 2 | 3 – 5 | 6 – 8 | >8 or increase in $O_2$ | |
| Brow Bulge (Sec) | None (<3) | Minimal (3 – 10) | Moderate (11 – 20) | Maximal (>20) | |
| Eye Squeeze (Sec) | None (<3) | Minimal (3 – 10) | Moderate (11 – 20) | Maximal (>20) | |
| Naso-Labial Furrow (Sec) | None (<3) | Minimal (3 – 10) | Moderate (11 – 20) | Maximal (>20)<br>*Sub-total Score: | |
| **Gestational Age (Wks + Days)** | >36 wks | 32 wks – 35 wks, 6 d | 28 wks – 31 wks, 6 d | <28 wks | |
| **Baseline Behavioural State** | Active and Awake | Quiet and Awake | Active and Asleep | Quiet and Asleep<br>†Total Score: | |

**SCORING INSTRUCTIONS**

**Step 1:** Observe infant for **15 seconds at rest** and assess vital sign indicators [highest heart rate (HR) and lowest $O_2$ Saturation ($O_2$ SAT)] and behavioural state.

**Step 2:** Observe infant for **30 seconds after procedure** and assess **change** in vital sign indicators (maximal HR, lowest $O_2$ SAT and duration of facial actions observed).

If infant requires an increase in oxygen at any point before or during procedure, they receive a score of 3 for the $O_2$ SAT indicator.

**Step 3:** Score for corrected gestational age (GA) and behavioural state (BS) if the sub-total score >0.

**Step 4:** Calculate total score by adding **Sub-total Score + BS Score**.

From Stevens, B.J., Gibbins, S., Yamada, J., et al.: The premature infant pain profile-revised (PIPP-R): Initial validation and feasibility. *Clinical Journal of Pain*, 30(3):238–243, 2014.

*Sub-total for physiological and facial indicators. If Sub-total score >0, add GA and BS indicator scores.

†Total Score: Sub-total Score + GA Score + BS Score.

**D. Neonatal Infant Pain Scale (Lawrence et al., 1993) (Fig. 16-1).**

1. Six-item scale. Five behavioral items (facial expression, crying, arms, legs, and state of arousal) and one physiologic indicator (breathing pattern). Each behavior except cry has descriptors for the two possible scores of 0 and 1. Cry is scored on a 3-point scale (0, 1, 2).
2. Originally tested in preterm and full-term neonates who required capillary, venous, or arterial punctures, but has also been used in research related to postoperative pain in neonates (Rouss et al., 2007; Suraseranivongse et al., 2006).
3. Total score can range from 0 to 7.

## NURSING CARE OF THE INFANT IN PAIN

Skilled observation, assessments, and interventions are the responsibility of the care providers. Pain intervention may be provided by both nonpharmacologic and pharmacologic methods.

**A. Nonpharmacologic approaches to pain management.**

1. Goals.
   a. To help minimize pain and stress while maximizing the infant's ability to cope with and recover from clinical procedures.
   b. To provide additive or synergistic benefits to pharmacologic therapy.

| | Before Time | | During Time | | | | | After Time | | |
|---|---|---|---|---|---|---|---|---|---|---|
| | 1 | 2 | 1 | 2 | 3 | 4 | 5 | 1 | 2 | 3 |
| **Facial expression**<br>0—Relaxed<br>1—Grimace | | | | | | | | | | |
| **Cry**<br>0—No cry<br>1—Whimper<br>2—Vigorous | | | | | | | | | | |
| **Breathing patterns**<br>0—Relaxed<br>1—Change in breathing | | | | | | | | | | |
| **Arms**<br>0—Relaxed/restrained<br>1—Flexed/extended | | | | | | | | | | |
| **Legs**<br>0—Relaxed/restrained<br>1—Flexed/extended | | | | | | | | | | |
| **State of arousal**<br>0—Sleeping/awake<br>1—Fussy | | | | | | | | | | |
| **Total** | | | | | | | | | | |

**Note: Time is measured in 1-minute intervals.**

FIGURE 16-1 ■ Neonatal Infant Pain Scale. (From Lawrence, J., Alcock, D., McGrath, P., et al.: The development of a tool to assess neonatal pain. *Neonatal Network*, 12[6]:59-66, 1993.)

2. Preventive measures.
   a. Reduce the total number of painful procedures to which the infant is exposed by:
      (1) Evaluating all aspects of caregiving.
      (2) Evaluating the number and grouping of laboratory and diagnostic procedures.
      (3) Scheduling clinical procedures based on medical necessity versus a routine schedule.
      (4) Using minimal amounts of tape/adhesives and using skin barrier products when possible.
      (5) Ensuring proper premedication prior to invasive procedures.
      (6) Using noninvasive monitoring devices when possible.
      (7) Establishing central venous/arterial access to minimize skin-breaking procedures.
      (8) Involving parents in caregiving by teaching signs and symptoms of pain and comfort that they can provide.
   b. Painful procedures should not be performed at the same time as other, nonemergency routine care (e.g., taking vital signs, changing a diaper) as this can cause sensory hypersensitivity (referred to as "wind-up" phenomenon) causing nonnoxious stimuli to be perceived as painful (Bouza, 2009; Holsti et al., 2005).
   c. Handling and immobilization in preparation for painful procedures should be minimized before a painful procedure as this may heighten activity in nociceptive pathways and accentuate the infants' pain responses.
   d. Use environmental interventions such as reduced lighting and noise levels to minimize infant stress.
3. Behavioral measures.
   a. Facilitated tucking (hand-swaddling technique that holds the infant's extremities flexed and contained close to the trunk) during a painful procedure may significantly reduce pain responses in preterm infants (Cignacco et al., 2007; Liaw et al., 2012).

b. Blanket swaddling following a painful procedure may help reduce physiologic and behavioral pain and distress in preterm neonates.
c. Pacifiers ranked by NICU nurses as the first choice of pain intervention.
   (1) Nonnutritive sucking (NNS) is thought to modulate the transmission or processing of nociception through mediation by the endogenous nonopioid system.
   (2) The efficacy of NNS is immediate but appears to terminate almost immediately upon cessation of sucking.
   (3) Pain relief is greater in infants who receive both NNS and sucrose (Naughton, 2013).
d. Studies demonstrate that a single 0.05- to 2-mL dose of 0.24 to 0.50 g (12% to 25%) sucrose given orally approximately 2 minutes before painful stimulus is associated with statistically and clinically significant reductions in PIPP scores and crying after a heel-stick procedure (Stevens et al., 2013b).
   (1) Interval coincides with endogenous opioid release triggered by the sweet taste of sucrose.
   (2) Safety of implementing repeated doses of sucrose in very low birth weight infants has not been confirmed; therefore, caution is advised before widespread use of repeated doses in preterm and critically ill neonates. Harrison and colleagues (2012) recommended using small volumes of sucrose for painful procedures only. The authors further recommended avoiding the use of sucrose for calming irritable infants who are not undergoing painful procedures, limiting the use of sucrose to less than 10 doses per 24 hours, and employing the use of other effective nonpharmacologic strategies during painful procedures when feasible.
   (3) A study by Stevens and colleagues (1999) noted no immediate adverse effects when administering a 24% sucrose-dipped pacifier during four random, consecutively administered, routine heel-stick procedures.
e. Breastfeeding may be used to alleviate procedural pain in neonates undergoing a single painful procedure (Shah et al., 2012).

**B. Pharmacologic approaches to pain management.**

1. Pharmacologic approaches to pain management should be used when moderate, severe, or prolonged pain is assessed or anticipated.
2. Pharmacologic therapy should maintain a balance between pain relief and adverse effects of analgesics.
3. IV opioids remain the most common class of analgesics administered in the NICU, particularly morphine sulfate and fentanyl citrate.
   a. Systemic opioids induce analgesia by acting at various levels of the CNS.
      (1) Spinal cord: Opioids impair or inhibit the transmission of nociceptive input from the periphery to the CNS.
      (2) Basal ganglia: Opioids activate a descending inhibitory system.
      (3) Limbic system: Opioids alter the emotional response to pain, making it more tolerable.
   b. Special considerations in neonates are as follows:
      (1) Longer dosing intervals are often required in neonates less than 1 month of age because of longer elimination half-lives and delayed clearance of opioids as compared with adults or children greater than 1 year of age.
      (2) Neonates should be monitored closely during opioid therapy and for several hours after opioids have been discontinued because enterohepatic recirculation in preterm and full-term neonates may result in higher plasma concentrations of opioids for longer periods as compared with older children.
      (3) Because of immature descending pain pathways, preterm infants may require significantly higher opioid concentrations to achieve adequate analgesia as compared with older children (Evans, 2001).
      (4) Efficacy of opioid therapy should be assessed using a valid and reliable neonatal pain scale. Sedation level should also be assessed regularly, monitoring for the attainment of desired sedation level or inadvertent oversedation.
      (5) Opioid-induced cardiorespiratory side effects in neonates are uncommon.
   c. Fentanyl is used as follows (NEOFAX, 2011):

(1) Bolus dose: 0.5 to 4 mcg/kg/dose every 2 to 4 hours by slow IV push.
(2) Continuous infusion: 1 to 5 mcg/kg/hr.
(3) Onset is almost immediately after IV administration.
(4) Adverse effects include respiratory depression, chest wall rigidity, tolerance and dependence, and urinary retention.

**d.** Morphine is used as follows (NEOFAX, 2011):
(1) Bolus dose: 0.05 to 0.2 mg/kg/dose by slow IV push, intramuscularly, or by subcutaneous route. Repeat as required, usually every 4 hours.
(2) Continuous infusion: Give loading dose of 0.1 to 0.15 mg/kg over 1 hour followed by a continuous infusion of 0.01 to 0.02 mg/kg/hr.
(3) Onset of action: beginning a few minutes after IV administration, with peak analgesia occurring at 20 minutes.
(4) Adverse effects: respiratory depression, hypotension, bradycardia, transient hypertonia, ileus, delayed gastric emptying, urinary retention, tolerance and dependence, and seizures.
(5) The potential for increased adverse neurologic outcomes exists in ventilated infants with hypotension receiving morphine. Therefore, all infants receiving morphine should be closely monitored for hypotension (Anand et al., 2004; Aranda et al., 2005; Hall et al., 2005).

**e.** Managing opioid tolerance and dependence.
(1) Tolerance is decreasing pain relief with the same dosage over time and is exhibited by increased wakefulness and increased sympathetic responses such as high-pitched crying and tremors when handled or disturbed. Tolerance to opioids is usually managed by increasing the dose, although adjunctive analgesics or sedatives may also be clinically beneficial.
(2) Neonates who require opioid therapy for more than several days should be weaned slowly to prevent withdrawal symptoms such as signs of neurologic excitability, gastrointestinal dysfunction, autonomic signs, poor weight gain, and skin excoriation due to excessive rubbing. The prevalence of opioid withdrawal is greater in infants who have received fentanyl as opposed to morphine. Similarly, infants who receive higher total doses or longer duration of infusion are significantly more likely to experience withdrawal (Dominguez et al., 2003). Data are insufficient to determine the optimal weaning rate of opioids to prevent withdrawal symptoms in neonates on opioid therapy (Hudak, Tan, and Committee on Drugs and Committee on Fetus and Newborn, 2012). Ducharme and colleagues (2005) reported that adverse withdrawal symptoms in children who received continuous infusions of opioids and/or benzodiazepines could be prevented when the daily rate of weaning did not exceed 20% for children who received opioids/benzodiazepines for 1 to 3 days, 13% to 20% for 4 to 7 days, 8% to 13% for 8 to 14 days, 8% for 15 to 21 days, and 2% to 4% for more than 21 days. Other opioid weaning protocols have been proposed by Roberston, Meyer and Berens, and Wolfson Children's Hospital (Hudak, Tan, and Committee on Drugs and Committee on Fetus and Newborn, 2012). A weaning scale such as the modified Neonatal Abstinence Scoring System should be used to manage opioid withdrawal in neonates exposed to prolonged opioid therapy (Finnegan, 1990) (see Chapter 3).

**4.** Nonopioid analgesics (NEOFAX, 2011).

**a.** Acetaminophen is a nonsteroidal antiinflammatory drug commonly used for short-term use with mild to moderate pain in neonates.
(1) Oral dose: 20- to 25-mg/kg loading dose followed by 12 to15 mg/kg/dose.
(2) Rectal dose: 30-mg/kg loading dose followed by 12 to 18 mg/kg/dose.
(3) Maintenance intervals are every 6 hours for term infants, every 8 hours for preterm infants ≥32 weeks, and every 12 hours for preterm infants younger than 32 weeks.
(4) Should not be used in infants less than 28 weeks as inadequate data exist on pharmacokinetics to permit calculation of appropriate dosages (American Academy of Pediatrics and Canadian Paediatric Society, 2006).

(5) Adverse effects: liver toxicity, rash, fever, thrombocytopenia, leukopenia, and neutropenia.
(6) Routine prophylactic use of acetaminophen at the time of vaccination is not recommended because of a potential reduction in antibody response.
(7) Although IV paracetamol has been demonstrated to lower postoperative morphine requirements in neonates and infants undergoing major noncardiac surgery (Ceelie et al., 2013), given its potential hepatotoxicity, a cautious approach should be employed, particularly in extremely preterm neonates (Cuzzolin et al., 2013).

5. EMLA cream (eutectic mixture of local anesthetics, lidocaine, and prilocaine).
   a. Approved in children at birth with a gestational age of 37 weeks or greater.
   b. EMLA cream reduces pain during venipuncture, circumcisions, arterial puncture, and percutaneous venous catheter placement.
   c. Local/topical dose: 1 to 2 g under occlusive dressing 60 to 90 minutes before procedure (NEOFAX, 2011).
   d. Adverse effects: methemoglobinemia, redness, and blanching.
6. Liposomal lidocaine cream (LMX 4%; Ferndale Laboratories, Michigan).
   a. Topical anesthetic for use in newborns.
   b. LMX may be a better choice than EMLA because of its faster onset of action and no risk of methemoglobinemia (Lehr et al., 2005).
   c. Few studies have evaluated the safety and efficacy of LMX for management of procedural pain in neonates. A study by Taddio and colleagues (2011) evaluating the effect of LMX and sucrose alone and in combination found that sucrose was more effective than LMX and LMX did not confer synergistic benefits for reducing pain when used in combination with sucrose during venipuncture in newborns. No adverse effects of LMX were observed.
7. Sedatives suppress the behavioral expression of pain and have no analgesic effects. Sedatives should only be used when pain has been ruled out. When administered with opioids, sedatives may allow more optimal weaning of opioids in critically ill, ventilator-dependent neonates who have developed tolerance from prolonged opioid therapy. The two most commonly used sedatives in neonates are midazolam and chloral hydrate. However, no research has been done to determine the safety or efficacy of combining sedatives and analgesics for the treatment of pain in infants.
8. Neuromuscular blocking agents. Chemical paralysis is often used for severely ill neonates. Because the use of paralytic agents masks the behavioral signs of agitation and pain, sedatives or analgesics should be used in conjunction with paralytics. Near-infrared spectroscopy (NIRS) shows promise as a tool to evaluate cortical pain somatosensory activation in the absence of behavioral measures and may be a future technology used to assess pain in infants who are receiving moderate to heavy sedation or paralytic agents (Holsti et al., 2011).

## PAIN MANAGEMENT AT END OF LIFE

**A. Although dying adults commonly receive opioids to relieve suffering at end of life, opioids are not routinely administered to critically ill or dying infants when life support is being withdrawn or withheld (Partridge and Wall, 1997).**

**B. As it is often difficult to accurately assess pain in neonates at end of life, caregivers should consider risk factors for pain and use physiologic measures to guide pain management decisions.**

**C. Opioid doses well beyond those described for standard analgesia are often required for infants who are in severe pain or who have developed tolerance after the prolonged use of opioids (Partridge and Wall, 1997). Therefore, continuous infusions of opioids should be titrated to desired clinical response (analgesia).**

**D. Physiologic comfort measures may palliate pain and distress in infants at end of life and include reduction of noxious stimuli, organization of caregiving, and positioning and containment strategies.**

## PARENTS' ROLE IN PAIN ASSESSMENT AND MANAGEMENT

**A. Parents have many concerns and fears about their infant's pain and about the medications used in the treatment of pain (Franck et al., 2005; Gale et al., 2004). Parents may fear the effects of pain on their child's development. They may also fear that their infant may become "addicted" to the analgesics (Franck et al., 2004).**

**B. Parents and health care professionals must talk openly and honestly about acute and chronic pain associated with medical diseases, as well as about pain associated with operative, diagnostic, and therapeutic procedures.**

**C. Parents should receive accurate and unbiased information about the risks and benefits of (as well as alternatives to) analgesia and anesthesia, so that they can make informed treatment choices (Harrison, 1993).**

**D. Parents' cultural and religious beliefs about pain should be taken into consideration when determining a pain management plan.**

**E. Parents should have the right to seek another medical opinion or to refuse a burdensome course of therapy (Harrison, 1993).**

**F. Parents should be taught to observe how their infant expresses pain through physiologic and behavioral cues.**

**G. Parents should be educated on how they can assist caregivers in providing nonpharmacologic pain relief during minor painful procedures their infant experiences.**

## REFERENCES


Ahn, Y.: The relationship between behavioral states and pain responses to various NICU procedures in premature infants. *Journal of Tropical Pediatrics*, 52 (3):201–205, 2006.

Akuma, A.O. and Jordan, S.: Pain management in neonates: A survey of nurses and doctors. *Journal of Advanced Nursing*, 68(6):1288–1301, 2012.

American Academy of Pediatrics and Canadian Paediatric Society: Prevention and management of pain in the neonate: An update. *Pediatrics*, 118(5):2231–2241, 2006.

American Academy of Pediatrics and Canadian Paediatric Society: Prevention and management of pain and stress in the neonate. *Pediatrics*, 105(2):454–461, 2000.

Anand, K.J. and Craig, K.D.: New perspectives on the definition of pain [editorial]. *Pain*, 67(1):3–6, 1996.

Anand, K.J., Hall, R.W., Desai, N., et al.: Effects of morphine analgesia in ventilated preterm neonates: Primary outcomes from the NEOPAIN randomized trial. *Lancet*, 363(9422):1673–1682, 2004.

Anand, K.J. and International Evidence-Based Group for Neonatal Pain: Consensus statement for the prevention and management of pain in the newborn. *Archives of Pediatrics and Adolescent Medicine*, 155 (2):173–180, 2001.

Aranda, J.V., Carlo, W., Hummel, P., et al.: Analgesia and sedation during mechanical ventilation in neonates. *Clinical Therapeutics*, 27(6):877–899, 2005.

Belda, S., Pallas, C.R., de la Cruz, J. and Tejada, P.: Screening for retinopathy: Is it painful? *Biology of the Neonate*, 86(3):195–200, 2004.

Bouza, H.: The impact of pain in the immature brain. *Journal of Maternal-Fetal and Neonatal Medicine*, 22 (9):722–732, 2009.

Brummelte, S., Grunau, R.E., Chau, V., et al.: Procedural pain and brain development in premature newborns. *Annals of Neurology*, 71(3):385–396, 2012.

Carbajal, R., Rousset, A., Danan, C., et al.: Epidemiology and treatment of painful procedures in neonates in intensive care units. *JAMA*, 300(1):60–70, 2008.

Ceelie, I., de Wildt, S.N., van Dijk, M., et al.: Effect of intravenous paracetamol on postoperative morphine requirements in neonates and infants undergoing major noncardiac surgery: A randomized controlled trial. *JAMA*, 309(2):149–154, 2013.

Cignacco, E., Hamers, J.P., Stoffel, L., et al.: The efficacy of non-pharmacological interventions in the management of procedural pain in preterm and term neonates: A systematic literature review. *European Journal of Pain*, 11(2):139–152, 2007.

Craig, K.D., Whitfield, M.F., Grunau, R., et al.: Pain in the preterm neonate: Behavioral and physiological indices. *Pain*, 52(3):287–299, 1993.

Cuzzolin, L., Antonucci, R. and Fanos, V.: Paracetamol (acetaminophen) efficacy and safety in the newborn. *Current Drug Metabolism*, 14(2):178–185, 2013.

Dominguez, K.D., Lomako, D.M., Katz, R.W. and Kelly, H. W.: Opioid withdrawal in critically ill neonates. *Annals of Pharmacotherapy*, 37(4):473–477, 2003.

Ducharme, C., Carnevale, F.A., Clermont, M.S. and Shea, S.: A prospective study of adverse reactions to the weaning of opioids and benzodiazepines among critically ill children. *Intensive and Critical Care Nursing*, 21(3):179–186, 2005.

Duhn, L. and Medves, J.: A systematic integrative review of infant pain assessment tools. *Advances in Neonatal Care*, 4(3):126–140, 2004.

El Sayed, M.F., Taddio, A., Faliah, S., et al.: Safety profile of morphine following surgery in neonates. *Journal of Perinatology*, 27(7):444–447, 2007.

Evans, J.C.: Physiology of acute pain in preterm infants. *Newborn and Infant Nursing Reviews*, 1(2):75–84, 2001.

Finnegan, L.P.: Neonatal abstinence. In N.M. Nelson (Ed.): *Current therapy in neonatal-perinatal medicine* (2nd ed.). Toronto, Ontario, 1990, BC Decker.

Fitzgerald, M. and Anand, K.J.S.: Developmental neuroanatomy and neurophysiology of pain. In N. Schechter, and D.B. Berde (Eds.): *Pain in infants, children and adolescents* Baltimore, 1993, Williams & Wilkins, pp. 11–32.

Franck, L.S.: Pain in the nonverbal patient: Advocating for the critically ill neonate. *Pediatric Nursing*, 15 (1):65–68, 90 1989.

Franck, L.S., Allen, A., Cox, S. and Winter, I.: Parent's views about infant pain in neonatal intensive care. *Clinical Journal of Pain*, 21(2):133–139, 2005.

Franck, L.S., Cox, S., Allen, A. and Winter, I.: Parental concern and distress about infant pain. *Archives of Disease in Childhood: Fetal and Neonatal Edition*, 89(1): F71–F75, 2004.

Gale, G., Franck, L.S., Kools, S. and Lynch, M.: Parents' perceptions of their infant's pain experience in the NICU. *International Journal of Nursing Studies*, 41 (1):51–58, 2004.

Hall, R.W., Kronsberg, S.S., Barton, B.A., et al.: Morphine, hypotension, and adverse outcomes among preterm neonates: Who's to blame? *Secondary results from the NEOPAIN trial. Pediatrics*, 115(5):1351–1359, 2005.

Harrison, D., Beggs, S. and Stevens, B.: Sucrose for procedural pain management in infants. *Pediatrics*, 130 (5):918–925, 2012.

Harrison, H.: The principles for family-centered neonatal care. *Pediatrics*, 92:643–650, 1993.

Holsti, L., Grunau, R.E., Oberlander, T.F. and Whitfield, M.F.: Prior pain induces heightened motor responses during clustered care in preterm infants in the NICU. *Early Human Development*, 81(3):293–302, 2005.

Holsti, L., Grunau, R.E. and Shany, E.: Assessing pain in preterm infants in the neonatal intensive care unit: Moving to a 'brain-oriented' approach. *Pain Management*, 1(2):171–179, 2011.

Hudak, M.L., Tan, R.C. and Committee on Drugs and Committee on Fetus and Newborn: Neonatal drug withdrawal. *Pediatrics*, 129(2):e540–e560, 2012.

Hummel, P. and van Dijk, M.: Pain assessment: Current status and challenges. *Seminars in Fetal & Neonatal Medicine*, 11:237–245, 2006.

International Association for the Study of Pain Subcommittee on Taxonomy: Pain terms: A list with definitions and notes on usage. *Pain*, 6(3):249–252, 1979.

Johnston, C., Barrington, K.J., Taddio, A., et al.: Pain in Canadian NICUs: Have we improved over the past 12 years? *Clinical Journal of Pain*, 27(3):225–232, 2011.

Johnston, C.C. and Stevens, B.J.: Experience in a neonatal intensive care unit affects pain response. *Pediatrics*, 98(5):925–930, 1996.

Krechel, S. and Bildner, J.: CRIES: A new neonatal postoperative pain measurement score: Initial testing of validity and reliability. *Paediatric Anaesthesia*, 5 (1):53–61, 1995.

Kumar, P., Denson, S.E., Mancuso, T.J. and Committee on Fetus and Newborn, Section on Anesthesiology and Pain Medicine, American Academy of Pediatrics: Premedication for nonemergency endotracheal intubation in the neonate. *Pediatrics*, 125(3):608–615, 2010.

Lago, P., Garetti, E., Merazzi, D., et al.: Guidelines for procedural pain in the newborn. *Acta Paediatrica*, 98 (6):932–939, 2009.

Lawrence, J., Alcock, D., McGrath, P., et al.: The development of a tool to assess neonatal pain. *Neonatal Network*, 12(6):59–66, 1993.

Lehr, V.T., Cepeda, E., Frattarelli, D.A., et al.: Lidocaine 4% cream compared with lidocaine 2.5% and prilocaine 2.5% or dorsal penile block for circumcision. *American Journal of Perinatology*, 22(5):231–237, 2005.

Liaw, J.J., Yang, L., Katherine Wang, K.W., et al.: Non-nutritive sucking and facilitated tucking relieve preterm infant pain during heel-stick procedures: A prospective, randomised controlled crossover trial. *International Journal of Nursing Studies*, 49(3):300–309, 2012.

McNair, C., Ballantyne, M., Dionne, K., et al.: Postoperative pain assessment in the neonatal intensive care unit. *Archives of Disease in Childhood: Fetal and Neonatal Edition*, 89(6):F537–F541, 2004.

Melzack, R.: Gate control theory: On the evolution of pain concepts. *Pain Forum*, 5:128–138, 1996.

Naughton, K.A.: The combined use of sucrose and non-nutritive sucking for procedural pain in both term and preterm neonates: An integrative review of the literature. *Advances in Neonatal Care*, 13(1):9–19, 2013.

*NEOFAX: A manual of drugs used in neonatal care*, (24th ed.). Montvale, NJ, 2011, Thomson Reuters.

Partridge, J.C. and Wall, S.N.: Analgesia for dying infants whose life support is withdrawn or withheld. *Pediatrics*, 99(1):76–79, 1997.

Plotsky, P., Bradley, C. and Anand, K.: Behavioral and neuroendocrine consequences of neonatal stress. In K.J.S. Anand, B.J. Stevens, and P.J. McGrath (Eds.): *Pain in neonates* (2nd revised and enlarged edition.). Amsterdam, 2000, Elsevier Science, pp. 77–101.

Ranger, M., Johnston, C.C. and Anand, K.J.S.: Current controversies regarding pain assessment in neonates. *Seminars in Perinatology*, 31:283–288, 2007.

Reynolds, M., Alvares, D., Middleton, J. and Fitzgerald, M.: Neonatally wounded skin induces NGF-independent sensory neurite outgrowth in vitro. *Developmental Brain Research*, 102:275–283, 1997.

Rouss, K., Gerber, A., Albisetti, M., et al.: Long-term subcutaneous morphine administration after surgery in newborns. *Journal of Perinatal Medicine*, 35(1):79–81, 2007.

Ruda, M., Ling, Q., Hohmann, A., et al.: Altered nociceptive neuronal circuits after neonatal peripheral inflammation. *Science*, 289:628–630, 2000.

Shah, P.S., Herbozo, C., Aliwalas, L.L. and Shah, V.S.: Breastfeeding or breastmilk for procedural pain in neonates. *Cochrane Database of Systematic Reviews* CD004950, 2012.

Simons, S.H., van Dijk, M., Anand, K.S., et al.: Do we still hurt newborn babies? A prospective study of procedural pain and analgesia in neonates. Archives of Pediatrics and Adolescent Medicine, 157:1058–1064, 2003.

Spence, K., Henderson-Smart, D., New, K., et al.: Evidenced-based clinical practice guideline for management of newborn pain. *Journal of Paediatrics and Child Health*, 46(4):184–192, 2010.

Stevens, B.J., Gibbins, S., Yamada, J., et al.: The premature infant pain profile-revised (PIPP-R): Initial validation and feasibility. *Clinical Journal of Pain, e-published ahead of print*, April, 17:, 2013.

Stevens, B., Johnston, C., Franck, L., et al.: The efficacy of developmentally sensitive interventions and sucrose for relieving procedural pain in very low birth weight neonates. *Nursing Research*, 48(1):35–43, 1999.

Stevens, B., Johnston, C., Petryshen, P. and Taddio, A.: Premature infant pain profile: Development and initial validation. *Clinical Journal of Pain*, 12(1):13–22, 1996.

Stevens, B., Johnston, C., Taddio, A., Gibbins, S. and Yamada, J.: The Premature Infant Pain Profile: Evaluation 13 years after development. *Clinical Journal of Pain*, 26(9):813–830, 2010.

Stevens, B., Yamada, J., Lee, G.Y. and Ohlsson, A.: Sucrose for analgesia in newborn infants undergoing painful procedures. *Cochrane Database of Systematic Reviews* CD001069, 2013.

Suraseranivongse, S., Kaosaard, R., Intaking, P., et al.: A comparison of postoperative pain scales in neonates. *British Journal of Anaesthesia*, 97(4):540–544, 2006.

Taddio, A., Goldbach, M., Ipp, M., et al.: Effect of neonatal circumcision on pain responses during vaccination in boys. *Lancet*, 345(1):291–292, 1995.

Taddio, A., Shah, V., Stephens, D., et al.: Effect of liposomal lidocaine and sucrose alone and in combination for venipuncture pain in newborns. *Pediatrics*, 127(4):e940–e947, 2011.

Walden, M. and Gibbins, S.: *Newborn pain assessment and management: Guideline for practice:* (3rd ed.). Glenview, IL, 2012, National Association of Neonatal Nurses.

CHAPTER

# 17 Families in Crisis

CAROLE KENNER AND MARINA BOYKOVA

**OBJECTIVES**

1. Define the concept of crisis.
2. Recognize the psychological tasks that the mother and family must accomplish to establish a healthy parent–child relationship after the crisis of the birth of a premature or sick infant.
3. Describe assessment strategies for identifying a family in crisis.
4. Identify the risks of teenage parenting on the adolescent and the infant.
5. Identify nursing interventions to support a family coping with stressful events surrounding the birth of their infant.
6. Evaluate maternal behaviors found to be predictive of specific parenting outcomes.
7. Recognize emotional characteristics related to grief.
8. Identify strategies for working with families experiencing perinatal or neonatal end-of-life issues.
9. Identify specific behaviors to be assessed that influence parental attachment to their infant.
10. Describe the nursing strategies to promote parental attachment.
11. Identify cultural influences that influence parenting a sick or dying neonate.

With current technological advances, even the most acutely ill or most premature infant has a good chance of going home. Neonates born as prematurely as 23 weeks of gestation are surviving. Although these advances are increasing the odds of having a live neonate, for parents, they also have brought on tremendous stress that lasts through the first years of the infant's life (Gray et al., 2012). When a newborn infant requires intensive care at birth because of illness, prematurity, or congenital malformations, or when an infant dies, the effects of these unexpected events on the parents can be overwhelming. The families of these infants may experience multiple crisis events during the infant's hospitalization and after discharge. The focus of this chapter is the psychosocial aspects of supporting parents who must cope with stressful events surrounding the birth of their infant. The chapter highlights various types of families who may experience a crisis when their infant undergoes a neonatal intensive care unit (NICU) stay or a perinatal/neonatal death.

## CRISIS AND THE BIRTH OF THE SICK OR PREMATURE INFANT

Pregnancy and transition to parenthood are periods of stress and change during which mothers and fathers are attempting to master the normal developmental process of parenthood (Emmanuel and St John, 2010; Miller and Sollie, 1980; Nelson, 2003). These major life changes are referred to as developmental or maturational stressors. In contrast, the birth of a premature or sick infant and the death of an infant are unexpected stressful life events for which a person or family is often psychologically unprepared (Watson, 2011). Such events are referred to as situational or accidental stressors. When such maturational and situational stressors occur simultaneously, the resulting pressure can overwhelm a person's usual coping resources and support system, thus leading to crisis.

A. **Definition of crisis.** Crisis is defined as a temporary disequilibrium that occurs when people face an important problem or transitional phase so stressful that they are unable to cope by using their customary problem-solving resources (Howland, 2007). If parents do not successfully work through the increased demands, ineffective coping may result. Ineffective coping causes personal and family psychological disequilibrium or crisis, which continues until new ways of coping can be developed and maintained (Caplan et al., 1965; Kaplan and Mason, 1960). Coping, however, is intimately tied to social support (Sheppard, 2009), resources available (Pinelli et al., 2008), cultural values and beliefs, and, in some instances, spirituality (Heidari et al., 2012; Holditch-Davis et al., 2009; Kenner et al., 2014), so these must be taken into account.

B. **Several psychological tasks** have been identified that the mother and family must accomplish to cope with the crisis of a premature birth or the birth of a sick infant and to establish a basis for a healthy parent–child relationship. These must take into consideration the psychological health of the mother and its impact on parent–infant interactions.

1. Acquisition of parental role. Alteration in parental role related to the infant's sickness and hospitalization leads to diminished parental feelings of attachment to the infant and decreased parental confidence in their own abilities to give care (Holditch-Davis et al., 2011; Miles et al., 2011; Zabielski, 1994). Alteration in parental role has been named as one of the major stressors for parents during the infant's/child's hospitalization (Miles et al., 1989), which in turn influences the parent–child relationship (Anderson et al., 2010; Miles et al., 2011).
2. Preparation for the possible loss of the infant. Parents often consider the possibility of disability or death of the infant while simultaneously hoping for the infant's survival (Bennett et al., 2005; Dyer, 2005; Fraley, 1990). This uncertainty about outcomes also influences parent–child relationships and parental well-being, leading to increased levels of anxiety.
3. Acknowledgment of failure to deliver a term infant. The mother struggles with feelings of guilt (Garel et al., 2007) and failure while grieving about the loss of an "ideal" infant. Often parents search for causes of the infant's condition. Family members may actually be, or be perceived as, blaming the mother for the premature infant (Golish and Powell, 2003; Shah et al., 2011). Family members may also feel guilty as if they too have contributed to the infant's condition.
4. Adaptation to the intensive care environment. Environmental stressors of the NICU (e.g., lights, noise, and equipment) influence parental well-being and perception of an infant. Parents struggle to develop secure relationships in the unfamiliar and stress-provoking setting of the intensive care unit (Bozzette et al., 2010; Korja et al., 2012; Lutz et al., 2009; Reyna and Pickler, 2009).
5. Resumption of interaction with the infant once the threat of loss has passed. Parents begin to make efforts to participate in the infant's care and gain confidence in their caregiving abilities (Raines and Brustad, 2012). Parental interactions may be adversely affected because of the effects of posttraumatic stress, depression, and fear that something might still happen to the infant (Cho et al., 2008; Jubinville et al., 2012; Placencia and McCullough, 2012; Vanderbilt et al., 2009).
6. Preparation for taking the infant home is another extreme task for parents (Smith et al., 2009, 2012). Parents must understand the special needs and characteristics of the premature or sick infant and the necessary precautions that must be taken and yet maintain a positive relationship with the infant, realizing that these needs are only temporary. Failure to resolve these tasks can contribute to such maladaptive parenting as being overprotective, resulting in the "vulnerable child syndrome" (Kokotos and Adam, 2009), or compensatory parenting (Miles and Holditch-Davis, 1995). Other negative parental outcomes include emotional disengagement and deprivation and low adherence to follow-up recommendations (Ballantyne et al., 2012) that may affect infant development and growth (Welch et al. for the Family Nurture Intervention [FTI] Trial Group, 2012). The psychological impact of having a sick infant often continues after a successful discharge, resulting in parental psychological distress postdischarge (Boykova and Kenner, 2012; Kenner et al., 2014; Meijssen et al., 2011a; Rowe and Jones, 2010).

C. **Discussion.** During the crisis periods, parents often display signs of anxiety, depression, increased levels of stress, fear, and powerlessness (Mackley et al., 2010; Nyström and Axelsson, 2002; Padovani et al., 2009; Solberg et al., 2011). They also may exhibit symptoms of acute posttraumatic stress disorder (PTSD), as well as physical or cognitive problems (Jubinville et al., 2012; Meijssen et al., 2011a; Vanderbilt et al., 2009; Wray et al., 2011). A family in crisis cannot effectively interact with their newly born infant because all their energy is going toward the crisis resolution. During the crisis period, parents are more receptive to overtures of help from other family members, friends, and the health care team. Nurses are in a key position because they work so directly with the parents to anticipate a family crisis and to promote positive coping and effective use of social supports. When interventions are put into place to promote effective coping and positive social support, the crisis will resolve and psychological equilibrium, a necessary step toward the establishment of a healthy parent–child relationship, will be restored. Factors that influence a family's return to equilibrium include the following (Kenner et al., 2014):

1. Understanding of the infant's health problem and the need for NICU care, and understanding of their parental role.
2. Resolving or at least lessening of the family's grief and guilt reactions to the need for NICU care.
3. Involving parents in caregiving activities as partners in care, and not visitors.
4. Changing the focus to patient-centered/family-centered care.
5. Using positive coping and social supports.

## Grief and Loss

A. **Introduction.** Unfortunately, not all pregnancies result in a healthy term infant. When adverse neonatal events occur, often the parents are overwhelmed by grief (Dyer, 2005; Golish and Powell, 2003). As the parents realize that their newborn is "less than perfect" and not the infant of their fantasies, acute grief reactions occur. Grief is also related to the loss of an experience of imagined parenting activities, such as if birth hospitalization did not occur, and the absence of symbolic rituals (i.e., baby shower). With neonatal death, the parents also grieve for the lost opportunity to parent the child. Because a lot of uncertainty about outcomes is present (as is the case with a preterm infant), the loss can be ambiguous, making parents physically and emotionally exhausted (Golish and Powell, 2003).

   One of the early tasks of parenting is to resolve the discrepancy between the idealized infant and the real infant. The acceptance of the perceived "loss" is vital for resolution of grief (Golish and Powell, 2003). To assist parents therapeutically in working through the feelings associated with loss, nurses working with high-risk infants must understand the grief process, recognize typical parental behaviors associated with grief, and provide appropriate nursing interventions. It also may be appropriate to help the parents actively plan the care of their yet-to-be-born or dying infant through use of an advance directive (Catlin, 2005). Much like in the adult, the advance directive during either the prenatal or the neonatal period allows the parents to say what they wish to be done and whether or not they want to "allow a natural death," a term much more acceptable than a do-not-resuscitate order.

B. **Definitions.**
   1. Grief: the response of sadness and sorrow to the loss of a valued object (Kenner, 2014).
   2. Anticipatory grief: grieving that occurs before an actual loss. If the outcome for the infant is healthy, then anticipatory grieving can lead to difficulties in attachment and problems in the parent–infant relationship.
   3. Chronic grief: unresolved or blocked grief; frequently seen in parents of a disabled child, who is a constant reminder of loss.
   4. Chronic sorrow: grief response associated with ongoing living loss that is permanent, progressive, recurring, and cyclic (Gordon, 2009).

C. **Signs of grief reaction include: sadness and despair, denial, numbness, shock, disbelief, and anger as well as fatigue and sleep disturbances (Golish and Powell, 2003).** Uncomplicated grief resolves through the stages of shock and disbelief, then developing awareness of the loss, and finally recovery in the form of reestablishment of well-being (Teel, 1991).

## SPECIFIC POPULATION OF PARENTS: ADOLESCENTS

Parents who are adolescent have some unique needs. They undergo the crises of parenthood and of having an infant in the NICU. In addition, these parents are dealing with the normal developmental tasks of adolescence. Sometimes these tasks seem to be in conflict with their needs as new parents. The nurse must be aware of these conflicts and realize their unique blending needs of taking on a new role and being at their developmental stage.

Adolescence is a turning point, or change period. It moves a child from childhood toward the maturation of the adult. Many physiologic changes are occurring, first at puberty and then in the move toward adulthood. Physical appearance changes and the adolescent is capable of childbearing. Maturation of the reproductive system now occurs much earlier than in the past. In the United States, girls are reaching menarche as young as 8 years of age. Adolescence is the time when childbearing becomes a potential reality for most individuals.

Development of the personality is tied to role attainment, much as for parents and the parenting role. Adolescents strive to have an identity unique from those of other family members. They are developing their self-concept and self-esteem. The peer group becomes important for validation of attitudes, values, and beliefs. However, adults can model this peer validation to enhance positive developmental outcomes for adolescent parents (Dishion et al., 2002). Adolescence is a time of constant change and usually turmoil—a period of maturational crisis.

A. **Some developmental tasks of this period are:**
   1. Independence from adults.
   2. Preparation for financial security.
   3. Gender identification.
   4. A stable, realistic, positive sense of self.

B. **In addition, adolescence:**
   1. Is characterized by high anxiety.
   2. Can be anticipated, and therefore preparation can be made.
   3. Requires normal social support for a successful transition.
   4. Is relatively easy to resolve because the individual's values usually do not conflict with societal expectations for the outcome, which is adult behavior.
   5. Is a period of vulnerability to a crisis occurrence if a traumatic event is added to the transitional state.

While adolescents have unique needs, they also are unique individuals. As health professionals, we often make assumptions of what they need or what type of parents they will be. The reality is they need to be assessed for their knowledge, level of crisis, and supports the same as any other individual or family. It has been shown that adolescents often underestimate the severity of their infant's illness (Boss et al., 2010) and require increased levels of informational and esteem/appraisal supports (Grassley, 2010; Logsdon and Koniak-Griffin, 2005). Perception is all there is—right or wrong—and health professionals should not perceive that all adolescents will be bad parents, or immature in their actions, or be more concerned with peers than with their child (Chittleborough et al., 2011). Health professionals must evaluate parental needs of adolescents certainly within the context of their developmental stage but also with consideration of their own personal, individualized needs (Riesch et al., 2010).

## THE FAMILY IN CRISIS

### Assessment

A. **Determine parents' understanding of the situation** (i.e., realistic vs. distorted). The parents' ability to resolve the crisis depends on their realistic perception of their situation: they need to be fully informed about their infant's condition and expected progress/outcome. An inability to understand the crisis may be related to low socioeconomic status, educational level, or cultural values and beliefs. Parents of a lower socioeconomic status or educational level may not fully understand what to expect of their infant or their role because they may lack good role models for themselves or the financial means to provide adequate, safe care for themselves or their infant. Older mothers may have difficulty in coping as they are used to being in control of their situations. They may actually blame the health professionals for the adverse outcomes of their pregnancy and delivery. Cultural values and beliefs also may play a role because different cultures view the infant in relationship to parents in different ways, and these parents' view of health and death may be different from the typical U.S. views; in addition, occurrence of depression might be influenced (Callister et al., 2010; Zauderer, 2009). In some countries, such as in India or China, only male offspring are valued, and girl babies are dismissed as nonessential; in some countries, such as Iran, the birth of infant that has been hospitalized in an NICU leads to stigmatization (Heidari et al., 2012). Whereas we often crave control over the environment in Western culture, other cultures may view this as fate. Native Americans usually accept what is. Blacks are more oriented to specific situations than time. Latinos value the inclusion of the extended family and view death as having rituals associated with it; touching an infant's head is seen as threatening by some Southeast Asians, Buddhists, and native Hawaiians; and Middle Eastern children make few independent decisions (a consideration when working with adolescent parents if their extended family is not present). When crucial conversations are necessary, the family's cultural values must be considered (Cone, 2007).

**B. Determine parents' grief response.** The extent to which parents are experiencing grief must be determined. Grief responses to death, premature birth, or the birth of an infant with a malformation are similar. These responses do not necessarily occur in the same sequence for all people. They are mediated by cultural beliefs and values as well as the parents' developmental stage (Whitaker et al., 2010). In addition, the responses may overlap and recur. PTSD often results from just having an infant in an NICU but is exacerbated if the child actually dies. Stages of grief such as shock, denial, anger, and acceptance may or may not be followed. Grief is very individualized and may be in the form of anticipatory grief because the parents fear the infant might die, even though the physical condition does not appear to warrant this fear. Consider this within the cultural context of the family, because it may not be acceptable to express grief or worries to outsiders. If the child is dying, then consider the parents' perspectives of what they need and want from us and of other end-of-life (EOL) issues, such as advance directives. One of the goals of the staff working with parents is to encourage the development of attachment, or an affectional tie, between the parents and infant. Consider too that dressing the infant in a diaper or loose clothing will allow the parents to have at least one image of their child as a baby and not a dying infant. Because the birth of a premature or a physically, psychologically, or neurologically challenged infant creates a sense of loss, the parents must first resolve their grief before attachment can be fully achieved.

**C. Determine parents' adaptation to and coping** with the stressful event.

1. Are the parents maintaining responsibilities related to activities of daily living (e.g., eating, personal grooming)?
2. To what degree has the family's normal lifestyle been affected by the crisis? (Are they able to return to work? Keep house? Care for other children in the household?)
3. Are the parents exhibiting positive coping skills within the context of their cultural values and beliefs?
4. To what extent has the financial status of the family been affected?

**D. Determine what support systems exist** for the parents and whether they are being used. It is also important to determine whether these supports are positive. The parents may have several people in their support network, but if these people are critical of how the parents are conducting themselves, then they may not be viewed as positive supports.

1. Who are the significant others in the lives of the parents? Consider biologic kinship (family) and/or emotional kinship (friends).
2. What professional supports are available?
3. Is a parent support group available?

**E. Understanding the origins of a crisis** and their links with the normal "ups and downs" of life is crucial to successful assessment and intervention. Events that stimulate the occurrence of a crisis, such as those of the teenage parent in the NICU, can originate from:

1. Being in a transitional state, such as
   a. Adolescence to adulthood.
   b. Childhood to parenthood.
2. Being a part of a social–cultural structure and
   a. Violating customs or cultural norms embedded in that structure, such as a teenager's becoming pregnant and having a newborn, or
   b. Behaving outside the accepted teenage social norms, as the role of parent would demand (although these examples are culture-specific): for example, being tied down to taking care of a newborn or having to arrange for child care at a time when peers are freely going to sports, games, and dances and having fun.
   c. Being exposed to hazardous or disturbing situations:
      (1) Birth of a first child. This is a disturbing situation because no one knows exactly what to expect of parenthood—a role never before experienced.
      (2) Lack of experience with parenthood.
      (3) Bearing of a sick newborn infant.

## Problems Associated With Adolescent Pregnancy

When teens become pregnant, they often experience the following problems:

A. **Loss of peer group.** Adolescents' peers often disappear, leaving them without support and feeling socially isolated. Their self-concept changes as they approach parenthood because, before the pregnancy, the peer group helped shape their self-perception.

B. **Disruption of family ties.** The pregnant adolescent and her boyfriend often bring on direct conflict with their parents. The rationale for this conflict is that the parents of the adolescents often believe that adolescence is an inappropriate time to start a family and that the adolescents need to live by the parental house rules. At the same time, the adolescent parents may be trying to take on adult responsibilities while feeling that they are being treated as children. This conflict removes a possible positive social support. It also disrupts the effort to assume a parental role if the adolescents' parents try to make decisions regarding the coming infant.

C. **Maternal health problems.** The pregnant female adolescent often has engaged in risky behaviors besides being sexually active. She may smoke, drink, or use drugs. She is at risk of having human immunodeficiency virus (HIV) infection and other sexually transmitted infections (STIs). This risk is not unique to adolescents but is possible because of the feelings of invincibility that accompany this age. The pregnant adolescent may be emotionally immature and may have to interrupt her education to bear the child. She may be forced into a marriage she does not want or is not ready for at this time. She may lack knowledge about normal fetal and infant growth and development. She may have very unrealistic expectations of an infant and of herself as a parent. She may have sought pregnancy as a way to have someone need her. She may not seek prenatal care or may try to hide the pregnancy by limiting weight gain. These actions may put her health and her infant's health at risk. She also often lacks parenting skills.

D. **Paternal problems.** The adolescent father may have engaged in risky sexual behaviors. He may have been smoking or used alcohol or drugs. He also may be at risk of having HIV infection or other STIs. If he is infected, the pregnant adolescent and the fetus are also at risk because these infections can be passed on to the maternal–fetal unit. The male adolescent may be generally stable psychologically, but he may not be thinking about future consequences of his sexual behavior, such as his inability to fulfill his parenting role. For example, because of his risky behaviors, he may have contracted HIV, which will take him away from the pregnant adolescent and his future child. If his family, his significant other, or her family views his behaviors as irresponsible, he may be isolated from an active role in future parenting. He may feel excluded from decisions regarding the continuation of the pregnancy or the placement of the child after birth. He may interrupt his own education to provide financial support to his new "family." He may be forced into a marriage he neither wants nor is ready for.

E. **Risks to the infant.** The infant is at risk of having a faulty, or negative, parent–infant interaction, generally because of the parents' lack of understanding of the normal growth and development process. The parents also often have unrealistic expectations of the child and their role as parents (Hess et al., 2004) and may lack parenting skills. The infant may be small for gestational age or premature and may require an expensive hospitalization that the parents are not ready financially or cognitively to accept. The infant may be less responsive or organized in cues for care by the parents. He or she may be more at risk of having slowed or delayed growth because of the parents' lack of understanding of normal infant care and feeding practices. The infant may not receive the type and amount of stimulation necessary for positive cognitive or behavioral development. An infant who is premature tends to be more irritable, to feed poorly, to have poor self-regulatory behaviors, and to be difficult to console. This seeming lack of responsiveness to parenting efforts often reinforces the adolescent parents' poor self-esteem and poor self-concept, which often accompany adolescent pregnancy. The infant may also be at risk of experiencing abuse or neglect.

   1. Prematurity, birth between 23 and 27 weeks of gestation, is more common among infants of adolescent mothers. The risk factors for delivering early are (Bowers, 2014):
      a. Low pregnancy weight.
      b. Lower socioeconomic status.
      c. Marital status: single.
      d. Tobacco use (smoking).

e. Narcotic or other substance use.
f. Anemia (hemoglobin concentration <11 g/dL).
g. First child.
h. Poor prenatal care.

2. Low birth weight (<2500 g) is also a risk factor for an adolescent's offspring. The risk can be as much as 6 times greater for 14-year-old and younger mothers.

## Intervention

Nursing care is generally concerned with both the physiologic and psychosocial needs of the patient and the family. However, nurses are the key health care providers who help parents to overcome the crisis. Assessment skills and appropriate interventions are of vital importance for well-being of family. It is the nurse who is viewed as the advocate for the family and who has the most continual interactions with parents. Importantly, mothers and health care professionals may view the child as medically fragile when this may or may not be the case. Also important, whereas most of the current research focuses on the maternal role and the mother's level of distress, fathers must be considered too. The father's perception of a crisis is just as important as the mother's, and interventions to ease their distress must be part of the preparation for taking an infant home (Boykova and Kenner, 2010). Many of the strategies or interventions are the same for all groups of parents because they represent parenting needs. Cultural influences must also be considered. Below are some interventions and strategies that can help alleviate the pressure of NICU hospitalization for parents.

A. **Be present with the physician or nurse practitioner at the initial meeting with the parents.**

B. **Talk with the mother and father together whenever possible.** Consider cultural values of each family. In some cultures, the father must receive the information first (Kenner et al., 2014).

C. **Determine and address the parents' perceptions of the infant's condition.** Talk with the parents and find out their concerns and perceptions. Too many times as health professionals we follow our perceptions and discuss the issues we deem important without validating if these views are shared by the parents.

D. **Be consistent with information given to parents by the staff.** If in an academic health care setting where the physicians or nurse practitioners rotate frequently, be sure that any changes in care that are reflective only of these staff changes are explained within that context. If parents do not understand the basis of these changes or are not told when their infant's condition really changes, then mistrust begins. Then the chance that the crisis will escalate is highly probable (Kenner et al., 2014).

E. **Do not overload parents with detailed information about their infant during their initial visits to the NICU;** provide basic facts and allow the parents some time to process the information. Help parents to understand the information given by repeating the information that is either given verbally or written. Often parents do not hear all of what is said due to their stress. Give them information on the disease process their infant is experiencing so they know what to expect.

F. **Assess the grief response.** Males and females express their grief in different ways. However, most, if not all, parents experience some form of grief by just having an infant who requires specialized care (Kenner et al., 2014). This reaction must be assessed throughout the hospital stay. Sometimes this response is directly tied to their understanding of the infant's condition. Other times it is related to cultural beliefs and values.

G. **Acknowledge any feeling of guilt that might be expressed** about the unexpected birth outcome. Let the parents know that these feelings are normal (Siegel et al., 2011).

H. **Facilitate adaptation of the parents' new role** by being a very good listener, by observing body language, and by helping them verbalize their feelings (Siegel et. al, 2011).

I. **Periodically assess the parents' understanding** of their infant's condition and their interpretation of the information that has been given to them. Information must be reinforced throughout the hospital stay. Whenever anyone is anxious, little information is actually heard or retained.

J. **Write notes from the infant to the parents** concerning the infant's status (e.g., equipment, feedings, oxygen concentration) and take pictures of the infant periodically. A notebook containing the notes and pictures can be kept at the infant's bedside for the parents. These can be memory books or scrapbooks that become especially important if the child dies. This intervention should be individualized because not all parents want this form of "communication." However, for some parents this is one strategy that promotes positive attachment (Siegel et al., 2011).

K. **Encourage the parents to keep a journal** concerning their experience of delivering a premature or sick infant. This action can assist families to work through their feelings as well as having memories to review what happened and reflect on issues that have been or have not been resolved (Howland, 2007).

L. **Give parents the freedom to express negative ideas without being judged.** Fear and frustration over the inability to control their infant's circumstances are often the basis for parental anger displaced to staff. Remember that control is not acceptable in all cultures, so it is important to ask what is making them uncomfortable. In addition, a positive way to approach this and possibly decrease their anger is to ask them what would help them to feel more comfortable.

M. **Encourage parents to participate in the care as they desire.** Parents need to understand and develop their roles as parents. If professionals provide all the care, a clear message is conveyed to the parents that they are not capable of helping their infant. They must understand all the things they have to contribute to the team approach to care. The role of parents at an NICU has been changed (Thomas, 2008), and now parents are a part of the health care team and as such should have a say in health care decisions. Dr. Bernadette Melnyk's COPE Program—Creating Opportunities for Parent Empowerment—has decreased stress, shortened length of stay, and increased coping by involving parents in their infant's care (Melnyk and Feinstein, 2009; Melnyk et al., 2004, 2006, 2008). Taking part in their infant's care helps parents to ease the crisis, decrease guilt and grief, increase parental attachment to a baby, and increase psychological well-being of parents. Examples are kangaroo care (skin-to-skin contact, done by placing the naked infant next to the parent's naked chest, with a blanket or gown draped over the parent and infant), calming care and comfort care for the infant, and feeding (Bigelow et al., 2012; Neu and Robinson, 2010; Skene et al., 2012; Welch et al. for the Family Nurture Intervention [FTI] Trial Group, 2012).

N. **Do not refer to parents as visitors.** Parents are not visitors. They are parents and are partners in the care of the infant. They are an integral part of the infant's care and should be a focus of nursing care. Parents as partners is a concept that is growing as part of the patient safety movement from the Institute of Medicine toward patient-focused and family-centered care. Many hospitals are creating Family Advisory Councils (FACs) that are either unit or hospital based (Sullivan and Altimier, 2007). These councils are composed of parents of former patients and representatives from many disciplines, which may include clergy and administration. The FACs guide the administration by giving input into policies that support family voices (Halm et al., 2006).

O. **Promote a developmentally supportive environment for the family.** Use of individualized family-centered care is important if the family is to be helped through this crisis (Kenner and McGrath, 2010). For example, kangaroo care, dimmed lights or cycled lights, private areas for parent interaction with the infant, and swaddling or cuddling of the infant promote positive development of the infant and family (McGrath, 2014).

P. **Determine parents' network of social support.** The social support network may include family, friends, clergy, and health professionals. Also determine whether the level of support is adequate from the parents' and the health professionals' standpoint. When possible, use new technologies such as mypatientline (www.mypatientline.com; by Jaduka, Dallas, TX), which allows the family a toll-free service with voice mail and connects the family to friends and other family members even at a distance. Online and telephone-based peer support and parent support groups are other examples of strategic interventions for NICU parents who require increased levels of social support (Ardal et al., 2011; Dennis et al., 2009; Lindberg et al., 2009; Liu et al., 2011; Preyde and Ardal, 2003).

Q. **Encourage parents to share their concerns and fears with each other.** Often it is not until the infant is discharged that parents share their feelings with each other. This is another area where culture plays a role. In some Asian cultures, expressions of concern are acceptable within the family unit but not with others. Health professionals may be viewed as authority figures and not ones to whom fears should be confided. It is important too to find out what this illness and hospitalization means to the family and to what degree they are viewed as stress (Howland, 2007).

R. **Assist parents in maintaining their relationship with one another.** Reinforce with them that they must take time for themselves as a couple. If the mother is alone, encourage her to maintain ties with other family members and her friends.
S. **Assist parents in maintaining their relationship with the infant's siblings** by helping them recognize the needs of the other children and identify how the needs can be met. Use resources such as coloring and activity books to help the siblings express their feelings.
T. **Assist the adolescent parents in defining their role with their own parents** by helping them learn how to talk with their parents.
U. **Encourage parents to attend a parent support group if desirable.** Involvement in a parent support group has been demonstrated to facilitate parental grieving, reduce fears, and increase feelings of parental competence. This intervention must be culture specific. In some cultures it is not acceptable to discuss family problems openly. It is also important to include the father's perspective. Some groups are for fathers only because this is a recognized growing need.
V. **Assist families of dying infants to tell you what they need.** EOL issues are never easy but are especially difficult in this population when celebration of a birth is the expectation. Asking the family what they need from us as health care professionals is important. Understanding what this death means to them is critical to plan individualized care. Finding out if they want siblings and extended family involved, and if clergy or spiritual healers are important, as well as what for them constitutes a good death are all important aspects of helping families cope (Kenner, 2014). Use of consistent information and the same message from all health care providers is important too. The use of a palliative care protocol is one method to ensure more consistency (Catlin, 2005; Catlin and Carter, 2002). Consideration of cultural differences once again is important (McGrath, 2014).

## Evaluation of Maternal Parenting Outcomes

A. **Predictors of good maternal parenting outcomes (Kenner et al., 2014).**
   1. Anxiety level is moderate to high: she worries about the infant's chances of surviving, the possibility of abnormality, and her competence as a mother.
   2. Seeks information about the infant.
   3. Demonstrates warmth toward infant and in other relationships.
   4. Has a support system (i.e., father of the infant, her mother, friends).
   5. Has had a previous successful experience with a premature infant (i.e., previous child, a sibling, other relative), which enables her to feel more experienced and confident.
   6. Recognizes positive attributes of the child (i.e., smiling).
   7. Views self positively.
   8. For an adolescent, has a centralized locus of behavioral control.
   9. Exhibits effective caregiving.
   10. Makes positive eye contact with the infant.

B. **Predictors of poor maternal parenting outcomes (Kenner et al., 2014).**
   1. Exhibits an inappropriately low anxiety level.
   2. Demonstrates passivity—does not actively seek out information related to infant's condition.
   3. Has limited verbal interaction.
   4. Visits infrequently and for short periods in the NICU. (Remember that sometimes infrequent visits are due to a lack of transportation and not self-determined parenting problems.)
   5. Is unaware of the infant's needs.
   6. Has unrealistic expectations of the infant or the parenting role.
   7. Personalizes the infant's behavior as a failure of her ability to parent or characterizes infant's behavior as "bad."
   8. During pregnancy, expressed little desire to have a child.
   9. Is more likely to express disappointment about the sex of the infant.
   10. Has no support system.
   11. Is an adolescent with little or no social supports.
   12. Exhibits role confusion.

## GRIEF AND LOSS

### Interventions for Facilitating Grief Resolution

A. **Listen.** Parents need to be given the opportunity to express their feelings.
B. **Acknowledge the pain of their loss.** This gives the parents permission to talk about their loss and provides support for acknowledging and working through their grief.
C. **Convey an attitude of acceptance, openness, and availability to the family.** Grieving people need permission to experience their feelings, regardless of how uncomfortable or unpleasant.
D. **Help the parents understand the individuality of the grieving process.** Mothers and fathers usually have "incongruent grieving": they do not grieve at the same pace. This incongruence frequently leads to marital discord because of misconceptions about feelings and an inability to communicate.

### Interventions for Parents Experiencing a Perinatal Loss

A. **Encourage the family to see, hold, and spend time with the infant** before and after death (Catlin and Carter, 2002; Kenner, 2014).
   1. Be sensitive to individual and cultural differences in rituals of saying goodbye.
   2. Physically bring the family together and offer privacy. Some hospitals have a neonatal hospice program in which the family is involved with the infant's care (Catlin and Carter, 2002; Kenner, 2014).
B. **Provide the parents with the following mementos if culturally acceptable:** photograph of the infant, identification bracelet, footprints, completed crib card, blanket, wisp of hair, and birth certificate. Keep these mementos in a file in the nursery for future retrieval should parents choose not to take the items at the time of the infant's death. This intervention must be individualized according to the needs and desires of each family (Catlin and Carter, 2002; Kenner, 2014). This is a very culturally sensitive topic and must be explored with the family.
C. **Provide information about support groups and/or grief counseling.** Consideration for individual family wishes is important. Not all families want or would benefit from support groups. Family follow-up, even if just a phone call from an NICU nurse or hospice nurse a few weeks after the loss, is very helpful to many families.
D. **Encourage the parents to name the infant.** This task is very important for many parents.
E. **Provide a booklet about perinatal loss for the parents and siblings.** Pediatric hospice and palliative care programs have a number of resources for parents and the left-behind siblings. There are many books and videos that are age appropriate. A good resource is Children's Hospice International at www.chionline.org or 1101 King Street, Suite 360, Alexandria, VA 22314; phone: 800-2-4-CHILD.
F. **Discuss options for autopsy, disposition of the body, and a memorial or funeral service.** It is important to ask parents what they need and what they would like. Some parents wish to be an active participant in the plans; other families want these arrangements to be done for them. Rituals surrounding death are culturally driven; for example, the taking of pictures after death is not acceptable to Native Americans, Eskimos, Amish, Russians, Hindus, and Muslims. It is the family's choice (Kenner, 2014).
G. **Offer the option for the infant to be baptized.** This option is not acceptable in all cultures.
H. **Assist parents in understanding the importance of informing siblings about the death of the infant.** Suggest that they use simple statements based on the children's level of understanding. Many times the siblings take the death much better than adults expect. Allowing them to see the infant after death may make the infant real to them. Of course, parental wishes are always to be the guiding principle for how the siblings are informed of the death and what part they play in the rituals following the death. Again, this is a culturally sensitive issue and beliefs must be explored with the family.
I. **Talk with parents about possible responses** from family and friends, who often minimize the infant's death in an attempt to offer comfort. Encourage them to delegate or give tasks to those who call them. If they need the laundry done or groceries bought, then these are simple tasks that can be delegated to others who truly want to help and do not know what to do. More

information on EOL issues can be obtained through the joint project of the American Association of Colleges of Nursing (AACN) and the City of Hope (COH) End-of-Life Nursing Education Consortium (ELNEC) found at www.aacn.nche.edu/ELNEC/index.htm. A pediatric-specific program is available.

## Interventions for Parents With a Preterm or Physically, Developmentally, or Psychologically Challenged Infant

These interventions have been incorporated into the interventions listed in the previous section (The Family in Crisis) and in the next section (Family–Infant Bonding).

## Family–Infant Bonding

Parents who have an infant who is born ill, prematurely, or physically or psychologically challenged are at risk of having parenting difficulties. These stressful events around the time of the infant's birth generate feelings of anxiety, disappointment, and grief in the parents. Moreover, early disruptions in the acquaintance and attachment process between parent and infant place these parents in a state of increased vulnerability for establishing a nurturing relationship with their infant. Opportunities for parents to learn to interpret their infant's unique needs and to develop reciprocal interaction through sensitivity to behavioral cues are also interrupted (Kenner et al., 2014). The relationship between parent–infant attachment and later parenting behaviors has been well established (Borghini et al., 2006; Fegran et al., 2008; Korja et al., 2009; Meijssen et al., 2011b). In addition, the parent–infant attachment is the basis for all the infant's subsequent attachments and is the relationship through which a sense of self is developed. Therefore, an important component of nursing care of the high-risk infant is facilitation of parent–infant interaction and attachment.

A. **Definitions.**
   1. *Bonding:* a gradual, reciprocal process that begins with acquaintance. It is a unique and specific relationship between two people and endures across time. Bonding occurs on a different timetable for mothers than for fathers. Although mothers experience a sharp increase in bonding around the fifth month of pregnancy and have intensifying feelings throughout the pregnancy, the father's feelings usually tend to develop more slowly than the mother's and become congruent after birth, when infant caregiving begins (McGrath, 2014).
   2. *Attachment:* the quality of the bond, or affectional tie, between parents and their infant, which begins early in the prenatal period, appears to increase when fetal movement is felt and is intensified with interaction between the parent and the infant after birth.

B. **Discussion.** The development of a warm, nurturing, and reciprocal relationship between infant and parent is essential for a healthy psychological outcome to the crisis of the birth of a premature, sick, or malformed infant (Kenner et al., 2014). "The parent 'at risk' cannot resolve a crisis surrounding birth of their infant and simultaneously establish warm attachment bonds while retaining his or her self-esteem without the support of others in the social system" (Mercer, 1977, p. 5). Neonatal nurses can provide this support by assessing the parents' responses to their infant and facilitating their acquaintance and attachment process with the infant.

C. **Assessment.**
   1. Note pattern of parental visiting to the NICU, duration of visits, and frequency of phone calls. This pattern, if abnormal, is predictive of maternal parenting difficulties. If parents are not visiting frequently, be careful to determine the reasons (i.e., cultural practices after childbirth, conflicting obligations between work and family roles, or lack of transportation to the hospital) before assuming that the parents are unconcerned or that parenting difficulties exist.
   2. Identify the development of attachment behaviors. Mothers' activity with their infants has been found to be indicative of the initial adjustment to the infant, important past and present interpersonal relationships, and involvement in taking care of the infant. Examples of attachment behaviors include the following:
      a. Touching: typical maternal progression of touching the premature infant is from fingertip touching of the infant's extremities to palmar stroking of the infant's trunk, to holding and embracing the infant. This progression of touch usually occurs during a period of several visits to the NICU.

b. Looking en face: aligning head with infant's head in the same plane to make eye-to-eye contact with the infant.
c. Talking to the infant, calling the infant by name.
d. Bringing pictures, toys, and/or clothes to the hospital.
e. Participating in caregiving activities, such as feeding, bathing, and clothing the infant.

## Interventions to Encourage Family–Infant Bonding

A. **If at all possible, show the infant to the parents in the delivery room and allow them to touch the infant, if only for a few moments.** This helps to establish the reality of the infant for the parents (Kenner et al., 2014).

B. **Encourage the parents to visit their infant in the intensive care nursery as soon as possible.**
   1. Before the first visit to the nursery, prepare the parents for what to expect by giving them written information about the unit, describing the atmosphere of the nursery (i.e., noise, high activity level, infants attached to various kinds of equipment) and discussing the normal aspects of their infant as well as deviations.
   2. If the mother is unable to visit because of conditions such as ordered bed rest or transport of the infant to another hospital, the father can be given pictures of the infant for the mother. In addition, the mother should be given the phone number of the nursery and encouraged to call as often as desired.
   3. For the parents of an infant born with a malformation, encourage the parents to see the infant together as soon as possible, but do not force them to interact. Point out to the family the normal qualities of the infant as well as the abnormalities (Kenner et al., 2014).

C. **Ensure that, during the family's first visit, the nurse assigned to the infant stays at the bedside** to explain equipment and the infant's condition, as well as to answer questions, provide emotional support, and encourage touching of the infant.

D. **Convey a positive, realistic attitude about the infant** rather than a negative or fatalistic viewpoint, which may alienate the parents and impair attachment (Kenner et al., 2014).

E. **Assist the parents with holding and cuddling their infant** as soon as possible, taking into consideration the infant's condition and the parents' readiness (e.g., assist in managing respiratory and monitoring equipment and intravenous lines). Some nurseries are implementing skin-to-skin care (kangaroo care) by parents as an alternative to the traditional modes of providing care to stable, hospitalized premature infants. This care consists of positioning the infant, dressed only in diapers, upright and prone between the mother's breasts. This vertical position in skin-to-skin contact provides tactile stimulation and warmth from the mother, as well as opportunities for eye-to-eye contact, auditory stimulation, and breastfeeding. Mothers usually wear their own front-opening blouses or dresses that are loosely fitted. Fathers can also be encouraged to engage in kangaroo care.

F. **Encourage the parents to participate in caregiving activities** as warranted by the infant's condition and tolerance for input. Explain to parents of very premature infants the relationship between neurologic maturity and the capacity for handling stimulation (Holditch-Davis and Blackburn, 2014).

G. **Model nurturing parenting behavior** such as stroking, touching, and talking to the infant for parents who may need assistance in developing positive parenting behaviors (Welch et al. for the Family Nurture Intervention [FTI] Trial Group, 2012).

H. **Give positive reinforcement** to parents as they interact with their infant. For example, say that "He seems to calm down when you talk with him," or "She really seems to sleep better after you have held her" (Kenner and McGrath, 2010). Assisting parents to recognize positive changes in the infant in response to their caregiving has a strong impact on the parents and increases their feelings of success.

I. **Use consistent caregivers for the premature or sick infant** to establish a rapport with the parents.

J. **Role-model caregiving techniques—one on one,** if possible, especially for adolescent parents.

K. **Avoid power struggles with parents by defining their role** and recognizing that they are the parents and that the infant is theirs, not the staff's.

L. **Suggest that the parents or siblings bring something for the infant,** such as a small toy, pictures of the family members to be taped on the infant's bed, and/or a tape recording of the parents' voices to be played for the infant. Share personalized information about the infant with the parents. This information can include statements such as "She really enjoys sucking on her pacifier" or "He was really active while I was giving him a bath," to assist the parents in individualizing and accepting the infant.
M. **Encourage sibling visitation** in the unit or window observation of the infant.
N. **Promote individualized, family-centered developmental care that includes the family unit** in the plan of care and an environment that supports the parents. Provide a private area, or a transitional care area, to encourage parental stays within a more homelike environment, and encourage developmental care that includes parents as an integral part of the health care team (Kenner and McGrath, 2010).
O. **After the mother's discharge from the hospital, maintain communication** with the parents by providing them with the phone number of the unit. For parents of transported infants, sending pictures and cards from their infant to show current status, arranging for transportation assistance through social service agencies for parents who lack means of travel, and maintaining frequent phone contact with parents can be helpful in promoting parent–infant attachment.
P. **Give the mother the opportunity to provide breast milk** for the infant should she so desire, and support her in this endeavor. However, be careful not to overemphasize the importance of breastfeeding. The rationale is that, if she should be unsuccessful or decide to stop breastfeeding, feelings of guilt or disappointment may occur if breastfeeding has been touted as the ideal infant feeding method.
Q. **Identify situations in which there are difficulties in parent–infant interaction or problems in the family's functioning.**
R. **Be sensitive to cultural practices** that may influence parent–infant behaviors while bonding and attachment remain strong.
S. **Identify infants who are at risk of having developmental difficulties (Kenner and McGrath, 2010).**
T. **Identify the unique needs of the parent with lower socioeconomic status.** This parent may want to provide the best possible care to the infant but either may not know how to do so (poor role models) or may not have the means to provide for the infant's perceived needs.
U. **Assess the cultural needs of minority parents.** This means to be culturally sensitive to what the parenting role means in that culture and then gear the interventions toward these cultural values and beliefs.

## Evaluation of Parent–Infant Bonding

Evaluation of parental behaviors should be based on ongoing patterns rather than on isolated incidents (Mercer, 1977).

A. **Positive attachment behaviors.** The parent:
   1. Visits frequently.
   2. Has named the infant.
   3. Makes positive comments when talking to or about the infant.
   4. Demonstrates increasing skill in holding the infant.
   5. Displays increasing eye and body contact between parent and infant (i.e., kissing, fondling, stroking, nuzzling).
B. **Behaviors of concern.** The parent:
   1. Is overly optimistic.
   2. Appears unconcerned about the infant's condition.
   3. Does not ask questions.
   4. Is passive or indifferent.
   5. Avoids close body contact by holding the infant at a distance, props the bottle whether or not the infant is held, positions the bottle in such a way that milk is unable to flow from the nipple.
   6. Is unable to describe any physical or behavioral features unique to the infant.

7. Attributes inappropriate characteristics to the infant, such as "she's lazy and stubborn just like her father."

C. **Make sure these areas of concern are considered within the context of the culture of the parents.** Different cultures approach parenthood and parent–infant interaction in different ways.

## SUMMARY OF PARENTAL NEEDS TO BE MET BY NICU STAFF

A. **Help the mother reconceptualize her image** of an "ideal" infant to the image of her premature, acutely ill, or malformed infant.
B. **Help the mother deal with feelings of guilt.**
C. **Help parents develop affectionate ties** with the infant through the infant's features (e.g., soft eyes; pretty, soft skin) and learn to read the infant's behavioral cues.
D. **Assist parents in gaining confidence** in holding the infant by encouraging them to participate in caregiving tasks.
E. **Promote communication** between the parents and, if they desire, extended family members.
F. **Be sensitive to the unique needs** of the individual families.
G. **Assist families in preparing for the transition** to home care after discharge (Kenner et al., 2014; Smith et al., 2012).
H. **Provide support for parents during the transition phase** after discharge of their infant from the NICU (Boykova and Kenner, 2012; Hutchinson et al., 2012; Kenner et al., 2014; Lopez et al., 2012).
I. **Assist parents in dealing with neonatal death** in a personally meaningful way.
J. **Assist parents in describing their cultural values and beliefs,** if applicable, to understand their views of the infant and their role as parents.

## REFERENCES


Anderson, L.S., Riesch, S.K., Pridham, K.A., et al.: Furthering the understanding of parent–child relationships: A nursing scholarship review series. Part 4: Parent–child relationships at risk. *Journal for Specialists in Pediatric Nursing*, 15(2):111–134, 2010.

Ardal, F., Sulman, J. and Fuller-Thomson, E.: Support like a walking stick: Parent-buddy matching for language and culture in the NICU. *Neonatal Network*, 30(2):89–98, 2011.

Ballantyne, M., Stevens, B., Guttmann, A., et al.: Transition to neonatal follow-up programs: Is attendance a problem? *Journal of Perinatal and Neonatal Nursing*, 26 (1):90–98, 2012.

Bennett, S.M., Litz, B.T., Lee, B.S. and Maguen, S.: The scope and impact of perinatal loss: Current status and future directions. *Professional Psychology: Research and Practice*, 36(2):180–187, 2005.

Bigelow, A., Power, M., MacLellan-Peters, J., et al.: Effect of mother/infant skin-to-skin contact on postpartum depressive symptoms and maternal physiological stress. *JOGNN: Journal of Obstetric, Gynecologic, & Neonatal Nursing*, 41(3):369–382, 2012.

Borghini, A., Pierrehumbert, B., Miljkovitch, R., et al.: Mother's attachment representations of their premature infant at 6 and 18 months after birth. *Infant Mental Health Journal*, 27(5):494–508, 2006.

Boss, R.D., Donohue, P.K. and Arnold, R.M.: Adolescent mothers in the NICU: How much do they understand? *Journal of Perinatology*, 30(4):286–290, 2010.

Bowers, B.: Prenatal, perinatal and postpartal risk factors. In C. Kenner, and J.W. Lott (Eds.): *Comprehensive neonatal nursing care* (5th ed.). New York, 2014, Springer Publishing.

Boykova, M. and Kenner, C.: Transition from hospital to home for parents of preterm infants. *Journal of Perinatal and Neonatal Nursing*, 26(1):81–87, 2012.

Boykova, M. and Kenner, C.: Partnerships in care: Mothers and fathers. In C.A. Kenner, and J.M. McGrath (Eds.): *Developmental care of newborns and infants* (2nd ed.). Glenview, IL, 2010, National Association of Neonatal Nurses, pp. 145–160.

Bozzette, M.A., Kenner, C.A. and Boykova, M.: The neonatal intensive care unit environment. In C. Kenner, and J. McGrath (Eds.): *Developmental care of newborns and infants* (2nd ed.). Glenview, IL, 2010, National Association of Neonatal Nurses, pp. 63–74.

Callister, L.C., Beckstrand, R.L. and Corbett, C.: Postpartum depression and culture: Pesado corazon. *MCN: American Journal of Maternal Child Nursing*, 35 (5):254–261, 2010.

Caplan, G., Mason, E.A. and Kaplan, D.M.: Four studies of crisis in parents of prematures. *Community Mental Health Journal*, 1(2):149–161, 1965.

Catlin, A.: Thinking outside the box: Prenatal care and the call for a prenatal advance directive. *Journal of Perinatal and Neonatal Nursing*, 19(2):169–176, 2005.

Catlin, A. and Carter, B.: Creation of a neonatal end-of-life palliative care protocol. *Journal of Perinatology*, 22 (3):184–195, 2002.

Chittleborough, C.R., Lawlor, D.A. and Lynch, J.W.: Young maternal age and poor child development: Predictive validity from a birth cohort. *Pediatrics*, 127(6):e1436–e1444, 2011.

Cho, J., Holditch-Davis, D. and Miles, M.S.: Effects of maternal depressive symptoms and infant gender on the interactions between mothers and their medically at-risk infants. *JOGNN: Journal of Obstetric, Gynecologic, & Neonatal Nursing*, 37(1):58–70, 2008.

Cone, S.: The impact of communication and the neonatal intensive care unit environment on parent involvement. *Newborn and Infant Nursing Reviews*, 7 (1):33–38, 2007.

Dennis, C.L., Hodnett, E., Kenton, L., et al.: Effect of peer support on prevention of postnatal depression among high risk women: Multisite randomised controlled trial. *BMJ*, 338:a3064, 2009.

Dishion, T.J., Bullock, B.M. and Granic, I.: Pragmatism in modeling peer influence: Dynamics, outcomes, and change processes. *Development and Psychopathology*, 14(4):969–981, 2002.

Dyer, K.A.: Identifying, understanding, and working with grieving parents in the NICU. *Part I: Identifying and understanding loss and the grief response. Neonatal Network*, 24(3):35–46, 2005.

Emmanuel, E. and St John, W.: Maternal distress: A concept analysis. *Journal of Advanced Nursing*, 66 (9):2104–2115, 2010.

Fegran, L., Helseth, S. and Fagermoen, M.S.: A comparison of mothers' and fathers' experiences of the attachment process in a neonatal intensive care unit. *Journal of Clinical Nursing*, 17(6):810–816, 2008.

Fraley, A.M.: Chronic sorrow: A parental response. *Journal of Pediatric Nursing*, 5(4):268–273, 1990.

Garel, M., Dardennes, M. and Blondel, B.: Mothers' psychological distress 1 year after very preterm childbirth: Results of the EPIPAGE qualitative study. *Child: Care, Health and Development*, 33(2):137–143, 2007.

Golish, T.D. and Powell, K.A.: 'Ambiguous loss': Managing the dialectics of grief associated with premature birth. *Journal of Social and Personal Relationships*, 20:309, 2003.

Gordon, J.: An evidence-based approach for supporting parents experiencing chronic sorrow. *Pediatric Nursing*, 35(2):115–119, 2009.

Grassley, J.S.: Adolescent mothers' breastfeeding social support needs. *JOGNN: Journal of Obstetric, Gynecologic, & Neonatal Nursing*, 39(6):713–722, 2010.

Gray, P.H., Edwards, D.M., O'Callaghan, M.J. and Cuskelly, M.: Parenting stress in mothers of preterm infants during early infancy. *Early Human Development*, 88(1):45–49, 2012.

Halm, M.A., Sabo, J. and Rudiger, M.: The patient-family advisory council. Keeping a pulse on our customers. *Critical Care Nurse*, 26(5):58–67, 2006.

Heidari, H., Hasanpour, M. and Fooladi, M.: The Iranian parents of premature infants in NICU experience stigma of shame. *Medicinski Arhiv*, 66(1):35–40, 2012.

Hess, C.R., Teti, D.M. and Hussey-Gardner, B.: Self-efficacy and parenting of high-risk infants: The moderating role of parent knowledge of infant development. *Journal of Applied Developmental Psychology*, 25 (4):423–437, 2004.

Holditch-Davis, D. and Blackburn, S.: Neurobehavioral development. In C. Kenner, and J.W. Lott (Eds.): *Comprehensive neonatal nursing care* (5th ed.). New York, 2014, Springer Publishing.

Holditch-Davis, D., Miles, M.S., Burchinal, M.R. and Goldman, B.D.: Maternal role attainment with medically fragile infants: Part 2: Relationship to the quality of parenting. *Research in Nursing and Health*, 34 (1):35–48, 2011.

Holditch-Davis, D., Miles, M.S., Weaver, M.A., et al.: Patterns of distress in African-American mothers of preterm infants. *Journal of Developmental and Behavioral Pediatrics*, 30(3):193–205, 2009.

Howland, L.C.: Preterm birth: Implications for family stress and coping. *Newborn and Infant Nursing Reviews*, 7(1):14–19, 2007.

Hutchinson, S.W., Spillett, M.A. and Cronin, M.: Parent's expereinces during their infant's transition from neonatal intensive care unit to home: A qualitative study. *Qualitative Report*, 17(Article 23):1–20, 2012.

Jubinville, J., Newburn-Cook, C., Hegadoren, K. and Lacaze-Masmonteil, T.: Symptoms of acute stress disorder in mothers of premature infants. *Advances in Neonatal Care*, 12(4):246–253, 2012.

Kaplan, D.M. and Mason, E.A.: Maternal reactions to premature birth viewed as an acute emotional disorder. *American Journal of Orthopsychiatry*, 30:539–552, 1960.

Kenner, C.: Palliative and end-of-life care. In C. Kenner, and J.W. Lott (Eds.): *Comprehensive neonatal nursing care* (5th ed.). New York, 2014, Springer Publishing.

Kenner, C., Boykova, M. and Ellerbee, E.: Postdischarge care of the newborn, infant, and families. In C. Kenner, and J.W. Lott (Eds.): *Comprehensive neonatal nursing care* (5th ed.). New York, 2014, Springer Publishing.

Kenner, and McGrath (Eds.): *Developmental care of the newborns and infants: A guide for health professionals* (2nd ed.). Glenview, IL, 2010, National Association of Neonatal Nurses.

Kokotos, F. and Adam, H.M.: The vulnerable child syndrome. *Pediatrics in Review*, 30(5):193–194, 2009.

Korja, R., Latva, R. and Lehtonen, L.: The effects of preterm birth on mother-infant interaction and attachment during the infant's first two years. *Acta Obstetricia et Gynecologica Scandinavica*, 91 (2):164–173, 2012.

Korja, R., Savonlahti, E., Haataja, L., et al.: Attachment representations in mothers of preterm infants. *Infant Behavior and Development*, 32(3):305–311, 2009.

Lindberg, B., Axelsson, K. and Öhrling, K.: Taking care of their baby at home but with nursing staff as support: The use of videoconferencing in providing neonatal support to parents of preterm infants. *Journal of Neonatal Nursing*, 15(2):47–55, 2009.

Liu, L.S., Hirano, S.H., Tentori, M., et al.: *Improving communication and social support for caregivers of high-risk infants through mobile technologies.* Paper presented at the ACM 2011 Conference on Computer Supported Cooperative Work, New York, NY. Available at http://dl.acm.org/citation.cfm?id=1958897

Logsdon, M.C. and Koniak-Griffin, D.: Social support in postpartum adolescents: Guidelines for nursing assessments and interventions. *JOGNN: Journal of Obstetric, Gynecologic, & Neonatal Nursing*, 34 (6):761–768, 2005.

Lopez, G.L., Anderson, K.H. and Feutchinger, J.: Transition of premature infants from hospital to home life. *Neonatal Network*, 31(4):207–214, 2012.

Lutz, K.F., Anderson, L.S., Riesch, S.K., et al.: Furthering the understanding of parent-child relationships: A nursing scholarship review series. Part 2: Grasping the early parenting experience—the insider view. *Journal for Specialists in Pediatric Nursing*, 14 (4):262–283, 2009.

Mackley, A.B., Locke, R.G., Spear, M.L. and Joseph, R.: Forgotten parent: NICU paternal emotional response. *Advances in Neonatal Care*, 10(4):200–203, 2010.

McGrath, J.: Family: Essential partner in care. In C. Kenner, and J.W. Lott (Eds.): *Comprehensive neonatal nursing care* (5th ed.). New York, 2014, Springer Publishing.

Meijssen, D., Wolf, M.J., Koldewijn, K., et al.: Maternal psychological distress in the first two years after very preterm birth and early intervention. *Early Child Development and Care*, 181(1):1–11, 2011a.

Meijssen, D., Wolf, M.J., van Bakel, H., et al.: Maternal attachment representations after very preterm birth and the effect of early intervention. *Infant Behavior and Development*, 34(1):72–80, 2011b.

Melnyk, B.M., Alpert-Gillis, L., Feinstein, N.F., et al.: Creating opportunities for parent empowerment: Program effects on the mental health/coping outcomes of critically ill young children and their mothers. *Pediatrics*, 113(6):e597–e607, 2004.

Melnyk, B.M., Crean, H.F., Feinstein, N.F. and Fairbanks, E.: Maternal anxiety and depression after a premature infant's discharge from the neonatal intensive care unit: Explanatory effects of the Creating Opportunities for Parent Empowerment program. *Nursing Research*, 57(6):383–394, 2008.

Melnyk, B.M. and Feinstein, N.F.: Reducing hospital expenditures with the COPE (Creating Opportunities for Parent Empowerment) program for parents and premature infants: An analysis of direct healthcare neonatal intensive care unit costs and savings. *Nursing Administration Quarterly*, 33 (1):32–37, 2009.

Melnyk, B.M., Feinstein, N. and Fairbanks, E.: Two decades of evidence to support implementation of the COPE program as standard practice with parents of young unexpectedly hospitalized/critically ill children and premature infants. *Pediatric Nursing*, 32 (5):475–481, 2006.

Mercer, R.T.: Nursing care for parents at risk. Thorofare, NJ, 1977, Charles B. Slack.

Miles, M.S., Carter, M.C., Hennessey, J., et al.: Testing a theoretical model: Correlates of parental stress responses in the pediatric intensive care unit. *Maternal Child Nursing Journal*, 18(3):207–219, 1989.

Miles, M.S. and Holditch-Davis, D.: Compensatory parenting: How mothers describe parenting their 3-year-old, prematurely born children. *Journal of Pediatric Nursing*, 10(4):243–253, 1995.

Miles, M.S., Holditch-Davis, D., Burchinal, M.R. and Brunssen, S.: Maternal role attainment with medically fragile infants: Part 1. *Measurement and correlates during the first year of life. Research in Nursing and Health*, 34(1):20–34, 2011.

Miller, B.C. and Sollie, D.L.: Normal stresses during the transition to parenthood. *Family Relations*, 29 (4):459–465, 1980.

Nelson, A.M.: Transition to motherhood. *JOGNN: Journal of Obstetric, Gynecologic, & Neonatal Nursing*, 32 (4):465–477, 2003.

Neu, M. and Robinson, J.: Maternal holding of preterm infants during the early weeks after birth and dyad interaction at six months. *JOGNN: Journal of Obstetric, Gynecologic, & Neonatal Nursing*, 39 (4):401–414, 2010.

Nyström, K. and Axelsson, K.: Mothers' experience of being separated from their newborns. *JOGNN: Journal of Obstetric, Gynecologic, & Neonatal Nursing*, 31 (3):275–282, 2002.

Padovani, F.H.P., Carvalho, A.E.V., Duarte, G., et al.: Anxiety, dysphoria, and depression symptoms in mothers of preterm infants. *Psychological Reports*, 104(2):667–679, 2009.

Pinelli, J., Saigal, S., Bill Wu, Y.-W., et al.: Patterns of change in family functioning, resources, coping and parental depression in mothers and fathers of sick newborns over the first year of life. *Journal of Neonatal Nursing*, 14(5):156–165, 2008.

Placencia, F.X. and McCullough, L.B.: Biopsychosocial risks of parental care for high-risk neonates: Implications for evidence-based parental counseling. *Journal of Perinatology*, 32(5):381–386, 2012.

Preyde, M. and Ardal, F.: Effectiveness of a parent "buddy" program for mothers of very preterm infants in a neonatal intensive care unit. *Canadian Medical Association Journal*, 168(8):969–973, 2003.

Raines, D.A. and Brustad, J.: Parent's confidence as a caregiver. *Advances in Neonatal Care*, 12(3):183–188, 2012.

Reyna, B.A. and Pickler, R.H.: Mother-infant synchrony. *JOGNN: Journal of Obstetric, Gynecologic, & Neonatal Nursing*, 38(4):470–477, 2009.

Riesch, S.K., Anderson, L.S., Pridham, K.A., et al.: Furthering the understanding of parent–child relationships: A nursing scholarship review series. Part 5: Parent–adolescent and teen parent–child relationships. *Journal for Specialists in Pediatric Nursing*, 15 (3):182–201, 2010.

Rowe, J. and Jones, L.: Discharge and beyond: A longitudinal study comparing stress and coping in parents of preterm infants. *Journal of Neonatal Nursing*, 16 (6):258–266, 2010.

Shah, P.E., Clements, M. and Poehlmann, J.: Maternal resolution of grief after preterm birth: Implications for infant attachment security. *Pediatrics*, 127 (2):284–292, 2011.

Sheppard, M.: Social support use as a parental coping strategy: Its impact on outcome of child and parenting problems—a six-month follow-up. *British Journal of Social Work*, 39:1427–1446, 2009.

Siegel, R., Gardner, S.L. and Dickey, L.A.: Families in crisis: Theoretical and practical considerations. In S.L. Gardner, B.S. Carter, M.I. Enzman-Hines, and J.A. Hernandez (Eds.): *Merenstein and Gardner's Handbook of neonatal intensive care* (7th ed.). St. Louis, 2011, Elsevier Mosby, pp. 849–897.

Skene, C., Franck, L., Curtis, P. and Gerrish, K.: Parental involvement in neonatal comfort care. *JOGNN:*

*Journal of Obstetric, Gynecologic, & Neonatal Nursing*, 41 (6):786–797, 2012.

Smith, V.C., Dukhovny, D., Zupancic, J.A., et al.: Neonatal intensive care unit discharge preparedness: Primary care implications. *Clinical Pediatrics*, 51 (5):454–461, 2012.

Smith, V.C., Young, S., Pursley, D.M., et al.: Are families prepared for discharge from the NICU? *Journal of Perinatology*, 29(9):623–629, 2009.

Solberg, Ø., Grønning Dale, M.T., Holmstrøm, H., et al.: Long-term symptoms of depression and anxiety in mothers of infants with congenital heart defects. *Journal of Pediatric Psychology*, 36(2):179–187, 2011.

Sullivan, P. and Altimier, L.: Creating a Family Advisory Council. *Newborn and Infant Nursing Reviews*, 7 (1):3–6, 2007.

Teel, C.S.: Chronic sorrow: Analysis of the concept. *Journal of Advanced Nursing*, 16(11):1311–1319, 1991.

Thomas, L.M.: The changing role of parents in neonatal care: A historical review. *Neonatal Network*, 27 (2):91–100, 2008.

Vanderbilt, D., Bushley, T., Young, R. and Frank, D.A.: Acute posttraumatic stress symptoms among urban mothers with newborns in the neonatal intensive care unit: A preliminary study. *Journal of Developmental and Behavioral Pediatrics*, 30(1):50–56, 2009.

Watson, G.: Parental liminality: A way of understanding the early experiences of parents who have a very preterm infant. *Journal of Clinical Nursing*, 20 (9–10):1462–1471, 2011.

Welch, M.G., Hofer, M.A., Brunelli, S.A., et al.: for the Family Nurture Intervention (FTI) Trial Group: Family nurture intervention (FNI): Methods and treatment protocol of a randomized controlled trial in the NICU. *BMC Pediatrics*, 12:14, 2012.

Whitaker, C., Kavanaugh, K. and Klima, C.: Perinatal grief in Latino parents. *MCN: American Journal of Maternal Child Nursing*, 35(6):341–345, 2010.

Wray, J., Lee, K., Dearmun, N. and Franck, L.: Parental anxiety and stress during children's hospitalisation: The StayClose study. *Journal of Child Health Care*, 15 (3):163–174, 2011.

Zabielski, M.T.: Recognition of maternal identity in preterm and fullterm mothers. *Maternal Child Nursing Journal*, 22(1):2–36, 1994.

Zauderer, C.: Maternity care for Orthodox Jewish couples: Implications for nurses in the obstetric setting. *Nursing for Women's Health*, 13(2):112–120, 2009.

CHAPTER

# 18 Patient Safety

JOAN RENAUD SMITH AND ANN DONZE

**OBJECTIVES**

1. Define and discuss organizational and individual approaches to developing a culture of safety.
2. Discuss the importance of teamwork, communication, and technology in providing safe care.
3. Discuss the role families have in promoting patient safety.
4. Discuss human factors and the relation to common errors.
5. Describe specific neonatal errors and recommended improvement strategies.
6. Describe the importance of discharge teaching to promote patient safety at home.

Patient safety has become a national priority, and improvement in patient safety has accelerated since an Institute of Medicine (IOM) report concluded that up to 98,000 lives are lost annually in U.S. hospitals as a result of error (Kohn et al., 1999). Many of these errors are preventable and have resulted in both death and an economic consequence as high as $29 billion annually (Kohn et al., 1999). Yet, more than a decade later, measurable improvement and sustainability are lacking, resulting in continued harm that remains common in today's complex health care system (Landrigan et al., 2010). Medically fragile infants are at high risk for encountering errors during their stay in the neonatal intensive care unit (NICU) and are defenseless compared with physiologically more mature newborns, leaving little margin for error. Infants receiving care in the NICU have been shown to experience wide variation in clinical care and outcomes (Profit et al., 2012). It is the responsibility of health care organizations and neonatal care providers to provide the best clinical care and ensure the safety of these vulnerable infants. While some errors occur at the point of service (e.g., a nurse administering the wrong medication), most errors occur as a result of flaws within the health care system or facility design (e.g., excessive noise levels or miscommunication) (Joseph and The Center for Health Design, 2006). Identifying and eliminating sources of patient harm are critical in delivering safe patient care. Mitigating harm is achieved by a line management approach, which means that *everyone* in the organization is responsible for the safety of the patient. To keep patients safe, all risk of hazards must be identified proactively by use of local resources, such as incident reports and near-miss reports, and external sources, such as Joint Commission Sentinel Events, networks such as the Vermont Oxford Network, and the literature. Once hazards are identified, it is important for the institution to commit resources to eliminate them (Handyside and Suresh, 2010).

Using evidence-based clinical practice interventions and strict adherence to protocols every time care is delivered, errors can be substantially reduced (Bizzarro et al., 2010). It is now possible to eliminate or nearly eliminate adverse events, and neonatal nurses are on the forefront of providing safe and efficient quality care. As neonatal nurses recognize and understand the causes of errors and rely on strict adherence to evidence-based interventions and improvement strategies, dramatic reductions of errors are possible. The knowledge and skills associated with safety must become routine nursing practice. Improving patient safety requires assimilation of knowledge from other disciplines and industries, and application of safety knowledge to health care. Since 2002, National Patient Safety Goals have been formulated by the Joint Commission to improve patient safety. These goals are drawn from recommendations by the Sentinel Event Advisory Group to spotlight problems in health care and focus on how to solve them. All Joint Commission–accredited health care organizations are surveyed for implementation of the goals (Table 18-1).

This chapter offers an introduction to basic patient safety principles and includes selected improvement strategies and resources for neonatal nurses to build a patient safety toolkit. Selected neonatal errors and improvement strategies are included and are by no means an exhaustive list. Box 18-1 includes definitions of selected improvement strategies. Neonatal nurses need to equip

■ TABLE 18-1
■ ■ **The Joint Commission's Hospital National Patient Safety Goals***

| Patient Safety Goal | Recommendations |
|---|---|
| **Goal 1** Improve the accuracy of patient identification | Use at least two ways to identify patients. For example, use the patient's name and date of birth. This is done to make sure that each patient gets the medicine and treatment meant for him. Make sure that the correct patient gets the correct blood type when he gets a blood transfusion. |
| **Goal 2** Improve the effectiveness of communication among caregivers. | Read back spoken or phone orders to the person who gave the order. Create a list of abbreviations and symbols that are not to be used. Quickly get important test results to the right staff person. Create steps for staff to follow when sending patients to the next caregiver. The steps should help staff tell about the patient's care. Make sure there is time to ask and answer questions. |
| **Goal 3** Improve the safety of using medications. | Create a list of medicines with names that look alike or sound alike. Update the list every year. Label all medicines that are not already labeled. For example, medicine in syringes, cups, and basins. Take extra care with patients who take medicines to thin their blood. |
| **Goal 7** Reduce the risk of health care–associated infections. | Use the hand cleaning guidelines from the World Health Organization or Centers for Disease Control and Prevention. Report death or injury to patients from infections that happen in hospitals. Use proven guidelines to prevent infections that are difficult to treat, and to prevent infections of the blood. Use safe practices to treat the part of the body where surgery was done. |
| **Goal 15** The hospital identifies safety risks inherent in its patient population. | This requirement applies only to psychiatric hospitals and patients being treated for emotional or behavioral disorders in general hospitals. |
| Universal Protocol for Preventing Wrong Site, Wrong Procedure | Create steps for staff to follow so that all documents needed for surgery are on hand before surgery begins. Mark the part of the body where the surgery will be done. Involve the patient in doing this. |

From The Joint Commission: *2013 Hospital national patient safety goals.* Oak Brook Terrace, IL, 2013, The Joint Commission. Reprinted with permission.

*This table includes the 2013 National Patient Safety Goals that apply to hospitals.

themselves with the best possible safety resources and knowledge in order to provide a safe and caring environment.

A. **Organizational and Individual Approaches to Developing and Sustaining a Culture of Safety.**

1. **Establish patient safety as a strategic priority (Botwinick et al., 2006).** The Joint Commission (2011) holds senior leaders accountable for routinely assessing the culture of safety within their organization. Each organization should have a Patient Safety Officer (PSO) who is a senior leader and should report directly to the organization's top executive (e.g., Chief Executive Officer [CEO], Chief Operating Officer [COO], Chief Medical Officer [CMO], etc.). The Board of Directors should be actively involved in patient safety reports and routinely track patient safety goals and areas needed for improvement. For safety to be seen as a priority for all staff members, senior leaders need to make safety a key focus for the organization. Senior leaders and frontline staff need to discuss adverse events and near misses and develop strategic plans for future safety.

   a. Selected strategies for incorporating a safe culture within the organization. (See Box 18-1 for selected definition of strategy terms.)
      - Executive walk rounds (used for the sole purpose of discussing safety with frontline staff).
      - Storytelling (inspires cultural change using real-life clinical experiences).

## BOX 18-1
## SELECTED NONTECHNOLOGICAL IMPROVEMENT STRATEGIES DEFINITIONS

1. **Five Rights:** rules traditionally thought to safeguard against errors. The five rights of medication administration (right patient, right drug, right dose, right route, and right frequency) are the basis of most education on drug administration and considered the "safe" way to administer medications. The five rights do not safeguard against major sources of error and may limit critical thinking.
2. **Forcing functions:** interventions that prevent error by "forcing" a safe action, such as removing concentrated potassium from the medication carts. Forcing functions are the strongest of interventions against human failure. A common example of a forcing function is designing oral syringes such that they cannot be connected to an intravenous port.
3. **Medication reconciliation:** the process of avoiding such inadvertent inconsistencies across transitions in care by reviewing the patient's complete medication regimen at the time of admission/transfer/discharge and comparing it with the regimen being considered for the new setting of care.
4. **Read-backs:** includes the listener repeating the key information, so that the transmitter can confirm its correctness.
5. **"Time Outs":** planned periods of quiet and/or interdisciplinary discussion focused on ensuring that key procedural details have been addressed. For example, the identification of a patient, for a surgical procedure, site, and other key aspects, often stating them aloud for double checking by other team members.
6. **Executive walk rounds:** used for the sole purpose of discussing safety with frontline staff.
7. **Storytelling:** a tool used to share events in the form of a story. It helps listeners remember facts and details that otherwise might be forgotten.
8. **Safety briefings:** an efficient tool used to share information and to increase safety awareness among frontline staff and foster a culture of safety into the daily routine, 24 hours a day 7 days a week.

Adapted from Agency for Healthcare Research and Quality: AHRQ's Glossary. 2013. Retrieved from http://psnet.ahrq.gov/glossary.aspx.

- Safety briefings (used to increase staff awareness of patient safety issues by creating an environment in which staff share information without fear of reprisal, and integrate the reporting of safety issues into daily work).
- Place patient safety on executive meeting agendas.
- Assign executives to performance improvement teams.
- Include safety in orientation programs.
- Design a communication plan when successful patient safety projects are implemented.
- Connect executive performance and compensation to improvements in patient safety.

It is important that leaders recognize that methods of improvement should be clearly outlined and a planned process should be in place to accelerate improvement in practice (Botwinick et al., 2006). Promoting a safe culture can begin by integrating multidisciplinary patient safety teams into preexisting committees at both the departmental and unit levels to implement safety initiatives at the bedside. NICU safety teams may include frontline professional and support staff, medical and nursing leadership, advanced practice nurses (APNs), pharmacy, and respiratory therapy. These interdisciplinary teams are responsible for identifying and responding to unit-specific safety concerns and risks, ensuring that safety efforts are integrated into the overall unit structure, and educating staff and faculty about the science of safety. One program designed to promote safety teams is the TeamSTEPPS program (Team Strategies and Tools to Enhance Performance and Patient Safety) (Samra et al, 2011).

2. **Establish a culture that supports safety** (Botwinick et al., 2006). It is the responsibility of individual health care organizations to assess their current state of patient safety. Fostering a culture of safety involves understanding and anticipating human limitations, anticipating the unexpected, and creating a nonpunitive learning environment for improvement and error reduction. Traditionally, health care organizations responded to errors by naming and blaming individuals, known as a *person-centered approach*. This approach is focused

on the individual and does not help to prevent future errors. An organization that seeks to blame and punish and lacks teamwork, communication, and transparency of errors is a culture that places patients in harm's way. A *systems approach* recognizes that the system is complex and that most errors reflect predictable human failings in the context of poorly designed systems. A shared accountability among health care organizations and individual practitioners is promoted in a just culture. A *just culture* recognizes that individuals should not be held responsible for system failures and that competent professionals make mistakes and may even adopt unhealthy shortcuts in their practice, but has a zero tolerance for their reckless behavior (Marx, 2001). It also provides a safe environment in which errors may be reported without fear of retribution in events in which there was no harm intended. In a just culture, individuals are encouraged to report errors that result in harm to patients as well as near misses, resulting in an environment in which to learn. Staff must experience a just culture in order to sustain self-disclosure of adverse events. Although a just culture seeks potential system failures and does not seek to blame individuals, it does include a well-established system of shared accountability.

3. **Engage key stakeholders.** Senior leaders need to engage key stakeholders in establishing a safe culture.
   a. **Nurses.** Neonatal nurses, APNs, and clinicians are highly educated, organized, skilled, and experienced and are typically the first line of defense in keeping patients safe. Frontline staff can identify firsthand the issues affecting patient safety and are the primary source of care. Their inclusion in the process is essential to the success of implementing patient safety factors.
   b. **Physicians.** Neonatologist and other physicians caring for infants should be involved in the process of establishing a safe culture. Physicians are highly trained, autonomous individuals with many time constraints. Engaging physicians early on with improvement projects related to their area of interest and encouraging active participation is important to establishing a culture of safety.
   c. **Additional stakeholders.** All members of the health care team are extremely valuable in improving quality and safety, and it is everyone's responsibility to promote a safe culture. Individual NICUs need to identify their own key members as part of their safety team: clinical pharmacists; respiratory therapists; social workers; chaplains; dietitians; support staff; laboratory technicians; lactation consultants; discharge coordinators; physical, occupational, and speech therapists; housekeeping; and any other members of the organization who have direct or indirect impact on patient care. A culture of safety requires effective communication and teamwork from all disciplines.
   d. **Board of trustees** (Botwinick et al., 2006). The Board plays a crucial role in moving the organization toward a higher level of patient safety and effectiveness. Board members may establish goals for organization improvements, integrate patient safety goals into the organization's strategic goals and business plans, review adverse reports and root cause analyses, and provide monetary resources for patient safety education and staffing.
   e. **Patients and families.** Patient-centered care is pivotal in the prevention of medical errors. Families are at the core of delivering patient-centered care in the NICU, and family-centered care (FCC) is vital to promoting patient safety. Families should be invited to collaborate with the health care team as partners. Improving quality and safety by bringing families into the planning, delivery, and evaluation of health care is the foundation of FCC (Institute for Family-Centered Care, 2008). The American Academy of Pediatrics' (AAP's) policy statement, *Patient- and Family-Centered Care and the Pediatrician's Role* (2003, reaffirmed in 2007 and 2012), provides a summary of the core principles of FCC and includes specific recommendations for how pediatricians can integrate FCC in hospitals, clinics, and their community. Studies have shown that, when health care providers and administrators partner with patients and families, the quality and safety of health care rise, the costs decrease, and provider and patient satisfaction increase (Institute for Family-Centered Care, 2008). The core concepts of FCC as outlined by the Institute for Family-Centered Care (2008) include the following:
      (1) *Dignity and respect*: Health care professionals need to listen, honor, value, and respect families as partners in the daily planning and delivery of care.

(2) *Information sharing*: Health care professionals need to provide families with unbiased, complete, accurate, and timely information in ways that are affirming and useful.
(3) *Participation*: Health care professionals should encourage and support families to participate in decision making and care at the level the family chooses.
(4) *Collaboration*: Families, practitioners, and organizational leaders should collaborate in policy and program development, implementation, and evaluation; facility design; professional education; and delivery of care.

Establishing a family-centered environment and empowering families to promote patient safety and quality takes a long-term commitment. This approach requires a transformation of the health care organization, including infusing FCC principles into the organization's mission statement and philosophy. Health care organizations can promote FCC by inviting families to participate in hospital and unit committees; setting up patient and family advisory councils; creating an environment that is welcoming and inviting to families and provides privacy, comfort, and the ability to access information; including families in education and training programs as well as research; and developing human resources policies to promote a family-friendly environment. Specific steps to assist health care organizations in developing an FCC environment are available (Institute for Family-Centered Care, 2008).

Both the AAP (AAP and Committee on Hospital Care and Institute for Patient- and Family-centered Care, 2012) and the Vermont Oxford Network's (VON) Neonatal Intensive Care Quality Improvement Collaborative (NIC/Q) (Dunn et al., 2006; VON, 2013) provide recommendations supporting the integration of families into high-quality patient care delivery. Families are encouraged to report concerns and to be actively involved in their infant's care as part of a patient safety strategy. National initiatives outlining strategies to encourage family participation in error prevention are available. Some of these initiatives include the Joint Commission's "Speak Up" initiatives (2013a), the National Patient Safety Foundation's "National Agenda for Action" (2013), and the Agency for Healthcare Research and Quality's "20 Tips" (2013).

4. **Teamwork and communication.** According to the IOM, health care providers tend to be trained as individuals even though they function almost exclusively as teams, and patient safety programs that promote team training and functioning need to be adopted (Kohn et al., 1999). Neonatal care has become increasingly complex, requiring teamwork and collaboration among multiple disciplines in order to achieve a common goal: to improve patient outcomes (Smith and Cole, 2009). Communication and teamwork are vital to creating and sustaining a culture of safety. More than two thirds of sentinel events reported to the Joint Commission were primarily caused by failures in communication (Joint Commission, 2013c). Communication among team members must flow freely regardless of their authority gradient. Patient care decision making should be shared among all members of the health care team. Mutual respect, trust, confidentiality, responsiveness, empathy, effective listening, and communication among all clinical team members are necessary for promoting shared decision making (Roberts and Perryman, 2007). Organizations need to adopt a zero-tolerance policy for abusive behaviors among all members of the health care team.

a. **Simulation and debriefing.** "Simulation refers to the recreation of an actual event that has previously occurred or could potentially occur" (Hunt et al., 2007, p. 306). Simulation and debriefing have been used in the Neonatal Resuscitation Program since its inception in 1987, but their use in the NICU has expanded to include many technical and interpersonal skills (Pilcher et al., 2012). The IOM suggests the use of simulation exercises focused on improving teamwork and communication as an important mechanism to improve patient safety (Kohn et al., 1999). Debriefing after a team simulation experience allows recognition of areas of appropriate performance and lessons learned as to where and how the errors could potentially be prevented. Simulation in conjunction with debriefing is necessary so errors can be identified and team members are made aware of their role in the error. Simulation can provide a replication of the neonatal environment, equipped with the technology and the models of equipment that will be encountered in the NICU as well as complex scenarios that require successful team interactions. Procedural and technical skills can also be simulated, allowing for teamwork and competency checks. Leadership skills during emergent situations can also be enhanced through the use of role simulation by improving communication skills as they relate to discussions about the futility of medical care, end-of-life decision making, and the chronicity of medical care. Rapid response teams, transport teams, and trauma teams are all high-functioning teams that rely on effective communication and have benefited from the use of simulation.

Incorporating simulation and debriefing methods into Neonatal Resuscitation Program training can promote effective communication and teamwork and potentially reduce the rate of errors (Thomas et al., 2007). There is now good evidence that simulation and debriefing improves self-confidence, knowledge, and operational performance in simulated settings. Emerging evidence supports that simulation and debriefing can improve performance in clinical settings and can result in safer patient outcomes (Griswold et al., 2012).

b. **Effective methods of teamwork and communication.**

(1) *Crew resource management (CRM).* CRM is a communication methodology used to promote team-centered decision making; it was developed by the aerospace industry to promote effective communication and teamwork (Sundar et al., 2007). CRM teaches team communication and highlights errors in a simulated setting in the hope of avoiding the same error in a real-life setting involving humans. It teaches that all members of a team are vital and that, if a team member at any level believes that something is not being done appropriately or in the best interest of the team or other people who have put their trust in the team, then that member must speak up (Hunt et al., 2007). Recent evidence shows CRM has the potential to positively impact the health care culture by producing safer patient care environments (Ricci and Brumsted, 2012).

(2) *SBAR (situation, background, assessment, and recommendation)* (Haig et al., 2006). SBAR is a method to improve hand-offs. The NICU is often chaotic and hurried, so critical information can fall through the cracks at hand-offs, and communication can be misunderstood. For example, a potential for error can occur when a verbal order for medication is written down by someone other than the order giver and transcribed onto an order form by a third person. Used extensively in medicine, and originating from the nuclear submarine service, SBAR is a communication tool to standardize discussion and information sharing among caregivers to ensure that patient information is consistently and accurately being delivered, especially during critical events, shift hand-offs, and patient transfers. As part of the National Patient Safety Goals, the Joint Commission (2013b) requires organizations to implement a standardized approach to hand-off communications. SBAR provides a shared mental model for all clinicians to use during hand-offs or transfers (Institute for Healthcare Improvement, 2011):

**S**ituation: What is happening at the present time?
**B**ackground: What are the circumstances leading up to this situation?
**A**ssessment: What do I think the problem is?
**R**ecommendation: What should we do to correct the problem?

5. **Human factor engineering and the environment.** Human factor engineering (HFE) is a science that studies the interactions between workers and their work system to determine if the workplace design meets the needs of the people working in it. Since 2002, human factors design has been promoted in NICUs through the VON's collaborative project to improve the quality and safety of neonatal care. A Human Factors Checklist Series was developed to allow NICUs to educate users on HFE principles and assess whether their units are optimally designed and to identify opportunities for improvement. The Checklist includes workplace topics such as staff alertness and fatigue, unit design and space, physical ergonomics, clinical alarms and warnings, labels and displays, procedures, devices, paper forms, and team performance (Handyside and Suresh, 2010). When units are well-designed using the science of HFE, the workplace facilitates efficient, accurate, and error-free performance by the health care team.

a. **Fatigue and shift work.** The IOM report *Keeping Patients Safe: Transforming the Work Environment of Nurses* identifies that research findings on overtime practices indicate that long work hours, without adequate and quality rest time, are associated with impaired performance and human errors (IOM and Committee on the Work Environment for Nurses and Patient Safety, 2004). The effects of fatigue as a result of long work hours, working at night, and insufficient sleep are often underestimated. Fatigue has been linked with slowed reaction time, lapses of attention, errors of omission, decreased ability to problem-solve, and reduced motivation and energy (American Nurses Association, 2013).

Studies linking fatigue with medical errors have been reported for pediatric critical care nurses and residents (Montgomery, 2007). Nurses who have good sleep habits, minimize their shift rotations and excessive work hours, and use strategic naps can reduce the adverse effects of fatigue that could potentially put patients at risk. Other strategies to reduce fatigue include rest breaks, exercise, and bright lights (Rogers, 2008). Although limited research has been conducted in the area of fatigue, specifically related to neonatal nurses and neonatal nurse practitioners, the National Association of Neonatal Nurses, separately (2011) and in conjunction with the National Association of Neonatal Nurse Practitioners (2012), has developed position statements recommending that all health care employers implement guidelines to minimize staff fatigue. These recommendations encourage close collaboration between staff and their employers in order to develop and implement risk reduction strategies to reduce the risk of fatigue-related incidents.

b. **NICU environment.** Human factors that have contributed to errors include fatigue, communication failure, poor hand-offs, problems with cross-coverage, workload, and staffing patterns. Addressing these factors can aid in reducing medical errors. The NICU environment is a complex adaptive system conducive to human error. Frequently, the NICU is chaotic and prone to many unanticipated interruptions and life-threatening events, leaving care providers with very little time to make thoughtful and sound decisions. Patients in the NICU often require complex multidisciplinary care; each layer of this complex system presents additional opportunities for error (Morriss, 2008).

(1) The physical environment (Braithwaite, 2008; Joseph and The Center for Health Design, 2006; White, 2005). The NICU directly affects not only the highly vulnerable and sensitive preterm infant but also the caregiver within the environment. Overcrowded and poorly designed workspaces and work flow areas, excessive noise, inadequate lighting, poor ventilation and air flow filtration systems, and insufficient family space can all affect patient and staff health and safety. Inadequate lighting, excessive noise, and a disorganized environment are likely to compound the burden of stress for nurses and lead to errors. Providing caregivers with a physical environment that lowers stress and improves job performance, safety, and satisfaction is the key for health care organizations. Lighting and sound levels often conflict for the neonate and caregiver. While dim lighting is appropriate for nighttime circadian cycles for the infant, dim lighting is difficult for night staff to provide direct physical care as well as to maintain a level of alertness and comfort. Providing night-shift workers with task lighting or short periods of bright-light exposure levels can improve mood, sleep, and levels of alertness. Many NICUs are designing or redesigning their units; efforts should focus on the individual needs of babies, families, and caregivers. Human engineers should be included in the design process to promote a safe environment.

(2) Social environment. The NICU is a complex, demanding environment and NICU nurses can experience high levels of stress resulting in burnout. Job satisfaction, emotional support, and self-care are important components for preventing burnout in staff (Braithwaite, 2008). Autonomy, supervisor and peer support, and inclusion of families and patients in the care process have been cited as aspects of the social environment that can contribute to staff satisfaction and decreased levels of burnout (Joseph and The Center for Health Design, 2006).

c. **Aging workforce.** Nurses are aging and their work is becoming more complex with changing technology, evolving work practices, and increasing documentation requirements. There is a need to redesign workplaces using ergonomic work principles in order to reduce the physical demands on nurses (Joseph and The Center for Health Design,

2006). Although the 2008 U.S. Department of Health and Human Services survey found that the share of registered nurses (RNs) less than 40 years of age grew for the first time since 1980, the mean age of a registered nurse in the United States is still 47 years. Ergonomic evaluation of the work area specific to the NICU may provide solutions to problems encountered by neonatal care providers. For instance, an ergonomic evaluation of the work area at an infant's bedside to reduce a care provider's neck and back problems may include a height-adjustable footstool and better monitor placement as potential solutions. More ergonomics research is needed in the area of computer workstations as they affect nurses' posture, readability, and level of fatigue (Joseph and The Center for Health Design, 2006).

d. **Staffing** (Kane et al., 2007). Increases in staff workload and age, coupled with a decrease in the number of RNs, can threaten patient safety. Nurses are vital in providing patients with high-quality and safe care. Researchers have examined the impact of nurse staffing levels and incidence of bloodstream infections and have found greater nurse-hours per patient day significantly reduce the incidence of infection in the NICU (Cimiotti et al., 2006; Leistner et al., 2013). In a meta-analysis of 94 observational studies, greater numbers of nursing staff members were associated with better patient outcomes in intensive care units and in surgical patients, but this association did not show a causal relationship and the majority of participating centers cared for adults (Kane et al., 2007). Staffing levels vary greatly across facilities, and methods for promoting safer staffing are needed. Skill mix and acuity are two additional factors that contribute to nurse staffing and its relationship to patient outcomes. A validated neonatal acuity tool is needed to determine appropriate nurse–patient ratios, followed by a large neonatal multicenter rigorous trial to conclude whether a relationship exists between increased nurse staffing (including skill mix and acuity) and improved patient outcomes.

6. **Health information technology** (Congressional Budget Office, 2008; Shekelle et al., 2006). In its 2001 report, *Crossing the Quality Chasm*, the IOM identified health information technology (HIT) as one of the most significant interventions to improve health care quality in the United States. Many national agencies support the use of HIT because of its promising improvement in the efficiency, cost-effectiveness, quality, and safety of medical care and delivery in the nation's health care system. Despite these recommendations, the majority of health care organizations have been slow to adopt HIT. Information technology strategies have proven effective in reducing human errors in industries such as aviation and banking. Technology eliminates duplicate work and illegible handwriting. HIT may improve care providers' decision making with integrating relevant automated decision-making and knowledge acquisition tools along with evidence-based clinical practice guidelines. Communication among caregivers, accessibility and availability of patient information, medication prescribing and use, and adherence to clinical practice guidelines can all be improved through the use of HIT. Some of the technologies that improve medication delivery and provide decision support for medication therapy include computerized provider order entry, bar coding, handheld computers, and a first generation of smart pumps and automated dispensing machines.

Limited evidence exists to support the use of HIT in the NICU and its effectiveness in reducing errors. Technology alone does not eliminate medication errors, and there are also concerns about the potential introduction of new errors or unintended consequences (Cochran et al., 2007). The cost of implementing HIT is a significant barrier for many health care organizations. Besides cost, there is also an element of human interface between good technology and user-friendly equipment. Health care professionals who adopt workaround strategies to override an inflexible system in order to achieve the desired task defeat the software-designed safeguards. Although HIT has grown exponentially, it may contribute to system complexity and additional opportunities for errors. Further research is needed to evaluate the efficacy of HIT and its impact on neonatal patient safety outcomes.

a. **Clinical Decision Support System (CDSS).** Clinical decision making has become extremely complex, requiring health care providers to use their knowledge and experience combined with rapidly emerging clinical diagnostic techniques, treatment regimens, drug therapies, and clinical practice guidelines. CDSS is an information system that can assist health care providers in making clinical decisions by providing standardized, evidence-based practice (EBP) resources to the bedside caregiver (Mack et al., 2009; Neonatology on the Web, 2010). Human errors increase when care providers rely on memory to complete a task. According to the IOM (2007), the growing amount of information required to make sound clinical and reliable decisions is surpassing unassisted human capacity, and CDSS offers a practical solution as an EBP resource.

b. **Computerized Provider Order Entry (CPOE).** CPOE is an electronic application for writing orders that provides clinical guidance during the ordering process and intercepts potential errors at the point of order origination. Implementation of a CPOE system is one of the 30 safe practices identified by the National Quality Forum (2009) to facilitate transfer of clear communication. The majority of CPOE systems interface with CDSS, which provides much of the value of implementing CPOE. The CDSS component provides clinical guidance such as notifying clinicians of inappropriate dosages through dose range checking, drug allergies, and the potential for adverse effects based on other known aspects of an infant's condition, such as concurrent medications or renal impairment. CDSS can also notify clinicians of high-cost laboratory tests and suggest alternatives, alert them that a redundant diagnostic test was performed recently, or bundle groups of orders based on best practice guidelines and evidence-based order sets (Palma et al., 2011). Both CPOE and CDSS promote safety by improving legibility; reducing or eliminating transcription errors; using standard names, catalogs, and dictionaries; automating calculations; providing alerts and reminders; monitoring for adherence to best practice; and screening for populations at risk (Lehmann and Kim, 2006). CPOE is one of the most frequently used systems for reducing error and managing patient care more safely. Many national organizational bodies recommend CPOE as a strategy to reduce medication errors; however, there is limited pediatric and neonatal-specific evidence with adequate power to support its ability to reduce errors and prevent adverse drug events (ADEs) in the NICU (Miller et al., 2007; Morriss, 2008; Walsh et al., 2008).

There are barriers in adopting CPOE within an organization. Barriers include cost for start-up and maintenance, changes to work flow process and design affecting all health care personnel and departments throughout the organization, and the challenge of implementing a system that is reliable and user-friendly. The majority of CPOE systems are designed for adult patients and require alteration in order to address the special needs of the NICU population. Many medications prescribed in the NICU are off-label or unlicensed (Kimland and Odlind, 2012), making it difficult to determine a CPOE standard based on best evidence. Although CPOE may decrease the frequency of ADEs, evidence suggests that computerized systems cannot prevent all errors or ADEs and may, in some cases, be responsible for new types of errors, such as juxtaposition errors, in which the clinician inadvertently chooses the incorrect patient or medication name from a drop-down menu (Abramson and Kaushal, 2012; Chuo and Hicks, 2008; Metzger et al., 2010; Palma et al., 2011). An evidence-based methodology for evaluating CPOE systems implemented and operating in hospitals does exist (Kilbridge et al., 2006). More research is needed to evaluate the efficacy of implementing CPOE in the NICU.

c. **Smart infusion pumps.** Medication errors related to intravenous (IV) infusion present the greatest potential for harm. Neonatal nurses program infusion pumps routinely in order to deliver parenteral fluids and high-risk medications such as dopamine, morphine, fentanyl, and insulin. Smart infusion pumps decrease the chance of error by using a drug formulary that is individualized for a particular patient population. Medications, advisories, usual concentrations, dosing units (e.g., mcg/kg/min, units/hr), and dosing limits are specific to that population. Smart pumps have both soft and hard alerts or stops. Soft alerts can be overridden based on unit guidelines; hard alerts are programmed in and cannot be changed without reprogramming the pump. Smart pumps can also collect and store data for many variables, such as alerts, medications given, and overrides (Lemoine and Hurst, 2012). Both continuous and bolus infusions can be programmed with the expanded drug dose calculator. The formularies or libraries are designed and managed by the hospital pharmacy department but require interdisciplinary collaboration to ensure safe and appropriate parameters are programmed.

IV pumps rely heavily on human factors and depend on error-free programming. Most smart pumps are not intuitive, and extensive training is required for proper implementation. Keypads allow double-value entry and are sometimes difficult to read from a distance. Smart pump technology contains computerized medication software to ensure appropriate dosage and flow rates based on safety parameters and is designed to reduce human fallibility and ADEs. However, overriding the soft alerts can also bypass the "smart" functionality. The storage function could be helpful in reviewing ADEs and near misses, but is rarely used in practice (Scanlon, 2012).

d. **Automated drug-dispensing units (ADUs) or automated dispensing machines (ADMs).** ADMs are computerized cabinets containing stock medications and supplies and are located on the patient unit. These automated machines provide quick access and tracking from the point-of-care entry to removal from the cabinet, leading to an elimination of possible errors within the phases of medication administration (from ordering to transcribing, dispensing, and administering). They are used for the purpose of automating access, distribution, management, and control of medications, fluids, and supplies. Guidelines for the safe use of ADMs have been developed by the American Society of Health-Care Pharmacists (2010). There are workaround or override concerns with the use of ADUs and ADMs; limiting the use of workarounds is necessary, otherwise the safety features become ineffective and staff may become complacent and not read the alert information when selecting overrides (Kester et al., 2006; Miller et al., 2008). Drug dose errors related to stocking are also a concern requiring the need for double checks.

e. **Bar-code medication administration (BCMA) technology or bar-code scanning medication administration (BSMA)** is used to prevent medication errors by placing a unique identifier (bar code) that is machine readable by an optical scanner on each medication. The effectiveness of BCMA to prevent medication errors before they reach the patient has been documented (Cochran et al., 2007). Before the medication is administered, BCMA matches the right medication with the right patient at the right time. BCMA has not yet been installed in many hospitals, and no reports exist regarding its effectiveness in preventing ADEs in the NICU.

Bar coding is associated with fewer patient identification errors by using a system of machine-readable codes that uniquely identify an item (Gray et al., 2006). Misidentification errors are not limited only to medication; these errors affect diagnosis and therapeutics and are also commonly seen when a mother's expressed breast milk has been given to the wrong infant (Suresh et al., 2004). Point-of-care bar coding systems have been identified as a technology used to decrease patient identification error. Radio frequency identification systems, which do not require line-of-sight access to patient identification bands, may also be reliable. Despite the potential benefits of either of these autoidentification technologies, it is the responsibility of the clinician to ensure that such technologies are adequately tested in the NICU environment (Gray et al., 2006).

f. **Radio frequency identification (RFID)** is expected to replace bar-code scanning because of its ability to read identification tags with greater versatility. RFID tags are used in newborn security systems and have the capability to track individuals in order to identify their location. Infant security systems are crucial to the design of both maternity and neonatal units, with the alarming mechanism at every point of entry to prevent infant abduction.

g. **Additional HIT.** Personal digital assistants, handheld computers, and cellular phones can integrate with electronic health records. Care providers work in a mobile environment, and these handheld devices can document and retrieve information at the point of care without delay, including evidence-based clinical practice guidelines (CPGs), pharmacy database and assessment guides, and diagnostic tests (Mack et al., 2009).

7. **Evidence-based practice (EBP).** According to the IOM's *Roundtable on Evidence-Based Medicine* (2007), EBP serves as a necessary and valuable tool for future progress; as a projected goal, by the year 2020, 90% of all clinical decisions will be supported by accurate, timely, and up-to-date clinical information that is supported by the best available evidence. EBP is the integration of the best available evidence with clinical expertise and patient values (Sackett et al., 2000). All three of these components are vital to the process. While nurses

may feel confident in their clinical expertise and, to some extent, patient/family values, many nurses are not aware of the most recent research findings available to optimize their nursing care (Brady and Lewin, 2007; Cadmus et al., 2008; Pravikoff et al., 2005). Neonatal nurses are encouraged to use EBP to guide daily decision making in order to provide the highest quality of care for individual patients and to decrease variations in practice (Smith et al., 2007). The EBP process requires nurses to be able to search for the evidence and apply the findings to practice. For nurses to integrate EBP into their practice, they need to value the importance of research and health care organizations need to commit to promoting EBP by allowing nurses time and the wherewithal to foster an EBP culture. Neonatal nurses need to be taught how to implement EBP and health care organizations need to accommodate convenient computer access to online EBP resources, including online journal articles and clinical practice guidelines (CPG) websites.

a. **Clinical practice guidelines.** One form of evidence increasing in volumes internationally, mainly in the adult patient population, is the use of CPGs (Kent and Fineout-Overholt, 2007). Evidence-based CPGs are systematically developed based on the strongest evidence, contain statements to guide practitioners, and include recommendations to assist in decision making (Kent and Fineout-Overholt, 2007). These evidence-based guidelines assist practitioners by reducing variability in practice and standardizing treatment. This standardization has been shown to improve quality in health care settings. Librarians or APNs trained in EBP can champion or mentor individual clinicians in using the EBP process.

   The following organizations foster development of high-quality evidence-based CPGs, Best Practice Sheets, or Potentially Better Practices (PBPs):

   - The Association of Women's Health, Obstetric and Neonatal Nurses (AWHONN) provides CPGs specific to newborns and their families, including breastfeeding support and neonatal skin care (www.awhonn.org/awhonn/category.products.do?catid=6).
   - The National Guideline Clearinghouse (NGC) is an initiative of the Agency for Healthcare Research and Quality (AHRQ) and is a free public resource for evidence-based CPGs. The NGC site contains abstracts and full-text CPGs, guideline comparisons, a searchable bibliography database for literature citations, and a discussion forum for exchanging ideas about guidelines (www.guideline.gov).
   - The Joanna Briggs Institute (JBI) is an interdisciplinary, not-for-profit, international research and development agency in Australia. The role of the JBI is to improve the feasibility, appropriateness, meaningfulness, and effectiveness of health care practices and health care outcomes by facilitating international collaborating centers, groups, expert researchers, and clinicians. Although their website targets the adult population, it does include good resources for neonatal nurses. Multiple EBP tools and resources as well Best Practice Sheets (or clinical practice guidelines) are also available on this website (www.joannabriggs.edu.au/pubs/best_practice.php).
   - The American Academy of Pediatrics offers an online practice management website, including a brief description of CPGs, their own developed CPG (specifically, *Management of Hyperbilirubinemia in the Newborn Infant 35 or More Weeks of Gestation*), and a list of CPG resources (http://www.aap.org/en-us/professional-resources/practice-support/quality-improvement/Pages/Guidelines-and-Policy-Development.aspx).
   - The Vermont Oxford Network offers PBPs, which are practices that are developed and tested by multidisciplinary neonatal teams that participate in the VON. The practices are considered "potentially better" because VON members believe that, until the practices can be evaluated, customized, and implemented into individual NICUs, it is unknown whether they are the best possible practice. Some practices may be controversial because there is limited or no evidence available. Members of the VON are given tools to assess the quality and strength of each PBP. PBPs are published and topics include, but are not limited to, neonatal pain management, family-centered care, reduction of bronchopulmonary dysplasia in very low birth weight infants, staffing in the NICU, and more. A list of publications related to the VON can be found at http://www.vtoxford.org/.
   - The National Association of Neonatal Nurses offers guidelines on the topics of pain, skin care, genetics, and peripherally inserted central catheters. A list of publications can be found at www.nann.org.

8. **Reporting methods.** A number of reporting methods exist and have been used to identify medical errors and adverse events (AEs), including chart review (both focused or trigger-based and nonfocused), direct observation, voluntary reporting by health care providers, and review of medical malpractice claims. Multiple methods may be necessary to effectively measure harm associated with hospital-based health care.
   a. **Voluntary reporting** systems are used by many health care organizations, although this is limited owing to its voluntary nature. Reporting systems can be performed at the unit level (incident reports) or at the national level (multi-institutional specialty-based reports). The majority of incident reporting systems in the NICU use a voluntary, non-punitive approach to incidents, and these reporting systems elicit many more incidents in the NICU than a mandatory system (Snijders et al., 2007). A voluntary system is key to reporting medical errors and AEs because health care providers may fear being stigmatized or punished for their actions. However, once a culture of safety is developed, reporting of errors and near misses by health care providers has been shown to increase (Snijders et al., 2009). It is important to include near misses when reporting in order to learn how to prevent errors. Automated reporting systems that allow quick and easy access are necessary for busy clinicians. Although voluntary reporting only provides a glimpse into a complex cause of error, system factors responsible for many errors can be identified in a voluntary reporting system. Using an Internet-based, voluntary, anonymous reporting system from 54 NICUs, members of the VON revealed large numbers of errors in virtually all domains in NICUs and identified factors contributing to the occurrence of errors. Among these factors, nearly half (47%) of reports were associated with a failure to follow a hospital policy or protocol, 27% with inattention, 22% with a communication problem, and 12% with distraction (Suresh et al., 2004). These findings suggest that adding new policies or protocols does not improve patient safety; rather, the responsibility lies within the system itself, monitoring processes, and identifying system-wide improvements to effectively understand errors and improve patient safety. Once errors are identified, improvement strategies are implemented, and future errors are prevented, health care providers will recognize the benefit of reporting.
   b. **Patient triggers.** Measuring the overall level of harm within a health care organization has been performed through the identification of "triggers," or clues, of AEs during manual chart review. A trigger is defined as an "occurrence, prompt, or flag" found on review of the medical chart that "triggers" a further investigation to determine the presence or absence of an AE. Historically, efforts to identify AEs have relied on voluntary reporting and tracking of errors. This method is often limited and may be unreliable because of a small percentage of errors ever being reported. Trigger methodology provides a more focused and efficient review of charts that may lead to identifying more AEs (Sharek, 2012). An example of a neonatal trigger would be the patient's use of naloxone, prompting a focused chart review for opioid-induced respiratory depression. In an effort to develop and test an NICU-specific trigger tool, members of the VON and the Child Health Corporation of America (CHCA) participated in a collaborative funded by the AHRQ. In a retrospective chart review, 749 charts from 15 different NICUs were examined for NICU-associated AEs. Results of this study identified low birth weight and early-gestational-age infants as most susceptible to AEs, with the most common AEs being nosocomial infections (27.8%), catheter infiltrates (15.5%), abnormal cranial imaging (10.5%), and accidental extubations requiring reintubation (8.3%) (Sharek et al., 2006). More than half of all identified AEs were classified as preventable, with 40% falling into the severe-harm group. Specific limitations of this study exist; however, the authors concluded that the NICU trigger tool is superior to identifying AEs compared with nontrigger methods, and the NICU trigger tool can potentially be automated, allowing identification of AEs in real time as well as providing the ability to track AE rates (Sharek et al., 2006). This kind of proactive search for problems is more effective than responding to reports of injuries and accidents after they occur.
   c. **Additional methods of identifying errors.** Traditional chart reviews or health care provider interviews are additional methods of identifying errors. Often these methods are labor intensive, costly, inefficient, and variable. Direct observation using real-time audits

during team rounds or routine nursing care can provide immediate feedback to frontline staff, which is key to behavior change for focused improvements in patient safety (Ursprung and Gray, 2010). Checklists with real-time surveillance methods identify care processes especially prone to error that are important safety areas, including mislabeled medications (tubing or syringes), absence of wristbands for patient identification, failure to follow hand hygiene practices, and inappropriate pulse oximeter settings (Ursprung and Gray, 2010). A culture of safety involves promoting practices that are evidence-based and safe and should be part of any NICU's quality improvement efforts. Families are also encouraged to participate in the process of identifying errors in order to provide a different perspective from most health care providers and to enhance the opportunity to learn about error prevention.

9. **Transparency and full disclosure** (Massachusetts Coalition for the Prevention of Medical Error [MCPME], 2006). Transparency is a process in which errors are fully disclosed to patients/families. It is a process that can be very challenging for health care providers. Disclosure refers to providing information to a patient and/or family about an incident. Data suggest that most patients/families wish to be informed of AEs; however, nurses and physicians may find it difficult to acknowledge their mistakes, whether due to fear of litigation or just an intense shame or guilt. Health care professionals hold themselves to very high standards and, as a result, may find it difficult to deal with failure. Because of the emotional effects of these events on both the patients/families and the caregiver, communication failures are often the reason patients/families file malpractice suits. Support to both families and caregivers are essential in disclosing errors. Error disclosure training has become part of the curricula at many medical schools and residency training programs (Stroud et al., 2013). It has also been incorporated in interprofessional training programs (University of Washington, 2013) and bedside nurses' training (Wayman et al., 2007). The Harvard teaching institutions have developed a consensus statement for use at the Harvard hospitals that provides a template for responding consistently and ethically to medical errors (MCPME, 2006).
   **a.** Strategies to support families after an AE through disclosure by care providers:
      - Provide prompt (within 24 hours after the event is discovered), compassionate, and honest communication with families following an incident, telling them what happened.
      - Take responsibility and openly acknowledge the incident, be sensitive, and provide good and skillful communication. The reactions of families to incidents are influenced both by the incident itself and the manner in which the incident is handled.
      - The initial communication should be by, or at least in the presence of, a caregiver with a prior relation of trust with the patients (this may be the attending physician or primary nurse).
      - Apologize when there has been an error. The attending physician responsible for the patient's care is the person most suitable to make the apology, along with the clinician responsible for carrying out the incident. However, in some situations, other health care professionals or administrators may be more appropriate for disclosing the error and apologizing. The apology helps to restore the family's dignity and begin the healing process.
      - Open communication by individual clinicians should be strongly supported by both institutional leaders and the health care team as a whole. (It is difficult for the clinician to be open and honest about problems that have occurred if he or she does not feel supported by management/leadership.)
      - Initial communication should focus on what happened and how it will affect the patient, including immediate effects and prognosis.
      - Commit to finding out why the event occurred, and how recurrences will be prevented from happening to others, and to conducting an ongoing investigation.
      - Follow-up care should also be provided for the families after the initial incident, with continued ongoing communication and support.

   **b.** Strategies to support caregivers following an AE. Similar to patients/families, caregivers are also affected, emotionally and functionally, following an AE and are frequently unrecognized as the "second victim." Caregivers should be provided with institutional support that enables them to recover. Adverse medical events are a time of charged emotions and hectic activity involving a variety of clinical services. A clearly defined process is required to assess, activate, and oversee an effective support response for clinicians in these situations. A trained group of individuals to provide emotional support to the caregivers who were involved in the AE is recommended. Organizations need to offer caregivers professional help to manage the stress of the AE so healing can occur and they can comfortably return to work and take better care of their patients. Caregivers should have structured assistance in debriefing the AE as a team and should be given instruction on documenting the event. Coaching in communicating with the family during the emotionally intense period immediately following an incident can be critical for maintaining the relationship of compassion and trust. Training programs, including simulation training, need to be developed to teach nurses, physicians, and other clinicians, as well as department chairs and managers, how to communicate AEs and how to provide support after experiencing an AE.

B. **Selected types of health care errors in the NICU.** Many selected improvement strategies are identified throughout this section. This is not an exhaustive list, and many of the same strategies can be used for each identified error. It is important to remember that the safety and efficacy of a new practice, protocol, or piece of equipment should be examined carefully prior to implementation.

1. **Patient misidentification** (Gray et al., 2006). Misidentification is a specific area of concern for NICU patients. Accurate patient identification is necessary for providing safe and effective services specifically related to medication and blood product administration, laboratory specimen collection, performance of diagnostic procedures, and administration of treatments. Unlike adults and many pediatric patients, neonates cannot participate in the process of identifying themselves. Methods used to differentiate individuals (age, size, sex, and hair color) are not readily available in the neonatal population. Frequently, names are similar and, in some cases, identical along with similar medical record numbers, resulting in an increased chance for misidentification. Wristbands are another tool used to verify patient identification in the NICU. However, wristbands are often inaccurate, incomplete, missing, or are affixed to the patient's bedside because of concern that they can lead to lacerations or abrasions to the preterm infant's fragile skin.
   a. Improvement strategies to reduce misidentification include:
      - Two patient identifiers
      - "Time out" immediately before starting the procedure
      - Bar codes
      - RFID
2. **Wrong administration of expressed breast milk (EBM) and blood products.** Multiple steps are involved in the process of administering EBM and blood products. Both EBM and blood products are body fluids and can carry infectious agents; because of the risk associated with potentially administering the wrong breast milk or blood products, methods need to be identified in order to reduce wrong administration.
   a. Improvement strategies (use the same strategies as used for misidentification and medication errors). Six Sigma is a process improvement strategy and has been used to reduce the incidence of incorrectly administering EBM (Drenckpohl et al., 2007). The Six Sigma methodology has been used in the manufacturing industry for years and its goal is performance excellence, stating that perfection is possible. The Six Sigma approach reduces variability within a process, ultimately reducing opportunities for failures. The steps are to define, measure, analyze, improve (DMAI), and control a problem (Kubiak and Benbow, 2009). Administration of human milk is complex and involves many people handling, transporting, storing, preparing, and administering the milk, resulting in the potential for error. The primary goal of Six Sigma is to eliminate the number of defects that can occur in a process (Kubiak and Benbow, 2009). This same method can be used as an effective strategy for improving other processes related to errors within an organization.
   b. Selected strategies to avoid wrong administration of human milk (Drenckpohl et al., 2007).
      (1) Label pumped breast milk.
         (a) Have mother label milk after pumping, using labels with the infant's first and last name, birth date, medical record number, and date and time pumped.

(2) Receive milk.
  (a) Read label to be sure it is complete.
  (b) If label is not complete, return bottle to mother/family member for completion.
  (c) Place human milk in labeled bin designated for the infant and store in freezer or refrigerator.
(3) Storage, preparation, and distribution of human milk according to institution protocol.
  (a) Each infant should have his or her own storage bin. In the case of multiple births and infants with similar names, consider specialized labels to alert staff of risk of misidentification.
(4) Verify milk for administration.
  (a) Never leave the milk at an infant's bedside unless the bedside RN has verified that this is the correct milk and the correct infant.
  (b) Before feeding, verify breast milk with another staff member, using two patient identifiers.
  (c) Many institutions have instituted bar coding for verification of patient identity prior to administration of breast milk (Dougherty and Nash, 2009; Fleischman, 2013).
(5) Develop an institution-specific policy outlining the steps to take if there is an error in breast milk administration.

3. **Medication errors.** Neonates are highly vulnerable to medication errors because of their extensive exposure to medications in the NICU, the lack of evidence on pharmacotherapeutic interventions in neonates, and the lack of neonate-specific formulations (Chedoe et al., 2007). Medication errors can occur throughout any stage of drug delivery and include preventable and nonpreventable ADEs. More research is needed regarding the epidemiology of medication errors in the NICU, and evidence-based interventions are needed to reduce medication errors and improve patient safety. In an effort to reduce the rate of pediatric medication errors, the AAP has developed recommendations uniquely pertinent to children and/or neonates (Stucky, 2003, reaffirmed 2007, retired 2011; AAP and Committee on Quality Improvement and Management and Committee on Hospital Care, 2011).
  **a.** Common stages of medication ordering and delivery where errors occur.
    (1) *Prescribing.* Incorrect dosing is the most common medication error in the NICU, related either to the prescribing phase or the administration phase (Chedoe et al., 2007). Deficiencies in prescribing medications contribute to nearly 14% of ADEs in hospitalized children (Sorrentino and Alegiani, 2012; Stavroudis et al., 2010). The most common cause of medication errors at the prescribing stage is the deficiency in performance or knowledge of the prescriber, physician, or nurse practitioner. Neonates are a heterogeneous group, and prescribing decisions must be made on an individual basis. Pharmacokinetic and pharmacodynamic parameters change continuously because of changes in the neonate's weight, length, and renal function (Chedoe et al., 2007; Dabliz and Levine, 2012). Incorrect recording of the patient's weight, dosage regimen, and units (e.g., milligrams and micrograms), and misplacement of decimal points when calculating, resulting in 10- or 100-fold overdoses, all contribute to dose errors at the prescribing phase (Chedoe et al., 2007). Specific to the NICU population is the rapid change in weights requiring frequent dosing recalculations in order to maintain therapeutic drug levels. The use of abbreviations, verbal orders, and poor handwriting can also lead to medication errors at the prescribing stage. Review of the prescribed orders, by a nurse or pharmacist, is critical at this stage of the medication process in order to detect or prevent an ADE (Dabliz and Levine, 2012).
    (2) *Transcribing.* CPOE has reduced or eliminated transcription errors for medications and other ordered treatments. However, as of 2010, only an estimated 21.7% of U.S. hospitals had CPOE (Abramson and Kaushal, 2012). Systems that continue to rely on multiple transcriptions and "hand-offs" of written information increase the chance of an error in the transcription phase. In handwritten processes, each transcription is an opportunity for error (Lehmann and Kim, 2006). Transcription accounts for as

■ TABLE 18-2
■ ■ **"Do Not Use" Abbreviations**

| Do Not Use | Potential Problem | Use Instead |
|---|---|---|
| U (unit) | Mistaken for "0"(zero), the number "4" (four) or "cc" | Write "unit" |
| IU (International Unit) | Mistaken for IV (intravenous) or the number 10 (ten) | Write "International Unit" |
| Q.D., QD, q.d., qd (daily) | Mistaken for each other | Write "daily" |
| Q.O.D., QOD, q.o.d., qod (every other day) | Period after the Q mistaken for "I" and the "O" mistaken for "I" | Write "every other day" |
| Trailing zero (X.0 mg) | Decimal point is missed | Write X mg |
| Lack of leading zero (.X mg) | | Write 0.X mg |
| MS | Can mean morphine sulfate or magnesium sulfate | Write "morphine sulfate" |
| $MSO_4$ and $MgSO_4$ | Confused for one another | Write "magnesium sulfate" |

Adapted from The Joint Commission: The official "Do Not Use" list. Retrieved from http://www.jointcommission.org/assets/1/18/Do_Not_Use_List.pdf. 

much as 18% of medication errors (Stavroudis et al., 2010). Errors related to similarly spelled drug names and similarly sounding drug names are common. Equally problematic are ambiguous abbreviations. The Joint Commission (2012) affirmed its official "Do Not Use" list of abbreviations (Table 18-2). Prior to dispensing medications, it is the responsibility of the pharmacist to review all orders confirming the name of the drug, patient, dose, quantity, directions for use, and route and time of administration.

(3) *Dispensing*. Control of drug preparation and dispensing is important in safeguarding children. Dispensing errors account for up to 11.8% of medication errors (Stavroudis et al., 2010). Errors can arise from inadequate medication order review; incorrect pharmacy computer order entry; incorrect drug selection; preparation and labeling; wrong dose, patient route, and formulation; and failure to note allergies or contraindications. Wrong base solution or diluents are also an issue when preparing parenteral drugs as well as in multiple preparation procedures (Lesar et al., 2006). Labeling and storage of look-alike and sound-alike drug names, or look-alike packaging, coupled with frequent interruptions and distractions, can lead to dispensing errors (Joint Commission, 2012). Pharmacist workload is another increased risk of dispensing a potentially unsafe medication (Malone et al., 2007). Ambiguous names, mistaken abbreviations, and miscommunication can also lead to adverse errors at this stage of the process.

(4) *Administration*. One third to one half of all medication errors in the NICU occur at the point of drug administration (Stavroudis et al., 2010; Suresh et al., 2004). Errors in the administration process could stem from administration to the wrong patient, incorrect administration technique or route, administration of expired drugs, incorrect preparation administered, omission of a dose, or administering an extra dose. Multiple distractions in the NICU, high workloads, and poor communication among health care providers can all lead to dosage calculation errors and delayed or missed drug administration. Errors in the route of administration, including IV infusions connected to nasogastric tubes, have also been reported (Joint Commission, 2006). Unfamiliarity or inexperience with medications and infusion devices, along with poorly designed programming functions, can also contribute to errors in administration.

b. High-alert medication: The Institute for Safe Medication Practices (2012) created a list of high-alert medications that bear a heightened risk of causing significant patient harm. The list provides health care professionals with specific medications that require special safeguards to reduce the risk of errors. Selected specific high-risk medications in the NICU (not an exhaustive list) are found in Box 18-2. The most commonly reported products to be associated with an error in the pediatric population are total parental nutrition and lipids, electrolytes, opioid analgesics (e.g., morphine and fentanyl),

BOX 18-2
**HIGH-ALERT MEDICATIONS**

- Antithrombotic agents (e.g., warfarin, heparin, and low molecular weight heparin)
- Adrenergic agonists, intravenous (IV) (e.g., EPINEPHrine, phenylephrine, norepinephrine)
- Adrenergic antagonists, IV (e.g., propranolol, metoprolol, labetalol)
- Anesthetic agents, general, inhaled, and IV (e.g., ketamine and propofol)
- Antiarrhythmics, IV (e.g., lidocaine and amiodarone)
- Dextrose, hypertonic, 20% or greater
- Inotropic medications, IV (e.g., digoxin and milrinone)
- Insulin, subcutaneous and IV
- Liposomal forms of drugs (e.g., liposomal amphotericin B)
- Moderate sedation agents, IV (e.g., midazolam, dexmedetomidine)
- Moderate oral sedation agents, for children (e.g., chloral hydrate)
- Narcotics/opioids, IV, transdermal, and oral (e.g., fentanyl and morphine)
- Neuromuscular blocking agents (e.g., vecuronium, succinylcholine, rocuronium)
- Parenteral nutrition preparations
- Potassium chloride for injection concentrate
- Sodium chloride for injection, hypertonic, greater than 0.9% concentration

Adapted from Institute for Safe Medication Practices: ISMP's high-alert medications. 2012. Retrieved from www.ismp.org/tools/highalertmedications.pdf.

antimicrobial agents (gentamicin, vancomycin, and ceftriaxone), and antidiabetic agents (insulin) (Hicks et al., 2006; Stavroudis et al., 2010).

(1) Selected safety measures to prevent high-alert medication errors.
- Limiting access to the high-alert medications.
- Special labeling of syringes and pumps infusing high-alert medications (e.g., color-coded).
- Standardized ordering, storage, preparation, and administration of products.
- Double checking/redundancies mechanisms (automated or independent double checks).
- Smart pump technology.
- System alerts.
- Standard concentrations.

**c.** Off-label medications (Conroy and McIntyre, 2005; Kimland and Odlind, 2012). Licensing procedures are performed to ensure the safety, effectiveness, and quality of medications. However, many medications intended to treat neonates are either prescribed outside the terms of the product license (off-label) or are not licensed (unlicensed) for this age group. Approximately 50% of medications prescribed in the NICU are used off label. Reference standards for doses of off-label and unlicensed medications are lacking, and clinicians are faced with different published reference standards for a single medication. As a result of the limited range of licensed medications in appropriate dosage forms and the need for weight-based dosing in neonates, more calculations and dilutions are involved prior to administration compared with those required in adults, leading to an increased number of opportunities for errors (Chedoe et al., 2007).

**d.** Selected medication improvement strategies:
- Instruct staff and practice mathematical calculations specific to neonates.
- Independently check calculations.
- Follow the "Five Rights" of medication safety.
- Ensure medication reconciliation.
- Have a clinical pharmacist on the unit.
- Implement a CPOE/CDSS with "forcing functions" (functions that limit routes and frequencies of drugs that are ordered and are specific to neonates, such as weight in kilograms and age in days of life).

- Use BCMA and ADUs.
- Standardize all medication infusions.
- Order sets or preprinted orders.
- Avoid or eliminate dangerous abbreviations; spell out dosage units.
- Use TALLman lettering.
- Remove certain high-alert drugs from "ward stock" and require dispensing only by pharmacy.
- Restrict verbal order.
- Require double checking by a second professional at each step of the medication process.
- Use a zero to the left of a dose less than 1 (e.g., use 0.1 rather than .1) and avoid a trailing zero (e.g., use 1 rather than 1.0).
- Require hand-off verification checks from one caregiver to the next for a patient receiving a high-alert drug infusion.
- Labeling precautions—Place labels on each medication dose that are specific to that single dose and contain all appropriate information. At a minimum, the label should include the patient name, room number, and identification number; the medication's generic and trade names when applicable; dosage, route, and frequency; and any alerts relating to the medication.
- Packaging—Separate drugs that look or sound alike and reduce or eliminate the availability of multiple drug strengths.
- Drug standardization—Provide a standardized order for all drugs.
- Storage and stocking—Limit the number of floor stock IV solutions. Remove all concentrated electrolytes from floor stock and never dispense them from the pharmacy.
- Use standardized abbreviations.
- Use a standardized formulary.
- Ensure that the medication reference manual includes multiple dilutions of the same drug.
- Store neonatal doses away from adult doses.
- Increase the availability of dilute forms of drugs used in neonatal areas.
- Preferentially use "neonatal" IV pumps.

4. **Health care–associated infections** (HAIs; nosocomial infections). (For detailed infectious disease information, see Chapter 32.) HAIs remain a major cause of morbidity, mortality, and cost for both adults and neonates despite concerted efforts of the Centers for Disease Control and Prevention (CDC) and infectious disease professionals (Klevens et al., 2007; Sharek et al., 2006; Siegel et al., 2007). An estimated 1.7 million HAIs occur in U.S. hospitals, among which 33,269 newborns in high-risk nurseries are affected (Klevens et al., 2007). Reducing the number of HAIs is a Joint Commission (2013b) National Patient Safety Goal (see Table 18-1) and one of the 30 safe practices identified by the National Quality Forum (2009). Treatment of these infections has become more complex because of an alarming rise in antibiotic resistance. Multidrug-resistant organisms, including methicillin-resistant *Staphylococcus aureus* (MRSA) and vancomycin-resistant enterococci (VRE), and certain gram-negative bacilli are problematic because they both are associated with increased mortality and their incidence has risen inexorably over the past decade. According to the CDC, MRSA now accounts for greater than 50% of hospital-acquired *S. aureus* infections, and there have been similar increases in VRE (Siegel et al., 2007). Selected improvement strategies have been effective in reducing the incidence of ventilator-associated pneumonia (VAP); however, additional prevention and surveillance efforts are needed along with strict adherence to these strategies in order to eliminate HAIs.

   a. **Central line–associated bloodstream infections (CLABSIs).** CLABSIs are primary bloodstream infections typically associated with the presence of a central line or an umbilical catheter in neonates at the time of or before the onset of the infection, resulting in an increased length of hospital stay, cost, and risk of mortality. Preterm infants are especially prone to infection and the presence of a central line increases the odds of an infection; the longer the catheter duration, the higher the odds of an infection (Malpiedi et al., 2013; Perlman et al., 2007). The most common organism associated with catheter-related sepsis is coagulase-negative *Staphylococcus*. Neonatal nurses can prevent CLABSI through proper central line management. Specific techniques are addressed in the CDC's *Guidelines for the Prevention of Intravascular Catheter-Related Infections* (2011), and the National Healthcare Safety Network annually publishes the incidence rate of CLABSI in preterm infants (Dudeck et al., 2013).

b. **Ventilator-associated pneumonia.** VAP is the second most common acquired HAI in the United States and is associated with significant morbidity and mortality (National Healthcare Safety Network [NHSN], 2013). VAP is a serious and common complication among intubated infants in the NICU, especially very low birth weight infants, and is associated with increased length of stay in the NICU and death. Neonatal nurses can help eliminate VAPs by following the CDC's *Guidelines for Preventing Health-Care-Associated Pneumonia* (2004; CDC and NHSN, 2013).The NHSN annually publishes the incidence rate of VAP in preterm infants (Dudeck et al., 2013).

c. **Surgical site infections (SSIs).** SSIs are the third most common nosocomial infection among hospitalized patients and contribute greatly to the mortality and morbidity associated with surgery, resulting in longer hospital stays and higher costs (NHSN, 2013). Compounding the problem of SSIs are the increased acuity of in-hospital surgical patients and the increasing numbers of patients with MRSA and VRE, leading to a greater morbidity, mortality, and cost (Barnett, 2007). The CDC's guidelines for the prevention of SSI were published a decade ago (Mangram et al., 1999), with a recent protocol edit of definitions (CDC, 2013). A recent update regarding antimicrobial prophylaxis during surgery has been developed jointly by the American Society of Health-System Pharmacists, the Infectious Diseases Society of America, the Surgical Infection Society, and the Society for Healthcare Epidemiology (Bratzler et al., 2013).

d. **Selected recommended improvement strategies reduce the risk of HAI.** The key to preventing transmission of organisms is highly correlated with the compliance rate with all practice interventions (Siegel et al., 2007). The majority of improvement strategies are taken from adult studies, and more research is needed to determine the effectiveness of these interventions in neonates.
   - Educate health care workers about multidrug-resistant organisms, CLABSI, VAPs, and SSIs and the necessity of prevention.
   - Educate families about basic infectious disease prevention, including the importance of adhering to hand hygiene practices and mode of transmission.
   - Maintain strict adherence to hand hygiene practices and use of Contact Precautions.
   - Implement a surveillance program to identify and track patients.
   - Aim for aggressive detection of carriers. Measure infection rates, monitor compliance with best practices, and evaluate the effectiveness of prevention efforts.
   - Share information with hospital senior leadership, physicians, nursing staff, and other clinicians.
   - Employ NICU-based infectious disease personnel.
   - Ensure rigorous isolation of colonized patients.
   - Make sure that the environment and personal equipment are thoroughly disinfected.
   - Elevate the head of the bed to a 30- to 35-degree angle.
   - Assess extubation readiness and the need for sedation daily.
   - Ensure proper oral and endotracheal tube (ETT) secretion care.
   - Change the ventilator circuit of drained and accumulated condensed water.
   - Evaluate central lines daily and remove nonessential catheters.
   - Limit the number of times a central line is opened for access.
   - Use a catheter checklist and a standardized protocol for central venous catheter insertion and daily maintenance (including routine cleaning and dressing changes).

5. **Unplanned extubations** (Barber, 2013). Unplanned endotracheal extubations requiring reintubation was in the top five of AEs reported using the NICU trigger methodology (Sharek et al., 2006). High-risk infants are at risk for hypoxia and hypercarbia with unintended extubation of the ETT, resulting in very dangerous and unsafe conditions and potentially a prolonged hospitalization. Limited data are available on the outcomes of unplanned ETT extubations in the NICU. Insufficient fixation of the ETT is reported as

the primary rationale for unexplained ETT extubations, followed by vigorous movement in the crib or incubator. However, limited evidence suggest that the majority of infants who experience unplanned ETT extubations do not require reintubation, signifying that many infants are remaining intubated who are ready for extubation. Additional research is needed to examine the relationship between unplanned ETT extubation and infant outcomes and potential strategies to reduce the incidence of unplanned ETT extubations.

**a.** Improvement strategies for unplanned extubations:
- Frequently assess ETT stability.
- Secure ETT (without oversecuring/taping or obscuring the measurement markings).
- Use two people when transferring or during excessive handling.
- Avoid excessive jarring or movement of incubator or crib.

**C. Discharge safety instruction.** Proactively implementing a comprehensive formalized discharge process is recognized as one of the 30 safe practices outlined by the National Quality Forum (2009) to reduce readmissions, promote more satisfied and informed patients/families, and promote better use of primary care services in the community after a hospital stay. Transitioning NICU families and their infants from hospital to home can be complex and challenging. Families need to be instructed on how to provide a safe environment at home (Boykova and Kenner, 2012; Forsythe and Kirchick, 2007). In addition to providing families with cardiopulmonary resuscitation instruction, immunization scheduling information, and developmental follow-up care, families also need to be aware of environmental and home safety precautions. Determining infant and family readiness for discharge and complete discharge instructions are provided in Chapter 19.

**1. Selected safety discharge topics** include the following:

**a.** *Medication reconciliation.* According to the Joint Commission's (2013b) National Patient Safety Goals (see Table 18-1), patients/families should be given a complete list of medications on discharge. The infant's primary care provider should also have a complete list of medications. At time of discharge, the list of home medications should be reconciled with medications the infant was receiving at time of discharge. Careful consideration should be given to which medications will be needed after discharge and which medications can be safely discontinued. Also, the care provider can determine whether additional medications may be needed at home.

**b.** *Environmental checklist.* To assess patient/family safe home environment (water, electricity, heat, smoke detectors, phone, heat/air source, fire evacuation plan, etc.).

**c.** *Car Seat Testing:* In 1990, the AAP recommended car seat challenges for infants ≤37 weeks of gestation. Due to relative hypotonia and risk of airway obstruction, these preterm infants are at risk for desaturation events, apnea, or bradycardia when placed in car seats. These recommendations were updated in 2009 (Bull, Engle, Committee on Injury, Violence, and Poison Prevention and Committee on Fetus and Newborn, American Academy of Pediatrics, 2009) and include:
- Hospital protocols should be developed for infants ≤37 weeks of gestation, but may also include more mature infants with poor tone.
- The period of observation should last for 90 to 120 minutes or the duration of travel to home, whichever is longer.
- The period of observation should be conducted by trained personnel.
- If the infant has documented desaturation and /or apnea and bradycardia events that are deemed significant, interventions to reduce the frequency of these events should be implemented before discharge. The infant should then be retested.
- Specific information regarding positioning in a car seat is included in recommendations, including the use of positioning devices and the angle of recline.
- Hospitals should provide teaching for families on positioning their infant in a car seat.
- Time spent in a car seat should be minimized. Car seats should only be used for travel.
- To improve observation of the infant, whenever possible, an adult should sit in the rear seat adjacent to the car seat.
- Car seat testing should also include inspection of the car seat to ensure that it meets current safety recommendations.

d. *Abusive Head Trauma (Shaken Baby Syndrome).* Infants who have required an NICU stay have been found to be at a higher risk of abuse than infants born at term. The National Center on Shaken Baby Syndrome (NCSBS) has developed a program adopted by many NICUs to educate parents about normal infant crying and the dangers of shaking an infant. The Period of PURPLE Crying Program focuses on helping the parent to understand that crying is normal and to develop a coping strategy when their infant is unconsolable. *PURPLE* is a mnemonic for *p*eak pattern (age when crying usually occurs), *u*npredictable, *r*esistant to soothing, *p*ain-like look on face, *l*ong bouts of crying, and *e*vening crying (NCSBS, 2013).

e. *Sleep-related death reduction strategies.* Studies have shown that there is an increased risk of sudden infant death syndrome (SIDS) among infants born preterm (AAP and Task Force on Sudden Infant Death Syndrome, 2011). Information and strategies designed to prevent sleep-related death need to be included as part of every NICU family's discharge teaching. Although many neonatal nurses provide specific back-to-sleep instructions at time of discharge, they frequently do not model safe sleep practices while infants are hospitalized (Grazel et al., 2010). Neonatal nurses are in influential positions and need to both instruct parents and model sleep-related death reduction strategies. Specific strategies include:
   - Model behavior practices prior to discharge, placing the bed in a flat position, positioning infants on their backs, and removing toys, blankets, and extra bedding.
   - Instruct parents to place baby on a firm sleeping surface. No soft bedding, including sheepskin, pillows, stuffed animals, and other soft products, should be in the crib.
   - Avoid overheating; babies should be clothed for sleep with a bedroom temperature that is comfortable for an adult with a light layer of clothing.
   - Avoid the use of sleep aid devices that are designed to keep babies in the side-lying position. There is no evidence to support the use of these devices and the prevention of SIDS. Consider using a sleeper or Halo SleepSack instead of blankets.
   - Encourage a smoke-free environment.
   - Avoid bed sharing. Babies should sleep in their own bed and close to their mother to promote breastfeeding.
   - Instruct parents to inspect crib to be used at home to ensure that it meets current safety requirements. The Consumer Product Safety Commission (CPSC) issues the safety standards for both full-size and non–full-size baby cribs. The most recent rules, at time of publication of this text, went into effect June 28, 2011. All cribs manufactured and sold in the United States must meet these standards. Standards relate to slat width, spacing, and strength; mattress size and composition; crib construction and hardware; and surface coatings used on the crib (CPSC, 2011).
   - Sleepware: Sleepware is also regulated by the CPSC. Infant sleepware should not be loose-fitting and should be flame resistant.

f. Home safety topics. Topics should include, but are not limited to, bathing; medication storage, preparation, and administration (both for the neonate going home and for any other children at home); general baby care (including oral feeding); and emergency phone numbers (e.g., pediatrician, 9-1-1, or the Poison Control Center).

## REFERENCES

Abramson, E.L. and Kaushal, R.: Computerized provider order entry and patient safety. *Pediatric Clinics of North America*, 59(6):1247–1255, 2012.

Agency for Healthcare Research and Quality: *20 tips to help prevent medical errors in children. Patient fact sheet*, 2013. Retrieved May 8, 2013, from http://www.ahrq.gov/consumer/20tipkid.htm.

American Academy of Pediatrics and Committee on Hospital Care and Institute for Patient- and Family-centered Care: Policy statement: Patient- and family-centered care and the pediatrician's role. *Pediatrics*, 129(2):394–404, 2012.

American Academy of Pediatrics and Committee on Quality Improvement and Management and Committee on Hospital Care: Policy statement: Principles of pediatric patient safety: Reducing harm due to medical care. *Pediatrics*, 127(6):1199–1210, 2011.

American Academy of Pediatrics and Task Force on Sudden Infant Death Syndrome. SIDS and other sleep-related deaths: Expansion of recommendations for a safe infant sleeping environment. *Pediatrics*, 128 (5):1030–1039, 2011.

American Nurses Association: *Health and safety: Nurse fatigue*, 2013. Accessed on May 10, 2013, from http://gm6.nursingworld.org/MainMenuCategories/WorkplaceSafety/Healthy-Work-Environment/Work-Environment/NurseFatigue.

American Society of Health-System Pharmacists: ASHP guidelines on the use of automated dispensing devices. *American Journal of Health-System Pharmacy*, 67:483–490, 2010.

Barber, J.A.: Unplanned extubation in the NICU. *JOGNN: Journal of Obstetric, Gynecologic, & Neonatal Nursing*, 42(2):233–238, 2013.

Barnett, T.E.: The not-so-hidden cost of surgical site infections. *AORN Journal*, 86(2):249–256, 2007.

Bizzarro, M.J., Sabo, B., Noonan, M., et al.: A quality improvement initiative to reduce central line–associated bloodstream infections in a neonatal intensive care unit. *Infection Control and Hospital Epidemiology*, 31(3):241–248, 2010.

Botwinick, L., Bisognano, M. and Haraden, C.: Leadership guide to patient safety. IHI Innovation Series white paper. Cambridge, MA, 2006, Institute for Healthcare Improvement.

Brady, N. and Lewin, L.: Evidence-based practice in nursing: Bridging the gap between research and practice. *Journal of Pediatric Health Care*, 21(1):53–56, 2007.

Braithwaite, M.: Nurse burnout and stress in the NICU. *Advances in Neonatal Care*, 8(6):343–347, 2008.

Bratzler, D.W., Dellinger, P., Olsen, K.M., et al.: Clinical practice guidelines for antimicrobial prophylaxis in surgery. *American Journal of Health-System Pharmacy*, 70(3):195–283, 2013.

Boykova, M. and Kenner, C.: Transition from hospital to home for parents of preterm infants. *Journal of Perinatal and Neonatal Nursing*, 26(1):81–87, 2012.

Bull, M.A., Engle, W.J. and Committee on Injury, Violence, and Poison Prevention and Committee on Fetus and Newborn, American Academy of Pediatrics: Safe transportation of preterm and low birth weight infants at hospital discharge. *Pediatrics*, 123 (5):1424–1429, 2009.

Cadmus, E., Van Wynen, E.A., Chamberlain, B., et al.: Nurses' skill level and access to evidence-based practice. *Journal of Nursing Administration*, 38(11):494–503, 2008.

Centers for Disease Control and Prevention: *Surgical site infection (SSI) event*. 2013. Retrieved May 8, 2013, from http://www.cdc.gov/nhsn/pdfs/pscmanual/9pscssicurrent.pdf Retrieved May 8, 2013, from http://www.cdc.gov/nhsn/pdfs/pscmanual/9pscssicurrent.pdf.

Centers for Disease Control and Prevention: *Guidelines for the prevention of intravascular catheter-related infections*, 2011. Accessed May 8, 2013, from http://www.cdc.gov/hicpac/pdf/guidelines/bsi-guidelines-2011.pdf.

Centers for Disease Control and Prevention: Guidelines for preventing health-care-associated pneumonia, 2003. Recommendations of CDC and the Healthcare Infection Control Practices Advisory Committee. *MMWR Recommendations and Reports*, 53(No. RR-3), 2004.

Centers for Disease Control and Prevention and National Healthcare Safety Network: *April 2013 CDC/NHSN Protocol Corrections, Clarification, and Additions*, 2013. Retrieved May 27, 2013, from http://www.cdc.gov/nhsn/pdfs/pscmanual/6pscvapcurrent.pdf.

Chedoe, I., Molendijk, H.A. and Dittrich, S.T.: Incidence and nature of medication errors in neonatal intensive care with strategies to improve safety. *Drug Safety*, 30 (6):503–513, 2007.

Chuo, J. and Hicks, R.W.: Computer-related medication errors in neonatal intensive care units. *Clinics in Perinatology*, 35(1):119–139, 2008.

Cimiotti, J.P., Haas, J.P., Saiman, L., et al.: Impact of staffing on bloodstream infections in the neonatal intensive care unit. *Archives of Pediatrics and Adolescent Medicine*, 160(8):832–836, 2006.

Cochran, G.L., Jones, K.J., Brockman, J., et al.: Errors prevented by and associated with bar-code medication administration systems. *Joint Commission Journal on Quality and Patient Safety*, 33(5):293–301, 2007.

Congressional Budget Office: *A CBO paper: Evidence on the costs and benefits of health information technology*, The Congress of the United States, Congressional Budget Office 2008. Retrieved May 8, 2013, from http://www.cbo.gov/sites/default/files/cbofiles/ftpdocs/91xx/doc9168/05-20-healthit.pdf.

Conroy, S. and McIntyre, J.: The use of unlicensed and off-label medicines in the neonate. *Seminars in Fetal and Neonatal Medicine*, 10(2):115–122, 2005.

Consumer Product Safety Commission: *A safer generation of cribs: New Federal requirements*, 2011. Retrieved May 8, 2013, fromhttp://www.cpsc.gov//PageFiles/115716/cribrules.pdf.

Dabliz, R. and Levine, S.: Medication safety in neonates. *American Journal of Perinatology*, 29:4956, 2012.

Dougherty, D. and Nash, A.: Bar coding from breast to baby: A comprehensive breast milk management system for the NICU. *Neonatal Network*, 28(5):321–328, 2009.

Drenckpohl, D., Bowers, L. and Cooper, H.: Use of the Six Sigma methodology to reduce incidence of breast milk administration errors in the NICU. *Neonatal Network*, 26(3):161–166, 2007.

Dudeck, M.A., Horan, T.C., Peterson, K.D., et al.: National Healthcare Safety Network (NHSN) report, data summary for 2011, device-associated module. 2013. Retrieved May 29, 2013, from http://www.cdc.gov/nhsn/PDFs/dataStat/NHSN-Report-2011-Data-Summary.pdf.

Dunn, M.S., Reilly, M.C., Johnston, A.M., et al.: Development and dissemination of potentially better practices for the provision of family-centered care in neonatology: The family-centered care map. *Pediatrics*, 188(Suppl. 2):S95–S107, 2006.

Fleischman, E.K.: Innovative application of bar coding technology to breast milk administration. *Journal of Perinatal and Neonatal Nursing*, 27(2):145–150, 2013.

Forsythe, P.L. and Kirchick, C.: Infant safety at home. *Advances in Neonatal Care*, 7(2):78–79, 2007.

Gray, J.E., Suresh, G., Ursprung, R., et al.: Patient misidentification in the neonatal intensive care unit: Quantification of risk. *Pediatrics*, 117(1):43–47, 2006.

Grazel, R., Pahlen, A.G. and Polomano, R.C.: Implementation of the American Academy of Pediatrics recommendations to reduce sudden infant death syndrome risk in NICUs: An evaluation of nursing knowledge and practice. *Advances in Neonatal Care*, 10(6): 332–342, 2010.

Griswold, S., Ponnuru, S., Nishisaki, A., et al.: The emerging role of simulation education to achieve patient safety. *Pediatric Clinics of North America*, 59 (6):1330–1340, 2012.

Haig, K.M., Sutton, S. and Whittington, J.: A shared mental model for improving communication between clinicians. *Joint Commission Journal on Quality and Patient Safety*, 32(3):167–175, 2006.

Handyside, J. and Suresh, G.: Human factors and quality improvement. *Clinics in Perinatology*, 37 (1):123–140, 2010.

Hicks, R.W., Becker, S.C. and Cousins, D.D.: Harmful medication errors in children: A 5-year analysis of data from USP's MEDMARX program. *Journal of Pediatric Nursing*, 21(4):290–298, 2006.

Hunt, E.A., Shilkofski, N.A., Stavroudis, T.A., et al.: Simulation: Translation to improved team performance. *Anesthesiology Clinics*, 25(2):301–319, 2007.

Institute for Family-Centered Care: *Advancing the practice of patient- and family-centered care: How to get started*, Bethesda, MD, 2008, Institute for Family-Centered Care.

Institute for Healthcare Improvement: *SBAR technique for communication: A situational briefing model*, 2011. Accessed on May 10, 2013, from http://www.ihi.org/knowledge/Pages/Tools/SBARTechniqueforCommunicationASituationalBriefingModel.aspx.

Institute for Safe Medication Practices: *ISMP's list of high-alert medications*, 2012. Retrieved May 8, 2013, from http://www.ismp.org/tools/highalertmedications.pdf.

Institute of Medicine: *The learning healthcare system: Workshop summary*, Washington, DC, 2007, National Academies Press.

Institute of Medicine: *Crossing the quality chasm: A new health system for the 21st century*, Washington, DC, 2001, National Academies Press.

Institute of Medicine and Committee on the Work Environment for Nurses and Patient Safety. Page (Ed.): *Keeping patients safe: Transforming the work environment of nurses* Washington, DC, 2004, National Academies Press.

Joint Commission: *Facts about Speak Up™ initiatives*, 2013a. Retrieved May 8, 2013, from http://www.jointcommission.org/assets/1/18/Facts_Speak_Up.pdf.

Joint Commission: *National patient safety goals 2013*, 2013b. Retrieved April 24, 2013, from http://www.jointcommission.org/assets/1/18/NPSG_Chapter_Jan2013_HAP.pdf.

Joint Commission: *Sentinel event statistics*, 2013c. Retrieved May 8, 2013, from http://www.jointcommission.org/SentinelEvents/Statistics/.

Joint Commission: *The official "Do Not Use" list*, 2012. Retrieved May 8, 2013, from http://www.jointcommission.org/facts_about_the_official_/.

Joint Commission: *Comprehensive accreditation manual for hospitals*, Chicago, IL, 2011, Joint Commission Resources.

Joint Commission: *Tubing misconnections: A persistent and potentially deadly occurrence. Sentinel Event Alert (Issue 36)*, 2006. Retrieved May 8, 2013, from http://www.jointcommission.org/sentinel_event_alert_issue_36_tubing_misconnections-a_persistent_and_potentially_deadly_occurrence/.

Joseph, A.: The Center for Health Design: The role of the physical and social environment in promoting health, safety, and effectiveness in the healthcare workplace. Concord, CA, 2006, Author. Issue paper #3.

Kane, R.L., Shamliyan, T., Mueller, C., et al.: Nurse staffing and quality of patient care. *Evidence Report/Technology Assessment*, 151:1–115, 2007.

Kent, B. and Fineout-Overholt, E.: Teaching EBP: Part 1. Making sense of clinical practice guidelines. *Worldviews on Evidence-Based Nursing*, 4(2):106–111, 2007.

Kester, K., Baxter, J. and Freudenthal, K.: Errors associated with medications removed from automated dispensing machines using override function. *Hospital Pharmacy*, 41(6):535–537, 2006.

Kilbridge, P.M., Welebob, E.M. and Classen, D.C.: Development of the Leapfrog methodology for evaluating hospital implemented inpatient computerized physician order entry systems. *Quality and Safety in Health Care*, 15(2):81–84, 2006.

Kimland, E. and Odlind, V.: Off-label drug use in pediatric patients. *Clinical Pharmacology & Therapeutics*, 91 (5):796–801, 2012.

Klevens, R.M., Edwards, J.R., Richards, C.L., et al.: Estimating healthcare-associated infections and deaths in U.S. hospitals, 2002. Atlanta, 2007, Centers for Disease Control and Prevention.

Kohn, L.T., Corrigan, J.M. and Donaldson, M.S.: To err is human: Building a safer health system. Washington, DC, 1999, National Academies Press.

Kubiak, T.M. and Benbow, D.W.: *The certified Six-Sigma black belt handbook:* (2nd ed.). Milwaukee, WI, 2009, ASQ Quality Press.

Landrigan, C.P., Parry, G.J., Bones, C.B., et al.: Temporal trends in rates of patient harm resulting from medical care. *New England Journal of Medicine*, 363:2124–2134, 2010.

Lehmann, C.U. and Kim, G.R.: Computerized provider order entry and patient safety. *Pediatric Clinics of North America*, 53(6):1169–1184, 2006.

Leistner, R., Thürnagel, S., Schwab, F., et al.: The impact of staffing on central venous catheter-associated bloodstream infections in preterm neonates—results of nation-wide cohort study in Germany. *Antimicrobial Resistance and Infection Control*, 2:11, 2013.

Lemoine, J.B. and Hurst, H.M.: Using smart pumps to reduce medication errors in the NICU. *Nursing for Women's Health*, 16(2):151–158, 2012.

Lesar, A., Mitchell, P. and Sommo, P.: Medication safety in critically ill children. *Clinical Pediatric Emergency Medicine*, 7(4):215–225, 2006.

Mack, E.H., Wheller, D.S. and Embi, P.J.: Clinical decision support systems in the pediatric intensive care unit. *Pediatric Critical Care Medicine*, 10(1):23–28, 2009.

Malone, D.C., Abarca, J., Skrepnek, G.H., et al.: Pharmacist workload and pharmacy characteristics associated with dispensing of potentially clinically important drug-drug interactions. *Medical Care*, 45(5):456–462, 2007.

Malpiedi, P.J., Peterson, K.D., Soe, M.M., et al.: National and state healthcare-associated infection standardized infection ratio report. 2013. Retrieved May 9, 2013, from http://www.cdc.gov/hai/national-annual-sir/index.html.

Mangram, A.J., Horan, T.C., Pearson, M.L., et al.: Guideline for prevention of surgical site infection. *American Journal of Infection Control Epidemiology*, 27(2):97–132, 1999.

Marx, D.: Patient safety and the "Just Culture": A primer for health care executives. 2001: New York, 2001, Columbia University Press. Retrieved May 10, 2013, from http://www.psnet.ahrq.gov/resource.aspx?resourceID=1582.

Massachusetts Coalition for the Prevention of Medical Error: *When things go wrong: Responding to adverse events*, Burlington, MA, 2006, Massachusetts Coalition for the Prevention of Medical Error.

Metzger, J., Welebob, E., Bates, D.W., et al.: Mixed results in the safety performance of computerized physician order entry. *Health Affairs (Millwood)*, 29 (4):655–663, 2010.

Miller, K., Shah, M., Hitchcock, L., et al.: Evaluation of medications removed from automated dispensing machines using the override function leading to multiple system changes. 2008: In K. Henriksen, J.B. Battles, and M.A. Keyes, et al, (Eds.): *Advances in patient safety: New directions and alternative approaches. Vol. 4: Technology and medication safety*. Rockville, MD, 2008, Agency for Healthcare Research and Quality. Retrieved May 13, 2013, from http://www.ncbi.nlm.nih.gov/books/NBK43777/.

Miller, M.R., Robinson, K.A., Lubomski, L.H., et al.: Medication errors in paediatric care: A systematic review of epidemiology and an evaluation of evidence supporting reduction strategy recommendations. *Quality and Safety in Health Care*, 16(2):116–126, 2007.

Montgomery, L.: Effect of fatigue, workload and environment on patient safety in the pediatric intensive care unit. *Pediatric Critical Care Medicine*, 8(Suppl. 2): S11–S16, 2007.

Morriss, F.H.: Adverse medical events in the NICU: Epidemiology and prevention. *NeoReviews*, 9(1):e8–e22, 2008.

National Association of Neonatal Nurses: Position Statement #3054*The effect of staff nurses' shift length and fatigue on patient safety*, July 2011. Retrieved April 24, 2013, from http://www.nann.org/uploads/files/The_Effect_of_Staff_Nurses_Shift_Length_and_Fatigue_on_Patient_Safety_2011.pdf.

National Association of Neonatal Nurses: National Association of Neonatal Nurse Practitioners: The impact of advanced practice nurses' shift length and fatigue on patient safety. Position Statement #3057. *Advances in Neonatal Nursing*, 12(3):189–200, 2012.

National Center on Shaken Baby Syndrome: *The period of purple crying*, 2013. Retrieved May 8, 2013, from http://www.purplecrying.info/.

National Healthcare Safety Network: *Patient safety component*, 2013. Retrieved May 8, 2013, at http://www.cdc.gov/nhsn/PDFs/pscManual/PSC-Manual-portfolio.pdf.

National Patient Safety Foundation's Patient and Family Advisory Council: *National agenda for action: Patients and families in patient safety; nothing about me, without me*, 2013. Retrieved May 6, 2013, from http://www.npsf.org/for-patients-consumers/tools-and-resources-for-patients-and-consumers/.

National Quality Forum: *Safe practices for better healthcare: 2009 Update: A consensus report*, Washington, DC, 2009, National Quality Forum.

Neonatology on the Web: *Computers in neonatology*, 2010. Retrieved May 10, 2013, from http://www.neonatology.org/neo.computers.html.

Palma, J.P., Sharek, P.W., Classen, D.C., et al.: Neonatal informatics: Computerized physician order entry. *NeoReviews*, 12:393–396, 2011.

Perlman, S.E., Saiman, L. and Larson, E.L.: Risk factors for late-onset health care-associated bloodstream infections in patients in neonatal intensive care units. *American Journal of Infection Control*, 35(3):177–182, 2007.

Pilcher, J., Goodall, H., Jensen, C., et al.: Special focus on simulation: Educational strategies in the NICU: Simulation-based learning: It's not just for NRP. *Neonatal Network*, 31(5):281–287, 2012.

Pravikoff, D.S., Tanner, A.B. and Pierce, S.T.: Readiness of US nurses for evidence-based practice. *American Journal of Nursing*, 105(9):40–51, 2005.

Profit, J., Etchegaray, J., Petersen, L.A., et al.: Neonatal intensive care unit safety culture varies widely. *Archives of Disease in Childhood: Fetal and Neonatal Edition*, 97(2):F120–F126, 2012.

Ricci, M.A. and Brumsted, J.R.: Crew resource management: Using aviation techniques to improve operating room safety. *Aviation, Space and Environmental Medicine*, 83(4):441–444, 2012.

Roberts, V. and Perryman, M.M.: Creating a culture for health care quality and safety. *The Health Care Manager*, 26(2):155–158, 2007.

Rogers, A.E.: The effects of fatigue and sleepiness on nurse performance and patient safety. In R.G. Hughes (Ed.): *Patient safety and quality: An evidence-based handbook for nurses*. Rockville, MD, 2008, Agency for Healthcare Research and Quality.

Sackett, D.L., Straus, S.E., Richardson, W.S., et al.: Evidence-based medicine: How to practice and teach EBM. Edinburgh, 2000, Churchill Livingstone.

Samra, H.A., McGrath, J.M. and Rollins, W.: Patient safety in the NICU: A comprehensive review. *Journal of Perinatal and Neonatal Nursing*, 25(2):123 132, 2011.

Scanlon, M.: The role of "smart" infusion pumps in patient safety. *Pediatric Clinics of North America*, 59:1257–1267, 2012.

Sharek, P.J.: The emergence of the trigger tool as the premier measurement strategy for patient safety. *AHRQ Web M&M*, 2012(5), pii:120, 2012.

Sharek, P.J., Horbar, J.D., Mason, W., et al.: Adverse events in the neonatal intensive care unit: Development, testing, and findings of a NICU-focused trigger tool to identify harm in North American NICUs. *Pediatrics*, 118(4):1332–1340, 2006.

Shekelle, P.G., Morton, S.C. and Keeler, E.B.: Costs and benefits of health information technology. Rockville, MD, 2006, Agency for Healthcare Research and

Quality. Evidence Report/Technology Assessment No. 132.

Siegel, J.D., Rhinehart, E., Jackson, M., et al.: for the Healthcare Infection Control Practices Advisory Committee: 2007 Guideline for isolation precautions: Preventing transmission of infectious agents in healthcare settings. Administrative responsibilities. Atlanta, 2007, Centers for Disease Control and Prevention.

Smith, J.R. and Cole, F.S.: Patient safety: Effective interdisciplinary teamwork through simulation and debriefing in the neonatal ICU. *Critical Care Nursing Clinics of North America*, 21(2):163–179, 2009.

Smith, J.R., Donze, A. and Magliaro, B.: A tool for guiding clinical decisions. *Neonatal Network*, 26(1):63–69, 2007.

Snijders, C., van Lingen, R.A., Klip, H., et al.: for the NEOSAFE Study Group: Specialty-based, voluntary incident reporting in neonatal intensive care: Description of 4846 incident reports. *Archives of Disease in Childhood: Fetal and Neonatal Edition*, 94:F210–F215, 2009.

Snijders, C., van Lingen, R.A., Molendijk, A., et al.: Incidents and errors in neonatal intensive care: A review of the literature. *Archives of Disease in Childhood: Fetal and Neonatal Edition*, 92(5):F391–F398, 2007.

Sorrentino, E. and Alegiani, C.: Medication errors in the neonate. *The Journal of Maternal-Fetal and Neonatal Medicine*, 25(54):91–93, 2012.

Stavroudis, T.A., Shore, A.D., Morlock, L., et al.: NICU medication errors: Identifying a risk profile for medication errors in the neonatal intensive care unit. *Journal of Perinatology*, 30:459–468, 2010.

Stroud, L., Wong, B.W., Hollenberg, E., et al.: Teaching medical error disclosure to physicians-in-training: A scoping review. *Academic Medicine*, 88(6):884–892, 2013.

Stucky, E.R.: American Academy of Pediatrics Committee on Drugs, and American Academy of Pediatrics: Prevention of medication errors in the pediatric inpatient setting. *Pediatrics*, 112(2):431–436, 2003; reaffirmed 2007; retired 2011.

Sundar, E., Sundar, S., Pawlowski, J., et al.: Crew resource management and team training. *Anesthesiology Clinics*, 25(2):283–300, 2007.

Suresh, G., Horbar, J.D., Plsek, P., et al.: Voluntary anonymous reporting of medical errors for neonatal intensive care. *Pediatrics*, 113(6):1609–1618, 2004.

Thomas, E.J., Taggart, B., Crandell, S., et al.: Teaching teamwork during the Neonatal Resuscitation Program: A randomized trial. *Journal of Perinatology*, 27 (7):409–414, 2007.

Ursprung, R. and Gray, J.E.: Random safety auditing, rootcause analysis, failure mode and effects analysis. *Clinics in Perinatology*, 37(1):141–165, 2010.

U.S. Department of Health and Human Services, Health Resources and Services Administration: *The registered nurse population. Findings from the 2008 National Sample Survey of Registered Nurses*, 2008. Retrieved April 24, 2013, from http://bhpr.hrsa.gov/healthworkforce/rnsurveys/rnsurveyfinal.pdf.

Vermont Oxford Network: NICQ 2007: Improvement in action. 2013: In J.D. Horbar, K. Leahy, and J. Handyside (Eds.): *System safety in the NICU* Retrieved May 3, 2013, from http://www.vtoxford.org/quality/ebook/ebook.aspx.

University of Washington, Institute for Simulation and Interprofessional Studies: Research. Retrieved October 8, 2013 from http://www.isis.washington.edu/research.

Walsh, K.E., Landrigan, C.P., Adams, W.G., et al.: Effect of computer order entry on prevention of serious medication errors in hospitalized children. *Pediatrics*, 121(3):e421–e427, 2008.

Wayman, K.I., Yaeger, K.A., Sharek, P.J., et al.: Simulation-based medical error disclosure training for pediatric healthcare professionals. *Journal of Healthcare Quality*, 29(4):12–19, 2007.

White, R.D.: The physical environment of the neonatal intensive care unit: Implications for premature newborns and their care-givers. *Business Briefing US Pediatric Care*, 2005. Retrieved May 10, 2013, from http://www.touchbriefings.com/pdf/1268/White.pdf.

CHAPTER

# 19 Discharge Planning and Transition to Home Care

PAT HUMMEL

**OBJECTIVES**

1. Describe current trends in the discharge of the high-risk infant.
2. Identify individualized clinical criteria for discharge.
3. Discuss the role of the family in the discharge of a high-risk infant.
4. Describe discharge planning and the transition-to-home process for the high-risk neonate.
5. Identify discharge teaching needs for parents of a high-risk infant.
6. Identify key components of infant and family care postdischarge.

## INTRODUCTION

Preterm birth rates have risen more than 20% since 1990. Nearly half a million babies are born preterm each year, and the numbers have risen steadily. The National Center for Health Statistics released final birth data for 2010, revealing that there were 478,790 preterm births; one in eight babies (12% of live births) were born preterm in the United States (Martin et al, 2012).

The preterm birth rate peaked at 12.8% in 2006, and fell slightly to 12% in 2010 (Table 19-1).

- 69% are born between 34 and 36 weeks of gestation, and are termed late-preterm births.
- 14% are born between 32 and 33 weeks of gestation.
- 17% are born at less than 32 weeks of gestation.

The infant mortality rate fell slightly to 6.6 deaths per 1000 live births in 2008, with prematurity the leading cause of death in the first month of life (Table 19-2).

Preterm birth cost the nation more than $26.2 billion in medical and educational costs and lost productivity in 2005. During the same year the average first-year medical costs, including both inpatient and outpatient care, were about 10 times greater for preterm ($32,325) than for term ($3325) infants. Average hospitalization cost between 2001 and 2004 for the moderately preterm infant, born at 32 to 34 weeks, was $31,000 (Kirkby et al., 2007). Many infants are discharged from the neonatal intensive care unit (NICU) with chronic conditions requiring ongoing medical care and increasing societal burden. Major morbidities tend to be highest in the smallest survivors (<1000 g at birth) and can include significant lifelong conditions such as cerebral palsy, cognitive delays, and visual or hearing loss (Wilson-Costello, 2007).

## GENERAL PRINCIPLES

A. **Coordinated, comprehensive discharge planning with a safe transition to home is critical for the health and well-being of high-risk infants and their families.**

B. **Discharge planning begins on admission to the intensive care nursery and continues throughout the hospitalization.**

C. **An interdisciplinary team of skilled professionals ensures successful transition to home (Box 19-1).**

D. **Parent–infant relationships and family dynamics are altered by emotional and financial stressors.** Maternal depression is common and negatively affects the parent–child relationship and infant development (Beck, 2003; Quevedo et al., 2012).

■ TABLE 19-1
■ ■ **Percentage of Preterm Births: United States, Final 1990, 2000, 2005, and 2010; and Preliminary 2011**

| Year | Preterm <37 weeks | Late Preterm 34 to 36 Weeks | 32 to 33 Weeks | Very Preterm <32 weeks |
|---|---|---|---|---|
| 2011 | 11.7 | Not available | Not available | Not available |
| 2010 | 12.0 | 8.3 | 1.70 | 2.0 |
| 2005 | 12.73 | 9.09 | 1.60 | 2.03 |
| 2000 | 11.64 | 8.22 | 1.49 | 1.93 |
| 1990 | 10.61 | 7.30 | 1.40 | 1.92 |

Data from National Center for Health Statistics: *Final natality data.* 2011. Retrieved from www.marchofdimes.com/peristats.

■ TABLE 19-2
■ ■ **Infant Mortality**

| Year | Percentage |
|---|---|
| 1998 | 7.2 |
| 2000 | 6.9 |
| 2005 | 6.9 |
| 2006 | 6.7 |
| 2007 | 6.8 |
| 2008 | 6.6 |

Data from National Center for Health Statistics: *Final mortality data, 1990-1994;* and *Period linked birth/infant death data, 1995-present.* 2008. Retrieved from www.marchofdimes.com/peristats.

■ BOX 19-1
■ **MEMBERS OF INTERDISCIPLINARY DISCHARGE PLANNING/TRANSITION-TO-HOME TEAM**

Parents
Neonatologist/neonatal nurse practitioner (NNP)/resident/bedside nurse
Primary pediatrician
Subspecialty physicians and advanced practice nurses, as applicable
Primary nurse
Social worker
Discharge planning coordinator/case manager
Developmental assessment and early intervention/follow-up team member
Home care nurse
Infant-specific support services as needed: occupational or physical therapist, nutritionist, lactation support, respiratory therapist, pharmacist
Durable medical equipment representative

E. **Parents, as the primary caregivers, must be educated to provide complex care for their infant and be empowered to advocate for their infant, facilitating transition to home and optimizing their child's health and development.**
F. **The medical home model for delivering primary care is particularly important for children with special health care needs.**
G. **The late preterm infant may have special needs at discharge, requiring vigilant follow-up (Whyte, 2010).**

## HEALTH CARE TRENDS

A. **Medical costs are rising rapidly.**
   1. The newborn period is a major source of uncompensated care and accounts for a high proportion of catastrophic cost cases, an increasing problem with the increased incidence and survival of premature infants (Kirkby et al., 2007).
   2. Economic pressures, including equitable reimbursement for services, and the utilization of costly medical resources, continue to challenge health care systems when caring for the very low birth weight (VLBW, $<1000$ g) infant in the hospital and home settings.

B. **Infants are discharged earlier from the NICU, requiring care of varying complexity, from nasogastric feedings, multiple medications, apnea monitors, and oxygen to ventilators, dialysis, and parenteral nutrition.**

C. **Infants are discharged with special needs on the premise that the home environment, as opposed to the hospital environment, is beneficial for the child and the family, and that health care costs will be decreased (Hummel and Cronin, 2004).**

D. **Early discharge of the VLBW infant can be accomplished in a safe and positive manner, benefiting the infant and family (Sajous et al., 2007a, 2007b; Sturm, 2005).**
   1. The infant must be physiologically stable before discharge.
   2. The parents must be able and willing to care for their infant in the home.
   3. Parental education must be complete before discharge, with parents demonstrating competency in the care of the infant.
   4. Skilled home nursing care by neonatal nurses contributes to the successful discharge of the high-risk infant. Sajous et al. (2007a, 2007b) describe an integrated neonatal home care program where preterm infants are discharged home safely to transition from nasogastric to oral feedings, and readmission rates were decreased for infants with bronchopulmonary dysplasia discharged with supplemental oxygen.

E. **Discharge planning includes the role of the case managers, whose roles include care coordination, utilization review, insurance reimbursement, and discharge planning.**

F. **Clinical pathways and care maps are effective tools for discharge planning and tracking outcomes.**

G. **The medical home model for delivering primary care is recognized as optimal in the care of the NICU graduate. The American Academy of Pediatrics developed the medical home model for delivering primary care that is accessible, continuous, comprehensive, family-centered, coordinated, compassionate, and culturally effective to all children and youth, including those with special health care needs.**

H. **NICU design is moving toward private rooms, enhancing family interaction and caregiving, facilitating preparation for discharge.**

I. **Electronic medical records are increasingly used, allowing improved documentation, retrieval, and interdisciplinary communication.**

J. **Evidence-based care is provided in the NICU and home care setting.**
   1. Resources include the Cochrane Neonatal Reviews, the Vermont Oxford Network, and the National Institute of Child Health and Development (NICHD) Neonatal Research Group.
   2. Additional organizations that publish guidelines for transition of the preterm infant to home include the American Academy of Pediatrics (AAP, 2008); the National Association of Neonatal Nurses (1999); Association of Women's Health, Obstetric and Neonatal Nurses; the March of Dimes; and the National Guideline Clearinghouse.

K. **Childhood disability is increasing and emotional, behavioral, and neurologic disabilities are now more prevalent than physical impairments.**
   1. Children and youth with special health care needs are defined by the Maternal and Child Health Bureau (MCHB) of the Department of Health and Human Services, Health Resources and Services Administration as *"those who have or are at increased risk for a chronic physical, development, behavioral, or emotional condition and who also require health and related services of a type or amount beyond that required by children generally."* This definition is broad and inclusive, and it emphasizes the characteristics held in common by children with a wide range of diagnoses (McPherson et al., 1998).

2. Approximately 10.2 million children in the United States, which represents 15% of all U.S. children, have special health care needs based on the MCHB definition.
3. More than a fifth of U.S. households with children have at least one child with special needs (Currie and Kahn, 2012).

## DISCHARGE CRITERIA MUST BE ESTABLISHED AND INDIVIDUALIZED TO THE INFANT AND FAMILY (BOX 19-2)

A. **Careful discharge planning, ensuring medical stability of the infant before discharge, is essential to the successful discharge and home care experience.** Medical stability is essential for a predetermined length of time before discharge. An infant who requires increasing support is not stable for discharge. Response to changes in care may not be apparent immediately in a child with a chronic illness; weaning and other major changes should not occur close to discharge.

B. **The required period of stability before discharge has not been studied or standardized.** Controversy and wide variations in practice exist in the apnea- or bradycardia-free length of time that an infant is observed before discharge (Hummel and Cronin, 2004; Zupancic et al., 2003). Discharge of a technology-dependent infant should be anticipated and planned, with the team agreeing on an end point and a stability point for discharge (Hummel and Cronin, 2004). Support should then be maintained and the infant prepared for discharge without changes.

C. **Assessment of the home and parental capabilities guide a safe discharge.** A multitude of factors contribute to the ability of a family to care for a medically complex infant in the home. Parent health, siblings, family support, financial difficulties, home facilities, proximity to health care, transportation options, child care or day care considerations, and other issues may prohibit discharge to the parent's home. Infant and parent needs must be balanced to achieve a safe discharge.

## PARENTAL NEEDS AND ROLE IN THE DISCHARGE AND TRANSITION-TO-HOME PROCESS

A. **Parents need emotional support as they struggle to cope with the ups and downs and uncertainties that accompany parenting an ill newborn (Eiser et al., 2005).** Social work, pastoral care, and parent-to-parent support groups may benefit parents and should be tailored to meet

### BOX 19-2
### INFANT READINESS FOR HOSPITAL DISCHARGE

- Sustained pattern of weight gain of sufficient duration.
- Adequate maintenance of normal body temperature.
- Competent feeding by breast or bottle without cardiorespiratory compromise.
- Physiologic maturity and stable cardiorespiratory function of sufficient duration.
- Appropriate immunizations administered.
- Appropriate metabolic screening performed.
- Hematologic status assessed and appropriate therapy instituted if indicated.
- Nutrition risks assessed and therapy and dietary modifications instituted if indicated.
- Hearing evaluation complete.
- Funduscopic examinations complete.
- Neurodevelopmental and neurobehavioral status assessed and demonstrated to parents.
- Car seat evaluation complete.
- Review of hospital course complete, unresolved medical problems identified, plans for follow-up monitoring and treatment instituted.
- Home care plan developed.

From The American Academy of Pediatrics, Committee on Fetus and Newborn: Hospital discharge of the high-risk neonate. *Pediatrics*, 122(5):1119-1126, 2008.

the family's needs. March of Dimes provides parent support online; local chapters may also provide support groups.

B. **Parenting an infant after discharge from the NICU presents many challenges, including multiple physician appointments, complex infant care, and the uncertainties of the infant's future (Bakewell-Sachs and Gennaro, 2004; Hummel and Cronin, 2004).** Effective interventions to promote mothering the high-risk infant include home nurse visits, skin-to-skin contact, individual infant-focused education and counseling, and theory-based group intervention (Gardner and Deatrick, 2006).

C. **Postpartum depression is common and exacerbated by mothering a high-risk infant (Beck and Indman, 2005).** NICU and home care nurses must remain vigilant, referring mothers for further care when depression is recognized (Beck, 2003, 2008a, 2008b).

D. **Cultural differences should be considered, as some cultures may expect that the infant stay in the hospital until the special needs are resolved.**

E. **The family is the constant in the infant's life and should be an active participant in care, starting at admission.** Continuing parental education involves assessment of knowledge and readiness to learn. Most parents desire an understanding of their infant's disease process and status. Caregivers should assist parents in learning their infant's behaviors and providing individualized care based on the responses (Cook et al., 2012; Heermann et al., 2005; Kleberg et al., 2007; Meijssen et al., 2011; Vandenberg, 2007; Westrup, 2007). Parents learn about parenting by observing caregivers and actively participating in their infant's care.

F. **Assessment of parental knowledge base and previous infant care experience contributes to an individualized teaching plan, established weeks prior to anticipated discharge.** Family educational, social, emotional, and financial needs must be assessed; discharge plans are individualized according to these needs (Giebe, 2007).
   1. Barriers to parental learning and participation in care need to be assessed and resources identified to alleviate the barriers. Recognition of parental needs and addressing each area in the discharge plan will ease the transition to home. Current caregiver knowledge level is assessed prior to teaching sessions, and each session is individualized according to the needs of the infant and family.
   2. Learning experiences can be offered through hands-on care, demonstration of specific care practices, and verbal reinforcement. Information can be obtained from a variety of sources, including individual demonstration, group teaching sessions with other parents, published teaching tools, videos, written materials, and Internet resources.

G. **Parents are active participants in care conferences and involved in discharge planning.**

H. **Parents should contact and meet a health care provider in the community and make follow-up appointments prior to the infant's discharge from the hospital.** The case manager, social worker, discharge coordinator, staff registered nurse, or advanced practice nurse can assist with the process. The health care provider should be capable of providing a medical home for the infant with special health care needs.

I. **Parents should be provided an opportunity to care for their infant in an overnight/transition room prior to discharge.** This is particularly important when the care is complex or questions remain regarding parental capabilities in caring for the infant.

## DISCHARGE PLANNING AND TRANSITION TO HOME

A. **Discharge planning begins at birth or when the infant's condition is no longer critical.**
   1. A long-term view of the infant's hospitalization is essential to discharge planning.
   2. A care map may assist in this process by cueing the team at specific intervals to plan for discharge.
   3. See Table 19-3 for planning for discharge with technology, related to complex medical issues.

B. **Discharge teaching should begin weeks prior to the projected discharge date.**
   1. Discharge education and home transition plans should be clearly outlined (Fig. 19-1).
   2. Planning should include a timeline to complete parent education and all steps necessary for home transition.

■ TABLE 19-3
■ ■ **Planning for Discharge With Technology**

| Potential Technology | Stability Criteria | Diagnosis/ Problem | Teaching Required | Home Nursing Needs | Supplemental Services |
|---|---|---|---|---|---|
| Oxygen<br>Apnea monitor<br>Pulse oximeter | Stable oxygen flow without changes for a defined number of days prior to discharge (varies from 5 to 10 days, per unit discretion) | BPD<br>Other CLD | Signs or symptoms of respiratory distress<br>DME<br>CPR demonstration<br>Medication administration | Intermittent skilled nursing visits | Occupational and physical therapy<br>Speech therapy<br>Nutrition |
| Nasogastric or gastrostomy tube feedings | Stable pattern of weight gain (15 to 30 g/day) | FTT<br>Severe GERD<br>Oral aversion | Nasogastric tube placement<br>Gastrostomy tube care<br>Tube feedings<br>High-caloric formula preparation<br>Bolus (gravity feedings)<br>Pump feedings | Intermittent skilled nursing visits | Speech therapy<br>Nutrition |
| Apnea monitor | Free of apnea/ bradycardia events requiring intervention, beyond gentle, tactile stimulation, for a defined number of days prior to discharge (varies from 2 to 7 days, per unit discretion) | Apnea of prematurity<br>GERD<br>Intrauterine growth restriction | DME<br>CPR demonstration<br>Medication administration<br>Thickened formula as ordered<br>Positioning | Intermittent skilled nursing visits | |
| Tracheostomy (with or without gastrostomy tube) | Stable oxygen requirement (room air or trach collar) | BPD<br>Pierre Robin syndrome<br>Tracheomalacia<br>Various disorders affecting airway competence | Signs or symptoms of respiratory distress<br>DME<br>CPR demonstration<br>Medication administration<br>Suction equipment<br>Tracheostomy change | Private duty nursing (approximately 8 hours/day) | Speech therapy<br>Occupational or physical therapy<br>Respiratory therapy (usually provided by DME vendor) |

■ TABLE 19-3
■ ■ **Planning for Discharge With Technology—cont'd**

| Potential Technology | Stability Criteria | Diagnosis/ Problem | Teaching Required | Home Nursing Needs | Supplemental Services |
|---|---|---|---|---|---|
| Ventilator | Stable respiratory condition without changes in ventilator support* or medication for an agreed-upon period prior to discharge (varies from 2 to 4 weeks, per unit discretion) | BPD<br>Central hypoventilation | Signs or symptoms of respiratory distress<br>DME<br>CPR demonstration<br>Medication administration<br>Gastrostomy tube placement and feeds<br>High-caloric formula preparation<br>Ventilator problem solving<br>Ventilator setting adjustments | Private duty nursing (approximately 12 to 24 hours/ day) | Occupational or physical therapy<br>Speech therapy<br>Respiratory therapy (usually provided by DME vendor)<br>Nutrition<br>Apply for handicapped parking permit |

*BPD*, Bronchopulmonary dysplasia; *CPR*, cardiopulmonary resuscitation; *CLD*, chronic lung disease; *DME*, durable medical equipment; *FTT*, failure to thrive; *GERD*, gastroesophageal reflux disease.
*Using a ventilator approved for in-home use.

3. Written information regarding the infant's care should be provided, particularly with complex discharges (Menghini, 2005).

C. **Family members are active participants in the home transition plan.** Parents should participate in infant care from birth and are essential team members in the care of their infant.

D. **Discharge planning and the transition-to-home process require a multidisciplinary approach.** Consistency in care providers is critical. Parents should be empowered to make decisions about their infant's care and discharge. The case manager, discharge planner, primary nurse, and social worker often coordinate the discharge process.

E. **Intermittent care conferences with the family throughout hospitalization ensure open communication, facilitating a smooth transition to home.** These can be formalized, including all team members, or simplified to include the parents and a few key team members.

F. **A comprehensive discharge-focused care conference should be completed several weeks prior to discharge.**
1. Parents are encouraged to bring a list of questions and needs to the conference.
2. All community providers should be invited to participate in the discharge care conference. If key personnel are unable to attend this conference, contact should be made to ensure that the practitioner is willing to care for the infant, and to communicate ongoing health issues and needs.
3. Criteria for discharge are discussed and the teaching plan is reviewed. The anticipated course of recovery and ongoing problems are outlined, and the home care/durable medical equipment needs are discussed.
4. Strategies to prevent rehospitalization are discussed (Smith et al., 2004).

G. **A comprehensive discharge summary, including resolved and ongoing problems, is given to the family on discharge, and sent to postdischarge caregivers.** See Box 19-3 for a list of

**NEONATAL DISCHARGE CHECKLIST**

***Things to do 1 week before discharge:***

- Mother's maiden name ____________
- Father's name ____________
- Pediatrician's name and phone number ____________
  ***Remind parents with HMOs that they need a referral from their primary physician for any specialty appointments.*
- Prescriptions (including for specialty formulas such as Neocate, Elecare, Pregestimil, Neosure, Enfacare) ____________
- Car seat testing ____________
- WIC form (if needed) ____________
- Home health equipment (DME) form/order and training scheduled (by Case Manager or Social Worker) ____________

***Things to do 1–3 days before discharge:***

- Blood pressure ____________
- Head circumference ____________
- Chest circumference ____________
- Weight ____________
- Length ____________
- Newborn screen ____________
- Appointments ____________
- Home health referral (if needed) ____________
- Discharge follow-up instructions ____________
- Medication schedule ____________

***Things to do the day of discharge:***

- Delayed infant discharge form (if infant is discharged home with mother) ____________
- Release of patient to person other than natural mother form (if infant is discharged home without mother) ____________
- EPIC discharge note ____________

***Things to send home with parents:***

- Gift pack
- Patient's belongings
- Digital thermometer
- Bulb syringe
- Oral medication syringes
- Additional supplies if necessary
- Discharge folder to include the following:
  - ☐ Discharge instructions
  - ☐ Scheduled appointments
  - ☐ Medication schedule
  - ☐ Medication teaching sheets
  - ☐ Formula preparation sheets
  - ☐ Completed immunization card
  - ☐ Admission and discharge summaries for parents
  - ☐ Additional teaching materials as needed

FIGURE 19-1 ■ Neonatal Discharge Checklist. (Copyright Loyola University Medical Center, Maywood, Ill.)

information to be included in the summary. An electronic summary and information can be provided on a disc or flash drive for computerized use.

**H. Infant care specifics to be completed prior to discharge includes:**

1. Perform parent and home evaluation, which may include a home visit if the infant has extensive needs.
2. Establish a realistic plan for care at home, including feeding schedules, medication schedules, and treatments.
3. Medications: Provide prescriptions several days before discharge for parents to fill and bring to the hospital for verification and teaching.
   a. Some medications need to be compounded by the pharmacy and may not be immediately available.

■ BOX 19-3
■ **PERTINENT INFORMATION FOR PARENTS AND CARE PROVIDERS AT TIME OF DISCHARGE**

Comprehensive discharge summary, including resolved and ongoing problems
List of follow-up appointments with timing, location, and phone numbers specified
Immunizations given
Respiratory syncytial virus (RSV) prophylaxis given
Written plan of care, particularly for complex discharge (could be electronic)
Medication schedule
Nutrition plan and formula recipe
Testing/imaging results: head ultrasound, renal ultrasound; computed tomography (CT), electroencephalogram (EEG), electrocardiogram (ECG); echocardiogram, magnetic resonance imaging (MRI), other pertinent testing
Additional test results such as pneumograms/sleep studies, eye examination findings, hearing screen results, newborn metabolic/state screen results
Pertinent laboratory values: recent complete blood count with hematocrit, hemoglobin, and reticulocyte count; bone health; medication levels

4. Assess that the parent is able to afford the medication.
5. Ensure that the medication is ordered and filled with the correct concentration, and that the container is properly labeled. Problems also occur when the generic name is used on the bottle and the trade name is mentioned in the medication list—be sure names match, or provide both names.
6. Round home medication doses to the nearest 1/10 (0.1) mL (except in extraordinary circumstances) to reduce the chance for error.
7. Verify that the medication label and instructions are documented in milliliters to be given, not with milligrams only.
8. Complete a medication sheet for home use, providing dosing and timing of each medication.

I. **Feeding/formula (Cooke, 2007; Pridham et al., 2004).**
   1. Facilitate acquisition of a high-quality breast pump early in hospitalization.
   2. Encourage breastfeeding; provide lactation consultation to promote continued breastfeeding and/or pumping of breast milk (Ayton et al., 2012; Isaacson, 2006; Vohr et al., 2006).
   3. Optimal nutrition is essential for improving developmental outcomes in preterm infants. Special formulas providing increased caloric and nutrient density are frequently necessary (Lapillonne et al., 2013; Tudehope et al., 2012).
   4. Provide prescriptions for formulas well before discharge. Special formulas may be difficult to find in the store and may need to be ordered.
   5. The Women, Infants, and Children (WIC) nutritional program may not provide special formulas, or may not provide enough formula for the infant's needs; this should be ascertained well before discharge.
   6. Assess the parent's ability to buy formula, especially expensive elemental formulas; provide assistance as needed with letters of necessity for payor coverage.
   7. Primary care practitioner chosen and follow-up appointments are made.
   8. Subspecialty appointments are made.
   9. Home care agency/nursing care ordered and arranged.
   10. Durable medical equipment ordered and teaching sessions arranged.
   11. Arrange circumcision per parental choice.
   12. Parents and all caregivers complete infant cardiopulmonary resuscitation (CPR) class.
   13. Audiology testing.
   14. Safe sleep practices are in place (Box 19-4).
   15. Car seat testing is completed (Box 19-5).
   16. Overnight stay in the transition room.
   17. Respite care is explored, including strategies to deal with stress.
   18. Emergency plan is formulated.

■ BOX 19-4
■ **SAFE SLEEP GUIDELINES**

1. Place infants to sleep on their backs, even though they may sleep more soundly on their stomachs. Infants who sleep on their stomachs and sides have a much higher rate of sudden infant death syndrome (SIDS) than infants who sleep on their backs.
2. Place infants to sleep in a baby bed with a firm mattress. There should be nothing in the bed but the baby—no covers, no pillows, no bumper pads, no positioning devices, and no toys. Soft mattresses and heavy covering are associated with the risk for SIDS.
3. Keep your baby's crib in the parents' room until the infant is at least 6 months of age. Studies clearly show that infants are safest when their beds are close to their mothers.
4. Do not place your baby to sleep in an adult bed. Typical adult beds are not safe for babies. Do not fall asleep with your baby on a couch or in a chair.
5. Do not overclothe the sleeping infant. Just use enough clothes to keep the baby warm without having to use cover. Keep the room at a temperature that is comfortable for you. Overheating an infant may increase the risk for SIDS.
6. Avoid exposing the infant to tobacco smoke. Don't have your infant in the same house or car with someone who is smoking. The greater the exposure to tobacco smoke, the greater the risk of SIDS.
7. Breastfeed babies whenever possible. Breast milk decreases the occurrence of respiratory and gastrointestinal infections. Studies show that breastfed babies have a lower SIDS rate than formula-fed babies do.
8. Avoid exposing the infant to people with respiratory infections. Avoid crowds. Carefully clean anything that comes in contact with the baby. Have people wash their hands before holding or playing with your baby. SIDS often occurs in association with relatively minor respiratory (mild cold) and gastrointestinal infections (vomiting and diarrhea).
9. Offer your baby a pacifier. Some studies have shown a lower rate of SIDS among babies who use pacifiers.
10. If your baby has periods of not breathing, going limp or turning blue, tell your pediatrician at once.
11. If your baby stops breathing or gags excessively after spitting up, discuss this with your pediatrician immediately.
12. Thoroughly discuss each of the above points with all caregivers. If you take your baby to daycare or leave him with a sitter, provide a copy of this list to them. Make sure they follow all recommendations.



■ BOX 19-5
■ **CAR SEAT GUIDELINES AND TESTING**

Discharge policies for newborns should include the following:

1. Determination of the most appropriate car safety seat for each newborn according to maturity and medical condition by a designated hospital employee.
2. Provision of information and training for parents and guardians should be presented before discharge on the generic issues related to correct use of car safety seats. Hands-on teaching including "return demonstration" should be a part of this instruction. The installation of a specific car seat in a specific car must be the parent's responsibility. Resources to address these issues are available from the AAP.
3. Increased frequency of oxygen desaturation and episodes of apnea or bradycardia while sitting in car safety seats suggests that preterm infants should have a period of observation in a car safety seat, preferably their own, before hospital discharge. This period of observation should be performed with the infant carefully positioned for optimal restraint and the car safety seat placed at an angle that is approved for use in the vehicle. A period of observation for a minimum of 90 to 120 minutes or the duration of travel, whichever is longer, is suggested. Hospitals should develop protocols to include car safety seat observation before discharge for infants born at less than 37 weeks of gestation. Protocols may also include testing for older at-risk infants such as those with hypotonia, micrognathia (Pierre Robin sequence), and infants who have undergone congenital heart surgery. Additional information is available at the AAP website, www.aap.org.

From Bull, M.J., Engle, W.A., Committee on Injury, Violence, and Poison Prevention and Committee on Fetus and Newborn, American Academy of Pediatrics: Safe transportation of preterm and low birth weight infants at hospital discharge. *Pediatrics*, 123(5):1424-1429, 2009.

J. **Selection of a primary health care practitioner, home nursing agency, and durable medical equipment company that will meet the needs of the infant and the family.**
   1. The discharge team should ideally be able to recommend a primary health care practitioner who is willing and able to care for the infant's complex medical needs (Kelly, 2006b). Parental requests and third-party payor restraints should be equally considered in this process. Ideally, parents should meet with the primary health care practitioner before discharge. Identify home nursing needs—intermittent or private duty.
   2. Plan home care after verification of third-party payor requirements and restraints.
   3. Home care personnel should be familiar with the infant's medical issues, with skilled, experienced personnel available for home visitation. An example of a successful home care program in place for more than 10 years includes NICU nurses cross-trained to provide intermittent home care nursing visits (Sajous et al., 2007a, 2007b).
   4. Criteria for selecting a durable medical equipment agency include the following (Gracey et al., 2004):
      a. Third-party payor restraints.
      b. Availability of appropriate supplies.
      c. Ability to respond to emergencies.
      d. Availability of back-up equipment.
      e. Experience of care providers.
      f. Location of the agency.

K. **Discharge to an alternative setting may be necessary because of medical necessity, social problems, or family dynamics.** If the NICU and parents are unable to coordinate and complete the discharge process, transfer to an interim facility that routinely transitions children with special needs into the home, or a facility geographically closer to the parent, may be optimal.
   1. Alternatives vary but can include specialized foster care, pediatric rehabilitation hospitals, pediatric nursing homes, or inpatient hospice care.
   2. Verify that the facility is able to provide care that meets the infant's needs, and that the costs are covered by third-party payors or through state Medicaid waivers.
   3. Parents should visit the facility prior to transfer. The parent should feel confident that the facility will provide appropriate, safe, and competent care for their child. Optimally, the parent should speak with another parent whose child received care currently or previously in the facility.

## NEONATAL TEACHING NEEDS

Teaching should be incorporated throughout the infant's stay. Written materials should be provided as much as possible, written at the sixth-grade reading level (Menghini, 2005). Teaching topics to be completed prior to discharge include the following:

A. **Back to sleep/safe sleep practices** (see Box 19-4).

B. **Car seat use.**

C. **Shaken baby syndrome prevention (Box 19-6).**

D. **Infant CPR training**
   1. Parents and other caregivers should be encouraged to attend an infant CPR class, often taught by a CPR nurse instructor, individually or in groups prior to discharge.
   2. The AAP, in coordination with the American Heart Association and using the technology of Laerdal Medical, developed *Infant CPR Anytime*, which contains everything needed for a lay individual to learn infant CPR and relief of choking. This is a self-directed learning product that allows those caring for infants to learn the core skills of infant CPR and relief of choking in just 22 minutes. For more information: http://www2.aap.org/family/infantcpranytime.htm.

E. **Basic infant care practices such as bathing, feeding, and diapering.**

F. **Medication teaching:**
   1. Observe the parent drawing up the medication.
   2. Provide a medication schedule, avoiding medication administration more than 3 times daily, and avoid nighttime dosing.

**BOX 19-6**
**SHAKEN BABY PREVENTION**

### What Is Shaken Baby Syndrome?

Shaken Baby Syndrome/Abusive Head Trauma (SBS/AHT) is a term used to describe a collection of signs and symptoms resulting from violent shaking or shaking and impacting of the head of an infant or small child. When a baby is vigorously shaken, the head moves back and forth. This sudden whiplash motion may or may not include a blow to the head, but does lead to a distinct pattern of injuries. Shaken Baby Syndrome occurs most frequently in infants younger than six months old, yet can occur up to the age of three. Although there are often no obvious outward signs of injury, serious bleeding may occur, particularly inside the head or behind the eyes. In reality, shaking a baby, if only for a few seconds, can injure the baby for life. These injuries can include brain swelling and damage, cerebral palsy, mental retardation, developmental delays, blindness, hearing loss, paralysis, or death.

Abusive head injuries are the most common cause of death in child abuse. These injuries are most common in infants under one year old, but the same injuries can be seen in children as old as age 4 or 5 years.

### How Does It Happen?

Everyone knows that babies cry, however medical research has shown that there is a time during an infant's first few weeks that crying becomes more intense, prolonged, and at times very difficult to soothe. This is recognized as a normal phase of infant development. Although normal, this inconsolable crying can become extremely challenging for parents. Often frustrated parents or other persons responsible for a child's care feel that shaking a baby is a harmless way to make a child stop crying. Professionals now feel that crying leads to most early traumatic brain injury or Shaken Baby Syndrome. About 25 percent of babies diagnosed with Shaken Baby Syndrome die.

### What Can You Do to Prevent a Tragedy?

If you or someone else shakes a baby, either accidentally or on purpose, call 9-1-1 or take the child to the emergency room immediately. Bleeding inside the brain can be treated. Immediate medical attention will save your baby many future problems . . . and possibly the baby's life.

### Other Suggestions for Parents

- Never throw or shake a baby
- Always provide support for the baby's head and neck
- Place the baby in a crib, leave the room for a few minutes
- Sit down, close your eyes and count to 20
- When you are frustrated, take time to calm yourself first
- Take a few slow, deep breaths
- Ask a friend to "take over" for a while
- Do not pick the baby up until you feel calm
- Take the baby for a stroller ride
- Play music, or sing to the baby
- Check for discomfort of diaper rash, teething, or fever
- Call the doctor if you think the baby is sick
- Make sure the baby is fed, burped, and dry
- Gently rock or walk the baby
- Offer a noisy toy or rattle
- Hug and cuddle the baby gently
- Make sure clothing is not too tight
- Give the baby a pacifier

From National Exchange Club Foundation: *National shaken baby syndrome campaign.* 2012. Retrieved from www.preventchildabuse.com/sbs.shtml.

3. Schedule medications carefully, as some medications cannot be mixed together or given concurrently.

G. **Formula/feeding teaching:**
1. Observe the parent mixing the formula—verify that the parent has correct measuring cups/spoons, blender, pitcher; these may need to be provided.
2. Written recipes for mixing formulas should be provided.
3. Observe parent feeding the infant, oral or by nasogastric or gastrostomy tube (Gracey and Morton, 2002; Thomas, 2007).

H. **Home oxygen teaching (Gracey et al., 2003):**
1. Hospital flow is usually in decimals (0.25 L/min), home flowmeters are in fractions (¼ L/min). Clarify hospital flow rate and verify in the home. Oxygen flow in the hospital should be rounded up to the next home flowmeter setting; increase, rather than decrease the oxygen flow in the home.
2. Increased flow may be needed in the home because of the long tubing, or when using a concentrator since the output is of slightly lower concentration than that from the tank.

3. Clarify that the parent knows how to adjust oxygen in case of an emergency; parents may think that they are increasing the oxygen when they are turning the flow ½ to ¼ L/min, since the denominator number is larger.

**I. Apnea monitor teaching:**
1. Monitor use, troubleshooting.
2. Alarm response and CPR.
3. Parents may remove the monitor when they are directly attending to the infant.

**J. Specialized teaching topics such as tracheostomy care, suctioning, ventilator, ostomy care, central line care, feeding alternatives, and any special equipment (Fiske, 2004).**
1. www.tracheostomy.com.
2. http://www.oley.org/links.html: education, outreach, and networking for those requiring home IV and tube feeding.

**K. Anticipatory guidance, educating parents regarding expectations postdischarge and tips on adapting to home (Box 19-7).**

**L. Infection prevention (Box 19-8).**

BOX 19-7
**TIPS FOR PARENTS**

**Home Readiness for Special-Needs Infant**
Place for infant to sleep safely
Car seat
Heat, electricity, telephone, running water
Normal baby supplies: diapers, clothing, bottles
Formula, measuring cups and spoons, blender, pitcher
Medications and syringes
Equipment—monitor, oxygen, etc.
Emergency phone numbers and plan
Flashlight with extra batteries
Thermometer and bulb syringe (provided on discharge)
Pediatrician appointment arranged within 1 week
Other appointments made before discharge

**Take Care of Yourself**
Ask for help, from family, friends, and health care providers.
Depression is common, get treatment—you want to be the best parent you can be.
Enjoy your infant.

**Infant Adjusting to the Home**
Realize that your baby will notice a difference in surroundings.
Try to get into a routine.
The baby may sleep better initially if there is a constant background noise (fan, soft music). Try to gradually lower the volume until your baby can sleep without noise.
Put your baby in bed when awake, when possible; allow him or her to learn how to get to sleep rather than depending on you. This will help with sleeping through the night.
Some babies cry more in the evening because they have received too much stimulation during the day—try decreasing the noise and activity throughout the day.

**Helping Your Infant Grow and Develop**
Hold your baby and respond to cries. Do not hold your baby constantly. Short periods of crying are fine if he or she is not hungry, or needs other attention. This helps your baby learn that you are there for him or her, but that she or he can also calm herself or himself.
Talk to your baby often.
Read books to your baby.
Turn off the television and videos—these hurt your baby's ability to pay attention for longer periods, and decrease their ability to calm themselves. Children should not watch TV until they are 2 years old.
Get therapies for your baby as the NICU or care provider recommends. Many infants need extra help for development. Therapies help your baby to develop the best he or she can, and therapy keeps your baby from developing or keeping abnormal developmental skills.
Avoid walkers, exersaucers, jumpers. These place a baby upright before they are ready and keep the baby from developing normally.
Babies need as much time as possible on their tummy, on a firm surface (playpen, floor), when they are awake and you are with them.
Make feeding time pleasant. Do not force-feed your baby. Ask for help if you have problems feeding your baby.

**Websites and Social Media for Parents**
www.preemies.org
www.prematurity.org
www.preemiecare.org/supportgroups.htm
www.nicuparentsupport.org
www.tracheostomy.com
www.facebook.com/lifeafterNICU

**BOX 19-8**
**INFECTION PREVENTION AFTER DISCHARGE**

Routine infant immunizations
Respiratory syncytial virus (RSV) protection: monthly injections November through March for certain preterm infants
Influenza injections: for infants more than 6 months old, given in the fall in two doses 1 month apart
Influenza injections: for all caregivers, all people in the home
Handwashing—the best method to prevent infection
Disinfectant hand gels used by caregivers
Avoid contact with ill people, especially children

M. **Infant temperament, developmental tasks, and milestones reviewed, including sleep patterns, feeding patterns, and infant state regulation.**
N. **Care issues such as vaccinations, traveling, and visitors should be reviewed.**

## FAMILY AND INFANT CARE POSTDISCHARGE (BOX 19-9)

A. **A successful discharge plan and transition to home facilitates collaborative care postdischarge.**
   1. Encourage the parents to choose a pediatrician or health care provider that has experience with the ongoing problems of premature infants (Kelly, 2006a). Coordination of care is essential for infants with complex medical needs and should be approached comprehensively and systematically.
   2. Primary health care provider and specialty follow-up appointments need to be coordinated and scheduled without conflicts, with the infant and family in mind. Medically complex infants can have four or more specialist appointments in addition to a primary care provider.
   3. Transportation should be planned for visits to the primary provider and subspecialists after discharge.
   4. Ongoing assessment and assistance with family financial needs should be addressed before discharge, with referrals to the appropriate agencies (i.e., WIC, Social Security, state governmental assistance, private charities). Families should be aware of community resources available to them, such as early intervention services, case management services, counseling, and transportation assistance. Volunteer agencies, local and national parent support groups, and Internet resources may be recommended, as appropriate.
   5. Immunizations, including respiratory syncytial virus (RSV) prophylaxis, are arranged for postdischarge care.
   6. Routine follow-up phone calls after discharge from the NICU can help with the transition and improve the discharge process as identified problems are addressed.

B. **Home care nursing may include intermittent home visits or in-home care for infants requiring complex around-the-clock care.**
   1. Transition from high-tech hospital setting to home environment may be facilitated by home care nursing.
   2. It is helpful if the home care nurse has met with the parents and infant before hospital discharge.
   3. The home care nurse reinforces the teaching and clarifies discharge instructions as needed.
   4. Intermittent home care is useful for infants who are medically stable, with parents able to provide care 24 hours a day without in-home direct nursing care. The home nurse assesses the infant, educates the parent, monitors medications and feedings, and communicates with the medical provider and the payor. Status updates are provided to the medical provider and a plan of care is formed in conjunction with the multidisciplinary team. The nurse assesses responses to changes in care on subsequent visits. Intermittent nursing visits conclude when the parent is independent with care and when the infant is stable medically and nutritionally, is not home-bound, and does not require frequent monitoring.
   5. Continuous in-home nursing care is another form of home care reserved for infants with complex needs that the parents cannot manage 24 hours a day. Continuous nursing care

■ BOX 19-9
■ **PREMATURITY-RELATED PROBLEMS THAT PRESENT OR CONTINUE AFTER DISCHARGE**

**Respiratory**
Ongoing oxygen dependency
Apnea
Reactive airway disease
Infections

**Cardiac**
Right ventricular hypertrophy
Cor pulmonale/pulmonary hypertension
Uncorrected congenital heart disease with cyanosis and/or congestive heart failure

**Gastrointestinal**
Emesis
Gastroesophageal reflux
Constipation
Strictures and bowel obstruction
Hernias (umbilical and inguinal)

**Nutritional**
Slow growth
Weight less than the 10th percentile on preterm growth curve
Feeding fatigue
Oral aversion
Need for nutritional supplements or hypercaloric formula
Need for adjunct feeding devices (e.g., tube feeding or gastrostomy)

**Hematologic**
Anemia

**Dentition**
Delayed tooth eruption
Altered oral and dental structures with arched palate secondary to dolichocephaly, exacerbated by prolonged oral intubation
Enamel defects

**Sensory**
Visual deficits secondary to retinopathy of prematurity (ROP): myopia, hyperopia, blindness
Strabismus and amblyopia
Cortical blindness
Hearing deficits
Speech and language delays
Hydrocephalus, ongoing shunt problems, such as infection and blockage

**Central Nervous System and Neurodevelopmental Differences**
Difficult temperament and behavior
Sensory integration problems
Tone and movement abnormalities
Cerebral palsy
IQ deficiencies
Learning disabilities
Attention deficits
School problems

is usually required for infants with a tracheostomy or home ventilation, or an infant requiring constant monitoring or care owing to special medical or nursing needs. Continuous nursing care may be provided 24 hours a day, or in shorter segments as needed. Twenty-four-hour-per-day nursing care is rarely possible because of financial and staffing constraints.

6. The primary long-term goal of home care nursing is to foster independence. This is achieved by educating the parent and by facilitating resource use and support services.

C. **Links to community agencies and resources facilitate coping with the changing needs of the child.**
   1. These links can start before discharge and are facilitated by the home care nurse and the primary provider.
   2. Parents caring for ventilated children at home report that their lives are highly complicated and frequently overwhelming. They also reported deep enrichments and rewarding experiences (Carnevale et al., 2006).

D. **Problems related to prematurity often continue after discharge from the NICU (Gracey et al., 2003; Stoll et al., 2010).** Hospital readmissions are not uncommon. Parents need education to recognize risk factors leading to readmission to the hospital and for the potential for ongoing problems (Kelly, 2006a, 2006b).

E. **Neurologic, developmental, neurosensory, and functional morbidities increase with decreasing birth weight.** Risk factors significantly associated with increased neurodevelopmental morbidity include a complicated NICU course, intracranial hemorrhage or cysts, and ongoing chronic illnesses such as bronchopulmonary dysplasia (Broitman et al., 2007;

Fanaroff et al., 2003; Kobaly et al., 2008; Stoll et al., 2010). Preterm infants have a higher incidence of cerebral palsy, mental retardation, and disorders of cortical function, including language disorders, visual perception problems, attention deficits, and learning disabilities. In addition, many infants less than 1000 g at birth have weights at less than the 10th percentile at 36 weeks of postmenstrual age. Particular attention needs to be focused on postnatal growth and developmental assessment postdischarge.

F. **Referrals to a developmental follow-up clinic and to the state early intervention program are essential components of follow-up care.** Follow-up clinics often have criteria that qualify the infant for inclusion, such as gestational age, birth weight, neurologic abnormalities, or other risk factors. The goals of the follow-up clinic include early identification of developmental disability, parent counseling (anticipatory guidance), and identification and treatment of medical complications, along with providing outcome data for the NICU. Clinics are usually staffed by a multidisciplinary team of professionals, including physician, nurse practitioner, occupational therapist, physical therapist, audiologist, psychologist, ophthalmologist, speech and language specialist, respiratory therapist, nutritionist, neurologist, and subspecialists. The first visit usually occurs 1 to 4 months after discharge; follow-up continues for months to years. The goals of a follow-up program may include the following:
   1. Developmental assessment, screening and/or diagnostic, is essential for the infant's well-being and for evaluation of NICU outcomes.
   2. Management of sequelae.
   3. Consultant follow-up assessment.
   4. Parent support.
   5. Early intervention (EI) services: A federal mandate requires that each state provide services up to the age of 3 years. The goal of EI is to enhance the development of infants and toddlers with disabilities and to minimize their potential for developmental delay. Each state establishes criteria for eligibility within parameters set by the federal government.
      a. Many infants discharged from the NICU will meet criteria for early intervention.
      b. Qualifying infants should be referred before discharge. Optimally, EI personnel would meet with the family before discharge, working with the NICU therapists and the follow-up clinic.
      c. Services may include screening and assessment, family training, counseling, home therapies (speech therapy; physical therapy, occupational therapy), psychological services, audiology services, vision services, social work services, and transportation.

G. **Palliative and hospice care**
   1. Infants with life-limiting conditions, without hope for a cure or recovery, require shift of the focus of treatment toward maximizing quality of life. End-of-life care, or hospice care, one aspect of palliative care, supports a peaceful, dignified death for the infant and the provision of loving support to the family and health care providers (National Association of Neonatal Nurses, 2010).
   2. Palliative care should be instituted well before discharge. The infant can be transitioned to the home setting or a palliative care/hospice setting. Referral to an agency or facility that is prepared to care for the infant and family should occur well before discharge. NICU personnel work closely with the agency caregivers and planners to ensure a seamless transition to the postdischarge setting.
   3. The End-of-Life Nursing Education Consortium (ELNEC) project is a national education initiative to improve palliative care. The project provides nurses with training in palliative care so they can teach this essential information to nursing students and practicing nurses (American Association of Colleges of Nursing, 2013).

## REFERENCES

American Association of Colleges of Nursing: The End-of-Life Nursing Education Consortium (ELNEC). 2013: Retrieved from www.aacn.nche.edu/elnec.

Ayton, J., Hansen, E., Quinn, S. and Nelson, M.: Factors associated with initiation and exclusive breastfeeding at hospital discharge: Late preterm compared to

37 week gestation mother and infant cohort. *International Breastfeeding Journal*, 7(1):16, 2012.

Bakewell-Sachs, S. and Gennaro, S.: Parenting the post-NICU premature infant. *MCN: American Journal of Maternal Child Nursing*, 29(6):398–403, 2004.

Beck, C.T.: State of the science on postpartum depression: What nurse researchers have contributed—part 1. *MCN: American Journal of Maternal Child Nursing*, 33(2):121–126, 2008a.

Beck, C.T.: State of the science on postpartum depression: What nurse researchers have contributed—part 2. *MCN: American Journal of Maternal Child Nursing*, 33 (3):151–156; quiz 157-158, 2008b.

Beck, C.T.: Recognizing and screening for postpartum depression in mothers of NICU infants. *Advances in Neonatal Care*, 3(1):37–46, 2003.

Beck, C.T. and Indman, P.: The many faces of postpartum depression. *JOGNN: Journal of Obstetric, Gynecologic, & Neonatal Nursing*, 34(5):569–576, 2005.

Broitman, E., Ambalavanan, N., Higgins, R.D., et al.: Clinical data predict neurodevelopmental outcome better than head ultrasound in extremely low birth weight infants. *Journal of Pediatrics*, 151(5):500–505, 2007.

Bull, M.J. and Engle, W.A., Committee on Injury, Violence, and Poison Prevention and Committee on Fetus and Newborn, American Academy of Pediatrics: Safe transportation of preterm and low birth weight infants at hospital discharge. *Pediatrics*, 123 (5):1424–1429, 2009.

Carnevale, F.A., Alexander, E., Davis, M., et al.: Daily living with distress and enrichment: The moral experience of families with ventilator-assisted children at home. *Pediatrics*, 117(1):e48–e60, 2006.

Cook, F., Bayer, J., Le, H.N., et al.: Baby Business: A randomised controlled trial of a universal parenting program that aims to prevent early infant sleep and cry problems and associated parental depression. *BMC Pediatrics*, 12:13, 2012.

Cooke, R.J.: Postdischarge nutrition of preterm infants: More questions than answers. Nestle Nutrition Workshop Series. *Paediatric Programme*, 59:213–224; discussion 224-228, 2007.

Currie, J.M. and Kahn, R.: Children with disabilities: Introducing the issue. *Children with Disabilities*, 22 (1):3–11, 2012.

Eiser, C., Eiser, J.R., Mayhew, A.G. and Gibson, A.T.: Parenting the premature infant: Balancing vulnerability and quality of life. *Journal of Child Psychology & Psychiatry & Allied Disciplines*, 46(11):1169 1177, 2005.

Fanaroff, A.A., Hack, M. and Walsh, M.C.: The NICHD Neonatal Research Network: Changes in practice and outcomes during the first 15 years. *Seminars in Perinatology*, 27(4):281–287, 2003.

Fiske, E.: Effective strategies to prepare infants and families for home tracheostomy care. *Advances in Neonatal Care*, 4(1):42–53, 2004.

Gardner, M.R. and Deatrick, J.A.: Understanding interventions and outcomes in mothers of infants. *Issues in Comprehensive Pediatric Nursing*, 29(1):25–44, 2006.

Giebe, J.M.: Safe discharge for infants with high-risk home environment. *Advances in Neonatal Care*, 7 (4):167–172, 2007.

Gracey, K., Hummel, P. and Cronin, J.: Family teaching toolbox: Choosing a home care provider. *Advances in Neonatal Care*, 4(6):365–366, 2004.

Gracey, K. and Morton, J.A.: Family teaching toolbox: Guide for breastfeeding your premature baby at home. *Advances in Neonatal Care*, 2(5):283–284, 2002.

Gracey, K., Talbot, D., Lankford, R. and Dodge, P.: Family teaching toolbox: Nasal cannula home oxygen. *Advances in Neonatal Care*, 3(2):99–101, 2003.

Heermann, J.A., Wilson, M.E. and Wilhelm, P.A.: Mothers in the NICU: Outsider to partner. *Pediatric Nursing*, 31(3):176–181, 2005.

Hummel, P. and Cronin, J.: Home care of the high-risk infant. *Advances in Neonatal Care*, 4(6):354–364, 2004.

Isaacson, L.J.: Steps to successfully breastfeed the premature infant. *Neonatal Network*, 25(2):77–86, 2006.

Kelly, M.M.: The medically complex premature infant in primary care. *Journal of Pediatric Health Care*, 20 (6):367–373, 2006a.

Kelly, M.M.: Primary care issues for the healthy premature infant. *Journal of Pediatric Health Care*, 20 (5):293–299, 2006b.

Kirkby, S., Greenspan, J.S., Kornhauser, M. and Schneiderman, R.: Clinical outcomes and cost of the moderately preterm infant. *Advances in Neonatal Care*, 7(2):80–87, 2007.

Kleberg, A., Hellstrom-Westas, L. and Widstrom, A.M.: Mothers' perception of Newborn Individualized Developmental Care and Assessment Program (NIDCAP) as compared to conventional care. *Early Human Development*, 83(6):403–411, 2007.

Kobaly, K., Schluchter, M., Minich, N., et al.: Outcomes of extremely low birth weight (<1 kg) and extremely low gestational age (<28 weeks) infants with bronchopulmonary dysplasia: Effects of practice changes in 2000 to 2003. *Pediatrics*, 121(1):73–81, 2008.

Lapillonne, A., O'Connor, D.L., Wang, D. and Rigo, J.: Nutritional recommendations for the late-preterm infant and the preterm infant after hospital discharge. *Journal of Pediatrics*, 162(3 Suppl.):S90–S100, 2013.

Martin, J.A., Hamilton, B.E., Ventura, S.J., et al.: Births: final data for 2010. *US Department of Health and Human Services National Vital Statistics Reports*, 61(1):1–71, 2012.

McPherson, M., Arango, P., Fox, H., et al.: A new definition of children with special health care needs. *Pediatrics*, 102(1 Pt. 1):137–140, 1998.

Meijssen, D.E., Wolf, M.J., Koldewijn, K., et al.: Parenting stress in mothers after very preterm birth and the effect of the Infant Behavioural Assessment and Intervention Program. *Child: Care, Health and Development*, 37(2):195–202, 2011.

Menghini, K.G.: Designing and evaluating parent educational materials. *Advances in Neonatal Care*, 5 (5):273–283, 2005.

National Association of Neonatal Nurses: Palliative care for newborns and infants (Position statement 3051). Glenview, IL, 2010, National Association of Neonatal Nurses.

National Association of Neonatal Nurses: Discharge guidelines for the technology dependent infant. (Unpublished manuscript.). Glenview, IL, 1999, National Association of Neonatal Nurses.

Pridham, K., Saxe, R. and Limbo, R.: Feeding issues for mothers of very low-birth-weight, premature infants through the first year. *Journal of Perinatal & Neonatal Nursing*, 18(2):161–169, 2004.

Quevedo, L.A., Silva, R.A., Godoy, R., et al.: The impact of maternal post-partum depression on the language development of children at 12 months. *Child: Care, Health and Development*, 38(3):420–424, 2012.

Sajous, C.H., Chybik, M.F. and Weiss, M.G.: Can infants be discharged home earlier from the neonatal intensive care unit without increasing their readmission? Paper presented at the Pediatric Academic Societies' Annual Meeting, Toronto, Canada, 2007a.

Sajous, C.H., Chybik, M.F. and Weiss, M.G.: Safety of home nasogastric feedings for healthy premature infants. Paper presented at the Pediatric Academic Societies' Annual Meeting, Toronto, Canada, 2007b.

Smith, V.C., Zupancic, J.A., McCormick, M.C., et al.: Rehospitalization in the first year of life among infants with bronchopulmonary dysplasia. *Journal of Pediatrics*, 144(6):799–803, 2004.

Stoll, B.J., Hansen, N.I., Bell, E.F., et al.: Neonatal outcomes of extremely preterm infants from the NICHD Neonatal Research Network. *Pediatrics*, 126 (3):443–456, 2010.

Sturm, L.D.: Implementation and evaluation of a home gavage program for preterm infants. *Neonatal Network*, 24(4):21–25, 2005.

Thomas, J.A.: A parent's guide to bottle feeding your premature baby. *Advances in Neonatal Care*, 7 (6):319–320, 2007.

Tudehope, D.I., Page, D. and Gilroy, M.: Infant formulas for preterm infants: In-hospital and post-discharge. *Journal of Paediatrics and Child Health*, 48(9):768–776, 2012.

Vandenberg, K.A.: Individualized developmental care for high risk newborns in the NICU: A practice guideline. *Early Human Development*, 83(7):433–442, 2007.

Vohr, B.R., Poindexter, B.B., Dusick, A.M., et al.: Beneficial effects of breast milk in the neonatal intensive care unit on the developmental outcome of extremely low birth weight infants at 18 months of age. *Pediatrics*, 118(1):e115–e123, 2006.

Westrup, B.: Newborn Individualized Developmental Care and Assessment Program (NIDCAP)—family-centered developmentally supportive care. *Early Human Development*, 83(7):443–449, 2007.

Wilson-Costello, D.: Is there evidence that long-term outcomes have improved with intensive care? *Seminars in Fetal and Neonatal Medicine*, 12(5):344–354, 2007.

Whyte, R.: Safe discharge of the late preterm infant. *Paediatrics and Child Health*, 15(10):655–666, 2010.

Zupancic, J.A., Richardson, D.K., O'Brien, B.J., et al.: Cost-effectiveness analysis of pre-discharge monitoring for apnea of prematurity. *Pediatrics*, 111(1):146–152, 2003.

CHAPTER

# 20 Genetics: From Bench to Bedside

JULIEANNE SCHIEFELBEIN

**OBJECTIVES**

1. Define birth defects and possible causes.
2. Become familiar with genetic terminology.
3. Identify the number of chromosomes in a normal human cell.
4. Describe the characteristics and causes of structural and numeric chromosomal abnormalities, modes of inheritance of single-gene disorders, and multifactorial inheritance.
5. Describe what prenatal diagnostic tests are available and which anomalies they detect.
6. Describe the components and benefits of genetic counseling.
7. Identify three patient care management issues in genetic counseling.
8. Verbalize the systematic process used to evaluate the malformed infant.
9. List common congenital malformations and possible mechanisms of cause.

The neonate born with a genetic defect or fetal anomaly presents a challenge to the neonatal intensive care unit (NICU) team. A definitive diagnosis is essential for management and care of the neonate and the neonate's family.

Congenital malformations commonly have multiple causes. This chapter includes information on basic genetics, characteristics, and causes of some common fetal anomalies, and a systematic process for the evaluation of the malformed infant. Commonalities of patient care management issues are addressed, with the understanding that every family requires individualized care.

## BASIC GENETICS

### Terminology

A. **Allele:** one of a series of alternate forms of a gene at the same locus on a chromosome (Jones, 2005; Jorde et al., 2010).
B. **Autosome:** one of 22 chromosomes that do not determine the sex of the individual.
C. **Birth defect:** an abnormality of structure, function, or metabolism, whether genetically determined or a result of environmental interference during embryonic or fetal life. A congenital defect may cause disease from the time of conception through birth or later in life (March of Dimes Foundation, 2008).
D. **Chromosome:** structural elements in a cell nucleus that carry the genes and convey genetic information.
   1. Each cell (except erythrocytes) in the body contains all the chromosomes received from both parents within its nucleus.
   2. There are 23 pairs of chromosomes, for a total of 46 chromosomes, with one maternal and one paternal chromosome creating each pair.
E. **Diploid:** containing a set of maternal and a set of paternal chromosomes, for a total of 46 chromosomes.
F. **Gamete:** one of two cells, containing 23 chromosomes (haploid number), with the union of a male gamete and a female gamete required during sexual production to create a new individual (with the diploid number of chromosomes).

G. **Gene:** the smallest unit of inheritance of a single characteristic, responsible for a physical, biochemical, or physiologic trait and located with other genes in linear sequence along the chromosome.
H. **Genotype:** hereditary composition of an individual.
I. **Haploid:** having half the number of chromosomes found in the person's cells; characteristic of the gametes.
J. **Locus:** the position that the gene occupies on a chromosome.
K. **Karyotype:** pictorial representation of the chromosomal characteristics of an individual or species.
L. **Penetrance:** The degree to which an inherited trait is manifested in the person who carries the affected gene (Nussbaum et al., 2007).
M. **Sex chromosomes:** the X and Y chromosomes which are responsible for sex determination—XX for female and XY for male.

## Dominance and Recessiveness

A. **Phenotype:** observable characteristics of an individual.
B. **Heterogeneous chromosomes:** differing pair of chromosomes, one from each parent, arraying differing genes for specific traits. When there are unlike genes on a locus, one gene dominates.
C. **Homologous chromosomes:** a matched pair of chromosomes, one from each parent, carrying the genes for the same traits.
D. **Dominant gene:** a gene that is expressed in the heterozygous state. In a dominant disorder, the mutant gene overshadows the normal gene. A dose of this gene is needed for expression.
E. **Recessive gene:** a gene whose effect is masked or hidden unless both genes of a set of homologous chromosomes at a given locus are abnormal, thus showing the disease. In a heterozygote (carrier), the normal gene overshadows the mutant gene.
F. **Possible combinations of chromosomes.**
   1. Both genes can be dominant—AA (homozygous).
   2. Both genes can be recessive—aa (homozygous).
   3. One gene can be dominant and one can be recessive—Aa (heterozygous).

## Autosomal Disorders

A. **Autosomal dominant disorders.**
   1. Characteristics of autosomal dominant disorders.
      a. Males and females are both affected equally; either parent can pass the gene on to sons or daughters.
      b. An affected offspring has an affected parent if the mutation is not new.
      c. Half the sons and half the daughters of an affected parent can be anticipated to have the disorder. There is a 50% chance with each pregnancy.
      d. Unaffected offspring of an affected parent will have all normal offspring if the mate is an unaffected person (assuming complete penetrance).
      e. If two affected people mate, three fourths of their offspring will be affected. A double dose of the mutant gene in any of the offspring will result in a lethal anomaly (except in the case of Huntington's disease).
      f. Family history of an anomaly indicates a vertical route of transmission through successive generations on one side of the family (if not a new mutation).
   2. Examples of autosomal dominant disorders: myotonic dystrophy, neurofibromatosis, and coronary artery disease (Allanson and Cassidy, 2010; Jones, 2005).
B. **Autosomal recessive disorders.**
   1. Characteristics of autosomal recessive disorders.
      a. Both males and females are affected equally.
      b. Parents of affected offspring are rarely affected and are usually heterozygous carriers.

c. After the birth of an affected offspring, there is a 25% chance, with each pregnancy, of having another affected offspring and a 50% chance that the offspring will be a carrier.
d. There may be a distant relative with the disorder.
e. Affected people who mate with unaffected people will have offspring who will be heterozygous carriers.
f. If two affected people mate, all offspring will be affected.
g. No family history indicates a horizontal route of transmission in the same generation.
h. There can be a difference in expression of the disorder: very mild in one member and extremely severe in another.

2. Examples of autosomal recessive disorders: cystic fibrosis, sickle cell anemia, Tay–Sachs disease, thalassemia major (Jones, 2005).

## X-Linked Disorders

**A. X-linked dominant disorders.**

1. Characteristics of X-linked dominant disorders.
   a. Both sexes can be affected; because females have a double chance of receiving the mutant X chromosome, they have twice the risk of being affected.
   b. Affected males will have all affected daughters and no affected sons.
   c. Affected females will transmit the disorders in the same manner as with autosomal dominant patterns.
   d. Two thirds of the time, affected females have an affected mother; one third of the time, they have an affected father.
   e. Family history shows no father-to-son transmissions.
2. Example: vitamin D–resistant rickets.

**B. X-linked recessive disorders.**

1. Characteristics of X-linked recessive disorders.
   a. Only male offspring are affected, with rare exceptions. A female offspring will be affected if she has both a carrier mother and an affected father.
   b. Carrier females transmit the disorder.
   c. All sons of affected males will be normal.
   d. All daughters of affected males will be carriers (with each pregnancy).
   e. Heterozygous females transmit the gene to half their sons, who will be affected, and to half their daughters, who will be carriers.
   f. Transmission is horizontal among males in the same generation; in addition, a generation will be skipped, and second-generation males will be affected.
2. Examples: Duchenne's muscular dystrophy, hemophilia, color blindness, and glucose-6-phosphate dehydrogenase deficiency (Kingston, 2002).

## Mitochondrial Disorders

**A. The great majority of genetic diseases are caused by defects in the nuclear genome. However, a small but significant number of diseases are the result of mitochondrial mutations.**

**B. Because of the unique properties of mitochondria, these diseases display characteristic modes of inheritance and a large degree of phenotypic variability (Jorde et al., 2010).**

**C. The mitochondria, which produce adenosine triphosphate (ATP), have their own unique deoxyribonucleic acid (DNA).** Mitochondrial DNA (mtDNA) is maternally inherited and has a high mutation rate. A number of diseases are known to be caused by mutations in mtDNA.

**D. Organ systems with large ATP requirements and high thresholds tend to be the ones most seriously affected by mitochondrial diseases; for example, the central nervous system (CNS) consumes 20% of the ATP the body produces and is often affected by mtDNA mutations.**

**E. Mitochondrial mutations are also involved in some common human diseases, for example, a form of deafness (Jorde et al., 2010).**

# CHROMOSOMAL DEFECTS

## Abnormal Number

A. **Polyploidy:** more than two sets of homologous chromosomes, showing multiples of the haploid number.
B. **Nonmultiples** are designated by the suffix "-somy"; monosomy is one less than the diploid number (45), and trisomy is one more than the diploid (47).
C. **Causes.**
   1. Nondisjunction: failure of paired chromosomes to separate during cell division.
   2. Chromosome lag: failure of a chromosome to travel to the appropriate daughter cell.
   3. Anaphase lag: chromosome lag during the third state of division of a cell nucleus in meiosis and mitosis.
   4. Mosaicism: nondisjunction of an anaphase lag that occurs during mitosis after fertilization, resulting in two different cell lines in the same person (Jones, 2005).

## Abnormal Structure

A. **Deletion:** loss of a chromosomal segment.
B. **Duplication:** any duplication of a region of DNA that contains a gene. It is a process that can result in a new mutation.
C. **Translocation:** occurrence of a chromosomal segment at an abnormal site, either on another chromosome or in the wrong position on the same chromosome (i.e., an inversion).
D. **Inversion:** occurs when a segment of the chromosome breaks off and reattaches in the reverse direction.
E. **Nonreciprocal translocation:** a one-way transfer of a chromosomal segment to another chromosome.
F. **Polygenic defects:** type of inheritance in which a trait is dependent on many different gene pairs with cumulative effects.
G. **Environmental influences.** Inadequate nutritional intake, certain drugs, irradiation, and viruses are examples that could alter the genetic makeup of an offspring while in vitro. Multifactorial: genes plus environment.
H. **Basic generalizations.**
   1. Loss of an entire autosome is usually incompatible with life.
   2. One X chromosome is necessary for life and development.
   3. If the male-determining Y chromosome is missing, life and development may continue but will follow female pathways.
   4. Extra entire chromosomes, the translocation of extra chromatin material, and the insertion of extra chromatin material are often compatible with life and development.
   5. Multiple congenital structural defects are present when gross aberrations are present (Blackburn, 2012).
I. **Incidence.**
   1. Autosomal aberrations: 5 in 1000 births.
   2. Sex chromosome aberrations: 2 in 1000 births.
   3. Spontaneous abortions: 60% are associated with chromosomal aberration (Jorde et al., 2010).

# PRENATAL DIAGNOSIS

Recent technological advances and marked progress in the understanding of the etiology and pathogenesis of many common disorders have allowed many families a prenatal diagnosis.

## Indications and Advantages of Prenatal Diagnosis

A. **Indications.**
   1. Advanced maternal age.
   2. Prior child with a chromosomal disorder.

3. Family history of neural tube defects.
4. Previous child with multiple malformations.
5. Carriers of X-linked diseases.
6. Carriers of chromosome translocation.
7. Couples at risk of having a child with a specific inborn error of metabolism (previous child or by carrier testing).
8. Ultrasonographic identification of major malformation, polyhydramnios, and/or intrauterine growth restriction (Jorde et al., 2010).

B. **Advantages.**
1. Knowledge that the fetus is unaffected.
2. Time to explore options and prepare for an affected newborn infant.
3. Opportunity electively to choose either to avoid starting a pregnancy or to abort an affected fetus.
4. Opportunity for the physician to plan delivery, management, and care of the infant when the disease is diagnosed in the fetus (Jorde et al., 2010).

## Prenatal Tests

### Triple and Quad Screen Tests.

A. **Screening test.** Performed at 15 to 20 weeks of gestation. The triple screen is a group of three tests that are used to screen pregnant woman in the second trimester of pregnancy. The quad screen adds a fourth test to the group. The test helps evaluate the risk that a fetus has certain abnormalities, including trisomy 21, and neural tube defects. Each test performed measures a different substance found in the blood: α-fetoprotein (AFP), human chorionic gonadotropin (hCG), unconjugated estriol ($uE_3$), and with the quad test, inhibin A. The newest marker, inhibin A, increases both the sensitivity and specificity of the screen. These tests have been established as a triple or quad screen because the power lies in their use together. A mathematical calculation involving the levels of these three or four substances and considerations of maternal age, weight, race, and diabetic status are used to determine a numeric risk for trisomy 21 and other selected chromosomal anomalies (i.e., trisomy 18). This risk is compared with an established cutoff. If the risk is higher than the cutoff value, then it is considered positive or increased.
1. **α-Fetoprotein** is a protein produced by fetal tissue. During development, AFP levels in fetal blood and amniotic fluid rise until about 12 weeks, then levels gradually fall until birth. Some AFP crosses the placenta and appears in the maternal blood.
2. **Human chorionic gonadotropin** is a hormone produced by the placenta. Levels rise in maternal blood for the first trimester of pregnancy and then fall to less than 10% by the end of pregnancy.
3. **Unconjugated estriol** is a form of estrogen that is produced by the fetus through metabolism. This process involves the liver, the adrenals, and the placenta. Some of the $uE_3$ crosses the placenta and can be measured in the mother's blood. Levels rise around the eighth week and continue to increase until shortly before delivery.
4. **Inhibin A** is a hormone also produced by the placenta. Inhibin is a dimer (has two parts) and is sometimes referred to as DIA or dimeric inhibin A. Levels in maternal blood decrease slightly from 14 to 17 weeks of gestation and then rise again.

B. **Screening test, not a diagnostic test.** Abnormal result does not indicate an abnormality but will indicate the possible need for a diagnostic test to rule out abnormalities.
1. **Trisomy 21:** the levels of AFP and $uE_3$ tend to be low and hCG and inhibin A levels high.
2. **Trisomy 18:** the levels of $uE_3$ and hCG levels are low and AFP levels are variable.
3. **Open neural tube defects:** where there is an opening in the infant's spine, head, or abdominal wall that allows higher than usual amounts of AFP to pass to the mother's blood.

C. **Shortfalls of this test.**
1. The test result is very dependent on the accurate determination of the gestational age of the fetus. If the gestational age of the fetus has not been accurately determined, the results may be falsely high or low.

2. In multiple-gestation pregnancies, calculation of the risk of trisomy 21 or trisomy 18 is difficult. For twin pregnancies, a "pseudo-risk" can be calculated comparing results to normal results in other twin pregnancies. For higher gestation pregnancies, risk cannot be calculated from these tests.
3. Evaluation of the risk of open neural tube defects in twin pregnancies can be determined, although it is not as effective as in singleton pregnancies.

D. **Results and further testing:** A multiple marker test or triple screen is used to determine if a fetus is at an increased risk of having certain congenital abnormalities. The test has a high rate of false positives; as few as 10% of women with abnormal results go on to have babies with congenital defects. The purpose of the test is to determine if further testing (such as ultrasound or amniocentesis) is warranted.

**Ultrasonography.**

A. **Procedure.** Transducer coated with ultrasonic gel is placed on the mother's abdomen, with high-frequency sound waves used to display sectional planes of the uterine contents on a monitor. Ultrasonography cannot detect all anomalies and cannot guarantee fetal outcome.

B. **Initial assessment** recommended by 16 to 20 weeks of gestation for the verification and evaluation of gestational age.

C. **Ultrasonography:** to detect abnormalities of fetus, placenta, amniotic fluid, and uterus; to monitor changes in anatomy and growth with serial ultrasonography.

D. **Diagnostic capability:** only as good as the person's training—not just contingent on the equipment.

E. **No known harmful effects.**

F. **Critical to safety of amniocentesis:** chorionic villus sampling and percutaneous blood sampling.

G. **Anatomic landmarks commonly observed:** fetal spine, kidneys, bladder, stomach, three-vessel cord, cord insertion, four-chambered heart, face, upper lip, biparietal diameter, head circumference, abdominal circumference, femur length, transcerebellar diameter, placenta, amount of amniotic fluid, uterus, and adnexa.

H. **Detectable anomalies:** many, including those indicative of various syndromes. Examples: anencephaly, atrial septal defect, cardiac anomalies, choroid plexus cyst, cleft lip, craniosynostosis, cystic hygroma, cystic kidneys, encephalocele, gastroschisis, hydrocephalus, microcephaly, myelomeningocele, omphalocele, skeletal dysplasia (Jorde et al., 2010).

**Amniocentesis ("Amnio").**

A. **Removal of 10 to 30 mL of amniotic fluid** through a needle placed into the woman's abdomen, for the purpose of chromosomal analysis and other biochemical tests as indicated.

B. **Procedure.** Normal results of amniocentesis do not guarantee a good fetal outcome. Obtain mother's blood type before procedure. If she is Rh negative, obtain father's blood type.

C. **Usual timing of procedure:** 16 to 18 gestational weeks, but amniocentesis can be performed later in gestation and as early as 14 weeks.

D. **Indications.**
1. Woman of advanced maternal age (>35 years at the time of expected delivery).
2. Previous fetus with Down syndrome.
3. Previous fetus with neural tube defect.
4. Both parents known as heterozygous carriers of autosomal recessive chromosome.
5. Both parents known as carriers of sex-linked recessive disorder.
6. Client or partner with balanced chromosomal translocation of his or her chromosomes.
7. A woman with an abnormal triple or quad screen.

E. **Fluid analysis:** requires 2 to 3 weeks for cells to grow adequately for accurate analysis.

F. **Risks:** Overall risk to mother or fetus is 1%.
1. Spontaneous abortion: approximately 0.5% of cases.
2. Hemorrhage.
3. Infection.
4. Premature labor.
5. Rh sensitization from fetal bleeding into maternal circulation.
6. Trauma to fetus or placenta.

G. **Analysis.**
   1. Fetal sex: determined through special staining techniques, karyotype, or amniotic fluid testosterone levels, providing risk information for X-linked disorder.
   2. $\alpha_1$-Fetoprotein: abnormally high or low levels raise concern (see earlier section on triple and quad screening, under Prenatal Tests).
   3. Biochemical: metabolism disorders, including Tay–Sachs disease (a lipid disorder) and amino acid, carbohydrate, and mucopolysaccharide metabolism disorders, can be discovered by 20 weeks of gestation.
   4. Chromosomes: abnormalities, including Down syndrome, other trisomies, and other chromosomal abnormalities, can be detected at 16 weeks of gestation by karyotyping.

H. **Postamniocentesis care.**
   1. It is important that the mother receive immune globulin (RhoGAM) if she is Rh negative and if father of fetus is either Rh positive or of unknown blood type. Do not give RhoGAM if Rh sensitization has occurred (Jenkins and Wapner, 2008).

**Chorionic Villus Sampling.**

A. **Transvaginal or transabdominal sampling** of the chorionic villi. Obtain fetal cells for the purpose of chromosomal analysis and other biochemical tests. Chorionic villus sampling (CVS) cannot identify neural tube defects.

B. **Preparation:** Review risks and benefits of the procedure, discuss options, and arrange to obtain CVS results. Obtain written consent for this procedure.

C. **Timing of procedure:** usually 8 to 10 weeks of gestation.

D. **Indications.**
   1. Mother prefers to make decisions regarding pregnancy in the first trimester.
   2. Severe oligohydramnios.

E. **Contraindications.**
   1. Multiple gestation.
   2. Uterine bleeding during this pregnancy.
   3. Active genital herpes infection or other cervical infection.
   4. Uterine fibroids.

F. **Fetal cell analysis:** requires 24 to 48 hours for initial results.

G. **Risks:** overall, 2% to 3%.
   1. Infection.
   2. Bleeding.
   3. Cervical lacerations.
   4. Miscarriage: 1% to 5%.

H. **Techniques of CVS.**
   1. Vaginal CVS: Catheter is inserted through the vagina and cervix into the chorion outer tissue of the embryonic sac, and a tiny amount of the chorionic villi is aspirated by suction or cut with forceps.
   2. Abdominal CVS: Needle is inserted through the abdomen into the chorion to obtain a sample of the chorionic villi.

I. **Post-CVS care.**
   1. Same recommendations as for postamniocentesis care.

**Percutaneous Umbilical Blood Sampling.**

A. **Sampling:** removal of fetal blood through a needle placed into the woman's abdomen and into the umbilical vein.

B. **Preparation:** same as that recommended for CVS.

C. **Timing:** 18 weeks to term.

D. **Indications.**
   1. Mother wants fast results to support her decision making regarding pregnancy.
   2. Abnormality is identified by ultrasonography late in pregnancy.
   3. Mother has been exposed to infectious disease that could affect development of fetus.
   4. Blood incompatibility (Rh disease).
   5. Drug or chemical level in fetal blood needs to be assessed.

E. **Risks.**
   1. Same as amniocentesis: infection, bleeding, isoimmunization, miscarriage, trauma to the fetus—overall 1% to 5% risk factor.
   2. Perforation of uterine arteries, clotting in fetal cord.
   3. Premature delivery.

F. **Results:** fetal blood analysis takes 3 days.

G. **Postsampling care:** same as postamniocentesis care (Drugan et al., 2005).

## POSTNATAL TESTING

A. **Chromosome analysis/karyotype:** an ordered display of an individual's chromosomes. This can be done on amniotic fluid prenatally. Chromosomes are analyzed by staining techniques that result in visibility of dark and light bands that are designated in a standardized way from the centromere.

B. **High-resolution banding/prometaphase banding:** Some disorders cannot be seen reliably on standard chromosome analysis and require special handling during processing. Prometaphase banding is used because the cell growth during culturing is adjusted to maximize the number of cells in prometaphase, where the chromosomes are much less condensed and therefore longer, rather than in metaphase, where the cell growth is stopped in standard chromosome studies. High-resolution banding can have from 550 to 800 bands and allows a much more detailed analysis.

C. **Fluorescence in-situ hybridization (FISH)** is a molecular cytogenetics technique that combines chromosome analysis with the use of fluorescence-tagged molecular markers (probes) that are applied after the chromosome preparation is produced. This method relies on the phenomenon of hybridization of complementary pieces of DNA. FISH is a powerful tool useful not only in diagnosing relatively common microdeletion or microduplication disorders but also for identifying the origin of extra chromosome material (Drugan et al., 2005).

D. **Polymerase chain reaction (PCR)** is a powerful technique in amplifying many copies of a segment of DNA so that it can be analyzed. PCR is useful in disorders with recurring mutation, for example, achondroplasia.

E. **Comparative genomic hybridization** microarray testing: This testing is an advancement in cytogenetic technology that is used for the detection of cytogenetic imbalances that are smaller than what can be detected through routine chromosome analysis. Testing will detect the loss (deletion) or gain (duplication) of chromosomal regions.

## HUMAN GENOME PROJECT

A. **What is the Human Genome Project?**
   1. The Human Genome Project was an international 13-year effort formally begun in October 1990 to discover all the estimated 30,000 to 35,000 human genes and make them accessible for further biologic study.
   2. The project started in the mid-1980s and is the single most important coordinated medical research initiative in the history of biomedical research. It culminated in the completion of the full human genome sequence in April 2000 (www.genome.gov).
   3. The goals of the project were to map genes on chromosomes and to determine the sequence of the nucleotides that make up human DNA, which is the basic genetic material. One of the top priorities was to generate complete sets of full-length chromosomal DNA (cDNA) clones and sequences for both human and model organism genes. It is expected that genome research will produce a ream of new information about the genes involved in inherited disorders, birth defects, and common conditions influenced by genetic factors.
   4. One insight already obvious is that even on a molecular level we are more than the sum of our 35,000 or so genes. However, surprisingly this new estimated number of genes is only one third of what was previously thought, although the numbers may be revised as more analyses are performed. This suggests to scientists that the genetic key to human complexity

lies not in the number of genes but in how gene parts are used to build different products in a process called alternative splicing.

5. In December 1999, the first human chromosome, chromosome 22, was sequenced. This is the location of defects that can cause DiGeorge syndrome, chronic myeloid leukemia, and neurofibromatosis. It is also the final autosome in the human sequence as outlined by the National Institutes of Health Human Genome Report in 2003 (Collins et al., 2003).
6. Though the outcome of the Human Genome Project itself is not ethically problematic, the use of the data generated presents major ethical questions that must be addressed. The future, then, presents the challenges of addressing the project's implications (Blackburn, 2012; Larsson, 2001).

B. **Ethical, legal, and social issues program.**
   1. Study is now under way on the ethical, legal, and social issues related to increasingly rapid progress in the field of human genetics. Four areas were identified for initial emphasis: privacy of genetic information, safe and effective introduction of genetic information in the clinical setting, fairness in the use of genetic information, and professional and public education.
   2. The program also emphasizes the importance of understanding the cultural, ethnic, social, and psychological influences that must inform policy development and service delivery issues.
   3. With time, these issues must be addressed to ensure that the maximal benefit is gained from the project (Blackburn, 2012; Larsson, 2001).

## GENETIC COUNSELING

A. **Definition:** Genetic counseling is a nondirective communication process that deals with the human problems associated with the occurrence, or the risk of occurrence, of a genetic disorder in a family. This process involves collaboration of people from multiple disciplines (physician, sonographer, nurse, genetic counselor, social worker, neonatologist, and pediatric specialist, as indicated) and family support.

B. **Principles of genetic counseling.**
   1. Based on correct diagnosis and pattern of inheritance.
   2. Nondirective.
   3. Reinforcement of information previously presented.
   4. Emphasis on communication with the primary care physician.

C. **Goal of genetic counseling** is to assist the family in comprehending the
   1. Diagnosis.
   2. Role of heredity.
   3. Recurrence risks and options.
   4. Possible courses of action.
   5. Methods of ongoing adjustment.

D. **Indications (Blackburn, 2012; Drugan et al., 2005).**
   1. Previously affected child, parent, or grandparent.
      a. Congenital malformation.
      b. Sensory defect.
      c. Metabolic disorder.
      d. Mental retardation.
      e. Known or suspected chromosome abnormality.
      f. Neuromuscular disorder.
      g. Degenerative CNS disease.
   2. Previously affected cousins.
      a. Muscular dystrophy.
      b. Hemophilia.
      c. Hydrocephalus.
   3. Consanguinity.
   4. Hazards of ionizing radiation.
   5. Recurrent miscarriages.
   6. Concern for teratogenic effect.

7. Advanced maternal age.
8. High or low maternal serum AFP.

E. **Methods of obtaining information needed.**
1. Questionnaire.
2. Pedigree.
3. Medical records.
4. Physical examination.
5. Laboratory tests.
6. Carrier detection.

F. **Provision of medical facts.**
1. Differential diagnosis.
2. Risks to fetus and mother.
3. Probable course of disorder.
4. Recommended management for prenatal course.
5. Type and timing of delivery.
6. Neonatal, pediatric, and long-term care requirements.

G. **Explanation of hereditary factors that contribute to the disorder.**

H. **Discussion with parents regarding all alternatives.**
1. Home care of newborn infant.
2. Institutionalization.
3. Adoption.
4. Appropriate method of termination for gestational age.
5. Objective information regarding fetal and neonatal status. Provide statistical risk factors as they relate to this individual fetus.
6. Identification of the normal characteristics that can exist in the affected fetus. Point these out in pictures to promote awareness of the total condition of the fetus.
7. Assistance to parents: understanding of causes, risks of recurrence, and limits of current treatments.
8. Discussion of options available for dealing with risk of recurrence.
9. Written information for parents and information regarding support groups.
10. Explanation of recommended obstetric care, mode and timing of delivery, and neonatal care (Jones, 2005).

# NEWBORN CARE

## Diagnosis

A. **Complete diagnosis:** important in planning care. Consideration for the infant's overall problems, in addition to the defect, is essential.

B. **Evaluation of infant with a birth defect.** A birth defect is a structural or functional abnormality of the body that is present from birth. The effects of a birth defect may be either immediate or delayed until later in life.

C. **Syndrome.**
1. Definition: a constellation of anomalies that cannot be explained otherwise and that result in similar patterns of expression.
2. Examples: fetal alcohol syndrome, trisomy 21.

D. **Sequence.**
1. Definition: a primary event or anomaly that sets a pattern of other events (anomalies). Designates a series of anomalies resulting from a cascade of events initiated from a single malformation.
2. Example: Pierre Robin sequence. Lannelongue and Menard first described Pierre Robin syndrome in 1891 in a report on two patients with micrognathia, cleft palate, and retroglossoptosis. In 1926, Pierre Robin published the case of an infant with the complete syndrome. Until 1974, the triad was known as Pierre Robin syndrome; however, the term *syndrome* is now reserved for those errors of morphogenesis with simultaneous presence of multiple anomalies caused by a single etiology. The term *sequence* has been introduced to include any condition that includes a series of anomalies caused by a cascade of events initiated

by a single malformation. The initial event, mandibular hypoplasia, occurs between the seventh and 11th week of gestation. This keeps the tongue high in the oral cavity, causing a cleft in the palate by preventing the closure of the palatal shelves. This explains the classic inverted U-shaped cleft and the absence of an associated cleft lip. Oligohydramnios could play a role in the etiology since the lack of amniotic fluid could cause deformation of the chin and subsequent impaction of the tongue between the palatal shelves.

**E. Association.**
1. Is a nonrandom occurrence in two or more individuals of multiple anomalies not known to represent a sequence or syndrome.
2. Example: *c*oloboma, *h*eart defect, *a*tresia choanae, *r*estricted growth and/or development, *g*enital anomalies, and *e*ar anomalies (CHARGE) association.

**F. Malformation.**
1. Definition: an abnormality of morphogenesis due to intrinsic problems within the developing structures.
2. Examples: neural tube defects, cleft lip and palate.

**G. Deformation.**
1. Definition: an abnormality of morphogenesis owing to intrinsic problems within the developing structures.
2. Examples: Pierre Robin sequence, uterine position defects, and oligohydramnios sequence.

**H. Disruption.**
1. Definition: an abnormality of morphogenesis due to disruptive forces acting on the developing structure. Can be due to pressure on developing structures.
2. Examples: amniotic bands, vascular accidents, and infections.

**I. Genetic heterogeneity.**
1. Definition: different causes may produce similar characteristics.
2. Examples: hydrocephalus, cleft lip and palate.

## History

**A. Family history.**
1. History of three generations.
2. Defects in the family history related to the problem in the child.
3. Medical records and/or photos of similarly affected relatives.
4. History of consanguinity.
5. Reproductive history, such as frequent spontaneous abortions.
6. Pattern of inheritance of the problems.

**B. Prenatal history.**
1. Length of gestation.
2. Fetal activity level.
3. Maternal exposures: infections, illness, high fevers, medications, x-ray examinations, known teratogens, alcohol, smoking, and use of street and prescription drugs.
4. Obstetric factors: uterine malformations, complications of labor, and presenting fetal part.
5. Neonatal factors: birth weight, length, head circumference, and Apgar scores.

## Examination and Care

**A. Physical examination.**
1. General: asymmetry, problems of relationship, and inappropriate size and strength.
2. Face: configuration; centered features with normal spacing; round, triangular, flat, birdlike, elfin, coarse, or expressionless characteristics.
3. Head: size of anterior fontanelle, prominence of frontal bone, flattened or prominent occiput, abnormalities in shape (proportionally large or small).
4. Skin: intact, or presence of skin tags, open sinuses, tracts.
5. Hair: texture, hairline, presence of whorls.
6. Eyes: structure and color of iris, presence of colobomas, centering and spacing of epicanthal folds (hypotelorism or hypertelorism), ptosis, slanting, eyelash length.

7. Ears: protruding or prominent shape, location, low-set, unilateral or bilateral defect, presence and/or degree of rotation.
8. Nose: beaked, bulbous, pinched, upturned, misshapen, number of nares, flattened bridge, patency, centered on face.
9. Oral: intact palate, presence of smooth philtrum, natal teeth; shape and size of tongue, mouth, jaw (micrognathia).
10. Neck: short and/or webbed, redundant folds.
11. Chest: symmetrical; presence of accessory nipples.
12. Abdomen: number of cord vessels, presence of abdominal wall defects and abdominal musculature, prune belly.
13. Genitourinary system (male): hypospadias—four degrees, dependent on placement of meatus; chordee; ambiguous genitalia; testes descended.
14. Anus: position, patency.
15. Spine: intact, scoliosis, lordosis, kyphosis.
16. Extremities: length, shape, absence of bones.
17. Hands and feet: broad, square, or spadelike shape; polydactyly, clinodactyly, syndactyly, abnormal creases in the palm of the hand (simian or Sydney creases), contractures, abnormally large or small size, overriding fingers, proximally placed thumb, rocker-bottom feet.

**B. Causation of defect.**

1. Identify the primary abnormality.
2. Recognize etiologic heterogeneity (a defect having more than one cause).
3. Determine category of congenital malformation, according to etiology.
   a. Malformation.
   b. Deformation.
   c. Disruption.
   d. Syndrome.
   e. Association
   f. Sequence.
   g. Genetic heterogeneity.

**C. Family care management for all genetic syndromes or disorders.**

1. Provide grief counseling. Acknowledge short- and long-term grief; promote awareness that each of the parents may be in a different stage of the grief process, creating additional stress. Recommend that parents communicate their needs to each other and ask for support when needed.
2. Encourage genetic counseling.
3. Facilitate family use of support systems: social services; Aid to Families with Dependent Children; Women, Infants, and Children (WIC) program; March of Dimes; clergy; mental health services; support groups; Internet information.
4. Provide unconditional emotional support. Allow parents and siblings to verbalize feelings.
5. Identify normal aspects of neonate that can coexist with the syndrome or disorder.
6. Promote parent involvement in care; offer choices in care and interventions.
7. Discuss treatment options and their risks and benefits.
8. Provide literature.
9. Obtain legal and ethical counsel when parents prefer not to pursue medical interventions (Nelson, 2012).

## Examples of Specific Disorders (for More Specific Disorders, See Chapter 35)

**VATER Association.** VATER is an acronym for *v*ertebral anomalies, *a*nal atresia, *t*racheo*e*sophageal fistula, and *r*adial and *r*enal dysplasia.

**A. Etiology and precipitating factors:** unknown.

**B. Incidence:** 1.6 in 10,000.

**C. Clinical presentation.** Three or more of the following defects are present:

1. Vertebral anomalies.
2. Anal atresia with or without fistula.
3. Tracheoesophageal fistula with esophageal atresia.

4. Radial dysplasia, including thumb or radial hypoplasia, polydactyly, and syndactyly.
5. Renal anomaly.
6. Single umbilical artery.

D. **Complications and outcome.**
1. Failure to thrive.
2. Possibility of normal life after slow mental development during infancy.

E. **Care management.**
1. Supportive: Prognosis and management depend on the extent and severity of the anomalies.
2. Surgery: surgical correction of anomalies.

**VACTERL Association.** VACTERL is an acronym for an association characterized by the sporadic, nonrandom association of specific abnormalities: *v*ertebral abnormalities, *a*nal atresia, *c*ardiac abnormalities, *t*racheoesophageal fistula and/or *e*sophageal atresia, *r*enal agenesis and dysplasia, and *l*imb defects.

A. **Etiology and precipitating factors.**
1. Unknown.
2. Injury between 4 and 6 weeks to a specific mesodermal area may produce simultaneous anomalies of the hindgut, lower vertebral column, lower urinary tract, and developing kidney.
3. Abnormalities: average of seven or eight per patient.

B. **Incidence:** rare (about 250 reported cases worldwide).

C. **Clinical presentation (Hockenberry, 2011; Jones, 2005).**
1. Vertebral anomalies.
2. Anal atresia with or without fistula.
3. Cardiac anomalies: commonly ventricular septal defects.
4. Tracheoesophageal fistula with or without esophageal atresia.
5. Radial dysplasia, including thumb or radial hypoplasia, polydactyly, and syndactyly.
6. Renal anomaly.
7. Single umbilical artery.

D. **Complications and outcome.**
1. Failure to thrive.
2. Normal life: minimal CNS anomalies with only occasional mental retardation.

E. **Care management (Hockenberry, 2011).**
1. Supportive: Prognosis and management depend on the extent and severity of the anomalies.
2. Surgery: surgical correction of anomalies.

## Common Trisomies

**Trisomy 21 (Down Syndrome).**

A. **Incidence and etiology.**
1. Incidence by maternal age is as follows:
   a. 15 to 29 years: 1 in 1500
   b. 30 to 34 years: 1 in 800
   c. 35 to 39 years: 1 in 270
   d. 40 to 44 years: 1 in 100
   e. 45 years or older: 1 in 50
2. Accounts for 15% to 20% of cases of severe mental retardation.
3. Risk increases with maternal age.
4. 25% of Down syndrome infants receive an extra chromosome from their father.
5. Person has 47 chromosomes (3 of chromosome 21).
6. Extra chromosome fits into group G21,22. Extra chromosome results from nondisjunction during meiosis. May occur unrelated to maternal risk factors and appear as follows:
   a. Chromosomes: 46.
   b. Translocation of chromosome 21.
   c. Familial transmission autosomal dominant.
   d. No abnormalities if chromosomes are balanced. There is one no. 21 and one no. 14 chromosome.
   e. Production of unbalanced gametes by balanced carriers: should consider prenatal diagnosis.

7. Some infants have mosaicism for trisomy 21 or translocation 14/21 or 21/22.
   a. Some have all the defects.
   b. Some have only a few.
   c. Some of this group may have normal intellectual ability.

B. **Clinical presentation (Jones, 2005).**
   1. Size: small; 20% are premature.
   2. Skull: short and round with a flat occiput.
   3. Eyes: slant upward and outward.
   4. Prominent epicanthal fold.
   5. Flat face.
   6. Brushfield's spots: iris may be speckled with a ring of round, grayish spots or flecks of gold in light-colored eyes.
   7. Cheeks: red.
   8. Palate: narrow and short.
   9. Nose: short with a flat nasal bridge.
   10. Tongue: protrudes; can become dry and wrinkled.
   11. Skin loose around lateral and dorsal aspects of the neck.
   12. Hands.
       a. Fingers: short.
       b. Hands: square.
       c. Single simian creases.
   13. Feet.
       a. Wide space between great toe and second toe.
       b. Deep crease that starts between the great toe and the second toe and curves.
   14. Muscular hypotonia.
   15. Narrow acetabular angle.
   16. Narrow iliac index.
   17. Broadened iliac bones.
   18. Delayed psychomotor development.
   19. Cardiac ventricular septal defects or other congenital heart defects found in 50% of infants.
   20. Duodenal atresia.

C. **Complications and outcome.**
   1. Congestive heart failure due to congenital heart disease.
   2. Upper respiratory tract infections.
   3. Delayed development: IQ ranges from 25 to 70.

## Trisomy 18

A. **Etiology and precipitating factors.**
   1. Nondisjunction most frequent; also possible partial trisomy, translocation, or mosaicism.
   2. Advanced parental age.

B. **Incidence:** 1 in 3500 births.

C. **Clinical presentation.**

   Characteristics 1 to 7 appear in most cases:

   1. Weight: low birth weight in term infant.
   2. Ears: low set and/or abnormal shape.
   3. Micrognathia and microstomia.
   4. Mental retardation.
   5. Hands.
      a. Clenched hand with flexed fingers.
      b. Flexion contraction of the two middle digits.
      c. Unfolded thumb.
   6. Cardiac: usually ventricular septal defect with patent ductal arteriosus.
   7. Feet: rocker bottom.

   Characteristics 8 to 14 may also appear:

   8. Eyes: ptosis of one or both eyelids.

9. Syndactyly.
10. Head: abnormally prominent occiput.
11. Genitourinary defects.
12. Hernias, especially umbilical.
13. Simian crease appears in 25%.
14. Arches on seven or more fingers in 80% of cases.

D. **Complications and outcome.**
1. Mortality rate: 30% die within 2 months of birth, usually of heart failure.
2. Survival: 10% survive past the first year with severe developmental delay.

E. **Care management.**
1. No treatment beyond supportive care.
2. Gavage/gastric tube feedings as needed for poor feeding.
3. Oxygen as needed for respiratory distress.
4. Parental support.

## Trisomy 13

A. **Etiology:** unknown; may be related to older maternal age.

B. **Incidence:** 1 in 15,000 births.

C. **Clinical presentation.**
1. Psychomotor delay.
2. Ears: malformed.
3. Hands: flexion deformities of hand, fingers, and wrist (postaxial polydactyly).
4. Cardiac: usually ventricular septal defect, patent ductus arteriosus, or rotational anomalies such as dextroposition.
5. Feet: rocker bottom.
6. Eyes: microphthalmos, colobomas of iris, cataracts.
7. Nose: broad and flattened, cleft lip and palate (not always).
8. Umbilicus: hernia, omphalocele.
9. Genitalia:
   a. Female: bicornuate or septate uterus.
   b. Male: cryptorchidism, small scrotum and anterior placement.
10. Kidneys: polycystic.
11. Skin: cutaneous hemangiomas, cutis aplasia.
12. Brain: gross defects, grand mal seizures, myoclonic jerks.
13. Hematologic abnormalities, such as increased frequency of nuclear projections in neutrophils and/or persistence of embryonic and/or fetal type of hemoglobin.

D. **Complications and outcome.**
1. Mortality rate: 44% die within the first month.
2. Survival: 18% survive the first year.
3. Severe mental retardation.

E. **Care management.**
1. No treatment beyond supportive care.
2. Parental support.

## REFERENCES


Allanson, J.E., and Cassidy, J.E., (Eds.): *Management of genetic syndromes* (3rd ed.). New York, 2010, Wiley-Blackwell.

Blackburn, S.T.: *Maternal, fetal & neonatal physiology: A clinical perspective*, (4th ed.). St. Louis, 2012, Elsevier Saunders.

Collins, F.S., Green, E.D., Guttmacher, A.E. and Guyer, M.S.: A vision for the future of genomics research. *Nature*, 422(6934):835–848, 2003.

Drugan, A., Isada, N.B. and Evans, M.I.: Prenatal diagnosis in the molecular age—indications, procedures, and laboratory techniques. In M.G. MacDonald, M.D. Mullett, and M.M.K. Seshia (Eds.): *Avery's neonatology: Pathophysiology & management of the newborn* (6th ed.). Philadelphia, 2005, Lippincott Williams & Wilkins, pp. 130–148.

Hockenberry, M.J.: *Wong's nursing care of infants and children*, (9th ed.). St Louis, 2011, Elsevier Mosby.

Jenkins, T.M. and Wapner, R.J.: Prenatal diagnosis of congenital disorders. In R.K. Creasy, R. Resnik, and J.D. Iams (Eds.): *Maternal-fetal medicine: Principles and practice* (6th ed.). Philadelphia, 2008, Elsevier Saunders, pp. 221–275.

Jones, K.: *Smith's recognizable patterns of human malformation*, (6th ed.). Philadelphia, 2005, Elsevier Saunders.

Jorde, L.B., Carey, J.C., Bamshed, M.J. and White, R.L.: *Medical genetics*, (4rd ed.). St Louis, 2010, Elsevier Mosby.

Kingston, H.M.: *ABC of clinical genetics*, (5th ed.). London, 2002, BMJ.

Larsson, A.: Neonatal screening for metabolic, endocrine, infectious and genetic disorders: Current and future directions. *Clinics in Perinatology*, 28 (2):449–461, 2001.

March of Dimes Foundation, White Plains, New York, 2008. Retrieved April 2, 2013, from www.marchofdimes.com/pnhec/.

Nelson, R.M.: Ethical decisions in the neonatal-perinatal period. In H.W. Taeusch, R.B. Ballard, and C.A. Gleason (Eds.): *Avery's diseases of the newborn* (9th ed.). Philadelphia, 2012, Elsevier Saunders, pp. 21–27.

Nussbaum, R.L., McInnes, R.R. and Willard, H.F.: *Thompson and Thompson genetics in medicine*, (7th ed.). Philadelphia, 2007, Elsevier Saunders.

CHAPTER

# 21 Intrafacility and Interfacility Neonatal Transport

S. LOUISE BOWEN

**OBJECTIVES**

1. Discuss planning for an intrafacility transport of a critically ill neonate.
2. Identify important considerations in the selection of transport vehicles.
3. Discuss the important factors to be considered in selecting team composition.
4. Describe the process of neonatal transport from the referring call, to transport of the patient, to arrival at the receiving hospital.
5. List four methods to increase safety in the transport environment.
6. Discuss legal and ethical considerations relating to neonatal transport.

In the late 1950s and early 1960s, intensive care for newborn infants first became available. As the scope of care for critically ill infants expanded, so did the number of hospitals offering this service. Unfortunately, because of the uneven distribution of these services, many areas remained without available resources. In the early 1970s, the need to regionalize perinatal care was recognized by health care providers. In 1976, the National Foundation-March of Dimes released the report "Toward Improving the Outcome of Pregnancy," which described regionalized care and identified criteria for level I, II, and III hospitals (Committee on Perinatal Health, 1976). The report also recommended the establishment of formal relationships between hospitals delivering different levels of care within a region so that every infant could receive appropriate care. The concept of regionalization led naturally to the need for the development of neonatal transport.

The U.S. Department of Health and Human Services reported almost 4 million live births in the United States in 2010, with 8.1% of low birth weight (less than 2500 grams) (Martin et al., 2010). Advances in neonatology and technology have led to increased survival rates of these low birth weight infants. These infants may be born outside a regional center and require transport to a neonatal intensive care unit. Infants with congenital anomalies or multisystem problems may also require transport to a regional neonatal intensive care center. The neonatal period is defined as the first 4 weeks of life and is the period of greatest mortality in childhood, with the highest risk occurring during the first 24 hours of life (March of Dimes, 2005). Intrafacility and interfacility transport of the critically ill neonate presents unique challenges. Transport of neonates occurs over 20,000 times annually in the United States (Shah et al., 2008). The transport environment does not provide optimal conditions. The goal is to transport these critically ill neonates in the most stable condition possible and to minimize adverse effects. The neonatal transport team must be knowledgeable about neonatal physiology and clinical requirements to provide optimal care and outcome. This chapter discusses various aspects of intrafacility and interfacility neonatal transport.

## HISTORICAL ASPECTS

A. **1899:** When most infants were born at home, the first ambulance incubator was developed to transport premature infants from home to Chicago's Lying-In Hospital (Butterfield, 1993; Cone, 1985).

B. **1935:** The Chicago Board of Health operated a special ambulance with incubator, oxygen, and humidity and was staffed with public health nurses (Chou and MacDonald, 1989).
C. **1948:** The New York City Department of Health, Maternity and Newborn Division established a well-organized transport service staffed with ambulance drivers, nurses, a pediatrician, and a transport clerk (Losty et al., 1950; Wallace et al., 1952).
D. **1966:** Dr. Sydney Segal published guidelines for neonatal transport (Segal, 1966) that were expanded in 1972 into a comprehensive transport manual (Segal, 1972).
E. **1970s:** The number of organized transport programs increased as a result of regionalization of perinatal care (Wood and Bose, 2005).

## PHILOSOPHY OF NEONATAL TRANSPORT

A. **The neonatal transport team is an extension of the neonatal intensive care unit (Ohning et al., 2012).**
   1. Interfacility neonatal transport is inherently different from typical emergency medical services (EMS) transport. Stabilization during interfacility transport is accomplished in the controlled setting of a medical facility, such as a hospital or medical clinic, in comparison with stabilization performed at the scene of an accident with limited support services. During interfacility transport, the patient is moved from a controlled setting (i.e., referring hospital) to the transport environment before arriving in the controlled setting of the receiving center. Scene-response systems move a patient from an uncontrolled setting to the controlled setting of a medical facility. The focus of EMS is on immediate short-term stabilization to sustain the patient until arrival at the medical facility. Interfacility transport systems focus on providing intensive care services from the referral facility and throughout the transport; thus more time is spent in stabilization at the point of origin.
   2. The level of care should remain the same or increase during neonatal interfacility transport.
B. **Crew and patient safety must be the highest priority of a transport program (American Academy of Pediatrics [AAP], 2007; Blumen, 2002; Levick, 2010).**
   1. Crew and patient safety must be the highest priority for both ground and air neonatal transport programs. The focus of a transport safety program is accident prevention. However, when an accident does occur, a systematic approach should be used to minimize the impact. Every team member is responsible for a safe program. Crew members' attitudes, participation, education, and judgment are variables that influence the safety program. Unsafe behaviors or practices are unacceptable in the transport environment.
C. **The neonate is a member of a family unit (Kenner and McGrath, 2010).**
   1. Parents and family of a critically ill neonate experience a mixture of emotions. Reactions of the parents may vary based on the condition of their infant and on their perception of the situation, past experiences, support systems, and coping mechanisms. The transport team plays a pivotal role assisting the family to cope with the crisis.
D. **Intrafacility and interfacility neonatal transport** should be planned and organized with appropriate transport staff and adequate equipment.
E. **Intrafacility and interfacility preparation, stabilization, and transport** should be performed as efficiently as possible using skilled staff and appropriate equipment. The continuum of care should not be interrupted during the transport process.

## INTRAFACILITY NEONATAL TRANSPORT (AAP, 2007; DEMMONS AND JAMES, 2008; NATIONAL ASSOCIATION OF NEONATAL NURSES, 2010a; SALYER, 2003)

A. **Preparation.**
   1. Neonates may require intrafacility transport for diagnostic and invasive procedures. The same concepts used for interfacility transport apply to intrafacility transport to avoid adverse outcomes.
   2. Level of care must be maintained or increased.

B. **Staffing.**
  1. Staff must be knowledgeable in neonatal physiology and pathophysiology and have excellent assessment skills. They must have the combined expertise and skills to provide safe transport.
  2. The type and number of personnel required is determined by patient acuity level and equipment.
  3. It is beneficial to have the bedside registered nurse as part of the transport staff because of patient knowledge. It may not be feasible with staffing shortages and patient care assignments.

C. **Effective communication** between staff of the neonatal intensive care unit, intrafacility transport team, and procedure department is critical. Formal hand-off process should be performed.

D. **Equipment.**
  1. Type of equipment selected is based on patient acuity level.
  2. Anticipate potential complications.
  3. Maintenance of a neutral thermal environment during the procedure presents challenges. The neonate may be transported to the procedure in a transport incubator or radiant warmer, depending on the patient's clinical condition and potential problems with hypothermia. Prevention of hypothermia during the procedure may require additional supplies.
     a. Radiant warming lights.
     b. Warm blankets.
     c. Hat.
     d. Crushable heat packs or thermal pad (do not place against fragile skin).
     e. Polyurethane wrap or bag.
  4. Monitoring devices should be compatible with the type of procedure performed.
  5. Equipment should have battery back-up capabilities. Plug in equipment to an electrical outlet to maintain the battery charge.

E. **Safety.**
  1. Use the most expeditious route between the unit and the procedure department.
  2. Anticipate and plan for potential problems (e.g., elevator not functioning).
  3. Supplies and equipment should be packaged for safe transport.
  4. Staff remaining with patient during the procedure should be provided with protective clothing and monitoring devices depending on type of procedure.
  5. The neonate and monitoring equipment should be positioned for optimal visualization.
  6. Staff may be required to stay with the neonate during the procedure given that other health care providers may not have the expertise to manage a neonate.
  7. The neonate should be assessed frequently during the procedure.

## INTERFACILITY NEONATAL TRANSPORT

### Types of Transports (AAP, 2007)

A. **One-way transport.**
  1. One-way transport uses services of personnel, equipment, and vehicles dispatched by the referral hospital to the receiving center.
  2. Advantages of one-way transport.
     a. Time-saving in patient arrival to the receiving center.
     b. Knowledge of the patient by referring staff.
  3. Disadvantages of one-way transport.
     a. Justification of the expense of maintaining experienced staff and equipment is difficult because of the small number of transports.
     b. May deplete the resources of local EMS or the referring hospital for the duration of the transport.
     c. Referring hospital and local EMS staff may not have appropriate equipment or training for transport of neonates. Studies have shown that there is an increased morbidity and mortality when neonates are transported by an untrained versus a trained neonatal team.

B. **Two-way transport.**
  1. Two-way transport uses the services of personnel, equipment, and vehicles dispatched by the receiving center.

2. Advantages.
   a. More cost-effective use of expensive equipment.
   b. More experienced transport staff trained specifically in neonatal transport.
   c. Improved neonatal stabilization techniques.
   d. Provide equipment specifically for neonatal transport.
3. Disadvantages.
   a. Time delay in moving patient from referring facility.
   b. Expense of maintaining transport program.

**C. Three-way transport.**

1. The neonate is transported from the referring facility to the receiving facility by a transport team from a third facility or air medical company.

**D. Back-/return transport (National Association of Neonatal Nurses [NANN], 2010a).**

1. Neonates are transferred back to the local or birth hospital when they no longer require the resources of the regional neonatal intensive care center. The family should be involved in the decision of transferring the infant.
   a. Parents should visit the local or birth hospital prior to the transfer.
2. Advantages.
   a. More efficient use of beds at regional center.
   b. Improved relations between community hospitals and tertiary care center.
   c. Greater opportunity for parental involvement.
   d. Familiarity of primary physician with infant before discharge home.
   e. Decreased cost during convalescence.
3. Disadvantages.
   a. Financial analysis of cost to keep infant at the regional facility versus cost of transport. Transfer of neonate back to referring hospital may depend on managed care or insurance contract.
   b. Potential need for transport back to higher-care facility if patient's condition deteriorates at community hospital.
   c. Parental anxiety and loss of continuity of care.

**E. Transfers out.**

1. Neonates are transferred for a specialized procedure or treatment not available at the current facility (i.e., extracorporeal membrane oxygenation, surgical procedure).
2. Neonate may be transported by a team from the receiving hospital, the referring hospital, or a third facility or company.
3. Receiving facility should consider back-transport after completion of the treatment or procedure.

## Selection of Transport Vehicles

**A. General considerations (AAP, 2007; Ohning et al., 2012).**

1. Appropriate vehicle selection may be dictated by diagnosis, clinical condition of the patient, available resources at the referring hospital, location of referring hospital, distance and duration of transport, geographic characteristics (road conditions, traffic conditions, construction detours), size of team, vehicle availability, weather, cost of the transport, and reimbursement.
2. Vehicles must be appropriately equipped, including power supplies, inverter, oxygen and air supply, suction, lighting, altitude pressurization where appropriate, means for securing incubators and all equipment, and room for adequate personnel.
3. An integrated system using multiple modes of transportation allows maximum flexibility to meet patient needs in a cost-effective manner.
4. Decisions regarding the appropriate vehicle for individual transport should be made by the medical control physician at the tertiary hospital, the transport team, and the referring physician in consideration of the impact on patient care and outcome, advantages and disadvantages of each vehicle, and cost.
5. Vehicle design and equipment placement must allow for continuation of patient care throughout the transport.
6. The vehicle must be equipped with appropriate locking devices and storage to secure the incubator and equipment.

**B. Specific vehicle considerations.**
 **1.** Ambulance (AAP, 2007; Ohning et al., 2012).
  **a.** Advantages.
   (1) Lower transport costs.
   (2) Operates in weather conditions that restrict air transport.
   (3) Does not require a landing zone or runway.
   (4) Ability to carry equipment and personnel for two incubators in specially equipped ambulances.
   (5) Increased space and patient more accessible.
   (6) Ability to stop vehicle or divert to the closest hospital in an emergency.
  **b.** Disadvantages.
   (1) Long response times due to speed limitations, road conditions, traffic congestion, and geographic location.
   (2) Delay of admission to tertiary care center because of long-distance ground transport.
 **2.** Helicopters (AAP, 2007; Ohning et al., 2012).
  **a.** Advantages.
   (1) Speed in response to calls and in returning patient to the receiving center for distances up to 150 miles.
   (2) Decreased response time to the referring facility.
   (3) Use of one-way helicopter transport to increase team's response time to referring hospital.
   (4) Avoid traffic delays and ground obstacles.
  **b.** Disadvantages.
   (1) Need for landing zone.
   (2) Increased noise and vibration levels.
   (3) Difficult to identify problems when they occur because of noise and vibration (e.g., pneumothorax, extubation).
   (4) High operational costs.
   (5) Space and weight limitations, including restricted patient access during flight.
   (6) Increased downtime because of weather.
   (7) May require ground transportation depending on landing zone location.
   (8) Securing the same incubator in a helicopter and an ambulance may not be possible because of different mounts and stretcher configurations. This must be evaluated prior to the transport.
 **3.** Fixed-wing aircraft (AAP, 2007; Ohning et al., 2012).
  **a.** Advantages.
   (1) Primarily beneficial for long-distance transports, usually greater than 150 miles.
   (2) Although fixed-wing transportation is expensive, favorable cost comparison possible over long distances when staff time is taken into consideration.
  **b.** Disadvantages.
   (1) If no contractual agreements with aircraft vendors, possible inadequate equipment and unfamiliarity of team with the aircraft or with general vendor operation.
   (2) Requires coordination of ground transportation on both ends of the flight.
   (3) Space limitations, and patient access may be limited.
   (4) Securing the same incubator in a fixed-wing aircraft and an ambulance may not be possible because of different mounts and stretcher configurations. This must be evaluated before the transport.
   (5) Requires an airport for landing and takeoff.
   (6) Multiple patient movements from aircraft and ambulances.

## Transport Personnel

**A. Composition of a neonatal transport team** varies with federal, state, and local regulations as well as budget, availability, professional standards, patient population, mission, referral area, expectations and available resources at referral hospital, skill and educational level of team, acuity, and volume of transports. The team must possess the combined expertise to assess, plan, implement, and evaluate actual and potential complications during transport of a critically ill neonate (Commission on Accreditation of Medical Transport Systems [CAMTS], 2012; NANN, 2010a; Woodward et al., 2002). The team may be staffed by using various combinations of personnel, with a minimum of two patient care providers trained in the management of critically ill neonates. These patient care providers are in addition to the ambulance drivers or pilots. At least one of the patient care providers should be a physician, registered nurse, or neonatal nurse practitioner. Team composition may remain constant or vary according to patient acuity (Woodward et al., 2002). When transporting two neonates in the same vehicle, specific patient care providers should be assigned to each infant. Cross-training staff within scope of practice and licensure increases efficiency of the team. Transport teams may be configured using a combination of the following personnel:

1. Physicians and neonatologists.
2. Fellows and residents.
3. Registered nurses.
4. Neonatal nurse practitioners.
5. Respiratory therapists.
6. Emergency medical technicians or paramedics.

B. **Roles for transport personnel,** including functions, responsibilities, qualifications, and competencies, must be clearly outlined in job descriptions.
   1. Transport personnel should function as a team.
   2. Cross-training personnel within scope of practice and licensure.
   3. The program should have a written policy specific to job performance for physical requirements and disqualifying mental conditions of team members.
      a. Weight and height requirements, especially in air transport.
      b. General physical condition.
      c. Notification to transport administration of use of prescription and over-the-counter medications (certain medications may delay mental function and reflexes).
   4. Staff should participate in neonatal transport with sufficient frequency to maintain expertise.

C. **Team composition considerations (AAP, 2007; CAMTS, 2012).**
   1. Physicians.
      a. Neonatologists should be utilized when their additional expertise is required.
      b. May limit resources in a busy neonatal practice.
      c. Residents provide less consistency as a result of rotations and lack of educational experience in neonatal intensive care.
      d. Fellows provide more consistency and increasing levels of expertise as they advance through their fellowship.
   2. Registered nurses.
      a. Requires advanced knowledge and experience in neonatal intensive care.
      b. May be the team leader.
      c. Educational requirements may include in-service programs and national certifications, including the Basic Life Support Course, the AAP/American Heart Association (AHA) Neonatal Resuscitation Program, the AAP/AHA Pediatric Advanced Life Support Course, the S.T.A.B.L.E. (Sugar and Safe Care, Temperature, Airway, Blood Pressure, Lab Work, Emotional Support) Program, the S.T.A.B.L.E. Program Cardiac Module, Certified Flight Registered Nurse (CFN), Certified Neonatal and Pediatric Transport (CNPT), and Certified Transport Registered Nurse (CTRN).
   3. Neonatal nurse practitioners.
      a. Licensed in most states to perform diagnostic and therapeutic procedures.
      b. Highly skilled, in addition to their advanced knowledge of neonatal intensive care therapies.
      c. Increased cost in comparison to a registered nurse; however, this may obviate the need for resident/fellow/neonatologist presence.
      d. Educational requirements may include in-service programs and national certifications, including the Basic Life Support Course, the AAP/AHA Neonatal Resuscitation Program, the AAP/AHA Pediatric Advanced Life Support Course, the S.T.A.B.L.E. Program, the S.T.A.B.L.E. Program Cardiac Module, CFN, CNPT, and CTRN.

4. Respiratory therapists.
   a. Frequent team members because the majority of neonates transported have a respiratory problem.
   b. Require advanced knowledge in neonatal intensive care.
   c. May assist with nursing functions as licensed by the state.
   d. Responsible for respiratory equipment, airway maintenance, and maintaining adequate oxygenation and ventilation during transport.
   e. Educational requirements may include in-service programs and national certifications, including the Basic Life Support Course, the AAP/AHA Neonatal Resuscitation Program, the AAP/AHA Pediatric Advanced Life Support Course, the S.T.A.B.L.E. Program, the S.T.A.B.L.E. Program Cardiac Module, CNPT, and Neonatal Pediatric Specialty (NPS).
5. Emergency medical technicians and paramedics.
   a. Role varies, depending on experience and education in neonatal care.
   b. Functions may include nursing or respiratory therapy responsibilities.
   c. Educational requirements may include in-service programs and national certifications, the Basic Life Support Course, the AAP/AHA Neonatal Resuscitation Program, the AAP/AHA Pediatric Advanced Life Support Course, the S.T.A.B.L.E. Program, the S.T.A.B.L.E. Program Cardiac Module, Certified CNPT, and Critical Care Paramedic (CCP).
6. Expertise required within the transport team (Demmons and James, 2008; NANN, 2010a).
   a. Assessment.
      (1) History taking.
      (2) Physical examination and gestational age assessment.
      (3) Interpretation of laboratory and radiologic findings.
   b. Knowledge of neonatal physiology and pathophysiology.
   c. Excellent communication and public relations skills.
   d. Technical and clinical competence.
   e. Leadership skills.
   f. Ability to work on a team.
   g. Physical examination and fitness criteria (physical agility and stamina).
   h. Knowledge of aviation physiology.
   i. Transport safety.
   j. Knowledge of transport environment and vehicles.
   k. Independence and flexibility.
   l. Procedures.
      (1) Bag-and-mask ventilation.
      (2) Endotracheal intubation.
      (3) Laryngeal mask airway insertion.
      (4) Arterial access (umbilical artery catheters, percutaneous artery catheters, arterial sampling).
      (5) Needle thoracostomy.
      (6) Thoracostomy tube insertion.
      (7) Venous access (umbilical venous catheters, peripheral intravenous [IV] lines).
      (8) Intraosseous insertion.
      (9) Administration of nitric oxide and nitrogen, as applicable.
      (10) Mobile extracorporeal membrane oxygenation, as applicable.
      (11) Administration of surfactant.
7. Justification for a neonatal team.
   a. Staffing: dedicated, unit based, on call.
   b. Use of personnel when there are no transports.
   c. Volume of transports.
   d. Review of other systems that could transport neonates. These systems should demonstrate appropriate clinical expertise and possess equipment to transport a critically ill neonate.
   e. Cost and reimbursement.

D. **Medical director** (AAP, 2007; Woodward et al., 2002). The role of the neonatal transport team medical director, including qualifications and responsibilities, must be clearly outlined in a job description.
   1. A neonatologist or a physician with acute care expertise or subspecialty training in neonatology.
   2. License to practice medicine in the transport program's state.
   3. Knowledgeable in transport medicine.
   4. Oversees medical aspects of the transport program.
   5. Involved in the quality management program.
   6. Involved in administrative aspects: selection of team members, orientation, education, program operation, policies, public relations, and outreach education.

## TRANSPORT EQUIPMENT (GERSHANIK, 2006; ORLANDO ET AL., 2007)

A. **Transport equipment and supplies must be checked regularly** to ensure that they are adequately stocked, functioning properly, and ready for immediate transport. Equipment should be scheduled for preventive maintenance programs regularly. A formal checklist may be used prior to each transport to ensure that correct equipment and correct number of supplies are secured for the transport.
B. **Recommended equipment must be operable on battery power.**
   1. Transport incubator.
   2. Cardiorespiratory monitor with pressure tracing and recorder.
   3. Pulse oximeter.
   4. Infant ventilator.
   5. Air–oxygen blender.
   6. End-tidal carbon dioxide monitor or adaptors.
   7. Airway humidification system.
   8. Invasive and noninvasive blood pressure monitors.
   9. IV infusion safety pumps.
   10. Transilluminator.
   11. Point-of-care testing, including portable blood gas analyzer and glucometer (state regulations vary regarding use and quality control checks in mobile intensive care environments).
   12. Defibrillator/pacer (minimum capacity, 2 watt-seconds).
   13. Liquid oxygen, oxygen tank in vehicle, or portable oxygen cylinders.
   14. Air tank in vehicle, portable air cylinders or air compressor.
   15. Inverter in vehicle. Equipment should have battery backup.
   16. Specialized equipment: nitric oxide, nitrogen, extracorporeal membrane oxygenation, and high-frequency ventilation during neonatal transport.
C. **Supplies for neonatal transport (Box 21-1).**
D. **Fixed-wing transports.**
   1. Ensure incubator fits through door of aircraft prior to transport.
E. **Evaluate type and grounding of electrical outlets in vehicles** prior to transport. Voltage and amperage differences may affect equipment.

## NEONATAL TRANSPORT PROCESS (AAP, 2007; DEMMONS AND JAMES, 2008; NANN, 2010a; SALYER, 2003)

A. **Referral call.** The initial transport request call may be taken by a dispatch center, transport team, neonatologist, or neonatal intensive care staff. The referring physician is responsible for selection of an appropriate receiving facility and contacting the receiving physician to request patient transfer. During the initial call, minimum information should be obtained to activate the appropriate team, select the mode of transport, and anticipate any special supplies or equipment that may be required during the transport. A neonatologist may provide consultation to the referring hospital as needed until the transport team arrives. Management given

■ BOX 21-1
■ **SUPPLIES FOR NEONATAL TRANSPORT**

**Respiratory Equipment**
Laryngoscope handle with blades, sizes Miller 00, 0, and 1
Spare laryngoscope bulbs and batteries
ET tube stylet (fits into the endotracheal tubes)
Anesthesia bag (not to exceed 750 mL) or self-inflating bag with oxygen reservoir
Manometer
Face mask (micropremie, premature, and term)
ET tubes, sizes 2.0, 2.5, 3.0, 3.5, and 4.0
Oral airways (sizes 000, 00, 0)
Suction catheter and glove sets, sizes 5 F, 6 F, 8 F, and 10 F
Portable suction
Meconium aspirator
Blood gas kit
CPAP neonatal prongs (extra small to large neonate)
Nasal cannula (premature, infant)
Ventilator circuit, nitric oxide circuit
Roll of waterproof tape or endotracheal tube securing device
Thoracentesis setups:
  Syringe, 60 mL
  Three-way stopcock
  IV catheters, 20 and 22 gauge
  Tubing T-connector
  Antiseptic solution
  Heimlich valves/closed drainage system
  Chest tubes, sizes 8 F, 10 F, and 12 F
  Oxygen hood
  Laryngeal mask airway (size 1 with 5-mL syringe)
  Bulb syringe
  End-tidal carbon dioxide monitor/carbon dioxide adapters

**IV Therapy Equipment**
Bags of $D_5W$, $D_{10}W$, 0.9% saline, 0.45% saline
IV pump tubing
IV filters
Platelet and blood infusion sets
Umbilical catheters, sizes 3.5 F and 5 F (single, double, triple lumen)
IV extension tubing
T-connectors, multiport connectors
Sterile drapes
Syringes, sizes 1 to 60 mL
Needleless connecting system
Three-way stopcock and stopcock plugs
Antiseptic wipes
Scalp vein needles, 23 and 25 gauge
IV catheters, 22, 24, and 26 gauge
Skin barrier
Safety razor
Medication additive labels
Tape measure
Armboards, sizes premature and infant
Intraosseous needles (intraosseous device)
Assorted tape
Umbilical tape
Antiseptic solution
Sizes 3-0 and 4-0 silk suture with curved needle
Umbilical catheter and thoracotomy set, including:
  Two sterile drapes
  Iris forceps
  Needle holders
  Scissors
  Curved forceps
  Tongue tissue forceps
  Sterile gauze pads, 2 × 2
  Scalpel and blade
  Blunt-end adapters, 17, 18, and 20 gauge

**Thermoregulation and Monitoring Equipment**
Hat
Polyurethane wrap or bag
Crushable heat packs and mattress
Space blankets
Thermometer
Neonatal electrocardiogram electrodes
Lead wires for heart monitor
Capillary tubes
Glucose level monitoring device
Lancets
Arterial transducer tubing

**Miscellaneous**
Camera
Parent information
Blood culture bottles
Scissors and hemostat
Flashlight
Gauze pads, 2 × 2
Limb restraints
Tourniquet
Pacifiers (various sizes)
Christmas tree adapters
Feeding tubes, sizes 5 F and 8 F
Salem sump tubes, sizes 10 F and 12 F
Dual-flow gastric tubes, sizes 10 F and 12 F
Sterile glove packs (assorted sizes)
Sphygmomanometer with blood pressure cuffs, sizes premature, neonate, and infant
Neonatal stethoscope
Trash bag; needle disposal system
Personal protective equipment (goggles, gowns, masks, gloves)
Visceral pack: normal saline solution, sterile gauze, sterile operating room drape, or sterile plastic bag

*Continued*

**BOX 21-1**
**SUPPLIES FOR NEONATAL TRANSPORT—CONT'D**

**Medications**

Epinephrine, 1:10,000
Sodium bicarbonate, 4.2%
Calcium gluconate, 10%
Dopamine
Dobutamine
Prostaglandin $E_1$ (Alprostadil)
Phenobarbital
Fosphenytoin
Diazepam (Valium)
Neuromuscular blocking agents
Analgesics
Lidocaine (Xylocaine), 1%
Heparin (1000 units/mL)
Normal saline diluent, 0.9%
Sterile water diluent
Flush solution
Broad-spectrum antibiotics
Albumin, 5%, and/or normal saline solution
$D_{50}W$ (for making higher-glucose-concentrated IV fluid)
Adenosine
Digoxin (Lanoxin)
Surfactant replacement therapy
Ophthalmic ointment
Vitamin K
Lorazepam (Ativan)
Sedative(s)
Milrinone
Reversals:
- Neostigmine (reverses neuromuscular blocking agents)
- Flumazenil (reverses benzodiazepine)
- Naloxone (reverses narcotic-induced respiratory depression)

*CPAP*, Continuous positive airway pressure; $D_5W$, $D_{10}W$, and $D_{50}W$, 5%, 10%, and 50% dextrose in water; *ET*, endotracheal; *IV*, intravenous.

via phone must be accurately documented and preferably recorded. Transport computer electronic medical record systems are available.

The initial call should be limited to 5 to 10 minutes. Information to be obtained during the initial referral call includes the following:

1. Time and date of referral call.
2. Patient name and gender.
3. Date and time of birth.
4. Gestational age, birth weight, and current weight.
5. Parent's name and demographic information (admissions may require for admitting patient to the hospital).
6. Referring physician.
7. Referring institution, including city, state, and phone number.
8. Reason for transfer request/preliminary diagnosis.
9. Current management (vital signs, respiratory support, fluid management [to prevent aspiration, the infant should receive nothing by mouth before transport], medications, significant findings of physical examination, pertinent laboratory and radiographic data).
10. Subsequent information may be obtained:
    a. Maternal prenatal, labor, and delivery history.
    b. Apgar scores.
    c. Other pertinent patient findings or medical management.
    d. Infection control issues.

**B. Selection and notification of team members.**

**C. Selection and dispatch of appropriate vehicle.**

**D. Selection of appropriate equipment and supplies.**

**E. Planning en route to referring hospital.**

1. Team members will discuss provisional and differential diagnoses, proposed plan of care, and division of responsibilities.
2. Referring hospital should be notified of time of team's dispatch, mode of transport, and estimated time of arrival to referring hospital.
3. Emergency and anticipated medication dosages and IV fluid amounts are calculated on the basis of weight.
4. Potential complications are anticipated and a plan of action formulated.
5. History and diagnostic study results to be obtained at referring hospital are identified.

F. **Stabilization at referral hospital.**

1. Introduce transport team members to referring physicians, staff, and family members. Check identification band on infant. All patients should be transported with identification band on. Parents' religious, cultural, and ethnic preferences should be incorporated into care if the care or safety of the neonate and/or crew are not compromised.
2. Maintain latex-safe environment.
3. Perform primary assessment of neonate to determine need for immediate interventions.
4. Obtain further details of history and current management.
5. Review previous radiographic images.
6. Obtain vital signs and glucose screening results. Determine blood gas values if clinical situation warrants.
7. Perform secondary assessment.
8. Complete pain assessment using a validated pain-scoring tool as part of the initial assessment and reassess during the transport (Blackburn, 2013).
   a. Recognition by the transport team that neonates feel pain.
   b. The neonate's response to pain becomes more defined with increased gestational age.
   c. Low birth weight and extremely low birth weight neonates display less organized and less vigorous response to pain.
   d. Transport team should observe for cues that the neonate is experiencing pain.
   e. The transport team should anticipate painful procedures to the neonate.
   f. The transport team should utilize nonpharmacologic techniques and/or administer pain medication or sedation as ordered or by protocol.
   g. The neonate should be reassessed for effectiveness of therapy after treatment of pain.
9. Initiate monitoring systems as appropriate; may include cardiorespiratory, peripheral blood pressure, arterial blood pressure monitoring, end-tidal carbon dioxide, and pulse oximetry.
10. Consult with designated transport physician regarding management plan and anticipated complications en route, or follow transport protocols.
11. Attempt to achieve normal or optimal blood gas values, blood pressure, temperature, perfusion, serum glucose level, and acid–base balance according to the plan of care.
12. Begin switching to transport equipment, including ventilator and IV pumps, carefully monitoring changes in patient status.
13. Notify receiving unit of estimated time of arrival, current patient status, family's status, and equipment needs on admission.
14. Family support (Kenner and McGrath, 2010). The transport team plays a pivotal role in recognizing the family in crisis, anticipating further crisis, intervening, and assisting the family through the transport process and admission to the receiving hospital.
   a. Identify members of the family unit, that is, parenting dynamics and extended family members. The family unit is often diverse. The "family" should be viewed as the object of care.
   b. If possible, provide the option of allowing the parents to remain in the room as their newborn is prepared for the transport.
   c. Update current patient status; discuss anticipated complications during transport and treatment plans. The parents should be involved in the plan of care.
   d. Assess the parents' understanding of the infant's condition, plans for traveling to the receiving center, and their needs for physical and emotional support.
   e. Provide information about the receiving center, including location, phone numbers, directions, attending physician, primary/admitting nurse, and visiting policy.
   f. Obtain written transport consents.
   g. Take a picture of the infant or provide a set of handprints or footprints of the infant to leave with the parents. Initiate the process for bedside video/webcam if available at the receiving hospital.
   h. The family may request that special objects, such as toys, pictures, or religious and cultural objects, be transported with their infant. The team should attempt to support the request if it does not interfere with safe transport and it is within the hospital policy.
   i. Leave a bonding agent (i.e., cloth) with a parent to keep against the skin that will be given to the infant during visitation.
   j. Discuss feeding options. If the mother is planning to breast-feed, discuss storage and transport of milk to receiving hospital.

k. Allow the parents to touch the infant prior to departure. This is helpful in bonding and in making the birth seem more real.
l. Depending on the team's policy and mode of transport, one parent may be allowed to accompany the infant.

15. Obtain copies of prenatal, maternal, and neonatal medical records. The records should be secured during the transport in accordance with the Health Insurance Portability and Accountability Act.
16. Distribute transport evaluation form(s) to referring hospital staff and/or parents.

**G. Planning en route to receiving hospital.**

1. Infant should be secured in incubator with a restraint device. Loose equipment must never be placed inside the incubator.
2. Continuously monitor temperature, pulse, respirations, blood pressure, oxygenation/ventilation, and pain status as indicated.
3. Documentation at regular intervals, as indicated by infant's condition:
   a. Vital signs, blood pressure, color, pain level.
   b. Readings of oxygenation and ventilation monitors and of respiratory support settings (including altitude if appropriate).
   c. Serum glucose screening.
   d. Important documentation times for status of infant, including arrival at referring hospital, departure from referring hospital, and time of transfer of care to receiving hospital staff.

**H. Arrival to receiving facility.**

1. Transport team should notify the parents/family.
2. Transport team provides report to hospital staff.
3. Follow-up may be provided to referring staff and physicians during the infant's hospitalization at the receiving center, maintaining patient confidentiality and following Health Insurance Portability and Accountability Act regulations.

**I. Neonates should be transported using individualized developmental care techniques.**

1. The sick premature infant experiences significant physiologic stress when incoming stimuli resulting from high noise levels and increased vibration, lighting, and handling exceed the immature nervous system's ability to respond. The infant responds with autonomic instability, hypoxia, and increased oxygen requirements. Incorporating developmental care techniques may decrease these maladaptive responses.
2. Shield the neonate's eyes from light or glare by placing an eye shield on the infant or covering the incubator with a flame-retardant incubator cover. The infant's eyes should be covered prior to use of lights in the vehicle. Limit use of overhead fluorescent lighting. Install and use dimmer switches in the vehicle. Indirect lighting should be directed away from the neonate to facilitate staff needs.
3. The neonate should be positioned in the incubator to support posture and movement and promote a calm, regulated behavioral state. Nesting or boundaries support the infant's position and conserve energy by containing movement. Positioning aids may be purchased or blanket rolls may be used.
4. Incubator portholes and doors should be closed with care. Objects should not strike the incubator.
5. A gel mattress may be used to decrease vibration and aid in positioning.
6. Decrease noise levels inside the vehicle by reducing speech levels, excluding radio or television use, and responding promptly to monitor alarms. An intercom system may be used for staff communication.
7. On ground transport, request that the ambulance driver avoid rough areas in road.

**J. Special transport stabilization considerations.**

1. Very low birth weight (VLBW) infant (AAP and American Heart Association, 2011; Thigpen, 2002).
   a. Ventilation.
      (1) Susceptibility to barotrauma with high peak inspiratory pressures.
      (2) Administration of surfactant replacement therapy by the transport team may be considered for infants meeting specific clinical criteria or for long-distance transports.

Ventilatory status must be closely monitored to prevent pulmonary air leaks because of changes in lung compliance after administration. Transport from the referring hospital may be delayed to stabilize the infant and monitor lung compliance changes prior to departure in the vehicle.

(3) The VLBW infant may experience increased incidence of hypoxia and oxygen requirements because of the stresses of transport. Developmental care techniques should be incorporated into care. Sedation prior to transport may be required.

(4) Continuous pulse oximetry and an air–oxygen blender should be used to monitor oxygen saturations and adjust oxygen concentrations to prevent hyperoxia.

**b.** Hypothermia.

(1) May require supplemental warming devices in addition to the prewarmed transport incubator: crushable heat packs or mattresses; hats; polyurethane wrap or bags especially designed for infants less than 28 weeks. Increase environmental temperature, warm objects prior to placing in contact with neonate.

(2) Because of the fragility of the skin, extreme care must be taken to not place warming devices in direct contact with skin.

(3) Transport incubator door and portholes should be kept closed as much as possible.

(4) Cover the outside of the incubator with a flame-retardant incubator cover.

(5) In cold weather, preheat the vehicle prior to loading the incubator.

**c.** Skin fragility.

(1) Minimal to gentle handling.

(2) Use monitoring devices designed for the VLBW infant.

(3) Minimize invasive procedures and placement of monitoring devices on skin.

(4) Maintain appropriate level of hydration. IV fluid administration is calculated on increased insensible water loss with decreased gestational age. Glucose should be closely monitored. Avoid rapid infusions of IV fluid.

(5) Application of a semipermeable polyurethane membrane or specific products designed for the VLBW infant may be placed on the skin to maintain integrity and decrease insensible water loss.

**2.** Spinal immobilization (Gomella, 2009).

**a.** Traumatic injuries to the neonatal spinal cord are rare.

**b.** Injuries may occur because of a congenital defect, birth injury, fall, or nonaccidental trauma. Most spinal cord injuries are caused by lateral or longitudinal stretching force of the neck or torsion of the neck.

**c.** The spinal column in the neonate is more susceptible to hyperextension injury as a result of increased elasticity.

**d.** Spinal immobilization may be required. Immobilization device should fit into the incubator.

**e.** Anticipate respiratory problems with higher spinal cord injuries.

**3.** Inhaled nitric oxide (iNO).

**a.** iNO may be initiated at the referring hospital or by the transport team. If initiated during transport, the treatment should continue for the duration of the transport.

**b.** Requires continuous monitoring of all iNO delivery equipment.

**c.** Follow Federal Aviation Administration regulations for rotor-wing and fixed-wing transports. The pilot should be informed when iNO is taken on board the aircraft and when started.

**d.** Ensure that a hand ventilation system is available.

**4.** Ventilation and airway assist devices.

**a.** Conventional ventilator.

**b.** T-piece resuscitator (AAP and AHA, 2011).

**c.** High-frequency jet ventilation (Gomella, 2009).

**d.** Heated humidified high-flow nasal cannula.

**e.** Noninvasive positive pressure ventilation.

**f.** Continuous positive airway pressure.

5. Transporting multiple births.
   a. If possible, transport at same time.
   b. Each neonate should have a minimum of one transport staff responsible for direct patient care (depending on the diagnosis and clinical condition). Additional transport staff should be available to assist in patient care as needed.
   c. Each neonate should have a set of transport equipment and supplies, including cardiorespiratory monitoring and airway equipment.
   d. Each neonate should have his or her own documentation records, including consent forms.
6. Therapeutic induced hypothermia using total body cooling or selective head cooling (Fairchild et al., 2010; Jacobs et al., 2011).
   a. Term or near-term infants with hypoxic–ischemic encephalopathy.
   b. Time-sensitive transport.
   c. Active cooling—use of total body cooling machine, cooling cap, cold packs, cooling mattress.
   d. Passive cooling—incubator temperature turned off.
   e. Continuous rectal temperature monitoring.
   f. Monitor for adverse effects of hypothermia.
   g. Sedation for comfort per protocol.

## DOCUMENTATION

A. **Necessity of documentation.** Patient status and the care provided must be documented throughout the transport.

B. **Logistical documentation.**
   1. Time of transport call.
   2. Time of departure en route to referring hospital.
   3. Time of arrival at referring hospital.
   4. Time of departure from referring hospital.
   5. Time of arrival at receiving hospital.
   6. Transport delays.
   7. Names of transport staff.
   8. Mode of transport.
   9. Names of referring facility and physician.

C. **Patient care documentation.**
   1. Significant maternal history, including medical history before pregnancy and prenatal, labor, and delivery history.
   2. Date and time of birth.
   3. Gestational age.
   4. Birth weight.
   5. Delivery room resuscitation, including Apgar scores.
   6. Care provided before the team's arrival at the referring hospital, including laboratory and radiographic findings and medications administered.
   7. Patient status on arrival of the transport team to the referring hospital, including physical assessment, vital signs, and current patient management.
   8. Problem list, including current and resolved problems.
   9. Ongoing documentation of patient assessment, management, and consultations with designated transport physician.
   10. Patient status on arrival of the transport team to the receiving hospital, including assessment, vital signs, and monitor readings.

## SAFETY (AAP, 2007; AIR AND SURFACE TRANSPORT NURSES ASSOCIATION, 2011; CAMTS, 2012; DEMMONS AND JAMES, 2008)

A. **Safety must be the highest priority in any transport program.**
   1. The transport program should develop a comprehensive safety program for team members and patients. Training should consist of orientation to the vehicle, emergency

and evacuation procedures, survival training, crew resource management, and quality management.

2. The number and names of all persons on board the transport vehicle must be documented and provided to dispatch before departing.
3. Any passenger(s), including parent(s) riding in a vehicle, should receive a safety briefing prior to the transport. The name(s) of any passengers must be provided to dispatch. Passenger(s) must meet all weight and/or height restrictions and must be able to be secured.
4. During each transport, the team should review evacuation procedures for the crew, the passenger(s), and the neonate.
5. Debriefing should be performed between crew members after each transport.
6. Critical incident stress management should be available for each crew member.

B. **Uniforms.**
1. Team members should be appropriately attired to the environmental conditions when on transport.
   a. Flame- and heat-resistant uniforms with reflective material or striping on uniforms for night operation.
   b. Garments such as jackets, gloves, socks, and underclothing should be made from fire-retardant or natural fibers.
   c. Protective footwear.
   d. Identification badge.
   e. Helmets should be worn during helicopter transports. Visors should be available to protect the eyes and face from projectile objects. Helmets may also be worn during fixed-wing and ground transport.
   f. Appropriate outer garments may be worn to protect against environmental conditions.
   g. Hearing protection should be worn by all crew who assist with patient loading and unloading while rotor blades are activated on the helicopter.

C. **Flotation vests should be worn by all crew members who fly over water.**

D. **Survival and first-aid kit should be located on each vehicle.**

E. **All equipment and articles in the ambulance or aircraft must be secured.**
1. The incubator may be mounted on a cart or stretcher.
2. The cart or stretcher must be locked into the vehicle.
3. Majority of vehicles use longitudinal placement of the incubator rather than horizontal placement.

F. **Restraint of all passengers, including the neonate, during transport.**
1. The neonate should be secured in the transport incubator with a restraint device. Owing to different gestational ages, the restraint device must adjust to fit various sizes and weights. The restraint must not constrict the thoracic cavity. A cushioned head pad should be placed in the incubator to provide protection to the neonate's head.
2. All staff and/or passengers should have seat belts/shoulder harnesses fastened.

G. **Establish a written policy on the use of lights and sirens.**
1. Follow state and local regulations.
2. Use only for life-threatening emergencies.

H. **Communication equipment.**
1. Communication devices are used between team members, dispatch and team, hospital and team, and team and medical control. All communication equipment must be maintained in full operating condition and in good repair.
2. Types of communication devices:
   a. Head sets.
   b. Pagers.
   c. Cell phone.
   d. Satellite phone.
   e. Global system for mobile communication (GSM).
   f. Radio.

I. **Preaccident planning.**
   1. Ground and air transport programs must have a policy outlining the procedure to follow if the vehicle, staff, and patient are in an accident.
      a. Notification of transport and hospital administration, risk management, public relations.
      b. Provision for staff to receive care.
      c. Provision for patient care and completion of the transport. The patient may return to the referring hospital for evaluation and treatment from the accident or go on to receiving hospital, whichever is most appropriate.
      d. Notification of transport team's emergency contact.
      e. Notification of the neonate's family.
      f. If appropriate, notification of other team members of the incident.
      g. If appropriate, lock-down of dispatch or transport office to limit the amount of personnel in the area.
      h. Assistance may be required to staff phones. Consider providing a separate phone number other than the team number to provide incident information and updates. A website may also be used to disseminate information.
   2. Staff must complete an emergency contact form that is updated annually or when there is a change of information. The form should include the following:
      a. Name of employee.
      b. Home address.
      c. Name, address, and phone, cell, and pager numbers of emergency contact.
      d. Alternate emergency contact information.
      e. Information on children.
      f. General directions to crew member's home.
      g. Current photograph in uniform.
      h. Fingerprints.
      i. Name, address, and phone number to obtain dental records.
   3. Contact local or state agencies for critical incident stress debriefing for the team. Immediate and long-term debriefing may be required.
   4. Staff should be aware of the benefits and services available prior to an incident. Benefits and services include but are not limited to worker's compensation, accident insurance, life insurance, and insurance coverage by vehicle vendor and organization. Staff should be knowledgeable if life insurance policy covers an accident while flying.

J. **Infection control.** Infection control and adherence to Universal Precautions should be planned because of the confined space of transport vehicle.

## DISASTER PREPARATION (GERSHANIK, 2006; ORLANDO ET AL., 2007)

A. **The neonatal transport team may have to assist in evacuating a neonatal intensive care unit.**
B. **Nontraditional transport equipment may be required** because of the time limitation of having one infant in a transport incubator; size and weight of transport incubator may be prohibitive in certain aircraft.
C. **Establish system of family notification of where the infant is being transported.**
D. **Establish system of patient tracking, patient identification, and medical record transfer.**
E. **Coordination with local, state, and federal agencies is essential. This may impact transport reimbursement.**

## AIR TRANSPORT CONSIDERATIONS

A. **Altitude.**
   1. Anticipate increased oxygen requirement or ventilatory support at higher altitudes.
   2. Provide supplemental oxygen for staff above 10,000 feet if in a nonpressurized aircraft.

3. Neonates are at increased risk of developing hypoxia as the partial pressure of alveolar oxygen decreases during ascent.
4. Slow ascent and descent are recommended to prevent rapid reexpansion of gas, which increases the risk for pneumothorax and air embolism in the neonate.

B. **Dysbarism.**
1. Increased atmospheric pressure results in expansion of gases.
2. Anticipate expansion of "trapped" gases in body spaces (pulmonary air leaks, necrotizing enterocolitis, bowel obstruction).
   a. Gastrointestinal tract: Insert orogastric tube and empty stomach of air.
   b. Pulmonary air leaks: Consider needle thoracentesis or tube thoracotomy for decompression prior to the transport.
   c. Equalization of pressures in the eustachian tubes may be restricted in the neonate or in staff with upper respiratory or sinus problems. Providing a pacifier to the infant during descent, if appropriate, can maintain patency of the eustachian tubes.

C. **Effects of motion.**
1. Staff should recognize and understand the stresses of transport and flight.
2. Anticipate patient instability on ascent and descent.
3. Staff should be able to differentiate monitor artifact from actual recordings.

D. **Noise and vibration.**
1. Provide ear protection for staff and for the neonate (especially in rotor-wing aircraft).
2. Provide routine hearing screens for staff.
3. Minimize noise levels in patient compartment of vehicle.
4. Anticipate patient instability.
5. Use mattress and padding to minimize vibration in incubator.

E. **Evaluation for extubation and pulmonary air leaks:** possibly difficult during transport, especially in rotor-wing aircraft. Anticipate problems during transport on the basis of diagnosis and clinical presentation.

F. **Out-of-state and international transport.**
1. **Prior to departing on international transports, the destination country should be investigated to ensure safety of the transport team.** Updated information on every country, including travel alerts and warnings, are available from the U.S. State Department's website at http://travel.state.gov.
2. **The team should be knowledgeable regarding out-of-state and international transport regulations and issues.**
   a. Language barriers.
   b. Time change issues.
   c. Landing permits and fees.
   d. Airport hours of operation.
   e. Fueling.
   f. Ground ambulance: availability, type, fees.
   g. Customs/immigration.
   h. Determine if there are any restrictions to transporting specific medications (i.e., narcotics) into a country. Some medications may be required to stay aboard the aircraft or are restricted in certain countries.
   i. Communication with regional neonatal intensive care center.
   j. Electrical systems vary in different countries and may not be able to accommodate equipment.
   k. Some countries require that a physician be present for the patient to be released from the country.

G. **Plan for crew hydration and nutrition on long-distance transports.**

H. **Plan for crew rest periods and overnight stays on long-distance transports.**

I. **Transport configuration and on-loading/off-loading procedures should be predetermined, documented, and practiced prior to an actual patient transport. Discuss securing of incubator and equipment in receiving state's/country's ambulance or mode of transportation prior to arrival.**

## LEGAL AND ETHICAL CONSIDERATIONS

**A. Legal issues (AAP, 2007; NANN, 2010a).**

1. Determination of the level of responsibility of the receiving and referring staffs and institutions during the transport process has not been clearly defined and is open to legal interpretations.
   a. Referring institution's level of responsibility gradually decreases as the receiving physician and transport team assume increasing responsibility for the management and care of the infant.
   b. Transport team should be aware of national and state regulations regarding transport and professional standards: Federal Aviation Administration; National Health, Transportation and Safety Administration; Department of Transportation; Federal Communications Commission; Health Care Financing Administration; The Joint Commission; the Clinical Laboratories Improvement Act; Health Insurance Portability and Accountability Act; and the Consolidated Omnibus Budget Reconciliation Act.
   c. Receiving institution acquires increasing responsibility from the time of the transport call and the initial consultation until the time of admission to the receiving hospital.
2. Parents or legal guardian must receive information regarding the infant's status, treatment options, the risks and benefits of transport, and the risk of not transferring.
   a. The transport program should have a policy on transporting a neonate in an emergency situation when the parent(s) are not able to provide consent.
3. Responsibilities of transport team members should be clearly outlined in their job functions and should be compatible with practice acts.
4. The transport nurse should be aware of federal and state regulations governing the transport and administration of controlled substances.
5. The transport program may not be able to perform neonatal transport for a specific period owing to external and internal factors.
   a. The program may not be able to perform transports due to weather (i.e., hurricanes, tornadoes, and snowstorms); transport accident; and neonatal intensive care bed status.
   b. Develop a plan on how to communicate this information to referral centers.
   c. If team is operational, develop a plan for performing three-point transports. Team and facility will maintain relationship with the referring hospital.
   d. If team is not operational, develop a plan for contacting another neonatal transport service.

**C. Ethical issues.** Dilemmas regarding the transport of neonates should be addressed by administrative, medical, and transport staff and should include information on the following (NANN, 2010b):

1. Infants with expected poor outcomes, including those with genetic disorders, severely asphyxiated infants, extremely low birth weight infants, and those with lethal anomalies.
2. Debriefing of the team may be required.

## QUALITY MANAGEMENT (CAMTS, 2012; NANN, 2010a)

Total quality management is a philosophy for continuously improving the quality of services and processes. The transport program should develop a quality management program to monitor, evaluate, and improve patient outcome and service. All members of the transport team and vendors should be involved in quality improvement planning and process.

- Regularly scheduled meetings.
- Written quality management plan with action plan and thresholds.

**A. Quality indicators may include but are not limited to the following:**

1. Transport statistics (number of completed transports, referral hospitals, referral physicians).
2. Equipment malfunction, failure, or supply.

3. Transport delays.
4. Stabilization times.
5. Crew and patient safety issues.
6. Number of transports per team member.
7. Procedures performed by crew on transport.
8. Documentation of patient care and medications.
9. Vehicle availability and out-of-service time.
10. Patient outcome (performance of cardiopulmonary resuscitation, death during transport, death within 24 hours of transport, intubation and/or extubation during transport, transport without vascular access due to inability to obtain).
11. Hypothermia, hyperthermia, hypotension during transport.
12. Appropriateness and timeliness of interventions and patient's response.
13. Family and referring hospital customer satisfaction.
14. Staff education and skills.
15. Number of aborted and canceled transports.
16. Review of transport policies and procedures a minimum of every 2 years.
17. Staff injuries.
18. Ground transports with red lights and sirens.
19. Trending of occurrences or near-miss occurrences.

B. **Quality improvement may be attained through a number of mechanisms.** A combination of these mechanisms is probably most effective.
   1. Case review by the team, medical director, and transport director.
   2. Use of peer review.
   3. Regular staff meetings.
   4. Case review with team members, which can be effectively accomplished by review of selected cases, including the following:
      a. Initial referral call.
      b. Transport logistics.
      c. Stabilization of the infant by the referring hospital as well as the transport team.
      d. Care provided during transport.
      e. Patient outcome.

C. **Peer review may be used to provide feedback to individuals.**
   1. Appropriateness of care provided.
   2. Clarity of treatment plan.
   3. Treatment plan rationale and outcome.
   4. Documentation.

D. **Issues identified through any of these mechanisms should be addressed with recommendations and plans for follow-up.**

E. **Outreach education.** Transport team members should meet with the health care providers from the referring hospitals to discuss transport stabilization, issues, and concerns.

F. **Policy manual.** Either electronic or hard copy is accessible to all personnel.

## REFERENCES


Air and Surface Transport Nurses Association: Position paper: Transport nurse safety in the transport environment. 2011. Retrieved February 13, 2013, from http://www.astna.org/PDF/ASTNASafetyPaper.pdf.

American Academy of Pediatrics: *Guidelines for air and ground transport of neonatal and pediatric patients:* (3rd ed.). Elk Grove Village, IL, 2007, American Academy of Pediatrics.

American Academy of Pediatrics and American Heart Association: *Textbook of neonatal resuscitation (NRP):* (6th ed.). Elk Grove Village, IL, 2011, American Academy of Pediatrics and American Heart Association.

Blackburn, S.T.: *Maternal, fetal & neonatal physiology:* (4th ed.). Maryland Heights, MO, 2013, Elsevier Saunders.

Blumen, I.: A safety review and risk assessment in air medical transport. Salt Lake City, 2002, Air Medical Physician Association.

Butterfield, L.J.: Historical perspectives of neonatal transport. *Pediatric Clinics of North America,* 40 (2):221–239, 1993.

Chou, M. and MacDonald, M.G.: Landmarks in the development of patient transport systems. In M.G. MacDonald, and M.K. Miller (Eds.): *Emergency transport of the perinatal patient* Boston, 1989, Little, Brown.

Commission on Accreditation of Medical Transport Systems: *Accreditation standards of the Commission on Accreditation of Medical Transport Systems* (9th ed.). Anderson, SC, 2012, Commission on Accreditation of Medical Transport Systems.

Committee on Perinatal Health: Toward improving the outcome of pregnancy. White Plains, NY, 1976, National Foundation-March of Dimes.

Cone, T.E.: History of the care and feeding of the premature infant. Boston, 1985, Little, Brown.

Demmons, L.L. and James, S.E.: *Standards for critical care and specialty ground transport* (2nd ed.). Lexington, KY, 2008, Air and Surface Transport Nurses Association.

Fairchild, K., Sokora, D., Scott, S. and Zanelli, S.: Therapeutic hypothermia on neonatal transport: 4-year experience in a single NICU. *Journal of Perinatology,* 30(5):324–329, 2010.

Gershanik, J.: Caring for and transporting very low birth weight infants during a disaster. *Pediatrics,* 117 (5):5365–5368, 2006.

Gomella (Ed.): *Neonatology: Management, procedures, on-call, problems, diseases, and drugs* (6th ed.). New York, 2009, McGraw-Hill.

Jacobs, S.E., Morley, C.J., Inder, T.E., et al.: Whole-body hypothermia for term and near-term newborns with hypoxic ischemic encephalopathy: A randomized controlled trial. *JAMA Pediatrics,* 165(11):692–700, 2011.

Kenner, C. and McGrath, J.M.: *Developmental care of newborns and infants:* (2nd ed.). Glenview, IL, 2010, National Association of Neonatal Nurses.

Levick, N.: Ambulance transport safety trends: Separating fact from fiction. 2010. Retrieved January 20, 2013, from http://www.objectivesafety.net.

Losty, M.S., Orlofsky, I. and Boles, T.: A transport service for premature babies. *American Journal of Nursing,* 50:10–12, 1950.

March of Dimes: Perinatal statistics. 2005. Retrieved January 14, 2008, from http://www.marchofdimes.com.

Martin, J., Hamilton, B., Ventura, S., et al.: Births: Final data. *National Vital Statistics Reports,* 61(1), 2010.

National Association of Neonatal Nurses: Neonatal nursing transport standards: Guidelines for practice. Glenview, IL, 2010a, National Association of Neonatal Nurses.

National Association of Neonatal Nurses: Position statement #3015: NICU nurses involvement in ethical decisions. 2010b: Retrieved January 20, 2013, from http://www.NANN.org.

Ohning, B.L., Rosenkrantz, T., Carter, B.S. and Springer, S.C.: Transport of the critically ill neonate. 2012: Retrieved March 23, 2013 from http://www.emedicine.medscape.com/article/978606.

Orlando, S., Bernard, M. and Mathews, P.: Neonatal nursing care issues following a natural disaster: Lessons learned from the Katrina experience. *Journal of Perinatal and Neonatal Nursing,* 22 (2):147–153, 2007.

Salyer, J.W.: Transport of infants and children. In M. Czervinske, and S. Barnhart (Eds.): *Perinatal and pediatric respiratory care* (2nd ed.) Philadelphia, 2003, W.B. Saunders, pp. 693–707.

Segal (Ed.): *Manual for the transport of high-risk newborn infants* Sherbrooke, Quebec, 1972, Canadian Paediatric Society.

Segal, S.: Transfer of a premature or other high-risk newborn infant to a referral hospital. *Pediatric Clinics of North America,* 13(4):1195–1205, 1966.

Shah, S., Rothberger, A., Caprio, M., et al.: Quantification of impulse experienced by neonates during inter- and intra-hospital transport measured by biophysical accelerometry. *Journal of Perinatal Medicine,* 36:87–92, 2008.

Thigpen, J.: Developmental considerations for resuscitation of the VLBW infant. *Neonatal Network,* 21 (4):21–26, 2002.

Wallace, H.M., Losty, M.A. and Baumgartner, L.: Report of two years' experience in the transportation of premature infants in New York City. *Pediatrics,* 22:439–447, 1952.

Wood, K.S. and Bose, C.: Neonatal transport. In M. MacDonald, M. Mullett, and M. Seshia (Eds.): *Avery's neonatology: Pathophysiology and management of the newborn* (6th ed.). Philadelphia, 2005, Lippincott Williams & Wilkins, pp. 40–53.

Woodward, G.A., Insoft, R.M., Pearson-Shaver, A.L., et al.: The state of pediatric interfacility transport: Consensus of the Second National Pediatric and Neonatal Interfacility Transport Medicine Leadership Conference. *Pediatric Emergency Care,* 18(1):38–43, 2002.

CHAPTER

# 22 Care of the Extremely Low Birth Weight (ELBW) Infant

JAN SHERMAN

**OBJECTIVES**

1. Discuss the mortality and morbidity associated with extreme prematurity.
2. Identify principles of nursing care specific to the ELBW infant population and their families.

## OVERVIEW

Care of premature infants with birth weights between 1000 and 1500 g has become almost routine in most neonatal intensive care units (NICUs) in the United States. The most recent challenge in neonatology is the care of ELBW infants (birth weight <1000 g). Although they represent a small percentage of overall births and NICU admissions, ELBW infants are often the most critically ill and at the highest risk for mortality and long-term morbidity of any NICU patient. They remain hospitalized for long periods of time, suffer the most acute and long-term complications of neonatal intensive care, and consume a disproportionate number of hospital days. The purpose of this chapter is to provide an overview of topics related to care of the ELBW infant. Detailed information on resuscitation, thermoregulation, ventilation, and fluids and electrolytes can be found in those specific chapters.

## EPIDEMIOLOGY (CENTERS FOR DISEASE CONTROL AND PREVENTION [CDC], 2013; MARCH OF DIMES, 2013)

A. **The premature birth rate has risen by 36% over the last 25 years and affects nearly 500,000 babies per year (1 of every 9 infants) born in the United States (Centers for Disease Control and Prevention [CDC]).**
B. **Preterm-related causes of death together accounted for 35% of all infant deaths in 2008, more than any other single cause.** Preterm birth is also a leading cause of long-term neurologic disabilities in children.
C. **Preterm birth costs the U.S. health care system more than $26 billion each year (CDC, 2013).** Women who are at increased risk of having a premature baby include African American women, women younger than 17, and women older than 35, as well as women who have a low income.
D. **Births at the threshold of viability, early preterm birth, or birth of an ELBW infant—especially those weighing less than 750 g or less than 26 weeks of gestation, pose a variety of complex medical, social, and ethical considerations.**
E. **The effect of such births on the infants, their families, the health care system, and society are profound.** Although the prevalence of such births is less than 1%, they account for nearly one half of all cases of perinatal mortality (American Academy of Pediatrics [AAP] and American College of Obstetricians and Gynecologists [ACOG], 2012).

## MORTALITY AND MORBIDITY (AAP AND ACOG, 2012)

A. **Mortality and survival with major neonatal morbidity for infants 501 to 1500 g decreased between 2000 and 2009.** Infants weighing 501 to 750 g had the greatest decrease in mortality but the least change in survival with major morbidity.
B. **In 2009, nearly half of all infants 501 to 1500 g and 89% of those weighing 501 to 750 g either died or survived after experiencing ≥1 major morbidity during their initial hospital stay, highlighting the continuing challenges facing these vulnerable patients, their families, and the health professionals who care for them.**
C. **There has been a dramatic increase in the number of multiple births in the United States over the past two decades, largely due to artificial reproductive technology and fertility-inducing drugs.**
D. **Perinatal risks that may be associated with assisted reproductive therapy include high-order multiple pregnancy, prematurity, low birth weight, small for gestational age, perinatal mortality, cesarean delivery, placenta previa, placental abruption, preeclampsia, and birth defects.**
E. **Recent studies have shown that triplet or higher-order births are associated with an increased risk of death or neurodevelopmental impairment at 18 to 22 months' corrected age when compared with ELBW singleton infants (Wadhawan et al., 2011).**
Table 22-1 details the rates for mortality and morbidity for 2000 and 2009 (Horbar et al., 2012).

## PERINATAL MANAGEMENT (AAP AND ACOG, 2012)

A. **Neonates born to women transported during the antepartum period have better survival rates and decreased risks of long-term sequelae than those transferred after birth.**
B. **Because ELBW and/or very preterm infants are at increased risk of predischarge mortality, they should be delivered at a level III facility unless this is precluded by the mother's medical condition or geographic constraints (Committee on Fetus and Newborn, 2012).**

■ TABLE 22-1
■ ■ **Comparison of Standardized Rates for Major Neonatal Morbidities in 2000 and 2009 for Surviving Infants 501 to 1500 g**

| | 2000 (%) | 2009 (%) |
|---|---|---|
| **Any Major Morbidity** | | |
| All 501 to 1500 g | 46.4 | 41.4 |
| 501 to 750 g | 84.5 | 82.7 |
| 751 to 1000 g | 63.1 | 57.4 |
| 1001 to 1250 g | 38.8 | 33.1 |
| 1251 to 1500 g | 23.3 | 18.7 |
| **Major Neonatal Morbidities** | | |
| Early bacterial infection | 2.0 | 1.7 |
| Late infection (bacterial or fungal) | 21.5 | 15.0 |
| NEC | 4.9 | 5.3 |
| CLD | 27.7 | 26.3 |
| Severe IVH (grades 3 and 4) | 6.5 | 6.1 |
| PVL | 3.0 | 2.7 |
| Severe ROP (stages 3 to 5) | 10.2 | 6.8 |

From Horbar, J.D., Carpenter, J.H., Badger, G.J., et al.: Mortality and neonatal morbidity among infants 501 to 1500 grams from 2000 to 2009. *Pediatrics*, 129(6):1019-1026, 2012.
*CLD*, Chronic lung disease; *IVH*, intraventricular hemorrhage; *NEC*, necrotizing enterocolitis; *PVL*, periventricular leukomalacia; *ROP*, retinopathy of prematurity.

C. **Antepartum transport avoids separation of mother and infant in the immediate postpartum period, allows mothers to communicate directly with NICU health care providers, and supports the goal of family-centered health care.**

## PERINATAL CONSULTATION (AAP AND ACOG, 2012)

A. **In general, parents of extremely preterm fetuses can be counseled that infants delivered before 24 weeks of gestation are less likely to survive and those who do are not likely to survive intact.**
B. **Whenever possible, data specific to the age, weight, and gender of the fetus should be used to aid management decisions made by obstetricians and parents of fetuses at risk of preterm delivery before 26 completed weeks of gestation.** This information may be developed by each institution and should indicate the population used in determining estimates of survivability.
C. **The Eunice Kennedy Shriver National Institute for Child Health and Development (NICHD) Neonatal Research Network's Extremely Preterm Birth Outcome Data website** provides a calculator to estimate infant outcomes based on birth weight, gestational age, gender, and antenatal corticosteroid administration. The calculator is available at http://www.nichd.nih.gov/about/org/der/branches/ppb/programs/epbo/pages/epbo_case.aspx.
D. **If the physicians involved believe that there is no chance of survival, resuscitation is not indicated and should not be initiated. If the physicians consider a good outcome to be very unlikely, then parents should be given the choice of whether resuscitation should be initiated and physicians should respect their preference.**
E. **When the physicians' judgment is that a good outcome is reasonably likely, physicians should initiate resuscitation and, together with the parents, continually evaluate whether intensive care should be continued.**

## ANTENATAL STEROIDS

Enhancement of fetal pulmonary function with the use of antenatal steroids lessens the prevalence and severity of neonatal respiratory distress syndrome. Current recommendations in the *Guidelines for Perinatal Care* (AAP and ACOG, 2012) include:

A. **A single course of corticosteroids (betamethasone or dexamethasone) is recommended for pregnant women between 24 weeks and 34 weeks of gestation who are at risk of preterm delivery within 7 days.**
B. **A single course of antenatal corticosteroids should be administered to women with premature rupture of membranes (PROM) before 32 weeks of gestation to reduce the risks of respiratory distress syndrome, perinatal mortality, and other morbidities.**
C. **The efficacy of corticosteroid use at 32 to 33 completed weeks of gestation for preterm PROM is unclear, but treatment may be beneficial, particularly if pulmonary immaturity is documented.** Sparse data exist on the efficacy of corticosteroid use before fetal age of viability, and such use is not recommended.
D. **A single rescue course of antenatal corticosteroids may be considered if the antecedent treatment was given more than 2 weeks prior, the gestational age is less than $32^{6/7}$ weeks, and the woman is judged by the physician to be likely to give birth within the next week.** However, regularly scheduled repeat courses or multiple courses (more than two) are not recommended.

## TIMING OF UMBILICAL CORD CLAMPING AFTER BIRTH (AAP, 2013)

A. **Evidence supports delayed umbilical cord clamping in preterm infants.** As with term infants, delaying umbilical cord clamping to 30 to 60 seconds after birth with the infant at a level below the placenta is associated with neonatal benefits, including improved transitional circulation, better establishment of red blood cell volume, and decreased need for blood transfusion.
B. **The single most important clinical benefit for preterm infants is the possibility for a nearly 50% reduction of intraventricular hemorrhage (IVH).** It is important to note that the timing of umbilical cord clamping should not be altered for the purpose of collecting umbilical cord blood for banking.

## DELIVERY ROOM CARE SPECIFIC TO ELBW INFANTS

A. **Careful adherence to details in the delivery room and during the first few hours after birth is essential to help avoid immediate and long-term complications of the ELBW infant.** NICUs should have a consistent approach to the initial care of the ELBW infant in the delivery room and upon admission to the NICU (Table 22-2).

B. *All neonatal resuscitations and delivery room management should follow the guidelines found in the* Textbook of Neonatal Resuscitation, *6th edition* (American Academy of Pediatrics and American Heart Association 2011). Also please see Chapter 5.

## THERMOREGULATION (SEE CHAPTER 6) (AAP AND ACOG, 2012)

A. **Very low birth weight (<1500-g) preterm babies are likely to become hypothermic despite the use of traditional techniques for decreasing heat loss.** Because infants younger than 28 weeks of gestation may become hypothermic while being dried, they should be immediately covered up to their necks in polyethylene wrap or a food-grade plastic bag and placed under a radiant warmer.

B. **The infant's temperature must be monitored closely because overheating has been described when plastic wrap is used in combination with an exothermic mattress.** The goal should be an axillary temperature of approximately 36.5° C (97.7° F).

## VENTILATORY PRACTICES IN THE DELIVERY ROOM (AAP AND ACOG, 2012)

A. **Administration of supplemental oxygen in the delivery room.**
   1. Current practice recommends supplemental oxygen administration be based on objective monitoring of oxygenation. It is recommended that pulse oximetry be used when resuscitation can be anticipated, supplemental oxygen is administered, positive pressure is administered for more than a few breaths, or cyanosis appears to persist.
   2. Because many babies born at less than 32 weeks of gestation will not reach target saturations when resuscitated with air, blended oxygen may be used. If blended oxygen is not available, resuscitation should be initiated with air.
   3. The use of room air for resuscitation of these infants has been proposed to protect from hyperoxia and damage to the lungs by oxygen free radicals. Many NICUs have developed their own policies regarding starting values of blended oxygen in the delivery room (Eichenwald, 2012).

B. **Assisted ventilation in the delivery room.**
   1. If positive pressure ventilation is required, it should be provided with low inspiratory pressure to prevent overdistention of the lungs, which can result in air leak and other lung injury. Adequate positive end-expiratory pressure (PEEP) will help to maintain lung volume (Eichenwald, 2012).

C. **Surfactant administration in the delivery room.**
   1. There continues to be uncertainty as to whether to give surfactant in the first few minutes of life to an ELBW newborn, apply nasal continuous positive airway pressure (NCPAP) without surfactant, or intubate giving surfactant and then extubate to CPAP. The potential benefits and risks of these strategies are still under study (Goldsmith and Karotkin, 2011).
   2. No matter the timing of the surfactant administration, it is only given after endotracheal tube position is confirmed (AAP and ACOG, 2012).
   3. Novel methods of surfactant administration are currently being studied. Klebermass-Schrehof et al. (2013) have described a new mode of surfactant administration without intubation, known as less invasive surfactant administration. CPAP is administered by a nasopharyngeal tube after delivery. At 20 to 30 minutes after birth, a thin catheter (1.3 mm diameter) is inserted into the trachea. Surfactant is then administered over 2 to 5 minutes via this catheter while the infant is breathing spontaneously. About 65% of the

■ TABLE 22-2
■ ■ **Treatment Guidelines for Initial Management of Extremely Low Birth Weight Infants**

| | **Delivery Room and NICU Admission** |
|---|---|
| Delivery room | Immediately place into polyethylene wrap or food-grade plastic bag up to the neck |
| | Ensure good thermoregulation |
| | "Gentle" ventilation as required |
| | Avoid hyperventilation and hyperoxia |
| | Administer surfactant (if prophylaxis approach) |
| | Initiate NCPAP (if early CPAP approach) |
| NICU admission | Obtain weight measurement |
| | Administer surfactant within first hour (if rescue approach) |
| | Establish vascular access: |
| | Peripheral intravenous catheter |
| | Umbilical arterial catheter |
| | Umbilical venous catheter (central, double-lumen) |
| | Start intravenous fluids as soon as possible with dextrose and amino acid solution |
| | Limit evaporative water losses (humidified incubator) |
| | Minimize stimulation |
| | Avoid hyperventilation and hyperoxia |
| | Maintain target oxygen saturations |
| | Obtain specimens for complete blood count with differential, blood culture, blood glucose measurement |
| | Give antibiotics as indicated |
| | Give parents information about their child |

| | **First 24 to 48 Hours** |
|---|---|
| Cardiovascular | Monitor blood pressure, give vasopressors as required |
| | Maintain vigilance for presence of patent ductus arteriosus |
| | Obtain echocardiogram as indicated |
| Respiratory | Give additional surfactant doses as indicated |
| | Maintain low tidal volume ventilation |
| | Avoid hyperventilation and hyperoxia |
| | Extubate infant and start on CPAP when possible |
| Fluid management | Obtain weight every 12 to 24 hours |
| | Monitor serum electrolyte, blood glucose, and calcium concentrations every 4 to 12 hours |
| | Use of humidity |
| | Limit evaporative water losses |
| | Administer skin care |
| Hematologic | Obtain second blood count |
| | Administer transfusion support as indicated |
| | Monitor bilirubin, begin phototherapy as indicated |
| Infection | Consider discontinuing antibiotics if blood culture results are negative at 48 hours |
| Nutrition | Start parenteral nutrition |
| | Discuss trophic feedings |
| Neurologic | Minimize stimulation |
| | Perform screening head ultrasonography |
| Social | Provide daily updates to the family |
| | Arrange to meet with family |

From Eichenwald, E.C.: Care of the extremely low-birthweight infant. In C.A. Gleason and S.U. Devaskar (Eds.): *Avery's diseases of the newborn* (9th ed.). Philadelphia, 2012, Elsevier Saunders, pp. 390–404.
*CPAP*, continuous positive airway pressure; *NCPAP*, nasal continuous positive airway pressure; *NICU*, neonatal intensive care unit.

extremely premature infants (23 to 25 weeks postmenstrual age) could be managed without mechanical ventilation (MV) during the first week of life, and 41% without any MV during the entire hospital stay. The authors found significantly higher survival rates (especially for the most immature infants), and less IVH, cystic periventricular leukomalacia (PVL), need for supplementary oxygen at day 28, and duration of MV compared to historical controls.

## ADMISSION TO THE NEONATAL INTENSIVE CARE UNIT

A. **General care.**
  1. All infants should be weighed upon admission; frequent determination of subsequent weights is a valuable tool in managing fluid and electrolyte balance. In many centers, ELBW infants are initially placed under a radiant warmer for easier access (i.e., for surfactant administration and catheter placement).
  2. Because of the high transepidermal fluid losses in these infants, intravenous (IV) fluids containing 5% to 10% dextrose should be started as quickly as possible after admission and efforts should be made to reduce evaporative water losses by increasing the relative humidity surrounding the infant.

B. **Ambient humidity.**
  1. **High humidity decreases transepidermal water loss (TEWL) and heat loss.** Humidity also decreases fluid requirements and electrolyte imbalances.
  2. 70% or higher humidity in the first week of life is needed to affect a difference in TEWL.

C. **Oxygen saturation range.**
  1. The optimal range for oxygen saturation continues to be controversial.
  2. The SUPPORT trial found that the risk of death during the initial hospitalization was increased among neonates randomly assigned to the lower-oxygen-saturation (85% to 89%) group as compared with those assigned to the higher-oxygen-saturation (91% to 95%) group. *The authors state that lower oxygen saturation targets cannot be recommended in these extremely preterm infants* (Vaucher et al., 2012).
  3. In general, oxygen is given for saturations less than 85% and weaned for saturations greater than 95%.

## VASCULAR ACCESS (SEE CHAPTER 15)

A. **Umbilical arterial catheter (UAC).**
  1. Close monitoring of blood pressure, arterial blood gases, and serum chemistries during the first few days after birth is necessary for high risk ELBW infants. Insertion of a UAC allows for reliable arterial access in critically ill infants. For infants greater than 1200 g, a 5 F catheter should be used. Infants less than 1200 g require a 3.5 F catheter (MacDonald and Ramasethu, 2007).

B. **Umbilical venous catheter (UVC).**
  1. Placement of a UVC at the same time the UAC is placed also provides the clinician with reliable venous access for infusion of fluids, medications, and blood products. Use of a double-lumen UVC helps to preserve IV sites and skin integrity.

C. **Percutaneous central venous catheter.**
  1. Before the UVC is removed, it is advisable to insert a PICC for infusion of parenteral nutrition and medications. PICC line sizes include 1.2 F, 1.9 F (single or double lumen), 2 F, and 3 F. The size PICC to be inserted should be determined by the size of the vein being used for cannulation.

## SKIN CARE (SEE CHAPTER 36)

A. **Gestational age is strongly linked to epidermal barrier function.** Poor epidermal barrier function in the extremely preterm infant leads to disturbances in temperature regulation and water balance. The skin barrier of premature infants is injured easily and can serve as a portal of entry for agents, causing serious bacterial infections (Telofski et al., 2012).

B. **Because of these risks, preservation of skin integrity should be incorporated into the care of the extremely preterm infant.** Objective tools such as the Association of Women's Health, Obstetric and Neonatal Nurses (AWHONN) Neonatal Skin Condition Score Tool can facilitate assessment of neonatal skin conditions (Lund et al., 2013).

C. **Limited use of adhesives and extreme care upon their removal, frequent repositioning of the infant to avoid pressure points on the skin, and use of soft bedding or a water mattress are the minimum requirements (Eichenwald, 2012).**

D. **Assessment of the overall skin condition involves evaluating all skin surfaces, head-to-toe, daily or more frequently**. Risk factors for skin injury include less than 32 weeks of gestation, edema, and adhesives applied to the skin to secure tubes, lines, and monitoring equipment.
E. **Turning the infant a minimum of every 4 hours is necessary, along with careful inspection of skin surfaces**. Even when turning side-to-side is not feasible, lifting the head, shoulders, and hips and supporting these areas with pressure-reducing surfaces is helpful (Harris et al., 2003; Lund, 2011; Telofski et al., 2012).

## ASSISTED VENTILATION (SEE CHAPTER 26)

A. **Noninvasive respiratory support** (NRS).
   1. NRS is becoming increasingly popular as a method of respiratory support in sick newborn infants. This support consists primarily of CPAP and noninvasive positive-pressure ventilation (NIPPV).
   2. A variety of CDP devices available today allow breaths to be delivered above the baseline CPAP pressure and to be synchronized or nonsynchronized to the infant's own breaths. The goal of such devices is to enhance $CO_2$ removal and stimulate breathing. Various CDP devices provide an adjunct to weaning infants off MV after they have been extubated and also help manage apnea of prematurity (Wiswell and Courtney, 2011).
   3. Marked bowel distention ("CPAP belly") is frequently seen. The air from the CPAP easily passes into the esophagus and is swallowed. Increased abdominal girth and visibly dilated intestinal loops may be seen. An increased risk of gastric perforation has been reported. An orogastric tube should always be placed whenever CPAP is used (Wiswell and Courtney, 2011).

B. **Mechanical ventilation**.
   1. MV is indicated when the ELBW infant is not exchanging gases sufficiently, or is acidotic, apneic, or bradycardic. In the first few days of life, surfactant administration is commonly needed.
   2. A variety of devices are now available for use: synchronized intermittent mandatory ventilation (SIMV), assist–control ventilation, volume-controlled ventilation, high-frequency jet ventilation (HFJV), and high-frequency oscillatory ventilation (HFOV).

C. **Methylxanthines**.
   1. Caffeine has been found to decrease the frequency of apnea of prematurity as well as decrease the need for MV.
   2. The Caffeine for Apnea of Prematurity Trial Group (Schmidt et al., 2007) reported on the short- and long-term effects of caffeine at 18 to 21 months in infants with very low birth weight. The study found a decreased rate of BPD, decreased death, less cerebral palsy, and decreased incidence of severe ROP in the treatment group.

## NUTRITIONAL MANAGEMENT (SEE CHAPTERS 8 AND 10) (DELL, 2011)

A. **ELBW infants are born with limited nutrient reserves, immature pathways for nutrient absorption and metabolism, and higher nutrient demands**. Medical conditions associated with extreme prematurity may complicate the adequate delivery of nutrients.
B. **All infants have a physiologic weight loss that is a reduction in extracellular water**. In very premature infants, the loss of extracellular fluid can be 15%.
C. **Fluid requirements**.
   1. Initial fluid therapy should be aimed at allowing a normal physiologic weight loss while preventing dehydration and electrolyte imbalances.
   2. Maintenance fluids required during the first week of life are displayed in Table 22-3. Fluids should be adjusted based upon the infant's clinical condition and any factors that may alter the fluid requirements.
D. **Parenteral nutrition**.
   1. ELBW infants are initially almost entirely dependent on parenteral nutrition. The extremely premature neonate is born with minimal glucose stores and can lose 1% of body protein per day when provided with IV glucose alone. Initiating fluids quickly is paramount in ELBW infants.

■ TABLE 22-3
■ ■ **Maintenance Fluid Requirements During the First Week of Life**

| Birth Weight (g) | Dextrose (g/100 mL) | Day 1 to 2 (mL/kg/day) | Day 3 to 7 (mL/kg/day) |
|---|---|---|---|
| <750 | 5 to 10 | 100 to 200 | 120 to 200 |
| 750 to 1000 | 10 | 80 to 150 | 100 to 150 |
| 1001 to 1500 | 10 | 60 to 100 | 80 to 150 |
| >1500 | 10 | 60 to 80 | 100 to 150 |

Adapted from Dell, K.M.: Fluid, electrolytes, and acid-base homeostasis. In R.J. Martin, A.A. Fanaroff, and M.C. Walsh (Eds.): *Fanaroff and Martin's neonatal-perinatal medicine: Diseases of the fetus and newborn* (9th ed.). St. Louis, 2011, Elsevier Mosby, pp. 669-684.

**E. Glucose.**

1. Glucose is the primary energy substrate for the brain. The normal glucose requirement is 4 to 8 mg/kg/min in preterm infants. Infants who weigh greater than 1000 g usually tolerate a 10% glucose solution initially, whereas infants weighing less than 1000 g should start on a 5% glucose solution.
2. ELBW infants are susceptible to hyperglycemia. Careful monitoring to avoid both hypoglycemia (plasma glucose level <40 mg/dL) and hyperglycemia (plasma level >150 mg/dL) is necessary, with adjustment of dextrose as necessary. Generally plasma glucose levels less than 200 mg/dL do not require treatment.

**F. Amino acids.**

1. Failure to provide adequate protein can significantly impact the long-term outcome of extremely premature infants.
2. Provision of 1 to 1.5 g/kg/day of IV amino acids, even when total caloric intake is low, can help limit catabolism, improve protein balance, and preserve endogenous protein stores.
3. Generally the maximum intake of IV amino acids is 3 to 4 g/kg/day for the ELBW infant.
4. Serum BUN and pH should be monitored since azotemia, hyperammononemia, and metabolic acidosis may be evidence of protein intolerance.
5. The appropriate balance of glucose and lipids in parenteral nutrition is critical. Nutrient and protein retention is maximal if the balance between carbohydrates and lipids is approximately 60:40.

**G. Lipids.**

1. IV lipids are important not only to prevent essential fatty acid deficiency but also as a significant source of nonprotein energy.
2. Essential fatty acid deficiency can develop in preterm infants within 72 hours. This deficiency can be avoided with a minimum of 0.5 to 1 g/kg/day of IV lipids.
3. IV lipids are available as 10%, 20%, and 30% emulsions. The 20% solutions are preferred because they have lower phospholipid-to-triglyceride ratios and liposomal content than the 10% solutions, resulting in lower plasma triglyceride, cholesterol, and phospholipid concentrations.
4. Lipid infusion rates in excess of 0.25 g/kg/hr can be associated with decreases in oxygenation.
5. Twenty percent lipids should be started at 0.5 to 1 g/kg/day and infused over 24 hours. Lipid concentrations can gradually be advanced to a maximum of 3 g/kg/day. Lipid infusion should not exceed 3 to 4 g/kg/day.
6. Triglyceride concentrations are most often used as an indication of lipid tolerance and should be maintained below 150 to 200 mg/dL.

**H. Complications of parenteral nutrition.**

1. The primary complications of parenteral nutrition are cholestasis (parenteral nutrition–associated liver disease) and complications related to the IV line. The exact cause of cholestasis remains unknown.
2. The most frequently identified risk factors in cholestasis are duration of parenteral nutrition, degree of immaturity, and delayed enteral feeding.

I. **Enteral nutrition.**
   1. Providing consistent enteral nutrition to ELBW infants is challenging. Issues of immature gut motility and function as well as the fear of necrotizing enterocolitis are prevalent.
   2. Human milk is the optimal food for infants because it provides immunologic and antibacterial factors, hormones, and enzymes not present in other infant food sources. The benefits of human milk for gastrointestinal function, host defense, and possibly neurodevelopmental outcome have been well documented.
   3. Early initiation (within the first few days after birth) of low-volume feedings (10 to 20 mL/kg/day) are not meant to give the infant significant nutrition, but only to promote continued functional maturation of the gastrointestinal tract.
   4. Small aliquots of human milk or premature formula may be provided at 1 to 2 mL/kg every 2 to 3 hours. Evidence suggests that these small trophic feedings may reduce or prevent intestinal atrophy in this high-risk population.
   5. One common approach is to advance feedings by 20 mL/kg/day if the infant tolerated the previous 24 hours of feeding; this typically results in full enteral feeding (150 mL/kg/day) in 7 to 10 days.
   6. Another approach is to prolong small feeding volumes (20 mL/kg/day) for a period of 5 to 10 days, especially in the high-risk ELBW infant population.
   7. As enteral feeds approach full volumes, usually 150 to 160 mL/kg/day, consideration should be given to using increasing caloric density.
   8. Feeding intolerance, indicated by gastric residuals that exceed 25% to 50% of the volume fed, abdominal distention, or microscopic blood in the stool, is common in ELBW infants and may be difficult to differentiate from early stages of necrotizing enterocolitis.

J. **Prebiotics and probiotics**: Several clinical trials of probiotics have been performed in neonates and have suggested that administration of probiotics may prevent necrotizing enterocolitis. There is currently no FDA-approved product for use in infants.

## MANAGEMENT AND PREVENTION OF INFECTION (SEE CHAPTER 32)

Bacterial and fungal infections are an important cause of illness and death among ELBW infants.

A. **Early-onset bacterial sepsis.**
   1. The incidence of neonatal sepsis ranges from 1 to 5 cases per 1000 live births with a case fatality rate of 5% to 10%.
   2. EOS is generally acquired vertically from bacteria colonizing the mother's lower genital tract or from infected amniotic fluid. The exception is transplacental transmission of *Treponema pallidum* and *Listeria monocytogenes* (Edwards, 2011).
   3. Risk factors for EOS.
      a. Maternal factors:
         (1) Intrapartum fever (>37.5° C).
         (2) Chorioamnionitis.
         (3) Prolonged rupture of membranes, greater than 18 hours.
         (4) Maternal colonization with group B streptococcus.
         (5) Colonization with genital mycoplasmas.
      b. Neonatal factors:
         (1) Less than 37 weeks of gestation.
         (2) Birth weight less than 2500 g.
         (3) The incidence is 10 times higher in infants with a birth weight less than 1000 g.

B. **Predominant organisms.**
   1. *Escherichia coli* is the most common cause of EOS in very low birth weight infants (Table 22-4).

C. **Clinical manifestations of sepsis and antimicrobial therapy** (**see Chapter 32**).

■ TABLE 22-4
■ ■ **Percentage of Organisms Associated with Early-Onset Sepsis**

| Early-Onset Sepsis | VLBW Early-Onset Sepsis |
|---|---|
| GBS = 46% | *Escherichia coli* = 49% |
| Other streptococci = 26% | CoNS = 17% |
| *E. coli* = 20% | GBS = 14% |
| *Enterococcus* = 4% | Other streptococci = 11% |
| *Staphylococcus aureus* = 4% | Other gram-positive = 9% |

Data from Falciglia, G., Hageman, J.R., Schreiber, M., and Alexander, K.: Antibiotic therapy and early onset sepsis. *NeoReviews*, 13:e86, 2012.
*CoNS*, Coagulase-negative *Staphylococcus*; *GBS*, group B *Streptococcus*; *VLBW*, very low birth weight.

# NEUROSENSORY COMPLICATIONS (EICHENWALD, 2012)

A. **The major neurosensory complications associated with extreme premature birth are IVH, periventricular white matter injury, and ROP.**
   1. Although the incidence of severe IVH has fallen with improvements in management and increased antenatal steroid use, it remains a major cause of brain injury with consequent abnormal neurodevelopment.
   2. ROP, a vascular proliferative disorder that affects the incompletely vascularized retina of preterm infants, is a major cause of blindness in these children. Severe retinopathy is 18-fold more likely to develop in infants delivered at less than 25 weeks of gestation compared with 28 weeks of gestation.

B. **NICUs should have a routine protocol of screening for neurosensory complications. Screening guidelines for common complications are shown in Table 22-5.**

# DEVELOPMENTAL INTERVENTIONS (EICHENWALD, 2012) (SEE CHAPTER 11)

A. **Infants born preterm are at increased risk of developing cognitive and motor impairments compared with infants born at term.** Early developmental interventions have been used in the clinical setting with the aim of improving the overall functional outcome for these infants.

■ TABLE 22-5
■ ■ **Recommended Screening for Common Complications of Extremely Low Birth Weight Infants**

| Complication | Screening |
|---|---|
| IVH | HUS on days 1 to 3; repeat on days 7 to 10 |
| Germinal matrix hemorrhage | Repeat HUS weekly until findings normal |
| IVH | Repeat HUS every 3 to 7 days until stable or resolved |
| IVH with ventricular dilatation or intraparenchymal bleeding | Repeat HUS every 3 to 7 days until stable or resolved<br>Consider measurement of resistive indices for progressive ventricular dilatation |
| Periventricular white matter disease | HUS at day 30; repeat at 36 weeks of postmenstrual age or at discharge<br>Consider magnetic resonance imaging if HUS findings are equivocal |
| ROP | Perform OE examination at 4 to 6 weeks of postnatal age<br>Repeat every 2 weeks if no ROP<br>Repeat weekly if ROP present<br>Repeat twice weekly for prethreshold disease or rapidly progressive ROP |
| Audiology screening | Hearing screen no earlier than 34 weeks of postmenstrual age, but before discharge home |

From Eichenwald, E.C.: Care of the extremely low-birthweight infant. In C.A. Gleason and S.U. Devaskar (Eds.): *Avery's diseases of the newborn* (9th ed.). Philadelphia, 2012, Elsevier Saunders, pp. 390-404.
*HUS*, Head ultrasonography; *IVH*, intraventricular hemorrhage; *OE*, ophthalmologic examination; *ROP*, retinopathy of prematurity.

**B.** Modification of the NICU environment to limit exposure of ELBW infants to negative stimuli by lowering ambient light and reducing noise, clustering caregiving periods and procedures to allow periods of uninterrupted sleep, and using positioning aids to promote containment is an intuitive part of their care.

**C.** Newer NICU designs, transitioning from open common rooms to private room settings, may also facilitate a better environment for vulnerable infants and enhance parental involvement.

## END-OF-LIFE CARE

**A. Noninitiation or withdrawal of intensive care for high-risk infants.**

1. Parents should be active participants in the decision-making process concerning the treatment of severely ill infants. This approach requires honest and open communication.
2. Ongoing evaluation of the condition and prognosis of the high-risk infant is essential. The health care provider must convey this information accurately and openly to the parents of the infant.
3. It is inappropriate for life-prolonging treatment to be continued when the condition is incompatible with life or when the treatment is judged to be harmful, of no benefit, or futile (AAP and ACOG, 2012).
4. Whenever nonresuscitation is considered an option, a qualified individual should be involved and present in the delivery room to manage this complex situation.
5. The decision to initiate or continue intensive care should be based only on the judgment that the infant will benefit from the intensive care (AAP and ACOG, 2012).

**B. Compassionate and comfort care.**

1. Comfort care should be provided to all infants for whom resuscitation is not initiated or is not successful.
2. Compassionate care to ensure comfort must be provided to all infants, including those for whom intensive care is not being provided.
3. When the extremely preterm newborn does not survive, support should be provided to the family by physicians, nurses, and other staff after the infant's death (AAP and ACOG, 2012).

## FUTURE DIRECTIONS

**A. The medical care of the ELBW infant is complex, and wide variability in approaches to care of these infants exists among practitioners and NICUs, as does variability in outcomes.** NICUs involved in treating ELBW infants should develop a coherent approach to the medical and ethical aspects of their care.

**B. New web-based tools may help with the development of individual "outcome trajectories" that may help with prediction of death or neurodevelopmental impairment in extremely premature infants.** The effects of various complications on long-term outcomes in ELBW infants would be useful to clinicians and parents in determining plans of care (Ambalavanan et al., 2012).

## REFERENCES


Ambalavanan, N., Carlo, W.A., Tyson, J.E., et al.: for the Generic Database and Follow-Up Subcommittees of the Eunice Kennedy Shriver National Institute of Child Health and Human Development Neonatal Research Network: Outcome trajectories in extremely preterm infants. *Pediatrics*, 130(1):e115–e125, 2012.

American Academy of Pediatrics: Timing of umbilical cord clamping after birth. *Pediatrics*, 131:e1323, 2013. Retrieved from http://www.acog.org/Resources_And_Publications/Committee_Opinions/Committee_on_Obstetric_Practice/Timing_of_Umbilical_Cord_Clamping_After_Birth.

American Academy of Pediatrics and American College of Obstetricians and Gynecologists: *Guidelines for perinatal care:* (7th ed.). Elk Grove Village, IL, and Washington, DC, 2012, American Academy of Pediatrics and American College of Obstetricians and Gynecologists.

American Academy of Pediatrics and American Heart Association: *Textbook of neonatal resuscitation (NRP):* (6th ed.). Elk Grove Village, IL, 2011, American Academy of Pediatrics and American Heart Association.

Centers for Disease Control, Prevention: Preterm birth. 2013: Retrieved from http://www.cdc.gov/

reproductivehealth/maternalinfanthealth/PretermBirth.htm.

Committee on Fetus and Newborn: Policy statement: Levels of neonatal care. *Pediatrics*, 130:587–597, 2012.

Dell, K.M.: Fluid, electrolytes, and acid-base homeostasis. In R.J. Martin, A.A. Fanaroff, and M.C. Walsh (Eds.): *Fanaroff and Martin's neonatal-perinatal medicine: Diseases of the fetus and newborn* (9th ed.). St. Louis, 2011, Elsevier Mosby, pp. 669–684.

Edwards, M.S.: Part 2: Postnatal bacterial infections. In R.J. Martin, A.A. Fanaroff, and M.C. Walsh (Eds.): *Fanaroff and Martin's neonatal-perinatal medicine: Diseases of the fetus and newborn* (9th ed.). St. Louis, 2011, Elsevier Mosby, pp. 793–829.

Eichenwald, E.C.: Care of the extremely low-birthweight infant. In C.A. Gleason, and S.U. Devaskar (Eds.): *Avery's diseases of the newborn* (9th ed.). Philadelphia, 2012, Elsevier Saunders, pp. 390–404.

Goldsmith, J.P. and Karotkin, E.H.: *Assisted ventilation of the neonate:* (5th ed.). St. Louis, 2011, Elsevier Saunders.

Harris, A.H., Coker, K.L. and Smith, C.G.: Case report of a pressure ulcer in an infant receiving extracorporeal life support: The use of a novel mattress surface for pressure reduction. *Advances in Neonatal Care*, 3:220–229, 2003.

Horbar, J.D., Carpenter, J.H., Badger, G.J., et al.: Mortality and neonatal morbidity among infants 501 to 1500 grams from 2000 to 2009. *Pediatrics*, 129 (6):1019–1026, 2012.

Klebermass-Schrehof, K., Wald, M., Schwindt, J., et al.: Less invasive surfactant administration in extremely preterm infants: Impact on mortality and morbidity. *Neonatology*, 103(4):252–258, 2013.

Lund, C.H.: Nursing care. In J.P. Goldsmith, and E.H. Karotkin (Eds.): *Assisted ventilation of the neonate* (5th ed.). St. Louis, 2011, Elsevier Saunders, pp. 126–139.

Lund, C.H., Kuller, J., Raines, D.A., et al.: Neonatal skin care: Evidence-based clinical practice guidelines. In AWHONN (Ed.): (3rd ed.). Washington, DC, 2013, AWHONN.

MacDonald, M.G. and Ramasethu, J.: *Atlas of procedures in neonatology:* (4th ed.). Philadelphia, 2007, Lippincott, Williams & Wilkins.

March of Dimes: Prematurity campaign. 2013: Retrieved from http://www.marchofdimes.com/mission/prematurity.html?link=botLeftTitle.

Schmidt, B., Roberts, R.S., Davis, P., et al.: for the Caffeine for Apnea of Prematurity Trial Group: Long-term effects of caffeine therapy for apnea of prematurity. *New England Journal of Medicine*, 357 (19):1893–1902, 2007.

Telofski, L.S., Morello, A.P., Mack Correa, M.C. and Stamatas, G.N.: The infant skin barrier: Can we preserve, protect, and enhance the barrier? *Dermatology Research and Practice*, 2012:198789, 2012.

Vaucher, Y.E., Peralta-Carcelen, M., Finer, N.N., et al.: for the SUPPORT Study Group of the Eunice Kennedy Shriver NICHD Neonatal Research Network: Neurodevelopmental outcomes in the Early CPAP and Pulse Oximetry Trial. *New England Journal of Medicine*, 367(26):2495–2504, 2012.

Wadhawan, R., Oh, W., Vohr, B.R., et al.: for the Eunice Kennedy Shriver National Institute of Child Health and Human Development Neonatal Research Network: Neurodevelopmental outcomes of triplets or higher-order extremely low birth weight infants. *Pediatrics*, 127(3):e654–e660, 2011.

Wiswell, T.E. and Courtney, S.E.: Noninvasive respiratory support. In J.P. Goldsmith, and E.H. Karotkin (Eds.): *Assisted ventilation of the neonate* (5th ed.). St. Louis, 2011, Elsevier Saunders, pp. 140–162.

CHAPTER

# 23 Care of the Late Preterm Infant

BARBARA ELIZABETH PAPPAS AND DEANNA LYNN ROBEY

**OBJECTIVES**

1. Review fetal development for the last 6 weeks of gestation.
2. Discuss the health and developmental risks for late preterm infants.
3. Describe emerging standards of care for the late preterm infant.
4. Identify short- and long-term outcome concerns for late preterm infants.

Neonates born between $34^{0/7}$ weeks and $36^{6/7}$ weeks of gestation continue to account for 8.28% of all deliveries and more than 70% of the preterm population (Hamilton et al., 2012). Outcome data continue to be collected, but mortality and morbidity risks have been found to be increased. The late preterm infant is at greater risk for medical problems; has a seven-fold increased risk of morbidity, and consumes more health care dollars than full-term infants (Shapiro-Mendoza et al., 2008). A standard of care that is evidence-based has been developed for these infants (Medoff-Cooper et al., 2010). Often not ill enough to justify care in the neonatal intensive care unit, the late preterm neonate is often cared for in the normal newborn nursery where policies and care models are focused toward the needs of the full-term infant. Thorough assessment of risk and health status, interventions, and parent education for these neonates should be individualized (Campbell, 2006). These infants will have a size, weight, and overall appearance similar to that of a full-term infant, and because of this, parents and professional caregivers may tend to treat them similarly to full-term infants. These late preterm infants may present with factors that increase their risk for morbidity (Mohan and Jain, 2011) (Box 23-1).

Communication among staff members is essential to provide optimal, high-quality care for these infants. There are a number of complications that can arise after birth while in the hospital and/or after discharge that require close observation (Medoff-Cooper et al., 2012) (Box 23-2).

## A. Hypothermia

1. Anatomy and physiology:
   a. Decreased brown and subcutaneous fat.
   b. Decreased glycogen stores and ability to convert stored glycogen.
   c. Neuromuscular immaturity with decreased ability to flex extremities and decrease surface area.
   d. Increased susceptibility to large temperature gradient between neonate and environment, especially during transition.
   e. Immature epidermal barrier, which leads to increased transepidermal water loss.
   f. High metabolic rate with decreased ability to generate heat.
2. Risk factors:
   a. Temperature may decrease as much as 2° to 3° C in the first 30 minutes of life; risk for temperature instability continues beyond first day of life.
   b. Increased susceptibility to heat loss.
   c. Increased comorbidities with hypothermia, such as hypoglycemia, respiratory distress, and respiratory and/or metabolic acidosis.
3. Clinical management (Medoff-Cooper et al., 2010):
   a. More frequent and prolonged assessment; after stable, continue to assess at feedings and as needed.

### BOX 23-1
### LATE PRETERM INFANT RISK FACTORS FOR INCREASED MORBIDITY

Younger than expected gestational age
Small for gestational age
Multiple gestation
No antenatal corticosteroid administration
Emergency or elective cesarean birth
Complicated vaginal birth
Antepartum hemorrhage
Gestational or chronic hypertension
Maternal diabetes
Maternal pulmonary, renal, or cardiac disorders
Maternal medications, illicit drug use
APGAR score of less than 7 at 5 minutes
Male gender
Racial or ethnic minority
Maternal smoking
Public insurance

From Mohan, S.S. and Jain, L.: Later preterm birth: Preventable prematurity? *Clinics in Perinatology*, 38:547-555, 2011.

### BOX 23-2
### POTENTIAL COMPLICATIONS OF THE LATE PRETERM INFANT

Hypothermia
Respiratory distress
Sepsis
Hyperbilirubinemia
Hypoglycemia
Feeding difficulties and associated dehydration
Apnea
Developmental, learning, and behavioral challenges

From Medoff-Cooper, B., Holditch-Davis, D., Verklan, M.T., et al.: Newborn clinical outcomes of the AWHONN late preterm infant research-based practice project. *JOGNN*: *Journal of Obstetric, Gynecologic, & Neonatal Nursing*, 41 (6):774-785, 2012.

(1) Assess axillary temperature within 30 minutes of life, and then every 30 minutes until the neonate's condition has remained stable for 2 hours. Axillary temperatures should be 36.5° C to 37.4° C (97.7° F to 99.3° F).
(2) Evaluate temperature every 4 hours for the first 24 hours of life, then if stable, once per shift until discharge.

**b.** Warm and humidify oxygen and keep infant away from drafts to decrease convective losses.
**c.** Encourage skin-to-skin holding, breastfeeding, and rooming-in.
**d.** Provide additional layers of clothing, prewarmed hats, and blankets.
**e.** May need additional support from incubator or radiant warmer—use servo-control to maintain normal temperature.
**f.** Utilize institutional protocol for weaning to open crib.
**g.** Delay first bath until transition is complete. Bath should be given under warming lights and last less than 10 minutes.
**h.** Observe for signs of cold stress: tachypnea, color change (pallor, mottling, cyanosis), and lethargy.

**B. Respiratory distress (see Chapter 24).**

1. Anatomy and physiology:
   a. Respiratory system is one of the last systems to mature.
   b. Normal lung fluid production and absorption for gestational age suggest difficulty with clearance of fluid, increased fluid retention, and delayed completion of transition.
   c. Surfactant production incomplete.
   d. Increased chest compliance, decreased muscle mass, and muscle immaturity.
   e. Central nervous system immaturity and increased risk for apnea and bradycardia.
   f. Decreased airway stability due to larger head size and decreased neck stability.
   g. Higher percentage of fetal hemoglobin and risk for tissue and end-organ hypoxia.
2. Risk factors:
   a. Altered metabolic stability and increased risk for hypothermia, hypoglycemia, acidosis, and anemia.
   b. More likely to require mechanical ventilation if delivered by cesarean section without labor (Jain and Dudell, 2006; Gyamfi-Bannerman, 2012).
3. Common conditions:
   a. Transient tachypnea of newborn.
   b. Respiratory distress syndrome.
   c. Pneumonia.
   d. Pulmonary hypertension of the newborn.
   e. Apnea and bradycardia of prematurity.
4. Clinical management (Medoff-Cooper et al., 2010):
   a. Evaluate the respiratory system—respiratory rate, type of respiration, muscle tone, and activity level—every 30 minutes. If stable for 2 hours, perform a respiratory assessment every 4 hours for the first 24 hours, and then once per shift until discharge.
   b. Evaluate the cardiac system: heart rate and perfusion every 4 hours in the first 24 hours, and then once per shift until discharge.
   c. Maintain a neutral thermal environment to prevent excessive energy consumption and increased oxygen requirements.
   d. Pulse oximeter: monitor oxygenation.
   e. Arterial blood gases: monitor ventilation and acid–base balance.
   f. Supplemental respiratory support as needed.

**C. Sepsis (see Chapter 32).**

1. Anatomy and physiology:
   a. Immature immune system despite normal cell counts.
   b. Decreased transference of maternal antibodies.
   c. Impaired skin integrity.
   d. Increased exposure to microorganisms due to prolonged hospitalization and invasive tests and procedures.
2. Risk factors:
   a. Maternal group β-hemolytic streptococcus (GBS) status positive or unknown.
   b. Previous delivery of a baby with GBS infection.
   c. Prolonged rupture of membranes (>18 hours).
   d. Inadequate antenatal antibiotic prophylaxis.
   e. Maternal temperature greater than 100.4° F and/or diagnosed chorioamnionitis.
3. Clinical management:
   a. Assess every 4 hours for signs and symptoms of infection for the first 24 hours, then once per shift until discharge.
      (1) Change in feeding behaviors, poor feeding.
      (2) Lethargy, hypotonia, irritability, jitteriness.
      (3) Temperature instability.
      (4) Respiratory distress.
      (5) Apnea and bradycardia.
      (6) Hypotension, poor perfusion.
      (7) Vomiting, diarrhea, gastric distention.
      (8) Hypoglycemia.

(9) Jaundice.
(10) Rashes, pustules, or other skin lesions.

b. If signs of infection are observed, obtain cultures and treat with antibiotics.
(1) Complete blood count.
(2) Vital signs monitored every 4 hours or more frequently as needed.

c. Identify if criteria for respiratory syncytial virus prophylaxis are met (Medoff-Cooper et al., 2010):
(1) Household contains more than five people.
(2) Small for gestational age.
(3) Presence of environmental pollutants, such as tobacco smoke.
(4) Preschool-age siblings.
(5) Child care attendance.
(6) Male gender.

**D. Hyperbilirubinemia (see Chapter 29).**

1. Anatomy and physiology:
a. Immature liver function.
b. Decreased gastric motility.
c. Increased normal breakdown of red blood cells.
d. Bilirubin levels generally peak by 5 to 7 days of life; increased risk for kernicterus (Askin et al., 2007).
e. Late preterm infants have an 8 times higher risk for total bilirubin level ≥20 (Medoff-Cooper et al., 2012).

2. Risk factors for hyperbilirubinemia requiring treatment or kernicterus (Medoff-Cooper et al., 2010):
a. Major risk factors:
(1) Jaundice appearing in first 24 hours.
(2) Presence of cephalohematoma or extensive ecchymosis.
(3) Exclusive breastfeeding, suboptimal feeding, and risk of dehydration.
(4) Blood group incompatibility.
(5) Previous sibling who required phototherapy.
(6) Predischarge total serum bilirubin (TSB) or transcutaneous bilirubin (TcB) in the high-risk zone on the bilirubin nomogram (Fig. 23-1).

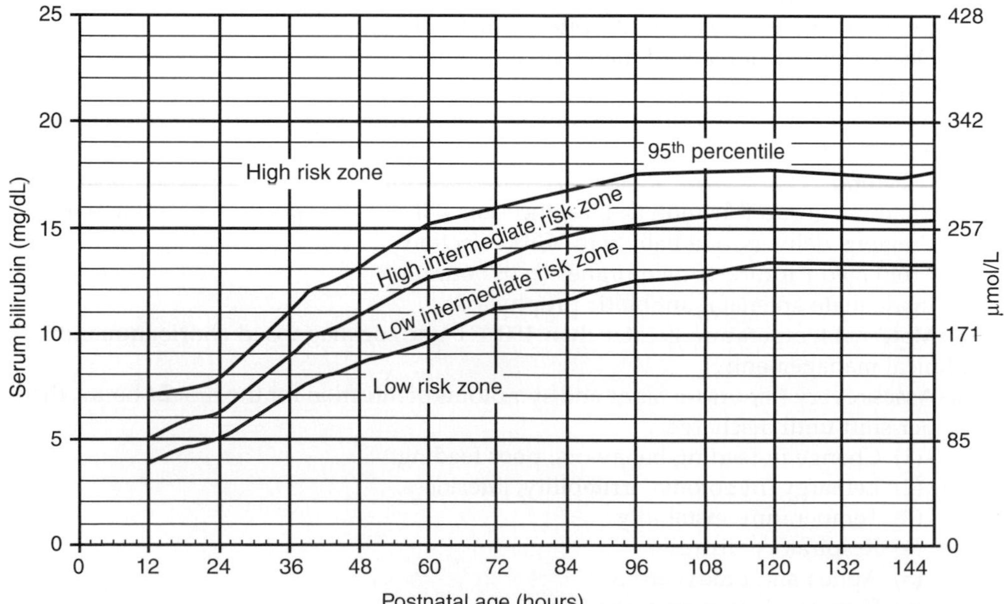


FIGURE 23-1 ■ Nomogram for designation of risk. (From American Academy of Pediatrics: Management of hyperbilirubinemia in the newborn infant 35 or more weeks of gestation. *Pediatrics*, 114[1]:297-316, 2004.)

b. Minor risk factors:
   (1) Jaundice observed before discharge.
   (2) Macrosomic infant of a diabetic mother.
   (3) Predischarge TSB or TcB in the high intermediate-risk zone on the bilirubin nomogram (see Fig. 23-1).
   (4) Previous sibling with jaundice.

3. Clinical management:
   a. Assess and ensure adequate feeding and hydration status. Provide support and encouragement for breastfeeding mothers.
   b. Assess for jaundice with each feeding and with routine physical assessment.
   c. Monitor for established stooling pattern.
   d. Screen for hyperbilirubinemia using TcB and/or TSB levels when jaundiced and/or prior to discharge. Repeat levels as indicated. Plot TSB levels on the nomogram to identify risk of developing severe hyperbilirubinemia (Fig. 23-2).
   e. Evaluate need for phototherapy and initiate per American Academy of Pediatrics (AAP, 2004) guidelines (see Figs. 23-1 and 23-2).
   f. Perform exchange transfusion as indicated per AAP guidelines.

E. **Hypoglycemia (see Chapter 9).**
1. Anatomy and physiology:
   a. Inadequate glycogen stores, decreased glucose production, and increased glucose utilization.
   b. Inadequate nutritional intake.
2. Risk factors:
   a. Feeding intolerance, including residuals and emesis.
   b. Excessive weight loss and/or dehydration.
   c. Failure to establish or maintain maternal breast milk.
   d. Three times more likely to have hypoglycemia than the term infant (Medoff-Cooper et al., 2012).
3. Clinical management:
   a. Evaluate for clinical conditions that increase risk of hypoglycemia (Medoff-Cooper et al., 2010).

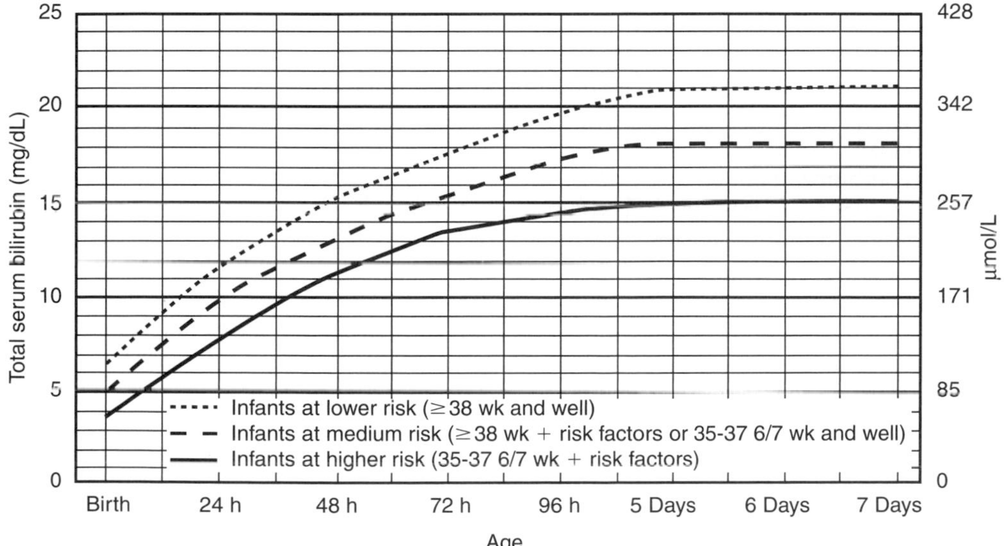


FIGURE 23-2 ■ Guidelines for phototherapy in hospitalized infants of 35 or more weeks of gestation. (From American Academy of Pediatrics: Management of hyperbilirubinemia in the newborn infant 35 or more weeks of gestation. *Pediatrics*, 114[1]:297-316, 2004.)

(1) Maternal: gestational diabetes/type 1 or type 2 diabetes, obesity, pregnancy-induced hypertension, intrapartum administration of intravenous glucose, use of tocolytics.
(2) Neonatal: temperature instability, respiratory distress, intrauterine growth restriction, twin gestation, 5-minute Apgar score $\leq 7$.

**b.** Monitor for adequate oral intake. If breastfeeding, feedings should be once every 2 to 3 hours, if formula feeding, 3 to 4 hours.
**c.** Evaluate for symptoms of hypoglycemia: change in feeding pattern, hypotonia, lethargy, abnormal cry, irritability, jitteriness, apnea, tachypnea, change in color, hypothermia, change in level of consciousness.
**d.** Monitor blood glucose levels per unit/hospital protocols or the AAP (Adamkin and AAP, Committee on Fetus and Newborn, 2011) guidelines for postnatal glucose homeostasis.
**e.** Initiate intravenous fluid support, as indicated: 27% of these infants need intravenous fluid support compared to 5% of full-term infants (Ramachandrappa and Jain, 2009).

**F. Feeding difficulties.**

**1.** Anatomy and physiology:
**a.** Immature oral motor development, including rooting and sucking reflexes; coordination of suck, swallow, and breathe.
**b.** Decreased gastric motility and absorption of nutrients.
**c.** Difficulty maintaining tone in large and small muscle groups: 41% of late preterm infants have been identified by bedside nurses to have difficulty feeding (Medoff-Cooper et al., 2012).
(1) Poor latch and inadequate milk transfer.
(2) Decreased suction and tongue tone.
(3) Increased drooling and gulping.
(4) Weak suck.
**d.** Immature neurobehavioral development:
(1) Immature brain development.
(2) Decreased ability to tolerate environment and stimulation and decreased ability to habituate.
(3) Cues inconsistent, unsustained, and subtle.
(4) Fatigues easily; increased sleep and decreased awake time.
(5) Disorganized and rapid change in behavior state.
**e.** Increased metabolic needs.

**2.** Risk factors:
**a.** Respiratory distress.
**b.** Immature neurodevelopment and oral feeding ability.
**c.** Hypoglycemia.
**d.** Hypothermia.
**e.** Hyperbilirubinemia.

**3.** Clinical management—breastfeeding:
**a.** Support skin-to-skin care.
**b.** Promote early lactogenesis.
**c.** Encourage pumping after each feeding. May need to pump before feeds as well.
**d.** Provide lactation support in the hospital and after discharge (Hallowell and Spatz, 2012).
**e.** Before- and after-feeding weights may be helpful in some populations.
**f.** Consider nursing assistance devices such as nipple shield.
**g.** May need fortified breast milk for increased calories.

**4.** Clinical management—formula feeding:
**a.** Assess for feeding readiness based on cues; use cues to direct feeding method (e.g., bottle/breast vs. gavage feeding; cessation of nippling effort).
**b.** Feed early in awakening; delay care and stimulation that tire infant.
**c.** May feed well first few feedings or days, and then fatigue.
**d.** Bottle feeding should not be pushed if infant is not awake or does not have sufficient energy; feeding relationship should be positive.
**e.** Provide external pacing if necessary.

f. Decrease overall stimulation during feeding (e.g., noises, light).
g. Utilize nonnutritive sucking between feedings and/or with gavage feedings.
h. Promote skin-to-skin care.
i. Avoid thermal stress.
j. May need transitional formula for increased calories.
k. Consider consultation with feeding team or lactation specialist.
l. If hospital stay 1 week or more, measure/plot weight, length, and head circumference.

5. General feeding considerations:
   a. Low-flow bottle nipple.
   b. May need supplementation with gavage feeding.
   c. Swaddle with hands to midline in tucked position.
   d. Hold close in crook of arm for feeding.
   e. Quiet, supportive feeding environment.
   f. Consider side-lying feeding.

G. **Neurologic development**.

1. Anatomy and physiology:
   a. Incomplete development of the central nervous system.
   b. Fifty percent decrease in cortical volume at 34 weeks of gestation compared to that of a full-term infant (Souto et al., 2011).
   c. Despite development of some sensory systems, continues to be vulnerable to stimulation as a result of illness and/or difficulty with habituation; may be especially sensitive with multiple stimuli.
   d. Ability to focus on visual stimuli limited.
   e. State system stability emerging as demonstrated by limited awake time, lack of smooth transition from sleep to awake, and rapid movement between sleep and awake states.
   f. Decreased stability of subsystems with illness and transition to extrauterine life.
2. Risk factors:
   a. At risk for apnea of prematurity and periodic breathing.
   b. Suck, swallow, and breathe coordination incomplete.
   c. Increased sleep requirements yet needs to awaken more frequently for oral feeds.
   d. Decreased muscle tone leading to need for supportive positioning care of airway and during feeds.
3. Clinical management:
   a. Provide developmentally supportive care practices (i.e., observe limited noise and light levels, developmental positioning tools, facilitated tucking, skin-to-skin care).
   b. Offer cue-based, individualized care; teaching parents cues and supportive measures.
   c. Offer voice or face stimulation separately, observing cues for tolerance before adding additional stimulation.
   d. Transition to increased lighting; promote dimmed light when alert, quiet. Support day–-night cycling of light and stimulation.
   e. Consider cranial ultrasound or other neuroimaging study as warranted.

H. **Discharge criteria**.

1. Normoglycemia.
2. Greater than 48 hours of age.
3. Normal vital signs for greater than 24 hours before discharge.
4. Voiding and stooling appropriately.
5. Stable or decreasing bilirubin.
6. Successful feeding for 24 hours with at least four consecutive successful feeds documented. Delay in discharge occurs due to feeding issues in up to 76% of late preterm infants (Adamkin, 2006).
7. Feeding plan in place and parent(s) educated on plan.
8. Weight loss of no more than 8% total (Souto et al., 2011) or no more than 3% per day (Engle, 2011).
9. Screenings completed: newborn metabolic screen, hearing screen, and car seat testing. Hepatitis B vaccine given.
10. Scheduled home care and follow-up appointments 24 to 48 hours after discharge (i.e., lactation support, weight checks, home treatment for hyperbilirubinemia).

**I. Parent education.**

1. When and how often to see primary health care provider (i.e., respiratory distress, jaundice, feeding, weight checks).
2. Temperature assessment and maintenance at home; avoid overdressing and underdressing.
3. Feeding plan (e.g., minimum number or volume of feeding per day).
4. Assessment for jaundice and dehydration (number of stools and wet diapers).
5. Offer instruction in infant cardiopulmonary resuscitation.
6. Education on sudden infant death syndrome (SIDS) prevention, "Back to Sleep," and safe sleeping environment.
7. Behavior expectations—amount of sleep–awake time to expect, cues.
8. Information on infection control, avoiding public places, and limiting visitors.
9. Information on developmental follow-up program and early intervention services.

**J. Long-term outcome.**

1. Increased risk for SIDS by as much as 50% (Darnall et al., 2006).
2. Increased risk for at least one hospital readmission within the first 6 to 12 months of life, especially if never admitted to neonatal intensive care unit (Cuevas et al., 2005; Jain and Cheng, 2006).
3. Increased incidence of developmental delay by 3 years of age (Engle, 2011; Souto et al., 2011).

## REFERENCES


Adamkin, D.H.: Feeding problems in the late preterm infant. *Clinics in Perinatology*, 33(4):831–837, 2006.

Adamkin, D.H.: and American Academy of Pediatrics Committee on Fetus and Newborn: Clinical report—postnatal glucose homeostasis in late-preterm and term infants. *Pediatrics*, 127(3):575–579, 2011.

American Academy of Pediatrics: Management of hyperbilirubinemia in the newborn infant 35 or more weeks' gestation. *Pediatrics*, 114(1):297–316, 2004.

Askin, D.F., Bakewell-Sachs, S., Medoff-Cooper, B., et al.: *Late preterm assessment guide*. Washington, DC, 2007, Association of Women's Health, Obstetric and Neonatal Nurses.

Campbell, M.A.: Development of a clinical pathway for near-term and convalescing premature infants in a level II nursery. *Advances in Neonatal Care*, 6 (3):150–164, 2006.

Cuevas, K.D., Silver, D.R., Brooten, D., et al.: The cost of prematurity: Hospital charges at birth and frequency of rehospitalizations and acute care visits over the first year of life. *American Journal of Nursing*, 105 (7):56–65, 2005.

Darnall, R.A., Ariagno, R.L. and Kinney, H.C.: The late preterm infant and the control of breathing, sleep, and brainstem development: A review. *Clinics in Perinatology*, 33(4):883–914, 2006.

Engle, W.A.: Morbidity and mortality in late preterm and early term newborns: A continuum. *Clinics in Perinatology*, 38:493–516, 2011.

Gyamfi-Bannerman, C.: Later preterm births: Management dilemmas. *Obstetrics and Gynecology Clinics of North America*, 39:35–45, 2012.

Hallowell, S.G. and Spatz, D.L.: The relationship of brain development and breastfeeding in the late-preterm infant. *Journal of Pediatric Nursing*, 27:154–162, 2012.

Hamilton, B.E., Martin, J.A. and Ventura, S.J.: and Division of Vital Statistics: Births: Preliminary data for 2011. *National Vital Statistics Reports*, 61(5):1–20, 2012. Retrieved from http://www.cdc.gov/nchs/data/nvsr/nvsr61/nvsr61_05.pdf.

Jain, S. and Cheng, J.: Emergency department visits and rehospitalizations in late preterm infants. *Clinics in Perinatology*, 33(4):935–945, 2006.

Jain, L. and Dudell, G.G.: Respiratory transition in infants delivered by cesarean section. *Seminars in Perinatology*, 30:296–304, 2006.

Medoff-Cooper, B., Holditch-Davis, D., Verklan, M.T., et al.: Newborn clinical outcomes of the AWHONN late preterm infant research-based practice project. *JOGNN: Journal of Obstetric, Gynecologic, & Neonatal Nursing*, 41(6):774–785, 2012.

Medoff-Cooper, B., Pedicord, K., Askin, D.F., et al.: *Assessment and care of the late preterm infant: Evidence-based clinical practice guideline*. Washington, DC, 2010, Association of Women's Health, Obstetric and Neonatal Nurses.

Mohan, S.S. and Jain, L.: Later preterm birth: Preventable prematurity? *Clinics in Perinatology*, 38:547–555, 2011.

Premji, S.S., Young, M., Rogers, C. and Reilly, S.: Transitions in the early-life of late preterm infants. *Journal of Perinatal & Neonatal Nursing*, 26(1):57–68, 2012.

Ramachandrappa, A. and Jain, L.: Health issues of the late preterm infant. *Pediatric Clinics of North America*, 56:565–577, 2009.

Shapiro-Mendoza, C.K., Tomashek, K.M., Kotelchuck, M., et al.: Effect of late-preterm birth and maternal medical conditions on newborn morbidity risk. *Pediatrics*, 121(2):223–232, 2008.

Souto, A., Prudel, M. and Hallas, D.: Evidence-based care management of the late preterm infant. *Journal of Pediatric Health Care*, 25(1):44–49, 2011.

CHAPTER

# 24 Respiratory Distress

DEBBIE FRASER

**OBJECTIVES**

1. Describe the anatomic and biochemical events associated with lung development.
2. Discuss the physiology of respiration.
3. Describe common respiratory disorders seen in the newborn infant.
4. Discuss common findings in respiratory distress syndrome, meconium aspiration syndrome, pneumonia, pulmonary hypertension, and bronchopulmonary dysplasia.
5. Describe nonpulmonary causes of respiratory distress.
6. Identify treatment strategies for common respiratory problems.
7. Formulate a plan of care for infants with respiratory disorders.

The most common life-threatening diseases in newborns are respiratory in origin. This is evidenced by the number of infants admitted to the neonatal intensive care unit (NICU) in respiratory distress. Respiratory distress syndrome (RDS), retained lung fluid syndromes, aspiration syndromes, air leaks, and congenital pneumonia account for approximately 90% of all respiratory distress in newborns. Pulmonary disease, however, is not the cause of all respiratory distress in newborn infants. Congenital malformations, metabolic abnormalities, central nervous system (CNS) disorders, and congenital heart disease may also present with respiratory distress. This chapter discusses common respiratory problems of the newborn infant, along with pathophysiology, clinical presentation, differential diagnosis, and management.

## LUNG DEVELOPMENT

A. **Anatomic events**. Five stages of lung development have been identified and are described as follows (Diehl-Jones, 2012):
   1. Embryonic development (weeks 1 to 5). The endoderm-derived embryonic foregut provides a single lung bud that begins to divide ventrocaudally through the mesenchyme surrounding the foregut. The pulmonary vein develops and extends to join the lung bud. The trachea develops at the end of the embryonic period. There are three divisions on the right side and two on the left side that will eventually become the lobes of the lungs.
   2. Pseudoglandular period (weeks 6 to 16). All conducting airways are formed. Cartilage appears; main bronchi are formed; demarcation of major lobes occurs; formation of new bronchi is complete; capillary bed is formed with connecting bronchial blood supply; no connection made with terminal air sacs. The lung at this time undergoes 14 more generations of branching and the formation of the terminal bronchioles. The lung resembles an exocrine organ because of surrounding loose mesenchymal tissues, hence the name *pseudoglandular*.
   3. Canalicular period (weeks 16 to 26). Formation of gas-exchanging acinar units (i.e., respiratory units). The appearance of glycogen-rich cuboidal cells and inclusions for surface-active material storage are seen; capillaries invade terminal airway walls; type II alveolar epithelial cells appear. Airway changes from glandular to tubular and increases in length and diameter. Vascular system proliferates and the capillaries are now closer to the epithelium-conducting airways. Respiratory bronchioles that will participate in gas exchange can be differentiated.
   4. Terminal sac period (weeks 26 to birth). Around week 26 alveolar sacs are formed; air–blood surface area is limited for gas exchange; and type II cells are unable to release surfactant in sufficient quantity to maintain air breathing. Capillary loops increase; type II cells cluster at

alveolar ducts, become numerous and mature; more budding occurs from alveolar ducts; and lung size increases rapidly because there is an exponential increase in surface area for gas exchange.

5. Alveolar period (week 32 to 8 to 10 years). This phase is characterized by continued alveolar proliferation and development.

**B. Biochemical events.**

1. Surface-active phospholipids line terminal air spaces and maintain alveolar stability by reducing surface tension.
2. Surfactant is a mixture of at least six phospholipids and four apoproteins.
   - **a.** Dipalmitoylphosphatidylcholine (DPPC) is the major surface-active lipid component of surfactant. DPPC reduces the surface tension at the air–water interface in the alveolus almost to zero (Diehl-Jones, 2012).
   - **b.** Surfactant includes cholesterol, proteins, complex carbohydrates, and glycolipids.
   - **c.** Phospholipids are responsible for the surface-active properties of surfactant. Surfactant proteins have recently been found to have important properties.
   - **d.** There are two groups of surfactant proteins: the hydrophilic surfactant proteins A and D (SP-A and SP-D) and the hydrophobic surfactant proteins B and C (SP-B and SP-C). SP-B and SP-C are known to enhance the surface tension–lowering properties of surfactant and facilitate its absorption and spread.
     - (1) SP-A with SP-B forms the tubular myelin lattice network. SP-A probably also has a role in the recycling of surfactant. SP-A activates alveolar macrophages and thus has a role in host defenses. SP-A is the most abundant of the surfactant proteins.
     - (2) SP-B is important in the formation of tubular myelin, enhances the uptake of phospholipids by the type II cell, and is also important in the recycling of surfactant.
     - (3) SP-C may have a role in surfactant dispersal and recycling, enhancing the rate of absorption and spreading of surfactant.
     - (4) SP-D may also have a role in host defense mechanisms and is upregulated during periods of acute lung inflammation (Gaunsbaek et al., 2013).
   - **e.** Surfactant reduces surface-tension forces in the alveoli that are capable of producing collapse at expiration (Diehl-Jones, 2012).
     - (1) Surfactant is produced in the type II pneumocyte beginning at 25 to 30 weeks of gestation and continuing to term (Diehl-Jones, 2012). Type II pneumocytes synthesize, store, secrete, and recycle surfactant (Blackburn, 2013).
     - (2) When the lungs are inflated, receptors in type II cells mobilize intracellular calcium, which causes the release of the contents of lamellar bodies into the air space. After secretion, surfactant may be taken back into type II cells with a turnover time of 10 hours.
3. The changing pattern of phospholipids in amniotic fluid can be used to assess surfactant production and maturation of pathways.
   - **a.** Material from the fetal lung contributes to amniotic fluid.
   - **b.** Concentrations of various phospholipids can be measured and will assist in determining lung maturity.
4. Sphingomyelin concentration remains stable, with a small peak at 28 to 30 weeks.
5. Lecithin and phosphatidylinositol concentrations remain low until 26 to 30 weeks, when an increase begins. A peak occurs at 36 weeks.
6. Phosphatidylglycerol (PG) appears at 30 weeks, peaks at 35 to 36 weeks, and increases as the phosphatidylinositol level falls.
   - **a.** When PG is present, the risk that RDS will develop in the infant is less than 1%.
   - **b.** PG is measured as absent or present.
   - **c.** Blood and meconium do not affect test results.
7. The lecithin/sphingomyelin (L/S) ratio has been used to assess fetal lung maturity.
   - **a.** An L/S ratio greater than 2:1 is considered to indicate fetal lung maturity.
   - **b.** An infant of a diabetic mother may develop RDS even with a mature L/S ratio (presence of PG ensures lung maturity).
   - **c.** Chronic fetal stress (e.g., maternal hypertension, retroplacental bleeding, maternal drug use, smoking) will tend to accelerate surfactant production, resulting in a mature L/S ratio in premature infants.

8. Fetal lung maturity.
    a. Measures ratio of surfactant to albumin.
    b. Sample should be free of blood and meconium.
    c. Less than 50 = immaturity; 50 to 70 = borderline maturity; greater than 70 = mature lungs.

C. **Role of antenatal steroids (American College of Obstetrics and Gynecology [ACOG], 2011).**
1. Antenatal corticosteroids and glucocorticoids (e.g., betamethasone or dexamethasone) affect lung maturation and present a strategy for preventing RDS. Betamethasone appears to significantly decrease neonatal death and morbidity (Mwansa-Kambafwile et al., 2010; Roberts and Dalziel, 2008). Steroids accelerate the normal pattern of lung growth by increasing the rate of glycogen depletion and glycerophospholipid biosynthesis. This leads to thinning of the intra-alveolar septa and increases the size of the alveoli. The number of surfactant-producing type II pneumocytes increases, as does the number of lamellar bodies inside the cells. This leads to increased synthesis of surfactant phospholipids. Steroids may also increase the amount of fibroblast pneumocyte factor, which increases surfactant production (Blackburn, 2013).
    a. Treatment with steroids is recommended for:
        (1) Maternal risk of preterm delivery between 24 and 34 weeks of gestation.
        (2) Treatment with corticosteroids less than 24 hours prior to delivery is still associated with a decrease in mortality, RDS, and intraventricular hemorrhage (IVH). It should be given unless delivery is imminent.
    b. Administration of corticosteroids in premature rupture of the membranes is not associated with a higher risk of chorioamnionitis.
    c. Two doses of betamethasone 12 mg should be given intramuscularly (IM) 24 hours apart, or four doses of dexamethasone 6 mg should be given IM every 12 hours in patients at risk for preterm delivery between 24 and 34 weeks of gestation. Repeated courses of glucocorticoids should not be routinely used; however, a single rescue course of steroids may be considered when birth is expected within 1 week if the previous treatment was more than 2 weeks prior and the gestational age of the fetus is less than 33 weeks.
2. Infants exposed to chronic stress in utero are usually small for gestational age and have more mature lungs (they also have small thymuses and large adrenal glands, suggesting high glucocorticoid levels in utero).

## PHYSIOLOGY OF RESPIRATION

Refer to Chapters 4 and 26.

## RESPIRATORY DISORDERS

### Respiratory Distress Syndrome

A. **Definition.**
1. Developmental disorder starting at or soon after birth and occurring most frequently in infants with immature lungs.
2. Increasing respiratory difficulty in the first 3 to 6 hours, leading to hypoxia and hypoventilation.
3. Progressive atelectasis.

B. **Incidence.**
1. Approximately 40,000 infants per year affected in the United States (Orlando, 2012).
2. The incidence of RDS is inversely related to gestational age, affecting 90% to 98% of all premature infants born between 22 and 27 weeks of gestation (Stoll et al., 2010).

C. **Etiology.**
1. Surfactant deficiency.
2. Pulmonary hypoperfusion.
3. Anatomic immaturity.
4. Precipitating factors associated with incidence and/or severity of RDS (Hamvas, 2011).
    a. Prematurity and low birth weight.
    b. Cesarean delivery without labor.

c. Maternal diabetes, especially if infant was born at less than 38 weeks of gestation.
d. Second twin (Gardner et al., 2011b).
(1) May be due to greater risk of asphyxia.
(2) First twin usually smaller, suggesting chronic stress leading to early lung maturation.
e. Perinatal hypoxia–ischemia.
f. Male/female ratio of 2:1.

D. **Pathophysiology**.
1. Production of surfactant is inadequate, occurring when the utilization of surfactant exceeds the rate of production. This leads to diffuse alveolar atelectasis, pulmonary edema, and cell injury (Jackson, 2012). Progressive worsening of these three factors will contribute to a loss of functional residual capacity, alteration in ventilation–perfusion ratio, and uneven distribution of ventilation (Hamvas, 2011).
2. Serum proteins, which inhibit surfactant function, leak into the alveoli. The increased water content, immature mechanisms for clearance of lung liquid, lack of alveolar–capillary apposition, and decreased surface area for gas exchange, typical of the immature lung, also contribute to the disease (Jobe and Ikegami, 2011).
3. Histologic findings are the presence of hyaline membranes and an eosinophilic material derived from injury to epithelial cells. The alveolar spaces are generally collapsed, with pulmonary edema, hemorrhage, and hemorrhagic edema noted (Hamvas, 2011).

E. **Clinical presentation**.
1. Almost exclusively in premature infants.
a. May appear to be a normally grown, healthy premature infant with good Apgar scores at birth.
b. Distress begins at or soon after birth.
2. Increasing respiratory difficulty related to progressive atelectasis. Symptoms are progressive.
a. Tachypnea (>60 breaths per minute) is usually the first sign; color may be initially maintained.
b. Audible expiratory grunt.
(1) Heard during first few hours.
(2) Caused by forcing of air past a partially closed glottis.
(3) Used to maintain positive end-expiratory pressure (PEEP) at the alveolar level in an attempt to prevent alveolar collapse.
(4) More pronounced with severe disease.
c. The chest wall in an infant is very compliant. When an infant breathes spontaneously, pleural pressure decreases during inspiration. When there is parenchymal disease, the chest wall produces greater negative pressure and the more compliant chest wall caves inward with a moderate decrease in pleural pressure, which results in retractions. Retractions are seen at the sternum and subcostal and intercostal spaces of the infant's chest and reflect a decrease in lung volume (Gardner et al., 2011b).
d. Nasal flaring.
e. Cyanosis due to increasing hypoxemia.
3. Oxygen requirements increase to maintain arterial $PO_2$ at 50 to 70 mm Hg because of decreased lung compliance secondary to decreased surfactant. Additional physical effort is needed to keep terminal airways open, resulting in increased work of breathing.
4. Paradoxical seesaw respirations may be seen.
5. If signs and symptoms are unattended, infant becomes obtunded and flaccid.
a. Pallor may obscure severe central cyanosis.
b. Poor capillary filling time (>3 to 4 seconds).
c. Progressive edema, usually seen in the face, palms, and soles.
6. Oliguria is common in the first 48 hours.
7. Breath sounds diminish and lung auscultation is usually described as "poor air entry" despite vigorous effort on the infant's part.
8. Crackles become audible as the disease progresses.
9. Cardiac murmurs are generally not heard until after 24 hours of age.

10. Tachycardia (heart rate >160 beats per minute [bpm]) is common and even more prevalent if acidosis and hypoxemia are present.

**F. Diagnosis.**

1. Signs and symptoms as previously described.
2. Hypoxemia (defined as arterial $Po_2$ level <50 mm Hg in room air) as a result of ventilation–perfusion mismatch and right-to-left intrapulmonary shunting, responding to supplemental inspired oxygen; respiratory failure secondary to alveolar hypoventilation ($Pco_2$ >50; pH ≤7.25).
3. Chest x-ray (CXR) reveals low lung volumes, hazy lung fields, and a fine reticulogranular pattern of density with air bronchograms. Occasionally the disease may appear worse in one lung than the other (Hamvas, 2011).
4. Diagnostic studies.
   a. CXR examination.
   b. Arterial blood gas (ABG) measurements.
   c. Blood cultures, complete blood cell count if risk factors are present. Pneumonia caused by group B streptococcus (GBS) has similar radiographic features; therefore, infection must be considered.
   d. Blood glucose level. Prematurity and increased work of breathing results in increased glucose consumption.

**G. Differential diagnosis.**

1. Pneumonia. Similar signs, symptoms, and radiologic features can be found in neonates with pneumonia and those with RDS.
2. Transient tachypnea of the newborn (TTN) can present with the same signs and symptoms, but these infants usually require ≤40% $Fio_2$, improve more quickly, and have larger lung volumes on CXR.
3. Pulmonary edema. A primary cardiac disorder with pulmonary edema (such as a patent ductus arteriosus [PDA]) can mimic RDS.

**H. Complications.**

1. Pulmonary.
   a. Air leaks.
   b. Pulmonary edema.
   c. Bronchopulmonary dysplasia (BPD).
2. Cardiovascular.
   a. PDA.
   b. Systemic hypotension.
3. Renal.
   a. Oliguria.
      (1) Most likely to follow hypoxia, hypotension, or shock ("prerenal" renal failure).
   b. Immature renal function with decreased glomerular filtration in very low birth weight infants.
   c. Natural diuresis will occur at approximately 48 to 72 hours of age, as infant's condition improves.
4. Metabolic.
   a. Acidosis. Atelectasis with increased work of breathing will lead to hypoxemia and acidemia, resulting in vasoconstriction of the pulmonary vasculature (Orlando, 2012). This then limits alveolar capillary blood flow, which further impedes the production of surfactant and compounds the problem.
   b. Hyponatremia or hypernatremia.
   c. Hypocalcemia.
   d. Hypoglycemia.
5. Hematologic.
   a. Anemia—may be iatrogenic due to blood loss required for diagnostic testing. Hematocrit should be corrected to near normal levels to ensure adequate oxygen-carrying capacity.
6. Neurologic.
   a. Seizures: may result from hypoglycemia or an IVH.

b. Hypoxia, positive pressure ventilation, rapid fluid infusions, rapid pH shifts, and acidosis are all factors causing changes in cerebral blood flow that may precipitate an IVH (Verklan and Lopez, 2011).

7. Other.
   a. Secondary nosocomial infections.
   b. Retinopathy of prematurity (ROP).
   c. Dislodged endotracheal tubes.
   d. Thrombus formation. Complication of umbilical catheters and peripheral central catheters needed to monitor respiratory status and provide adequate nutrition.

I. **Management**. RDS is a disease that is self-limited and transient. Adequate surfactant can be produced by the premature infant within 48 to 72 hours.

1. Goal of treatment is supportive until disease resolves and to prevent further lung injury (Orlando, 2012).
2. Surfactant replacement therapy.
   a. Benefits include the following (Engle and Committee on Fetus and Newborn, 2008):
      (1) Reduced morbidity and mortality rates.
      (2) Improved compliance and decreased resistance in surfactant-poor acini, thereby reducing the pressure needed to inflate the lungs and decreasing work of breathing.
      (3) Improved ventilation in low-volume lung units, which increases the $Pa_{O_2}$, decreases the right-to-left intrapulmonary shunt, and improves overall oxygenation of the infant.
   b. Surfactants approved by U.S. Food and Drug Administration (FDA) for treatment of RDS:
      (1) Natural surfactants: beractant (Survanta), poractant alfa (Curosurf), and calfactant (Infasurf). Composed of minced bovine, porcine, or calf lung with added lipids.
      (2) A synthetic form of surfactant (Surfaxin) was approved in 2012.
   c. Three treatment approaches are related to timing.
      (1) Prophylaxis. Treatment within 15 minutes of birth: infants born at less than 27 to 30 weeks of gestation, especially if the mother did not receive antenatal steroids; dose given via endotracheal tube after initial resuscitation. Additional doses may be given if necessary. Prophylactic use of surfactant has been shown to decrease the incidence and severity of RDS and to reduce the risk of air leak, BPD, and death (Bahadue and Soll, 2012; Engle and Committee on Fetus and Newborn, 2008). Because of the risks associated with intubation, controversy exists as to which infants should be selected for prophylactic surfactant (Jackson, 2012).
      (2) Early rescue. Treatment of infants within 1 to 2 hours of life with signs of RDS; multiple doses can be given. The goal of intervention is to avoid progressive alveolar atelectasis leading to respiratory failure requiring intermittent positive pressure ventilation (IPPV) (Jackson, 2012).
      (3) Late rescue: treatment at 4 to 6 hours of age for infants requiring mechanical ventilation and more than 40% $Fi_{O_2}$. Early or prophylactic therapy has been shown to confer more benefit than late rescue treatment (Bahadue and Soll, 2012); however, by delaying intubation and surfactant administration, some infants who otherwise may have been intubated and treated may be successfully managed with noninvasive treatment methods such as nasal continuous positive airway pressure (CPAP) (Rojas-Reyes et al., 2012).
      (4) Combining surfactant administration and CPAP: In an effort to avoid intubation and mechanical ventilation, many centers are now using an approach that combines intubation and surfactant administration with immediate extubation to nasal CPAP. This approach, referred to as INSURE, has been shown to reduce the need for subsequent mechanical ventilation in low birth weight infants (Kandraju et al., 2013; Pfister and Soll, 2012; Sandri et al., 2010).
      (5) Administering surfactant without intubation: In an effort to provide the benefit of early surfactant administration while avoiding the hazards of intubation, some centers are studying the administration of surfactant through small catheters inserted into the trachea (Dargaville et al., 2013) or via a laryngeal mask

(Attridge et al., 2013). The development of less invasive methods of surfactant delivery is likely to result in increased utilization and potential benefit to the very low birth weight infant.

(6) Beractant (Survanta): Dose is 4 mL/kg through the endotracheal tube above the carina. Four doses can be given during the first 48 hours of life (Gardner et al., 2011b).

(7) Poractant alfa (Curosurf): Initial dose is 2.5 mL/kg given in two aliquots via the endotracheal tube. Two subsequent doses of 1.25 mL/kg can be administered at 12-hour intervals if needed (Gardner et al., 2011b).

(8) Calfactant (Infrasurf): Given via the endotracheal tube, dose is 3 mL/kg divided in two aliquots, every 12 hours for a total of three doses if needed (Gardner et al., 2011b).

(9) Lucinactant (Surfaxin): Dose is 5.8 mL/kg given via the endotracheal tube. Up to four doses can be given in the first 48 hours if needed (Gardner et al, 2011b).

3. Provide warm, humidified oxygen to maintain normal $PaO_2$.
4. Provide CPAP via nasal prongs or endotracheal tube if indicated.
5. Use assisted ventilation for profound hypoxemia ($PaO_2$ <50 mm Hg) and/or hypercapnia ($PaCO_2$ >60 mm Hg).
6. Monitor oxygenation by pulse oximetry and/or transcutaneous monitoring.
7. Monitor pulmonary status with CXR examination, as clinically indicated.
8. Other measures.
   a. Stabilize temperature.
   b. Provide adequate fluid and electrolyte intake. Monitor intake and output, blood urea nitrogen, and serum creatinine.
   c. Monitor arterial/capillary blood gases, electrolytes, calcium, bilirubin, and glucose.
   d. Monitor blood pressure for hypotension. Give pharmacotherapeutic agents (e.g., dopamine, dobutamine, or hydrocortisone) as indicated.
   e. Maintain hematocrit.
   f. Administer antibiotics for associated pneumonia/rule out sepsis.
   g. Optimize nutrition with early introduction of total parenteral nutrition with protein and initiation of minimal enteral feeds as soon as the infant is medically stable.

**J. Prevention of RDS.**

1. Maternal glucocorticoid administration prenatally.
2. Use of L/S ratio, fetal lung maturity, and PG determination for timing labor induction or elective cesarean delivery.
3. Perinatal management to avoid situations leading to pulmonary circulation compromise in the fetus or newborn infant.
   a. Obstetric.
      (1) Maternal hypotension.
      (2) Oversedation.
      (3) Maternal hypoxia.
      (4) Fetal distress without prompt delivery.
   b. Neonatal.
      (1) Delayed resuscitation.
      (2) Uncorrected hypoxia or acidosis.
      (3) Hypothermia, hypoglycemia, and hypovolemia.

**K. Outcome.**

1. Infants with chronic lung disease improve slowly and progressively if they can be kept infection free. May have episodes of bronchiolitis and pneumonia (especially pneumonia caused by respiratory syncytial virus [RSV]); long-term sequelae are related to specific complications (e.g., BPD, IVH, ROP).
2. Infants who weigh greater than 1500 g who have mild to moderate RDS have the same developmental outcome as infants of the same gestational age without RDS.
3. Factors associated with poorer neurodevelopmental outcome include chronic lung disease, neonatal infection, severe ROP, periventricular leukomalacia (Horbar et al., 2012), grade 3 or 4 IVH (Payne et al., 2013), poor postnatal growth (Belfort et al., 2011), younger gestational age, and male sex (Moore et al., 2012).

## Pneumonia

A. **Definition**. Infection of the fetal or newborn lung; may be intrauterine or neonatal.
   1. Intrauterine infection.
      a. Passage of infecting agent by infection of fetal membranes.
      b. Transplacental transmission.
      c. Aspiration of meconium or infected amniotic fluid during delivery.
   2. Neonatal infection.
      a. Acquired during nursery stay.
      b. Pathogens are generally different from those acquired in utero.
      c. Results from passage from other infants, equipment, or caregivers.

B. **Incidence**.
   1. Neonatal pneumonia occurs in 1% of term infants and in 10% of preterm infants (Abu-Shaweesh, 2011). The incidence varies by institution and according to causative agent.
   2. The incidence of ventilator-acquired pneumonia (VAP) is more difficult to determine because of the difficulty in applying diagnostic criteria to newborn infants; however, estimates place the rates of VAP at 0.7 to 2.2 per 1000 ventilator days (Edwards et al., 2009).

C. **Etiology**.
   1. Risk of infection greatest in premature infants because of immature immune system and lack of protective maternal antibodies. Pneumonia can occur by several routes: transplacental, amniotic fluid, at delivery, and nosocomially (Abu-Shaweesh, 2011).
   2. Immature ciliary system in the tracheobronchial tree, leading to suboptimal removal of inflammatory debris, mucus, and pathogens. The number of pulmonary macrophages is insufficient for bacterial clearance (Orlando, 2012).
   3. Multiple organisms cause neonatal pneumonia (Box 24-1).

BOX 24-1

**COMMON ORGANISMS ASSOCIATED WITH NEONATAL PNEUMONIA**

| **TRANSPLACENTAL** | **AMNIOTIC FLUID** |
|---|---|
| Rubella | Cytomegalovirus |
| Cytomegalovirus | Herpes simplex virus |
| Herpes simplex virus | Enteroviruses |
| Adenovirus | Genital mycoplasma |
| Mumps virus | *Listeria monocytogenes* |
| *Toxoplasma gondii* | *Chlamydia trachomatis* |
| *L. monocytogenes* | *Mycobacterium tuberculosis* |
| *M. tuberculosis* | Group B streptococcus (GBS) |
| *Treponema pallidum* | *Escherichia coli* |
| | *Haemophilus influenzae* (nontypeable) |
| | *Ureaplasma urealyticum* |
| **AT DELIVERY** | **NOSOCOMIAL** |
| GBS | *Staphylococcus aureus* |
| *E. coli* | *Staphylococcus epidermidis* |
| *S. aureus* | GBS |
| *Klebsiella* spp. | *Klebsiella* spp. |
| Other streptococci | *Enterobacter* spp. |
| *H. influenzae* (nontypeable) | *Pseudomonas* spp. |
| *Candida* spp. | Influenza viruses |
| *C. trachomatis* | Respiratory syncytial virus |
| *U. urealyticum* | Enteroviruses |

From Weisman, L.E. and Hansen, T.N. (Eds.): *Contemporary diagnosis and management of neonatal respiratory diseases* (3rd ed.). Newtown, Pa., 2003, Handbooks in Health Care (division of AMM Co.), p. 142.

**D. Pathophysiology.**

1. Congenital pneumonia.
   a. Infant may be born critically ill or stillborn to a mother with a history of chorioamnionitis. Evidence of pulmonary inflammation is found in 15% to 38% of stillborn infants at autopsy (Abu-Shaweesh, 2011). Other factors linked to congenital pneumonia include excessive obstetric manipulation, prolonged labor with intact membranes, maternal fever, and maternal urinary tract infection (Orlando, 2012).
   b. Prolonged rupture of membranes (>18 hours); ascending organisms may infect amniotic fluid. If mother is in active labor, contamination occurs more rapidly.
   c. Infective organisms may cross the placenta and enter the fetal circulation, causing septicemia that may present as pneumonia.
   d. Infants usually show signs of generalized illness from birth, but signs of illness may be delayed hours to days if the infective fluid is aspirated during delivery.
2. Neonatal pneumonia.
   a. Infection occurs days to weeks after birth.
   b. Pathogenic organism is acquired from hospital personnel, parents, or other infected infants.
   c. Both bacterial and viral pathogens are associated with neonatal pneumonia. The most common bacterial organisms include GBS, *Escherichia coli*, *Klebsiella*, *Pseudomonas*, *Proteus*, *Staphylococcus epidermidis*, group A streptococci, *Listeria*, *Enterobacter*, *Staphylococcus aureus*, *Mycoplasma*, and *Ureaplasma*. Viral infections such as herpes, cytomegalovirus, *Toxoplasma gondii*, varicella-zoster virus, RSV, enterovirus, adenovirus, and parainfluenza virus are also seen (Abu-Shaweesh, 2011; Orlando, 2012).

**E. Clinical presentation.**

1. Labor greater than 24 hours.
   a. Prolonged rupture of membranes (>18 hours).
   b. Maternal fever/chorioamnionitis.
   c. Foul-smelling or purulent amniotic fluid.
   d. Fetal tachycardia.
   e. Decreased fetal heart rate variability.
2. Signs and symptoms.
   a. Often indistinguishable from other forms of respiratory distress and sepsis.
   b. Tachypnea, grunting, retractions, cyanosis, hypoxemia, hypercapnia, and hypoglycemia.
   c. With severe involvement, shock-like syndrome, usually in the first 24 hours of life, with recurrent apnea followed by cardiovascular collapse, profound hypoxemia, and persistent pulmonary hypertension. These signs represent a poor prognosis.
3. Physical examination.
   a. Physical signs are variable.
   b. Diminished breath sounds may be present over one or more areas.
   c. In addition, localized dullness, harshness, or rales may be audible.
   d. Radiologic findings can mimic those seen with RDS. In addition, pleural effusions may be seen on CXR with GBS pneumonia.

**F. Diagnostic evaluation.**

1. History of any previously mentioned contributing factors is suggestive.
2. Infant may require resuscitation in the delivery room.
3. CXR findings are variable.
   a. Unilateral or bilateral alveolar infiltrates.
   b. Diffuse interstitial pattern.
   c. Pleural effusions.
4. Blood culture because septicemia may present as pneumonia.
5. A complete blood cell count may show neutropenia/leukopenia or may have an abnormal ratio of immature to total neutrophils.
6. Polymerase chain reaction (PCR) to detect herpes viruses.
7. ABG values should be obtained because metabolic acidosis may be severe.

8. Tracheal aspirate culture should be obtained, especially if the infant has an endotracheal tube in place.
9. Cerebrospinal fluid cultures should be obtained when infant is stable, because meningitis often accompanies pneumonia.

G. **Differential diagnosis**.
1. RDS.
2. Sepsis/meningitis.
3. TTN.
4. Meconium aspiration.
5. Lung hypoplasia.
6. Pulmonary hemorrhage.
7. Congenital heart disease.

H. **Complications**.
1. Cardiopulmonary complications similar to those of RDS.
2. Systematic inflammatory response syndrome.
3. Disseminated intravascular coagulopathy (DIC).
4. Persistent pulmonary hypertension.
5. Meningitis.

I. **Management**.
1. Antibiotic therapy (see Chapter 32).
2. Maintain normal temperature.
3. Monitor glucose levels.
4. Monitor blood pressure and treat hypotension.
5. Use oxygen with or without assisted ventilation to maintain normal ABG values.
6. Correct respiratory and metabolic acidosis.
7. Provide adequate fluid and electrolyte intake.
8. Monitor for evidence of DIC.
9. High-frequency ventilation, nitric oxide, and extracorporeal membrane oxygenation (ECMO) have been used for patients who are critically ill with pneumonia, with variable outcomes.
10. Provide support for the family.

## Retained Lung Fluid Syndromes—Transient Tachypnea of the Newborn

A. **Definition**. Delayed clearance of the fetal lung fluid—TTN.

B. **Incidence**
1. TTN occurs at a rate of 5.7 per 1000 live births (Abu-Shaweesh, 2011).

C. **Clinical presentation**.
1. Term and near-term infants.
2. In first few hours, tachypnea results in respiratory rates of 60 to 120 breaths per minute; grunting and retractions may also be present.
3. Hypercapnia and respiratory acidosis.
4. Duration may be 1 to 5 days.

D. **Etiology**.
1. Delay in removal of lung fluid.
2. Excessive amount of lung fluid.

E. **Pathophysiology**.
1. Fetal lung fluid has a higher chloride concentration than plasma, interstitial fluid, or amniotic fluid. During labor, a surge of fetal catecholamines occurs resulting in the cessation of active transport of chloride and reabsorption of fetal lung fluid via a protein gradient and removal by the lymphatic system. Approximately two thirds of the lung fluid is removed before birth. Infants born without labor or prematurely may not have the time to reabsorb the fetal lung fluid.
2. Infants at highest risk for retained fetal lung fluid include the following:
   a. Birth near or at term.
   b. Cesarean delivery without labor.

c. Breech delivery.
d. Second twin.
e. Maternal asthma.
f. Precipitous delivery.
g. Delayed cord clamping (results in a transfusion of blood, which may transiently elevate the central venous pressure).
h. Macrosomia.
i. Male sex.
j. Maternal sedation.

3. TTN may originate from reduced lung compliance because of delayed reabsorption of lung fluid at the time of birth and/or the distention of interstitial spaces by fluid, leading to alveolar air trapping and decreased lung compliance (Whitsett et al., 2005).
4. Delayed clearance of lung fluid by pulmonary lymphatic system. The retained fetal lung fluid accumulates in the peribronchiolar lymphatics and bronchovascular spaces and interferes with forces promoting bronchiolar patency, and results in bronchiolar collapse with air trapping or hyperinflation. Hypoxemia results from continued perfusion of poorly ventilated alveoli, and hypercarbia results from mechanical interference with alveolar ventilation. Decreased lung compliance results in tachypnea and increased work of breathing (Abu-Shaweesh, 2011).

F. **Diagnosis**.
1. Early signs and symptoms may be difficult to distinguish from those of other respiratory problems; however, they are usually milder.
2. CXR examination reveals diffuse haziness and streakiness in both lung fields, with clearing at the periphery. Fluid may be present in the interlobar fissures, and mild hyperinflation may be present.
3. Diagnosis is frequently one of exclusion.

G. **Differential diagnosis**.
1. RDS.
2. Pneumonia/sepsis.

H. **Management**.
1. Because diagnosis is not conclusive, other disorders should be ruled out.
2. Supportive management.
   a. CPAP with or without supplemental oxygen.
   b. Temperature regulation.
   c. Adequate fluid intake and nutritional support.
   d. Maintain ABGs within acceptable levels.
   e. Maintain blood glucose at normal levels.
3. If respiratory rate is greater than 60 breaths per minute, delay feedings to avoid possible aspiration.
4. If history indicates risk of infection, broad-spectrum antibiotics (e.g., ampicillin and gentamicin) should be administered until culture results are negative.

I. **Outcome**.
1. Self-limited.
2. Need for respiratory support and tachypnea decreases steadily over several days. Infant may remain mildly tachypneic beyond the need for CPAP.
3. Some infants with TTN have high pulmonary artery pressures documented by echocardiography. If hypoxemia and tachypnea persist, persistent pulmonary hypertension of the newborn (PPHN) may be present.

## Persistent Pulmonary Hypertension of the Newborn

A. **Definition**. PPHN is caused by right-to-left shunting through the fetal shunts at the atrial and ductal levels. It is secondary to persistent elevation of pulmonary vascular resistance (PVR) and pulmonary artery pressure (Parker and Kinsella, 2012). Seventy-seven percent of infants are diagnosed in the first 24 hours of life, 93% diagnosed by 48 hours of life, and 97% of the infants by 72 hours of life (Gardner et al., 2011b). Incidence is 1.9 per 1000 live births (Roofthooft et al., 2011).

**B. Pathophysiology.**

1. After delivery, adequate oxygenation depends on lung inflation, closure of fetal shunts, decreased PVR, and increased pulmonary blood flow.
2. Over the first 12 to 24 hours of life, PVR normally falls by 50% of its total decline (Delaney and Cornfield, 2012).
3. When PVR remains high, adaptation from fetal to neonatal circulation is impaired.
4. Neonatal pulmonary vessels have greater vasoactive properties than adult pulmonary vessels and respond to hypoxia and acidosis with vasoconstriction. Numerous factors increase and decrease PVR.
5. Development of increased vascular smooth muscle contributes to vasospasm. Development of pulmonary artery musculature occurs late in gestation, making PPHN generally a condition of the term and post-term infant.
6. High PVR and pulmonary hypertension impede pulmonary blood flow, which promotes hypoxemia, acidemia, and lactic acidosis.
7. Newborns with persistent elevation of PVR share several characteristics, including abnormal pulmonary vasoreactivity, diminished response to vasodilating stimuli, and increased circulating levels of endothelin, a vasoconstrictor (Delaney and Cornfield, 2012).
8. Studies have described low plasma arginine and nitric oxide metabolites in infants with PPHN, suggesting that a genetic link of the urea cycle may contribute to this process of PPHN (Pearson et al., 2001).

**C. Etiology.**

1. Maladaptation. The pulmonary vascular bed is structurally normal, but PVR remains high. Maladaptation generally results from active vasoconstriction, which may be transient or persistent (Delaney and Cornfield, 2012).
   a. Hypoxia/asphyxia. This is the most common precipitating factor in PPHN. It is correlated with abnormal muscularization and remodeling of small pulmonary arteries. Acute asphyxia may induce persistent pulmonary vasospasm.
   b. Pulmonary parenchymal disease (RDS, meconium aspiration, pneumonia, other aspiration syndromes) can cause pulmonary vasospasm and may be associated with vascular remodeling.
   c. Bacterial sepsis. The underlying mechanism may be endotoxin-mediated myocardial depression or pulmonary vasospasm associated with high levels of thromboxanes and leukotrienes.
   d. Prenatal pulmonary hypertension.
      (1) Fetal systemic hypertension.
      (2) Premature closure of ductus arteriosus, associated with maternal use of aspirin, prostaglandin inhibitors (nonsteroidal antiinflammatory drugs [NSAIDs]), phenytoin (Dilantin), lithium, or indomethacin. However, some studies have shown no increase in PPHN rates in infants exposed to NSAIDs in utero (Van Marter et al., 2013).
      (3) Maternal selective serotonin reuptake inhibitors use in late pregnancy is associated with a two-fold increase in the risk of PPHN in the newborn (Kieler et al., 2012).
      (4) Maternal conditions including diabetes, asthma, preeclampsia, and smoking.
   e. Any condition preventing normal circulatory transition at delivery (CNS depression, delayed resuscitation, hypothermia).
   f. Hypothermia and hypoglycemia contributing to acidosis, which will potentiate pulmonary vasoconstriction.
   g. Hyperviscosity/polycythemia. This may lead to a functional obstruction of the pulmonary vascular bed.
2. Maldevelopment: abnormal pulmonary vessels. Musculature is hypertrophied and extends into normally nonmuscularized arteries. The excessive muscularization affects lumen size, which increases vascular resistance. Causes of maldevelopment include the following:
   a. Intrauterine asphyxia: increases systemic arterial blood pressure in the fetus and diverts more blood to the lung, resulting in pulmonary vessel development.
   b. Fetal ductal closure: forces cardiac output from the right ventricle through the lungs, resulting in maldevelopment.
   c. Congenital heart disease: abnormal pulmonary vessels resulting from various defects.

3. Underdevelopment: decreased number of pulmonary vessels. Blood is shunted because there are too few vessels for blood to flow through the lungs. There is a decreased cross-sectional area available for gas exchange. Severity depends on the timing of the interruption of lung development in utero: reduced numbers of bronchial generations if early (<16 weeks) and decreased number of alveoli if later in gestation. Contributing conditions include the following:
   a. Pulmonary hypoplasia (i.e., Potter sequence).
   b. Space-occupying lesions or lung masses (e.g., diaphragmatic hernia, cystic adenomatoid malformation) that prevent normal development of lung tissue and the capillary bed.
   c. Congenital heart disease. Pulmonary atresia or tricuspid atresia may lead to decreased blood flow and vascular underdevelopment.

D. **Clinical presentation**.
1. Near-term, term, or post-term infants.
2. History of hypoxia or asphyxia at birth.
   a. Low Apgar scores.
   b. Infant usually slow to breathe or difficult to ventilate.
   c. Meconium-stained fluid, nuchal cord, abruptio placentae or any acute blood loss, and maternal sedation.
3. Respiratory abnormalities.
   a. Symptoms seen before 12 hours of age.
   b. Tachypnea.
   c. Retractions if airway is obstructed (e.g., because of aspiration).
   d. Cyanosis out of proportion to degree of distress; cyanosis of sudden onset that often is intractable.
   e. Low $Pa{O_2}$ despite high oxygen concentration administration because of right-to-left shunting. Differences are seen between preductal and postductal oxygenation.
   f. CXR may be normal unless aspiration or pneumonia present (will see infiltrates in these cases).
4. Cardiovascular abnormalities.
   a. Blood pressure is usually lower than normal.
   b. Electrocardiogram will show a right axis deviation.
   c. Systolic murmur is frequently heard, usually from a PDA, foramen ovale, or tricuspid insufficiency. Single loud second heart sound ($S_2$), resulting from high pulmonary pressures, may be heard.
   d. Echocardiogram shows dilated right side of the heart and evidence of pulmonary hypertension and shunting across the foramen ovale.
   e. Congestive heart failure has been reported occasionally.
5. Metabolic abnormalities.
   a. Hypoglycemia.
   b. Hypocalcemia.
   c. Metabolic acidosis.
   d. Decreased urine output or coagulopathy caused by kidney and liver damage from asphyxia may occur.

E. **Diagnosis**.
1. PPHN will be suspected on the basis of history and clinical course.
2. Pre- and postductal arterial blood samples or oxygen saturation monitoring. Because of the right-to-left shunting at the level of the ductus arteriosus, there will be a preductal and a postductal $Pa{O_2}$ difference. Difference in $Pa{O_2}$ of 15 mm Hg or greater documents ductal shunting (Orlando, 2012).
3. Hyperoxia test. A right-to-left shunt is demonstrated if $P{O_2}$ does not increase in 100% oxygen. Cause may be either PPHN or congenital heart disease.
4. An echocardiogram will rule out structural heart disease, evaluate myocardial function, measure pulmonary artery pressures, and diagnose right-to-left shunting at the level of the PDA or foramen ovale.
5. CXR may or may not be helpful, but should be taken to rule out other lung pathology.

6. Electrolytes, calcium, serum lactate, and glucose levels and complete blood cell count should be obtained.
7. An ABG measurement is done to determine degree of acidosis and hypoxemia.

F. **Differential diagnosis**.
1. Congenital heart disease.
2. Pulmonary disease.
    a. Severe disease may mimic PPHN.
    b. Disease may coexist with PPHN.

G. **Complications**.
1. Pulmonary.
    a. Air leaks. Related to high mean airway pressures used in ventilator management.
    b. BPD.
2. Cardiovascular.
    a. Systemic hypotension.
    b. Congestive heart failure.
3. Renal.
    a. Decreased urine output related to asphyxia and hypotension.
    b. Acute tubular necrosis caused by asphyxia.
    c. Hematuria, proteinuria.
4. Metabolic.
    a. Hypoglycemia, hypocalcemia.
    b. Metabolic acidosis.
5. Hematologic.
    a. Thrombocytopenia.
    b. DIC: depends on precipitating cause of PPHN.
    c. Hemorrhage (e.g., gastrointestinal, pulmonary).
6. Neurologic.
    a. CNS irritability.
    b. Neurodevelopmental delay.
7. Iatrogenic.
    a. Thrombus formation or complications of invasive monitoring equipment.
    b. Dislodged endotracheal tube.
8. Other.
    a. Edema due to "third spacing."
    b. Side effects of pharmacologic agents used for treatment.

H. **Management**.
1. Main goal is to correct hypoxia and acidosis (major contributing factors) and promote pulmonary vascular dilation, as well as support extrapulmonary systems.
2. Management will depend on the cause of PPHN.
3. Supportive care.
    a. Monitor vital signs.
    b. Temperature stabilization. Avoid exposure to cold drafts, which can trigger pulmonary vasoconstriction (diving reflex).
    c. Adequate intravenous (IV) fluid infusion.
    d. Monitor electrolytes, glucose, calcium, complete blood cell count, ABGs.
    e. Correction of metabolic abnormalities.
    f. Blood cultures and antibiotics.
4. Specialized monitoring.
    a. Umbilical catheters.
        (1) Arterial: blood gas access, arterial pressure monitoring.
        (2) Venous: infusion of vasopressors.
    b. Right radial arterial line: monitor preductal blood gases.
    c. Pulse oximetry. Preductal and postductal applications can be helpful.
5. Oxygen: most potent pulmonary vasodilator.
6. Ventilation.
    a. Conventional mechanical ventilation.

b. High-frequency ventilation (HFV), high-frequency oscillatory ventilation (HFOV), or high-frequency jet ventilation (HFJV). Used when conventional mechanical ventilation fails or when excessive barotrauma is a concern. Meta-analysis has failed to demonstrate a consistent benefit of HFV over conventional ventilation in term infants (Henderson-Smart et al., 2009).
   (1) Oxygenation.
      (a) Goal is to keep $Pa_{O_2}$ at greater than 50 mm Hg.
      (b) Danger of ROP is minimal because most infants are born at or near term.
   (2) Adequate ventilation to keep $Pa_{CO_2}$ values in normal range. Low normal $CO_2$ levels aid in reducing acidosis and pulmonary artery pressure caused by the vasoconstriction effects of hypercapnia. Previous practices of hyperventilation to induce hypocarbia are less commonly used because of the adverse effects of low $CO_2$ levels (Orlando, 2012).
c. Inhaled nitric oxide (iNO) reduces death or the need for ECMO in infants with PPHN. Oxygenation improves in about 50% of infants receiving iNO. A similar benefit of iNO for infants with congenital diaphragmatic hernia has not been demonstrated (Finer and Barrington, 2006).
   (1) iNO is a selective pulmonary vasodilator.
      (a) Potent and short acting, with a half-life of 3 to 5 seconds.
      (b) Combines with hemoglobin and becomes inactivated.
      (c) Inactivation results in formation of methemoglobin; levels need to be monitored during treatment.
   (2) A starting doses of 20 parts per million (ppm) in term newborn infants with PPHN is commonly used (Dhillon, 2012). Weaning should be aimed at reducing the dose to less than 10 ppm by 4 hours of age (Kinsella and Abman, 2011).
   (3) iNO withdrawal (weaning) needs to be systematic; in some infants abrupt discontinuation may result in rebound increased PVR (Kinsella and Abman, 2011).
   (4) Infants with severe parenchymal lung disease/underinflation and PPHN respond better to iNO when it is combined with HFOV.
d. Surfactant replacement: especially for etiology based on significant parenchymal disease (Orlando, 2012).
e. ECMO may be used when conventional therapies are unsuccessful.

7. Minimal stimulation and handling.
   a. Infants will show marked fluctuation (generally decreases) in their $Pa_{O_2}$ if handled or manipulated.
   b. The pulmonary arteries are very reactive to changes in $Pa_{O_2}$; therefore, any action that causes a decrease in $Pa_{O_2}$ (e.g., suctioning, blood sampling, vital signs, ventilator changes) will cause further vasoconstriction.
   c. Suction only as needed to maintain a patent airway.
   d. Sedatives and analgesics are used for procedures and treatments.
   e. The bedside nurse must be a strong advocate for these patients and keep noise and environmental stimuli to a minimum.
8. Pharmacologic support
   a. Vasopressors.
      (1) Goal is to keep the systemic pressure above pulmonary pressure to decrease right-to-left shunting.
      (2) Dopamine is the drug of choice. Dopamine is an endogenous catecholamine with a short half-life and must be given by constant infusion. Dosage: 5 to 10 mcg/kg/min of continuous IV infusion. Begin at lowest dose and titrate by monitoring effects (i.e., blood pressure, urine output, capillary refill, perfusion, and heart rate) (Roig et al., 2011).
      (3) Dobutamine is a synthetic catecholamine with primary $\beta_1$-adrenergic receptor effects to support blood pressure in patients with shock and hypotension related to myocardial ischemia, pulmonary hypertension, and cardiomyopathy. Dosage: 10 mcg/kg/min by continuous infusion; titrate by monitoring effects (i.e., blood pressure, urine output, capillary refill, perfusion, and heart rate) (Gardner et al., 2011b).

(4) Nitroprusside increases cardiac output by decreasing left ventricular preload and afterload, acting on the arterial and venous smooth muscle. Dosage: 0.4 to 5 mcg/kg/min. Closely follow thiocyanate and cyanide levels (Gardner et al., 2011b).

(5) Epinephrine is an adrenergic agonist that increases systemic blood pressure, improves cardiac contractility, and elevates heart rate. Dosage: 0.05 to 0.5 mcg/kg/min given as a continuous infusion (Roig et al., 2011).

**b.** Pulmonary vasodilators.

(1) iNO (previously described).

(2) Sildenafil may be as effective as iNO in improving pulmonary vasodilation (Gardner et al., 2011b). It has been suggested as adjunctive therapy to facilitate weaning of iNO. A Cochrane review of this therapy suggests the need for additional research before widespread adoption (Shah and Ohlsson, 2011).

(3) Milrinone improves oxygenation without decreasing systemic blood pressure. Loading dosage: 75 mcg/kg given over 1 hour followed by 0.5 to 0.75 mcg/kg/min (Roig et al., 2011).

**c.** Analgesics and sedatives.

(1) Fentanyl citrate. In addition to analgesic effect, fentanyl produces a sedative effect. Dosage: 0.3 to 2 mcg/kg per dose by slow IV push. Repeat as required (usually every 2 to 4 hours). Frequently used as a constant infusion at 0.3 to 5 mcg/kg/hour. Tolerance may develop rapidly, requiring weaning to prevent significant withdrawal symptoms (Gardner et al., 2011a).

(2) Morphine sulfate. Dosage: 0.05 to 0.2 mg/kg per dose IV. Repeat as required, usually every 4 hours. For continuous infusion, usual dose is 10 to 15 mcg/kg/hour. Tolerance may develop with prolonged use, requiring slow weaning to prevent significant withdrawal symptoms (Gardner et al., 2011a; Roig et al., 2011).

**I. Outcome**.

1. PPHN survival rate is dependent on the center and the underlying disease process.
2. Residual chronic lung disease is common, although recently low-dose iNO has reduced the need for ECMO and has reduced the occurrence of chronic lung disease in neonates with hypoxemic respiratory failure (Finer and Barrington, 2006).
3. Sensorineural hearing loss is higher among children treated for PPHN.
4. The need for remedial assistance in school is increased in PPHN survivors (Eriksen et al., 2009).

## Meconium Aspiration Syndrome

**A. Definition and etiology of meconium aspiration syndrome (MAS)**.

1. Meconium is a mixture of epithelial cells and bile salts found in the fetal intestinal tract.
2. With intrauterine stress or asphyxia, peristalsis is stimulated and relaxation of the anal sphincter occurs, releasing meconium into the amniotic fluid. Postmature fetuses pass meconium more readily than those that are less mature.
3. Aspiration may occur whenever meconium passes into the amniotic fluid, but the risk increases when repeated episodes of severe asphyxia lead to gasping respirations in utero.

**B. Incidence**. Meconium-stained amniotic fluid is present in approximately 8% to 29% of all newborns delivered. Of these, 5% develop MAS (Orlando, 2012).

**C. Pathophysiology**.

1. Complete or partial airway obstruction can occur.
2. Atelectasis or ball–valve air trapping leads to hyperinflation.
3. A chemical pneumonitis develops (probably caused by bile salts). Inflammation develops that is mediated by neutrophils and macrophages, resulting in edema in the alveoli that interferes with surfactant production and increases surface tension (Edwards et al., 2013; Mokra and Calkovska, 2013).
4. Meconium decreases the levels of surfactant proteins SP-A and SP-B, and large numbers of phospholipids (Mokra and Calkovska, 2013).
5. The hypoxia associated with meconium aspiration increases PVR.

D. **Clinical presentation/diagnosis.**
   1. MAS is a disease of term or post-term infants. MAS is rarely seen in infants born at less than 36 weeks of gestation.
   2. Asphyxia and the results of chronic hypoxia may predispose these infants to PPHN.
   3. Vigorous resuscitation is frequently needed in the delivery room because of central depression.
   4. Respiratory distress signs are nonspecific and may include tachypnea, nasal flaring, and retractions.
   5. Respiratory distress may range from mild and transient to severe and prolonged.
   6. If there has been prolonged placental insufficiency, infants may appear to be wasted, with hanging skinfolds (usually around knees, buttocks, and axillae).
   7. Nail beds and skin may be stained a yellow-green.
   8. The chest may appear to be hyperinflated or barrel shaped.
   9. CXR shows hyperexpanded lucent areas mixed with areas of atelectasis throughout lung fields.
   10. Expiration phase of respirations may be prolonged.
   11. Coarse crackles are common on auscultation.
   12. No specific laboratory data are useful for diagnosis of MAS.
   13. ABGs will show the following:
      a. Respiratory and metabolic acidosis in severe cases.
      b. Low $Pao_2$ even with 100% oxygen administration.

E. **Complications.**
   1. Pulmonary.
      a. Air leaks (pneumothorax and pneumomediastinum) due to ball–valve phenomenon leading to overinflation and air trapping and high ventilator pressures.
      b. Pneumonia.
      c. PPHN.
   2. Metabolic.
      a. Acidosis.
      b. Hypoglycemia.
      c. Hypocalcemia.
   3. Neurologic: will depend on degree of hypoxia, if any.

F. **Management and prevention.**
   1. Delivery room management.
      a. If the infant is depressed with no respiratory effort and poor muscle tone, and/or has a heart rate less than 100 bpm, direct suctioning of the trachea soon after delivery is indicated, before respirations are established. Clear the mouth and posterior pharynx with a suction catheter to facilitate visualization of the glottis. Tracheal suctioning with an endotracheal tube is recommended. Using a meconium aspirator, suction as you slowly withdraw the endotracheal tube. This procedure should be repeated, if necessary (American Academy of Pediatrics [AAP], 2011).
   2. Respiratory care.
      a. ABGs to determine degree of respiratory compromise and type of therapy needed.
      b. Assisted ventilation.
         (1) May need to use a lower level of PEEP to avoid inadvertent PEEP and a higher respiratory rate to induce alkalosis and prevent PPHN.
         (2) May choose HFV.
         (3) iNO if PPHN develops.
      c. Surfactant replacement therapy every 6 hours for up to four doses has been shown to reduce the risk of air leaks, lessen the need for ECMO, and improve gas exchange (El Shahed et al., 2007; Gizzi et al., 2010). More recently, lung lavage with surfactant has been shown to improve clinical outcome in MAS. Further research in this area is needed to confirm the optimal approach to lung lavage (Choi et al., 2012).

G. **Outcome.**
   1. The prognosis for infants with mild cases of MAS is generally excellent unless complications such as PPHN or severe asphyxia occur during the course of the disease.

2. In more severe cases, neurologic sequelae are common and death may occur despite vigorous, maximal support.

## Bronchopulmonary Dysplasia

**A. Definition.**

1. In 1967, Northway, Rosan, and Porter originally described the four stages of BPD based on the time that the change occurred (from birth to 30 days of life) and on the type of alveolar and bronchial damage and repair that occurred.
2. A more clinically useful definition now focuses on the need for oxygen or ventilatory support. The subjectivity of x-ray changes or clinical symptoms has been removed from this definition (Groothuis and Makari, 2012).
3. A new proposed definition is an infant less than 32 weeks of gestation who has reached 36 weeks of postmenstrual age, was treated with oxygen for greater than 28 days, and requires oxygen or positive pressure at 36 weeks of postmenstrual age (Table 24-1). This definition also established criteria for mild, moderate, and severe BPD (Jobe and Bancalari, 2001).

**B. Incidence.**

1. Statistics vary because of the difference in diagnostic criteria and practices in individual centers.
2. The estimated incidence of BPD varies widely and is related to birth weight and gestational age. Estimates suggest that the rate of BPD is 42% in infants 501 to 750 g, 25% in infants 751 to 1000 g, and 11% in infants 1001 to 1250 g at birth (Kugelman and Durand, 2011).
3. Genetic variations in surfactant proteins, toll-like receptors, and vasoendothelial growth factor are thought to contribute to BPD (Gien and Kinsella, 2011; Mailaparambil et al., 2010).

**C. Etiology.**

1. The etiology of BPD is multifactorial, resulting from acute lung injury, arrested lung development, and abnormal repair processes that occur in the lung.
2. Maternal chorioamnionitis has been implicated in the development of BPD (Lahra et al., 2009; Zhang et al., 2011).
   a. Prior to delivery, chorioamnionitis triggers an inflammatory response that may alter cell signaling pathways critical to development of lung alveoli and capillaries (Gien and Kinsella, 2011; van der Meer et al., 2010).

■ TABLE 24-1

■ ■ **Definition of Bronchopulmonary Dysplasia: Diagnostic Criteria**

| | Gestational Age at Birth | |
|---|---|---|
| | **<32 Weeks** | **>32 Weeks** |
| Time point of assessment | 36 weeks PMA or discharge to home, whichever comes first | >28 days but <56 days of postnatal age or discharge to home, whichever comes first |
| | Treatment with oxygen >21% for at least 28 days **plus** | |
| Mild BPD | Breathing room air at 36 weeks PMA or discharge, whichever comes first | Breathing room air by 56 days postnatal age or discharge, whichever comes first |
| Moderate BPD | Need* for <30% oxygen at 36 weeks PMA or discharge, whichever comes first | Need* for <30% oxygen at 56 days' postnatal age or discharge, whichever comes first |
| Severe BPD | Need* for ≥30% oxygen and/or positive pressure (PPV or nCPAP) at 36 weeks PMA or discharge, whichever comes first | Need* for ≥30% oxygen and/or positive pressure (PPV or nCPAP) at 56 days' postnatal age or discharge, whichever comes first |

Adapted from Jobe, A.H. and Bancalari, E.: Bronchopulmonary dysplasia. *American Journal of Respiratory and Critical Care Medicine*, 163 (7):1723-1729, 2001.

*BPD*, Bronchopulmonary dysplasia; *nCPAP*, nasal continuous positive airway pressure; *PMA*, postmenstrual age; *PPV*, positive pressure ventilation.

*A physiologic test confirming that the oxygen requirement at the assessment time point remains to be defined. This assessment may include a pulse oximetry saturation range.

b. The relationship between inflammation and BPD is difficult to interpret because of the variability of the fetal response to inflammation, the organism involved, and the concomitant exposure to antenatal steroids (Jobe, 2011).

3. Oxygen toxicity plays a role in the development BPD (Kugelman and Durand, 2011).
   a. The preterm infant has lower levels of antioxidant mediators as well as vitamins C and E, which have antiinflammatory properties. These together make the premature pulmonary system especially vulnerable to oxygen toxicity (Gien and Kinsella, 2011).
   b. High inspired oxygen concentrations cause the production of reactive oxygen species (ROS) and the release of chemotactic factors that attract neutrophils to the lung, initiating the inflammatory cycle. An ongoing inflammatory process in the lung ensues that causes and continues parenchymal damage (Bancalari and Walsh, 2011).
   c. The correlation between initial oxygen exposure and subsequent development of BPD is generally linear; however, low birth weight infants receiving little or no oxygen in the first week of life are still at risk of developing BPD (Laughon et al., 2009).
   d. When ROS injure epithelial and endothelial cells, pulmonary edema and activation of inflammatory cells results (Bancalari and Walsh, 2011).
   e. Pulmonary edema results in a leak of proteins into the alveoli, which inactivates surfactant, exacerbating the surfactant deficiency of prematurity (Bancalari and Walsh, 2011).
4. Assisted ventilation with positive pressure results in lung damage (barotrauma and volutrauma), which contributes to BPD development.
   a. Intubation interrupts normal pulmonary function (mucociliary function is damaged; dead space is increased, leading to increased pressure needs).
   b. Barotrauma is related to the intensity and amount of time exposed to elements of positive pressure ventilation (peak inspiratory pressure, inspiratory time, and PEEP). Repeated distention of distal airways during mechanical ventilation of infants with poor alveolar compliance results in ischemia. Because of the immaturity of the pulmonary system, the alveolar capillary unit is further disrupted by mechanical ventilation, leading to pulmonary edema. Many factors contribute to barotrauma, such as the structure of the tracheobronchial tree and the physiologic effects of surfactant deficiency.
   c. Ventilation using volumes that are too low results in cycles of alveolar collapse (atelectrauma), which is as damaging as overventilation (van Kaam, 2011).
5. Increased shunting (left to right) via a PDA has been described as a possible cause of BPD (Jobe, 2011). Medical or surgical treatment of the PDA, however, does not decrease rates of BPD and may increase the rate of other morbidities (Kugelman and Durand, 2011).
6. Excessive fluid intake contributes to the development of BPD (Bell and Acarregui, 2008).
7. Gestational age plays an important role in the development of BPD.
   a. Damage to the developing lung is more likely in infants weighing less than 1500 g.
   b. Damage may occur with less exposure to the previously noted factors in the infant less than 1250 g.
8. Nutritional deficits contribute to the risk for developing BPD.
   a. Adequate caloric and protein intake is required for cell growth and division.
   b. Vitamin A is essential for differentiation, integrity, and repair of respiratory epithelial cells (Moreira et al., 2012; Young, 2007). Vitamin A supplementation in neonates has been shown to reduce the incidence and severity of BPD (Moreira et al., 2012).
   c. Poor nutrition may impair macrophages and neutrophil and lymphocyte function (Biniwale and Ehrenkranz, 2006). Infants who develop BPD are more likely to have had a lower protein intake and received fewer calories in the first week of life than preterm infants who do not develop BPD (Ehrenkranz et al., 2011).

D. **Pathophysiology**. All levels of the tracheobronchial tree are involved.

1. Large airways.
   a. Submucosal glandular hypertrophy.
   b. Increased bronchial smooth muscle.
   c. Bronchial mucosa hyperplasia.
   d. Submucosal fibrosis.
   e. Inflammatory infiltrates.
   f. Granulation tissue.

   g. Loss of cilia.
   h. Tracheomalacia or bronchomalacia frequently develops.
2. Small airways.
   a. Bronchiolar smooth muscle hypertrophy.
   b. Focal mucosal squamous metaplasia.
   c. Chronic inflammation.
   d. Peribronchial edema.
   e. Peribronchiolar fibrosis.
   f. Necrosis with intraluminal debris.
   g. Luminal narrowing.
   h. Excessive production of mucus.
3. Alveoli.
   a. Decreased number of alveoli.
   b. Enlarged alveoli.
   c. Alveolar septal destruction, which leads to emphysematous blebs.
4. Pulmonary vascular bed.
   a. Muscular hypertrophy of the medial layer of pulmonary arterioles leads to increased pulmonary pressures.
   b. Dysgenesis resulting in fewer capillaries.
   c. Endothelial cell hyperplasia, which leads to a decreased cross-sectional area.

**E. Clinical presentation.**

1. Predisposing risk factors.
   a. Oxygen, intubation, and assisted ventilation.
   b. Gestational age less than 32 weeks.
   c. Nutritional deficiencies.
   d. Underlying lung disease.
   e. Air leaks.
   f. Infection.
   g. PDA.
2. Increase in ventilatory requirements or inability to be weaned from ventilator.
3. Hypoxia, hypercapnia, and respiratory acidosis.
4. Audible crackles and wheezing.
5. Retractions.
6. Increased secretions.
7. Bronchospasm.
8. Electrocardiogram showing right ventricular hypertrophy and right axis deviation.
9. CXR showing hyperinflation, infiltrates, blebs, and cardiomegaly.
10. Fluid intolerance, as evidenced by increase in weight, edema, and decrease in urine output, despite no change in fluid intake.

**F. Diagnosis.**

1. Diagnosis of exclusion.
2. CXR findings (see Chapter 14).
3. Clinical signs (e.g., tachypnea, hypercapnia, hypoxia, crackles) help make diagnosis.

**G. Complications.**

1. Intermittent bronchospasm.
2. Inability to be weaned from ventilator and/or oxygen supplementation.
3. Recurrent infections.
   a. Pneumonia.
   b. Upper respiratory tract infections.
   c. Otitis media.
4. Congestive heart failure from cor pulmonale.
5. BPD "spells."
   a. Infant becomes irritable, agitated, and dusky; has increased respiratory effort, hypoxia, and hypercapnia.
   b. Cause is unknown but may be bronchospasm or increased PVR.
6. Gastroesophageal reflux.
7. Developmental delays.

**H. Prevention.**

1. Prevention of preterm birth is the single most important strategy to prevent morbidity and mortality, including BPD (Kugelman and Durand, 2011).
2. Administration of antenatal steroids reduces the incidence of RDS and the need for mechanical ventilation by 50%; however, studies have failed to show a reduction in BPD rates (Gien and Kinsella, 2011).
3. Prophylactic surfactant therapy has been shown to reduce the risk of BPD (Bahadue and Soll, 2012).
4. Routine use of steroids (e.g., dexamethasone) for prevention or treatment of chronic lung disease in preterm infants is not recommended (Watterberg and AAP, Committee on Fetus and Newborn, 2010).
5. Gentle ventilation, permissive hypercapnia, and early extubation have all been suggested as ways to decrease BPD. Synchronized intermittent mandatory ventilation is associated with less severe BPD because the incidence of pulmonary air leaks decreases.
6. HFV does not have a significant benefit compared to conventional ventilation, but this finding is difficult to interpret because many studies of HFV did not use an optimal lung volume strategy (Cools et al., 2009, 2010; van Kaam, 2011).
7. Aggressive nutrition is needed to promote lung growth, maturation, and repair, and protect the damaged lung from infection (Ehrenkranz et al., 2011). Early introduction of protein and human milk has been shown to improve growth and overall outcome in preterm infants (Dani and Poggi, 2012).

**I. Management.**

1. Minimize length of exposure to mechanical ventilation.
2. Intubation for surfactant administration and extubation to nasal CPAP (nCPAP) has been shown to reduce the length of mechanical ventilation and reduce the rate of BPD (Stevens et al., 2007).
3. Continue respiratory support as needed.
   - a. nCPAP.
     - (1) Some very low birth weight infants can be supported by nCPAP, avoiding intubation and mechanical ventilation (Morley et al., 2008; SUPPORT Study Group, 2010).
   - b. Assisted ventilation.
     - (1) Weaning should be attempted as quickly as the infant's condition allows.
     - (2) Use synchronized modes of ventilation with the minimal amount of pressure and volume needed to deliver adequate tidal volumes, but always assess each infant individually.
   - c. Oxygen is administered as needed to prevent hypoxia and avoid cor pulmonale.
     - (1) The appropriate target for oxygen saturation ($Spo_2$) has not been established. Current recommendations suggest an initial target of 88% to 92% pending further research (Kugelman and Durand, 2011).
     - (2) Avoid large variations in oxygen saturation, which can contribute to lung injury and the development of BPD (Ratner et al., 2009).
     - (3) Weaning can usually be accomplished by use of pulse oximetry and occasional monitoring of blood gas.
4. Diuretics may be used to control fluid retention leading to pulmonary edema. Furosemide (Lasix) is used most often. Despite the benefits of diuretics in decreasing edema and interstitial water, a meta-analysis of diuretics for the treatment of infants with BPD found that "there is no strong evidence for routine chronic use of tubular diuretics in preterm infants with chronic lung disease" (Stewart et al., 2011). Decreased calcium reabsorption leads to hypercalciuria, bone demineralization, and renal calcifications (Segar, 2012). Metabolic alkalosis may result in compensatory hypoventilation. Ototoxicity may occur in infants receiving diuretic therapy (Oh, 2012). Follow serum electrolyte values to monitor for hyponatremia, hypokalemia, and metabolic alkalosis.
5. Caffeine
   - a. Caffeine has been shown to have both a lung protective and brain protective effect, perhaps in part due to the shorter duration of mechanical ventilation in infants receiving caffeine (Schmidt et al., 2007).

6. Fluid restriction may help reduce pulmonary edema and right-sided heart failure.
7. Cardiac evaluation for complications.
   a. Cor pulmonale (right ventricular hypertrophy) due to prolonged pulmonary hypertension.
   b. Electrocardiography and echocardiography should be performed periodically to evaluate the progression/development of right ventricular hypertrophy.
8. Optimal nutrition. Adequate protein and calorie intake in the first week of life reduces the incidence and severity of BPD (Ehrenkranz et al., 2011). Provide increased calories to compensate for increased work of breathing and fluid restriction. Infant may need 150 to 180 kcal/kg/day.
9. Use of steroids.
   a. High-dose dexamethasone (0.05 mg/kg/day) has not been shown to have any benefit compared to low-dose therapy and has an increased risk of adverse neurodevelopmental outcomes (Watterberg and AAP, Committee on Fetus and Newborn, 2010).
   b. Low-dose dexamethasone (0.02 mg/kg/day) may facilitate extubation in low birth weight infants without the increased risk seen in high-dose therapy. Selective use of a short course of low-dose steroids may have a role in infants older than 1 or 2 weeks who cannot be weaned from the ventilator (Kugelman and Durand, 2011).
   c. Complications include impairment of growth, possible increase in neurodevelopmental abnormalities, hypertension, myocardial hypertrophy, gastrointestinal hemorrhage and perforation, gastric ulcerations, nosocomial sepsis, hyperglycemia, and transient adrenal suppression.
   d. Has not been found to have a substantial impact on long-term outcomes such as duration of supplemental oxygen requirement, length of hospital stay, or mortality.
   e. Early treatment with inhaled corticosteroids in very low birth weight infants has no discernible benefits in the prevention and treatment of chronic lung disease and is not recommended (Watterberg and AAP, Committee on Fetus and Newborn, 2010).
10. RSV: BPD infants are at high risk for RSV outbreaks and account for many readmissions, with 25% of BPD infants needing assisted ventilation. Treatment modalities include the following:
   a. Benefits of RSV prophylaxis:
      (1) Palivizumab (Synagis): humanized monoclonal antibody against RSV. Administration of Synagis results in a 55% decrease in hospital admissions for RSV (AAP, Committee on Infectious Diseases and Committee on Fetus and Newborn, 2009).
   b. AAP recommendations include the following:
      (1) Five doses of RSV prophylaxis to infants who are less than 2 years of age with chronic lung disease requiring medical therapy within 6 months before the anticipated start of the RSV season, infants born at 29 to 32 weeks of gestation (prophylaxis up to 6 months of age), and infants born at 28 weeks of gestation and younger (prophylaxis until 12 months of age). A total of five doses is completed for all infants in this risk category.
      (2) Infants 32 to 35 weeks: prophylaxis in the first 3 months of life for infants at highest risk of RSV exposure. That is either those attending day care or those with one or more children less than 5 years of age living in the home. Prophylaxis for this group is only given until 3 months of age with a maximum of three doses.
      (3) Infants with severe chronic lung disease may benefit from prophylaxis during a second RSV season if they continue to require medical therapy.
   c. Palivizumab dose is 15 mg/kg, IM route, given monthly during RSV season, with the first dose to be given at the start of the season (AAP, Committee on Infectious Diseases and Committee on Fetus and Newborn, 2009).

J. **Outcome.**
1. Mortality rate:
   a. The prognosis for infants with BPD is dependent on the severity of the disease and the infant's overall health status.
      (1) Death is uncommon and is usually caused by respiratory failure (Bancalari and Walsh, 2011).
      (2) Complications such as cor pulmonale or infection may also be a cause of mortality in infants with BPD.

2. Some infants will be discharged home with oxygen supplementation.
3. Pulmonary function:
   a. Long-term follow-up of BPD infants suggests that, while there is some normalization of lung mechanics, abnormalities of the chest wall, alveoli, and small airways persist (Balinotti et al., 2009; Fakhoury et al., 2010; Filippone et al., 2009; Jobe, 2011).
   b. Asthma is more prevalent in premature infants with BPD compared to those without (Fawke et al., 2010).
4. Neurologic and developmental sequelae.
   a. Infants with BPD demonstrate deficits compared with and term children in intelligence; reading, mathematics, and gross motor skills; and special education services may be required. Cerebral palsy is also more common (Doyle and Anderson, 2009; Karagianni et al., 2011).
   b. Sensorineural hearing loss and visual difficulties are more common in premature infants with BPD compared to those without BPD (Doyle and Anderson, 2009).

## PULMONARY AIR LEAKS (PNEUMOMEDIASTINUM, PNEUMOTHORAX, PNEUMOPERICARDIUM, PULMONARY INTERSTITIAL EMPHYSEMA)

A. **Definition**. Alveolar overdistention and rupture. May occur spontaneously or as a secondary cause, usually when assisted ventilation is used.

B. **Incidence**. Air leaks occur in 1% to 2% of all newborns; however, many are asymptomatic (Fraser, 2012). In infants receiving CPAP, bag-and-mask ventilation, or mechanical ventilation, the incidence ranges from 16% to 36% (Gardner et al., 2011b).

C. **Pathophysiology**.
1. Iatrogenic, resulting from the use of excessive airway pressure during resuscitation or with assisted ventilation.
2. Can occur spontaneously if there is uneven air distribution at birth.
   a. Some areas are expanded, whereas others remain collapsed.
   b. Infant will generate pressure to expand unopened areas, leading to greater pressure in already expanded areas, which results in the air leak.
3. Frequently, underlying lung disease is present.
   a. Obstructive: such as ball–valve trapping of air, seen with MAS.
   b. Poor lung compliance: such as seen with RDS.
4. Overdistention of alveoli leads to rupture, with gas moving into nonventilated tissues. Air travels via vascular sheaths to the lining of the lung. Interstitial air can dissect around blood vessels or along lymphatics, becoming pulmonary interstitial emphysema (PIE). Air can move from the lining to the mediastinum, resulting in pneumomediastinum, through to the thoracic cavity and visceral pleura, resulting in a pneumothorax. When the air moves along the great vessels to the pericardium, a pneumopericardium results. If air dissects down from the mediastinum through the sheaths of the great vessels, pneumoperitoneum results.

D. **Clinical presentation and diagnosis** (**see Chapter 14 for x-ray findings**).
1. Pneumothorax.
   a. Sudden deterioration if air leak is large.
   b. Decreased breath sounds on the affected side, hypotension, skin mottling, and shift of the mediastinum (detected by shift of the point of maximal cardiac impulse on auscultation) to the unaffected side.
   c. Obtain CXR.
   d. Transillumination (translucent glow when fiberoptic light is placed against the skin) of the chest wall may confirm presence of pneumothorax, without having to wait for a CXR.
   e. If the air leak is small, may be asymptomatic.
2. Pneumomediastinum.
   a. Should be anticipated with MAS.
   b. Signs include increased anteroposterior diameter of chest and indistinct heart sounds.
   c. CXR may show "sail sign," indicating elevation of the thymus surrounded by air.

3. Pneumopericardium.
   a. Immediate presentation with hypotension, muffled heart sound, and bradycardia from cardiac tamponade.
   b. Life-threatening.
   c. CXR will show air encircling the heart, halo appearance.
4. PIE.
   a. Difficult to interpret.
   b. Limited to infants with poor lung compliance who are receiving CPAP or positive pressure ventilation.
   c. CXR shows microcystic areas throughout one or both lungs; may show hyperinflated lungs and flattened diaphragm.
   d. May progress to pneumomediastinum and/or pneumothorax.
   e. Hypoxia and hypercapnia commonly present.

E. **Management**.
1. Pneumothorax.
   a. If asymptomatic, will often resolve without treatment.
   b. Symptomatic (tension) pneumothorax requires emergency removal of air. Associated with hypoxia, hypotension, and cardiopulmonary arrest.
      (1) Thoracentesis (needle aspiration to remove air) may be necessary until a chest tube can be placed, if infant's condition has acutely deteriorated, or until adequate pain, pharmacologic support can be administered.
      (2) Thoracostomy tube is placed in the anterior chest and connected to underwater seal drainage system, with continuous negative pressure of 10 to 15 cm $H_2O$, and left in place until air ceases to bubble from the chest tube for at least 24 hours and pneumothorax is resolved by CXR examination. The chest tube may be left in place for a period of time after the suction is discontinued.
      (3) In infants with minimal symptoms, administration of supplemental oxygen may aid the absorption of the air in the pneumothorax by the pleural capillaries. Because of the toxic effects of oxygen, this treatment is not recommended for preterm infants.
2. Pneumomediastinum.
   a. Usually not treated.
   b. If associated with pneumothorax (common occurrence), supplemental oxygen may help resolve condition, as described previously.
3. Pneumopericardium. Emergency treatment is required by placement of a long catheter or chest tube into the pericardial sac with constant application of gentle negative pressure.
4. PIE.
   a. If unilateral and persistent, intubation of mainstem bronchus supplying opposite lung may show improvement in condition.
   b. If bilateral, supportive treatment is given (e.g., oxygen, ventilation, fluids).
   c. Minimize positive inspiratory pressure and shorten inspiratory time.
   d. High-frequency ventilation.
   e. Place affected side in dependent position.

F. **Outcome**.
1. Outcome depends on underlying lung pathology.
2. Mortality rate is high with pneumopericardium, bilateral pneumothoraces, and bilateral PIE.
3. In survivors of bilateral PIE, the risk of chronic lung disease is high.

## PULMONARY HYPOPLASIA

A. **Definition**. Defective or inhibited growth of the lungs, either unilateral or bilateral. Developmental disorder that results in decreased numbers of alveoli, bronchioles, and arterioles.

B. **Pathophysiology**.
1. Conditions that compress the lungs or limit lung growth (e.g., diaphragmatic hernia, cystic adenomatoid malformation) are one etiology of pulmonary hypoplasia.

2. Conditions that result in oligohydramnios (e.g., renal disorders, amniotic fluid leakage) are associated with pulmonary hypoplasia caused by thoracic compression.
3. Associated congenital malformations, such as renal dysgenesis (Potter syndrome), phrenic nerve absence, and vertebral and chromosomal anomalies, should be considered.

C. **Diagnosis**.
1. Often very difficult to diagnose.
2. Any of the above conditions are suggestive of pulmonary hypoplasia.
3. Usually present with severe respiratory distress.
4. Higher than usual pressures needed for ventilation; pneumothorax common.
5. Hypercapnia difficult or impossible to treat early in disease course.
6. CXR will usually show decreased volume of the thorax.
7. Symptoms of PPHN possible.

D. **Management**. Treatment is supportive and directed at respiratory failure.
1. Assisted ventilation/HFV.
2. Treatment of PPHN.
3. iNO.
4. ECMO.

E. **Outcome**.
1. Degree and etiology of hypoplasia determine outcome.
2. Mortality rate is high.
3. Management is difficult, but infant can function adequately if treatment and support can be continued until lung growth occurs, although this outcome is rare.

## PULMONARY HEMORRHAGE

A. **Definition**.
1. Localized areas of bleeding into alveoli (generally found at autopsy); also known as hemorrhagic pulmonary edema.
2. Can be a massive generalized bleeding event.

B. **Etiology and pathophysiology**.
1. Usually occurs as a complication of other disorders such as prematurity, erythroblastosis, intracranial hemorrhage, asphyxia, aspiration, heart disease, sepsis, hypothermia, PDA, and surfactant replacement.
2. May be due to trauma from improper suctioning technique.
3. Usually due to large increase in pulmonary microvascular pressure; results in capillary rupture and fluid transudation from other capillaries (Fraser, 2012).

C. **Clinical presentation**.
1. May present with sudden, severe respiratory distress.
2. Bright red blood or frothy pink secretions may be suctioned from the trachea.

D. **Management**.
1. Use of assisted ventilation is necessary to maintain gas exchange and provide PEEP.
2. Transfusion of packed red blood cells if large hemorrhage with decreased hematocrit/hemoglobin.
3. Identify any clotting abnormalities and treat.
4. Assess for and treat PDA.
5. Treat other underlying diseases.

E. **Outcome**.
1. If bleeding is massive, death will occur quickly despite vigorous management.
2. If hemorrhage is small or isolated, infant will recover and outcome will be dependent on underlying disease.

## OTHER CAUSES OF RESPIRATORY DISTRESS

A. **Upper airway disorders**.
1. Choanal atresia.
   a. Incidence is 1 in 8000 births. Ninety percent of choanal atresia results from bony occlusion while 10% of infants have a membranous occlusion (Arensman, 2011).

b. Bone or membrane protrudes into nasal passages, causing blockage or narrowing.
c. If condition is bilateral, gasping respirations and cyanosis occur immediately after birth because neonates are obligate nose breathers. Many infants have associated anomalies (Treacher Collins syndrome, tracheoesophageal fistula, palatal abnormalities, CHARGE association [*c*oloboma, *h*eart disease, choanal *a*tresia, *r*estricted growth and development, *g*enital hypoplasia, and *e*ar anomalies]), congenital heart disease.
d. Signs of distress are intermittent when condition is unilateral.
e. These infants usually present with pink color when crying but become blue when not crying due to the fact that the mouth is open and provides a patent airway during crying.
f. Failure to pass a catheter through the nasal passages to the posterior oropharynx will make the diagnosis.
g. Initially treat by placing infant in prone position with a large oral airway taped securely in place (an endotracheal tube can be used if placement of an oral airway is difficult).
h. Surgical correction of the problem is necessary and consists of perforation of the obstruction and serial dilation by use of obturators.

2. Micrognathia.
   a. Defined as mandibular undergrowth.
   b. Occurs with certain syndromes and sequences such as Pierre Robin syndrome, trisomy 18, trisomy 22, and cri-du-chat syndrome (deletion of the short arm of chromosome 5).
   c. Airway distress may be alleviated by prone positioning.
   d. Use of an oral airway or endotracheal tube will provide an open airway.
   e. If an endotracheal tube is in place, humidification will be needed to prevent the drying of secretions.
   f. Tracheostomy may be necessary in rare cases.
   g. Generally mandibular growth "catches up" by 6 to 12 months of age.
   h. Mandibular distraction osteogenesis is considered for infants with significant respiratory or feeding compromise (Cicchetti et al., 2012).
3. Cystic hygroma.
   a. Form of cystic lymphangioma, with benign water cysts occurring most frequently in the neck (80%); can also be found in the groin, axilla, and mediastinum.
   b. Usually seen at birth.
   c. Mass will occupy the submandibular region and may compromise the airway in 25% of cases.
   d. Symptoms depend on the size and location.
   e. Treatment is related to complications.
      (1) If infant is free of symptoms, surgical excision is performed between 4 and 12 months of age.
      (2) Excision must be performed at an earlier age if the airway is compromised or if infections are recurrent.
      (3) Multiple excisions are usually performed to prevent damage to nerves and vascular structures.
4. Obstruction of larynx or trachea.
   a. Stridor is a major symptom and usually requires no specific treatment, but mechanical causes must be ruled out.
   b. Direct laryngoscopy will reveal structural abnormalities such as polyps, webs, and granulomas.
   c. Hemangiomas of the larynx or trachea may cause obstruction.
   d. Extrinsic compression of the upper airway occurs with thyroglossal duct cyst, cervical neuroblastoma, vascular ring, and double aortic arch.
   e. Laryngotracheomalacia results from collapse of the larynx and cervical trachea, which produces stridor; condition is usually self-limiting and resolves by 6 to 12 months of age, when the tracheal diameter increases and the cartilage matures.
5. Tracheoesophageal fistula (refer to Chapter 29).

**B. Congenital thoracic disorders.**

1. Cystic adenomatoid malformation (CAM).

a. Primary pulmonary tissue dysplasia with failure of terminal bronchioles to canalize, which leads to intrapulmonary mass consisting of multiple small cysts.
b. Confusion exists regarding the nomenclature used to describe CAM (Keller et al., 2012).
   (1) Type 0 CAM is also referred to as acinar dysplasia and accounts for fewer than 2% of CAM cases.
   (2) Type 1 CAM is the most common, occurring in 60% to 65% of cases. It presents as a single or a few large (3- to 10-cm) cysts that communicate with the bronchi.
   (3) Type 2 CAM is found in 15% to 20% of cases. It is composed of multiple small, evenly distributed cysts that resemble terminal bronchioles (0.5 to 2.0 cm); 50% of these infants have other anomalies, and only 56% survive. Most common associated anomalies are sirenomelia, renal agenesis, and extralobar pulmonary sequestration.
   (4) Type 3 CAM is found in 5% to 10% of cases. It is a large bulky solid lesion composed of evenly distributed small (<0.2 cm in size) cysts. This type resembles the early canalicular stage of fetal lung development and may be the result of an insult at the time of lung bud branching.
   (5) Type 4 CAM has been added to the CAM types and describes a lesion similar to type 1 CAM. Type 4 CAM consists of larger cysts, usually in the periphery of one lobe. The presentation of type 4 CAM often consists of mild respiratory distress and may be detected incidentally.
c. Respiratory distress may be seen at birth, or the malformation may cause no symptoms.
d. Prenatal hydrops is predictive of a poor outcome (Kotecha et al., 2012; Witlox et al., 2011).
e. May be confused with diaphragmatic hernia or pulmonary sequestration on x-ray.
f. One percent to 2% of type I CAMs develop malignant changes; therefore, long-term follow-up is necessary (Kotecha et al., 2012).
g. Some lesions regress and disappear spontaneously.
h. Treatment of choice is surgical excision of the involved lobe.

2. Bronchogenic cyst.
   a. Mucus-producing cyst.
   b. May cause tracheal, bronchial, or esophageal obstruction.
   c. Distress usually not severe.
   d. Treatment is surgical excision.
3. Congenital lobar emphysema.
   a. Overdistention of one or more lobes of the lung (upper lobes generally affected; 10% in right middle lobe).
   b. Inability of the lung to deflate properly, possibly because of a defect in bronchial cartilage.
   c. Possibility of severe respiratory distress within hours of birth but usually delayed for weeks or months.
   d. CXR examination is diagnostic (refer to Chapter 14).
   e. Treatment of choice: surgical resection.
4. Chondrodystrophies.
   a. Group of disorders of bone growth, resulting in short stature.
   b. Possible respiratory distress because of small thoracic cavities.
   c. Treatment: based on degree of distress.
5. Neuromuscular disorders.
   a. Conditions resulting in hypotonia, such as spinal muscular atrophy and myotonic dystrophy, result in varying degrees of respiratory distress.
   b. Management will depend on degree of distress.

C. **CNS disorders**.
   1. Seizures.
   2. Hypoxic–ischemic injury.
   3. Intracranial hemorrhages.
   4. Drugs.
   5. Meningitis.

D. **Cardiovascular and hematologic disorders**.
   1. Congenital heart disease.

2. Anemia.
3. Polycythemia.
4. Shock.
5. Sepsis.

E. **Diaphragmatic disorders (see also Chapter 14).**
1. Diaphragmatic hernia.
2. Diaphragmatic paralysis.
3. Diaphragmatic eventration.

F. **Renal disorders.**
1. Pulmonary hypoplasia results from renal agenesis or renal dysgenesis.

## REFERENCES


Abu-Shaweesh, J.M.: Respiratory disorders in preterm and term infants. In R.J. Martin, A.A. Fanaroff, and M.C. Walsh (Eds.): *Fanaroff and Martin's neonatal-perinatal medicine: Diseases of the fetus and newborn* (9th ed.). St. Louis, 2011, Elsevier Mosby, pp. 1141–1170.

American Academy of Pediatrics: Initial steps in resuscitation. In J. Kattwinkel (Ed.): *Textbook of neonatal resuscitation* (6th ed.). Elk Grove Village, IL, 2011, American Academy of Pediatrics.

American Academy of Pediatrics, Committee on Infectious Diseases and Committee on Fetus and Newborn: Revised indications for the use of palivizumab for the prevention of respiratory syncytial virus infections. *Pediatrics*, 124(6):1694–1701, 2009.

American College of Obstetrics and Gynecology: Committee opinion: Antenatal corticosteroid therapy for fetal maturation. 2011. Accessed March 27, 2013 at http://www.acog.org/Resources_And_Publications/Committee_Opinions/Committee_on_Obstetric_Practice/Antenatal_Corticosteroid_Therapy_for_Fetal_Maturation.

Arensman, R.M.: Surgical interventions for respiratory distress and airway management. In J.P. Goldsmith, and E.H. Karotkin (Eds.): *Assisted ventilation of the neonate* (5th ed.). St. Louis, 2011, Elsevier Saunders, pp. 435–451.

Attridge, J.T., Stewart, C., Stukenborg, G.J., and Kattwinkel, J.: Administration of rescue surfactant by laryngeal mask airway: Lessons from a pilot trial. *American Journal of Perinatology*, 30 (3):201–206, 2013.

Bahadue, F.L. and Soll, R.: Early versus delayed selective surfactant treatment for neonatal respiratory distress syndrome. *Cochrane Database of Systematic Reviews*, (11):CD001456, 2012.

Balinotti, J.E., Tiller, C.J., Llapur, C.J., et al.: Growth of the lung parenchyma early in life. *American Journal of Respiratory and Critical Care Medicine*, 179:134–137, 2009.

Bancalari, E.H. and Walsh, M.C.: Bronchopulmonary dysplasia. In R.J. Martin, A.A. Fanaroff, and M.C. Walsh (Eds.): *Fanaroff and Martin's neonatal-perinatal medicine: Diseases of the fetus and newborn* (9th ed.). St. Louis, 2011, Elsevier Mosby, pp. 1179–1191.

Belfort, M.B., Rifas-Shiman, S.L., Sullivan, T., et al.: Infant growth before and after term: Effects on neurodevelopment in preterm infants. *Pediatrics*, 128:e899–e906, 2011.

Bell, E.F. and Acarregui, M.J.: Restricted versus liberal water intake for preventing morbidity and mortality in preterm infants. *Cochrane Database of Systematic Reviews*, (3):CD000503, 2001. Update in: *Cochrane Database of Systematic Reviews*, (1):CD000503, 2008.

Biniwale, M.A. and Ehrenkranz, R.A.: The role of nutrition in the prevention and management of bronchopulmonary dysplasia. *Seminars in Perinatology*, 30 (4):200–208, 2006.

Blackburn, S.T.: *Maternal, fetal, and neonatal physiology: A clinical perspective* (4th.). St. Louis, 2013, Elsevier Saunders.

Choi, H.J., Hahn, S., Lee, J., et al.: Surfactant lavage therapy for meconium aspiration syndrome: A systematic review and meta-analysis. *Neonatology*, 101 (3):183–191, 2012.

Cicchetti, R., Cascone, P., Caresta, E., et al.: Mandibular distraction osteogenesis for neonates with Pierre Robin sequence and airway obstruction. *Journal of Maternal-Fetal & Neonatal Medicine*, 25(Suppl. 4):141–143, 2012.

Cools, F., Askie, L.M., Offringa, M., et al.: for the PreVILIG Collaboration: Elective high-frequency oscillatory versus conventional ventilation in preterm infants: a systematic review and meta-analysis of individual patients' data. *Lancet*; 375:2082–2091, 2010.

Cools, F., Henderson-Smart, D.J., Offringa, M., et al.: Elective high frequency oscillatory ventilation versus conventional ventilation for acute pulmonary dysfunction in preterm infants. *Cochrane Database of Systematic Reviews*, (3):CD000104, 2009.

Dani, C. and Poggi, C.: Nutrition and bronchopulmonary dysplasia. *Journal of Maternal-Fetal & Neonatal Medicine*, 25(Suppl. 3):37–40, 2012.

Dargaville, P.A., Aiyappan, A., De Paoli, A.G., et al.: Minimally-invasive surfactant therapy in preterm infants on continuous positive airway pressure. *Archives of Disease in Childhood: Fetal and Neonatal Edition*, 98(2):F122–F126, 2013.

Delaney, C. and Cornfield, D.N.: Risk factors for persistent pulmonary hypertension of the newborn. *Pulmonary Circulation*, 2(1):15–20, 2012.

Dhillon, R.: The management of neonatal pulmonary hypertension. *Archives of Disease in Childhood: Fetal and Neonatal Edition*, 97(3):F223–F228, 2012.

Diehl-Jones, W.: Physiologic principles of the respiratory system. In D. Fraser (Ed.): *Acute respiratory care of the neonate* (3rd ed.). Santa Rosa, CA, 2012, NICU INK Books, pp. 1–28.

Doyle, L.W. and Anderson, P.J.: Long-term outcomes of bronchopulmonary dysplasia. *Seminars in Fetal and Neonatal Medicine*, 14(6):391–395, 2009.

Edwards, J.R., Peterson, K.D., Mu, Y., et al.: National Healthcare Safety Network (NHSN) report: Data summary for 2006 through 2008, issued December 2009. *American Journal of Infection Control*, 37 (10):783–805, 2009.

Edwards, M.O., Kotecha, S.J. and Kotecha, S.: Respiratory distress of the term newborn infant. *Paediatric Respiratory Reviews*, 14(1):29–36, 2013.

Ehrenkranz, R.A., Das, A., Wrage, L.A., et al., for the Eunice Kennedy Shriver National Institute of Child Health and Human Development Neonatal Research Network: Early nutrition mediates the influence of severity of illness on extremely LBW infants. *Pediatric Research*, 69(6):522–529, 2011.

El Shahed, A.I., Dargaville, P., Ohlsson, A, and Soll, R.F.: Surfactant for meconium aspiration syndrome in full term/near term infants. *Cochrane Database of Systematic Reviews*, 3:CD002054, 2007.

Engle, W.A.: and Committee on Fetus and Newborn: Surfactant-replacement therapy for respiratory distress in the preterm and term neonate. *Pediatrics*, 121(2):419–426, 2008.

Eriksen, V., Nielsen, L.H., Klokker, M, and Greisen, G.: Follow-up of 5- to 11-year-old children treated for persistent pulmonary hypertension of the newborn. *Acta Paediatrica*, 98(2):304–309, 2009.

Fakhoury, K.F., Sellers, C., Smith, E.O., et al.: Serial measurements of lung function in a cohort of young children with bronchopulmonary dysplasia. *Pediatrics*, 125:e1441–e1447, 2010.

Fawke, J., Lum, S., Kirkby, J., et al.: Lung function and respiratory symptoms at 11 years in children born extremely preterm: The EPICure study. *American Journal of Respiratory and Critical Care Medicine*, 182:237–245, 2010.

Filippone, M., Bonetto, G., Cherubin, E., et al.: Child hood course of lung function in survivors of bronchopulmonary dysplasia. *JAMA*, 302:1418–1420, 2009.

Finer, N.N. and Barrington, K.J.: Nitric oxide for respiratory failure in infants born at or near term. *Cochrane Database of Systematic Reviews*, (4):CD000399, 2006.

Fraser, D.: Complications of positive pressure ventilation. In D. Fraser (Ed.): *Acute respiratory care of the neonate* (3rd ed.). Santa Rosa, CA, 2012, NICU INK Books, pp. 195–238.

Gardner, S.L., Enzman-Hines, M, and Dickey, L.A.: Pain and pain relief. In S.L. Gardner, B.S. Carter, M. Enzman-Hines, and J.A. Hernandez (Eds.): *Merenstein & Gardner's handbook of neonatal intensive care* (7th ed.). St. Louis, 2011a, Elsevier Mosby, pp. 223–269.

Gardner, S.L., Enzman-Hines, M, and Dickey, L.A.: Respiratory diseases. In S.L. Gardner, B.S. Carter, M. Enzman-Hines, and J.A. Hernandez (Eds.): *Merenstein & Gardner's handbook of neonatal intensive care* (7th ed.). St. Louis, 2011b, Elsevier Mosby, pp. 581–677.

Gaunsbaek, M.Q., Rasmussen, K.J., Beers, M.F., et al.: Lung surfactant protein D (SP-D) response and regulation during acute and chronic lung injury. *Lung*, 191(3):295–303, 2013.

Gien, J. and Kinsella, J.P.: Pathogenesis and treatment of bronchopulmonary dysplasia. *Current Opinion in Pediatrics*, 23:305–313, 2011.

Gizzi, C., Papoff, P., Barbàra, C.S., et al.: Old and new uses of surfactant. *Journal of Maternal-Fetal & Neonatal Medicine*, 23(Suppl. 3):41–44, 2010.

Groothuis, J.R. and Makari, D.: Definition and outpatient management of the very low-birth-weight infant with bronchopulmonary dysplasia. *Advances in Therapy*, 29(4):297–311, 2012.

Hamvas, A.: Pathophysiology and management of respiratory distress syndrome. In R.J. Martin, A.A. Fanaroff, and M.C. Walsh (Eds.): *Fanaroff and Martin's neonatal-perinatal medicine: Diseases of the fetus and newborn* (9th ed.). St. Louis, 2011, Elsevier Mosby, pp. 1106–1116.

Henderson-Smart, D.J., De Paoli, A.G., Clark, R.H., et al.: High frequency oscillatory ventilation versus conventional ventilation for infants with severe pulmonary dysfunction born at or near term. *Cochrane Database of Systematic Reviews*, (3):CD002974, 2009.

Horbar, J.D., Carpenter, J.H., Badger, G.J., et al.: Mortality and neonatal morbidity among infants 501-1500 grams from 2000 to 2009. *Pediatrics*, 129 (6):1019–1026, 2012.

Jackson, J.C.: Respiratory distress in the preterm infant. In C.A. Gleason, and S.U. Devaskar (Eds.): *Avery's diseases of the newborn* (9th ed.). Philadelphia, 2012, Elsevier Saunders, pp. 633–646.

Jobe, A.: The new bronchopulmonary dysplasia. *Current Opinion in Pediatrics*, 23(2):167–172, 2011.

Jobe, A.H. and Bancalari, E.: Bronchopulmonary dysplasia. *American Journal of Respiratory Care Medicine*, 163(7):1723–1729, 2001.

Jobe, A.H. and Ikegami, M.: Pathophysiology of respiratory distress syndrome and surfactant metabolism. In R.A. Polin, W.W. Fox, and S.H. Abman (Eds.): *Fetal and neonatal physiology* (4th ed.). Philadelphia, 2011, Elsevier Saunders, pp. 1137–1150.

Kandraju, H., Murki, S., Subramanian, S., et al.: Early routine versus late selective surfactant in preterm neonates with respiratory distress syndrome on nasal continuous positive airway pressure: A randomized controlled trial. *Neonatology*, 103(2):148–154, 2013.

Karagianni, P., Tsakalidis, C., Kyriakidou, M., et al.: Neuromotor outcomes in infants with bronchopulmonary dysplasia. *Pediatric Neurology*, 44(1):40–46, 2011.

Keller, R.L., Guevara-Gallardo, S. and Farmer, D.L.: Surgical disorders of the chest and airways. In C.A. Gleason, and S.U. Devaskar (Eds.): *Avery's diseases of the newborn* (9th ed.). Philadelphia, 2012, Elsevier Saunders, pp. 672–697.

Kieler, H., Artama, M., Engeland, A., et al.: Selective serotonin reuptake inhibitors during pregnancy and risk of persistent pulmonary hypertension in the newborn: Population based cohort study from the five Nordic countries. *BMJ*, 344:e8012, 2012.

Kinsella, J.P. and Abman, S.H.: Special ventilatory techniques III. In J.P. Goldsmith, and E.H. Karotkin (Eds.): *Assisted ventilation of the neonate* (5th ed.). St. Louis, 2011, Elsevier Saunders, pp. 249–264.

Kotecha, S., Barbato, A., Bush, A., et al.: Antenatal and postnatal management of congenital cystic adenomatoid malformation. *Paediatric Respiratory Reviews*, 13:162–171, 2012.

Kugelman, A. and Durand, M.: A comprehensive approach to the prevention of bronchopulmonary dysplasia. *Pediatric Pulmonology*, 46:1153–1165, 2011.

Lahra, M.M., Beeby, P.J., and Jeffery, H.E.: Intrauterine inflammation, neonatal sepsis, and chronic lung disease: A 13-year hospital cohort study. *Pediatrics*, 123:1314–1319, 2009.

Laughon, M., Allred, E.N., Bose, C., et al.: Patterns of respiratory disease during the first 2 postnatal weeks in extremely premature infants. *Pediatrics*, 123:1124–1131, 2009.

Mailaparambil, B., Krueger, M., Heizmann, U., et al.: Genetic and epidemiological risk factors in the development of bronchopulmonary dysplasia. *Disease Markers*, 29:1–9, 2010.

Mokra, D. and Calkovska, A.: How to overcome surfactant dysfunction in meconium aspiration syndrome? *Respiratory Physiology & Neurobiology*, 187(1):58–63, 2013.

Moore, T., Hennessy, E.M., Myles, J., et al.: Neurological and developmental outcome in extremely preterm children born in England in 1995 and 2006: The EPI-Cure studies. *BMJ*, 345:e7961, 2012.

Moreira, A., Caskey, M., Fonseca, R., et al.: Impact of providing vitamin A to the routine pulmonary care of extremely low birth weight infants. *Journal of Maternal-Fetal & Neonatal Medicine*, 25(1):84–88, 2012.

Morley, C.J., Davis, P.G., Doyle, L.W., et al., for the COIN Trial Investigators: Nasal CPAP or intubation at birth for very preterm infants. *New England Journal of Medicine*, 358:700–708, 2008. Erratum in: New England Journal of Medicine, 358(14):1529, 2008.

Mwansa-Kambafwile, J., Cousens, S., Hansen, T., and Lawn, J.E.: Antenatal steroids in preterm labour for the prevention of neonatal deaths due to complications of preterm birth. *International Journal of Epidemiology*, 39(Suppl. 1):i122–i133, 2010.

Northway, W.H., Rosan, R.C., and Porter, D.Y.: Pulmonary disease following respiratory therapy of hyaline membrane disease. *New England Journal of Medicine*, 276(7):357–368, 1967.

Oh, W.: Fluid and electrolyte management of very low birth weight infants. *Pediatrics and Neonatology*, 53 (6):329–333, 2012.

Orlando, S.: Pathophysiology of acute respiratory distress. In D. Fraser (Ed.): *Acute respiratory care of the neonate* (3rd ed.). Santa Rosa, CA, 2012, NICU INK Books, pp. 29–50.

Parker, T.A. and Kinsella, J.P.: Respiratory failure in the term newborn. In C.A. Gleason, and S.U. Devaskar (Eds.): *Avery's diseases of the newborn* (9th ed.). Philadelphia, 2012, Elsevier Saunders, pp. 647–657.

Payne, A.H., Hintz, S.R., Hibbs, A.M., et al., for the Eunice Kennedy Shriver National Institute of Child Health and Human Development Neonatal Research Network: Neurodevelopmental outcomes of extremely low-gestational-age neonates with low-grade periventricular-intraventricular hemorrhage. *JAMA Pediatrics*, 167(5):451–459, 2013.

Pearson, D.L., Dawling, S., Walsh, W.F., et al.: Neonatal pulmonary hypertension: Urea-cycle intermediates, nitric oxide production, and carbamoyl-phosphate synthetase function. *New England Journal of Medicine*, 344(24):1832–1838, 2001.

Pfister, R.H. and Soll, R.F.: Initial respiratory support of preterm infants: The role of CPAP, the INSURE method, and noninvasive ventilation. *Clinics in Perinatology*, 39(3):459–481, 2012.

Ratner, V., Slinko, S., Utkina-Sosunova, I., et al.: Hypoxic stress exacerbates hyperoxia-induced lung injury in a neonatal mouse model of bronchopulmonary dysplasia. *Neonatology*, 95:299–305, 2009.

Roberts, D. and Dalziel, S.R.: Antenatal corticosteroids for accelerating fetal lung maturation for women at risk of preterm birth. *Cochrane Database of Systematic Reviews*, (4):CD004454, 2008.

Roig, J.C., Fink, J., and Burchfield, D.J.: Pharmacologic adjuncts I. In J.P. Goldsmith, and E.H. Karotkin (Eds.): *Assisted ventilation of the neonate* (5th ed.). St. Louis, 2011, Elsevier Saunders, pp. 347–370.

Rojas-Reyes, M.X., Morley, C.J., and Soll, R.: Prophylactic versus selective use of surfactant in preventing morbidity and mortality in preterm infants. *Cochrane Database of Systematic Reviews*, (3):CD000510, 2012.

Roofthooft, M.T., Elema, A., Bergman, K.A., and Berger, R.M.: Patient characteristics in persistent pulmonary hypertension of the newborn. *Pulmonary Medicine*, 2011:858154, 2011.

Sandri, F., Plavka, R., Ancora, G., et al.: Prophylactic or early selective surfactant combined with nCPAP in very preterm infants. *Pediatrics*, 125(6):e1402–e1409, 2010.

Schmidt, B., Roberts, R.S., Davis, P., et al.: for the Caffeine for Apnea of Prematurity Trial Group: Long-term effects of caffeine therapy for apnea of prematurity. *New England Journal of Medicine*, 357:1893–1902, 2007.

Segar, J.: Neonatal diuretic therapy: Furosemide, thiazides, and spironolactone. *Clinics in Perinatology*, 39:209–220, 2012.

Shah, P.S. and Ohlsson, A.: Sildenafil for pulmonary hypertension in neonates. *Cochrane Database of Systematic Reviews*, (8):CD005494, 2011.

Stevens, T.P., Harrington, E.W., Blennow, M., and Soll, R.F.: Early surfactant administration with brief ventilation vs. selective surfactant and continued mechanical ventilation for preterm infants with or at risk for respiratory distress syndrome. *Cochrane Database of Systematic Reviews*, (4):CD003063, 2007.

Stewart, A., Brion, L.P., and Ambrosio-Perez, I.: Diuretics acting on the distal renal tubule for preterm infants with (or developing) chronic lung disease. *Cochrane Database of Systematic Reviews*, (9): CD001817, 2011.

Stoll, B.J., Hansen, N.I., Bell, E.F., et al., for the Eunice Kennedy Shriver National Institute of Child Health and Human Development Neonatal Research Network: Neonatal outcomes of extremely preterm infants from the NICHD Neonatal Research Network. *Pediatrics*, 126(3):443–456, 2010.

SUPPORT Study Group of the Eunice Kennedy Shriver NICHD Neonatal Research Network, Finer, N.N., Carlo, W.A., Walsh, M.C., et al.: Early CPAP versus surfactant in extremely preterm infants. *New England Journal of Medicine*, 362:1970–1979, 2010. Erratum in: New England Journal of Medicine, 362(23):2235, 2010.

van der Meer, P., Blackwell, T.S., Lawrence, S., et al.: Fibroblast growth factor-10 expression through inhibition of Sp1-mediated NF-κB activation limits airway branching. *Journal of Immunology*, 185:4896–4903, 2010.

van Kaam, A.: Lung-protective ventilation in neonatology. *Neonatology*, 99(4):338–341, 2011.

Van Marter, L.J., Hernandez-Diaz, S., Werler, M.M., et al.: Nonsteroidal antiinflammatory drugs in late pregnancy and persistent pulmonary hypertension of the newborn. *Pediatrics*, 131(1):79–87, 2013.

Verklan, M.T. and Lopez, S.M.: Neurologic disorders. In S.L. Gardner, B.S. Carter, M. Enzman-Hines, and J.A. Hernandez (Eds.): *Merenstein & Gardner's handbook of neonatal intensive care* (7th ed.). St. Louis, 2011, Elsevier Mosby, p. 781.

Watterberg, K.L., and American Academy of Pediatrics, Committee on Fetus and Newborn: Policy statement—postnatal corticosteroids to prevent or treat bronchopulmonary dysplasia. *Pediatrics*, 126 (4):800–808, 2010.

Whitsett, J.A., Rice, W.R., Warner, B.B., et al.: Acute respiratory disorders. In M.G. MacDonald, M.D. Mullett, and M.M.K. Seshia (Eds.): *Avery's neonatology: Pathophysiology and management of the newborn* (5th ed.). Philadelphia, 2005, Lippincott, pp. 553–577.

Witlox, R.S., Lopriore, E., Oepkes, D., and Walther, F.J.: Neonatal outcome after prenatal interventions for congenital lung lesions. *Early Human Development*, 87:611–618, 2011.

Young, T.E.: Nutritional support and bronchopulmonary dysplasia. *Journal of Perinatology*, 27(Suppl. 1): S75–S78, 2007.

Zhang, H., Fang, J., Su, H, and Chen, M.: Risk factors for bronchopulmonary dysplasia in neonates born at $\leq$ 1500 g (1999-2009). *Pediatrics International*, 53 (6):915–920, 2011.

CHAPTER

# 25 Apnea

MARTHA GOODWIN

**OBJECTIVES**

1. Define types of apnea seen in the newborn infant.
2. Identify three causes of apnea.
3. Describe the pathogenesis of apnea in the premature infant.
4. Describe the evaluation process for the infant with apnea.
5. Discuss management techniques for controlling apnea.
6. Discuss the current status of home monitoring.

Apnea represents one of the most frequently encountered respiratory problems in the premature infant. It is not known why some infants are affected and others are not, although certain factors have a good predictive value. Apnea in the term infant is not ever a normal finding and must always be investigated. In the preterm infant, apnea that presents in the first 24 hours has historically been perceived as pathologic, whereas that occurring later has most often been attributed to immaturity. The mechanism of action is not fully understood but can be characterized as an immature respiratory system faced with demands it is ill equipped to handle. This chapter will provide a comprehensive review of apnea of the newborn infant, including causes, evaluation, treatment, and long-term home follow-up.

## DEFINITIONS OF APNEA

A. **Periodic breathing.**
   1. Definition: recurrent sequences of pauses in respiration lasting 5 to 10 seconds followed by 10 to 15 seconds of rapid respiration.
   2. Seen in less than 2% of healthy term infants and in 30% to 95% of healthy preterm infants more than 24 hours of age.
   3. Not accompanied by cyanosis or changes in heart rate.
   4. Episodes of periodic breathing in the preterm infant decrease significantly by 39 to 41 weeks of postmenstrual age (Miller et al., 2010).
   5. Studies do not support a link between periodic breathing and significant apnea or sudden infant death syndrome (SIDS) (Miller et al., 2010).

B. **Apnea.**
   1. Definition: cessation of respiration for at least 20 seconds, or less if complicated by cyanosis, pallor, hypotonia, or bradycardia.
   2. Most apnea occurs in the healthy preterm infant without organic disease. Up to 80% of infants weighing less than 1000 g and 25% weighing less than 2500 g at birth will have apnea during their neonatal course (Miller, Fanaroff, and Martin, 2011).

## TYPES OF APNEA

A. **Primary apnea.**
   1. Definition: initial cessation of respiratory movements after a period of rapid respiratory effort as a result of asphyxia during the delivery process.
   2. Exposure to stimulation and/or oxygen will usually induce spontaneous respiratory effort.

B. **Secondary apnea.**
   1. Definition: apnea occurring after a period of deep, gasping respirations and fall in blood pressure and heart rate, brought about by prolonged asphyxia during the delivery process. The gasping becomes slower and weaker and then ceases.

2. Infant will not respond to stimulation and will require more vigorous resuscitation.
3. For each minute in secondary apnea before resuscitation, there is a 2-minute delay before gasping is reestablished and another 2 minutes before the onset of regular respirations.
4. It is not usually possible to distinguish primary from secondary apnea at birth (Kattwinkel, 2010).

C. **Central apnea.**
1. Definition: absence of airflow and respiratory effort.
2. Cause of central apnea in the preterm infant is not fully understood.
3. Contributing factors are thought to include the following:
   a. Chest wall afferent neuromuscular signals and chest wall instability.
   b. Diaphragmatic fatigue.
   c. Immature, paradoxic response of neonate to hypoxia and hypercapnia.
   d. Altered levels of local neurotransmitters in the brainstem region of the central nervous system (CNS).
4. Fifteen percent of apnea episodes are central in origin.
5. Closure of upper airway occurs in about half of cases of central apnea (Al-Sufayan et al., 2009).

D. **Obstructive apnea.**
1. Definition: absence of airflow with continued respiratory effort, associated with blockage of airway at the level of pharynx and/or larynx (Kattwinkel, 2010).
2. Hyperextension or flexion of the neck may induce obstruction of the airway.
3. May be caused by obstruction of airflow at the mouth or nose as a result of anatomic abnormalities such as macroglossia (Beckwith–Wiedemann syndrome, congenital hypothyroidism) or micrognathia (Pierre Robin sequence).
4. Up to 30% of apnea episodes are obstructive in origin.

E. **Mixed apnea.**
1. Definition: a combination of central and obstructive apnea, obstruction usually at the level of the pharynx.
2. Fifty percent to 60% of neonatal apnea episodes are mixed.

F. **Idiopathic apnea, or apnea of prematurity.**
1. Diagnosis after exclusion of pathologic processes in the premature infant.
2. Not necessarily associated with the presence of periodic breathing.
3. Recurrent apnea seen in preterm infants who show no other abnormalities.
4. Onset within the first week of life, usually at 24 to 48 hours. If not present within the first week of life, will usually not appear unless later illness develops. If mechanically ventilated, apnea may not present until postextubation.
5. More likely to be obstructive than central in the first 2 days of life.
6. Episodes of apnea cease by term in 95% of infants; may persist longer in infants born at less than 28 weeks of gestational age (Scott et al., 2011).

## PATHOGENESIS OF APNEA IN THE PREMATURE INFANT

A. **Immature central respiratory center.**
1. Decreased afferent traffic occurs as a result of
   a. Poor CNS myelinization,
   b. Decreased number of synapses, and
   c. Decreased dendritic arborization.
2. Decreased amounts of neurotransmitters have been measured in infants with apnea and may play an important role in respiratory control (Kattwinkel, 1977).
3. Fluctuating respiratory center output has been implicated.

B. **Chemoreceptors.**
1. Located in the medulla (central) and the carotid and aortic bodies (peripheral), chemoreceptors relay information to the respiratory center in the brain regarding pH, $Po_2$, and $Pco_2$ via the vagus and glossopharyngeal nerves.
   a. Hypoxemia is sensed in the carotid and aortic bodies and results in an increase in alveolar ventilation. Premature infants with apnea do not respond to hypoxemia as effectively as infants who do not have apnea (MacFarlane et al., 2013).

b. Hypercapnia is sensed centrally. The normal response to an increased arterial $P_{CO_2}$ is an increase in minute ventilation. Neonates can increase ventilation by only 3 or 4 times the baseline values, in comparison with the 10- to 20-fold increase that adults can obtain. Premature infants exhibit a blunted response to elevated $P_{CO_2}$, resulting in ongoing hypoventilation and hypercapnia. This diminished response predisposes them to apnea (MacFarlane et al., 2013).

2. Biphasic response of the premature infant to hypoxia.
   a. During the first minute of hypoxia, a brief increase in respiratory effort occurs. It is followed in the next 2 to 3 minutes by a decrease in respiratory rate and by periodic breathing, respiratory depression, and apnea. Initial stimulation of the peripheral chemoreceptors is followed by overriding depression of the respiratory centers as a result of hypoxia (Kattwinkel, 2010).
   b. At 7 to 18 days of postnatal age, an infant can maintain the adult response to hypoxia of sustained hyperventilation.
3. Depressed response to hypercapnia. The premature infant exhibits decreased sensitivity to increased levels of carbon dioxide, requiring higher levels of carbon dioxide to stimulate respirations (Gauda et al., 2013).

**C. Thermal afferents.**
1. Apnea is increased in an environment that may be too warm for the infant.
2. Thermal receptors in the trigeminal area of the face produce an apneic response to stimulation by a cold or hot gas mixture.

**D. Mechanoreceptors.**
1. Stretch receptors alter the timing of respiration at various lung volumes.
   a. Head's paradoxic reflex: a gasp followed by apnea after abrupt lung inflation.
   b. Hering–Breuer reflex.
      (1) Vagally mediated, it acts to inhibit inspiration and/or prolong expiration.
      (2) Lung inflation initiates inhibitory impulses that terminate inspiration and prolong expiratory time.
      (3) Mechanoreceptors are very active in the neonate but rarely seen in the adult.
2. Pharyngeal collapse and airway obstruction are produced by negative pharyngeal pressure generated during inspiration.
3. Intercostal phrenic inhibitory reflex, an inward movement of the rib cage during inspiration, prematurely ends inspiration (Mathew, 2011).

**E. Protective reflexes.**
1. Stimulation of the posterior portion of the pharynx with suctioning, endotracheal or gavage tube placement, or gastroesophageal reflux can stimulate apnea.
2. Pulmonary irritant receptors can produce an apneic response to direct bronchial stimulation.
3. Laryngeal taste receptors can produce an apneic response to various chemical stimuli (Kattwinkel, 1977).

**F. Sleep state.**
1. Eighty percent of the neonate's day is spent in sleep.
2. Respiratory depression occurs predominantly in rapid eye movement (REM) or transitional sleep.
   a. May be influenced by central mechanisms at the level of the brainstem.
      (1) May be due to a defect in a sleep-related feedback loop or respiratory command.
      (2) Variability of respiratory rhythmicity is seen in active sleep.
   b. May be related to paradoxical respirations in which chest wall movements are out of phase, resulting in rib cage collapse with abdominal expansion during inspiration. This would lead to a decrease in lung volume and functional residual capacity.
   c. May be related to decreased skeletal muscle tone of the tongue and pharynx during sleep, which could lead to increased resistance and obstruction in the upper airway (Mathew, 2011; Zhao et al., 2011).

## CAUSES OF APNEA

**A. Prematurity.**

**B. Hypoxia.**

C. **Respiratory disorders.**
   1. Respiratory distress syndrome.
   2. Pneumonia.
   3. Aspiration.
   4. Acidosis.
   5. Airway obstruction.
   6. Pneumothorax.
   7. Atelectasis.
   8. Pulmonary hemorrhage.
   9. Postextubation status.
   10. Congenital anomalies of the upper airway.

D. **Cardiovascular disorders.**
   1. Hypotension.
   2. Arrhythmias.
   3. Congestive heart failure.
   4. Patent ductus arteriosus.

E. **Infection.**
   1. Sepsis.
   2. Pneumonia.
   3. Meningitis.
   4. Viral infections.
   5. Necrotizing enterocolitis.

F. **CNS disorders.**
   1. Congenital malformations.
   2. Seizures.
   3. Asphyxia.
   4. Intracranial hemorrhage.
   5. Kernicterus.
   6. Tumors.

G. **Drugs.**
   1. Maternal drugs.
      a. Narcotics.
      b. Analgesics.
      c. Anesthesia.
      d. β-Blocker antihypertensive agents.
      e. Magnesium sulfate.
   2. Neonatal drugs.
      a. Anticonvulsants: phenobarbital, pentobarbital.
      b. Cardiovascular drugs: prostaglandin $E_1$.
      c. Narcotics/analgesics.
         (1) Fentanyl.
         (2) Morphine.
         (3) Midazolam hydrochloride.
         (4) Lorazepam.

H. **Metabolic disorders.**
   1. Hypocalcemia.
   2. Hypoglycemia.
   3. Hypomagnesemia.
   4. Hyponatremia.
   5. Acidosis.
   6. Hyperammonemia.

I. **Hematopoietic disorders.**
   1. Polycythemia.
   2. Anemia.

J. **Reflex stimulation.**
   1. Posterior pharyngeal stimulation.

2. Gastroesophageal reflux—controversial, recent studies do not support a link. Some studies have shown apnea precedes reflux when the two are linked (Omari, 2009).

K. **Environmental factors.**
1. Rapid warming.
2. Hypothermia.
3. Hyperthermia.
4. Elevated environmental temperature.
5. Feeding.
6. Stooling.
7. Painful stimuli.

## EVALUATION FOR APNEA

A. **History.**
1. Perinatal risk factors.
   a. Maternal bleeding, drugs, fever, hypertension, prolonged rupture of membranes, polyhydramnios, chorioamnionitis, decreased fetal movements, abnormal fetal presentation.
   b. Fetal hypoxia, trauma.
2. Neonatal risk factors.
   a. Prematurity.
   b. Cardiorespiratory disease.
   c. Metabolic abnormalities.
   d. Temperature instability.
   e. Infection.
   f. Environmental causes.
   g. CNS disorders.

B. **Physical examination.** A complete physical and neurologic examination should be performed. Evaluate for congenital malformations, especially those involving the airway. Evaluate for signs of respiratory distress and heart disease. Abnormal behavior, tone, or posturing may be associated with a neurologic focus. An abdominal examination should be performed, which may reveal symptoms related to obstruction, infection, necrotizing enterocolitis, or congestive heart failure.

C. **Documentation of apnea episodes.** A record of apneic episodes should be maintained as part of the infant's record. This allows the caregiver to determine a pattern, if any, to the apnea. It may also provide information about precipitating events or specific events associated with the apnea. Information documented should include the following:
1. Duration of apnea episode.
2. Time of apnea episode and any relation to feeding, activity, stooling, sleep, or procedures.
3. Infant's position: prone or supine, with head of bed elevated or flat.
4. Associated bradycardia/heart rate.
5. Associated color change and/or oxygen desaturation.
6. Type of stimulation required to resolve the episode:
   a. None, self-resolved.
   b. Gentle tactile stimulation.
   c. Vigorous tactile stimulation.
   d. Oxygen.
   e. Bag-and-mask ventilation.

D. **Laboratory evaluation.**
1. Basic evaluation to look for infection, respiratory deterioration, and metabolic problems.
   a. Complete blood cell count, with differential cell and platelet counts.
   b. Blood gases.
   c. Serum glucose, electrolytes, calcium, magnesium.
   d. Blood culture, lumbar puncture for evaluation of cerebrospinal fluid, and urine culture.
2. Extensive laboratory evaluation for less common causes of apnea.
   a. Toxicology screen.
   b. Urine collection for detection of amino acids and organic acids.

c. Serum ammonia.
d. State screen and expanded neonatal screen for metabolic disease.

E. **Other.**
1. Echocardiogram or electrocardiogram: may detect cardiac abnormality or conduction disorders.
2. Electroencephalogram: may confirm suspected seizures.
3. Chest x-ray: may demonstrate respiratory or cardiac abnormalities.
4. Cranial ultrasound, computed tomography, or magnetic resonance imaging: may demonstrate structural abnormalities or hemorrhages.
5. Barium swallow and pH study: to evaluate pharyngeal structure and function or gastroesophageal reflux.
6. Pneumogram.
a. Measures chest wall movement, heart rate, oxygen saturation, and nasal airflow by thermistor or carbon dioxide probe (4 channel); measures esophageal pH if needed (5 channel if esophageal probe is used).
b. No predictive value for SIDS; recording monitors are as effective at detecting apnea over a prolonged period.

## MANAGEMENT TECHNIQUES

A. **Treat underlying cause if determined.**
B. **Provide needed medical or surgical intervention.**
C. **Maintain environmental temperature at the low end of the neutral thermal zone.**
D. **Avoid triggering reflexes:**
1. Vigorous catheter suctioning.
2. Hot or cold to the face.
3. Sudden gastric distention.

E. **Positioning.** Prone positioning is associated with higher oxygen saturation, shorter gastric emptying time, and decreased incidence of regurgitation and aspiration. Historical data suggested prone positioning to decrease apneic episodes. A recent systematic review found no decrease in apnea, bradycardia, or desaturation with body positioning in the prone position (Bredemeyer and Foster, 2012). The only infants for whom prone positioning is recommended are those with upper airway disorders or impaired airway protective mechanisms for whom the risk of death due to gastroesophageal reflux is greater than the risk of SIDS or other sleep-related death (Task Force on Sudden Infant Death Syndrome, 2011).
F. **Maintain the neck in a neutral position, not flexed or hyperextended. Use of a neck roll is recommended.**
G. **Avoid vigorous manual ventilation to prevent intermittent hyperoxia, hypocapnia, and blunting of the $CO_2$ response.**
H. **Attempt to control apnea by avoiding painful stimuli, loud noises, extremely vigorous tactile stimulation, or potent odors.** No evidence supports effectiveness of kinesthetic stimulation in reduction of apnea.
I. **Consider providing continuous positive airway pressure.**
1. Increases end expiratory lung volumes and splints the upper airway and weak chest wall, thereby improving compliance and oxygenation and decreasing respiratory muscle work so that diaphragmatic movements are less tiring and more effective.
2. Complicates gavage feedings and may increase risk of aspiration. Increases risk of air leak.

J. **Pharmacologic therapy.**
1. Methylxanthine (aminophylline, theophylline, caffeine), administered orally or intravenously. Used to treat apnea of prematurity after pathologic causes have been eliminated.
a. Mechanisms of action include the following:
(1) Stimulation of central respiratory chemoreceptors.
(2) Increased ventilatory response to carbon dioxide.
(3) Increased oxygenation.
(4) Increased minute ventilation (theophylline).
(5) Stabilization of oscillations in breathing (theophylline).

(6) Improved diaphragmatic contractility.
(7) Relaxation of bronchial smooth muscle (theophylline).
(8) CNS excitation.
(9) Increased respiratory drive.
(10) Increased respiratory muscle activity.
(11) Increased skeletal muscle activity.

**b.** Pharmacokinetics.
(1) Half-life of aminophylline and theophylline is approximately 30 hours.
(2) Half-life of caffeine is approximately 100 hours.
(3) Both theophylline and caffeine are rapidly absorbed intravenously. Oral absorption of caffeine is rapid, and oral absorption of theophylline is variable.
(4) Metabolism of caffeine and theophylline takes place in the liver. This is slower in the neonate than in the adult.
(5) Theophylline is metabolized to caffeine by a metabolic pathway unique to the preterm infant.
(6) Serum concentrations must be checked to avoid toxic levels.

**c.** Dosage:
(1) Aminophylline.
(a) Route: intravenous (IV).
(b) Loading dose: 5 to 8 mg/kg.
(c) Maintenance dose: 2 to 6 mg/kg/day divided every 8 to 12 hours.
(d) Therapeutic level: 5 to 15 mcg/mL.
(2) Caffeine.
(a) Route: IV or by mouth.
(b) Loading dose: 10 mg/kg, caffeine base; 20 mg/kg, caffeine citrate.
(c) Maintenance dose: 2.5 mg/kg, caffeine base; 5 mg/kg, caffeine citrate; every 24 hours beginning 24 hours after loading dose (Lexi-Comp, 2011).
(d) Avoid use of caffeine benzoate preparation, which can displace bilirubin from albumin-binding sites.
(e) Therapeutic level: 5 to 20 mcg/mL.
(f) Higher doses and therapeutic levels have been studied, with no reported adverse effects, but are not commonly used.

**d.** Side effects.
(1) Caffeine: tachycardia, cardiac dysrhythmias, increased wakefulness, increased active sleep, gastrointestinal distention, gastrointestinal bleeding, and diuresis with sodium loss.
(2) Theophylline: tachycardia, cardiac dysrhythmias, seizures, jitteriness, feeding intolerance, gastroesophageal reflux, dehydration, hyperglycemia, and hypotension.

**e.** Caffeine versus theophylline.
(1) Theophylline is a more potent vasodilator.
(2) Theophylline causes a more rapid and sustained tachycardia.
(3) Caffeine diffuses more rapidly in the CNS.
(4) Caffeine is given only once a day.
(5) Caffeine has a wider therapeutic index.
(6) Caffeine may be effective in apnea not responsive to theophylline and vice versa.
(7) Caffeine has a longer half-life, resulting in smaller changes in its plasma concentration.
(8) On the basis of its higher therapeutic ratio, more reliable enteral absorption, and longer half-life, caffeine is recommended over theophylline for treatment of apnea of prematurity (Henderson-Smart and Steer, 2010).

**2.** Doxapram.
**a.** Potent respiratory stimulant for apnea refractory to methylxanthine therapy.
**b.** Mechanism of action thought to be stimulation of the peripheral chemoreceptors at low doses (0.5 mg/kg/hr) and of the CNS at higher doses.
**c.** Increases minute ventilation, tidal volume, and mean inspiratory flow and decreases $P_{CO_2}$ (Dani et al., 2006).

d. Pharmacokinetics.
   (1) Half-life is approximately 10 hours in the first few days of life and 8 hours at 10 days of age.
   (2) Steady-state levels are reached within 24 hours.
e. Dosage.
   (1) Route: IV.
   (2) Loading dose: 2.5 to 3 mg/kg followed by (3).
   (3) Continuous infusion of 1/mg/kg/hr, titrate to lowest effective dose. Maximum 2.5 mg/kg/hr.
   (4) Controversy exists over therapeutic and toxic plasma levels. Guidelines include the following:
      (a) Therapeutic level: 1.5 to 5 mg/L.
      (b) Toxic level: 5 mg/L. Levels greater than 3.5 mg/L may produce side effects.
f. Side effects.
   (1) Jitteriness, irritability, vomiting, seizures, abdominal distention, increased gastric residuals, hyperglycemia, and glycosuria.
   (2) Hypertension, tachycardia, and increased cardiac output.
   (3) Increased work of breathing resulting from respiratory stimulation, consequent increased oxygen consumption and carbon dioxide production, and increased tidal volume and respiratory rate.
   (4) Increased risk of intraventricular hemorrhage if used in the first few days of life.
g. Contraindication: use in newborn infant not routinely recommended because preparation contains benzyl alcohol.
   (1) Benzyl alcohol is associated with "gasping syndrome," characterized by metabolic acidosis, renal failure, liver failure, and cardiovascular collapse.
   (2) Cumulative doses might be toxic for the liver, kidney, or brain.
   (3) Insufficient data exist on clinical benefit and long-term effects (Lexi-Comp, 2011; Spitzer, 2012).

K. **Assisted ventilation.** Used for apnea resistant to other methods of therapy.

## HOME MONITORING

A. **Effectiveness of home monitoring.** The American Academy of Pediatrics states that cardiorespiratory monitoring is effective in preventing death from apnea for certain selected infants but is clearly inappropriate for others, with the primary objective being to serve the best interest of the infant based on the infant's history (Task Force on Sudden Infant Death Syndrome, 2011).

B. **Indications for home monitoring.**
   1. Premature infant with symptoms of idiopathic apnea of prematurity who is otherwise ready for hospital discharge.
   2. A survivor of an apparent life-threatening event defined as apnea, cyanosis, altered muscle tone, choking, or gagging.
   3. Sibling death due to SIDS.
   4. Tracheostomy, mechanically supported ventilation.
   5. A sleep apnea syndrome caused by a neurologic disorder, periodic breathing, upper airway abnormality, or idiopathic syndromes.
   6. Other conditions of ill or high-risk infants, as determined on an individual basis.

C. **Home monitoring is not indicated in prevention of SIDS in symptom-free, healthy infants.**

D. **Monitoring technology.**
   1. Transthoracic impedance combined with electrocardiography is current standard.
      a. Electrodes are placed on infant's chest or inside an adjustable belt worn around the chest.
      b. A small electric current passes between the electrodes. The impedance to this current is measured as the chest wall diameter changes. The monitor senses this change and equates it with respiration.
      c. Electrocardiograph reads cardiac activity.
      d. High and low limits for respirations and heart rate are set by the clinician.

   e. Monitor is compact and portable, weighing less than 5 pounds. A battery pack is available for use outside the home.
2. Technical problems include artifacts from signal interference, false alarms caused by shallow breathing, and the monitor's inability to detect obstructive apnea. Incorrect placement of leads can result in false alarms as well.
3. Advances in technology allow recording of home monitor events for evaluation by the clinician.
   a. Recording of events allows monitoring of compliance.
   b. True events can be distinguished from false alarms.
   c. Fewer rehospitalizations are needed.
   d. Recording is as sensitive as a pneumogram for evaluating whether monitoring can be discontinued.
   e. Fewer monitor days are needed for infants without events.

E. **Follow-up care.**
1. Multidisciplinary team includes physician, nurse, social worker, case manager, and equipment company representatives.
2. Family and other caregivers of the infant are trained in cardiopulmonary resuscitation before hospital discharge. Thorough education in use of the monitor is also provided before discharge.
3. Care includes close telephone contact—within 24 hours after discharge and every week to 2 weeks afterward as needed.
4. Visiting nurse makes home visit within the first week and then as needed.
5. A team member is available 24 hours a day for answering questions and solving problems. Equipment company representative is available as needed for problems and information.
6. Home follow-up does not replace clinic visits.
7. In 80% of infants, apnea of prematurity will cease between 40 and 44 weeks of postmenstrual age; in asymptomatic infants, home monitoring can be stopped at 45 weeks of postmenstrual age (Silvestri, 2009).

## REFERENCES


Al-Sufayan, F., Bamehrez, M., Kwiatkowski, K., and Alvaro, R.E.: The effects of airway closure in central apneas and obstructed respiratory efforts in mixed apneas in preterm infants. *Pediatric Pulmonology*, 44:253–259, 2009.

Bredemeyer, S.L. and Foster, J.P.: Body positioning for spontaneously breathing preterm infants with apnea. *Cochrane Database of Systematic Reviews*, (6):CD004951, 2012.

Gauda, E.B., Shirahatab, M., Masona, A., et al.: Inflammation in the carotid body during development and its contribution to apnea of prematurity. *Respiratory Physiology & Neurobiology*, 185:120–131, 2013.

Henderson-Smart, D.J., and Steer, P.A.: Caffeine versus theophylline for apnea in preterm infants. *Cochrane Database of Systematic Reviews*, (1):CD000273, 2010.

Kattwinkel, J.: *Textbook of neonatal resuscitation* (6th ed.). Elk Grove Village, IL, 2010, American Academy of Pediatrics and American Heart Association.

Kattwinkel, J.: Neonatal apnea: Pathogenesis and therapy. *Journal of Pediatrics*, 90(3):342–347, 1977.

Lexi-Comp: Pediatric & Neonatal Lexi-Drugs Online™. Hudson, OH, 2011, Lexi-Comp, Inc.

MacFarlane, P.M., Ribeiro, A.P. and Martin, R.J.: Carotid chemoreceptor development and neonatal apnea. *Respiratory Physiology & Neurobiology*, 185:170–176, 2013.

Mathew, O.P.: Apnea of prematurity: Pathogenesis and management strategies. *Journal of Perinatology*, 31:302–310, 2011.

Miller, M.J., Fanaroff, A.A., and Martin, R.: Respiratory disorders in preterm and term infants. In R. Martin, A.A. Fanaroff, and M.C. Walsh (Eds.): *Fanaroff and Martin's neonatal-perinatal medicine: Diseases of the fetus and infant* (9th ed.). Philadelphia, 2011, Elsevier Mosby, pp. 1141–1169.

Omari, T.I.: Apnea-associated reduction in lower esophageal sphincter tone in premature infants. *Journal of Pediatrics*, 154:374–378, 2009.

Silvestri, J.M.: Indications for home apnea monitoring (or not). *Clinics in Perinatology*, 36(1):87–99, 2009.

Spitzer, A.R.: Evidence-based methylxanthine use in the NICU. *Clinics in Perinatology*, 39:137–148, 2012.

Task Force on Sudden Infant Death Syndrome: SIDS and other sleep-related infant deaths: Expansion of recommendations for a safe infant sleeping environment. *Pediatrics*, 128:1030, 2011.

Zhao, J., Gonzalez, F., and Dezhi, M.: Apnea of prematurity: From cause to treatment. *Journal of Pediatrics*, 170:1097–1105, 2011.

CHAPTER

# 26 Assisted Ventilation

DEBBIE FRASER AND WILLIAM DIEHL-JONES

**OBJECTIVES**

1. Identify the concepts of FRC, $V_T$, VC, and TLC and describe their importance in the physiology of ventilation.
2. Describe the concepts of elastic recoil, compliance, resistance, and gas trapping and their importance in ventilating the lungs of the newborn infant.
3. Explain the relationship of fetal hemoglobin, pH, and temperature to the oxyhemoglobin dissociation curve.
4. List potential causes of respiratory and metabolic acid–base disturbance in the newborn infant. Identify ranges of pH, $Pao_2$, $Paco_2$, $HCO_3^-$, and base excess/deficit in various respiratory disease states in the newborn infant.
5. Identify treatment modalities for neonates in respiratory distress.
6. Describe various types of mechanical ventilation devices available for the neonate.
7. List nursing interventions required to care for ventilated infants, based on the theories of mechanical ventilation.
8. Differentiate between high-frequency jet ventilation and high-frequency oscillatory ventilation.
9. Identify the nursing interventions required for high-frequency ventilation that differ from those required for conventional ventilation.
10. Identify changes in patient status that indicate potential complications with assisted ventilation.
11. Describe various medications used to enhance lung status in the ventilated patient.

Caring for an infant requiring assisted ventilation is a challenge. It is necessary for the nurse to understand the normal pulmonary physiology as well as the pathophysiology of pulmonary diseases in the neonate. An understanding of the basic mechanical principles of various ventilators is important to providing optimal care for a neonate. New ventilation techniques are being developed rapidly, and the choices for ventilating the neonate are greater now than ever before. The focus of this chapter is to provide the basic knowledge needed to care for the infant requiring oxygen therapy or mechanical ventilation.

## PHYSIOLOGY

A. **Definitions (Blackburn, 2013).**
   1. Tidal volume ($V_T$): the amount of air that moves into or out of the lungs with each single breath at rest (4 to 6 mL/kg).
   2. Vital capacity (VC): the volume of air maximally inspired and maximally expired (40 mL/kg).
   3. Functional residual capacity (FRC): the volume of gas that remains in the lungs after a normal expiration (30 mL/kg).
   4. Total lung capacity (TLC): the amount of air contained in the lung after a maximal inspiration (63 mL/kg).
   5. Physiologic dead space: anatomic plus alveolar dead space.
      a. Anatomic dead space: the volume of gas within the area of the pulmonary conducting airways that cannot engage in gas exchange.
      b. Alveolar dead space: the volume of inspired gas that reaches the alveoli but does not participate in gas exchange because of inadequate perfusion to those alveoli.
   6. Mechanical dead space: gas that fills the ventilator circuit for availability in inspiration, as well as exhaled gas. Minimal dead space is desirable. Excessive dead space can cause increased retention of carbon dioxide.

B. **Concepts (Keszler and Abubakar, 2011).**
   1. Elastic recoil: the natural tendency for a stretched object to return to the original resting volume. With inhalation, alveoli stretch to a certain point, and during exhalation the alveoli return to their original size in an infant with normal lungs.

2. Lung compliance: the change in volume that occurs with a change in pressure (elasticity of the lung). It also refers to the relationship between a given change in volume and the pressure required to produce that change. An infant with severe hyaline membrane disease will have decreased compliance (because of lack of surfactant) requiring increased pressure to overcome the resistance generated by the surface tension in the alveoli. The major force contributing to elastic recoil of the lung is surface tension at the air–liquid interface in distal bronchioles and alveoli. The amount of distal airway pressure needed to counteract the tendency of the alveoli and bronchioles to collapse is demonstrated by the Laplace relationship: the relationship between pressure, surface tension, and the radius of a structure. The pressure needed to stabilize an alveolus is directly proportional to twice the surface tension and inversely proportional to the radius of that alveolus.
3. Lung resistance: the result of friction between moving parts. Airway resistance is determined by the flow rate, viscosity, and density of the respiratory gases as well as the length and diameter of the airways (Keszler and Abubakar, 2011). An increase in airway resistance increases the time needed for air to reach the alveoli. High rates of airflow increase airway resistance by creating turbulence. Resistance to gas in a 2.5-mm endotracheal tube (ETT) is higher than in a 3.5-mm ETT because of the narrow lumen of the smaller tube. It takes greater pressure to force air through a small tube. Anatomic sources of resistance in the newborn infant include nasal passages, the glottis, the trachea, and the main bronchi. During intubation, the ETT is also a source of resistance.
4. Gas trapping: more gas entering the lung than leaving the lung. A partially occluded ETT can cause gas trapping. Debris from meconium can allow gas into the lung but may occlude the airway during exhalation (known as a ball–valve effect).
5. Inadvertent positive end-expiratory pressure (PEEP): a result of gas trapping in which volume and pressure increase in the distal airways through end-expiration. Providing oxygen by nasal cannula can result in inadvertent PEEP in the small premature infant.
6. Ventilation–perfusion ratio ($\dot{V}_A/\dot{Q}$) (Fig. 26-1). Matching pulmonary ventilation and perfusion is necessary for efficient gas exchange. The relationship between ventilation and perfusion is expressed as a ratio and describes the relationship between alveolar ventilation and capillary perfusion of the lungs. A 1:1 ratio indicates that the alveoli are in perfect contact with the pulmonary capillaries, allowing exchange of $O_2$ and $CO_2$. A $\dot{V}_A/\dot{Q}$ ratio of zero indicates a shunt whereby no ventilation occurs during passage of blood through the lungs. Abnormalities of the $\dot{V}_A/\dot{Q}$ ratio may be due to:
   a. Too little ventilation with normal blood flow.
   b. Too little blood flow with normal ventilation.
   c. A combination of the above.
7. Mean airway pressure (MAP): mean or average pressure transmitted to the airways throughout an entire respiratory cycle (Gardner et al., 2011). MAP is dependent on the ventilator rate, gas flow through the ventilator circuit, peak inspiratory pressure (PIP), PEEP, and inspiratory time. Increasing MAP can greatly influence the management of respiratory distress in decreasing atelectasis and true intrapulmonary shunting and is a useful tool in determining oxygenation.
8. Permissive hypercapnia: ventilation strategy that allows carbon dioxide levels to remain elevated. This strategy is designed to minimize barotrauma by avoiding the use of mechanical ventilation or by using minimal ventilatory rates and pressures.

C. **Oxygen transport.**
1. The amount of oxygen that can be delivered to the tissues is dependent on cardiac output and the oxygen content of the blood.
2. Oxygen is transported to tissue cells bound reversibly to hemoglobin and dissolved in plasma $O_2$. The amount of $O_2$ that is dissolved in the plasma is small (0.3 mL of $O_2$ dissolved in 100 mL of plasma per 100 mm Hg of $O_2$) compared with the amount that is bound to hemoglobin (1.34 mL of $O_2$ per gram of 100% saturated hemoglobin).
3. The amount of oxygen carried in the blood by hemoglobin depends on the hemoglobin concentration and the percent saturation of the hemoglobin. Adequate saturation is affected by the amount of hemoglobin available. Hemoglobin is almost fully saturated at a $Po_2$ of 80 to 100 mm Hg.

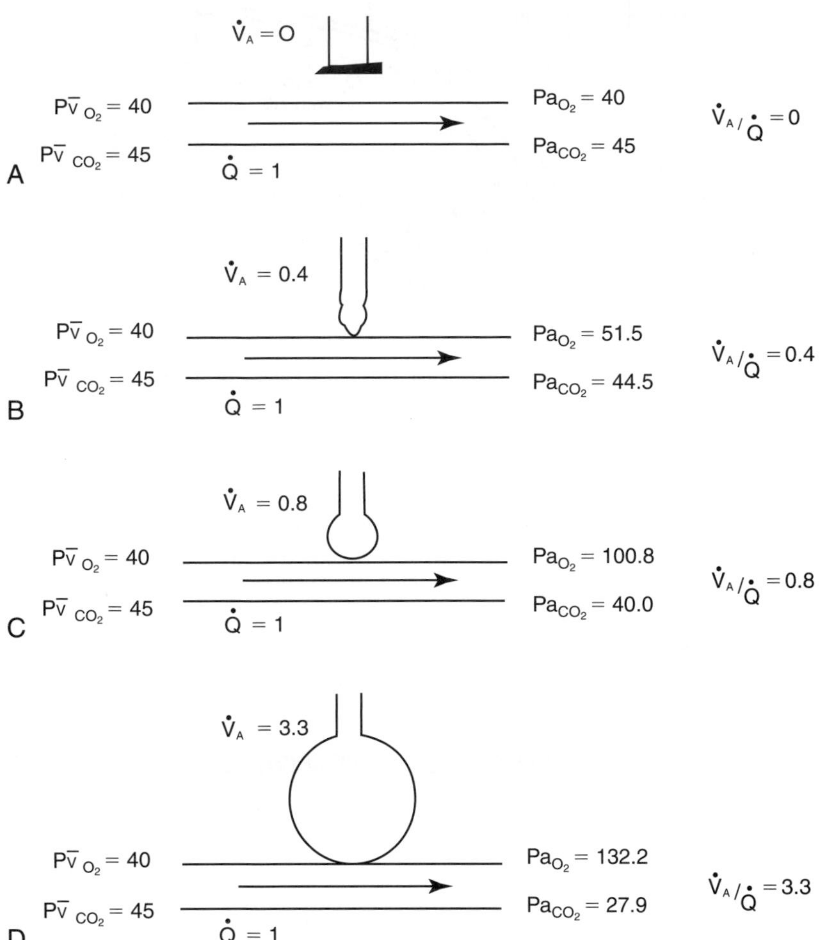


FIGURE 26-1 ■ Effects of various ventilation–perfusion ($\dot{V}_A/\dot{Q}$) ratios on blood gas tensions. **A,** Direct venoarterial shunting ($\dot{V}_A/\dot{Q}=0$). Venous gas tensions are unaltered, and arterial blood has the same tension as venous blood. **B,** Alveolus with a low $\dot{V}_A/\dot{Q}$ ratio. Only partial oxygenation and $CO_2$ removal take place in this alveolus because of underventilation in relation to perfusion. **C,** Normal alveolus. **D,** Underperfused alveolus with high $\dot{V}_A/\dot{Q}$ ratio. Note that although the oxygen tension is 32 mm Hg greater than in normal alveolus (**C**), this results in only a slightly higher saturation and $O_2$ content. (From Thibeault, D.W. and Gregory, G.A.: *Neonatal pulmonary care*. Norwalk, Conn., 1986, Appleton-Century-Crofts.)

4. The binding of oxygen to hemoglobin varies with the $Pa{O_2}$. The relationship is nonlinear and gives rise to an S-shaped curve—the oxyhemoglobin dissociation curve. The amount of oxygen that combines with hemoglobin at a given $P{O_2}$ depends on the position of the hemoglobin–oxygen dissociation curve (Fig. 26-2). Factors that determine the position of the dissociation curve are:
   a. Concentration of 2,3-diphosphoglycerate and the proportion of hemoglobin A (adult) to hemoglobin F (fetal).
   b. Temperature.
   c. $P{CO_2}$.
   d. pH.
5. With decreased affinity (shift to the right), hemoglobin releases $O_2$ more easily to the tissues.
6. With increased affinity (shift to the left), oxygen is unloaded less rapidly and efficiently in the peripheral tissues.

D. **Control of breathing** (Gardner et al., 2011). Control of ventilation (Box 26-1) is affected by both neurologic and chemical factors. The neurologic factors include central nervous system (CNS)

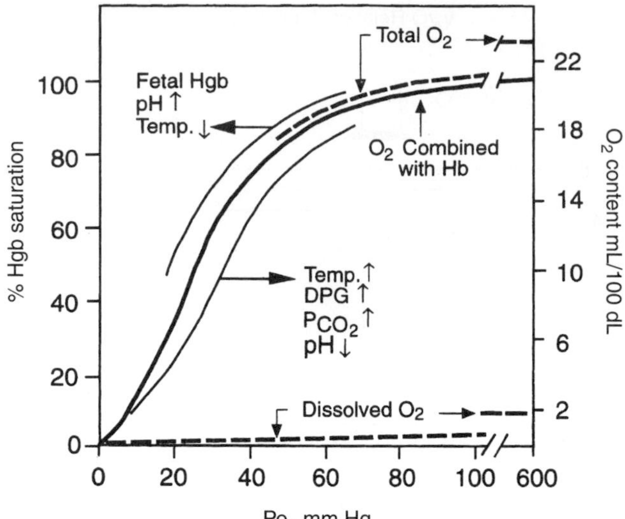


FIGURE 26-2 ■ Hemoglobin–oxygen dissociation curve. Nonlinear or S-shaped oxyhemoglobin curve and the linear or straight-line dissolved $O_2$ relationships between the $O_2$ saturation ($Sa_{O_2}$) and the $P_{O_2}$. Total blood $O_2$ content is shown with division into a portion combined with hemoglobin and a portion physically dissolved at various levels of $P_{O_2}$. Also shown are the major factors that change the $O_2$ affinity for hemoglobin and thus shift the oxyhemoglobin dissociation curve either to the left or to the right. *DPG,* 2,3-diphosphoglycerate. (Modified from West, J.B.: *Respiratory physiology: The essentials* [2nd ed.]. Baltimore, 1979, Williams & Wilkins, pp. 71, 73.)

## BOX 26-1

## FACTORS AFFECTING CONTROL OF VENTILATION IN THE SPONTANEOUSLY BREATHING NEONATE

**A. Neurologic Factors**

1. "Maturity" of the CNS.
   a. Degree of myelination, which largely determines speed of impulse transmission and response time to stimuli affecting ventilation.
   b. Degree of arborization, or dendritic interconnections (synapses) between neurons, allowing summation of excitatory potentials coming in from other parts of the CNS, and largely setting the neuronal depolarization threshold and response level of the respiratory center.
2. Sleep state (i.e., REM sleep vs. quiet or non-REM sleep).
   a. REM sleep is generally associated with irregular respirations (both in depth and frequency), distortion, and paradoxic motion of the ribcage during inspiration, inhibition of Hering–Breuer and glottic closure reflexes, and blunted response to $CO_2$ changes.
   b. Quiet sleep is generally associated with regular respirations, a more stable ribcage, and a directly proportional relationship between $P_{CO_2}$ and degree of ventilation.
3. Reflex responses.
   a. Hering–Breuer reflex, whereby inspiratory duration is limited in response to lung inflation sensed by stretch receptors located in major airways. Not present in adult humans, this reflex is very active during quiet sleep of newborn babies but absent or very weak during REM sleep.
   b. Head reflex, whereby inspiratory effort is further increased in response to rapid lung inflation. Thought to produce the frequently observed "biphasic sighs" of newborn infants that may be crucial for promoting and maintaining lung inflation (and therefore breathing regularity) after birth.
   c. Intercostal–phrenic reflex, whereby inspiration is inhibited by proprioception (position-sensing) receptors in intercostal muscles responding to distortion of the lower ribcage during REM sleep.
   d. Trigeminal–cutaneous reflex, whereby tidal volume increases and respiratory rate decreases in response to facial stimulation.
   e. Glottic closure reflex, whereby the glottis is narrowed through reflex contraction of the laryngeal adductor muscles during respiration, "breaking" exhalation and increasing subglottic pressure (as with expiratory "grunting").

## BOX 26-1
## FACTORS AFFECTING CONTROL OF VENTILATION IN THE SPONTANEOUSLY BREATHING NEONATE—CONT'D

**B. Chemical Drive Factors (Chemoreflexes)**

1. Response to hypoxemia (falling $Pa_{O_2}$) or to decrease in $O_2$ concentration breathed (mediated by peripheral chemoreceptors in carotid and aortic bodies):
   a. Initially there is increase in depth of breathing (tidal volume), but subsequently (if hypoxia persists or worsens), there is depression of respiratory drive, reduction in depth and rate of respiration, and eventual failure of arousal.
   b. For the first week of life, at least, these responses are dependent on environmental temperature (i.e., keeping the baby warm).
   c. Hypoxia is associated with an increase in periodic breathing and apnea.
2. Response to hyperoxia (increase in $Fi_{O_2}$) breathing causes a transient respiratory depression, stronger in term than in preterm infants.
3. Response to hypercapnia (rising $Pa_{CO_2}$ or $[H^+]$) or to increase in $CO_2$ concentration breathed (mediated by central chemoreceptors in the medulla):
   a. Increase in ventilation is directly proportional to inspired $CO_2$ concentration (or, more accurately stated, to alveolar $CO_2$ tension), as is the case in adults.
   b. Response to $CO_2$ is in large part dependent on sleep state: in quiet sleep, a rising $Pa_{CO_2}$ causes increase in depth and rate of breathing, whereas during REM sleep the response is irregular and reduced in depth and rate. The degree of reduction closely parallels the amount of ribcage deformity occurring during REM sleep.
   c. Ventilatory response to $CO_2$ in newborn infants is markedly depressed during behavioral activity, such as feeding, and easily depressed by sedatives and anesthesia.

From Goldsmith, J.P. and Karotkin, E.H.: *Assisted ventilation of the neonate* (3rd ed.). Philadelphia, 1996, W.B. Saunders, p. 26.
*CNS*, Central nervous system; *REM*, rapid eye movement.

maturity, sleep state, and reflexes. The chemoreflexes include responses to hypoxemia, hyperoxia, and hypercapnia.

**E. Hypoxia.** Delivery of $O_2$ to tissues is inadequate. Causes include the following:
1. Heart failure.
2. Anemia. Hemoglobin available to transport oxygen is reduced, although completely saturated. $Pa_{O_2}$ levels are usually normal.
3. Abnormal hemoglobin. $O_2$ is not released to the tissues.
   a. Methemoglobin.
   b. Bart hemoglobin.
4. Cardiogenic or hypovolemic shock.

**F. Hypoxemia.** $O_2$ content of arterial blood is low because of extrapulmonary or intrapulmonary shunts. The blood has bypassed adequately ventilated alveoli.
1. Intrapulmonary shunt.
   a. Ventilation–perfusion mismatch caused by lung diseases such as atelectasis, respiratory distress syndrome, or pneumonia.
   b. Can occur whenever alveoli are inadequately ventilated (hypoventilation).
2. Extrapulmonary shunt.
   a. Cyanotic congenital heart disease. Abnormal heart structure causes blood to bypass the lungs for oxygenation.
   b. Pulmonary artery hypertension. Blood shunts from the right side of the heart to the left side via a patent foramen ovale or ductus arteriosus, or both, causing blood to bypass the lungs.
      (1) Comparison of the $Pa_{O_2}$ or $O_2$ saturation of preductal and postductal blood can help determine whether or not a right-to-left shunt is present.
      (2) In the presence of shunting, preductal blood obtained from the right radial artery has a greater than 5% difference in saturation from postductal blood obtained from the umbilical artery or posterior tibial artery.

## TREATMENT MODALITIES

A. **Blow-by oxygen.** Free flow of $O_2$ from a bag and mask or flow of $O_2$ through $O_2$ tubing near the infant's face may be useful for short-term $O_2$ delivery to an infant who is breathing but needs an $O_2$-enriched atmosphere for oxygenation (i.e., in the delivery room following a trial of room air, during caregiving activities, during placement of an intravenous [IV] line, during weighing). There is no way to determine the exact content of $O_2$ delivered to the infant. Oxygen content depends on $O_2$ concentration, flow rate, the distance of the $O_2$ source from the infant, and the ventilatory efforts of the infant.

B. **Nasal cannula. Humidified $O_2$ is delivered at a set flow rate via a cannula, with the flow directed into the nares. The exact concentration of oxygen delivered by nasal cannula cannot be measured.**
   1. Conventional nasal cannula. Oxygen is delivered through the cannula and is regulated by the flow (measured in liters). Low-flow meters are capable of delivering amounts as small as 0.02 L/min. The concentration of oxygen used may be 100% or may be regulated with the use of a blender system.
   2. High-flow nasal cannula (HFNC). Flow is greater than 1.5 to 2 L/min, with oxygen blended to a known concentration. High flow rates result in the delivery of various levels of continuous positive airway pressure (CPAP) depending on the type of cannula, size of the infant, whether the infant's mouth is open or closed, and the flow rate used (Mosca et al., 2012). Adequate humidification is essential with the use of high flow to prevent drying and damage to the nasal passages. HFNC may be comparable to nasal CPAP in level of respiratory support supplied (Miller and Dowd, 2010).
   3. A blender should be used to adjust the concentration of oxygen being delivered by cannula, although the amount of oxygen entering the infant's lungs cannot be accurately determined because of the entrainment of room air around the cannula.
   4. Indications. A nasal cannula is used when there is a need for prolonged oxygen therapy, as in chronic lung disease, transfer or transport, and increased mobility of the infant for feedings or for other developmental activities.
   5. Complications. Pressure-related tissue damage may occur because of improper or infrequent changing, $O_2$ concentration may vary, hypoxemia may result from a displaced cannula, and the cannula may be occluded by nasal secretions (may cause significant respiratory distress). Flow through the cannula may result in drying of the nasal mucosa, predisposing the infant to tissue damage and thickened nasal secretions.

C. **CPAP.**
   1. Mask CPAP: delivery of positive pressure (5 to 8 cm $H_2O$ pressure) with variable amounts of $O_2$ via face or nasal mask. Requires appropriate-sized mask and tight seal around the nose or, in the case of face mask CPAP, the nose and mouth.
      a. Indications: atelectasis, apnea, respiratory distress, and pulmonary edema.
      b. Advantages: short-term use to assist with alveolar expansion and to inhibit alveolar collapse (atelectasis); intubation not required. May be useful in infants whose nares are too small to accommodate CPAP prongs. Alternating between nasal prong CPAP and nasal mask CPAP may help to reduce skin breakdown around the nares in low birth weight (LBW) infants (Wisewell and Courtney, 2011).
      c. Complications: carbon dioxide retention in the dead space of the mask, pulmonary hyperexpansion potentially leading to air leaks (i.e., pneumothorax, pneumomediastinum), aspiration of stomach contents, and gastric distention.
   2. Nasal CPAP: generally started at 5 to 6 cm $H_2O$ pressure and titrated up to 8 cm $H_2O$ pressure (Bingham and Fraser, 2012) delivered by prongs that fit into the nares, in addition to a measured concentration of oxygen.
      a. Indications: atelectasis, apnea, mild to moderate respiratory distress, and pulmonary edema.
      b. Advantage: intubation not required.
      c. Complications: ineffective ventilation, pneumothorax, variable pressure delivery when infant's mouth is open, molding of the head from securing straps, erosion of the septum from poorly fitting prongs, nasal obstruction as a result of increased

secretions, agitation, dislodging of prongs by an active infant, and gastric distention and perforation.

3. Nasopharyngeal CPAP: delivered by ETT or long nasal prongs, passed through the nares and positioned with the tip of the tube in the oropharynx.
   a. Indications: atelectasis, apnea, respiratory distress, pulmonary edema, and to assist in weaning from mechanical ventilation.
   b. Advantage: stable placement of tube, which an infant is less likely to dislodge than with nasal CPAP.
   c. Disadvantages: need for a skilled provider to place the tube, possible damage to the nasal septum and oropharynx, more invasive than other forms of CPAP, variable pressure delivery when infant's mouth is open, and gastric distention. Research has demonstrated that short nasal prongs are more effective in preventing reintubation than nasopharyngeal tubes (De Paoli et al., 2008).
4. Bilevel CPAP: provides continuous positive pressure at two separate CPAP levels. The background or baseline CPAP is set at 4 to 7 cm $H_2O$ with sighs or brief periods of increased pressure set at 2 to 4 cm of $H_2O$ higher than baseline.
   a. Indications: atelectasis, apnea, moderate respiratory distress, and pulmonary edema. May facilitate extubation in very low birth weight infants (Lista et al., 2010).
   b. Advantage: intubation not required. Higher MAPs may stabilize airways and assist in the recruitment of alveoli (Bingham and Fraser, 2012).
   c. Complications: ineffective ventilation, pneumothorax, variable pressure delivery when infant's mouth is open, erosion of the septum from poorly fitting prongs, agitation, dislodging of prongs by an active infant, feeding intolerance, and gastric distention.
5. Nasal intermittent positive pressure ventilation (NIPPV): combines nasal CPAP with ventilator breaths delivered at a set peak pressure are delivered through nasal CPAP prongs or nasal CPAP mask.
   a. Indications: apnea, atelectasis, moderate respiratory distress.
   b. Advantages: Compared to nasal CPAP, NIPPV has been shown to reduce work of breathing and decrease the need for mechanical ventilation in the first 72 hours of life (Chang et al., 2011; Meneses et al., 2012).
   c. Complications: ineffective ventilation, pneumothorax, variable pressure delivery when infant's mouth is open, erosion of the septum from poorly fitting prongs, agitation, dislodging of prongs by an active infant, feeding intolerance, and gastric distention.
6. Mechanical ventilation: respiratory support of infant using mechanical assistance.
   a. Gas-exchange mechanisms in spontaneous and conventional mechanical ventilation.
      (1) Convection (bulk flow) in large airways goes to approximately the eighth bronchial generation. Gas moves along a negative pressure gradient from the upper airways to the alveoli.
      (2) Molecular diffusion occurs in terminal airways and alveoli. This is the exchange of gases in adjacent spaces.
      (3) The status of alveolar ventilation is determined as follows: Alveolar ventilation = respiratory rate × (tidal volume delivered – anatomic dead space volume).
   b. Indications: respiratory failure (hypoxemia, hypercapnia, and/or acidemia), pulmonary insufficiency, need for surfactant administration, severe apnea and bradycardia episodes, cardiovascular support, CNS disease, and surgery.
   c. Advantages: consistent delivery of assisted ventilation and oxygen therapy, decreases the work of breathing, and stabilizes the airway.
   d. Disadvantages: intubation by skilled provider, x-ray examination to confirm placement, possible intermittent x-ray examinations to verify placement or lung status, continuous monitoring of vital signs and oxygen saturation. Exposes the neonate to potential volutrauma/barotrauma of the lung tissue and increases the risk of chronic lung disease.
   e. Complications: tube malposition or dislodgment, underventilation or overventilation, tracheobronchial injury, pulmonary air leaks, infection, intracranial hemorrhage, bronchopulmonary dysplasia (BPD), and retinopathy of prematurity.

## Types of Assisted Ventilation

**A. Positive pressure devices.**

1. Bag-and-mask ventilation. Positive pressure and $O_2$ are delivered via face mask applied with an adequate seal around the mouth and nose. Maximal pressure relief valves should be present to prevent administration of excessive pressure. A manometer should measure pressure delivered to the patient. Device does not require intubation and can be very effective for short-term use, including initial resuscitation.
2. T-Piece resuscitator. Levels of positive pressure and PEEP are preset. Breaths are delivered by occluding the PEEP cap on the T-piece. A gas source is required to operate the T-piece resuscitator. Has the advantage of controlling the amount of pressure applied with each breath, thus eliminating variable pressure delivery inherent in bag-and-mask ventilation. A meta-analysis comparing the T-piece resuscitator to other self-inflating bags found no difference in morbidity or mortality (Hawkes et al., 2012).
3. Pressure-cycled ventilator. Inspiratory phase ends when a preset pressure is reached within the ventilator circuit, regardless of the volume of gas delivered during inspiration.
4. Time-cycled, pressure-limited, continuous-flow ventilator. A predetermined pressure of gas is administered; the duration of inspiration and expiration can be adjusted. Ventilator also allows for the infant's spontaneous respiratory efforts, facilitating a gradual reduction of support. The operator determines the rate, PIP, PEEP, inspiratory time, and flow.
5. Volume-cycled ventilator. Inspiration ends when a preset volume of gas is delivered, regardless of the pressure reached within the ventilator circuit. The pressure used to deliver the breath will vary inversely with the infant's lung compliance and respiratory effort. An increase in ventilation is achieved by increasing $V_T$ or rate; oxygenation is improved by increasing PEEP, $FiO_2$, or $V_T$ (Harris and Fraser, 2012).
6. Pressure support ventilator. PSV supports breaths initiated by the infant by delivering a mechanical breath to a preset volume, and it uses a variable inspiratory time to allow the infant greater control and synchrony with the ventilator. PSV is flow cycled such that, when inspiratory flow decreases by a certain percentage, inspiration ends. PSV ventilators usually have a maximum inspiratory time that is preset. PSV is often used as a weaning mode of ventilation (Keszler, 2012).

## Ventilator Modes

**A. Intermittent mandatory ventilation.** "Breaths" are delivered at a predetermined rate, regardless of where the patient is in the respiratory cycle. The ventilator continues to deliver fresh gas, which allows spontaneous respirations as well. It is possible to stack a ventilator breath on top of a spontaneous breath during either inspiration or expiration. This may lead to air trapping, air leaks, CNS dysfunction, and irregularity of blood pressure and cerebral blood flow.

**B. Patient-triggered ventilation.** Mechanical breaths are delivered in response to a signal derived from the patient and detected as a spontaneous respiratory effort. The signal may be derived from a sensor that detects airflow, airway pressure, chest wall movement, or esophageal pressure (Keszler, 2012). The goal of patient-triggered ventilation is to avoid asynchrony of breathing by the patient and breaths given by the ventilator. Asynchrony may lead to air trapping, air leaks, CNS dysfunction, and irregularity of blood pressure and cerebral blood flow. Patient-triggered ventilation has been shown to improve gas exchange, decrease the need for and duration of ventilation, reduce the incidence of air leaks, and provide ventilation that better matches the infant's own efforts (Brown and DiBlasi, 2011; Keszler, 2012).

1. Synchronized intermittent mandatory ventilation.
   a. Preset number of ventilator breaths is synchronized with the onset of spontaneous breaths. When the infant initiates a breath, the ventilator supports that breath according to the preset PIP and inspiratory time.
   b. Unassisted breaths occur between ventilator breaths, with continuous flow of gas from the ventilatory circuit.
   c. Partial asynchrony may occur if the patient attempts to terminate the inspiratory effort while the ventilator is in the inspiratory phase.

2. Assist/control (A/C) mode of ventilation.
   a. A synchronized breath is delivered each time a spontaneous patient breath meeting the threshold criteria is detected, or mechanical breaths are delivered at a preset regular rate if the patient does not exhibit spontaneous respiratory effort (i.e., if the patient has apnea).
   b. A detection system signals the start of inspiratory effort, which allows for synchronous initiation of inspiration.
   c. Asynchronous expiratory-phase breaths may still occur.
3. PSV.
   a. PSV is pressure limited and flow cycled. The ventilator supports each breath and terminates the breath when the inspiratory flow drops below a preset threshold. This termination mechanism avoids prolonged inspiration and maximizes synchrony (Keszler, 2012).
4. Neurally assisted ventilation (neurally adjusted ventilatory assist [NAVA]).
   a. Relatively new, NAVA uses measured electrical activity in the diaphragm to detect the onset of a breath and trigger the ventilator to support the breath.
   b. Each breath is supported in proportion to the intensity of the infant's inspiratory effort in an attempt to optimize synchrony (Biban et al., 2010).
5. Volume-targeted ventilation.
   a. Volume-targeted ventilation can be used in conjunction with synchronized intermittent mandatory ventilation or A/C modes in patient-triggered ventilation.
   b. A $V_T$ is set by the operator based on the infant's weight and disease condition.
   c. The benefits of volume-targeted ventilation include reduced risk of death or chronic lung disease, reduced risk of air leaks, and a reduced duration of mechanical ventilation when compared to pressure-limited ventilation (Wheeler et al., 2010).

## NURSING CARE OF THE PATIENT REQUIRING RESPIRATORY SUPPORT OR CONVENTIONAL MECHANICAL VENTILATION

A. **Care of $O_2$ delivery devices.**
   1. Oxygen hood. Warm, humidified (to prevent heat loss) $O_2$, delivered via head hood, is usually blended to select the appropriate amount needed. The percentage of $O_2$ in the hood must be monitored by a properly calibrated $O_2$ analyzer placed in the hood near the infant's nose. Ensure a hood of correct size for each infant. To prevent buildup of $CO_2$, do not block openings in the hood and ensure an adequate flow of 5 to 7 L/min. Clean and change per unit protocol.
   2. Nasal cannula. Remove and clean secretions every 4 to 6 hours as needed. Inspect surrounding tissue for pressure-related injury. If sudden onset of respiratory distress occurs, inspect cannula for secretions and suction nasopharynx for mucus. Change cannula according to unit protocol. Some infants receiving oxygen by nasal cannula benefit from the administration of saline drops to moisten the mucosa. These should be administered according to unit protocol. In addition, oxygen/air flow should be warmed and humidified.
   3. Nasal prong CPAP. Ensure that CPAP device is of the correct size to decrease the incidence of pressure necrosis of the nares. Nasal CPAP units come in a variety of sizes and should be short and wide, with thin walls to allow for maximal airflow. They should be soft and flexible and should be easy to secure and maintain. Humidification of 90% to 100% should be provided in the CPAP system to prevent drying out of the mucous membranes and subsequent formation of thick secretions. Evaluate the need for suctioning every 2 to 4 hours. Inspect surrounding tissue for pressure-related injury. Secure the device to a stockinette cap or with soft straps provided by some manufacturers. Lightweight tubing is helpful for ease in securing the device and in keeping the unit in the nose. The infant can be positioned supine, on either side, or prone, generally with the head of the bed at approximately a 30-degree angle. Observe for abdominal distention resulting from excessive air entering the stomach from the CPAP device. Consider aspirating every few hours from an orogastric tube or leaving it open to continuously vent gas from the stomach. Feeding is not contraindicated during delivery of CPAP. The clinical condition must be evaluated before institution of feedings. Change prongs according to unit protocol, generally every 2 or 3 days.

4. ETT. After correct placement has been determined, note the depth of the tube at the gum or lip and post at the bedside. This is important for future reference in case the tube slips, if reintubation is needed, or to determine suction catheter length. Secure the ETT with tape or other method. Each institution generally develops a method that works well for the staff and patients. Observe for evidence of slipping or tape loosening and secure again when necessary to prevent accidental extubation. Position the infant supine, on either side, or in the prone position, with the head in a neutral position. Be aware that the tube moves with the chin and can move several centimeters with flexion or extension of the head. Signs of extubation include sudden deterioration in clinical status, abdominal distention, crying, decreased chest wall movement, breath sounds in the abdomen, agitation, cyanosis, and bradycardia. Notify the physician or neonatal nurse practitioner if extubation is a concern and prepare for reintubation as soon as possible. Intubation equipment should be readily available. A bag and mask with pressure manometer or a T-piece resuscitator should also be available at each bedside and should be tested during each shift. Suction the ETT when necessary. Complications of an ETT include palatal grooves (consider a palate protector, which can be made by a pediatric dentist or is commercially available), nasal erosion, subglottic stenosis, tracheoesophageal perforation during insertion of the tube, aspiration, infection, and tracheal granuloma.
5. Tracheostomy tube. Daily changing of the dressing and weekly changing of the tube are usually adequate. Inspect the site for signs of tissue pressure and/or necrosis. Suctioning is necessary to keep the airway clear of secretions. Family members need to be included in this procedure, thus facilitating discharge.

**B. Suctioning the airway.**

1. Nontracheal tubes.
   - **a.** Suctioning of the mouth, nose, and tubes should be performed on an as-needed basis. The presence of a foreign body in the mouth or nose will cause an increase in secretions.
   - **b.** Suctioning can coincide with the cleaning or changing of the tubes or with routine caregiving.
2. Endotracheal tubes.
   - **a.** The amount of secretions will be disease related. Infants with resolving respiratory distress syndrome, patent ductus arteriosus (PDA), BPD, and pneumonia are more likely to require suctioning because of an increased production of mucus. Patients with early-stage respiratory distress syndrome and those with most types of congenital heart disease will not have much mucus and will require less suctioning. Suctioning is done on an as-needed basis, never on a routine schedule (Gardner et al., 2011). Criteria for suctioning include evidence of secretions (audible or visible), changes in vital signs, agitation or restlessness, and changes in oxygenation or ventilation.
   - **b.** Protocols for suctioning vary from one institution to another. Administering manual breaths with the ventilator before and after suctioning may be necessary to maintain lung volumes during the procedure. Hyperoxygenation prior to suctioning is generally not appropriate.
   - **c.** In-line suction devices allow suctioning while ventilation continues and are associated with a decrease in episodes of hypoxia and smaller changes in heart rate; however, differences in long-term outcomes have not been demonstrated (Taylor et al., 2011).
   - **d.** Do not advance the suction catheter farther than the distance of the ETT, and do not suction too vigorously.
   - **e.** Vacuum pressure range should be 60 to 100 mm Hg (Gardner et al., 2011). A 5 F or 6 F suction catheter for a 2.5- to 3.5-mm ETT, or an 8 F suction catheter for a 4- to 4.5-mm ETT, is usually appropriate.
   - **f.** Complications of suctioning include hypoxemia, bradycardia, barotrauma, changes in blood pressure, alterations in cerebral blood flow, intraventricular hemorrhage, tracheal damage, atelectasis, infection, and pneumothorax.

**C. Initiating mechanical ventilation.** The goal of mechanical ventilation is to assist in providing adequate tissue oxygenation and eliminating $CO_2$.

1. Establish an airway. Endotracheal intubation should be performed by a skilled provider (see Chapter 15).

2. Ventilator selection. The ventilator selected for use is based on the patient's condition and disease process, the patient's response to previous ventilatory support, and staff experience and comfort with the device. Patient-triggered or synchronized ventilation is now the preferred method of mechanically ventilating neonates in most NICUs. There are a number of devices and ventilator modalities that allow the operator to control the PIP or volume delivered to the neonate, as well as the rate, PEEP, flow, and inspiratory time.
3. Parameters to be set and/or monitored during mechanical ventilation.
   a. Rate of intermittent mandatory ventilation. Infants without respiratory failure have a resting respiratory rate of approximately 40/minute, whereas infants with respiratory failure may have a respiratory rate of 0/minute to more than 100/minute. A beginning ventilator rate of 30 to 40/minute for an infant with respiratory failure should be adequate. For infants without respiratory failure, a rate of 20 to 30/minute should be adequate. The ventilator rate will affect the ability to remove $CO_2$. The rate is adjusted to maintain the arterial tension of $CO_2$ in the range of 40 to 50 mm Hg and to avoid excessive respiratory effort, which would exhaust the infant. A rate greater than 40/minute may shorten the expiratory phase of ventilation and cause air trapping.
   b. PIP. PIP is the primary factor used for determining VT and affecting $Pa{O_2}$ (Harris and Fraser, 2012). Determining the appropriate PIP requires careful and skilled assessment. The complications of excessive PIP include air leaks, decreased venous return, intraventricular hemorrhage, and decreased cardiac output. Factors such as weight, gestational age, disease process, lung compliance, and airway resistance must be considered. Auscultation of breath sounds to assess aeration and compliance is necessary. Visual inspection of chest wall movement should guide your assessment. A beginning PIP of 20 cm $H_2O$ is appropriate for most preterm infants. The lowest PIP that will provide adequate ventilation is ideal, with the goals of preventing barotrauma and volutrauma and decreasing the incidence of air leaks and chronic lung disease (Dargaville and Tingay, 2012). Certain conditions may warrant use of high PIP, including poor compliance, atelectasis, or pulmonary hypertension. Before connecting the patient to the ventilator, ensure that the inspiratory pressure is correct. Recheck after the connection has been made, and adjust as necessary.
   c. VT. VT is the primary factor affecting both oxygenation and ventilation. When using volume-targeted ventilation, the operator determines the desired volume to be delivered with each breath rather than setting the PIP. Based on averaging a series of breaths, the ventilator determines the PIP needed to deliver the desired volume of gas. An upper limit for the PIP should be set by the operator to prevent the delivery of excessive pressure.

      An increase in ventilation is achieved by increasing the volume of gas to be delivered (VT) or the rate. Increased oxygenation is achieved by increasing the $Fi{O_2}$, the PEEP, or the VT (Harris and Fraser, 2012). Determination of VT is based on the infant's weight, with a beginning VT of 4 to 5 mL/kg being most common.
   d. PEEP. This measure aids in maintaining FRC, stabilizing and recruiting atelectatic areas for gas exchange, improving compliance, and improving ventilation–perfusion matching in the lung (Gardner et al., 2011). PEEP is important in assisted ventilation for infants with surfactant deficiency because of the likelihood of alveolar collapse. Physiologic PEEP is estimated at 2 cm $H_2O$. Levels lower than 2 cm $H_2O$ are not generally recommended. In most instances, medium levels, about 4 to 7 cm $H_2O$, are recommended. Levels greater than 8 cm $H_2O$ are associated with pulmonary air leaks and reduction of cardiac output.
   e. Inspiratory/expiratory (I/E) ratio: ratio of time spent in inspiration to time spent in expiration. Determining this time should be based on the underlying reason for ventilation. A physiologic I/E ratio in a nondisease state is equal to 1:2 or 1:3, meaning a short inspiratory time with a longer expiratory time. Prolonged expiratory time is useful during weaning, when oxygenation is not as problematic. The I/E ratio will affect the $Pa{O_2}$ and $Pa{CO_2}$. Changes affect MAP and oxygenation.
   f. Flow rate: flow of gas (measured in liters per minute) through the patient's circuit. The flow rate determines the ability of the ventilator to deliver the desired amount of PIP,

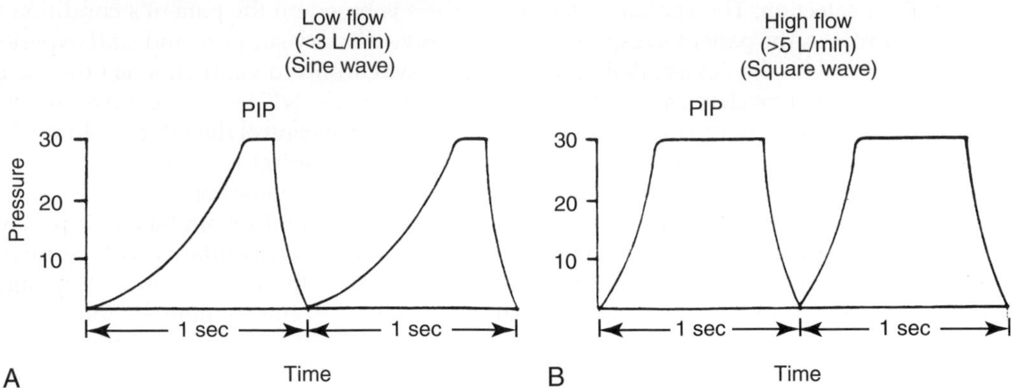


FIGURE 26-3 ■ Comparison of ventilator waveforms. **A,** Relative sine wave. **B,** Relative square wave. (From Goldsmith, J.P. and Karotkin, E.H. [Eds.]: *Assisted ventilation of the neonate* [3rd ed.]. Philadelphia, 1996, W.B. Saunders, p. 169.)

waveform, I/E ratio, and respiratory rate. A flow rate of at least twice the infant's minute ventilation ensures that the ventilator can reach the desired pressure. Flow rates of 4 to 10 L/min are usually adequate (Harris and Fraser, 2012). With low flow rates (<3 L/min), inspiratory pressure gradually builds to a peak just before expiration, closely resembling a sine waveform (normal breaths are shaped like a sine waveform). There may be less barotrauma to the airways with a sine waveform. High flows of 4 to 10 L/min or higher are necessary with square waveform ventilation or when high rates are used. A square waveform pattern moves the ventilator breath rapidly from the resting or expiratory pressure level to the PIP. Because the PIP is reached sooner than with a sine waveform, the PIP is held for a longer period (Fig. 26-3). This may be advantageous with atelectatic areas of the lung. It may also contribute to barotrauma.

**g.** MAP: average distending pressure throughout a complete respiratory cycle. It is the major determinant of oxygenation. MAP is most affected by changes in PEEP, PIP, and I/E ratio. Increases in oxygenation are directly related to increases in MAP, and increased barotrauma to the lungs can result with high MAP. Close attention to the MAP during ventilation is essential, especially once the underlying disease begins to resolve.

**4.** For effects of different ventilator changes, see Box 26-2.

## HIGH-FREQUENCY VENTILATION

High-frequency ventilation (HFV) is any of several forms of mechanical ventilation that use small $V_T$ at rates of at least 150 breaths per minute (Truog and Golombek, 2005) to ventilate patients with severe respiratory failure. The advantage of HFV over conventional mechanical ventilation is the ability to deliver adequate minute volumes using small $V_T$ with lower distal airway pressures.

**A. Gas-exchange mechanisms in HFV.** The $V_T$ used may be less than or equal to anatomic dead-space volume. According to gas-exchange theories for conventional ventilation, alveolar ventilation during HFV should be zero.

**B. Theories of gas exchange during HFV.**

1. Augmented (facilitated) diffusion: Gas molecules diffuse higher in the airways.
2. Coaxial diffusion: Fresh gases travel down the center of the airway, and $CO_2$ elimination occurs along the periphery of the airway (Fig. 26-4).
3. Entrainment: Gas molecules from higher in the airway are pulled into the area of low pressure created behind a high-velocity gas entry point, such as a jet cannula port (Fig. 26-5).
4. Interregional gas mixing ("pendelluft"): Because of the different time constants of the respiratory units, gases in the periphery of the lung may move between alveolar units to provide better matching of ventilation and perfusion.

■ BOX 26-2
■ **SPECIFIC EFFECTS OF DIFFERENT VENTILATOR CHANGES**

**Increasing PIP**
1. Increases $V_T$ and Ve
2. Adds little to MAP unless combined with a reversal of I/E ratio or prolongation of IT
3. Affects maximum dilation of alveoli already open, contributing to barotrauma
4. Opens alveoli with high critical opening pressures

**Reversing I/E Ratio (for Lengthening IT while Respiratory Rate is Kept Constant)**
1. Has little effect on $V_T$ or Ve beyond the minimum IT needed to deliver $V_T$ or reach desired PIP level (or both)
2. Can contribute on more than one-to-one basis to MAP, depending on original PIP and degree of reversal of I/E ratio
3. Allows expansion of atelectatic alveoli at lower PIP
4. May cause inadvertent PEEP, overinflation of alveoli, and reduction of pulmonary blood flow

**Increasing Background CPAP or PEEP**
1. Decreases $V_T$ and Ve unless significant atelectasis is overcome
2. Adds to MAP on a one-to-one basis
3. Holds open alveoli and terminal airways on end-expiration, thus raising closing volume and aiding in equal distribution of ventilation
4. Reduces likelihood of inadvertent PEEP

From Goldsmith, J.P. and Karotkin, E.H. (Eds.): *Assisted ventilation of the neonate* (3rd ed.). Philadelphia, 1996, W.B. Saunders, p. 62.
*CPAP*, Continuous positive airway pressure; *I/E*, inspiratory/expiratory; *IT*, inspiratory time; *MAP*, mean airway pressure; *PEEP*, positive end-expiratory pressure; *PIP*, peak inspiratory pressure; *$V_T$*, tidal volume; *Ve*, expired volume per unit time.

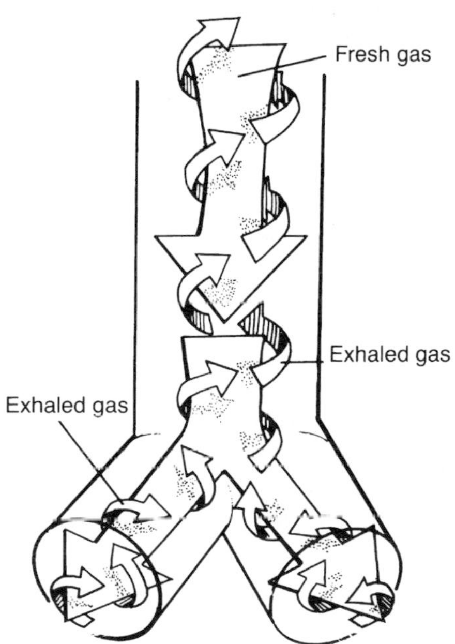

FIGURE 26-4 ■ Coaxial diffusion.

C. **Effectiveness of gas exchange.** All forms of HFV produce gas exchange with lower distal PIPs and small tidal volumes, theoretically reducing the risk of barotrauma and volutrama.
D. **Types of high-frequency ventilators.**
   1. High-frequency jet ventilation (HFJV): Bunnell Life Pulse Jet Ventilator (Bunnell Inc., Salt Lake City, Utah).

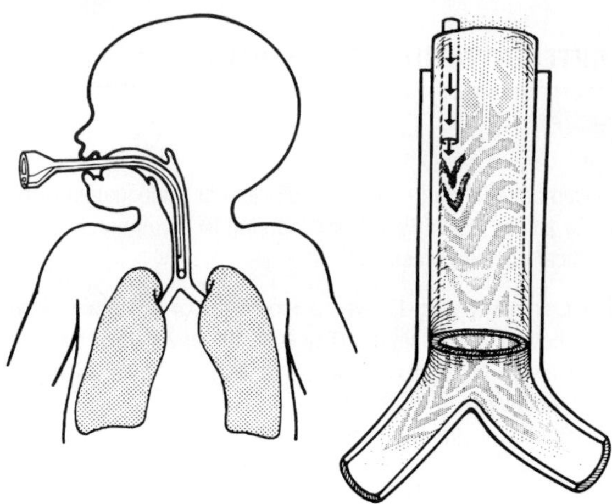

FIGURE 26-5 ■ Entrainment during high-frequency jet ventilation. Gas molecules near the jet orifice are "entrained," or dragged along with the jet pulse, whereby additional volume is delivered to the patient without substantially increasing static airway pressure. (From Harris, T.R.: Physiologic principles. In J.P. Goldsmith and E.H. Karotkin [Eds.]: *Assisted ventilation of the neonate* [2nd ed.]. Philadelphia, 1988, W.B. Saunders.)

**a.** A jet injector delivers short, rapid, high-velocity pulses from a humidified, pressurized gas source directly into the trachea via a special jet ETT adapter ("jet nozzle") that attaches to a standard ETT.

**b.** Servo-controlled driving pressure: continuously adjusts the pressure of the gas supply to the jet nozzle to maintain desired peak airway pressure. Solenoid valve: opens and closes gas supply to the jet nozzle.

**c.** Humidification system: built in-line.

**d.** Proximal airway pressures: monitored and continuously displayed; used in servo-control of pressure delivery.

**e.** Conventional ventilator: used in tandem to provide gas for patient's spontaneous breathing, PEEP, and background ventilation (sighs).

**f.** Exhalation: passive.

**g.** Ventilation ($CO_2$ removal) is primarily determined by the amplitude (PIP – PEEP) or size of the breath.

**h.** Oxygenation is related to MAP, which is generated primarily by the tandem conventional ventilator PEEP but includes all the pressure sources (HFJV PIP, Rate, and I-time) and the rate, PIP, PEEP, and inspiration time (I-time) provided by the conventional ventilator (Fraser, 2012).

**i.** Indications for use: effective with disorders in which $CO_2$ elimination is the major problem. Severe atelectatic disorders such as respiratory distress syndrome may also benefit from HFJV, as do obstructive disorders such as meconium aspiration syndrome and restrictive lung diseases and air leaks (Fraser, 2012).

**j.** Parameters to be set and/or monitored:

(1) PIP: set on both the HFJV and the conventional ventilator.

(a) HFJV PIP is usually initially set at the same PIP required during conventional ventilation, and the conventional ventilator PIP is set based on the lowest PIP needed to achieve lung inflation. There is no fixed relationship between the two PIPs.

(b) A higher conventional PIP may cause interruption of the HFJV breaths.

(2) Servo-controlled pressure: internal adjustment of driving pressure by the ventilator as patient compliance and pressure settings change.

(a) Lower servo-pressure reflects worsening lung disease, airway obstruction, pneumothorax, or kinked ventilator tubing.

(b) Higher servo-pressure indicates improved lung compliance or a leak in the patient/system.

(3) PEEP: set on conventional ventilator; displayed on HFJV ventilator. Value displayed may be lower than value set, because of where and how it is measured. The PEEP provided by the conventional ventilator assists in lung recruitment when atelectasis is a problem.
(4) Jet valve "on" time is the time that the jet valve is open; similar to inspiratory time, usually 0.02 second.
(5) Rate set on jet and conventional ventilators:
  (a) The HFJV rate is usually 240 to 420 breaths per minute; Bunnell default setting of 420/minute is a typical starting rate for this ventilator. Decreasing the HFJV rate lengthens the exhalation time and improves the I:E ratio. Slower HFJV rates are critical for larger patients (>2 kg) and patients with hyperinflation.
  (b) The rate for conventional intermittent mandatory ventilation is usually set between 0 and 5 breaths per minute to provide background ventilation (sigh breaths), which helps to recruit lung volume and to prevent atelectasis.
(6) $FiO_2$: set on HFJV and conventional ventilators.

**k.** Weaning from HFJV is usually accomplished as the acute phase of the illness resolves. Air leaks should be resolved for 1 or 2 days before switching back to Nasal CPAP or conventional mechanical ventilation. Weaning is accomplished by decreasing the PIP and reducing the HFJV rate to 240 to 300 breaths per minute. Support from conventional mechanical ventilation is increased using small $V_T$ breaths if the patient cannot be supported on Nasal CPAP.

**l.** Patient assessment and care.
(1) Patient will require a special jet ETT adapter that is attached to the standard ETT (Fig. 26-6).
(2) Suctioning may be performed with HFJV on or off.
  (a) Placing HFJV ventilator on stand-by mode during suctioning is the preferred method because it eliminates the potential for pressure fluctuations.
  (b) Suctioning with the HFJV ventilator running may help decrease respiratory decompensation during the procedure in some patients.
(3) Humidification of gases is important with HFJV in preventing obstruction of the ETT.
  (a) Main port of ETT is suctioned as usual.
(4) Tubing to the conventional ventilator must never be kinked because overpressurization of the circuit and alveolar rupture may occur if expiratory gas cannot escape.

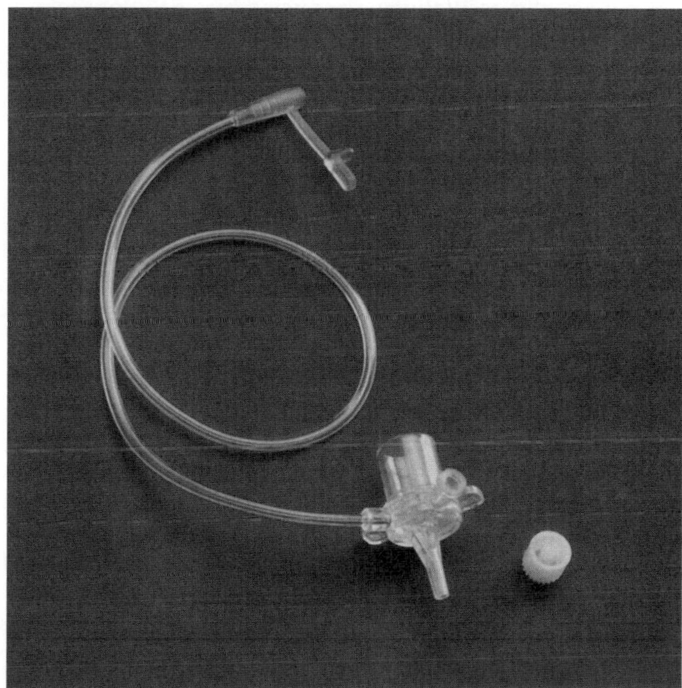

FIGURE 26-6 ■ LifePort endotracheal tube adapter. (Courtesy Bunnell, Inc., Salt Lake City, Utah.)

(5) Vibration of the chest wall is an indicator of lung compliance, airway patency, and effectiveness of ventilator settings.
   (a) Chest wall vibration must be assessed after head position changes to ensure that the jet port of the ETT has not been occluded by the tracheal wall.
   (b) Sudden decrease in chest wall vibration may indicate a plugged ETT or a pneumothorax.

(6) Vibration may interfere with electrical monitoring of heart rate and respiratory rate.
   (a) Use pulse from arterial line or pulse oximeter to monitor heart rate if necessary.
   (b) Spontaneous respiratory rate can be counted and trended if breathing effort is adequate.

(7) HFJV ventilation is efficient at $CO_2$ elimination and at oxygenation.
   (a) MAP is the major determinant of oxygenation.
   (b) Increasing the PEEP to raise MAP improves oxygenation. Conventional ventilator breaths can be used to recruit lung volume, but PEEP must be high enough to maintain lung volume.
   (c) Pressure difference between PIP and PEEP is the major determinant of ventilation.

(8) Patients are generally weaned to a low PIP and adequate MAP before being switched to nasal CPAP. Some patients are switched back to conventional ventilation before extubation if nasal CPAP is not tolerated.

**m.** Complications and problems:
   (1) Airway obstruction, which may be indicated by decreased chest wall vibration, increased $P_{CO_2}$, and decreased servo-pressure.
   (2) Air trapping occurs when HFJV rate is too fast or when too many conventional breaths are used (> 5 bpm) or the conventional breaths are too large or both.

**2.** HFOV. In the United States, the majority of HFOV is provided by the SensorMedics 3100 (Sensor Medics Inc., Yorba Linda, Calif.). In Canada and the United Kingdom, the Dräger Babylog (Dräger Medical, Lübeck, Germany) HFOV is more commonly used.

**a.** Piston, or vibrating diaphragm, moves a small volume of gas toward and then away from the patient.

**b.** The amount of gas moved is referred to as the amplitude.

**c.** Oscillators deliver very little bulk gas. A continuous flow of fresh gas flows past the source that powers the oscillations, producing bias gas flow in a resulting push–pull fashion and thereby eliminating $CO_2$ buildup and delivering $O_2$. A low-pass filter allows gas to exit the system while maintaining vibration of gas in the airway.

**d.** MAP is governed by the rate of gas flow into the circuit and the resistance to flow out of the circuit (Fraser, 2012).

**e.** Amplitude is determined by the driving pressure or stroke volume of the piston or vibrating diaphragm.

**f.** Proximal airway pressure is monitored by the ventilator, but clinical relevance is questionable because it probably does not reflect alveolar pressure.

**g.** HFOV allows for the use of higher MAP with less barotrauma, in comparison with conventional mechanical ventilation and ventilation with small $V_T$.

**h.** Exhalation is active, assisted by the oscillating device.

**i.** Oxygenation is determined by MAP. Ventilation ($CO_2$ removal) is governed by amplitude or MAP.

**j.** Indications for use are as follows:
   (1) Severe lung disease that is unresponsive to conventional ventilation.
   (2) Pulmonary air leaks, pulmonary interstitial emphysema, pneumothorax, and bronchopleural fistula.
   (3) Pulmonary hypoplasia and diaphragmatic hernia: treated with limited success. HFV can be used to stabilize the condition of these patients.
   (4) Persistent pulmonary hypertension and meconium aspiration syndrome: treated with mixed results. The improved $CO_2$ exchange may lead to a respiratory alkalosis that would result in dilation of the pulmonary vascular bed.
   (5) Failure of conventional mechanical ventilation.

k. Parameters to be set or monitored:
   (1) MAP: affects oxygenation.
   (2) Amplitude or stroke volume: size of pressure wave produced by oscillator (another way to describe volume delivered).
   (3) $FiO_2$: set on the ventilator as with conventional ventilation.
   (4) Frequency: 180 to 900 "breaths" per minute (3 to 15 Hz where 1 Hz = 60 breaths).

l. Patient care and assessment:
   (1) No special ETT is required.
   (2) Suctioning procedure is performed as usual. Infants on high-frequency ventilation often benefit from the use of an in-line suctioning device to minimize postsuctioning atelectasis.
   (3) Chest wall vibration is assessed, rather than breath sounds, to determine the effectiveness of ventilator settings and lung compliance changes. Breath sounds are not audible during HFOV.
   (4) Vibration may interfere with electrical monitoring of heart rate and respiratory rate.
      (a) Use pulse from arterial line or pulse oximeter for heart rate monitoring if necessary.
      (b) Respiratory rate cannot be monitored.
      (c) Sighs help reduce microatelectasis and improve oxygenation.
   (5) Complications and problems are:
      (a) Microatelectasis, poor oxygenation.
      (b) Increased incidence of intraventricular hemorrhage in the collaborative trial of HFV using oscillators for treatment of respiratory distress syndrome in preterm infants (HIFI Study Group, 1989; Moriette et al., 2001). Recent studies have failed to demonstrate an increased risk.

m. Studies evaluating the use of HFOV have demonstrated mixed results depending on the volume strategy used. Henderson-Smart and colleagues (2009) completed a Cochrane Review of HFOV for term or near-term infants and found no data to support the routine use of HFOV. A Cochrane Review comparing HFOV to conventional ventilation for preterm infants found that elective HFOV resulted in a reduction in chronic lung disease at term. Results were inconsistent across studies and some short-term neurologic morbidity was found, but this did not reach statistical significance (Cools et al., 2009). Other benefits include decreased need for surfactant replacement (Moriette et al., 2001) and decreased days on oxygen and ventilation (Rimensberger et al., 2000).

## NURSING CARE DURING THERAPY

### A. Physical assessment.

1. Observation. One of the most valuable tools in assessing an infant's respiratory status is observation. Does the infant appear to be comfortable while breathing, or does the infant show signs and symptoms of distress by grunting, flaring, and retracting? The Silverman–Andersen score is a screening tool that uses five signs or symptoms to assess respiratory distress in the newborn infant (Fig. 26-7). Assess the skin color of the infant. It should be uniformly pink. Skin color that is blue, dusky, or pale needs to be evaluated further. A dramatic change in skin color needs to be investigated immediately to rule out a pneumothorax versus a mechanical obstruction. Observe the infant's respiratory rate. Is it within the normal range (40 to 60 breaths per minute)? When observing the respiratory rate, consider variables such as environment, temperature, and the infant's state of activity or inactivity, which can increase or decrease the respiratory rate. Observe whether the chest rises symmetrically; if asymmetrical, suspect a possible pneumothorax, diaphragmatic hernia, or phrenic nerve palsy. With accidental extubation, chest movement may not be observable or may be decreased from previous observations.
2. Auscultation. Listen to the breath sounds carefully to determine differences in the upper and lower lung fields and differences in the left and right lung fields. Is aeration equal bilaterally? Are fine coarse crackles evident? Are other abnormal sounds audible? A finding in a ventilated infant may be louder breath sounds on the right; if so, suspect that the ETT may

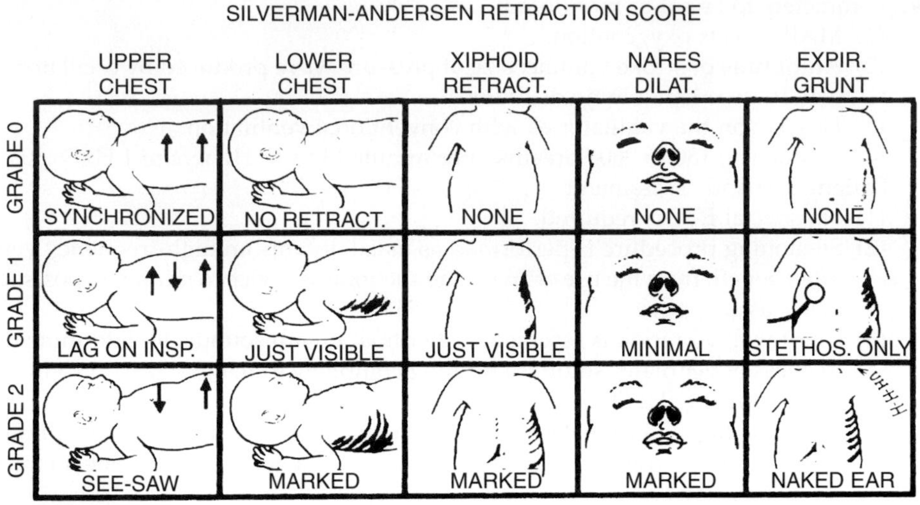

SILVERMAN-ANDERSEN RETRACTION SCORE

| | UPPER CHEST | LOWER CHEST | XIPHOID RETRACT. | NARES DILAT. | EXPIR. GRUNT |
|---|---|---|---|---|---|
| GRADE 0 | SYNCHRONIZED | NO RETRACT. | NONE | NONE | NONE |
| GRADE 1 | LAG ON INSP. | JUST VISIBLE | JUST VISIBLE | MINIMAL | STETHOS. ONLY |
| GRADE 2 | SEE-SAW | MARKED | MARKED | MARKED | NAKED EAR |

FIGURE 26-7 ■ Silverman–Andersen scale to assess respiratory distress in the newborn infant. (Adapted from Silverman, W.A. and Andersen D.H.: A controlled clinical trial of effects of water mist on obstructive respiratory signs, death rate, and necropsy findings among premature infants. *Pediatrics*, 17[1]:1-10, 1956.)

have slipped into the right bronchus or that a pneumothorax may have occurred, necessitating evaluation. Rule out other noises and their points of origin. Bowel sounds heard in the chest are an indication of a diaphragmatic hernia. In the patient receiving HFV, chest wall vibration is an indicator of lung compliance, airway patency, and effectiveness of ventilator settings. Chest wall vibration must be assessed after repositioning. Sudden decrease in chest wall vibration may indicate a plugged ETT or a pneumothorax.

3. ETT observation. Fogging or condensation in the ETT is a sign that the infant is intubated. The condensation occurs on exhalation and is visible in the ETT. Observation of the tube position more than 1 cm from its desired location may indicate extubation or placement in the right mainstem bronchus.
4. Signs of extubation:
   a. Audible crying.
   b. Absent or decreased breath sounds.
   c. Cyanosis.
   d. Bradycardia.
   e. Hypoxemia.
   f. Agitation, restlessness.
   g. Increased abdominal distention.

B. **Equipment function.** All ventilators used for conventional mechanical ventilation should have been approved by the U.S. Food and Drug Administration (FDA) and should display rate (intermittent mandatory ventilation), PIP, PEEP, VT (where applicable), inspiratory time, I/E ratio, MAP, and $O_2$ concentration. Ventilators must be plugged into an electrical outlet that provides emergency power in the event of a power failure.

1. All mechanical ventilators should have:
   a. Alarms activated to alert caregivers to ventilator malfunction or disconnection,
   b. Preset pressure-relief valves to ensure against administration of excessive PIP and PEEP,
   c. Frequently scheduled inspections by licensed respiratory therapists,
   d. Ventilator tubing changed routinely per unit policy,
   e. $O_2$ concentration analyzed routinely and documented in the patient record, and
   f. Routine cleaning between patient use.
2. The following equipment, to be located in the immediate area of all infants requiring mechanical ventilation, should be checked for proper functioning and replaced as needed:
   a. Laryngoscope with blade.
      (1) Size 0 for infants weighing less than 3 kg.
      (2) Size 1 for infants weighing more than 3 kg.

b. Sterile ETTs.
   (1) Size 2.5 for infants weighing less than 1000 g.
   (2) Size 3 for infants weighing 1000 to 2000 g.
   (3) Size 3.5 for infants weighing 2000 to 3000 g.
   (4) Size 3.5 or 4 for infants weighing more than 3000 g.
c. Sterile stylet (plastic coated).
d. Magill forceps (nasal intubation).
e. Suction tubing and catheters (suction control gauge set at 60 to 100 mm Hg).
f. Sterile orogastric tubes.
   (1) Size 5 F or 6 F for infants weighing less than 1 kg.
   (2) Size 8 F for infants weighing more than 1 kg.
g. Anesthesia bag with manometer and mask or T-piece resuscitator, capable of delivering blended $O_2$, and $O_2$ source.
h. Tape, scissors.
i. Carbon dioxide detector.

C. **Noninvasive monitoring.**
1. All infants receiving $O_2$ therapy should be considered as potential candidates for mechanical ventilation and should be monitored with the following:
   a. Heart rate monitor: audible beat-to-beat capability and alarm device for bradycardia (<100 beats per minute [bpm]) or tachycardia (>180 bpm); should provide a visual display of electrocardiogram and actual heart rate.
   b. Respiratory monitor: visual display of respiratory wave pattern and actual respiratory rate; should include alarm device for apnea and tachypnea. Respiratory rate trend mode is preferred.
   c. Blood pressure monitoring: peripheral (cuff) blood pressure or arterial blood pressure monitoring, performed on a scheduled interval, and documented on the permanent record.
   d. $O_2$ analyzer: continuous monitoring of $O_2$ content of the gas delivered to the patient, with mandatory alarm device for $O_2$ concentration greater than or less than the desired range.
   e. Pulse oximetry: continuous monitoring for critically ill infants; intermittent checks with documentation of peripheral $O_2$ saturations indicated for infants not critically ill.
   f. Additional requirements for all infants requiring mechanical ventilation, based on clinical condition:
      (1) Arterial access (usually via umbilical artery catheter) for:
         (a) Blood gas sampling.
         (b) Blood pressure monitoring.
      (2) Transcutaneous $Po_2$ and $Pco_2$ monitoring as indicated by clinical status.
2. Pulse oximetry.
   a. Pulse oximetry is a noninvasive and continuous method of measuring hemoglobin $O_2$ saturation. With the use of red and infrared light, the saturation of hemoglobin bound to $O_2$ is determined and displayed by a digital readout on the monitoring device. The main advantage of pulse oximetry is the short response time in determining $O_2$ saturation in a neonate. It also reduces the number of invasive blood gas measurements necessary for a particular infant. It can be used in various settings outside the NICU (e.g., in neonatal transport, delivery room care, and surgery). The alarm device will alert attendants if $O_2$ saturations are at less or greater than the desired range. **Pulse oximetry does not eliminate the need for blood gas analysis because clinical signs of ventilation and acid–base balance must still be evaluated.**
   b. An accurate reading is dependent on several factors, a primary factor being the perfusion status of the infant. The accuracy of pulse oximetry decreases with low perfusion states. Phototherapy, motion artifact, dyes (ink from footprints), and vasoconstricting drugs (dopamine) can affect saturation readouts. Research has shown that the incidence of severe retinopathy of prematurity in LBW infants can be reduced by lowering the oxygen saturation alarm limits and implementing oxygen targeting guidelines and educational programs (Martinelli et al., 2012).
3. End-tidal $CO_2$ monitoring.
   a. Measures $CO_2$ tension through gas analysis during respiration.

b. Most accurate when infants have normal lung function and a normal $\dot{V}_A/\dot{Q}$ ratio.
c. Markedly less accurate in infants with severe lung disease (large alveolar–arterial gradient) and cannot be relied on for accuracy.
d. May be useful in premature infants with mild to moderate lung disease and in infants with normal lung function.
e. Transcutaneous $CO_2$ monitoring is more accurate in the infant with severe lung disease.

D. **Blood gas measurement.** Blood gas measurement is the standard method for monitoring oxygenation, ventilation, and acid–base balance in the ill neonate. Different methods are available for obtaining the blood sample, with umbilical arterial catheterization being the most common. Other methods for sampling include the use of indwelling peripheral arterial catheters, intermittent arterial puncture, and capillary sampling. Arterial samples are preferred over capillary samples (heel stick) because arterial samples are more reliable in obtaining an accurate $Pao_2$ value. Capillary samples are useful for measuring $Pco_2$ and pH in infants with chronic lung disease. All these methods are invasive, with potential for complications (see Chapter 15).

## MEDICATIONS USED DURING VENTILATION THERAPY

A. **Surfactant:** A deficiency of surfactant in the lungs of premature infants results in impaired gas exchange and increased work of breathing. Administration of exogenous surfactants is routine in preterm infants with evidence of respiratory distress syndrome. Surfactant therapy may also be indicated for more mature infants with meconium aspiration or pulmonary hypertension (American Academy of Pediatrics, Committee on Fetus and Newborn, 2008). Exogenous surfactant may be in a natural form taken from the lungs of pigs or calves (Beractant [Survanta], Bovine Lung Exogenous Surfactant, Curosurf, Infasurf) or synthetic surfactant (Surfaxin). Exogenous surfactant is a liquid preparation administered directly into the endotracheal tube.
   1. Dose: depends on the product used; approximately 4 or 5 mL/kg.
   2. Administration: Ensure that the ETT is in proper position prior to beginning surfactant administration. Follow the manufacturer's recommendations regarding positioning for administration.
   3. Monitor: continuous cardiac, respiratory, and oxygen saturation monitoring during and after administration; frequent vital signs and blood pressure; and ongoing assessment of air entry and chest excursion.
   4. Considerations: infants may become hypoxic, bradycardic, or distressed during surfactant administration. Rapid changes in lung compliance may occur during and immediately following dosing. Changes in lung compliance increase the risk of pulmonary hemorrhage in infants with a PDA.
   5. Endotracheal suctioning is delayed for at least 1 to 2 hours after dosing to avoid removing the drug.
   6. Results: Cochrane Review of natural surfactant use in preterm infants found an improvement in respiratory status, a decreased risk of pneumothorax, a decrease in pulmonary interstitial emphysema, a decreased risk of BPD, and a decreased mortality (Seger and Soll, 2009).

B. **Bronchodilators.**
   1. Methylxanthines: Theophylline and caffeine citrate are used to stimulate respirations in preterm neonates (see Chapter 25). In addition to improving respiratory drive, methylxanthines also increase the contractility of the diaphragm and enhance chemoreceptor sensitivity to carbon dioxide. Theophylline has largely been replaced by caffeine, which has a lower risk of toxicity.
      a. Caffeine: preferred by many clinicians over theophylline because it is given once daily and has fewer adverse effects. Caffeine does not have as great a bronchodilator or diuretic effect as theophylline.
         (1) Dose: loading dose, 10 mg/kg of caffeine base; maintenance 2.5 to 5 mg/kg of caffeine base every 24 hours beginning 24 hours after loading dose (Johnson, 2011).
         (2) Serum drug concentrations are not routinely monitored.
         (3) Adverse effects: usually well tolerated. Tachycardia, jitteriness, and mild glycosuria may occur at higher serum concentrations.

**C. Diuretics.**

1. Furosemide (Lasix): affects chloride transport in the loop of Henle, causes loss of chloride, sodium, potassium, and calcium. Diuresis may decrease pulmonary blood flow, decrease vascular resistance, and increase pulmonary compliance.
   - **a.** Dose: 1 to 2 mg/kg intravenously or by mouth (Roig et al., 2011); a higher oral dose may be required because of reduced bioavailability. Interval: premature infant, every 24 hours; term, every 12 hours; full-term greater than 1 month, every 6 to 8 hours. Long-term therapy: consider a dose every other day.
   - **b.** Monitor: accurate intake and output; specific gravity to evaluate response; frequent electrolyte values to monitor losses and replacement.
   - **c.** Considerations: ototoxic, with transient and permanent hearing losses reported; renal calculi reported with long-term use.
2. Spironolactone (Aldactone): exerts inhibitory effect of aldosterone on the tubules, with resultant increase in sodium losses and sparing of potassium.
   - **a.** Dose: 1 to 2 mg/kg by mouth every 24 hours (Roig et al., 2011).
   - **b.** Monitor: accurate intake and output; specific gravity to evaluate response; electrolyte values after 48 to 72 hours to detect hyperkalemia.
   - **c.** Considerations: may cause rash, vomiting, and diarrhea. Use with caution in infant with impaired renal function.
3. Hydrochlorothiazide with spironolactone (Aldactazide): Thiazides inhibit sodium reabsorption in the distal nephron, resulting in increased excretion of sodium chloride. Spironolactone is an aldosterone antagonist that helps to prevent potassium excretion and hypokalemia.
   - **a.** Dose: 1 to 3 mg/kg/day given as a single daily dose or divided every 12 hours.
   - **b.** Monitor: accurate intake and output when first starting spironolactone, signs of dehydration, serum electrolytes.
   - **c.** Considerations: may cause hyperglycemia or altered glucose tolerance; hypokalemia may result despite the potassium-sparing effect of spironolactone.
4. Chlorothiazide (Diuril) acts on the distal tubule to inhibit chloride reabsorption. It also decreases calcium excretion.
   - **a.** Dose: 10 to 20 mg/kg/day (Roig et al., 2011).
   - **b.** Monitor: accurate intake and output when first starting chlorothiazide, serum electrolytes.

**D. Corticosteroids.**

1. Dexamethasone (Decadron): a long-acting antiinflammatory medication used in the treatment of chronic lung disease and tracheal edema before and after extubation. Studies have documented an increased risk of adverse neurodevelopmental outcomes in infants receiving systemic steroid therapy. These findings have resulted in the following recommendations developed by the American Academy of Pediatrics, Committee on Fetus and Newborn, (2010):
   - **a.** Routine use of corticosteroids for the prevention or treatment of chronic lung disease in LBW infants is not recommended.
   - **b.** Therapy with high-dose dexamethasone is not recommended.
   - **c.** There is not enough evidence to make a recommendation regarding low-dose dexamethasone therapy.
2. Monitor serum and urine glucose, blood pressure, and gastric aspirates for blood. Echocardiogram is indicated if treatment continues longer than 7 days.
3. Considerations: adverse effects hyperglycemia, glycosuria, hypertension, cardiac effects, sodium and water retention, poor weight gain, hypokalemia, hypocalcemia, and increased risk of sepsis.

**E. Paralytic agents.**

1. Pancuronium (Pavulon): pharmacologic relaxation/paralysis of the skeletal muscle to promote improved mechanical ventilation with improved oxygenation/ventilation, decreased barotrauma, decreased fluctuations in cerebral blood flow.
   - **a.** Dose: 0.04 to 0.15 mg/kg IV push. Interval: every 1 to 4 hours as needed for paralysis (Roig et al., 2011).

b. Monitor: vital signs, including blood pressure, continuously.
c. Considerations: mandatory use of mechanical ventilation, adequate pulmonary toilet mandatory because no swallow or gag reflex is present, eye lubricant necessary. Signs of toxicity: tachycardia, hypertension, or hypotension.

2. Vecuronium (Norcuron): similar to pancuronium, but shorter acting. Dose: 0.03 to 0.15 mg/kg IV push every 1 to 2 hours as needed for paralysis. Can be given by infusion at a dose of 0.1 mg/kg/hr (Roig et al., 2011).

F. **Pain control/sedation (see Chapter 16).**

G. **Inhaled nitric oxide (iNO):** Endogenous nitric oxide is released from the endothelium and is responsible for vascular smooth muscle relaxation. iNO is used to promote relaxation of the pulmonary smooth muscle to facilitate perfusion of the lung and gas exchange. iNO has been approved by the FDA for the treatment of near-term and term infants with persistent pulmonary hypertension of the newborn (Gardner et al., 2011). Use of iNO in preterm infants remains experimental.

1. Dose: initial 20 parts per million (ppm); after 4 hours, reduce dose to 6 ppm. iNO is then weaned by 20% in a stepwise fashion to a dose of 1 ppm before discontinuation (Bell, 2012; Kinsella and Abman, 2011).
2. Duration of therapy: usually less than 5 days.
3. Monitor: vital signs, including blood pressure, continuously; complete blood count, methemoglobin levels, and environmental levels of nitric oxide.
4. Considerations: may cause methemoglobinemia, decreased platelet aggregation.
5. Term and late preterm infants—significant reduction in the need for ECMO (Finer and Barrington, 2006). Cochrane Review concluded that enough evidence exists to recommend iNO for this population of infants with hypoxic respiratory failure who do not have diaphragmatic hernia (Finer and Barrington, 2006).
6. Premature infants: A meta-analysis of iNO in preterm infants demonstrated a 7% reduction in the combined risk of death or BPD at 36 weeks for infants treated with iNO, but no reduction in death alone or BPD. The authors concluded that there was insufficient evidence to recommend the use of iNO in preterm infants with respiratory failure (Donohue et al., 2011).

## WEANING FROM CONVENTIONAL VENTILATION

A. **Indications.**

1. Clinical status of infant consistent with beginning resolution of pulmonary condition.
2. Ventilation becomes easier with less support and may result in hypocapnia.
3. Less inspiratory pressure is required to achieve desired $V_T$.

B. **Techniques.**

1. Physical assessment of respiratory status: breath sounds, aeration, chest wall excursion, and spontaneous respiratory rate. Physical assessment of cardiovascular status: color, perfusion, heart rate, pulses, blood pressure, and presence or absence of murmur. Physical assessment of neurologic status: presence of spontaneous respirations, tone, irritability, and reflexes.
2. Radiographic evaluation: useful in documenting improved lung status and absence of pathologic changes.
3. Laboratory analysis: fluid, electrolyte, and hematologic stability.
4. Blood gas analysis: primary information for weaning an infant from conventional mechanical ventilation. If all other assessments indicate improvement, blood gas analysis provides information about the appropriate ventilator settings to adjust. To decrease the $Pao_2$, alter the $Fio_2$ or the MAP: reduce PIP, inspiratory/expiratory time ratio, or PEEP. To increase $Paco_2$, decrease ventilation: decrease rate or $V_T$. During weaning, it is important to try to decrease the most injurious parameters first. Oxygen toxic effects from free $O_2$ radicals damage lung tissue, and $O_2$ is associated with retinopathy of prematurity. Therefore, it is important to keep $O_2$ use at a minimum. PIP, PEEP, I/E time ratio, and rate are all associated with barotrauma, so weaning should be achieved as soon as possible.

C. **Extubation from mechanical ventilation.** When low ventilator parameters have been achieved (intermittent mandatory ventilation, 10 to 20/minute; PIP, 14 to 18 cm $H_2O$; $V_T$ 3.5 to 5 mL/kg; $Fio_2$, 21% to 30%), the infant should be evaluated for extubation. Some infants may need a transition to nasal CPAP, nasal prong, cannula, or $O_2$ hood.

## Nursing Care During Weaning Process

A. **Airway management, equipment function, and monitoring of the infant do not change during the weaning process.**
B. **Frequent assessment of the infant's vital signs, blood pressure, $O_2$ saturation, and neurologic status is essential.** Documentation of this assessment will facilitate appropriate changes in ventilator support.
C. **Be alert for decompensation of respiratory or cardiovascular status during this time, and notify the appropriate personnel when necessary.**
D. **Preparation for extubation.**
   1. Equipment for reintubation available at the bedside.
   2. Suction of ETT and oropharynx.
   3. Postextubation equipment ready for use.
   4. Blood gas determination after extubation.
   5. X-ray examination of chest to rule out atelectasis if decompensation occurs.
   6. Frequent physical assessment every 1 to 2 hours after extubation for 24 hours.
   7. Frequent position changes; suctioning as needed.
   8. Explanation of the plan and process to the family before extubation.

# INTERPRETATION OF BLOOD GAS VALUES

The purpose of obtaining blood gas values is to determine whether the patient has adequate ventilation and perfusion. Blood gas values also facilitate analysis of oxygenation and acid–base status. Oxygenation is determined by the $PaO_2$ value. The $PaO_2$ is the amount of $O_2$ dissolved in the serum—3% of the total $O_2$ content. The remainder of the body's $O_2$ is bound to hemoglobin. Acceptable arterial blood gas values are illustrated in Table 26-1. Capillary $PaO_2$ reliability is uncertain. The value is lower than with an arterial specimen. Acid–base balance is indicated by the pH and the base deficit or excess. Ventilation is measured by $PCO_2$.

A. **Acidosis and alkalosis.** Changes in the pH from the normal range indicate a change in the acid–base status of the infant. An elevated pH, greater than 7.45, is alkalosis, which is caused by excess base or decreased acid level in the blood. A decreased pH, less than 7.35, is acidosis, which is caused by decreased base or increased acid level in the blood.
   1. Respiratory acidosis ($PaCO_2$ >45 mm Hg; pH <7.35), caused by the accumulation of $CO_2$, the respiratory acid, results from hypoventilation.
   2. Respiratory alkalosis ($PaCO_2$ <35 mm Hg; pH >7.45), caused by the decrease of $CO_2$, results from hyperventilation.
   3. Metabolic alkalosis ($HCO_3^-$ >26 mEq/L, base excess > +2, pH >7.45) is caused by a failure to excrete $HCO_3^-$, which is controlled by kidney function.
   4. Metabolic acidosis ($HCO_3^-$ <22 mEq/L, base deficit > −2, pH <7.35) is caused by failure to retain $HCO_3^-$ or by an increase in blood acid, which is controlled by the kidney.
   5. For causes of acidosis and alkalosis, see Table 26-2.
B. **Disorders of acid–base balance (see Chapter 8).**
C. **Interpreting a blood gas value.**
   1. Evaluate the pH. Is there an acidosis or an alkalosis?
   2. Evaluate the $PaCO_2$. If it is not normal, does it contribute to the acid–base status? Or is it a compensating factor?

**TABLE 26-1**
**Normal Arterial Blood Gas Values**

| | |
|---|---|
| pH | 7.35 to 7.45 |
| $PaCO_2$ | 35 to 45 mm Hg |
| $PaO_2$ | 50 to 80 mm Hg |
| $HCO_3^-$ | 22 to 26 mEq/L |
| Base excess | −2 to +2 |

■ TABLE 26-2
■ ■ **Causes of Acidosis and Alkalosis**

| Cause | Mechanism |
|---|---|
| | **Respiratory Acidosis (↑ $Paco_2$, ↓ pH)** |
| CNS depression | Maternal narcotics during labor, asphyxia, intracranial hemorrhage, neuromuscular disorder, CNS dysmaturity (apnea of prematurity) |
| Decreased ventilation–perfusion ratio | Obstructed airway, meconium aspiration, choanal atresia |
| Decreased lung compliance | Respiratory distress syndrome, pulmonary insufficiency, diaphragmatic hernia |
| Injury to the thorax | Phrenic nerve paralysis, pneumothorax |
| | **Metabolic Acidosis (↓ $HCO_3^-$, pH, and Base Deficit [Negative Value])** |
| Decreased tissue perfusion | Increased lactic acid production |
| Sepsis, congestive heart failure | Increased lactic acid production |
| Renal failure | Increased organic acids |
| Renal tubular acidosis | Renal loss of base |
| Diarrhea | Gastrointestinal loss of base |
| | **Respiratory Alkalosis (↓ $Paco_2$, ↑ pH)** |
| Iatrogenic | Excessive mechanical ventilation |
| Hypoxemia | Increase in alveolar ventilation |
| CNS irritation (pain) | Increase in alveolar ventilation |
| | **Metabolic Alkalosis (↑ $HCO_3^-$, pH, and Base Excess [Positive Value])** |
| Gastric suction | Loss of acid |
| Vomiting | Loss of acid |
| Diuretic therapy | Renal losses of $H^+$ ion |
| Iatrogenic | Administration of $HCO_3^-$ (base added) |

*CNS*, Central nervous system.

3. Evaluate the $HCO_3^-$ and the base excess or deficit. If they are not normal, do they contribute to the acid–base status? Or are they compensating factors?
4. Evaluate the $Pao_2$. Is there hypoxia or hyperoxia?
5. From this information, you can attempt to identify the specific cause of the abnormal acid–-base status and treat as indicated.

## REFERENCES


American Academy of Pediatrics, Committee on Fetus and Newborn: Policy statement: Postnatal corticosteroids to prevent or treat bronchopulmonary dysplasia. *Pediatrics*, 126(4):800–808, 2010.

American Academy of Pediatrics, Committee on Fetus and Newborn: Surfactant-replacement therapy for respiratory distress in the preterm and term neonate. *Pediatrics*, 121(2):419–432, 2008.

Bell, S.G.: Neonatal respiratory pharmacology. In D. Fraser (Ed.): *Acute respiratory care of the neonate* (3rd ed.). Santa Rosa, CA, 2012, NICU INK Books, pp. 239–275.

Biban, P., Serra, A., Polese, G., et al.: Neurally adjusted ventilatory assist: A new approach to mechanically ventilated infants. *Journal of Maternal-Fetal & Neonatal Medicine*, 23(Suppl. 3):38–40, 2010.

Bingham, D. and Fraser, D.: Noninvasive ventilation for neonates. In D. Fraser (Ed.): *Acute respiratory care of the neonate* (3rd ed.). Santa Rosa, CA, 2012, NICU INK Books, pp. 159–181.

Blackburn, S.T.: *Maternal, fetal, and neonatal physiology: A clinical perspective:* (4th ed.). Maryland Heights, MO, 2013, Elsevier Saunders.

Brown, M.K. and DiBlasi, R.M.: Mechanical ventilation of the premature neonate. *Respiratory Care*, 56 (9):1298–1311, 2011; discussion: 56(9):1311-1313, 2011.

Chang, H.Y., Claure, N., D'ugard, C., et al.: Effects of synchronization during nasal ventilation in clinically stable preterm infants. *Pediatric Research*, 69(1):84–89, 2011.

Cools, F., Henderson-Smart, D.J., Offringa, M., and Askie, L.M.: Elective high frequency oscillatory ventilation versus conventional ventilation for acute pulmonary dysfunction in preterm infants. *Cochrane Database of Systematic Reviews*, (3): CD000104, 2009.

Dargaville, P.A. and Tingay, D.G.: Lung protective ventilation in extremely preterm infants. *Journal of Paediatrics and Child Health*, 48(9):740–746, 2012.

De Paoli, A.G., Davis, P.G., Faber, B., and Morley, C.J.: Devices and pressure sources for administration of nasal continuous positive airway pressure (NCPAP) in preterm neonates. *Cochrane Database of Systematic Reviews*, (1): CD002977, 2008.

Donohue, P.K., Gilmore, M.M., Cristofalo, E., et al.: Inhaled nitric oxide in preterm infants: A systematic review. *Pediatrics*, 127(2):e414–e422, 2011.

Finer, N.N. and Barrington, K.J.: Nitric oxide for respiratory failure in infants born at or near term. *Cochrane Database of Systematic Reviews*, (4): CD000399, 2006.

Fraser, D.: High-frequency ventilation: The current challenge to neonatal nursing. In D. Fraser (Ed.): *Acute respiratory care of the neonate* (3rd ed.). Santa Rosa, CA, 2012, NICU INK Books, pp. 277–297.

Gardner, S.L., Enzman-Hines, M., and Dickey, L.A.: Respiratory diseases. In S.L. Gardner, B.S. Carter, M. Enzman-Hines, and J.A. Hernandez (Eds.): *Merenstein & Gardner's handbook of neonatal intensive care* (7th ed.). St. Louis, 2011, Elsevier Mosby, pp. 581–677.

Harris, T.R. and Fraser, D.: Principles of mechanical ventilation. In D. Fraser (Ed.): *Acute respiratory care of the neonate* (3rd ed.). Santa Rosa, CA, 2012, NICU INK Books, pp. 137–158.

Hawkes, C.P., Ryan, C.A., and Dempsey, E.M.: Comparison of the T-piece resuscitator with other neonatal manual ventilation devices: A qualitative review. *Resuscitation*, 83(7):797–802, 2012.

Henderson-Smart, D.J., De Paoli, A.G., Clark, R.H., and Bhuta, T.: High frequency oscillatory ventilation versus conventional ventilation for infants with severe pulmonary dysfunction born at or near term. *Cochrane Database of Systematic Reviews*, (3): CD002974, 2009.

HIFI Study Group: High-frequency oscillatory ventilation compared with conventional mechanical ventilation in the treatment of respiratory failure in preterm infants. *New England Journal of Medicine*, 320(2):88–93, 1989.

Johnson, P.J.: Caffeine citrate therapy for apnea of prematurity. *Neonatal Network*, 30(6):408–412, 2011.

Keszler, M.: Synchronized and volume-targeted ventilation. In D. Fraser (Ed.): *Acute respiratory care of the neonate* (3rd ed.). Santa Rosa, CA, 2012, NICU INK Books, pp. 183–194.

Keszler, M. and Abubakar, M.K.: Physiologic principles. In J.P. Goldsmith, and E.H. Karotkin (Eds.): *Assisted ventilation of the neonate* (5th ed.). St. Louis, 2011, Elsevier Saunders, pp. 19–46.

Kinsella, J.P. and Abman, S.H.: Special ventilatory techniques III. In J.P. Goldsmith, and E.H. Karotkin (Eds.): *Assisted ventilation of the neonate* (5th ed.). St. Louis, 2011, Elsevier Saunders, pp. 249–264.

Lista, G., Castoldi, F., Fontana, P., et al.: Nasal continuous positive airway pressure (CPAP) versus bi-level nasal CPAP in preterm babies with respiratory distress syndrome: A randomised control trial. *Archives of Disease in Childhood: Fetal and Neonatal Edition*, 95(2):F85–F89, 2010.

Martinelli, S., Gatelli, I., and Proto, A.: $SpO_2$ and retinopathy of prematurity: State of the art. *Journal of Maternal-Fetal & Neonatal Medicine*, 25(Suppl. 4):108–110, 2012.

Meneses, J., Bhandari, V., and Alves, J.G.: Nasal intermittent positive-pressure ventilation vs nasal continuous positive airway pressure for preterm infants with respiratory distress syndrome: A systematic review and meta-analysis. *Archives of Pediatrics and Adolescent Medicine*, 166(4):372–376, 2012.

Miller, S.M. and Dowd, S.A.: High-flow nasal cannula and extubation success in the premature infant: Comparison of two modalities. *Journal of Perinatology*, 30 (12):805–808, 2010.

Moriette, G., Paris-Llado, J., Walti, H., et al.: Prospective randomized multi-center comparison of high-frequency oscillatory ventilation and conventional ventilation in preterm infants of less than 30 weeks with RDS. *Pediatrics*, 107(2):363–372, 2001.

Mosca, F., Colnaghi, M., Agosti, M., and Fumagalli, M.: High-flow nasal cannula: Transient fashion or new method of non-invasive ventilatory assistance? *Journal of Maternal-Fetal and Neonatal Medicine*, 25 (Suppl. 4):68–69, 2012.

Rimensberger, P., Beghetti, M., Hanquinet, S., et al.: First intention high-frequency oscillation with early lung volume optimization improves pulmonary outcome in VLBW infants with RDS. *Pediatrics*, 105 (6):1202–1208, 2000.

Roig, J.C., Fink, J., and Burchfield, D.J.: Pharmacology adjuncts I. In J.P. Goldsmith, and E.H. Karotkin (Eds.): *Assisted ventilation of the neonate* (5th ed.). St. Louis, 2011, Elsevier Saunders, pp. 347–370.

Seger, N. and Soll, R.: Animal derived surfactant extract for treatment of respiratory distress syndrome. *Cochrane Database of Systematic Reviews*, (2): CD007836, 2009.

Taylor, J.E., Hawley, G., Flenady, V., and Woodgate, P. G.: Tracheal suctioning without disconnection in intubated ventilated neonates. *Cochrane Database of Systematic Reviews*, (12): CD003065, 2011.

Truog, W.E. and Golombek, S.G.: Principles of management of respiratory problems. In M.G. MacDonald, M.D. Mullett, and M.M.K. Seshia (Eds.): *Avery's neonatology: Pathophysiology and management of the newborn* (6th ed.). Philadelphia, 2005, Lippincott Williams & Wilkins, pp. 553–577

Wheeler, K., Klingenberg, C., McCallion, N., et al.: Volume-targeted versus pressure-limited ventilation in the neonate. *Cochrane Database of Systematic Reviews*, (11): CD003666, 2010.

Wiswell, T.E. and Courtney, S.E.: Noninvasive respiratory support. In J.P. Goldsmith, and E.H. Karotkin (Eds.): *Assisted ventilation of the neonate* (5th ed.). St. Louis, 2011, Elsevier Saunders, pp. 140–162.

CHAPTER

# 27 Extracorporeal Membrane Oxygenation

LEIGH ANN CATES

**OBJECTIVES**

1. Examine briefly common neonatal ECMO pathophysiology.
2. Discuss indications and contraindications for neonatal ECMO.
3. Discuss the criteria used to determine an infant's need for neonatal ECMO.
4. Examine common perfusion techniques in neonatal ECMO.
5. Review the technical and mechanical aspects of the neonatal ECMO procedure.
6. Review the physiology of neonatal extracorporeal circulation.
7. Discuss the general care given to infants undergoing the ECMO procedure and the support provided to their families.
8. Review follow-up and outcome of neonatal ECMO survivors.

## ECMO: A HISTORICAL PERSPECTIVE

Extracorporeal life support (ECMO) was developed initially by surgeon John Gibbon as a heart–lung bypass machine for use in adult open heart surgeries. Currently, neonatal ECMO has been in use for over three decades, and has transitioned from a rarely utilized lifesaving modality to a routine practice in major children's centers across the nation. Employed initially to manage newborn respiratory failure in 1975 (Bartlett, 2010), neonatal ECMO presently aids in the management of multiple pathologies from cardiac anomalies to overwhelming sepsis. In fact, the Extracorporeal Life Support Organization (ELSO), founded in 1989, has created a national registry for ECMO cases; ELSO reported in 2010 that 20,000 of the over 40,000 ECMO cases were newborns (Bartlett, 2010). With this increase in use and understanding, survival rates have improved and there has been an ushering in of new neonatal ECMO technology, including membrane lungs, safe centrifugal pumps, and vascular access.

A. **ELSO International Registry Report** (*Neonatal ECMO Registry Report*, **2008**).
    1. A total of 92 ECMO centers reported. Survival by diagnosis was as follows: meconium aspiration syndrome (MAS), 94%; persistent pulmonary hypertension of the newborn (PPHN)/persistent fetal circulation, 78%; respiratory distress syndrome/hyaline membrane disease, 84%; pneumonia, 59%; sepsis, 75%; air leak syndrome, 74%; congenital diaphragmatic hernia (CDH), 51%; and other diagnoses, 63%.
    2. After a peak of ECMO cases during the years 1989 to 1995 (927 to 1181 cases per year), the number of ECMO cases for neonates has decreased (472 to 571 cases per year) for the years 2003 to 2008, while the survival rate has declined to 63% to 68%. This decline in both cases and survival reflects a change in the kinds of neonates who require ECMO support, having failed the more sophisticated ventilator management, surfactant, and use of inhaled nitric oxide that is currently standard practice (Ford, 2006).

B. **New technology** (**2008**).
    1. Roller pumps began to be replaced by safer centrifugal pumps (Bartlett, 2010).
    2. A new generation of membrane lungs developed.
    3. Increased capabilities of vascular access.

## COMMON NEONATAL ECMO PATHOPHYSIOLOGY

When discussing neonatal ECMO, the practitioner must keep in mind a strong understanding of fetal circulation, including the three primary shunts: the ductus venosus, patent ductus arteriosus (PDA), and patent foramen ovale (PFO). Additionally, the practitioner should also have a firm understanding of the most common disease processes associated with the utilization of neonatal ECMO, including but not limited to the management of the underlying pulmonary hypertension, related to sepsis, MAS, pneumonia, CDH, or idiopathic PPHN (Shelley and Rees, 2010). Pulmonary hypertension in the newborn period is characterized by elevated pulmonary vascular resistance forcing deoxygenated blood to shunt right to left through a PDA or PFO. Subsequently, there is mixing of oxygenated and deoxygenated blood in the aorta followed by systemic hypoxia and acidosis resulting in a persistent state of increased pulmonary vascular resistance (Short, 2010). Pulmonary vascular resistance can be decreased primarily through an increase in arterial oxygenation ($Pao_2$), use of nitric oxide, and a correction in acidosis. Additionally, the patient may require correction of polycythemia, hypocalcemia, and systemic hypotension, as well as the need for gentle ventilation and sedation. Once these methods have been employed and failed, the patient may require being placed on ECMO (Short, 2010).

## CRITERIA FOR USE OF ECMO

The goal is to properly identify patients who would benefit from ECMO while simultaneously limiting those patient populations in which the potential risks outweigh the benefits. Thus, inclusion criteria were developed to aid centers in ECMO candidate selection. These criteria are guidelines and are not mandates (Shelley and Rees, 2010).

A. **Neonatal ECMO patient criteria.**
   1. Gestational age greater than 34 weeks.
   2. Birth weight greater than 2000 g; small-for-gestational-age infants should not be excluded.
   3. Reversible lung disease.
   4. No significant coagulopathy or uncontrolled bleeding—should be corrected prior to initiating ECMO, if possible.
   5. Intracranial hemorrhage grade 2 or less.
   6. Failure of optimal medical management.
   7. No lethal anomalies or brain injuries.
   8. No major cardiac malformations (except in infants requiring stabilization and life support before or after surgery).
   9. Must have decision to provide "full support" (Shelley and Rees, 2010).

B. **Acute and reversible pathology.**
   1. Respiratory distress syndrome.
   2. MAS.
   3. PPHN.
   4. CDH.
   5. Sepsis.
   6. Pneumonia.
   7. Life support before or after cardiac surgery.
   8. Acute respiratory distress syndrome.

C. **Cranial and cardiac ultrasonography findings** ruling out severe intracranial hemorrhage and cyanotic congenital heart disease.

D. **Objective criteria for final selection predictive of greater than 80% mortality rate (Box 27-1).** To achieve specificity, each ECMO center must determine its own mortality indicators and criteria. Criteria may differ in different disease states, such as septic shock, CDH, or severe air leak caused by barotrauma.

E. **Pre-ECMO stabilization, including optimal ventilatory management and trial of high-frequency ventilation, volume support, vasopressors, vasodilator medications, surfactant, and nitric oxide if indicated.** These should be used at a center where ECMO can be initiated quickly if the infant does not respond adequately (Shelley and Rees, 2010).

**BOX 27-1**
**NEONATAL ECMO PATIENT QUALIFYING CRITERIA**

**Alveolar–Arterial Difference in Partial Pressure of Oxygen ($AaDo_2$):**
600 to 624 mm Hg for 4 to 12 hours at sea level

$$AaDo_2 = \frac{\text{Atmospheric pressure} - 47 - (Paco_2 + Pao_2)}{Fio_2}$$

Note: 47 is the partial pressure of water vapor.

**Oxygenation Index (OI):**
25 to 60 for 30 minutes to 6 hours

$$OI = \frac{MAP \times Fio_2 \times 100}{Pao_2}$$

where MAP is mean airway pressure.

**$Pao_2$:**
35 to 50 mm Hg for 2 to 12 hours

**Acute Deterioration**
$Pao_2 \leq 30$ to 40 mm Hg
pH $\leq 7.25$ for 2 hours
Intractable hypotension

From Rosenberg, E. and Seguin, J.: Selection criteria for use of ECLS in neonates. In J. Zwischenberger and R.H. Bartlett (Eds.): *ECMO: Extracorporeal cardiopulmonary support in critical care*. Ann Arbor, Mich., 1995, Extracorporeal Life Support Organization.

## ECMO PERFUSION TECHNIQUES

Prior to placing a patient on ECMO, a multidisciplinary team must decide what modality of perfusion delivery will be best for the patient and the patient's particular disease process. The two most common approaches are venoarterial (VA) and venovenous (VV). VA support, the most widely used ECMO modality in the United States, is a technique whereby the cannulas are inserted to permit drainage of deoxygenated blood from a large vein or veins (Heard et al., 2010a). Subsequently, the blood is circulated through an artificial lung for oxygenation, and returned to the body through a major artery such as the aorta. Conversely, VV ECMO, which is gaining ground in the neonatal population, utilizes only the venous system for both drainage and return of blood to the patient.

### Venoarterial Perfusion

**A. Technique for VA perfusion.**
1. Deoxygenated blood is drained from the right side of the heart through a cannula placed in the right atrium via the right internal jugular vein.
2. Venous cannula must be a size that is capable of delivering total cardiac output (120 to 150 mL/kg/min) to the membrane lung; cannulas of largest possible internal diameter (8 F to 14 F) are inserted.
3. Oxygenated blood is returned through a cannula placed into the ascending aorta via the right common carotid artery.
4. Achieves approximately 60% to 80% of normal cardiac output (Heard et al., 2010a).

**B. Advantages.**
1. Technique provides both respiratory and cardiac support by decompressing pulmonary circulation, decreases pulmonary artery and pulmonary capillary filtration pressure, and supports circulation by augmenting the pumping action of the heart.

2. Positive pressure ventilation can be reduced to minimal parameters: peak inspiratory pressure, 15 to 25 cm $H_2O$; positive end-expiratory pressure, 5 to 10 cm $H_2O$; respiratory rate, 10 to 20/minute; and fractional concentration of oxygen in inspired gas ($FiO_2$), 21% to 30%.

C. **Disadvantages.**
1. Emboli (air or particulate) could be infused directly into the arterial circulation.
2. Ligation of carotid artery may be permanent and subsequently affect cerebral perfusion.
3. Greater potential for left ventricular "cardiac stun" (Fukuda et al., 1999).

## Venovenous Perfusion

A. **Technique for VV perfusion.**
1. Double-lumen cannula is used (size 12 F, 14 F, or 15 F). Deoxygenated blood is drained from the venous limb, positioned in the right atrium.
2. Blood is returned through the arterial limb, also located in the right atrium, with side holes positioned at the tricuspid valve.
3. Blood flow is directed across the valve, into the right ventricle, and through the pulmonary circulation. It returns to the left atrium before entering the systemic circulation via the aorta.

B. **Advantages (Heard et al., 2010b).**
1. No ligation of the carotid artery is necessary.
2. Oxygenated blood flows through pulmonary circulation, which may help reverse pulmonary hypertension.
3. Oxygenated blood is provided to the coronary arteries.
4. Emboli (air or particulate) are less likely to result in severe compromise to the infant because blood is not returned directly to the arterial circulation.
5. May eliminate potential for left ventricular cardiac stun.

C. **Disadvantages.**
1. VV perfusion can be used only with adequate cardiac function because systemic flow is dependent on cardiac output. In the event of cardiac stun, or decreased function, emergent conversion to VA ECMO may be needed.
2. Recirculation of oxygenated blood can occur. Oxygenated blood returned to the right atrium may be emptied again into the venous side of the double-lumen cannula, rather than across the tricuspid valve.
3. Use of somewhat higher ventilatory support may be required because lower flow rates are achieved with the smaller lumens of the double-lumen cannula.
4. Vasopressor therapy may need to be continued to support blood pressure and ECMO flow.
5. Greater potential for right ventricular cardiac stun.

# CIRCUIT COMPONENTS AND ADDITIONAL DEVICES

Neonatal care and equipment are constantly being modified and improved, and neonatal ECMO equipment is not different. Rather than use the circuits utilized for short runs of cardiac bypass, novel biocompatible circuits and improved centrifugal pumps controlled by highly advanced computerized servo-regulated systems are emerging. Additionally, vascular access cannulas are being improved to provide reliable care and enhance outcomes (Harris et al., 2010).

A. **ECMO circuit (Fig. 27-1)**
1. The ECMO circuit consists of polyvinyl chloride tubing, Luer-Lock connectors, stopcocks, and infusion sites.
2. Some manufacturers have developed surface bonding materials for circuit tubing and cannulas, in an effort to minimize the activation of complement, platelets, and inflammatory mediators, and these are thought to be less thrombogenic (Harris et al., 2010).
3. Blood circulates throughout all components of the ECMO circuit; parenteral fluids, medications, and blood products are administered into the venous side of the circuit (before the membrane oxygenator).

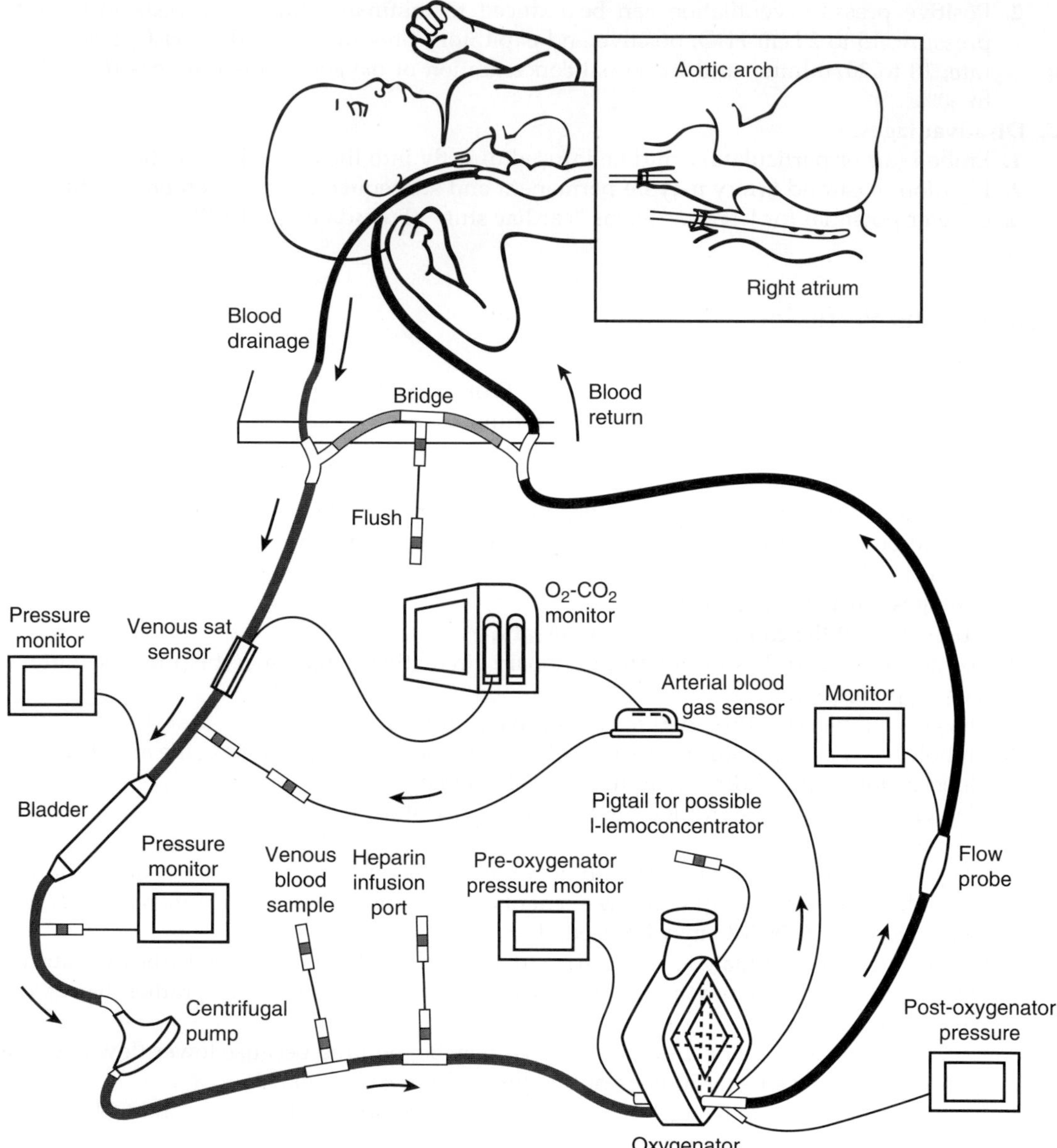


FIGURE 27-1 ■ Configuration of neonatal centrifugal ECMO circuit. (Adapted with permission from Short, B., and Williams, L. (Eds.): *ECMO specialist training manual* (3rd ed.). Ann Arbor, Mich., 2010, Extracorporeal Life Support Organization.)

4. Only platelets are infused on the arterial side of the circuit, or into the patient directly, to prevent adherence to the membrane oxygenator.
5. Precautions and guidelines for placing medications and blood products into the circuit are the same as those for safely administering medications and blood products directly to patients.

**B. Pumps.**

1. Roller/occlusive: uses the principle of fluid displacement utilizing two rollers placed opposite of one another to pull blood from the right atrium and push blood forward through the circuits tubing (Harris et al., 2010).
   a. Servo-regulation of venous return: bladder reservoir, pressure monitoring with roller pump.
   b. Collapsible silicone bladder distends with returning venous blood.

c. If using a roller head pump, inadequate flow (decreased venous return) into the ECMO circuit causes the bladder to collapse, which triggers a microswitch and an audible alarm and stops the roller head pump.
d. When the bladder reexpands, the microswitch engages the pump and normal pump operation continues.
e. Adequate venous return is critical for maintaining cardiorespiratory support; therefore, the cause of decreased return must be recognized and corrected immediately.
f. Servo-mechanism regulation of ECMO flow can also be achieved by transducers placed in the circuits. Premembrane (venous) pressure and postmembrane (arterial) pressure may be monitored continuously to signal extracorporeal flow problems before collapse of the silicone bladder. This allows for early detection and timely intervention.
   (1) Fall in premembrane pressure indicates decreased venous return.
   (2) Rise in postmembrane pressure indicates malfunction of membrane oxygenator or heat exchanger.
g. Other devices have been recently introduced to regulate venous flow, including a thin-walled section of tubing encased in rigid housing that is mounted vertically in the circuit, and does not have the clotting issues associated with the conventional silicone bladder (Hansell, 2005).
h. Advantages.
   (1) Can be operated manually in case of power failure.
   (2) Lower cost.
   (3) Less initial volume of blood needed to prime circuit.
   (4) Flow not dependent on patient's afterload status.
   (5) Used for more than 20 years and can equate to greater experience and comfort level of ECMO providers.
i. Disadvantages.
   (1) The discharge of plastic particles into the patient's circulatory system resulting in embolization.
   (2) Requires use of servo-regulated bladder box or pressure servo-regulator.
   (3) Total pressure delivered by the rollers to the circuit is critical in delivery calculations.
   (4) Limited availability of circuits due to transition of many ECMO centers to the centrifugal pump.

2. Centrifugal/constrained vortex/nonocclusive pump: works on the principle of a constrained vortex in which an object spins in a fluid environment. The spinning results in an area of low pressure at the nucleus of the vortex, and an area of high pressure results at the periphery. The centrifugal pump contains a plastic housing composed of a single inlet located in the center low-pressure region and outlet positioned along the high-pressure outer border (Harris et al., 2010).
   a. Advantages.
      (1) Flow manipulated by the device's revolutions per minute (RPMs [the rate at which the pump spins]).
      (2) If the patient's volume fluctuates, the RPMs remain steady, resulting in less negative (volume decrease) or positive pressure (volume increase) on the atrium.
      (3) Can be operated by hand or short-term battery backup.
   b. Disadvantages.
      (1) Inaccuracy of flow measurements at low RPMs.

C. **Gas-exchange devices.**
   1. Silicone membrane oxygenator—made of a solid silicone polymer membrane envelope with a plastic space screen that is wrapped spirally around a spool; encased in a silicone rubber sleeve.
      a. Maximizes gas exchange across the membrane.
      b. Only oxygenator currently approved by the U.S. Food and Drug Administration for long-term use.
      c. No direct blood-to-gas interface.
   2. Polypropylene (microporous) hollow-fiber oxygenator—contains small tubes with tiny pores through which gas exchange takes place (Harris et al., 2010).

a. Potential advantage during priming; can have bioactive coating.
b. Direct blood-to-gas interface.
c. Designed for short-term use (~2 hours).
d. Good for rapid response scenarios.

3. Polymethylpentene (PMP) hollow-fiber oxygenator—contains microporous tubes with tiny pores through which gas exchange takes place (Harris et al., 2010).
   a. Potential advantage during priming; can have bioactive coating.
   b. Direct blood-to-gas interface.
   c. Can be used for up to 6 hours.
   d. Good for rapid response scenarios.

D. **Heat exchanger.**
1. Located after the oxygenator, or incorporated into the oxygenator.
2. Can add or subtract heat from the blood before returning it to the infant's circulation.
3. Heat loss occurs from cooling effect of ventilating gases inside the oxygenator and circuit exposure to ambient air temperature.
4. Important for maintenance of homeostasis of clotting functions and physiologic functions.

E. **ECMO console.**
1. Monitors circuit pressure on both the venous and arterial sides of the circuit.
2. Provides bubble detection.
3. Thorough automated alarm system, including servo-regulation of the pump when aberrant conditions are discovered.

F. **Bubble detector.**
1. Placed beyond heat exchanger to detect air in blood flowing through arterial side of pump as the blood is returned to the patient.
2. In some systems, when air is detected, the roller head pump is shut off and flow to the patient ceases.
3. Critical importance in VA ECMO.

G. **Activated clotting time (ACT) monitoring.**
1. Because heparin is used to prevent clotting, ACT is the most common bedside method to measure anticoagulation in the ECMO patient (Harris et al., 2010).
2. Use to titrate heparin infusion based on ECMO center's desired ACT ranges and required effects.
3. Initial bolus of heparin during cannulation (usually 100 units/kg).
4. Infusion pump for continuous infusion of heparin solution at 25 to 100 units/kg/hr into ECMO circuit.
5. Titration of heparin solution to keep ACT within the desired range (usually 180 to 220 seconds, but acceptable at 160 to 250 seconds).
6. For control of heparin administration, no heparin added to any other medications or fluids (an exception may be the fluids being infused into umbilical or peripheral arterial lines).
7. Factors that influence heparin requirements: thrombocytopenia, abnormal clotting studies, urinary output, and infusions of blood products that contain clotting factors.

H. **Blood gas monitoring.**
1. Mixed venous oxygen saturation ($SvO_2$), monitored continuously, is the optimal parameter to assess tissue oxygen delivery. It can be measured through fiberoptic catheters or by using optical reflectance technology. Correlation with co-oximeter values measured by a blood gas machine is required.
2. Arterial blood gas measurements obtained beyond the membrane oxygenator in the ECMO circuit reflect the function of the membrane lung.
3. Patient blood gas values and noninvasive oxygen saturation monitoring are used to assess the recovery of lung function and the infant's acid–base balance.

I. **Cannulas.**
1. Cannulas are surgically placed in large blood vessels to remove deoxygenated venous blood and return oxygenated blood to the circulation.
2. Before insertion of the cannulas, the infant is paralyzed and given opiates to prevent respiratory movement and air embolism, and systemic heparin is given to prevent clotting of the

cannulas and the circuit; this is because when circulating blood comes into contact with artificial surfaces, coagulation is activated (Annich and Miskulin, 2005).
3. In VA ECMO, the venous cannula tip is positioned in the right atrium to drain blood flow from the inferior vena cava and the superior vena cava. The arterial cannula tip reaches just to the aortic arch.
4. In VV ECMO, the double-lumen cannula is commonly placed in the internal jugular vein, and is positioned in the right atrium, with the arterial side directed toward the tricuspid valve.
5. Double-lumen cannulas are now available that could potentially avoid cannulation of two vessels in order to avoid the carotid artery (Harris et al., 2010).

## PHYSIOLOGY OF EXTRACORPOREAL CIRCULATION

The primary goal behind ECMO is to sufficiently supply the body with oxygen so that metabolic requirements are met while removing the body of subsequent waste by-products (Rees and Waldvogle, 2010). The body naturally exchanges gases at the alveolar and tissue levels. Oxygenation of the blood is achieved during ECMO through the use of a membrane oxygenator. The arterial partial pressure of oxygen ($Pa{O_2}$) and carbon dioxide ($CO_2$) are the primary forces in diffusion of gases across the membrane. $CO_2$ exchange is independent of blood flow, and dependent on gas diffusion gradient, sweep gas flow rate, and membrane surface area. Conversely, $Pa{O_2}$ is independent of sweep gas flow rate, yet dependent on blood flow rate, blood path thickness, membrane diffusion thickness, $Pa{O_2}$ concentrations, and membrane surface area. ECMO improves $Pa{O_2}$ delivery by improving $Pa{O_2}$ content through stabilization of the saturation of hemoglobin, taking 60% of the cardiac output away from native lung, and providing a stable source of delivery via the membrane oxygenator (Rees and Waldvogle, 2010).

A. **Blood flow.**
   1. VA bypass is instituted by draining venous blood into the ECMO circuit; a like amount of oxygenated blood is returned to the arterial circulation.
   2. As bypass flow increases, flow through the pulmonary artery decreases faster than bypass flow and reduces total flow in the systemic circulation, causing peripheral and pulmonary hypotension.
   3. Blood volume replacement is required for optimal tissue perfusion.
   4. ECMO perfusion is nonpulsatile (pulse contour decreases as flow rate increases); kidneys interpret this as inadequate flow and promote the release of renin and aldosterone, which causes sodium retention, extracellular fluid expansion, and a decreased total body potassium concentration.
   5. Total patient flow is the sum of ECMO flow and pulmonary blood flow; adequate flow is reached when oxygen delivery and tissue perfusion result in normoxia, normal pH, normal $Sv{O_2}$, and normal organ function.
   6. Total gas exchange and support are achieved at a flow rate of 120 to 150 mL/kg/min.

B. **Gas exchange.**
   1. Oxygen diffuses into the blood because of a pressure gradient between the elevated oxygen pressure in the gas compartment and the low oxygen pressure in the venous blood.
   2. Carbon dioxide diffuses from the blood compartment to the gas compartment as a result of a pressure gradient between venous carbon dioxide pressure and the ventilating gas. The carbon dioxide transfer rate is 6 times greater than that of oxygen transfer. The ventilating gas mixture is usually enriched with carbon dioxide to prevent hypocapnia.

C. **Blood–surface interface.**
   1. During ECMO, up to 80% of the cardiac output is exposed to a large artificial surface each minute.
   2. Clot formation is prevented by systemic heparinization; platelet destruction is minimized by preexposure of the circuit to albumin.
   3. Platelets show the greatest effect of exposure to a foreign surface, as evidenced by decreased platelet count (thrombocytopenia) and function.
   4. Hemolysis is monitored regularly by measuring plasma free hemoglobin levels. The level is usually not significantly altered by ECMO flow, although increases may indicate problems with red blood cell destruction in the membrane oxygenator or small-lumen cannula.

5. All types of white blood cells decrease in concentration, and phagocytic activity is significantly decreased.
6. After cessation of ECMO, platelets and white blood cell counts return to normal.

## CARE OF THE INFANT REQUIRING ECMO

The neonate requiring ECMO requires a collection of highly trained personnel each with unique skills and training. The team composition minimally consists of the pediatric surgical team, neonatologist specializing in the management of ECMO, and an ECMO specialist (physician [MD], registered nurse [RN], registered respiratory therapist [RRT], or perfusionist) to operate and manage the circuit, as well as the bedside nurse (Williams and Short, 2010). The following is an outline of the responsibilities of the ECMO specialist and the bedside nurse in the care of the infant during ECMO (Nugent and Matranga, 1997; Rais-Bahrami and Powell, 2010; Remenapp et al., 2005; Sheehan, 1999).

**A. Cannulation.**

1. Cannulation requires the initiation of systemic anesthesia and analgesia; the operating room staff is in attendance.
2. See Table 27-1 for nursing responsibilities and interventions.
3. ECMO specialist responsibilities:
   a. Maintain and monitor ECMO circuit.
   b. Assess physiologic stability.
   c. Maintain physiologic parameters such as blood gas values, blood pressure, platelet count, $Svo_2$ and arterial oxygen saturation ($Sao_2$), and ACT.
   d. Assist nurse in the general care of the infant.
   e. Be prepared for circuit emergencies.

■ TABLE 27-1
■ ■ **Nursing Responsibilities and Interventions for ECMO**

| Responsibility | Intervention |
|---|---|
| **BEFORE CANNULATION** | |
| Obtain and document baseline physiologic data. | Record weight, length, and head circumference.<br>Draw blood samples for CBC, electrolytes, calcium, glucose, BUN, creatinine, PT/PTT, platelet count and function, ABGs, ACT.<br>Record vital signs: heart rate; respiratory rate; systolic, diastolic, and mean blood pressure; and temperature. |
| Ensure adequate supply of blood products for replacement. | Draw, type, and cross-match samples for 2 units of packed red blood cells and fresh frozen plasma.<br>Keep 1 unit of packed cells and fresh frozen plasma always available in the blood bank and a separate set at the bedside. |
| Diagnostic exams. | Pre-ECMO CXR.<br>Pre-ECMO HUS.<br>Pre-ECMO ECHO. |
| Maintain prescribed pulmonary support. | Maintain ventilator parameters.<br>Administer muscle relaxants if indicated. |
| Assemble and prepare equipment. | Prepare infusion pumps to maintain arterial lines and infusion of parenteral fluids and medications into the ECMO circuit.<br>Place the infant on a radiant warmer with the head positioned at the foot of the bed to provide thermoregulation and access for cannulation.<br>Attach infant to physiologic monitoring devices to monitor heart rate, intra-arterial blood pressure, transcutaneous oxygen, and other parameters. |
| Circuit priming meds and fluids. | To be added to circuit for priming: 2 units PRBCs; Plasmalyte A, 1000 mL; albumin 25%, 50 mL; heparin, 200 units; sodium bicarbonate, 20 mEq; calcium gluconate, 200 mg. |

■ TABLE 27-1
■ ■ **Nursing Responsibilities and Interventions for ECMO—cont'd**

| Responsibility | Intervention |
|---|---|
| Labs drawn from prime. | ABGs, whole blood sodium, whole blood potassium, whole blood ionized calcium, whole blood glucose, hemoglobin, and hematocrit. |
| | Insert urinary catheter and NG tube; place to gravity drainage. |
| | Remove IV lines just prior to heparinization (optional). |
| | Prepare loading dose of heparin (50 to 100 units/kg). |
| | Prepare heparin solution for continuous infusion (100 units in 30-mL syringe to be infused into circuit at 25 units/kg/hr). |
| | Prepare and infuse pain medication: morphine sulfate 0.03 mg/kg/hr or fentanyl 1 mcg/kg/hr. |
| | Prepare paralyzing drug (pancuronium bromide, 0.1 mg/kg, or succinylcholine, 1 to 4 mg/kg). |
| | Assist in insertion of arterial line (umbilical or peripheral). |
| | Administer prophylactic antibiotics. |
| Additional meds/fluids to have on hand. | $D_{10}W$, 250-mL bag; $D_5W$, 250-mL bag; NS, 250-mL bag. |
| | Optional to be administered by surgeon—cryoprecipitate, 10 mL; calcium chloride 10%, 5 mL; bovine thrombin, 5000 units/5 mL. |
| Be prepared to administer cardiopulmonary support. | Have medications and blood products available to correct hypovolemia, bradycardia, acidosis, and cardiac arrest. |
| **DURING CANNULATION** | |
| Monitor cardiopulmonary status during procedure. | Monitor heart rate and intra-arterial blood pressure continuously. |
| | Obtain blood gas values after paralysis and during cannulation, as indicated by the infant's response to the procedure. |
| Administer medications. | Give loading dose of heparin systemically when vessels are dissected free and are ready to be cannulated. |
| | Give paralyzing drug systemically just before cannulation of internal jugular vein if infant has not been previously paralyzed. Give analgesia for anesthetic effect. |
| Reduce ventilator parameters to minimal settings. | Once adequate bypass is achieved, reduce PIP to 16 to 20 cm $H_2O$, PEEP to 4 cm $H_2O$, ventilator rate to 10 to 20 breaths per minute, and $Fio_2$ to 21% to 30%. Patients undergoing VV bypass may require greater respiratory support. |
| **DURING ECMO RUN** | |
| Monitor and document physiologic parameters. | Record hourly and PRN: heart rate, blood pressure (systolic, diastolic, mean), respirations, temperature, oxygen saturation, ECMO flow. |
| | Measure hourly accurate intake and output of all body fluids (urine, gastric contents, blood); test all stools for occult blood. |
| | Assess hourly: color, breath sounds, heart tones, murmurs, cardiac rhythm, arterial pressure waveform, peripheral perfusion. |
| | Assess hourly: level of consciousness, reflexes, tone, and movement of extremities. |
| | Assess every 8 to 12 hours: neurologic examination, including fontanelle tension, pupil size, and reaction. |
| | Assess weight and head circumference daily. |
| | Circuit check per ECMO perfusion flow sheet. |
| Routine labs. | All other blood specimens are drawn from ECMO circuit by ECMO specialist: hourly ABGs until stable; ACT every 2 hours, platelets every 6 hours, aPTT every 6 hours × 48 hours, then daily. |
| | Daily: plasma-free hemoglobin, heparin assay, fibrinogen, D-dimer; electrolytes, calcium, platelets, Chemstrip, creatinine, total and direct bilirubin. |
| | Record ventilator parameters hourly. |
| Administer medications. | Remove air bubbles and double-check dosages before infusion. |
| | Place all medications and fluids (except heparin drip) into the venous side of the ECMO circuit or |

*Continued*

■ TABLE 27-1
■ ■ **Nursing Responsibilities and Interventions for ECMO—cont'd**

| Responsibility | Intervention |
|---|---|
| | central venous line.<br>Prepare and administer the arterial line (umbilical or peripheral) infusion.<br>NPO, OG to gravity, and administer parenteral alimentation. |
| Provide pulmonary support. | Perform gentle endotracheal suctioning according to individual assessment and need.<br>Maintain patent airway; be alert to extubation or plugging.<br>Obtain daily chest films, head ultrasounds, and tracheal aspirate cultures as indicated.<br>Maintain ventilator parameters. |
| Heparin (bleeding) precautions. | ***Avoid*** all of the following: rectal probes, injections, venipunctures, heel sticks, NG tubes (oral only), nasal suctioning, administration of medications intramuscularly or by venipuncture.<br>Avoid invasive procedures. Do not change OG tube, urinary catheters, or endotracheal tube unless absolutely necessary; use gentle premeasured endotracheal tube suction technique.<br>Observe for blood in urine, stools, and endotracheal OG tubes. |
| Maintain excellent infection control. | Change all fluids and tubing daily.<br>Change dressings daily and as needed.<br>Maintain closed system for urinary catheter drainage.<br>Maintain strict aseptic and handwashing techniques.<br>Use universal barrier precautions. |
| Provide physical care. | Keep skin dry, clean, and free of pressure points.<br>Monitor blood loss from cannula site.<br>Give mouth care as needed.<br>Provide ROM every 8 hours or as indicated.<br>Turn side to side every 1 to 2 hours.<br>Nonnutritive sucking every 4 hours. |
| Provide pain management, sedation, stress reduction. | Minimize noise level.<br>Cluster patient care to maximize sleep period.<br>Administer analgesia: fentanyl or morphine as continuous IV drip.<br>Manage iatrogenic physical dependency by following dose reduction regimen. |
| Be alert to complications and emergencies. | See text.<br>Social services consult. |
| **AFTER ECMO RUN** | |
| | Head CT and MRI prior to discharge. |

Adapted from Nugent, J. and Matranga, G.: Extracorporeal membrane oxygenation. In D.F. Askin (Ed.): *Acute respiratory care of the newborn* (2nd ed.). Petaluma, Calif., 1997, NICU Ink, pp. 341-368.

*ABGs*, Arterial blood gases; *ACT*, activated clotting time; *aPTT*, activated partial thromboplastin time; *BUN*, blood urea nitrogen; *CBC*, complete blood cell count; *CT*, computed tomography; *CXR*, chest x-ray; $D_5W$, 5% dextrose in water; $D_{10}W$, 10% dextrose in water; *ECHO*, echocardiogram; $FiO_2$, fractional concentration of oxygen in inspired gas; *HUS*, hemolytic–uremic syndrome; *IV*, intravenous; *MRI*, magnetic resonance imaging; *NPO*, nothing by mouth; *NG*, nasogastric; *NS*, normal saline; *OG*, orogastric; *PEEP*, positive end-expiratory pressure; *PIP*, peak inspiratory pressure; *PRBCs*, packed red blood cells; *PRN*, as needed; *PT/PTT*, prothrombin time/partial thromboplastin time; *ROM*, range of motion; *VV*, venovenous.

**B. During ECMO "run."**

1. Bypass is gradually instituted until approximately 80% (120 to 150 mL/kg/min) of cardiac output is diverted through the ECMO circuit.
2. At maximal flow, blood gas values should normalize and $SvO_2$ is maintained at greater than 70%.
3. $SvO_2$ is an excellent indicator of adequate flow during VA ECMO because it is a measure of tissue perfusion and efficiency of extracorporeal circulation in meeting metabolic demands.
4. Oxygenation during VV ECMO is assessed by infant's arterial blood gas values and continuous oxygen saturation monitoring via pulse oximetry. $SvO_2$ is not an accurate reflection of deoxygenated blood because of recirculation; $SvO_2$ is used as a trending parameter during VV ECMO.

5. Ventilator settings are reduced to a minimum; vasopressor therapy and chemical paralysis are usually discontinued; enteral feedings are generally withheld because of concern about hypoxic injury to the gastrointestinal tract; and blood loss is quantified and replaced.
6. Emergencies during ECMO (DeBerry et al., 2005; Heard et al., 2010b):
   a. Circuit emergencies.
      (1) Air embolism.
      (2) Tubing rupture.
      (3) Oxygenator malfunction.
      (4) Accidental decannulation.
      (5) Power failure.
      (6) Gas source failure.
      (7) Equipment malfunction.
   b. Responsibilities of the nurse during a circuit emergency (Williams and Short, 2010):
      (1) Notification of physician.
      (2) Ventilation.
      (3) Anticoagulation.
      (4) Chemical resuscitation.
      (5) Blood loss replacement.
   c. Responsibilities of the ECMO specialist during a circuit emergency (Williams and Short, 2010):
      (1) Clamp catheters.
      (2) Open bridge.
      (3) Remove gas source.
      (4) Repair circuit.

**C. ECMO patient complications (DeBerry et al., 2005).**

1. Electrolyte/glucose/fluid imbalance: Sodium requirements decrease; potassium requirements increase because of the action of aldosterone. Calcium replacement may be needed if citrate–phosphate–dextrose anticoagulated blood is used. Hyperglycemia may necessitate a decrease in the glucose concentration of IV fluids.
2. CNS deterioration: cerebral edema, intracranial hemorrhage, and seizures. Deterioration results from initial hypoxia, acidosis, hypercapnia, or vessel ligation.
3. Generalized edema: The extracellular space is enlarged by the distribution of crystalloid solution and the action of aldosterone and antidiuretic hormone. The use of diuretics or hemofiltration may be necessary if edema causes brain or lung dysfunction.
4. Renal failure: Acute tubular necrosis results from pre-ECMO hypotension and hypoxia. Indicators of renal failure are abnormal blood urea nitrogen and creatinine values. Low-dose dopamine therapy and/or hemodialysis may be necessary.
5. Hemorrhage due to thrombocytopenia, coagulopathy.
6. Decreased venous return and/or hypovolemia due to inadequate circulating blood volume, pneumothorax, and/or partial venous catheter occlusion or malposition.
7. Hypertension due to overinfusion of blood products, renal ischemia, and excretion of renin–angiotensin.
8. PDA: Left-to-right shunting may cause increased blood flow to the lung, necessitating high pump flows without the expected increase in $Pa_{O_2}$. Ligation may be necessary.
9. Cardiac stun: Transient loss of ventricular contractility (1 to 3 days) is manifested by hypotension, decrease in aortic pulse pressure, poor peripheral perfusion, and decreased $Pa_{O_2}$. It is possibly due to mismatch between afterload and ventricular contractility during ECMO.
10. Mechanical complications: These include incorrect catheter placement or accidental displacement, oxygenator failure, power failure, air entrainment, and accidental decannulation.

**D. Weaning/decannulation.**

1. Signs of improvement and indicators that the infant is ready to be weaned are as follows:
   a. Improvement of lung fields on chest x-ray examination.
   b. Clinical findings: improved breath sounds, rising $Pa_{O_2}$ on fixed ECMO flow, improvement in lung compliance.

2. Once improvement has been ascertained, flow rate is decreased slowly in 10- to 20-mL increments until ECMO support is no longer needed to maintain adequate gas exchange at low ventilator settings (Bartlett, 2005). Ventilator settings are usually increased during weaning from the settings used during ECMO.
3. When flow rate is 50 to 100 mL/kg/min, a state of "idling" is achieved, the infant remains at this lowest possible flow rate for 4 to 8 hours.
4. If improvement in lung function remains stable, cannulas are clamped, heparin is infused directly into the infant, and the circuit is recirculated via a bridge. If blood gas values deteriorate, the cannulas are unclamped and ECMO support is resumed.
5. In VV ECMO, the cannulas are not clamped during the "trial off" procedure; gas flow to the membrane oxygenator is discontinued. Low flow rates are maintained, and patient response is assessed by measurement of blood gases.
6. Decannulation proceeds if blood gas values remain satisfactory.
7. Before decannulation, the infant undergoes chemical paralysis and ventilator parameters are increased to compensate for loss of spontaneous respiratory function.
8. After adequate anesthesia and analgesia has been administered, the cannulas are removed. Both the internal jugular vein and the carotid artery are ligated. In some ECMO centers, carotid reconstruction is attempted (Cheung et al., 1997; Levy et al., 1995). The efficacy of this procedure is debatable because of clot formation at the site of reconstruction.
9. After decannulation, the infant is weaned as tolerated from the ventilator and routine NICU care is resumed.

## POST-ECMO CARE

A. **Lung recovery is achieved through weaning of the infant from assisted ventilation.** Occasionally the use of steroids and/or diuretics is necessary to improve recovery.

B. **Assessment of neurologic recovery involves clinical evaluation and computed tomography scan.** It may be difficult to assess neurologic status during opiate use or while the infant is recovering from significant illness, so assessment may be deferred until the infant is ready for discharge.

C. **Weaning from opiate analgesics and sedatives involves a gradual reduction of doses and careful monitoring for withdrawal symptoms.** Infants receiving ECMO therapy require opiate infusions or scheduled dosing of opiates and sedatives throughout their course of ECMO to prevent excessive movement, which can dislodge the cannulas (Arnold et al., 1990; Caron and Maguire, 1990; Franck and Vilardi, 1995).

D. **Establishing oral feedings may be difficult.** Prolonged respiratory compromise, the effect of opiates on state control, alterations in swallowing caused by neck dissection during cannula placement, and gastroesophageal reflux, particularly in infants with CDH, are some of the causes of feeding problems in the post-ECMO infant. Feeding difficulties are generally more common in infants with CDH than in those with other diagnoses such as MAS or PPHN.

## PARENTAL SUPPORT

A. **The ECMO candidate's parents are in crisis.** They are aware that ECMO is a method of last resort with no guarantee of positive result, and the technology is overwhelming.

B. **Parents need concise, accurate, understandable information about their child's condition and the required procedures.**

C. **Parent-to-parent support, using parents of "ECMO graduates," is efficacious and a positive experience.**

D. **Parents should have access to their infant.** ECMO candidates have an increasingly positive outcome, and every effort should be made to encourage involvement and bonding.

## FOLLOW-UP AND OUTCOME

For some neonatal ECMO patients, their postcannulation status mirrors that of an infant with moderate to severe hypoxic–ischemic encephalopathy, thus appearing, hypotonic, lethargic, and hyporeflexive (Glass, 2010). Additionally these infant may require weaning from narcotics or sedative medications. The following is a discussion of the follow-up and outcome of neonates previously requiring ECMO (Bernbaum et al., 1995; Boggs and LaPrade-Wolf, 1992; Boykin et al., 2003; Glass, 2010; Glass and Brown, 2005; Glass et al., 1989, 1995; Hofkosh et al., 1991; Kanto, 1994).

A. **Critical scrutiny of survivors is essential to assess the value and safety of ECMO.** Survivors should be evaluated at 4 to 6 months, and then yearly until school age. The following are assessed:
   1. Growth and development.
   2. Cardiorespiratory development.
   3. Cerebrovascular status.
   4. Neurologic and psychological functioning.

B. **Medical morbidity includes poor somatic growth, feeding problems, chronic lung disease, and rehospitalizations.** Predictors include diagnosis of CDH, lower birth weight, and age at initiation of ECMO.

C. **Rate of bilateral hearing loss requiring amplification is approximately 5%.** By 5 years of age, the majority of ECMO-treated neonates are functioning in normal range for IQ, although lower than control children who were not ill in the neonatal period (Glass et al., 1995). Risk for developmental disability is similar to pre-ECMO mortality risk, irrespective of whether they receive cardiopulmonary resuscitation, the degree of prematurity, and presence of neuroimaging abnormality (Glass and Brown, 2005).

D. **School-age ECMO survivors are twice as likely as other children to have neuropsychological deficits and are at risk of having academic problems.** Predictors include lower birth weight, abnormal findings on neurologic imaging, chronic lung disease, and failure to thrive. However, even children who do not have these risk factors can have neuropsychological testing to predict the need for special education services.

E. Psychological morbidity, including behavioral problems, is also reported and may be due to altered parenting styles and family stress. Early trauma from severe illness may set the stage for problems in parent–child interactions, highlighting the need for early parental support and involvement.

## REFERENCES


Annich, G. and Miskulin, J.: Coagulation, anticoagulation, and the interaction of blood and artificial surfaces. In K. Van Meurs, K.P. Lally, G. Peek, and J.B. Zwischenberger (Eds.): *ECMO: Extracorporeal cardiopulmonary support in critical care* (3rd ed.). Ann Arbor, MI, 2005, Extracorporeal Life Support Organization, pp. 29–58.

Arnold, J., Truog, R., Orav, E.J., et al.: Tolerance and dependence in neonates sedated with fentanyl during extracorporeal membrane oxygenation. *Anesthesiology*, 73(6):1136–1140, 1990.

Bartlett, R.: The history of extracorporeal life support. In B. Short, and L. Williams (Eds.): *ECMO specialist training manual* (3rd ed.). Ann Arbor, MI, 2010, Extracorporeal Life Support Organization, pp. 1–6.

Bartlett, R.: Physiology of ECLS. In K. Van Meurs, K. Lally, G. Peek, and J. Zwischenberger (Eds.): *ECMO: Extracorporeal cardiopulmonary support in critical care* (3rd ed.). Ann Arbor, MI, 2005, Extracorporeal Life Support Organization, pp. 5–27.

Bernbaum, J., Schwartz, I.P., Gerdes, M., et al.: Survivors of extracorporeal membrane oxygenation at 1 year of age: The relationship of primary diagnosis with health and neurodevelopmental sequelae. *Pediatrics*, 96(5 Pt. 1):907–913, 1995.

Boggs, K. and LaPrade-Wolf, P.: Beyond survival: Strategies for establishing a follow-up program for infants with extracorporeal membrane oxygenation. *Neonatal Network*, 11(1):7–13, 1992.

Boykin, A., Quivers, E., Wagenhoffer, K., et al.: Cardiopulmonary outcome of neonatal extracorporeal membrane oxygenation at ages 10-15 years. *Critical Care Medicine*, 31(9):2380–2384, 2003.

Caron, E. and Maguire, D.: Current management of pain, sedation and narcotic physical dependency of the infant on ECMO. *Journal of Perinatal & Neonatal Nursing*, 4(10):63–74, 1990.

Cheung, P.Y., Vickar, D.B., Hallgren, R.A., et al.: Carotid artery reconstruction in neonates receiving extracorporeal membrane oxygenation: A 4-year follow-up study. Western Canadian ECMO Follow up Group. *Journal of Pediatric Surgery*, 32 (4):560–564, 1997.

DeBerry, B., Lynch, J., Chung, D. and Zwischenberger, J.: Emergencies during ECLS and their management. In K. Van Meurs, K.P. Lally, G. Peek, and J.B. Zwischenberger (Eds.): *ECMO: Extracorporeal cardiopulmonary support in critical care* (3rd ed.). Ann Arbor, MI, 2005, Extracorporeal Life Support Organization, pp. 133–156.

Ford, J.: Neonatal ECMO: Current controversies and trends. *Neonatal Network*, 25(4):229–238, 2006.

Franck, L. and Vilardi, J.: Assessment and management of opioid withdrawal in ill neonates. *Neonatal Network*, 14(2):39–48, 1995.

Fukuda, S., Aoyama, M., Yamada, Y., et al.: Comparison of venoarterial versus venovenous access in cerebral circulation of newborns undergoing extracorporeal membrane oxygenation. *Pediatric Surgery International*, 15:78–84, 1999.

Glass, P.: Outcome after neonatal ECMO. In B. Short, and L. Williams (Eds.): *ECMO specialist training manual* (3rd ed.). Ann Arbor, MI, 2010, Extracorporeal Life Support Organization, pp. 239–244.

Glass, P. and Brown, J.: Outcome and follow-up of neonates treated with ECMO. In K. Van Meurs, K.P. Lally, G. Peek, and J.B. Zwischenberger (Eds.): *ECMO: Extracorporeal cardiopulmonary support in critical care* (3rd ed.). Ann Arbor, MI, 2005, Extracorporeal Life Support Organization, pp. 319–328.

Glass, P., Miller, M. and Short, B.: Morbidity for survivors of extracorporeal membrane oxygenation: Neurodevelopmental outcome at 1 year of age. *Pediatrics*, 83(1):72–78, 1989.

Glass, P., Wagner, A., Papero, P., et al.: Neurodevelopmental status at age five years of neonates treated with extracorporeal membrane oxygenation. *Journal of Pediatrics*, 127(3):447–457, 1995.

Hansell, D.: ECLS equipment and devices. In K. Van Meurs, K.P. Lally, G. Peek, and J.B. Zwischenberger (Eds.): *ECMO: Extracorporeal cardiopulmonary support in critical care* (3rd ed.). Ann Arbor, MI, 2005, Extracorporeal Life Support Organization, pp. 107–119.

Harris, W., Darling, E. and Lawson, S.: ECMO equipment and devices. In B. Short, and L. Williams (Eds.): *ECMO specialist training manual* (3rd ed.). Ann Arbor, MI, 2010, Extracorporeal Life Support Organization, pp. 77–98.

Heard, M., Davis, J. and Fortenberry, J.: Principles and practice of venovenous and venoarterial extracorporeal membrane oxygenation. In B. Short and L. Williams (Eds.): *ECMO specialist training manual* (3rd ed.). Ann Arbor, MI, 2010a, Extracorporeal Life Support Organization, pp. 59–76.

Heard, M., Lynch, J. and Zwischenberger, J.: ECMO mechanical complications. In B. Short and L. Williams (Eds.): *ECMO specialist training manual* (3rd ed.). Ann Arbor, MI, 2010b, Extracorporeal Life Support Organization, pp. 99–112.

Hofkosh, D., Thompson, A., Nozza, R., et al.: Ten years of extracorporeal membrane oxygenation: Neurodevelopmental outcome. *Pediatrics*, 87(4):549–555, 1991.

Kanto, W.P.: A decade of experience with neonatal extracorporeal membrane oxygenation. *Journal of Pediatrics*, 124(3):335–347, 1994.

Levy, M.S., Share, J.C., Fauza, D.O., et al.: Fate of the reconstructed carotid artery after extracorporeal membrane oxygenation. *Journal of Pediatric Surgery*, 30(7):1046–1049, 1995.

*Neonatal ECMO Registry Report*, Ann Arbor, MI, 2008, Extracorporeal Life Support Organization.

Nugent, J. and Matranga, G.: Extracorporeal membrane oxygenation. In D.F. Askin (Ed.): *Acute respiratory care of the newborn* (2nd ed.). Petaluma, CA, 1997, NICU Ink, pp. 341–368.

Rais-Bahrami, K. and Powell, D.: Extracorporeal membrane oxygenation cannulation and decannulation. In B. Short, and L. Williams (Eds.): *ECMO specialist training manual* (3rd ed.). Ann Arbor, MI, 2010, Extracorporeal Life Support Organization, pp. 49–58.

Rees, N. and Waldvogel, J.: Extracorporeal life support (ECLS) physiology. In B. Short, and L. Williams (Eds.): *ECMO specialist training manual* (3rd ed.). Ann Arbor, MI, 2010, Extracorporeal Life Support Organization, pp. 37–48.

Remenapp, R., WinklerPrins, A. and Mossberg, I.: Nursing care of the patient on ECMO. In K. Van Meurs, K.P. Lally, G. Peek, and J.B. Zwischenberger (Eds.): *ECMO: Extracorporeal cardiopulmonary support in critical care* (3rd ed.). Ann Arbor, MI, 2005, Extracorporeal Life Support Organization, pp. 595–607.

Sheehan, A.: Bedside nursing care and ECMO specialist responsibilities. In K. Van Meurs (Ed.): *ECMO specialist training manual* (2nd ed.). Ann Arbor, MI, 1999, Extracorporeal Life Support Organization, pp. 199–206.

Shelley, C. and Rees, N.: Management of the neonate on ECMO. In B. Short, and L. Williams (Eds.): *ECMO specialist training manual* (3rd ed.). Ann Arbor, MI, 2010, Extracorporeal Life Support Organization, pp. 119–134.

Short, B.: Neonatal pulmonary physiology and pathophysiology. In B. Short, and L. Williams (Eds.): *ECMO specialist training manual* (3rd ed.). Ann Arbor, MI, 2010, Extracorporeal Life Support Organization, pp. 7–16.

Williams, L. and Short, B.: Responsibilities of the ECMO specialists and RN staff. In B. Short, and L. Williams (Eds.): *ECMO specialist training manual* (3rd ed.). Ann Arbor, MI, 2010, Extracorporeal Life Support Organization, pp. 219–226.

CHAPTER

# 28 Cardiovascular Disorders

SHARYL L. SADOWSKI

**OBJECTIVES**

1. Describe how to differentiate between cyanosis that is cardiac in origin and that which is pulmonary in origin.
2. Discuss implementation of a universal pulse oximetry screening protocol.
3. Name the major classifications of congenital heart disease; list two anomalies in each.
4. Discuss the link between congenital heart disease and genetics, including use of available tests.
5. Define and describe the anatomy, clinical manifestations, and the possible medical and/or surgical treatment of tetralogy of Fallot (TOF), coarctation of the aorta, patent ductus arteriosus (PDA), ventricular septal defect (VSD), atrial septal defect (ASD), and hypoplastic left heart syndrome (HLHS).
6. Describe the basic medical rationale for care of the newborn infant with a suspected or identified cardiac defect.
7. Describe the basic surgical rationale for treatment of major cardiovascular defects.
8. List signs and symptoms of congenital heart abnormalities in the newborn infant.
9. Discuss available diagnostic modalities and the congenital cardiac defects they are used to diagnose.
10. List the signs and symptoms of PDA and the current medical, transcatheter, and surgical interventions.
11. Discuss the treatment modalities used in congestive heart failure, including the risks and benefits to the neonate.
12. Define the three classifications of shock, and list one cause under each category.
13. Discuss the major complications and sequelae of open heart surgery and list two factors that contribute to the sequelae.

Until the 20th century, there was limited clinical interest in congenital heart disease. In the majority of cases, the cardiac anomaly was incompatible with life; in the others, no treatment existed either to remedy the condition or to relieve its symptoms. Today, with advances in prenatal and early postnatal diagnosis and treatment of congenital heart defects (CHDs), the survival and quality of life of infants with congenital heart disease have markedly improved. Yet, anywhere from 20% to 30% of neonates with critical heart defects are not diagnosed prior to discharge from the hospital following birth (Mahle et al., 2009). A delay in diagnosis leads to increased morbidity and mortality (Altman, 2013). Due to the prevalence of missed diagnosis before discharge, the U.S. Department of Health and Human Services made a recommendation for universal pulse oximetry screening prior to discharge from the hospital. The American Academy of Pediatrics Section on Cardiology and Cardiac Surgery endorsed the recommendation in 2012.

Advances in fetal echocardiography have resulted in a significant increase in the prenatal diagnosis of many CHDs, allowing for extensive parental counseling, thus providing time for parents to make decisions about treatment options prior to birth (Dorfman et al., 2008; Kaplan et al., 2005) and delivery at a tertiary hospital (Donofrio et al., 2013). Telemedicine has also made a big impact on CHD, allowing for accurate diagnosis at remote hospitals, thus quicker implementation of care (Grant et al., 2010). In addition, advancements in angiography, interventional catheterization, and the advent of three-dimensional (3-D) echocardiography (Friedberg et al., 2010), coupled with a more complete understanding of newborn physiology, have led to improvements in diagnostic and treatment capabilities with decreased risk. In addition, newer surgical techniques that limit time spent in deep hypothermia with circulatory arrest or on continuous cardiopulmonary bypass, use of normothermic cardiopulmonary bypass, and surgery on beating hearts not only permits the total correction of many forms of CHDs in the neonatal period but increases survival and decreases morbidities (Newazhay et al., 2012). In most cases, early intervention is essential to minimize and prevent long-term morbidity or early death (Knowles et al., 2012).

Whereas these advances have allowed for correction of many CHDs with dramatic decreases in mortality, neurodevelopmental morbidities are still found (Stone, 2010). Multiple clinical trials reported in the literature substantiate earlier findings of neurodevelopmental impairments in patients following neonatal cardiac surgery (Newburger et al., 2012). Although overall intelligence has been spared, only 21% of school-age patients function at age-appropriate levels, 37% have moderate disabilities, and 6% have severe disabilities. The disabilities were identified as motor and cognitive impairments, including speech and language delays, gross and fine motor deficiencies, and visual–motor delays. Many studies have linked these outcomes to deep hypothermic cardiac arrest and continuous cardiopulmonary bypass that is used during open heart surgery.

# CARDIOVASCULAR EMBRYOLOGY AND ANATOMY

## Cardiac Development

Fetal cardiac development occurs rapidly from day 18 to the 12th week of fetal life (Sedmera, 2011).

**A. Cardiac tube.**

1. Heart development is first identified at 18 to 19 days of fetal life with formation of a heart tube (Table 28-1; Fig. 28-1, *A*).
2. The heart tube elongates and develops dilatations and contractions that will later form the ventricles, bulbus cordis, and outflow tracts (Fig. 28-1, *B*). Molecular studies are beginning to identify that the heart tube actually becomes the left ventricle, but more studies are needed (van de Berg and Moorman, 2009).
3. The pairs of aortic arches develop from the cephalic, extracardial portion of the heart tube. The caudal end will form the early ventricle (Fig. 28-1, *C*).
4. Abnormal development during this time will include corrected transposition and dextrocardia (Collins-Nakai and McLaughlin, 2002).

**B. Cardiac septation:** begins in the middle of the fourth week and is complete by the end of the fifth week of fetal life (Fig. 28-1, *D*).

1. Atrial septum and foramen ovale are formed from two septa and endocardial cushions.
   - a. Atrial septum primum is formed by unidirectional growth from the top of the atrium toward the endocardial cushions, resulting in formation of the septum.
   - b. A second septum (septum secundum) appears to the right of the septum primum and grows to overlap the ostium secundum. Thus the flapped opening, the foramen ovale, is created (Fig. 28-2).

■ TABLE 28-1
■ ■ **Timeline for Fetal Heart Development**

| Age (Days) | Cardiovascular Morphogenesis |
|---|---|
| 18 | Angiogenic tissue appears |
| 19 to 20 | Endothelial heart tubes appear |
| 21 | Fusion of endothelial heart tubes |
| 23 to 25 | Differentiation of atria, ventricles, and bulbus cordis; heart begins to beat |
| 25 | Fusion of atria, dorsal mesocardium regresses, formation of bulboventricular loop |
| 26 to 27 | Circulation is established |
| 32 | Appearance of septum primum |
| 33 | Intraventricular septum begins to form |
| 35 | Foramen secundum present |
| 36 to 37 | Fusion of atrial endocardial cushions |
| 43 | Ridges form in the bulbus cordis |
| 46 | Closure of ventricular septum, formation of coronary arteries |
| 47 | Septum secundum appears |

Data from Collins-Nakai, R. and McLaughlin, P.: How congenital heart disease originates in life. *Cardiology Clinics*, 20(3):367-383, 2002; Park, M.K.: *Pediatric cardiology for practitioners* (5th ed.). Philadelphia, 2008, Elsevier Mosby; Theorell, C.: Cardiovascular assessment of the newborn. *Newborn and Infant Nursing Reviews*, 2(2):111-127, 2002.

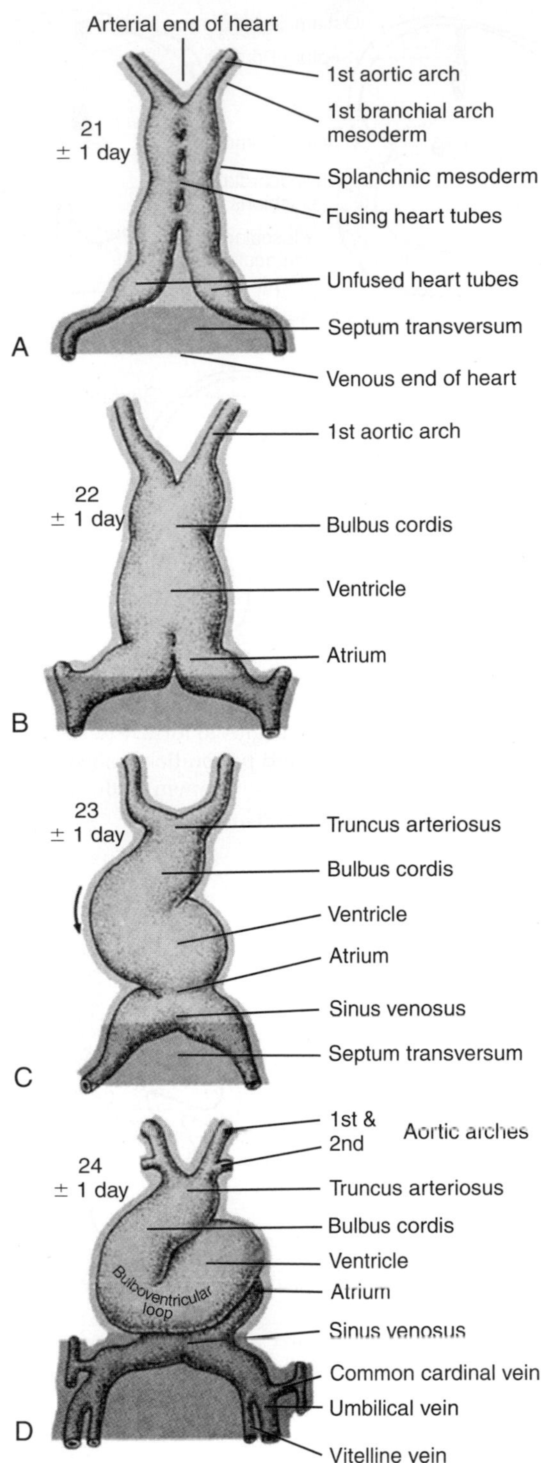


FIGURE 28-1 ■ Sketches of ventral views of the developing heart (at 20 to 25 days), showing fusion of endocardial heart tubes to form a single heart tube. Bending of the heart tube to form a bulboventricular loop is also illustrated. (Adapted from Moore, K.L. and Persaud, T.V.N.: *The developing human: Clinically oriented embryology* [8th ed.]. Philadelphia, 2008, Elsevier Saunders.)

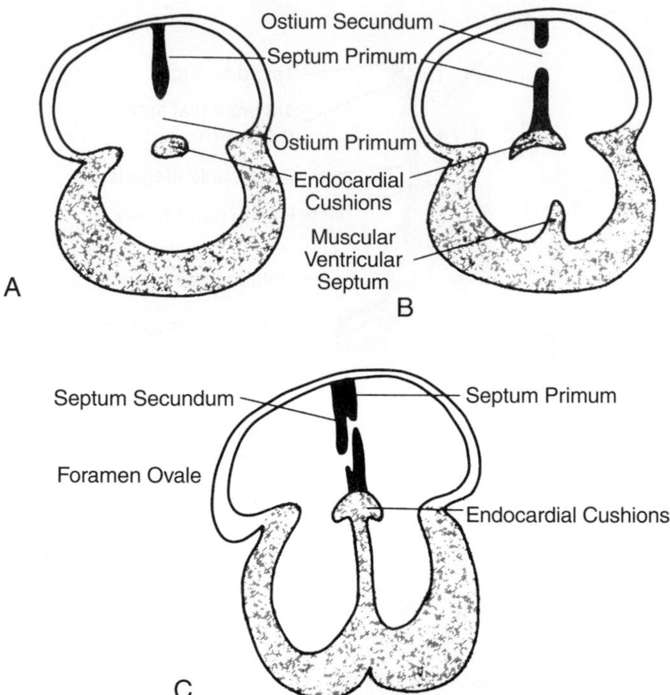


FIGURE 28-2 ■ Atrial septation. **A**, Septum primum begins to form, extending toward endocardial cushion (note ostium primum). **B**, Ostium primum is closed and perforation (called ostium secundum) forms in the septum primum. **C**, Septum secundum forms, creating the foramen ovale. (From Hazinski, M.F.: Congenital heart disease in the neonate. *Neonatal Network*, 21[3]:31-42, 1983.)

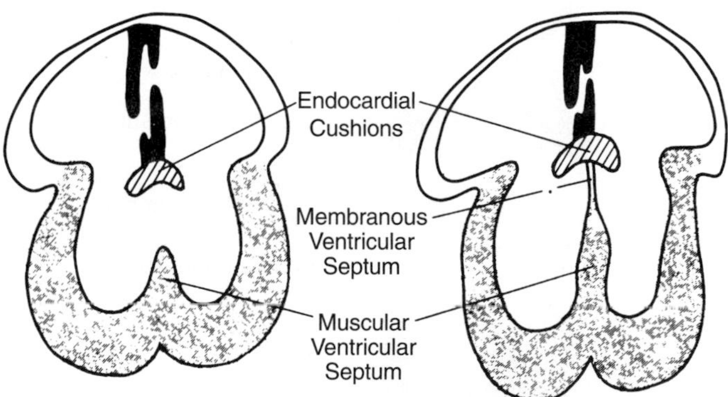


FIGURE 28-3 ■ Ventricular septation (with muscular and membranous septum). (From Hazinski, M.F.: Congenital heart disease in the neonate. *Neonatal Network*, 21[3]:31-42, 1983.)

2. Ventricular septation results from fusion of the endocardial cushions and dilation and fusion of the ventricles (Fig. 28-3).
3. Tissue of endocardial cushion forms the atrioventricular valves (Fig. 28-4).
   a. Tricuspid valve: between right atrium and ventricle.
   b. Mitral valve: between left atrium and ventricle.
4. Abnormal development during cardiac septation can lead to the following:
   a. VSD, ASD, and endocardial cushion defect (atrioventricular canal).
   b. Absence, deformation, stenosis, or atresia of the tricuspid and/or mitral valves.

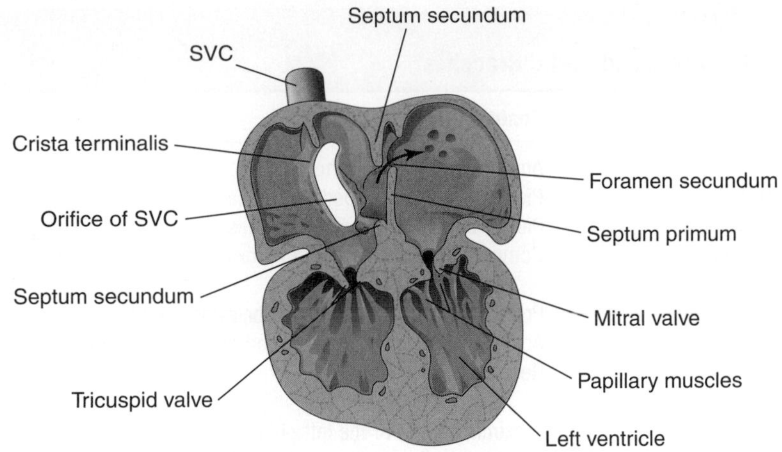


FIGURE 28-4 ■ The developing heart at about 8 weeks, showing the heart after it is partitioned into four chambers. *Arrow* indicates flow of well-oxygenated blood from right to left atrium. *SVC*, superior vena cava. (From Moore, K.L. and Persaud, T.V.N.: *The developing human: Clinically oriented embryology* [8th ed.]. Philadelphia, 2008, Elsevier Saunders.)

## Great Vessel Development

A. **Single vessel (truncus arteriosus)** extends from the ventricles until the fourth week of fetal life. It will then separate into the aorta and the pulmonary artery (Fig. 28-5).
   1. The semilunar valves (aortic and pulmonic valves) develop from three ridges of tissue at the opening to the aorta and pulmonary trunk.
B. **Development of aorta and aortic branches** (Table 28-2). The truncus arteriosus connects with the aortic sac, which in turn connects with the paired aortic branches. A series of six paired aortic arches then form in succession (Fig. 28-6).
   1. The third arches become part of the common carotid arteries.
   2. The right fourth arch becomes the proximal portion of the right subclavian artery.
   3. The left fourth arch becomes the aortic arch segment between the left common carotid artery and left subclavian artery.
   4. The left sixth arch becomes part of the left pulmonary artery and the ductus arteriosus.
   5. The right sixth arch forms the right pulmonary artery.
   6. Abnormalities include interrupted aortic arch and coarctation of the aorta.
C. **Developmental abnormalities of truncal septation include (Collins-Nakai and McLaughlin, 2002):**
   1. Truncus arteriosus.

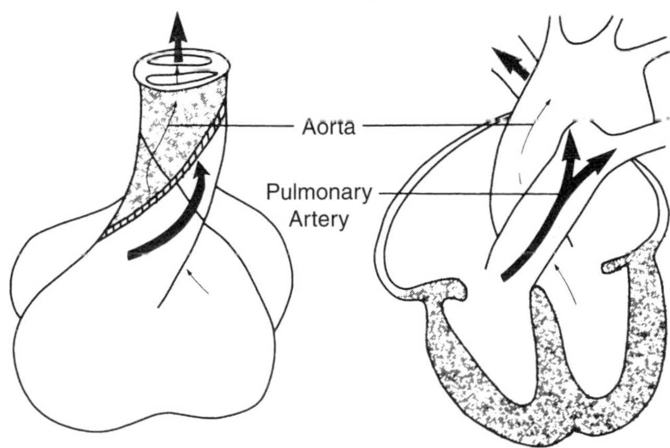


FIGURE 28-5 ■ Closing of the truncus arteriosus and division into the pulmonary artery and aorta. (From Hazinski, M.F.: Congenital heart disease in the neonate. *Neonatal Network*, 21[3]:31-42, 1983.)

■ TABLE 28-2
■ ■ **Development of Aorta and Aortic Branches**

| Embryonic Vessel | Results In |
|---|---|
| Truncus arteriosus | Aorta and pulmonary artery |
| First pair of aortic arches | Pieces remain as stapedial arteries |
| Second pair of aortic arches | Pieces remain as stapedial arteries |
| Third pair of aortic arches | Common carotid arteries and proximal portion of internal carotid arteries |
| Fourth pair of aortic arches | |
| Right | Proximal portion of the right subclavian artery |
| Left | Aortic arch segment between left common carotid and left subclavian artery |
| Fifth pair of aortic arches | Regresses totally |
| Sixth pair of aortic arches | |
| Left | Proximal portion of the left pulmonary artery and ductus arteriosus |
| Right | Proximal portion of the right pulmonary artery |

Data from Collins-Nakai, R. and McLaughlin, P.: How congenital heart disease originates in life. *Cardiology Clinics*, 20(3):367-383, 2002; Park, M.K.: *Pediatric cardiology for practitioners* (5th ed.). Philadelphia, 2008, Elsevier Mosby; Theorell, C.: Cardiovascular assessment of the newborn. *Newborn and Infant Nursing Reviews*, 2(2):111-127, 2002.

2. TOF.
3. Pulmonary and/or aortic valve atresia or stenosis.
4. Transposition of the great vessels (dextroposition).
5. Double-outlet right ventricle.

## Circulatory Development

A. **Heart contractions begin around 21 days;** the atrium and ventricle muscle layers are continuous. Contractions result in a rhythmic peristalsis.
B. **Electrical conduction system** is functional around 10 weeks, with normal sinus rhythm seen by 16 weeks (Blackburn, 2013).
C. **Establishment of fetal circulation:** With completion of atrial and ventricular septation, development of valves between chambers and outflow tracks, and separation of the truncus arteriosus into the great vessels, fetal circulation is established.
D. **Fetal circulation is anatomically and physiologically different from adult circulation,** and adaptation after birth is necessary (Blackburn, 2013). For a full discussion of fetal circulation and cardiopulmonary adaptation at birth, see Chapter 4.

## Cardiovascular Physiology

A. **Normal circulation (see Fig. 4-2).**
   1. Oxygen-poor blood enters the right atrium and passes through the tricuspid valve into the right ventricle, where it is pumped through the pulmonary artery to the lungs.
   2. As the blood flows through the lungs, it gives up carbon dioxide and gains oxygen.
   3. Oxygen-rich blood returns from the lungs through the pulmonary veins. It enters the left atrium and then passes through the mitral valve into the left ventricle, which pumps it through the aortic valve and into the aorta.
   4. The aorta then delivers oxygenated blood to all body organs and tissues.
B. **Cardiac depolarization**
   1. Results from the electrical discharge across the myocardial cell (total net movement of ions across the cell wall) and is measured by the electrocardiograph.
   2. Shortening of muscle fibers (contraction) usually follows cardiac depolarization. Strength of cardiac (ventricular) contraction is measured by blood pressure or arterial pulse palpation.
   3. Cardiac electrical activity does not ensure adequate cardiac function.
      a. Congenital defects or surgical injury to the conduction system may result in arrhythmias or heart block.

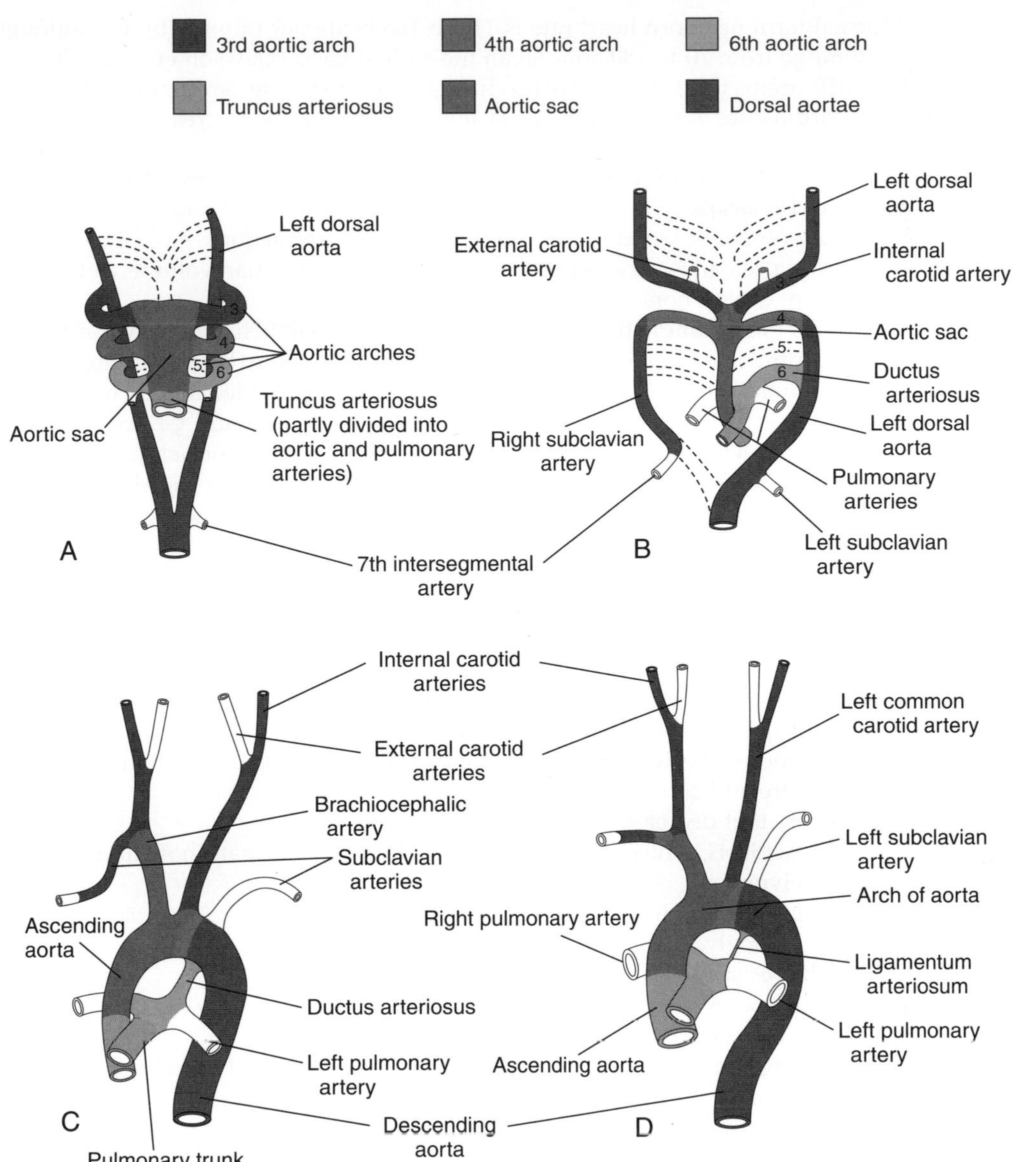


FIGURE 28-6 ■ Schematic drawings illustrating arterial changes that result during transformation of the truncus arteriosus, aortic sac, aortic arches, and dorsal aortas into the adult arterial pattern. **A**, Aortic arches at 6 weeks. **B**, Aortic arches at 7 weeks. **C**, Arterial arrangement at 8 weeks. **D**, Sketch of arterial vessels of 6-month-old infant. (From Moore, K.L., Persaud, T.V.N., and Torchia, M.G.: *The developing human: Clinically oriented embryology* [9th ed.]. Philadelphia, 2013, Elsevier Saunders.)

**b.** Electrolyte disturbance (i.e., altered fluid composition surrounding the cells) can affect electrical activity.
(1) Hypokalemia and hyperkalemia.
(2) Hypocalcemia and hypercalcemia.
(3) Hypoxia.
(4) Acidosis.

**C. Cardiac output.**

**1.** Cardiac output is the volume of blood ejected by the heart in 1 minute. Approximations vary from 120 to 200 mL/kg/min.

**2.** Cardiac output = stroke volume × heart rate (in liters per minute).

**a.** As heart rate fluctuates, so will cardiac output.

(1) Normal term newborn heart rate is 110 to 166 beats per minute (bpm), although it may range from 70 to 180 bpm on an individual basis (Dawson et al., 2010).

**b.** Tachycardia seems to be an effective mechanism for improving cardiac output as long as the tachycardia does not compromise diastolic filling time and decrease coronary artery perfusion.

**3.** Stroke volume is relatively fixed at 1.5 mL/kg and is affected by three factors: preload, contractility, and afterload.

**a.** Preload: the volume of blood in the ventricles before contraction.

(1) Clinically, preload is a measurement of pressure, rather than volume, in the ventricles before contraction.

(2) Increasing the volume in the ventricles, consequently lengthening the myocardial fibers before contraction, should result in improved stroke volume (Frank–Starling law). The newborn infant is capable of increasing stroke volume provided there is no increase in systemic vascular resistance (SVR) or rapid rise in aortic pressure. Given the neonate's smaller contractile mass, less compliant myocardium, and normal maximization of myocardial fiber length, volume infusions are likely to increase aortic pressure and afterload, resulting in a decline in stroke volume (Wernovsky and Gruber, 2005).

**b.** Contractility: speed of ventricular contraction.

(1) Cardiac cycle consists of ventricular contraction (systole), followed by ventricular relaxation (diastole). As contraction time decreases, relaxation time (diastole) increases, with an increase in ventricular filling volume (preload) before contraction.

(2) Ventricular contractility cannot be directly measured. Measurements of cardiac shortening fractions and ejection fraction provide an indirect assessment of contractility.

(3) Contractility in neonates is influenced by the following:

(a) Exogenous catecholamine (dopamine/dobutamine) use, which increases blood pressure and cardiac output.

(b) Factors that decrease contractility:

(i) Acidosis, which impairs myocardial response to catecholamines.

(ii) Hypoxia.

(iii) Electrolyte disturbances.

(iv) Hypoglycemia.

**c.** Afterload: the resistance to blood leaving the ventricle.

(1) Dependent on SVR and pulmonary vascular resistance (PVR); if SVR or PVR increases, afterload increases.

(2) The neonate's myocardium is very sensitive to increased afterload; with small increases in afterload, stroke volume can fall significantly.

(3) Afterload can be reduced by intravenous (IV) infusion of vasodilators (e.g., nitroglycerin, amrinone, and nitroprusside). Dobutamine can be used to decrease PVR (Young and Mangum, 2008).

**4.** Concepts of blood flow.

**a.** Flow is directly proportional to pressure/resistance.

**b.** Blood flow will always take the path of least resistance.

**c.** If heart action (pressure) remains unchanged but vasoconstriction or dilation or obstruction to flow (resistance) changes, flow will change (i.e., cardiac output will vary).

**d.** PVR starts to fall by almost 80% after delivery, resulting in a dramatic increase in pulmonary blood flow and subsequent increase in systolic blood pressure (Blackburn, 2013). This normal decline is influenced by prematurity, low birth weight, and hypoxia episodes.

## CONGENITAL HEART DEFECTS

For a list of abbreviations used for cardiac defects, see Table 28-3.

### Occurrence

**A. Incidence:** 3 to 9 per 1000 live births (Miller et al., 2011); the incidence in premature infants is 2 to 3 times that of term infants (Altman, 2013).

■ TABLE 28-3
■ ■ **Abbreviations Used for Cardiac Defects**

| | |
|---|---|
| AS | Aortic stenosis |
| ASD | Atrial septal defect |
| CoA | Coarctation of the aorta |
| HLHS | Hypoplastic left heart syndrome |
| IAA | Interrupted aortic arch |
| PA | Pulmonary atresia |
| PDA | Patent ductus arteriosus |
| PFO | Patent foramen ovale |
| PS | Pulmonary stenosis |
| TA | Truncus arteriosus |
| TAPVR | Total anomalous pulmonary venous return |
| TGV or TGA | Transposition of the great vessels or arteries |
| VSD | Ventricular septal defect |

1. 85% of cases are due to multifactorial causes.
2. 10% to 12% are due to chromosomal factors.
3. 1% to 2% are due to genetic factors.
4. 1% to 2% are due to exposure to maternal or environmental teratogens (Lott, 2014).
5. 14.5% to 66% are in conjunction with other structural anomalies.

**B. Genetic factors:** Chromosomal abnormalities: overall incidence of CHD in patients with a chromosome aberration is 30%. Isolated cardiac defects result from multiple genes and their interaction with factors in the environment. Advances in technology have identified genetic factors for many of these defects.

1. Incidence of CHD varies with chromosomal abnormality. Syndromes with an entire extra chromosome or syndromes with a missing chromosome are detected with normal chromosomal studies (van der Born et al., 2011):
   - **a.** Trisomy 21: approximately 45%.
   - **b.** Trisomy 18: 90% to 100%.
   - **c.** Trisomy 13: 90%.
   - **d.** Turner's syndrome: 25% to 45% (45,X0 karyotype or mosaic 46,XX).
2. Syndromes requiring fluorescence in-situ hybridization (FISH) analysis include those with mosaicism and those with deletions in a chromosome.
   - **a.** Chromosome deletion syndromes 18, 13, 5, and 4: 25% to 50%.
   - **b.** Mosaic Turner's syndrome: X and Y chromosome. FISH probe needed to rule out Y chromosome (Bishara and Clericuzio, 2008).
3. Microdeletions that are detected through FISH:
   - **a.** 22q11 deletion syndrome: 80% to 85%.
   - **b.** Williams syndrome: 50% to 70% (deletion of elastin gene at 7q11.23).
   - **c.** Alagille syndrome: 90% (*JAG1* deletion on 20p12).
   - **d.** Noonan's syndrome: greater than 50% (12q24.1, *PTPN11* gene).
   - **e.** DiGeorge deletion: greater than 50% (22q11.2) (Hartman and Medoff-Cooper, 2012).
4. Single-mutant-gene syndromes: 1% to 2% of all cardiovascular abnormalities in newborn infants. Both autosomal dominant and recessive syndromes have been associated with CHD. According to Bishara and Clericuzio (2008), the tests for these syndromes include gene mutation analysis via array comparative genomic hybridization (aCGH). This type of testing can detect smaller imbalances in the genome, allowing for detection of mutations, insertions, deletions, and imprinting abnormalities.
   - **a.** Holt–Oram syndrome: greater than 85% to 95% (*TBX5* gene found at 12q24.1).
   - **b.** X-linked situs inversus Xq25, *ZIC3* gene.
   - **c.** Kartagener's syndrome (Fleiner, 2006): 100% (*DNAI1* on 9p21-p13, *DNAH5* on 5p15-p14).

   d. Beckwith–Wiedemann syndrome: 10% to 35%, imprinting defects of *KIP2/LIT1* and paternal *IGF2* genes at 11p15.5 (Jonas and Demmer, 2007).
5. Multifactorial: approximately 90% due to genetic predisposition coupled with a causative factor.
   a. Cornelia de Lange's syndrome: approximately 30%.
   b. VACTERL (*v*ertebral anomalies, *a*nal atresia/stenosis, *c*ardiac defects [50%], *t*racheo*e*sophageal fistula, *r*adial defects, *l*imb anomalies) (Wechsler and Wernovsky, 2004).
   c. CHARGE (*c*oloboma, *h*eart defects [50% to 70%], choanal *a*tresia, *r*estriction of growth and development, *g*enital anomalies, *e*ar anomalies) (Wechsler and Wernovsky, 2004).
6. Genetic counseling is done to evaluate cause and recurrence risk. The risk of having another child with a cardiac lesion is 3% to 4% if the cause is unknown (Beck and Hudgins, 2003). However, this risk may be as much as 13% higher in specific syndromes.
   a. DiGeorge syndrome: Chromosomal microarray analysis should be recommended as first-line test if the infant has developmental disabilities (Hartman, et al., 2011).
      (1) 7% of parents carry the deletion.
      (2) Recurrence risk is up to 50% (Bishara and Clericuzio, 2008).
      (3) Prenatal diagnosis in future pregnancies via chorionic villus sampling (CVS) or amniocentesis, with FISH requested specifically.
   b. Trisomies 13, 18, and 21 all carry recurrence risk of 1%, and prenatal diagnosis in future pregnancies is done using CVS or amniocentesis. The recurrence risk for trisomy 21 increases after maternal age 40.

C. **Environmental factors and teratogens** can include fetal exposure to drug, chemical, infectious, or physical agents; maternal disease or altered metabolic state with the period of greatest risk at 14 to 50 days of fetal life (Lott, 2014).
1. Cardiac teratogenesis is associated with maternal ingestion of the following:
   a. Thalidomide: dramatically illustrated the extraordinarily deleterious effects of prescribed drug on a developing fetus; included PDA, ASD, VSD, and pulmonary stenosis (Smithells and Newman, 1992).
   b. Anticonvulsants: 2% to 3% of infants exposed to anticonvulsants will have associated congenital cardiac defects such as pulmonary stenosis, coarctation of the aorta, and PDA. Glickstein (2007) reported the following defects with use of specific anticonvulsants in pregnancy:
      (1) Phenytoin (fetal hydantoin syndrome): VSD, D-transposition of the great vessels (D-TGV), TOF, HLHS, pulmonary atresia, ASD, aortic stenosis, and pulmonic stenosis.
      (2) Carbamazepine (Tegretol): VSD, TOF.
      (3) Valproic acid: VSD, coarctation of the aorta, interrupted aortic arch, TOF, HLHS, aortic stenosis, ASD, pulmonary atresia.
      (4) Trimethadione (fetal trimethadione syndrome): VSD, TGV, TOF, HLHS, double-outlet right ventricle, pulmonary atresia, ASD, aortic stenosis, pulmonic stenosis.
      (5) Pentobarbital: no confirmed specific embryopathy but may potentiate the effects of other drugs taken concurrently.
   c. Anticoagulants.
      (1) Warfarin (Coumadin): abortion or fetal embryopathic development in weeks 6 to 9 of gestation. Cardiac malformations have been identified, but no consistent cardiac defect has been noted.
      (2) Heparin: because of its larger molecular weight, does not cross the placenta.
   d. Antineoplastic medications.
      (1) Aminopterin: cardiac manifestations include dextroposition but are not as prominent as other defects resulting from drug ingestion.
      (2) In general, the disorders for which antineoplastic agents are used are serious enough to preclude pregnancy (Glickstein, 2007).
   e. Lithium: approximately 10% of infants exposed will have defects such as Ebstein's anomaly, ASD, and tricuspid atresia.
   f. Retinoic acid: aortic arch abnormalities, other congenital heart malformations.
   g. Isotretinoin.

h. Alcohol: fetal alcohol syndrome (FAS) is accompanied by a variety of cardiac lesions (e.g., VSD with or without subpulmonic and subaortic stenosis, ASD, coarctation of the aorta, TOF).
i. Amphetamine: 5% to 10% will have congenital cardiac defects such as VSD, PDA, ASD, and TGV (Kensey et al, 2011).
j. Selective serotonin reuptake inhibitors: increased risk of VSD if used in first trimester (Koren and Nordeng, 2012).
k. Tobacco and smoking: correlation between first-trimester smoking and defects such as pulmonary valve stenosis, TGV, ASD, right ventricular outflow tract defects, and PDA in term newborns (Alverson et al., 2011).

2. Exposure to environmental hazards such as radiation, heat, and gases may produce teratogenic effects, but there are no specific associated cardiac malformations.
3. Assisted reproductive technology highly linked to cardiac defects such as outflow tract abnormalities, VSD, TGV, and ASD (Tararbit et al., 2011).

D. **Maternal disease and viral infections (Box 28-1).**

1. Women with diabetes mellitus, especially insulin-dependent, have a 5 times greater risk of their children being born with cardiac anomalies than the general population of pregnant women have. Disorders include hypertrophy of the septum and myocardium, VSD, double-outlet right ventricle, TGV, truncus arteriosus, and coarctation of the aorta.
2. Maternal lupus erythematosus may be linked to complete congenital heart block and dilated cardiomyopathy.

BOX 28-1

**CLASSIFICATION OF MATERNAL DISEASES AFFECTING THE FETAL CARDIOVASCULAR SYSTEM**

**Category I: Maternal Diseases That Directly Affect the Fetal Cardiovascular System (Excluding Teratogenic Effects)**

Pheochromocytoma
Hyperthyroidism
Diabetes mellitus
Collagen vascular disease (e.g., Ro antibody)
Rubella
Cytomegalovirus
Enterovirus infection
Toxoplasmosis
Listeriosis
Maternal group B streptococcal colonization with fetal invasion
Syphilis
Inherited metabolic diseases

**Category II: Maternal Diseases That May Indirectly Affect the Fetal Cardiovascular System as a Result of Abnormalities of Uteroplacental Function**

Neoplastic diseases
Diabetes mellitus
Maternal cardiac disease
Anemia (including the hemoglobinopathies)
Hypertensive disorders
Collagen vascular disease (e.g., lupus anticoagulant and systemic lupus erythematosus)
Renal disease (associated with hypertension)
Asthma
Cholestatic jaundice of pregnancy
Cytomegalovirus
Bacterial infections

From Katz, V. and Bowes, W.: Maternal diseases affecting the fetal cardiovascular system. In W. Long (Ed.): *Fetal and neonatal cardiology*. Philadelphia, 1990, W.B. Saunders, p. 135.

3. Rubella and cytomegalovirus produce clinically significant heart disease (Kensey et al, 2011). Disorders seen are PDA, pulmonary stenosis and branch pulmonary artery stenosis, VSD, and ASD.
4. Maternal obesity has been linked to congenital heart disease (Glickstein, 2007).
5. Maternal fever and influenza are linked to right ventricular outflow tract and atrioventricular defects (Oster et al., 2011).

## RISK ASSESSMENT AND APPROACH TO DIAGNOSIS OF CARDIAC DISEASE

### Sex Preferences Associated With Cardiac Lesions

A. **Males.**
   1. Coarctation of the aorta.
   2. Aortic stenosis.
   3. TGV.
   4. HLHS.

B. **Females.**
   1. ASD.
   2. PDA.

### History (Kensey et al, 2011)

A. **Gestational age.**
   1. Preterm. Infants born prematurely are much more likely to have pulmonary problems resulting in cyanosis than to have congestive heart failure (CHF), but they do have a higher incidence of:
      a. PDA.
      b. Left-to-right shunts (e.g., VSD or atrioventricular canal).
   2. Term. The majority of infants with CHF are term infants.

B. **Maternal history (see Box 28-1).**
   1. Infants of mothers with uncontrolled diabetes have an increased risk of:
      a. TGV.
      b. VSD.
      c. Cardiomyopathy.
      d. Complex congenital heart disease.
   2. Lupus may cause congenital heart block and cardiomyopathy.
   3. Viral and bacterial illnesses may directly and indirectly affect the fetal cardiovascular system.
   4. Seizures or coagulation disorders can be linked to CHDs because the medications used may be teratogens.
   5. Maternal congenital heart disease can lead to an increased risk of same defect in infant.
   6. Maternal age greater than 35 years increases risk.
   7. Alcohol consumption: increase in cardiac defects seen with FAS.

C. **Familial.**
   1. Incidence of CHDs increases by 3- to 4-fold when a first-order relative (parent or sibling) has CHD (Oyen et al., 2009; Park, 2008). Risk increases by 10-fold if two first-order relatives have congenital heart disease (Table 28-4).

D. **Perinatal history.**
   1. Intrauterine growth pattern and birth weight.
   2. Prenatal diagnosis with ultrasound.
   3. Mode of delivery.
      a. Vaginal delivery most common for CHD, and initial Apgar scores are usually good.
      b. History of cesarean section and poor Apgar scores more indicative of asphyxia and respiratory distress.

■ TABLE 28-4
■ ■ **Familial Recurrence Risks**

| Cardiac Anomaly | Family Member with Congenital Heart Defect | Risk (%) |
|---|---|---|
| Overall | Parent | 3.2 |
| | Grandparent | 1.8 |
| | Aunt/Uncle/Cousin | 1.1 |
| PDA—patent ductus arteriosus | Mother | 3.5 to 4 |
| | Father | 2.5 |
| | Sibling | 3 |
| VSD—ventricular septal defect | Mother | 6 |
| | Father | 2 |
| | Sibling | 3 |
| ASD—atrial septal defect | Mother | 4 to 4.5 |
| | Father | 1.5 |
| | Sibling | 2-3 |
| AVC—atrioventricular canal | Mother | 14 |
| | Father | 1 |
| | Sibling | 3-4 |
| Tetralogy of Fallot | Mother | 6 to 10 |
| | Father | 1.5 |
| | Sibling | 2.5 |
| Aortic stenosis | Mother | 13 to 18 |
| | Father | 3 |
| | Sibling | 2 |
| Pulmonary stenosis | Mother | 4 to 6.5 |
| | Father | 2 |
| | Sibling | 2 |
| Coarctation of the aorta | Mother | 4 |
| | Father | 2 |
| | Sibling | 2 |
| Other defects (TGA, tricuspid atresia, truncus arteriosus, HLHS) | Sibling | 1.4 (average) |

Data from Park, M.K.: *Pediatric cardiology for practitioners* (5th ed.). Philadelphia, 2008, Elsevier Mosby; Theorell, C.: Cardiovascular assessment of the newborn. *Newborn and Infant Nursing Reviews*, 2(2):111-127, 2002; Altman, C.A.: Congenital heart disease (CHD) in the newborn: Presentation and screening for CHD. *UpToDate*. 2013. Available at www.uptodate.com
*HLHS*, Hypoplastic left heart syndrome; *TGA*, transposition of the great arteries.

**E. Universal pulse oximetry screening (American Academy of Pediatrics, Section on Cardiology and Cardiac Surgery, 2012).**

1. Recommended by U.S. Department of Health and Human Services.
2. Endorsed by American Academy of Pediatrics.
3. Used to identify newborns at risk for HLHS, TOF, TGV, total anomalous pulmonary venous return (TAPVR), pulmonary atresia, critical aortic stenosis, truncus arteriosus.
4. Implementation (Kemper et al., 2011).
   a. Should not be done until >24 hours of age in well-baby and intermediate care nurseries.
      (1) Earlier screening may lead to false-positive results.
   b. Monitor pulse oximetry of both the right hand (RH; preductal) and either foot (postductal).
      (1) Negative screen—discharge home.
         (a) If pulse oximeter reading is >95% in RH or foot and difference between RH and foot is <3%.
      (2) Suspicious screen—repeat screen in 1 hour.

(a) If reading is 90% to 95% in RH and foot or there is ≥3% difference between RH and foot, repeat in 1 hour.
(b) If second reading is the same, then repeat again in 1 hour. If pulse oximeter readings indicate positive test, then refer for further testing.
(3) Positive screen—refer for further testing
(a) If pulse oximeter reading in RH or foot is less than 90%, further testing warranted.

## Clinical Presentation

A. **Cyanosis** (in the first week may be sole evidence of a heart lesion).
1. With cardiovascular problems, cyanosis is unexpected or gradual in onset.
2. Cyanosis observation.
a. Dependent on hemoglobin levels; at least 5 g of desaturated hemoglobin/dL is necessary before cyanosis becomes apparent.
b. Will be influenced by presence of anemia or polycythemia and the levels of 2,3-diphosphoglycerate.
3. Differentiation between central and peripheral cyanosis.
a. Peripheral or acrocyanosis results from sluggish movement of blood through the extremities and increased tissue oxygen extraction.
(1) Persists from birth and can last several days.
(2) Does not involve mucous membranes.
(3) May be caused by peripheral vasomotor instability.
b. Central cyanosis results from desaturated blood leaving the heart.
(1) Seen as bluish discoloration of tongue and mucous membranes, reflecting arterial desaturation.
(2) Central cyanosis may present difficulties in making a differential diagnosis between respiratory and cardiac origin.

B. **Respiratory pattern.**
1. Useful in the differentiation of cyanosis.
2. Tachypnea (respiratory rate >60) without dyspnea is an important, often subtle, clue to cardiac anomalies. In the absence of cyanosis, it may indicate a left-to-right shunt lesion. Tachypnea is significant if coupled with feeding difficulty. It is suggestive of CHF if the infant must stop feeding to catch its breath.
3. Hyperpnea (increased respiratory depth) is observed in congenital heart lesions resulting in diminished pulmonary blood flow.
4. Crying may exacerbate cyanosis in neonates with CHD because of increased oxygen consumption by the tissues.

C. **Heart sounds.**
1. First heart sound ($S_1$) represents closure of the mitral and tricuspid valves at the onset of ventricular systole.
a. Best heard at the fourth intercostal space in the left midclavicular line (mitral) and at the fourth intercostal space at the sternal borders (tricuspid).
b. $S_1$ is accentuated with the following:
(1) Increased cardiac output.
(2) Increased flow across atrioventricular valves.
(3) Specific conditions such as the following:
(a) PDA.
(b) VSD with increased mitral flow.
(c) TAPVR.
(d) Arteriovenous malformation.
(e) TOF.
(f) Anemia.
(g) Fever.
c. Conditions decreasing $S_1$ include the following:
(1) Decreased atrioventricular conduction.
(2) CHF.
(3) Myocarditis.

2. Second heart sound ($S_2$) occurs at the end of ventricular systole from closure of aortic and pulmonic valves.
   a. Heard best at upper left sternal border.
   b. Split $S_2$ is a normal occurrence, reflecting closure of aortic valve before the pulmonic valve.
      (1) Increases on inspiration.
      (2) Single $S_2$ is often heard in the first 2 days of life because of increased PVR.
      (3) Splitting of $S_2$ is influenced by:
         (a) Abnormalities of aortic or pulmonic valves.
         (b) Conditions altering PVR or SVR.
   c. Conditions widening the $S_2$ are influenced by the following:
      (1) ASD.
      (2) TAPVR.
      (3) TOF.
      (4) Pulmonary stenosis.
      (5) Ebstein anomaly.
   d. Absent $S_2$ splits occur in the following:
      (1) Pulmonary atresia and severe pulmonary stenosis.
      (2) Aortic stenosis/atresia.
      (3) Persistent pulmonary hypertension.
      (4) *l*-TGV.
      (5) Truncus arteriosus.
3. Third heart sound ($S_3$) is due to increased flow across the atrioventricular valves from rapid, passive ventricular filling from the atria.
   a. Follows $S_2$ and is a low-pitched, broad sound.
   b. Prominent in situations of increased atrioventricular flow and increased ventricular filling (Altman, 2013).
      (1) Left-to-right shunts (e.g., ASD, VSD, PDA).
      (2) Anemia.
      (3) Mitral valve insufficiency.
4. Fourth heart sound ($S_4$) occurs at the final phase of ventricular filling and active atrial contraction during late diastole.
   a. Occurs just before $S_1$ and is low pitched.
   b. Rarely heard in the newborn infant.
   c. Always pathologic and indicates decreased ventricular compliance.
5. Ejection clicks are heard as snapping sounds just after the first heart sound in the first 24 hours of life.
   a. Abnormal (except during first 24 hours of life) and indicate cardiac disease.
   b. Audible for short duration after $S_1$.
   c. Associated with dilation of the great vessels or deformity of aortic or pulmonic valve.
   d. Other conditions associated with ejection clicks include the following:
      (1) Aortic valve stenosis.
      (2) Truncus arteriosus.
      (3) TOF (severe).
      (4) Pulmonary valve stenosis.
      (5) HLHS.
      (6) Coarctation of the aorta.
6. Murmurs.
   a. Murmurs are audible vibrations resulting from turbulence of blood flow and may be due to:
      (1) Abnormal valves.
      (2) Septal defects.
      (3) Regurgitated flow through incompetent valves.
      (4) High blood flow across normal structures.
   b. Physiologic murmurs have been noted in 50% of neonates in the first 48 hours of life (Altman, 2013). Generally, these murmurs are due to:
      (1) Transient left-to-right flow via the ductus arteriosus.

(2) Increased flow over the pulmonary valve associated with a fall in PVR.
(3) Mild bilateral peripheral pulmonary arterial stenosis because of size and pressure differences between the main pulmonary trunk and the left and right pulmonary arterial branches.

**c.** Absence of murmur does not indicate absence of significant cardiac disease.

**d.** Evaluation of murmurs includes the following:

(1) Intensity of sound.
(a) Murmurs are graded I through VI. Grade III or less generally present no hemodynamic problems (Lott, 2014).
(i) Grade I: barely audible, only after careful auscultation.
(ii) Grade II: soft, easily audible on auscultation.
(iii) Grade III: moderately loud, not associated with a thrill.
(iv) Grade IV: loud murmur associated with a thrill.
(v) Grade V: very loud. May be heard with stethoscope just touching the chest wall.
(vi) Grade VI: extremely loud. Can be heard with stethoscope off the chest wall.
(b) Presence of a thrill on palpation is associated with a loud murmur of at least grade IV.

(2) Timing within cardiac cycle.
(a) Systolic: heard during ventricular systole (i.e., between $S_1$ and $S_2$) or, if feeling the pulse during auscultation, at the upstroke of the pulse.
(i) Identified as early, mid-, or late systolic.
(ii) Pansystolic (holosystolic): heard throughout systole. Heard in mitral or tricuspid insufficiency and VSD.
(iii) Ejection murmurs: turbulence of blood flow leaving the heart; noted in aortic or pulmonic valve stenosis, TOF, ASD, and TAPVR. The majority of innocent murmurs are systolic ejection murmurs (Lott, 2014).
(b) Diastolic: heard during period of ventricular filling (i.e., between $S_2$ and $S_1$) and are usually indicative of a cardiac disorder.
(i) Early: results from aortic or pulmonic valve insufficiency.
(ii) Mid: increased blood flow across normal mitral or tricuspid valve.
(iii) Late: associated with stenotic mitral or tricuspid valve.
(c) Continuous: audible throughout cardiac cycle but can be louder in systole or diastole (e.g., PDA).

(3) Quality and pitch.
(a) Pitch: reflects frequency of vibrations.
(i) High-pitched sound from turbulent blood flow from a high-pressure area to a low-pressure area. Generally reflects valve insufficiency on the left side of the heart, whereas a low-pitched sound reflects right-sided valve insufficiency.
(ii) Low-pitched sound is from a low-pressure difference in turbulent blood flow reflecting right-sided valve insufficiency.
(b) Quality is described as:
(i) Harsh.
(ii) Blowing.
(iii) Musical.

(4) Location: in terms of maximal intensity described by anatomic location on chest wall.

(5) Radiation if present.

**D. Peripheral pulses (Altman, 2013).**

**1.** Pulses should be synchronous with equal intensity.

**2.** Upper and lower extremity pulses should be palpated simultaneously and differences documented.

**3.** Discrepancies (e.g., pulses that are greater in upper than in lower extremities) raise the possibility of an abnormal aortic arch.

4. Right brachial artery pulse should be compared with pulses in lower extremities because the right subclavian is always preductal.
5. Pulse volume graded from 0 to 4.
   a. 0 = absent.
   b. 1+ = weak.
   c. 2+ = weak to average.
   d. 3+ = strong.
   e. 4+ = bounding.
6. Weak pulses indicate low cardiac output, as seen in:
   a. Left heart outflow obstructive lesions.
   b. Myocardial failure.
   c. Shock.
7. Bounding pulses indicate aortic runoff.
   a. PDA.
   b. Aortic insufficiency.
   c. Systemic-to-pulmonary shunts.
8. Visible precordial impulse persisting after the first 12 hours of life occurs in defects with volume overload and is suggestive of left-to-right shunt (Wechsler and Wernovsky, 2004).

E. **Blood pressure.**
1. Normal values are dependent on birth weight and gestational age. The mean arterial pressure (MAP) is reported as being the same as the gestational age of the infant (Seri and Evans, 2001).
   a. Healthy term infant: average systolic pressure is 56 to 77 mm Hg; average diastolic pressure is 33 to 50 mm Hg. MAP is 42 to 60 mm Hg (Sansoucie and Cavaliere, 2007).
   b. Premature infant's blood pressure varies with size and gestational age; the lower limit of the MAP is similar numerically to the gestational age for infants of 26 to 32 weeks of gestation. For neonates weighing less than 800 g, the MAP may be lower than the gestational age (Frost et al., 2011).
2. Blood pressure values may also be affected by postnatal age, body temperature, infant's behavioral state, and cuff size.
3. Cuff width should be 25% greater than the width of the extremity. If the width is too narrow, the blood pressure will have a false high reading. If the cuff width is too wide, the blood pressure will have a false low reading (Frost et al., 2006).
4. Compare upper and lower extremity pressures. Systolic blood pressure of the upper extremities 20 mm Hg above that of lower extremities is suggestive of the following:
   a. Coarctation of the aorta. PDA may mask these pressure differences.
   b. Aortic arch abnormalities.
      (1) In addition, blood pressure differences between the upper extremities are seen with aortic arch abnormalities.
      (2) To evaluate, simultaneously measure blood pressure in both arms and one leg. Either leg can be evaluated because the blood supply to both legs comes from the descending aorta below the level of the defect.
5. In a term infant, neonatal hypertension is defined as a systolic blood pressure greater than 90 mm Hg and a diastolic pressure greater than 60 mm Hg.
   a. In a premature infant, systolic pressure greater than 80 mm Hg and diastolic pressure greater than 50 mm Hg indicate hypertension.
   b. Structural and/or functional renal abnormalities are the most common causes of hypertension.

## Diagnostic Adjuncts

A. **Arterial blood gas values** are used primarily to help differentiate lung disease versus heart disease as the cause of cyanosis.
1. $Paco_2$: generally normal in CHD and elevated in pulmonary parenchymal disease.
2. Hyperoxia test: should be performed on all neonates with suspected CHD.

a. Sample arterial $Po_2$ with infant breathing room air if tolerated. Have the patient breathe 100% oxygen for at least 10 minutes and repeat the arterial $Po_2$. Measurements should be at both pre- and postductal sites (Altman, 2013).
   (1) Umbilical artery sample may detect right-to-left shunts via PDA. The lowered $Pao_2$ is usually a reflection of lung disease and not of primary heart disease.
   (2) Administration of oxygen to infants with cardiac disease resulting in high pulmonary blood flow and CHF will improve oxygen levels (i.e., increased $Pao_2$) through decreased PVR and increased pulmonary blood flow.
   (3) Most accurate assessment of cardiac versus pulmonary disease can be made if the right radial or temporal (preductal) and umbilical artery samples (postductal) are taken simultaneously.
   (4) Monitoring of preductal and postductal transcutaneous oxygen pressure or pulse oximetry provides a noninvasive evaluation for cardiac versus pulmonary disease.

b. Preductal $Pao_2$ will rise to greater than 100 mm Hg with pulmonary disease, whereas an increase to less than 100 mm Hg is consistent with cardiac disease. The response of arterial $Po_2$ in the hyperoxia test should be interpreted in view of the clinical picture (Altman, 2013).

**B. Pulse oximetry is noninvasive and cost-effective.**

1. The combination of pulse oximetry and clinical examination has a sensitivity of 76.5% and specificity of 99.9% in detecting CHD (Mahle et al., 2009).

**C. Chest x-ray examination is used to (Satou, 2013).**

1. Rule out pulmonary parenchymal disease,
2. Identify increased pulmonary vascular markings, as seen in lesions with left-to-right shunting,
3. Evaluate aortic arch, and
4. Evaluate cardiac size, shape, and position.
   a. Cardiomegaly: defined as cardiac/thoracic ratio greater than 0.6.
   b. See Chapter 14 for chest x-ray findings in heart disease.

**D. Electrocardiography (ECG).**

1. Reflects abnormal hemodynamic burdens placed on the heart.
2. Used to determine severity of disease by assessing the degree of atrial or ventricular hypertrophy. Right ventricular predominance is normal shortly after birth. (In utero, the right ventricle does most of the cardiac work.)
3. Changes in ST segments or T waves may suggest myocardial ischemia.
   a. Tall, peaked P waves are common in right-sided heart failure.
   b. Wide, notched P waves are seen with left-sided heart failure.
4. ECG is the major diagnostic tool for evaluating arrhythmias and the impact of electrolyte imbalances (e.g., potassium and calcium) on electrical conductivity.
5. Normal ECG values in term neonates (Flanagan et al., 2005; Kensey et al, 2011):
   a. Heart rate: 120 to 160 bpm in first week.
   b. Normal sinus rhythm: P wave precedes QRS complex.
   c. P wave: duration 0.04 to 0.08 second.
   d. P-R interval: 0.09 to 0.12 second. Prolonged interval is seen in first-degree heart block and is usually benign.
   e. Rightward deviation of the QRS complex with a maximum of −180° and duration of 0.03 to 0.07 second. Prolonged complex indicates interventricular conduction delay.
   f. Occasional Q waves in $V_1$.
   g. Premature infants have higher resting heart rates with greater variation. Duration of P wave is shorter. P-R and QRS intervals are decreased (0.10 and 0.04 second, respectively).

**E. Echocardiography (Prakash et al., 2010).**

1. Provides rapid, noninvasive, and relatively painless evaluation of cardiovascular anatomy and function by use of ultrasonic sound waves. Used to estimate pressures, measure gradients, and evaluate cardiac function. The soft tissue and fluids that comprise the heart provide clear windows for cardiac imaging using echocardiography. Although advances in technology and decrease in size of transducers have increased the sensitivity of echocardiography, it does have some limitations.

a. There are three types of echocardiograms (ECHO).
   (1) Transthoracic echo: most common.
   (2) Transesophageal echo: small transducer is placed in the esophagus in neonates weighing ≥2.5 kg. Used to visualize structures in the posterior chest such as the pulmonary veins. It is also used to guide interventional procedures.
   (3) Fetal echo: conducted on the pregnant mother to examine the fetal heart and major blood vessels for structural defects and arrhythmias prior to birth. A family history of CHD, fetal abnormalities detected during routine obstetric ultrasound, abnormal amniocentesis, abnormal fetal heart rhythm, maternal insulin-dependent diabetes mellitus, and exposure to known teratogens are all indications for a fetal echocardiogram. Detects 30% to 50% of severe CHD before birth (Prakash et al., 2010).
b. M-mode (single-dimension) echocardiography permits evaluation of anatomic relationships of heart and vessels, including relative sizes of each. It is also used to evaluate the motion of the cardiac valves and detect pericardial fluid. Most commonly used to determine ventricular function.
c. Two-dimensional (real-time) echocardiography provides more specific information regarding anatomic relationships. This mode is used to diagnose PDA, or ventricular dysfunction in premature infants.
d. Color-flow Doppler echocardiography shows:
   (1) Patterns of blood flow (i.e., right-to-left vs. left-to-right shunting).
   (2) Location of restrictions and/or regurgitation.
   (3) Direction of motion (i.e., warm colors indicate movement toward the transducer and cool, away from the transducer).
e. Continuous-wave Doppler echocardiography shows the quantity of flow across an obstruction, giving an estimate of pressure gradients, which is beneficial in aortic, pulmonary, and mitral stenosis (Kipps and Silverman, 2005). It is used to detect the direction of shunting, to estimate cardiac output, and to assess ventricular diastolic function.
f. Contrast echocardiography is accomplished by rapid injection of sterile contrast solution, saline or dextrose in water solution in a vein while conducting an ultrasonographic examination. It allows for greater evaluation of flow patterns throughout the heart and identifies the presence of shunts.
g. 3-D echocardiography provides a great number of cross-sectional images. The newest technique in pediatric echocardiography is matrix-array 3-D, which enhances the ability to identify spatial relationships and assess function, and can record a large amount of image data using limited examination times (Parra and Vera, 2012).

**F. Magnetic resonance imaging (MRI):**

1. Three-dimensional, providing high-resolution images of the heart and great vessels. Used in conjunction with echocardiograms and cardiac catheterization to evaluate pulmonary arteries and veins, and systemic veins. It has become the gold standard to quantify mass, volume, and function of both ventricles. Newer modalities that combine both echocardiography and contrast-enhanced MRI are being used to assess ventricular function and volumes (Parra and Vera, 2012).

**G. Cardiac catheterization (Ofori-Amanfo and Cheifetz, 2013):**

1. The focus of this invasive procedure has changed over the past 10 years from a diagnostic modality to an interventional procedure. However, noninterventional cardiac catheterization remains an important tool in presurgical hemodynamic evaluation, and reevaluation of previously repaired defects and biopsies of transplanted hearts to detect rejection.
   a. Measures pulmonary artery pressure, detects pulmonary artery stenosis.
   b. May be used in palliative treatment (e.g., in the use of balloon atrial septostomy to treat TGV).
   c. Radiofrequency perforation of atrial septum and atretic valves.
   d. Balloon valvuloplasty.
   e. Acyanotic heart lesions; catheterization can be delayed until the full effect of medical management of CHF is seen.
   f. Treatment modalities during catheterization include coil placement to close the ductus arteriosus, placement of stents following balloon dilation of stenotic heart valves or

narrow vessels, and implantation of devices to close ASDs and VSDs, valvuloplasty, and recently, percutaneous valve implantation, as well as post–cardiac transplantation biopsy.

2. Procedure: advancement of a catheter through the umbilical, subclavian, femoral, or right internal jugular vessels and into the heart.
   a. If balloon septostomy is anticipated, a large vessel will be needed.
   b. Pressure measurements are made of all chambers and outlet tracts.
3. Concomitant angiography (injection of contrast medium): often performed to achieve maximal cardiac information.
4. Interventional techniques have replaced conventional surgery for many lesions.
   a. Objective is improvement or preservation of cardiac function and improvement in quality and quantity of life.
   b. Common procedures.
      (1) Dilation of valvular lesions (mitral stenosis).
      (2) Balloon valvuloplasty for critical aortic or pulmonary valve stenosis.
      (3) Dilation and stent placement of coarctation of the aorta.
      (4) Dilation and stent placement of pulmonary artery stenosis.
      (5) Balloon atrial septostomy.
      (6) Transcatheter defect occlusion for PDA.
      (7) Catheter-delivered devices for ASD closure and certain muscular VSD closures.
      (8) Percutaneous valve implantation.
5. Complications.
   a. Mortality risk is related to the defect, severity of symptoms, and the patient's condition.
   b. High sodium content of contrast medium contributes to myocardial depression and exerts an osmotic effect, temporarily increasing intravascular volume.
   c. Hemorrhage with catheter insertion or removal may lead to hypotension, shock, and cardiac tamponade if bleeding is in the pericardial sac.
   d. Dysrhythmias are not uncommon (e.g., premature atrial and ventricular beats, heart block, and tachycardia), because of catheter manipulation.
   e. In infants younger than 4 months of age, the rate of nonfatal serious complications is 12%.
   f. Need for increased awareness of a possible link between diagnostic procedures using ionizing radiation and increase in biomarkers of genetic damage for carcinogenesis (Andreassi et al., 2006).

H. **Laboratory data (Kunanithy, 2011).**
1. Arterial blood gases.
   a. Arterial $PO_2$ to confirm central cyanosis.
   b. $PCO_2$ to rule out pulmonary or CNS disorders.
2. Complete blood cell count with differential cell count.
   a. Rules out anemia or polycythemia as cause of CHF.
   b. Decreased number of neutrophils and presence of left shift: possible indication of sepsis. Group B β-hemolytic streptococci can mimic HLHS.
3. Blood glucose concentration. Used to evaluate hypoglycemia as potential cause.
4. Electrolytes (especially potassium and calcium). Both potassium and calcium are major cations in electrical conductivity. Alterations can adversely affect cardiac contractility.

## DEFECTS WITH INCREASED PULMONARY BLOOD FLOW

### Patent Ductus Arteriosus

A. **Incidence:** fourth most common lesion.
1. Isolated PDA in term gestations: 1 per 2000 live births.
2. In preterm gestations (Mezu-Ndubuisi et al., 2012):
   a. Incidence is inversely related to gestational age and weight.
   b. Appears in 30% of infants weighing less than 1500 g at birth.
   c. Is apparent in 40% of infants weighing 751 to 1000 g at birth.
   d. Seen in 50% of infants weighing 500 to 750 g at birth.

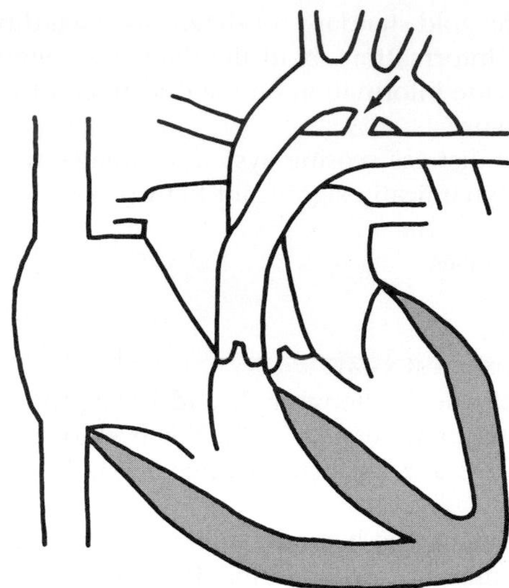

FIGURE 28-7 ■ Patent ductus arteriosus (PDA).

3. Occurs 3 times more commonly in females than in males.

B. **Anatomy:** persistent patency of the ductus arteriosus or failure of the ductus arteriosus to close within 72 hours after birth (Fig. 28-7).
   1. In-utero patency of this structure is functional, diverting blood to the placenta for gas exchange. About 90% of right ventricular outflow is through the ductus arteriosus.
   2. Persistent patency is influenced by several factors.
      a. Improvement in oxygenation causes the pulmonary vascular resistance to drop rapidly. Although increased oxygen tension is a potent stimulant of smooth muscle contraction, which should decrease patency, premature infants have an immature response to oxygen; thus the PDA remains open.
      b. Lack of ductal smooth muscle (e.g., in premature infants) prolongs patency.
      c. Prostaglandins inhibit closure of ductus.

C. **Hemodynamics.**
   1. As PVR falls and SVR rises, a left-to-right shunt via the PDA results in blood flow from the aorta into the pulmonary artery, increasing pulmonary blood flow. The increased pulmonary artery pressure and increased left ventricular pressure and volume lead to bilateral CHF.
   2. Because left-to-right flow is dependent on a drop in PVR, infants with pulmonary disease (e.g., respiratory distress syndrome) will show symptoms when lung disease improves. Before this time, PVR greater than SVR leads to a right-to-left shunt via the patent ductus (commonly referred to as persistent pulmonary hypertension of the neonate).

D. **Clinical manifestations.**
   1. Presents at 4 to 7 days of life with inability to wean from the ventilator or has a need for increased ventilatory and oxygen support. May present with apneic and/or bradycardic spells if not on a ventilator.
      a. Increased pulmonary vasculature and cardiomegaly.
      b. Bounding peripheral pulses and hyperactive precordium.
      c. Widening pulse pressure (>20 mm Hg).
      d. Low diastolic blood pressure.
      e. Unexplained metabolic acidosis.
   2. Continuous murmur may be present at the upper left sternal border but may be "silent" in 10% to 20% of the preterm infants despite hemodynamically significant shunt.
   3. Radiographic findings consist of normal size or mild cardiomegaly (cardiothoracic ratio >0.60), pulmonary edema, and increased pulmonary vascularity. These "typical" signs may be absent if the infant is receiving positive pressure ventilation.

4. Echocardiography is the gold standard for diagnosis. Two-dimensional echocardiography will provide anatomic information about the diameter, length, and shape of the ductus. Doppler flow will provide information on the ductal shunt magnitude and patterns, and pulmonary artery pressure.
5. Clinical cardiovascular distress scoring system evaluates five variables, and score $\geq 3$ is associated with hemodynamically significant PDA (Mezu-Ndubuisi et al., 2012).
   a. Heart rate.
   b. Peripheral arterial pulses.
   c. Precordial pulsations.
   d. Duration of murmur.
   e. Cardiac silhouette on chest x-ray.
6. B-type natriuretic peptide levels between 70 and 100 pg/mL are used to identify a symptomatic PDA (Mezu-Ndubuisi et al., 2012). Some studies have reported specificity of 100% and sensitivity of 93% using a cutoff value of 132.5 pg/mL (Davlouros et al., 2011).

E. **Management.**
1. Dependent on whether shunt is hemodynamically significant. In premature infants, the PDA may prolong ventilator use beyond the dictates of the initial lung disease.
2. Hemodynamically significant ductus arteriosus includes the following:
   a. Heart rate greater than 170 bpm.
   b. Respiratory rate greater than 70/minute.
   c. Hepatomegaly greater than 3 cm below costal margin.
   d. Bounding pulses.
3. Conservative measures are generally employed initially, which may minimize exposure to pharmacologic agents. However, delaying treatment may decrease response to nonsteroidal antiinflammatory drugs (NSAIDs).
   a. Fluid restriction.
   b. Diuretics: used cautiously with fluid restriction, may lead to electrolyte imbalance, dehydration, and caloric deprivation.
   c. Positive end-expiratory pressure: useful in reducing left-to-right shunt via PDA.
4. Medical management using an NSAID that inhibits cyclooxygenase-1 (COX-1) and/or cyclooxygenase-2 (COX-2). Treatment choices are indomethacin and ibuprofen lysine, both manufactured by Ovation Pharmaceuticals, Inc. Ductal recurrence rate may approach 40% (Mezu-Ndubuisi et al., 2012).
   a. Ibuprofen lysine gained U.S. Food and Drug Administration approval in 2006 for treatment of clinically significant PDA in neonates with birth weight 500 to 1500 g and gestational age $\leq 32$ weeks at time medication is given (Overmeire, 2007). Inhibits both COX-1 and COX-2 enzymes but has less COX-1 inhibition than indomethacin.
      (1) Initial dose 10 mg/kg intravenously (IV), followed by two doses of 5 mg/kg IV at 24 and 48 hours after the first dose.
      (2) Significantly lower incidence of oliguria as compared to indomethacin (Hermes-DeSantis and Aranda, 2007).
      (3) Does not decrease cerebral blood flow (Corff and Sekar, 2007).
      (4) Does not reduce mesenteric blood flow (Capparelli, 2007).
      (5) According to Aranda and Thomas (2005), ibuprofen lysine is equally safe and effective as indomethacin, with maintenance of cerebral, mesenteric, and renal blood flow favoring ibuprofen lysine.
      (6) Monitor serum creatinine, blood urea nitrogen, platelet count, and urine output during treatment course.
   b. Indomethacin management includes the following:
      (1) As a prostaglandin inhibitor, indomethacin can constrict and close the PDA in some premature infants.
      (2) Initial dosage is 0.2 mg/kg IV, followed by 2 doses of 0.1 mg/kg IV every 12 to 24 hours, for a total of three doses (Corff, 2007).
      (3) Prophylactic treatment in the extremely low birth weight premature neonate in the first 24 hours after birth showed a decrease in intraventricular hemorrhage when compared to placebo (Markham, 2006).

(4) Complications related to indomethacin being a stronger COX-1 inhibitor are as follows:
   (a) Transient oliguria and decreased renal blood flow.
   (b) Increased incidence of gastrointestinal bleeding.
   (c) Inhibition of platelet aggregation for 7 to 9 days, with potential for intracerebral hemorrhage.

(5) Contraindications are (Corff, 2007):
   (a) Renal failure (blood urea nitrogen concentration >30 mg/dL, serum creatinine concentration >1.8 mg/dL, urine output <0.5 mL/kg/hr).
   (b) Active bleeding or platelet count < 50,000.
   (c) Suspected necrotizing enterocolitis.
   (d) Thrombocytopenia.
   (e) Sepsis: suspected or proven.

5. Paracetamol is a new drug that has been trialed in patients in Turkey who have failed to respond to ibuprofen (Oncel et al., 2013).
6. Surgical management: ligation of the PDA should be reserved for those patients with need for escalating respiratory support or inotrope-dependent hypotension (Clyman, 2012).
   a. Standard approach is surgical ligation via posterolateral thoracotomy incision risk.
   b. New techniques include placement of a stainless-steel spring coil or Amplatzer PDA occlusion device via interventional cardiac catheterization, with complete occlusion rates of approximately 90% at 24 hours after the procedure and 98% at 6 months. Minimally invasive video-assisted thoracoscopic surgery allows for PDA closure using two titanium clips that are placed using a trocar (Dutta and Albanese, 2006).

F. **Prognosis:** Surgical mortality is less than 1%. If the defect is asymptomatic or medically or surgically ligated, prognosis is excellent, but there is now some evidence that surgical ligation is a morbidity by itself (Clyman, 2012).

## Ventricular Septal Defect

A. **Incidence:** At 2 per 1000 live births, VSDs are the most common of all CHDs, accounting for almost 50% (Altman, 2013).

B. **Anatomy:** Abnormal opening in the septum between the right and left ventricles. Sizes range from pinhole to almost complete absence of the ventricular septum (Fig. 28-8).

C. **Hemodynamics.**
   1. The degree of hypertrophy of ventricles and the pressure relationships are dependent on the size of the defect. A small defect allows pressure differences between ventricles.

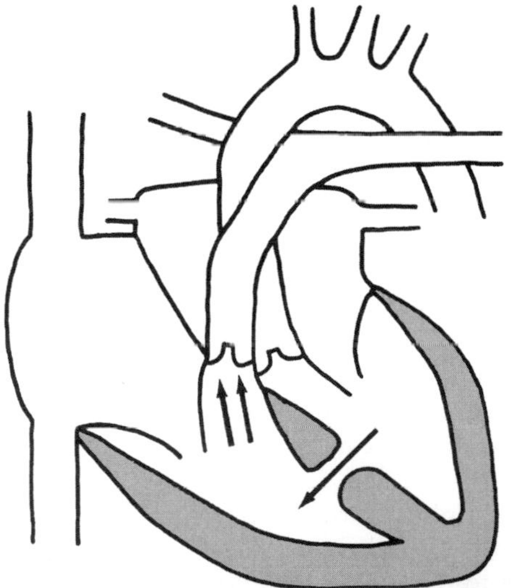

FIGURE 28-8 ■ Ventricular septal defect (VSD).

2. PVR less than SVR results in a left-to-right shunt, producing increased pulmonary blood flow and leading to decreased pulmonary compliance and pulmonary edema.
3. Excessive pulmonary artery blood flow eventually results in pulmonary artery hypertrophy and stenosis.
4. High pulmonary artery pressure can delay maturation of pulmonary arterioles.

D. **Clinical manifestations.**
1. Size dependent.
2. Small VSD.
   a. Asymptomatic.
   b. High-pitched pansystolic murmur along the left sternal border 4 to 10 days after birth.
3. Moderate VSD: asymptomatic except for murmur, fatigue with feeding, and recurrent respiratory infections.
4. Large VSD.
   a. Present at 1 to 2 months of age with CHF, hepatomegaly, recurrent pulmonary infections, and increased precordial activity.
   b. Loud, blowing pansystolic murmur at the left lower sternal border.
   c. Chest x-ray examination: cardiomegaly and increased pulmonary vascular markings.
   d. Two-dimensional echocardiography is capable of identifying 90% of VSDs. Doppler and/or color-flow mapping increases the accuracy of diagnosis of VSD. Color flow is extremely useful in identifying multiple VSDs and the direction of blood flow across the VSD.

E. **Management.**
1. Fifty percent to 75% of small defects will close spontaneously; 20% of large defects become smaller or close.
2. Plasma B-type natriuretic peptide is useful in the diagnosis of CHF in pediatrics (Davlouros et al, 2011). With mild CHF, treatment consists of digoxin and diuretics.
3. Surgery is indicated if patient has failure to thrive or intractable CHF.
   a. Palliative: surgical banding of pulmonary artery to reduce pulmonary blood flow, decrease CHF, and prevent pulmonary vascular resistance.
   b. Surgical: repair by suturing defect or patching defect through a median sternotomy. The defect is approached via the right atrium and tricuspid valve through ventriculotomy. Indicated when closure is necessary in the first 6 to 12 months of life. If the infant is less than 2000 g, it may be necessary to perform pulmonary artery banding to decrease blood flow to the lungs. Surgical closure is then done when the infant is greater than 2000 g. Newer approaches include a combination of surgery with cardiopulmonary bypass, echocardiography, and intraoperative device placement in multiple and complex muscular VSDs (Mo et al., 2011).
   c. Transcatheter devices such as the clamshell, double-umbrella, and buttoned devices, and patch may be used (Webb et al., 2011).

F. **Prognosis:** excellent. Mortality rate is less than 5% in infants. Complications from surgical closure may include right bundle-branch block, third-degree heart block, and aortic and/or tricuspid insufficiency. Earlier surgical repair, rather than palliative banding with delayed repair, is associated with better results. If VSD remains open with a large left-to-right shunt after 9 months of age, complications may result in pulmonary vascular disease (Tao et al., 2010).

## Atrial Septal Defect

A. **Incidence:** 1 per 5000 live births, 7% to 10% of all cardiac defects. Female to male ratio 2:1.

B. **Anatomy:** defect in formation of septum, resulting in a communication between right and left atria. Defect may be an ostium primum defect, an ostium secundum defect (most common), or a partial endocardial cushion defect (Fig. 28-9). By definition, a patent foramen ovale is generally excluded, although symptoms can be the same.

C. **Hemodynamics.**
1. Immediately after birth, right ventricular pressure is greater than left ventricle pressure, so there is no shunt or only a small right-to-left shunt.
2. As PVR decreases, left-to-right shunt develops with concomitant right ventricular volume overload and hypertrophy.

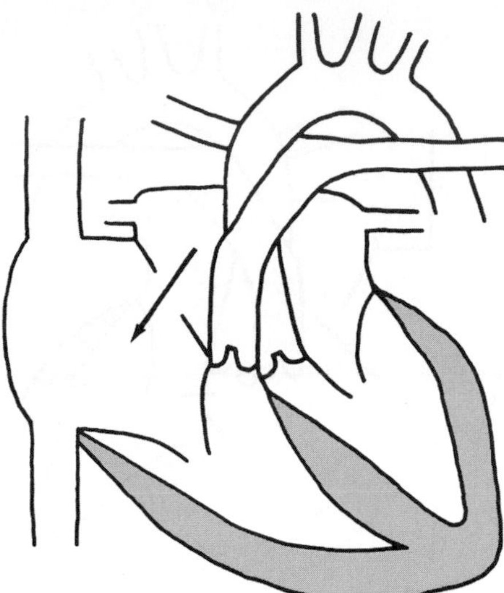

FIGURE 28-9 ■ Atrial septal defect (ASD).

D. **Clinical manifestations.**
 1. The isolated defect is generally asymptomatic and unrecognized. If ASD is diagnosed in infancy, greater than 50% of the patients will be symptomatic.
 2. CHF from left-to-right shunt with mitral valve insufficiency.
 3. Failure to thrive.
 4. Recurrent respiratory infections.
 5. Systolic murmur at the second intercostal space at the left sternal border, persistent split $S_2$ if shunt is large, diastolic murmur heard at the left lower sternal border.
 6. Chest x-ray examination: increased pulmonary vascular markings with enlarged right atrium and ventricle (Kensey et al, 2011).

E. **Management.**
 1. If defect is small, clinical follow-up is indicated; the defect may close spontaneously.
 2. ASD with CHF: medical treatment of CHF and delay surgical repair.
 3. ASD with intractable CHF or if defect is very large or lacks significant borders for positioning of closure device: early surgical repair (i.e., suturing or patching of defect).
 4. Surgical repair is done by placement of a patch using the patient's own pericardium, a bovine pericardium, Gore-Tex, or Dacron. All surgical repairs are done with the patient on cardiopulmonary bypass. Complications include residual shunting, arrhythmias, and embolization of the device (American Heart Association, 2008).
 5. Transcatheter closure devices are now commonly used for ASD closure. Device sizes range from 6 to 48 mm. The larger the device, the larger the infant needs to be. Implantation of the device is guided by transthoracic echocardiography. One type of device has two sides, with one side of the device placed on the left side of the septum and the other on the right, which forms a sandwich over the defect. This acts as a framework for normal tissue to grow over the defect (Chen et al., 2012).

F. **Prognosis.**
 1. Spontaneous closure occurs in up to 20% of ASDs during the first year of life.
 2. If left unrepaired, lifetime mortality risk is 25% (Moake and Ramaciotti, 2005).
 3. Perioperative mortality rate is less than 1%, with good long-term results in survivors. Survival at 5 years of age is 97% and at 10 years, 95% (Chen et al., 2012).

## Endocardial Cushion Defect (Atrioventricular Canal)

A. **Incidence:** 1 per 9000 live births. Most common heart defect found in Down syndrome.

B. **Anatomy.**

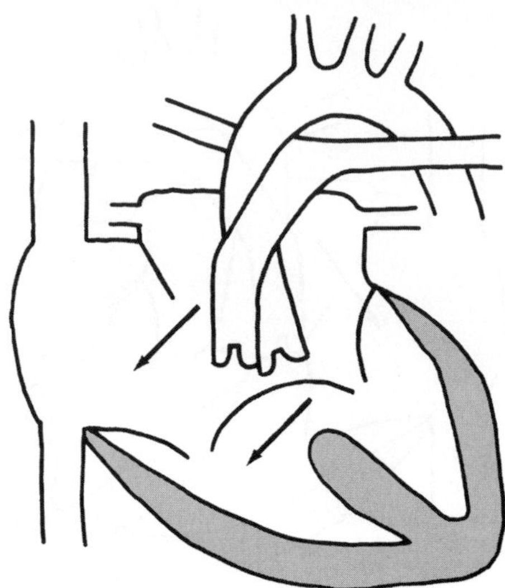

FIGURE 28-10 ■ Atrioventricular canal (AVC).

1. Endocardial cushions form the lower portion of the atrial septum, the upper portion of the ventricular septum, and septal portions of the mitral and tricuspid valves.
2. A wide range of defects is possible, from simple cleft of the mitral and/or tricuspid valves to complete absence of the lower atrial and upper ventricular septa with common atrioventricular valve (i.e., atrioventricular canal) (Fig. 28-10).

C. **Hemodynamics.**
   1. With PVR less than SVR, blood dependently shunts left to right via the ASD and the VSD.
   2. Higher pressure of the left ventricle creates obligatory left-to-right shunting via the atrioventricular valve (atrioventricular valve regurgitation). Blood flows from the left ventricle to the mitral portion of the atrioventricular valve to the left atrium to the ASD, and to the right atrium.

D. **Clinical manifestations.**
   1. Isolated ostium primum atrial defect: rarely identified in the neonatal period.
   2. Isolated ventricular defect: see clinical features of VSD.
   3. Complete atrioventricular canal.
      a. Atrioventricular valve regurgitation controls age at presentation.
         (1) Severe: seen at 1 to 2 weeks of age with CHF.
         (2) Valves competent: seen in first or second month of life.
      b. Respiratory distress.
      c. Active precordium, with a thrill at the left lower sternal border.
      d. Variable murmurs; usually loud pansystolic murmur at the lower left sternal border, radiating to left back.
      e. Recurrent respiratory infections.
      f. Chest x-ray examination: cardiomegaly, bilateral atrial and ventricular hypertrophy, increased pulmonary markings.

E. **Management.**
   1. Objective: avoid development of pulmonary vascular obstructive disease.
   2. Medical management: prevent or control CHF with digoxin and diuretics.
   3. Palliative pulmonary artery banding to decrease pulmonary overload. Does not influence obligatory shunting of the atrioventricular valve.
   4. Pulmonary artery banding with later repair is an alternative strategy to primary repair with closure of atrial and ventricular septal defects and mitral and tricuspid valve reconstruction (Dhannapuneni et al., 2011). If complete atrioventricular canal, surgery is done before 6 months of age; if partial, surgery is done between 6 and 12 months.

F. **Prognosis.**
   1. Prognosis is dependent on details of anatomic form and on the presence of significant associated noncardiac anomalies and significant pulmonary obstructive vascular disease.
   2. Best results are seen with ostium primum defect or common atrium; long-term prognosis is good.
   3. Outlook for complete atrioventricular canal without operation is poor.
   4. Mortality rate for surgical repair is under 5%. A 4% incidence in repeat surgery within the first 6 months was needed for left atrioventricular residual regurgitation (Atz et al., 2011).

## OBSTRUCTIVE DEFECTS WITH PULMONARY VENOUS CONGESTION

### Coarctation of the Aorta

A. **Incidence:** 7% of congenital heart lesions (Punukollo et al., 2011).
   1. Most common presentation between 5 and 14 days of life.
   2. Male dominance: 2:1.
   3. Thirty percent of those with Turner's syndrome will have this defect.
B. **Anatomy:** constriction of aorta at the junction or the transverse aortic arch or the vicinity of the ductus arteriosus (Fig. 28-11).
   1. Most common site is below the origin of the left subclavian artery.
   2. Preductal coarctation is associated with hypoplasia of the aortic arch. Defects such as VSD, PDA, and transposition of the great arteries will be found in 40%.
   3. Up to 60% of infants with coarctation will have a bicuspid aortic valve.
C. **Hemodynamics.**
   1. Isolated coarctation: obstruction to left ventricular outflow, leading to increased left ventricular, left atrial, and pulmonary venous pressures. Pulmonary venous congestion develops.
   2. Coarctation with VSD: elevated left ventricular pressure, shunting blood left to right via VSD and causing pulmonary overload.
   3. Preductal coarctation: dependent on PDA for distal aorta and lower body blood flow.
D. **Clinical manifestations.**
   1. CHF as a result of pressure overload on the left ventricle.
      a. If severe, will result in cardiovascular collapse after ductus closes.
   2. Decreased or absent pulses in the lower extremities in 92%.
   3. Lower extremities cool to touch.
   4. Higher blood pressure (>15 mm Hg) in upper extremities is the most consistent factor in critical coarctation and is present in 97%. If blood pressures are lower in the upper extremities, the following applies:

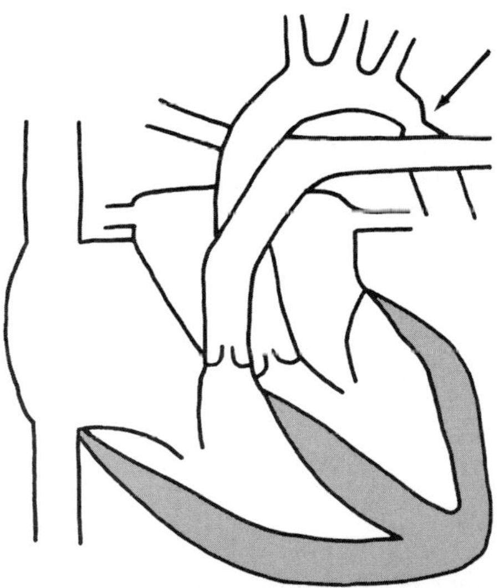

FIGURE 28-11 ■ Coarctation of aorta.

   a. Decreased blood pressure in left arm: indicative of left subclavian artery as site of coarctation.
   b. Decreased blood pressure in right arm: right subclavian artery arises below coarctation (rare).
   c. Pulses that "wax and wane": related to increase or decrease in PDA blood flow.
5. Heart sounds.
   a. Postductal: no murmur or short systolic ejection click in axilla or back.
   b. Preductal with VSD: harsh pansystolic murmur at the left lower sternal border.
   c. Gallop rhythm possible.
6. Systolic thrill heard at the suprasternal notch.
7. Chest x-ray examination: enlarged heart with left ventricular hypertrophy and increased pulmonary vascular markings.
8. Transthoracic echocardiography is the standard tool used to detect coarctation of the aorta and has a sensitivity of 91%.
9. MRI to determine the location of the coarctation and whether it affects any other vessels (Mayo Clinic Staff, 2006).
10. Cardiac catheterization is diagnostic and usually performed prior to surgical management to evaluate for other anomalies.

E. **Management.**
   1. Aggressive medical management of CHF.
   2. Prostaglandin $E_1$ ($PGE_1$) to dilate ductus arteriosus (preductal lesion).
      a. Dose: 0.05 to 0.1 mcg/kg/min IV infusion, titrate dose.
      b. Response: Ductus arteriosus will reopen 30 to 120 minutes after infusion starts.
      c. Adverse effects: apnea, fever, hypotension.
   3. Palliative balloon angioplasty in critically ill neonates has been documented in infants less than 1000 g (Dryzek et al., 2012).
   4. Isolated postductal coarctation: control of CHF first, then delayed surgical correction.
   5. Correction: three common repairs.
      a. Balloon angioplasty to open the narrowing.
         (1) Has highest rate of injury to the aortic wall.
      b. Percutaneous stent placement has lower acute complications (Forbes et al., 2011).
         (1) More likely to need reintervention.
      c. Surgical correction.
         (1) Either resection of abnormal segment and reanastomosis, or
         (2) Subclavian patch across area of obstruction.

F. **Prognosis.**
   1. Outcome is dependent on complexity of coarctation, with mortality rates at 1 month ranging from zero for simple coarctation to 10%; can be higher for complex coarctation associated with VSD or other left-sided obstruction (Reade et al., 2006).
   2. Long-term prognosis after coarctation repair is determined by the presence of residual or recurrent coarctation, persistence of pulmonary hypertension, and residual cardiovascular lesions (Sakurai et al., 2012).
      a. Incidence of recurrence of 5% to 10% after midline sternotomy approach resection and end-to-end anastomosis has been reported after repair in infancy (Sakurai et al., 2012).
      b. Overall surgical mortality is less than 5% in infancy; however, earlier detection and use of $PGE_1$ has reduced mortality.
      c. The most common complication is hypertension.

## Aortic Stenosis

A. **Incidence:** 1 per 24,000 live births, accounts for 5% to 6% of all cardiac anomalies.
   1. Four times more likely in males.

B. **Anatomy:** may be subvalvular, valvular, or supravalvular, with valvular stenosis being the most common form. The myocardium of the left ventricle is hypertrophied (Fig. 28-12).
   1. Valvular stenosis usually has a bicuspid aortic valve.
   2. Supravalvular stenosis is the least common and is seen with Williams syndrome.

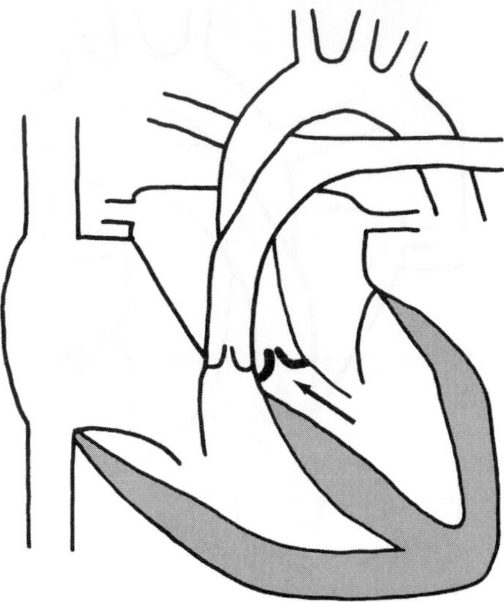

FIGURE 28-12 ■ Aortic stenosis.

C. **Hemodynamics:** Obstruction to left ventricular outflow leads to increased left ventricular pressures and hypertrophy. If aortic stenosis is severe in utero, blood flow through the ventricle is decreased, resulting in left ventricular hypoplasia and left-sided heart syndrome.

D. **Clinical manifestations.**
   1. Usually asymptomatic at birth (Kensey et al, 2011).
   2. Acrocyanosis.
   3. Heart sounds include a grade II to IV/VI harsh systolic murmur in upper right sternal border, radiating to the neck and lower left sternal border.
   4. Suprasternal notch thrill may be present.
   5. CHF symptoms may be delayed by weeks but progress rapidly after onset.
   6. Chest x-ray examination shows cardiomegaly with normal pulmonary vascular markings.
   7. If critical aortic stenosis is present, sudden deterioration is likely.

E. **Management.**
   1. Medical management is usually not successful.
   2. Initially, CHF is treated with fluid restriction, diuretics, digoxin, acidosis management, and antibiotic prophylaxis.
   3. If stenosis is critical, use $PGE_1$ to prevent hypoxia.
   4. The treatment of choice in neonates is balloon valvuloplasty. Early mortality rate is 5%. However, 20% will develop significant aortic insufficiency at 2 years (Rossi et al., 2011).
   5. Surgery is reserved for patients who fail balloon valvuloplasty and involves open aortic valvotomy or valve replacement, with mortality less than 10% (Hraska et al., 2012). The number of aortic valvotomies has declined substantially since balloon valvuloplasty has gained favor.
   6. The modified Ross–Konno procedure may be used in children with complex left ventricular outflow obstruction (Fadel et al., 2013).

F. **Prognosis.**
   1. Success rate of balloon valvuloplasty is very high.
   2. Aortic stenosis accounts for 1% of all sudden death in children with heart disease.

## OBSTRUCTIVE DEFECTS WITH DECREASED PULMONARY BLOOD FLOW

### Tetralogy of Fallot

A. **Incidence:** 1 per 5000 live births. Most common cyanotic heart lesion, accounting for 10% of all defects.

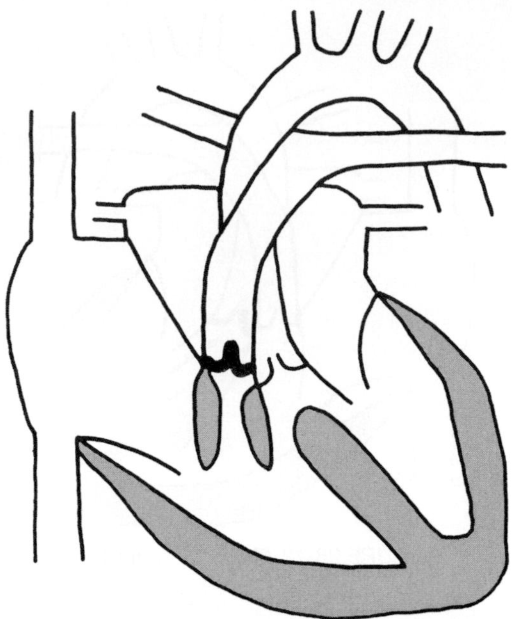

FIGURE 28-13 ■ Tetralogy of Fallot (TOF).

B. **Anatomy:** classified as a combination of four defects, although numbers 3 and 4, below, are consequences of numbers 1 and 2, below (Fig. 28-13).
   1. Pulmonary stenosis: obstruction of outflow tract.
   2. VSD.
   3. Aorta overriding VSD.
   4. Right ventricular hypertrophy.

C. **Hemodynamics.**
   1. Dependent primarily on degree of pulmonary stenosis and to a lesser extent on VSD size.
   2. In severe pulmonary stenosis, blood flow passes from right to left via the VSD, with resulting hypoxia and cyanosis.
   3. In mild pulmonary stenosis, blood flows from left to right via the VSD, with CHF resulting.
   4. In mild to moderate pulmonary stenosis, blood flow via the VSD may be minimal as long as PVR and SVR are balanced. With crying, right-to-left shunting occurs.

D. **Clinical manifestations.**
   1. Presentation is a function of the degree of pulmonary stenosis.
   2. Severe obstruction presents in the first days of life with severe cyanosis, hypoxia, and dyspnea.
   3. Milder pulmonary obstruction presents in the first days of life with mild cyanosis.
   4. Harsh grades II to IV/VI systolic murmur with thrill present at mid- to upper left sternal border.
   5. Chest x-ray examination shows normal-sized boot-shaped heart with normal or decreased pulmonary vascular markings.
   6. Traditional "Tet spells" (paroxysmal dyspnea and severe cyanosis) are common in infants and can occur in neonates.

E. **Management.**
   1. Medical (Kensey et al, 2011).
      a. Propranolol is the drug of choice for treating hypercyanotic infants.
      b. $PGE_1$ is used to maintain patency of the ductus arteriosus until the infant can be taken to surgery in severe TOF.
   2. Corrective surgery involves closure of the VSD with a patch and eliminating the pulmonary stenosis by resection. The pulmonary outflow tract may be enlarged by a patch. This procedure is done while the infant is on cardiopulmonary bypass. Controversy still remains over the best approach in neonates (Kanter et al., 2010).

a. Surgical correction is now preferred before 6 months of age (Habib et al., 2010).
b. If the neonate has severe pulmonary stenosis or atresia, a Blalock–Taussig procedure is generally performed, with full correction at a later time (Ahmad et al., 2007).
c. Primary total repair has been done on infants under the age of 3 months with no increase in number of reinterventions and may be better for pulmonary artery growth than staged repair (Park et al., 2010).

**F. Prognosis.**

1. Prognosis without surgery is very poor. Mortality rate in infancy is about 6% in those with palliation.
2. Complications/residual effects include arrhythmias, decreased or absent pulses in affected arm, inadequate shunt, and CHF resulting from large shunt.
3. Postoperative mortality for complete repair is about 8%. This rate increases with the more severe forms of TOF.

## Pulmonary Stenosis

**A. Incidence:** 1 per 14,000 live births, 5% to 8% of all CHDs.

**B. Anatomy:** narrowed opening either in pulmonary valve as a consequence of pulmonary valve cusp fusions (Fig. 28-14) or above or below the valve because of tissue hypertrophy.

**C. Hemodynamics.**

1. In utero, right ventricular hypoplasia can develop, depending on the degree of pulmonary valve stenosis and subsequent decrease in right ventricular blood flow.
2. After birth, the combination of right ventricular hypoplasia and severe pulmonary valve stenosis redirects blood flow from right to left at the atrial level via the foramen ovale. Pulmonary blood becomes dependent on a left-to-right flow via the PDA.
3. In mild stenosis, the pulmonary blood flow is not excessively restricted and is PDA independent. As PVR decreases, atrial right-to-left shunt will decrease, improving systemic hypoxia.

**D. Clinical manifestations.**

1. Mild pulmonary stenosis: loud systolic murmur at left upper sternal border is the only finding.
2. Moderately severe stenosis.
   a. Murmur is less prominent. Murmur of tricuspid insufficiency may be noted.
   b. Cyanosis is present and increases with PDA closure.
   c. Generally, hepatomegaly is present.
3. Chest x-ray examination: mild cardiomegaly with bulging right heart border and decreased pulmonary vascular markings.

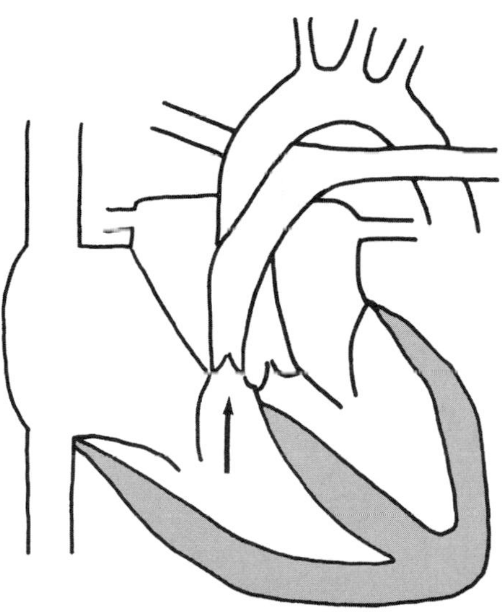

FIGURE 28-14 ■ Pulmonary stenosis (PS).

4. Two-dimensional echocardiography used to make anatomic and physiologic diagnosis (Wechsler and Wernovsky, 2004).

E. **Management.**
   1. Cyanotic neonate.
      a. Initial management: oxygen, bicarbonate, and $PGE_1$.
      b. Nonsurgical treatment with transcatheter balloon valvuloplasty.
         (1) Few complications; effective.
         (2) Treatment of choice for most lesions.
         (3) Is 96% successful in neonatal patients (Holzer et al., 2012).
      c. Surgical valvotomy or tissue excision is reserved for specific cases or when valvuloplasty fails and patient is symptomatic.
   2. Noncyanotic neonate: conservative management includes catheterization at 6 to 12 months if stenosis is severe, with subsequent surgery if right ventricular pressure exceeds systemic.

F. **Prognosis:** excellent. Operative mortality rate for valvuloplasty is less than 1%.

## Pulmonary Atresia

A. **Incidence:** 1 per 14,000 live births, accounting for less than 1% of cardiac defects.

B. **Anatomy:** complete obstruction of the pulmonic valve, resulting in a hypoplastic right ventricle and tricuspid valve (Fig. 28-15). In the presence of a VSD, the right ventricle may be of adequate size.

C. **Hemodynamics.**
   1. Venous blood returning to the right atrium goes across the foramen ovale into the left atrium, into the left ventricle, and out the aorta.
   2. Blood flow to the lungs is derived entirely from a left-to-right shunt at the ductus arteriosus, which is generally small and tortuous. As the PDA closes, severe hypoxemia ensues.
   3. Regurgitant blood flow occurs at the tricuspid valve.

D. **Clinical manifestations.**
   1. Mild cyanosis at birth, progressing to intense cyanosis by 24 hours.
   2. Tachypnea.
   3. Heart sounds.
      a. PDA murmur is present.
      b. Soft systolic murmur is heard at the upper left sternal border, and harsh systolic murmur at the lower right and upper left sternal border if tricuspid insufficiency is present.
   4. Chest x-ray examination shows increased heart size with decreased pulmonary markings. Right atrial hypertrophy is seen in 70%.

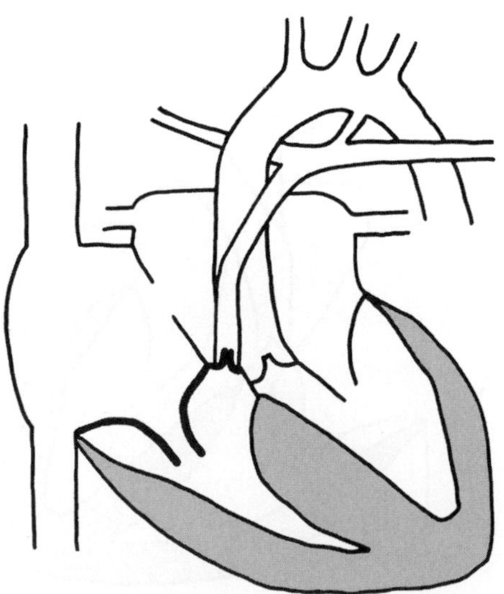

FIGURE 28-15 ■ Pulmonary atresia.

5. Two-dimensional echocardiography with Doppler and color-flow mapping and 3-D echocardiography are used to determine absence of blood flow across the pulmonary valve and are standard for diagnosis (Parra and Vera, 2012).

E. **Management.**
1. Initial treatment is use of oxygen and bicarbonate for metabolic acidosis and $PGE_1$ to maintain patency of the ductus arteriosus.
2. Cardiac catheterization is done with balloon atrial septostomy in infants with pulmonary atresia.
3. Balloon valvuloplasty with or without stent placement is used in small neonates and infants (Chubb et al., 2012).
4. Percutaneous valve placement is a newer treatment option with favorable outcomes (Balzer, 2012).
5. Mild right ventricle hypertrophy: surgical valvotomy may be effective.
6. With severe hyperplasia of right ventricle and tricuspid valve, usually a Blalock–Taussig shunt to provide systemic-to-pulmonary shunting in the neonatal period that may be converted at 3 to 6 months to a bidirectional Glenn procedure. These infants will later require definitive repair via completion of the Fontan procedure, resulting in communication between the right atrium and pulmonary artery. Closure of ASD or VSD is done at this time (Zahorec et al., 2011).

F. **Prognosis.**
1. Without surgery, the mortality rate is 100%. If reconstruction of the right ventricular outflow tract is needed and the ductus arteriosus is closed, the mortality rate is 25%.
2. Long-term complications are arrhythmias, CHF, and sudden death.
3. Increased mortality following Blalock–Taussig shunt with ductal closure is noted.

## Tricuspid Atresia

A. **Incidence:** 1 per 18,000 live births. Most are diagnosed prenatally via ultrasound and fetal echocardiography.

B. **Anatomy:** agenesis of the tricuspid valve development with associated patent foramen ovale or ASD (Fig. 28-16).
1. VSD is often associated with the hypoplastic right ventricle.
2. Pulmonary atresia or stenosis typically present.
3. TGV occurs in 30% of the cases.

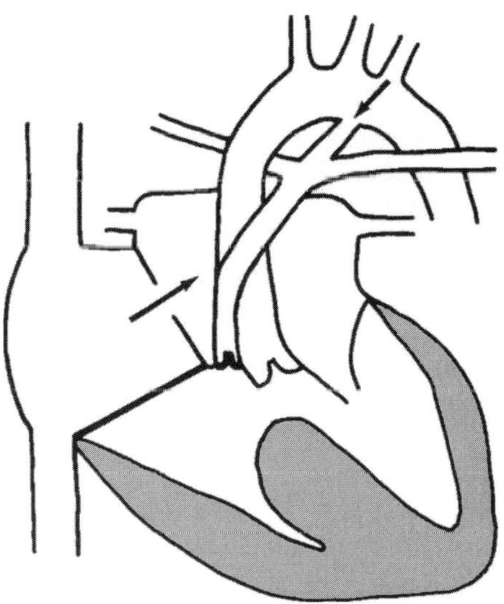

FIGURE 28-16 ■ Tricuspid atresia. *Arrows* identify shunting through the patent foramen ovale and the patent ductus arteriosus.

C. **Hemodynamics.**
   1. Systemic venous blood is shunted from the right atrium across the foramen ovale or ASD into the left atrium. With an isolated defect, the pulmonary blood flow is supplied by the left ventricular outflow via the PDA.
   2. In the presence of a VSD, some of the blood entering the left ventricle shunts across into the hypoplastic right ventricle and out the pulmonary artery—or out the aorta in the case of coexisting transposition. If severe pulmonary stenosis or atresia is present, blood does not flow through the VSD (see also item C.1, above).

D. **Clinical manifestations.**
   1. Cyanosis usually presents soon after birth with an isolated defect or coexisting VSD and pulmonary outflow tract obstruction. Increasing cyanosis occurs with closure of the ductus.
   2. Dyspnea; tachypnea may be present.
   3. CHF ensues with large VSD and absent pulmonary stenosis, usually within the first month of life.
   4. Murmur is absent unless associated with pulmonary stenosis, VSD, or PDA.
   5. Chest x-ray examination shows variable heart size, depending on the degree of pulmonary stenosis; size is generally nondiagnostic.
   6. Cardiac catheterization to perform a balloon septostomy to improve intra-atrial mixing of blood.

E. **Management.**
   1. Primary treatment: oxygen, bicarbonate, and $PGE_1$ for severe hypoxia.
   2. Palliative treatment.
      a. Systemic-to-pulmonary artery shunt, including Blalock–Taussig procedure.
      b. Large VSD with no pulmonary stenosis: pulmonary artery banding is performed to control CHF.
   3. Reparative surgery.
      a. Right atrium is connected to either the right ventricular outflow tract or the pulmonary artery (Fontan or modified Fontan procedure), so that the right atrium forces blood into the lungs. Closure of the ASD and VSD is done at this time if they are present.
      b. Modified Fontan procedure separates oxygenated and unoxygenated blood inside the heart but does not restore normal hemodynamics or anatomy.
      c. Bidirectional Glenn procedure on or off cardiopulmonary bypass is a safe alternative (LaPar et al., 2012).

F. **Prognosis:** Survival is 82% at 1 year, 75% at 5 years, and 70% at 20 years. Complications include heart failure, persistent shunts, and dysrhythmias.

# MIXED DEFECTS

## Transposition of the Great Vessels

A. **Incidence:** 1 per 5000 live births; male predominance, 2:1. Most common cardiac cause of cyanosis in neonates (Thammineni et al., 2011).

B. **Anatomy:** positions of the great arteries are reversed (i.e., the pulmonary artery arises from the left ventricle and the aorta from the right ventricle). Without other intracardiac defects (e.g., VSD, ASD), an independent, parallel circuit exists (Fig. 28-17). In dextroposition (D-presentation), the aorta is situated to the left of the pulmonary artery.

C. **Hemodynamics.**
   1. Oxygenated blood returns from the lungs to enter the left atrium and ventricle, then recirculates to the lungs by way of the pulmonary artery.
   2. Unoxygenated blood returns to the right atrium and ventricle and is returned through the aorta to the body.
   3. Mixing of oxygenated and unoxygenated blood occurs at the ductus arteriosus (as long as patency exists) or through any existing septal defects (ASD, VSD).
      a. Mixing is required for survival.
      b. Shunting occurs from left to right through septal defects or the PDA, ameliorating the degree of cyanosis and hypoxia.

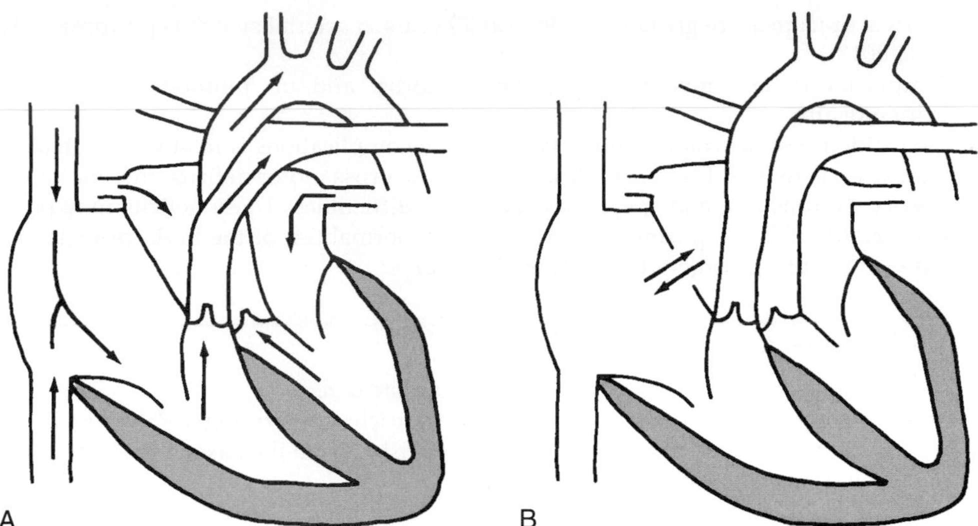


FIGURE 28-17 ■ Transposition of great vessels (TGV). **A**, Normal anatomy. **B**, Appearance of heart with TGV.

**D. Clinical manifestations.**

1. Cyanosis is present within the first 24 hours of life and becomes progressively more intense.
2. Prominent murmurs are uncommon; VSD (if present) will have a loud murmur.
3. Chest x-ray findings are usually normal; the heart may have an "egg-on-a-string" appearance. Pulmonary vasculature may be increased or decreased.
4. Echocardiography is the standard diagnostic test, with speckle tracking echocardiography to determine myocardial segment contraction timing (Parra and Vera, 2012).

**E. Management: TGA is a cardiac emergency.**

1. Correction of metabolic acidosis.
2. $PGE_1$ to maintain patency of the PDA until palliative surgery can be performed (Hiremath et al., 2011).
3. Palliation of choice: catheter-introduced balloon atrial septostomy.
   a. Balloon catheter is inserted into the femoral or umbilical vein; it is advanced across the foramen ovale into the left atrium. The balloon is inflated and pulled across the atrium, creating an ASD.
   b. Procedure rapidly improves systemic and pulmonary circulation admixing, thus increasing $Pa{O_2}$ (40s) and saturation (80s).
4. Blade septostomy: if balloon septostomy is unsuccessful, surgical excision of the posterior aspect of the septum is done during cardiac catheterization (Kensey et al., 2011; Lott, 2014) technique, and a hole is excised in the atrial septum.
5. Pulmonary artery banding: to prevent pulmonary vascular disease, to decrease CHF, or to exercise the left ventricle before surgery by increasing the ventricular workload.
6. Corrective surgery.
   a. Arterial switch operation (Jatene procedure) is the treatment of choice: detaches aorta, coronary arteries, and pulmonary artery, reattaching to correct ventricles. Procedure is generally performed within the first 2 weeks of life and provides both anatomic and physiologic correction.
   b. Mustard or Senning procedure: creates a baffle at the atrium to divert systemic venous blood into the left ventricle and pulmonary artery and pulmonary venous blood into the right ventricle and aorta.
   c. Rastelli procedure: intraventricular repair combined with placement of an extracardiac shunt from the right ventricle to the pulmonary artery. Used for TGV with large VSD and extensive left ventricular outflow tract obstruction.

**F. Prognosis.**

1. Without surgery, 90% will die within the first year.

2. Survival outcomes are greater than 98% at 20 years, if arterial switch is performed (Khairy et al., 2013).
3. Complications are myocardial ischemia, aortic and/or pulmonary stenosis, and sudden death.
4. The incidence of neurologic and developmental complications is relatively high after neonatal arterial switch. These complications include gross motor deficits, fine motor deficits, sensory dysfunction, and speech and language difficulties. These deficits may be a combined result of the hypoxemia before repair, abnormalities of the brain prior to surgery, and events during surgery (Tabbutt et al., 2012).

## Truncus Arteriosus

A. **Incidence:** 1 per 33,000 live births, 1% to 2% of cardiac defects.
B. **Anatomy:** a single great artery arises from both ventricles, overriding a VSD (Fig. 28-18).
   1. Type I: most common, short pulmonary artery arising from the base of the common trunk, then divides into the right and left arteries.
   2. Type II: right and left pulmonary arteries arise from the posterior surface of the common trunk.
   3. Type III: right and left pulmonary arteries have separate origins in the lateral walls of the common trunk (Jones et al., 2006).
C. **Hemodynamics.**
   1. Both ventricles pump blood into the common trunk supplying the systemic and pulmonary circulation. As PVR drops, preferential shunting to the pulmonary circulation occurs, increasing blood flow to the lungs and workload of the left ventricle.
   2. If pulmonary arteries are stenotic or hypoplastic, blood flow to the lungs is restricted.
D. **Clinical manifestations.**
   1. CHF with bounding pulses and widened pulse pressure.
   2. Intermittent cyanosis: severe cyanosis with pulmonary artery stenosis.
   3. Heart sounds: harsh systolic murmur at the mid- to lower left sternal border and systolic ejection click with single $S_2$.
   4. Chest x-ray examination: cardiomegaly with increased pulmonary vascular markings. (Exception: if pulmonary artery stenosis exists, decreased pulmonary markings are seen.)
   5. Echocardiography with cross-section, and Doppler flow and color mapping is the standard diagnostic test and is used to identify the number of truncal valve leaflets and presence of pulmonary stenosis, and to assess the aortic arch. The newer matrix-array 3-D echocardiography is of benefit (Friedberg et al., 2010).

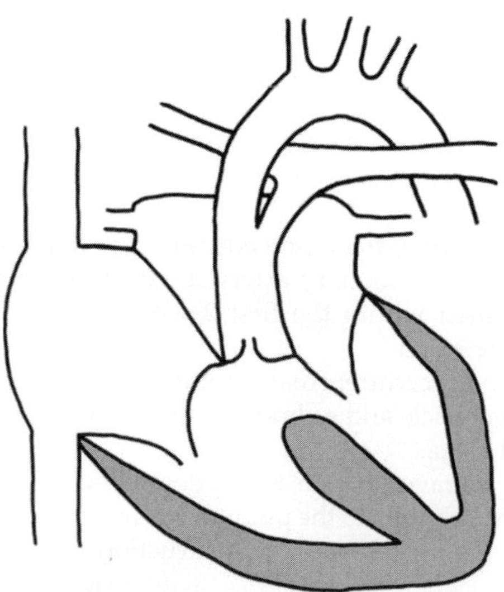

FIGURE 28-18 ■ Truncus arteriosus.

E. **Management.**
   1. Medical management is temporary and is directed toward treating CHF.
      a. Diuretics, digoxin, and angiotensin-converting enzyme inhibitors are used to control pulmonary overload and decrease systemic resistance, which leads to a decrease in PVR.
   2. Surgical repair at a few days to 4 weeks of age is the treatment of choice.
      a. Homograft between the right ventricle and the pulmonary artery.
      b. VSD closure using a patch.
      c. Separation of the pulmonary arteries from the truncus (Cowles, 2012).
   3. Homografts are preferred to synthetic because they are more flexible, easier to use during surgery, and less prone to obstruction.
   4. A newer therapy still undergoing research is tissue-valve engineering to find the ideal conduit for the right ventricular outflow tract (de Siena et al., 2011).

F. **Prognosis.**
   1. Mortality rate ranges from 70% to 95% in the first year of life if left unrepaired.
   2. Postsurgical long-term mortality is 10% to 30% (Russell et al., 2012).

## Total Anomalous Pulmonary Venous Return

A. **Incidence:** 1 per 17,000 live births, 1% of all cardiac defects.

B. **Anatomy:** Pulmonary veins drain into the right atrium either directly or indirectly via a systemic venous channel (Fig. 28-19).
   1. Presence of a patent foramen ovale or true ASD is required for survival.
   2. Varying degrees of pulmonary venous obstruction occur.
   3. Three types of TAPVR occur.
      a. Supracardiac: pulmonary veins attach above the diaphragm, often to the superior vena cava (common form).
      b. Cardiac: pulmonary veins attach directly to the coronary sinus and drain into the right atrium.
      c. Infracardiac: pulmonary veins attach below the diaphragm into the portal venous system, draining into the inferior vena cava (most severe form).

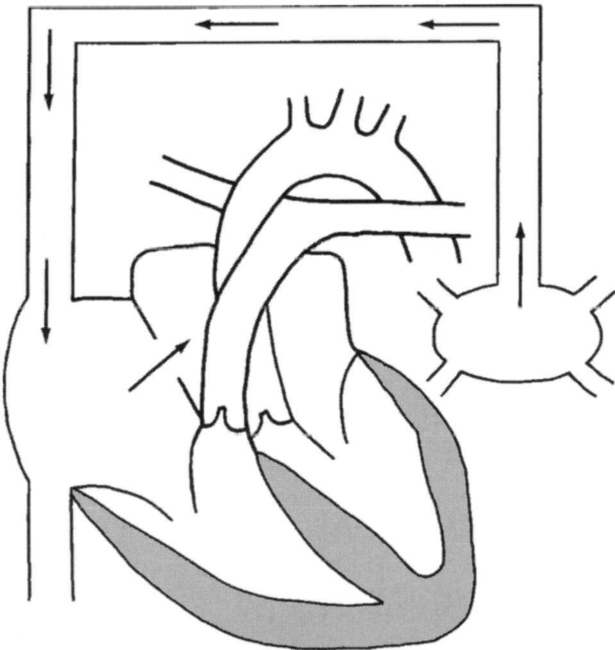

FIGURE 28-19 ■ Total anomalous pulmonary venous connection (TAPVR).

C. **Hemodynamics.**
 1. Oxygenated blood from the lungs drains into the right atrium, mixing with the systemic venous return. Part of this flow passes into the left atrium via the patent foramen ovale or ASD, into the left ventricle, and out the aorta. With the normal decrease in PVR, pulmonary blood flow will increase.
 2. If obstruction to pulmonary venous return exists, the resulting increase in PVR leads to pulmonary edema and diversion of blood from the pulmonary artery to the aorta via the PDA. Closure of the PDA then increases right-to-left atrial shunting.

D. **Clinical manifestations.**
 1. Nonobstructed.
  a. CHF.
  b. Mild cyanosis.
  c. Heart sounds: systolic murmur at the upper left sternal border, diastolic rumble at the lower left sternal border. Wide split $S_2$ may be present but is generally nonspecific.
  d. Chest x-ray examination: right ventricle dilation, increased pulmonary vascular markings, and "snowman" appearance after 4 months of age.
  e. Echocardiography will demonstrate a right ventricular dilation (Stein, 2007).
 2. Obstructed.
  a. Profound cyanosis present.
  b. Respiratory distress, may not respond to mechanical ventilation. This form may require emergent surgical repair (Cowles, 2012).
  c. Electrocardiography will show right ventricular hypertrophy with a right-axis deviation.
  d. Chest x-ray examination: normal size, with pulmonary edema.
 3. Echocardiography with color-flow mapping reveals an extra cavity behind the left atrium, a right-to-left shunt across the atrial septum, and the anomalous return as the blood enters the atrium, superior vena cava, or coronary sinus. Blood speckle imaging allows for better visualizations of the pulmonary veins (Nyrnes et al., 2010).
 4. MRI provides anatomic and functional data useful in planning repair.
 5. Computed tomography is superior at identifying spatial resolution with short imaging times, but carries the risk of ionizing radiation (Vyas et al., 2012).

E. **Management: Surgical treatment of obstructed TAPVR is an emergency.**
 1. Medical management of nonobstructed TAPVR is only a temporary measure and is aimed at preventing or treating CHF.
 2. Cardiac catheterization may be omitted to speed time to operation, with surgery based on echocardiography.
 3. Anomalous veins are detached and transplanted to the left atrium; the ASD is repaired.

F. **Prognosis.**
 1. Mortality rate for infants with TAPVR who undergo surgery is 6% to 20% in infancy (Kelle et al., 2010); the highest mortality is in the supracardiac type.
 2. Long-term prognosis is excellent because TAPVR is closer to a surgically "curable" condition (~90%) than are most congenital cardiac lesions.

## Hypoplastic Left Heart Syndrome

A. **Incidence:** 2 to 2.6 per 10,000 live births; 2% of all cardiac defects; 28% have chromosomal abnormalities. HLHS is the most common cardiac cause of death in the first week of life (Stumper, 2010).

B. **Anatomy.**
 1. Hypoplastic left ventricle, aortic arch, and ascending aorta.
 2. Atretic or hypoplastic mitral and aortic valves (Fig. 28-20).

C. **Hemodynamics.**
 1. Obstruction of blood flow through the left side of the heart due to hypoplastic aorta and ventricle leads to pulmonary venous congestion and edema.
 2. Blood supply to the descending aorta and to the aortic arch and coronary arteries (retrograde flow) is dependent on the PDA.
 3. Coarctation of the aorta is present in 75% of patients.

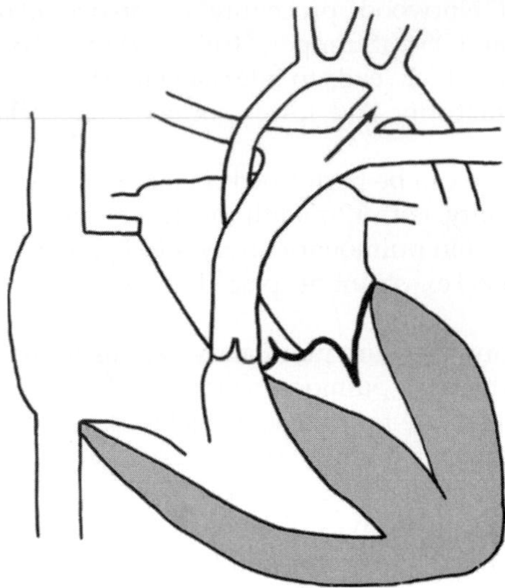

FIGURE 28-20 ■ Hypoplastic left heart syndrome (HLHS).

D. **Clinical manifestations.**
   1. Asymptomatic at birth.
   2. Tachypnea and dyspnea with increasing pulmonary blood flow.
   3. CHF: usually presents at 24 to 48 hours of life.
   4. Cyanosis: rarely permanent despite mixing of systemic and pulmonary circulations.
   5. Rapid deterioration as PDA closes (Stumper, 2010).
      a. Severe mottling.
      b. Gray pallor of skin.
      c. Markedly diminished pulses.
      d. Cardiovascular collapse and shock.
      e. Systolic murmur present in two thirds.
   6. Chest x-ray examination: cardiomegaly with increased pulmonary blood flow and pulmonary edema.
   7. Prenatal diagnosis by fetal echocardiography at 18 to 22 weeks in about 60% of cases (Stumper, 2010). Fetal interventions to prevent development of the syndrome are being studied, using ultrasound-guided percutaneous approach to perform balloon dilation and stent placement in areas of restriction, or aortic valvuloplasty. Results have shown that the majority of fetuses will have increased aortic and mitral valves, but not growth of the left ventricle. This does allow for improved left heart physiology. About 10% of the fetuses will either die or be delivered prematurely (McElhinney et al., 2010). Fetal diagnosis allows for counseling of parents and planning delivery at a center with a pediatric cardiology surgical center with an expert multidisciplinary team for neonatal management (Donofrio et al., 2013). These centers often take the newborn directly to the operating room for palliation. Postnatal diagnosis with echocardiography to determine size of interatrial communication, atrioventricular valve function, and ascending aorta size should include tissue Doppler imaging and 3-D echocardiography (Parra and Vera, 2012).

E. **Management.**
   1. Treatment options include a multistaged surgical approach, cardiac transplantation, and, though it is not as common in the present decade, comfort care.
   2. Initial management.
      a. $PGE_1$ to maintain ductus arteriosus patency and systemic circulation.
      b. Systemic afterload-reducing agents.
      c. Aggressive management of acidosis.
      d. Transcatheter balloon atrial septostomy to decompress the left atrium if not taken to surgery immediately following birth.

3. Staged surgical repair ("Norwood" procedure) has an overall mortality rate at ages 1, 5, and 10 years of 25%, 30%, and 35% (Stumper, 2010). Arrhythmias are found in 57% of patients between stages 1 and 2, which leads to interstage mortality rates ranging from 2% to 20%. Other factors are prematurity and lower socioeconomic class (Ghanayem et al., 2012; Trivedi et al., 2011).
   a. First (Norwood) stage can be performed on infants with birth weights as low as 1.5 kg and has a 15% mortality, with 12-month survival around 61% (Karamichalis et al., 2010).
      (1) Division of the main pulmonary artery and ligation of the ductus arteriosus.
      (2) Minimized Gore-Tex shunt is placed to maintain pulmonary blood flow and prevent CHF.
      (3) Atrial septectomy to ensure pulmonary venous return to the right atrium.
      (4) Connection of the right pulmonary artery and the aorta using an aortic allograft.
      (5) Newer Sano procedure for first stage includes placement of a conduit between the right ventricle and left and right pulmonary arteries. This has led to improved early survival, and improved coronary and systemic perfusion (Stumper, 2010).
      (6) "Hybrid" approach: involves placement of a stent in the ductus arteriosus along with bilateral pulmonary artery banding. This is done in a special suite that has catheterization and surgery capabilities. Complications include narrowing of the ductus, which requires balloon dilation, and increased pulmonary blood flow.
   b. Second stage: bidirectional Glenn procedure (anastomosis of the superior vena cava to the right pulmonary artery) done between 4 and 6 months of age to reduce volume overload to the right ventricle. Most infants will have developed severe cyanosis from limited pulmonary circulation. Mortality rate for this stage is less than 7%.
   c. Third stage, or modified Fontan procedure, with a mortality rate of less than 5% (Stumper, 2010).
      (1) Involves completion of Fontan procedure between 12 and 24 months of age to connect the inferior vena cava to the pulmonary artery and close the atrial communication using a conduit made of polytetrafluoroethylene.
      (2) Completion of stages 2 and 3 separates the pulmonary from the systemic circulation.
   d. Disadvantages.
      (1) Two or three open surgeries in the first 2 years of life.
      (2) Single right ventricle supplies the systemic circulation.
      (3) Higher systemic venous pressures resulting in liver dysfunction.
      (4) Some of these patients will go on to need a transplant.
   e. Contraindication: significant tricuspid valve or pulmonic valve dysplasia associated with functional disturbances.
4. Cardiac transplantation.
   a. Provides a structurally and physiologically normal heart in one operation.
   b. About 23% of infants die while waiting for a donor heart (U.S. Food and Drug Administration, 2011). This number still remains high, but newer modalities to provide support while waiting for a heart include extracorporeal membrane oxygenation (ECMO), and the Berlin Heart. ECMO may only be used for short-term support. About 45% of the infants placed on ECMO will survive to transplantation (Almond et al., 2011).
   c. Complications include the following:
      (1) Increased susceptibility to infections as a result of immunosuppression.
      (2) Allograft rejection, with acute rejection as the leading cause of death in the first year following transplantation.
      (3) Systemic hypertension: usually seen only in the first year after transplantation.
      (4) Recurrent or residual coarctation: managed with angioplasty or surgical repair.
      (5) Abnormal neurologic findings in as many as 19%, including seizures.
      (6) Post-transplantation death, with 1 in 9 infants dying before discharge, seen primarily in those who needed ECMO or ventilator support (Gandhi et al., 2011).

**F. Prognosis.**

1. Comparison of staged repair versus heart transplantation outcomes requires evaluation of numbers of surviving children who completed procedures and numbers of those "lost" through death awaiting procedure or death between stages of the procedure.

2. According to websites that list survival data, survival following transplantation has improved to 89% at discharge from hospital, 80% to 85% at 1 year, and 70% to 80% at 3 years, not including deaths while awaiting transplant, which can approach 25%. Recent advancements in ABO-incompatible transplant and use of ventricular assist devices have increased survival rates (Tweddell et al., 2012).
3. Overall, 1-year survival after completion of the staged procedure is 75%.

# CONGESTIVE HEART FAILURE

## Etiology

A. **CHF is a set of clinical signs and symptoms** that reflect the heart's inability to deliver adequate oxygen to meet the metabolic requirements of the body.
   1. Cardiac output is unable to meet the body's metabolic requirements.
   2. Right and/or left ventricular end-diastolic pressures are elevated, impeding systemic and/or pulmonary venous returns.

B. **Although structural heart defects are the most common cause of CHF** in neonates, other causes such as birth asphyxia, severe anemia, dysrhythmias, and sepsis should be considered.
   1. Timing of detection is often helpful in predicting causes because the diseases causing CHF characteristically show up at certain ages. Table 28-5 indicates conditions associated with CHF and their time of onset.
   2. CHF in utero that is detected at birth may be due to the following:
      a. Profound anemia: erythroblastosis fetalis or twin-to-twin transfusion.
      b. Arrhythmia: supraventricular tachycardia or congenital heart block.
      c. Intrauterine infection with myocarditis.
      d. Arteriovenous malformations.
      e. Absent pulmonary valve.
      f. Premature ductus arteriosus closure: maternal use of prostaglandin inhibitor (e.g., aspirin, ibuprofen).
      g. Volume overload: twin-to-twin or mother-to-infant transfusion.

## Clinical Manifestations

A. **Common signs (Satou, 2013).**
   1. Tachypnea (60 to 100 respirations per minute at rest) is the first clinical sign of pulmonary edema.
   2. Tachycardia (160 to 180 bpm at rest) from compensation for decreased cardiac output.
   3. Four-limb blood pressure may yield a higher blood pressure in the right arm than in either leg, indicating an aortic obstruction.
   4. Central or prolonged peripheral cyanosis due to poor perfusion.

■ TABLE 28-5
■ ■ **Causes of Congestive Heart Failure and Time of Onset**

| Age at Onset of Symptoms | Underlying Cause |
|---|---|
| At birth | Hypoplastic left heart syndrome (HLHS) |
| | Severe tricuspid or pulmonary regurgitation |
| | Systemic arteriovenous fistula |
| In first week of life | Patent ductus arteriosus (PDA) in premature infants |
| | Transposition of the great vessels (TGV) |
| | Total anomalous pulmonary venous return (TAPVR) with pulmonary venous obstruction |
| 1 to 4 weeks after birth | Coarctation of the aorta |
| | Critical aortic or pulmonary stenosis |
| | All other lesions listed above |

Data from Park, M.K.: *Pediatric cardiology for practitioners* (5th ed.). Philadelphia, 2008, Elsevier Mosby.

5. Arrhythmias.
6. Poor feeding—may take up to 45 minutes to complete a feeding.
7. Cardiomegaly on x-ray.
   a. Dilational or hypertrophic cardiomyopathy.
   b. Diminished or engorged pulmonary vasculature.
8. Hepatomegaly (3 to 5 cm below coastal margin): one of the most useful signs.
9. Pulmonary fine rales and coarse rales (rhonchi).

**B. Less common signs.**
1. Peripheral edema: usually not obvious unless CHF is present for some time.
2. Diaphoresis.
3. Gallop rhythm.
4. May have mottling of the extremities from redistribution of blood flow to vital tissues.
5. Electrocardiogram indicating the following:
   a. Hypertrophy of one or more chambers.
   b. Abnormal mean QRS axis.
   c. Rhythm disturbances.
6. Grading the severity of CHF is difficult and not standardized. Several tools have been reported in the literature but lack testing to suggest reliability.

## Management of Congestive Heart Failure

**A. General measures** (appropriate for any heart disease).
1. Use semi-Fowler's or prone position to achieve maximal diaphragmatic excursion and lung expansion.
2. Decrease oxygen consumption.
   a. Maintain neutral thermal environment.
   b. Minimize stimulation (e.g., heel sticks, radial sticks).
   c. Provide sedation with morphine or fentanyl for agitated infant.
   d. Consider assisted ventilation to reduce work of breathing and decrease pulmonary edema if present.
3. Provide supplemental oxygen. The amount is dictated by the $Pao_2$ and the presence of CHD with admixing of arterial and venous blood.
4. Correct acidosis and any metabolic derangements (e.g., hypoglycemia or hypocalcemia).

**B. Specific measures.**
1. Fluid and nutritional support.
   a. During acute phase, volume intake is reduced, generally to two thirds of maintenance levels.
   b. Use of glucose polymers (Polycose) or medium-chain triglycerides (MCT oil) enhances caloric content without significant volume increase.
   c. IV infusions of up to 50% fat emulsions can also be used to increase caloric intake with minimal intake volume.
2. Pharmacologic therapy.
   a. Digoxin therapy (Table 28-6).
      (1) Inotrope to achieve maximal cardiac output; use in patients with left-to-right shunt is controversial.
      (2) Digitalize patient and observe for bradycardia (discontinue if heart rate <100 bpm).
         (a) Arrhythmias or heart block.
         (b) Hypokalemia.
         (c) Toxic effects: increased in premature infants because of a longer serum half-life (61 to 170 hours) for digoxin than in term or older infants (18 to 45 hours) (Takemoto et al., 2011).
   b. Diuretic therapy.
      (1) Used to eliminate excess intravascular fluid.
      (2) Furosemide (Lasix), 1 to 2 mg/kg every 12 hours IV, or 1 to 3 mg/kg every 12 hours by mouth, may increase to four times a day if needed (Satou, 2013).
         (a) In severe CHF, the IV route is preferable for its rapid onset of action.

■ TABLE 28-6
■ ■ **Digoxin Dosages and Common Side Effects**

| Digitalizing Schedule | Common Side Effects |
|---|---|
| Preterm infant<br>Oral (PO) route: 20 mcg/kg total dose*<br>Term infant<br>PO route: 30 mcg/kg total dose* | Total dose is usually divided into three doses giving one half, then one fourth, then one fourth of the total dose every 8 hours. Check electrocardiogram rhythm strip for rate, P-R interval, and dysrhythmias before each dose. |
| **Maintenance Schedule** | |
| Preterm infant<br>PO route: 5 to 10 mcg/kg/day* | Total dose should be divided to give twice daily. Allow 12 to 24 hours between last digitalizing and first maintenance doses. It takes about 6 days to "digitalize" a patient with maintenance doses alone. The sign of digitalis effect is usually prolongation of the P-R interval. The first sign of digitalis toxicity is usually vomiting, dysrhythmia, or bradycardia. |
| Term infant<br>PO route: 5 to 10 mcg/kg/day | Drugs such as quinidine, amiodarone, and diuretics predispose to digoxin toxicity. The clearance of digoxin is directly related to renal function. Dosage must be reduced in patients with impaired renal function. |

*Intravenous dose is 75% of PO dose.

(b) Hypokalemia and hypochloremia are side effects that can result in metabolic alkalosis.
(c) May cause hypocalcemia, with urinary loss of calcium leading to nephrocalcinosis.
(d) Use is contraindicated in renal failure.

(3) Chlorothiazide (Diuril), 20 to 40 mg/kg/day in two divided oral doses (Takemoto et al., 2011).
(a) Administered when less acute oral diuresis is required.
(b) IV dose 2 to 8 mg/kg/day divided in two doses.
(c) Does not produce the profound potassium losses seen with furosemide; may reduce urinary calcium losses seen with furosemide.

(4) Spironolactone (Aldactone), 1 to 3.3 mg/kg/day by mouth.
(a) Potassium sparing; must monitor for hyperkalemia.

c. Inotropic agents.
(1) May be necessary in severe CHF or cardiogenic shock.
(2) Most commonly used are dopamine, dobutamine, and isoproterenol.
(3) Milrinone (short-term, <48 hours only)
(a) IV dose 0.3 to 1 mcg/kg/min.
(b) Loading dose of 50 to 75 mcg/kg IV over 15 minutes if needed.
(4) Nesiritide has shown promise in pediatric patients older than 1 month who have low cardiac output and those with CHF who have not responded to traditional therapy (Behera et al., 2009). Further investigation is needed.

C. **Cardiology consultation to rule out or establish presence of congenital heart lesion.** Cardiac catheterization, angiocardiography, and surgery may be indicated.

## POSTOPERATIVE CARDIAC MANAGEMENT

### Noninvasive Monitoring

A. **Electrocardiography.**
1. Continuous display of a limb lead, which shows P wave and QRS complex, should be monitored.
a. Tachycardia.
b. Bradycardia.

   c. Fibrillation.
   d. Asystole.
2. Lead II: assessment of amplitude, axis, and presence and absence of P waves.
3. Lead $V_5$ changes: septal or lateral wall ischemia.

B. **Blood pressure: manual.**
1. Cuff can be used to occlude an arterial catheter leak.
2. Measurement of upper and lower extremities after repair of coarctation of the aorta gives pressure gradient across repair site.
3. Avoid extremity for blood pressure measurement when an artery has been used for surgical repair (e.g., subclavian patch for coarctation of the aorta, Blalock–Taussig shunt).

C. **Pulse oximetry.**
1. Decreasing oxygen saturations may indicate:
   a. Decreased cardiac output.
   b. Increasing intracardiac shunting.
   c. Increased intrapulmonary shunting.
2. Continuous monitoring is useful in pulmonary hypertension. Small decreases in saturation may be the first sign of increased pulmonary artery pressure with onset of right-to-left shunting.

D. **Urinary output.**
1. Hourly output rate of 1 to 2 mL/kg/hr is a good clinical indicator of renal perfusion (Spence, 2007).
   a. Invalid in first 2 hours postoperatively after diuretic administration.
   b. Urinary retention can be induced by analgesics.
   c. A sudden decrease in urine output may indicate renal failure.
2. Oliguria may persist for up to 48 hours following cardiopulmonary bypass.
3. It is common to see increased urine output secondary to osmotic diuresis in the initial postoperative period, followed by decreased urine output after 6 to 8 hours (Pike and Falco, 2002).

E. **Cerebral near-infrared spectroscopy (Bronicki and Chang, 2011).**
1. Assesses cerebral oxygenation.
2. Use for tracking patient trends.

## Invasive Monitoring

For pressure values from cardiac catheterization, see Table 28-7.

A. **Arterial pressure.**
1. Mandatory for timely vasoactive medication adjustments.
2. Arterial tracing provides information for analysis of waveform and calculation of pulse pressure.
3. Pronounced phasic variations during mechanical ventilation may indicate hypovolemia or heart failure.

B. **Right-sided cardiac pressures.**
1. In patients with normal cardiac anatomy: right atrial pressure = right ventricular end- diastolic pressure = central venous pressure.

■ TABLE 28-7
■ ■ **Pressure Values From Cardiac Catheterization**

| Pressure | Normal Neonatal Values |
|---|---|
| Systemic arterial pressure | 60 to 90/20 to 60 mm Hg (birth to 5 days of age) |
| Right atrial pressure | 3 mm Hg |
| Right ventricular pressure | 30/3 mm Hg |
| Pulmonary artery occlusion pressure/pulmonary wedge pressure | 6 to 10 mm Hg |
| Left atrial pressure | 8 mm Hg |
| Left ventricular pressure | 100/6 mm Hg |

2. Increasing values seen with (Bronicki and Chang, 2011):
   a. Right ventricular overload.
   b. Poor ventricular function.
   c. Elevated pulmonary artery pressure, resulting from reactive pulmonary hypertension.
   d. Tricuspid regurgitation.
   e. Cardiac tamponade.
   f. Residual shunting.
3. Particularly useful for evaluating the following:
   a. Right-sided cardiac lesions.
      (1) Pulmonic stenosis.
      (2) TOF.
   b. Those lesions requiring high right atrial pressures, such as in the Fontan procedure.
4. Right-sided line may be used to give vasoactive and inotropic medications, and to provide parenteral nutrition.

C. **Pulmonary artery pressure.**
1. Surgical placement using a purse-string structure or transthoracic placement of a pulmonary artery catheter into the right ventricular outflow tract is indicated for those neonates at risk for pulmonary hypertension (Bronicki and Chang, 2011).
2. Measurements guide the medical management of pulmonary hypertension and are most frequently used in conditions in which postoperative pulmonary hypertension is anticipated, as in endocardial cushion repair, TAPVR, and mitral valve stenosis (Wernovsky and Gruber, 2005). Incidence of severe pulmonary hypertension following pediatric cardiac surgery found to be 2%.
3. Mixed venous oxygen saturation ($S\bar{V}O_2$) monitoring can be obtained from pulmonary artery catheters with continuous oximetry capabilities.
   a. $S\bar{V}O_2$ reflects a balance between oxygen delivery and consumption.
   b. Alterations are seen in:
      (1) Anemia.
      (2) Shock.
      (3) Left-to-right or right-to-left shunts.
   c. Change in $S\bar{V}O_2$ generally precedes detectable hemodynamic changes by several minutes.

D. **Left-sided cardiac pressures are monitored using a left atrial line.**
1. In patients with normal cardiac anatomy: left ventricular end-diastolic pressure = left atrial pressure = pulmonary artery occlusion pressure = pulmonary artery wedge pressure.
2. Used to monitor systemic ventricular function and pulmonary shunting (Bronicki and Chang, 2011).
3. Useful in patients with mitral valve dysfunction, as seen in post–endocardial cushion repair.
4. Requires meticulous line care because the risk of air or particulate embolization is high.
5. Usually removed 1 to 2 days postoperation.

E. **Epicardial pacing wires.**
1. Usually attached to right atrium and/or right ventricle.
2. Provide temporary back up pacing for up to 10 days.
3. Access to dual-chamber pacing is most important after surgical repairs near the cardiac conduction system. For example:
   a. Cardiac resynchronization.
   b. VSD.
   c. Transposition of the great arteries.
   d. Truncus arteriosus.
   e. Endocardial cushion defects.

## Hemodynamic Management

Neonates experience wide swings in physiologic responses, namely, heart rate, temperature, glucose metabolism, and systemic and pulmonary vascular resistance.

A. **Bradycardia.**
   1. Common result of intraoperative cooling; proportional to degree of hypothermia.
   2. After extensive atrial surgery, such as arterial switch procedure, TAPVR repair.
   3. After injury to sinoatrial node.
   4. With conducting problems:
      a. Sinoatrial block.
      b. Sinus asystole.
      c. Atrioventricular block is of most concern in the postoperative period.
   5. As a consequence of edema around conduction system (generally resolves in 3 to 4 days).

B. **Tachycardia:** Observed as a consequence of or in response to the following:
   1. Pain.
   2. Anxiety/agitation.
   3. Fever.
   4. Hypovolemia.
   5. Junctional conduction disturbance.

# POSTOPERATIVE DISTURBANCES

## Heart Failure

### Etiology

A. **Most common postoperative event** resulting from decreased neonatal cardiac reserve, limited by
   1. Decreased myofilament numbers;
   2. Decreased ventricular compliance;
   3. Greater oxygen consumption, cardiac output, and resting heart rate in the neonate; and
   4. Nearly maximal neonatal cardiac performance in the absence of stress.

B. **Causes (Bronicki and Chang, 2011):**
   1. Cardiopulmonary bypass adversely affects myocardial performance.
      a. Causes inflammatory response, which may be decreased by pre-bypass glucocorticoids.
   2. Residual anatomic lesions.
      a. Transesophageal echocardiography in the operating room has minimized the incidence.
   3. Pulmonary artery hypertensive crisis.
      a. Life-threatening right heart failure may be caused by an acute increase in pulmonary artery pressure.
   4. Arrhythmias.

C. **Preload or diastolic filling:**
   1. Hypovolemia.
      a. Inadequate volume replacement.
      b. Inadequate mechanical hemostasis.
      c. Impaired clotting.
   2. Iatrogenic volume overload.
   3. Left ventricular dysfunction.
   4. Cardiac compression.

D. **Afterload:**
   1. In the postoperative period, the neonatal heart is extremely sensitive to increased afterload.
   2. Evidenced by peripheral vasoconstriction.
      a. Vasodilators are used to enhance the reduction of ventricular afterload.

E. **Contractility:**
   1. Decreased peripheral perfusion.
   2. Decreased urine output.
   3. Treat with inotropic medications.

F. **Inadequate systemic venous return:**
   1. Excessive positive end-expiratory pressure.
   2. Tension pneumothorax.
   3. Atrial baffle obstruction.
   4. Postpericardial effusions.

G. **Increased pulmonary vascular resistance.**
H. **Decreased cardiac contractility,** resulting from the following:
   1. Accidental discontinuation of vasoactive drugs.
   2. Electrolyte disturbances.
   3. Hypoglycemia.
   4. Surgical manipulation or damage.

**Recognition of Low Cardiac Output**

A. **Frequently seen with changes in preload, afterload, and contractility** in the postoperative period, identified by impaired multiorgan system perfusion and elevated filling pressures (Bronicki and Chang, 2011).
B. **Factors that influence the severity of low cardiac output:**
   1. Age less than 1 month.
   2. Weight less than 2.5 kg.
   3. Preoperative condition.
   4. Type of defect.
C. **Observation: "just not doing well."**
   1. Noninteractive or becoming less interactive with environment.
   2. Lack of/or decreasing vigor of cry.
   3. Awake but "floppy."
D. **Color:**
   1. Violet color of mucosa.
   2. Gray skin or mottling of skin.
E. **Extremities:**
   1. Cool to touch.
   2. Lack of or decrease in pedal pulses.
   3. Capillary refill time longer than 3 seconds.
   4. Edema: often seen postoperatively as "third spacing," but also indicative of fluid overload.
F. **Oliguria (urine output <0.5 to 1 mL/kg/hr).**
   1. Transient acute renal failure may occur in 5% of neonates who require cardiopulmonary bypass during cardiac surgery.
G. **Tachycardia.**
   1. Gallop rhythm.
   2. Distant heart sounds: possible indication of pericardial effusions.
H. **Low arterial blood pressure.**
I. **Respiratory distress.**
   1. Retractions, tachypnea, grunting, and/or stridor in infant after extubation.
   2. Rales: often heard after bypass procedure.
J. **Weight gain disproportionate to caloric intake.**
   1. May be early indicator of fluid retention.
K. **X-ray findings.**
   1. Excessive cardiac size or enlargement of specific chamber.
   2. Large cardiac silhouette or "bag-of-waters" appearance may indicate pericardial effusions.
   3. Increased fluffy densities; these are not seen if elevated positive end-expiratory pressure is used in ventilation.
L. **Metabolic derangement.**
   1. Metabolic acidosis, generally resulting from low bicarbonate levels and lactic acid buildup that results from diminished tissue perfusion.
   2. Low sodium value, in part due to excessive free water.

**Management of Low Cardiac Output**

A. **Use blood for volume replacement.**
   1. Maintain hemoglobin greater than 12 g/dL for noncyanotic lesions and greater than 15 g/dL for cyanotic lesions (Cuadrado, 2002).
B. **Volume challenge is appropriate in light of cardiopulmonary bypass third spacing.**
   1. Close monitoring required.
   2. Strict intake and output.
   3. Neonates are easily fluid overloaded when given excessive fluids (Spence, 2007).

C. **Provide correction of metabolic disorders.**
   1. Hypocalcemia, hyponatremia, and hypoglycemia.
   2. Acid–base balances.
      a. Acidosis may result from poor tissue perfusion, prolonged hypovolemia, or impaired renal function. Correction depends on the underlying cause.

D. **Reduce right ventricular afterload.**
   1. Hyperventilation.
   2. Pulmonary vasodilating agents.
      a. $PGE_1$.
      b. Nitroglycerin.
      c. Nitroprusside is a mixed vasodilator frequently used with dopamine or dobutamine.
      d. Inhaled nitric oxide.
   3. Provide sedation and analgesia.

E. **Treat rate or rhythm disturbance.**
   1. Increased heart rate.
      a. Rate of 200 to 210 bpm is tolerated well, with acceptable myocardial work and oxygen consumption.
      b. Cardioversion can be used for supraventricular tachycardia, atrial flutter/fibrillation, and ventricular tachycardia (Hay et al., 2003).
   2. Atrial or atrioventricular pacing is often necessary.

F. **Consider pharmaceutical agents.**
   1. Isoproterenol (Isuprel): acts to decrease pulmonary and systemic vascular resistance (decreases afterload).
   2. Nitroprusside or nitroglycerin: a venodilator that reduces afterload.
   3. Milrinone: increases heart rate and contractility with some vasodilatory properties. Does not affect platelet function (Young and Mangum, 2008).
   4. Nesiritide is a venous and arterial dilator with diuretic properties (Bronicki and Chang, 2011).
   5. Volume replacement: often necessary because of vasodilation (maintain preload). Central venous pressure is useful in determining volume needs.
   6. Vasopressors (i.e., dopamine >10 mcg/kg/min, or dobutamine). Potential for increasing PVR. Careful monitoring of effects is necessary.

G. **Mechanical circulatory support (Bronicki and Chang, 2011).**
   1. Berlin Heart Excor can be used as bilateral or single ventricular support.
   2. Centrifugal ventricular assist device.
   3. ECMO.

H. **Monitor blood pressure.**

**Bleeding**

A. **Provide sedation.** Avoid agitation, prevent hypertension and pressure at active and potential bleeding sites, which may aggravate or disrupt clot formation.

B. **Assess and treat coagulopathy.**
   1. Coagulation factors are 30% to 40% lower in neonates with CHDs than in neonates without defects (Pike and Falco, 2002).
   2. Use fresh whole blood less than 48 hours old for volume and clotting.
      a. Maintain hematocrit greater than 40% to 45% (Artman et al., 2002).
   3. Use cryoprecipitate for fibrinogen (aids clotting).
   4. Evaluate platelets: count is low and function is inadequate because of "bypass" and deep hypothermia.
      a. Give platelet infusion.
      b. Give desmopressin (DDAVP), 0.3 mcg/kg, to increase levels of von Willebrand's factor, which stimulates platelets to aggregate.

**Pulmonary Hypertension/Pulmonary Vasospasm (see Chapter 24)**

A. **Avoid hypoxemia and acidosis.**
   1. Hypoxia increases PVR and acidosis.
   2. Neonates at risk for postoperative pulmonary hypertension need to be identified on return from the recovery room (Bronicki and Chang, 2011).

a. Large VSD.
b. Complete atrioventricular canal.
c. Truncus arteriosus.
d. TAPVR.
e. D-Transposition of the great arteries.

**Maintenance of Fluid and Electrolyte Balance (see Chapter 8)**

A. **Hypoglycemia, hypokalemia, and hypocalcemia are potential problems.**
  1. All result in decreased myocardial function.
  2. Potential for seizures is present.
    a. Poor cardiac output to the brain may cause seizures.
    b. Cardiopulmonary bypass and circulatory arrest also predispose an infant to seizures.

## Shock

### Etiology

A. **Shock is a complex state of inadequate circulating blood volume,** resulting in insufficient perfusion, oxygenation, and nutrients to the tissues. Several varieties of shock are recognized.
B. **Hypovolemic shock** may be caused by (Karlsen and Tani, 2003):
  1. Blood loss from placental abnormalities (e.g., umbilical cord rupture, abruptio placentae, placenta previa, and twin-to-twin transfusion syndrome).
  2. Acute blood loss postnatally (such as intracranial or pulmonary hemorrhage).
  3. Acute or chronic blood loss postsurgically.
  4. Plasma and fluid losses.
    a. Skin integrity losses (e.g., myelomeningocele, gastroschisis).
    b. Pleural effusions (e.g., erythroblastosis fetalis or nonimmune hydrops).
    c. Body water loss from persistent vomiting/continuous gastric suctioning, diarrhea, or evaporative skin losses.
    d. Capillary leak syndrome resulting in third spacing.
C. **Cardiogenic shock** may be caused by (Karlsen, 2006):
  1. Myocardial failure due to severe hypoxemia, hypoglycemia, hypocalcemia, or acidosis.
  2. Congenital heart lesions.
  3. Cardiac arrhythmias.
    a. Sustained supraventricular tachycardia.
    b. Complete atrioventricular block (third degree).
  4. Restriction of cardiac function by:
    a. Tamponade.
    b. Tension pneumothorax.
    c. Excessive levels of ventilatory distending pressures.
  5. Myocarditis: often associated with sepsis.
D. **Distributive shock** (septic shock):
  1. Results from impaired peripheral arterial resistance usually caused by sepsis (i.e., release of bacterial toxins). The toxins cause capillary leak, which then leads to hypovolemic shock (Karlsen, 2006).
  2. Typically is associated with gram-negative organisms; however, gram-positive organisms may be the causative agent.

### Clinical Indicators

A. **Signs of shock are frequently nonspecific.** (Cardiogenic shock may be indistinguishable from CHF.)
B. **Cardiopulmonary status changes.**
  1. Tachycardia at rest.
  2. Bradycardia.
  3. Tachypnea, increased work of breathing, dyspnea.
  4. Poor peripheral perfusion.
    a. Pallor (especially with acute blood loss).
    b. Capillary refill time longer than 3 seconds.
    c. Mottling.

d. Weak, thready pulses.
e. Cool extremities.

5. Hypotension (blood pressure may be normal in early stages).
6. Hypotonia, lethargy that may progress to a comatose state.

C. **Decreased urinary output.**

D. **Metabolic disturbances.**
1. Metabolic acidosis.
2. Hypoglycemia.
3. Hypothermia.

E. **Evidence of coagulation defects.**
1. Oozing from IV sites, suture lines, etc.
2. Coagulopathy: abnormal prothrombin time, partial thromboplastin time, fibrinogen.

F. **Indicators of blood volume** (or effective blood volume):
1. Change in hemoglobin and hematocrit values.
2. Response to fluid challenge of 10 mL of saline solution per kilogram of body weight, while blood pressure and urine output are monitored.
3. Positive Kleihauer–Betke test result indicates fetal-to-maternal transfusion in utero. This test examines the maternal blood for the presence of fetal erythrocytes.

G. **Indicators of cardiac function.**
1. See B. Cardiopulmonary Status Changes, above.
2. Echocardiogram establishes anatomic defects and/or specific myocardial function abnormalities.
3. Central venous pressure is generally elevated, except during hypovolemic shock.

H. **Indicators of septic shock.**
1. Clinical signs of sepsis or positive culture results.
2. Normal blood pressure in the face of prominent hypoperfusion.
3. Edema or sclerema from capillary protein and fluid leakage.
4. Oliguria, proteinuria.
5. Persistent pulmonary hypertension of the neonate (common).

**Management of Shock**

A. **Depends largely on prevailing pathogenesis.** A large proportion of the care is supportive.

B. **Supportive care.**
1. Maintain oxygenation and ventilation as dictated by arterial blood gas values.
   a. Give ventilatory support if concurrent pulmonary disease exists.
   b. Provide neutral thermal environment to decrease oxygen consumption.
   c. Decrease external stress (i.e., handling, peripheral blood sampling).
   d. Consider sedatives, analgesics, and neuromuscular blockade to decrease stress.
2. Promptly treat acidosis to avoid adverse effects on myocardial contractility. Sodium bicarbonate is often necessary.
3. Maintain fluid and electrolyte balance.

C. **Specific therapies.**
1. Increase blood volume and erythrocyte mass.
   a. Maintain blood pressure and maximize oxygen content.
   b. Treatment of acute blood loss may require large volume transfusion.
   c. Monitoring arterial blood pressure is essential; monitoring of central venous pressure ideally should be included.
   d. Caution: In cardiogenic shock, added volume may increase the myocardial workload.
2. Treat the infectious process in septic shock.
   a. Antibiotic therapy should be initiated.
   b. Consider use of granulocyte colony-stimulating factor, giving 5 to 10 mcg/kg/day for 3 to 5 days for infants who are in septic shock and have an absolute neutrophil count less than $1000/mm^3$ (Takemoto et al., 2011).
3. Maximize cardiac output.
   a. Inotropic agents such as epinephrine are useful in cardiogenic shock to increase cardiac output and support circulation. Start early in septic shock if evidence of oliguria, hypotension, or acidosis exists. Monitor for hypertension and edema (Takemoto et al., 2011).

Norepinephrine may prove useful in dopamine-resistant shock. According to Takemoto and colleagues (2011), the usual dose is 0.5 mcg/kg/min.

b. Isoproterenol (Isuprel): increases heart rate and contractility ($\beta_1$-adrenergic effects). Simultaneous effects produce bronchodilation and smooth muscle relaxation ($\beta_2$-adrenergic effects). Usual dose is 0.05 to 2 mcg/kg/min. Observe for ventricular arrhythmias and tachycardia.

c. Dopamine: increases cardiac contractility and cardiac output, affecting preload, contractility, and afterload, all three components of cardiovascular function (Evans and Seri, 2005). Effects are dose dependent. At low doses (1 to 3 mcg/kg/min IV), selective vasodilation of the renal, mesenteric, cerebral, and coronary vascular beds occurs, with little effect on heart rate or blood pressure. With moderate doses (5 to 10 mcg/kg/min), increased blood pressure and improved tissue perfusion can be observed. Beneficial effects are dependent largely on adequate blood volume. Correct hypovolemia before the dopamine infusion. At higher doses (>10 mcg/kg/min IV), vasoconstriction occurs, and includes vasoconstriction of the pulmonary vasculature, increased right ventricular afterload, reduction in pulmonary blood flow, right-to-left shunting through fetal structures, increased blood pressure, and increased hypoxemia. Tachycardia, dysrhythmias, and ectopic beats can occur as a consequence of dopamine infusion.

d. Dobutamine (Dobutrex): increases cardiac contractility and heart rate while exerting limited effects on vasculature. Cardiac output increases, depending on myocardial catecholamine stores. Dose is 5 to 10 mcg/kg/min as a continuous IV infusion (Satou, 2013).

e. Milrinone has proven beneficial in pediatric patients who continue to have increased vascular resistance after cardiac output is corrected to a low normal state (Wechsler and Wernovsky, 2004). Milrinone should be given for less than 72 hours (Takemoto et al., 2011). In term neonates, a loading dose of 75 mcg/kg IV is given over 60 minutes, followed by an infusion of 0.5 to 0.75 mcg/kg/min. In preterm neonates of less than 30 weeks of gestational age, loading dose is 0.75 mcg/kg/min for 3 hours, followed by 0.2-mcg/kg/min IV infusion.

f. Corticosteroids have been used in premature infants to treat hypotension when volume expanders and standard modalities have failed. Recent studies have shown that steroids do improve blood pressure in this population. It is unclear if corticosteroid use in preterm neonates is safe and effective.

g. Digitalis should be considered and used selectively, especially in the face of hypoxia or toxic myocardiopathy.

4. Correct any tension pneumothorax or cardiac tamponade.

D. **Treatment goals.**
1. Reduce morbidity.
2. Normalize hemodynamic status.
3. Halt progression of the shock state.

## Pain Control and Sedation (see Chapter 16)

A. **Pain assessment is the fifth vital sign;** however, assessment of pain in newborn infants remains a major challenge for health care providers. Of even greater concern is assessment of pain in critically ill neonates. These infants have marginal organ system reserves, which leads to lack of adequate compensatory mechanisms (Wernovsky et al., 2005).

## Developmental Care (see Chapter 11)

A. **Measures taken to facilitate developmentally appropriate care.**
1. Decrease noise and lighting.
2. Decrease hands-on care; cluster tasks.
3. Provide nonnutritive sucking.
4. Use positional devices and facilitated tucking.
5. Administer analgesics and sedatives.
6. Involve the family (Pridham et al., 2010).

## Long-Term Outcomes

A. **There are more than a million adults now living with complex congenital heart disease who required surgery in the first month of life.**
B. **Mortality has decreased dramatically over the last decade;** however, mortality remains higher in low birth weight infants with the same defects (Marino et al., 2012).
C. **Neurodevelopmental outcomes.**
   1. Adverse outcomes are well documented in the literature.
      a. Infancy.
         (1) Feeding issues are present in 50% of infants.
         (2) Delay in milestones by several months.
   2. Damage to central nervous system, including new white matter injury (Beca et al., 2013).
      a. 44% of all who had surgery before 8 weeks of age.
      b. Equally common with or without cardiopulmonary bypass during surgery.
      c. Most frequently seen in patients who had circulatory arrest or arch surgery.
D. **Factors associated with poor outcomes.**
   1. Preoperative factors (Khoshnood et al., 2012).
      a. Gestational age (inversely related) (Goff et al., 2012).
      b. Type of defect; increased risk of aneurysms with coarctation of the aorta.
      c. Brain anomaly or injury.
      d. Age at time of repair.
      e. Presence of syndrome or chromosomal abnormality.
      f. Non-white race and ethnicity (Oster et al., 2011).
      g. Lower socioeconomic class (Tabbutt et al., 2012).
      h. Parental distress (Brandlistuen et al., 2011).
   2. Operative factors.
      a. Type of circulatory support during surgery (Caputo et al., 2011).
         (1) Deep hypothermic circulatory arrest.
            (a) Period of cerebral ischemia followed by reperfusion leading to inflammatory response.
         (2) Continuous cardiopulmonary bypass.
      b. Hemodilution.
      c. Degree of cooling.
   3. Postoperative.
      a. Seizures within 48 hours of surgery.
         (1) Linked to increase in cerebral palsy and neurodevelopmental delays.
         (2) Hypoxemia, low cardiac output; cardiac arrest.
         (3) CHF.
      b. Lower Neonatal Intensive Care Unit Network Neurobehavioral Scale (NNNS) (Massaro et al., 2011).

## Parental Support and Education (see Chapter 17)

### General Information

Whether made prenatally or postnatally, the diagnosis of a CHD or disease is stress-inducing for parents and other family members. Having the diagnosis made prenatally does not lessen the stress experienced after birth. It is imperative that families be given support, accurate education, and skills to care for their newborn. Postoperatively, parents focus on feeding, weight gain, and caregiver sleep deprivation. Education must be directed toward these issues and may be facilitated by a family-centered approach to care (Hartman and Medoff-Cooper, 2012).

## REFERENCES

Ahmad, U.A., Fatimi, S.H., Naqvi, I., et al.: Modified Blalock-Taussig shunt: Immediate and short-term follow-up results. *Heart Lung Circulation*, 17:54–58, 2007.

Almond, C.S., Singh, T.P., Gauvreau, K., et al.: Extracorporeal membrane oxygenation for bridge to heart transplantation among children in the United States. *Circulation*, 123:2975–2984, 2011.

Altman, C.A.: Congenital heart disease (CHD) in the newborn: Presentation and screening for critical CHD. *UpToDate*. 2013. Available atwww.uptodate.com; accessed April 2, 2013.

Alverson, C.J., Strickland, M.J., Gilboa, S.M., and Correa, A.: Maternal smoking and congenital heart defects in the Baltimore-Washington Infant Study. *Pediatrics*, 127:e647–e653, 2011.

American Academy of Pediatrics, Section on Cardiology and Cardiac Surgery: Endorsement of Health and Human Services recommendation for pulse oximetry screening for critical congenital heart disease. *Pediatrics*, 129:190, 2012.

American Heart Association: Surgical management of atrial septal defect. *AHA News*. 2008. Retrieved January 26, 2008, from www.americanheart.org.

Andreassi, M.G., Ait-Ali, L., Botto, N., et al.: Cardiac catheterization and long-term chromosomal damage in children with congenital heart disease. *European Heart Journal*, 27:2703–2704, 2006.

Aranda, J.V. and Thomas, R.: Pharmacology review: Pharmacokinetic considerations with intravenous ibuprofen lysine. *NeoReviews*, 12(3):e516–e523, 2005.

Artman, M., Mahony, L. and Teitel, D.F.: *Neonatal cardiology*. New York, 2002, McGraw-Hill, pp. 196-199, 231-243.

Atz, A.M., Hawkins, J.A., Lu, M., et al.: Surgical management of complete atrioventricular septal defect: Associations with surgical technique, age, and trisomy 21. *Journal of Thoracic and Cardiovascular Surgery*, 141(6):1371–1379, 2011.

Balzer, D.T.: Percutaneous pulmonary valve implantation: fixing the problems and pushing the envelope. *Current Opinions in Pediatrics*, 24(5):565–568, 2012.

Beca, J., Gunn, J.K., Coleman, L., et al.: New white matter brain injury after infant heart surgery is associated with diagnostic group and the use of circulatory arrest. *Circulation*, 127:971–979, 2013.

Beck, A.E. and Hudgins, L.: Congenital cardiac malformations in the neonate: Isolated or syndromic? *NeoReviews*, 4(4):e105–e110, 2003.

Behera, S.K., Zuccaro, J.C., Wetzel, G.T. and Alejos, J.C.: Nesiritide improves hemodynamics in children with dilated cardiomyopathy: A pilot study. *Pediatric Cardiology*, 30:26–34, 2009.

Bishara, N. and Clericuzio, C.L.: Common dysmorphic syndromes in the NICU. *NeoReviews*, 3(1):e29–e38, 2008.

Blackburn, S.T.: Cardiovascular system. In S.T. Blackburn (Ed.): *Maternal, fetal, and neonatal physiology: A clinical perspective* (4th ed.). St. Louis, 2013, Elsevier Saunders, pp. 267–314.

Brandlistuen, R.E., Stene-Larsen, K., Holmstrom, H., et al.: Occurrence and predictors of developmental impairments in 3-year old children with congenital heart defects. *Journal of Developmental and Behavioral Pediatrics*, 32:526–532, 2011.

Bronicki, R.A. and Chang, A.C.: Management of the postoperative pediatric cardiac surgical patient. *Critical Care Medicine*, 39:1974–1984, 2011.

Capparelli, E.V.: Pharmacologic, pharmacodynamic, and pharmacokinetic considerations with intravenous ibuprofen lysine. *Journal of Pediatric Pharmacology and Therapeutics*, 12(3):158–170, 2007.

Caputo, M., Patel, N., Angelini, G.D., et al.: Effect of normothermic cardiopulmonary bypass on renal injury in pediatric cardiac surgery: A randomized controlled trial. *Journal of Thoracic and Cardiovascular Surgery*, 142:1114–1121, 2011.

Chen, Q., Cao, H., Zhang, G.C., et al.: Safety and feasibility of intra-operative device closure of atrial septal defect with transthoracic minimum invasion. *European Journal of Cardio-Thoracic Surgery*, 41(1):121–125, 2012.

Chubb, H., Pesonen, E., Sivasubramanian, S., et al.: Long-term outcome following catheter valvotomy for pulmonary atresia with intact ventricular septum. *Journal of the American College of Cardiology*, 59 (16):1468–1476, 2012.

Clyman, R.I.: Surgical ligation of the patent ductus arteriosus: Treatment or morbidity? *Journal of Pediatrics*, 161(4):583–584, 2012.

Collins-Nakai, R. and McLaughlin, P.: How congenital heart disease originates in life. *Cardiology Clinics*, 20(3):367–383, 2002.

Corff, K.E.: Clinical considerations in the management of PDA in premature infants. Symposium presented at National Association of Neonatal Nurses Conference, 2007.

Corff, K.E. and Sekar, K.C.: Clinical considerations for the pharmacologic management of patent ductus arteriosus with cyclooxygenase inhibitors in premature infants. *Journal of Pediatric Pharmacology and Therapeutics*, 12(3):147–157, 2007.

Cowles, R.A.: Congenital heart defect—corrective surgery. *Medline Plus Medical Encyclopedia*. 2012. Available at http://www.nlm.nih.gov/medlineplus/ency/article/002948.htm.

Cuadrado, A.R.: Management of postoperative low cardiac output syndrome. *Critical Care Nursing Quarterly*, 25(3):63–71, 2002.

Davlouros, P.A., Karatza, I., Xanthopoulou, G., et al.: Diagnostic role of plasma BNP levels in neonates with signs of congenital heart disease. *International Journal of Cardiology*, 147(1):42–46, 2011.

Dawson, J.A., Kamlin, C.F.C., Wong, C., et al.: Changes in heart rate in the first minutes after birth. *Archives of Disease in Childhood: Fetal and Neonatal Edition*, 95: F177–F181, 2010.

de Siena, P., Ghorbel, M., Chen, Q., et al.: Common arterial trunk: Review of surgical strategies and future research. *Expert Review of Cardiovascular Therapy*, 9(12):1527–1538, 2011.

Dhannapuneni, R.R.V., Gladman, G., Kerr, S., et al.: Complete atrioventricular septal defect: Outcome of pulmonary artery banding improved by adjustable device. *Journal of Thoracic and Cardiovascular Surgery*, 141(1):179–182, 2011.

Donofrio, M.T., Levy, R.J., Schuette, J.J., et al.: Specialized delivery room planning for fetuses with critical congenital heart disease. *American Journal of Cardiology*, 111(5):737–747, 2013.

Dorfman, A.T., Marino, B.S., Wernovsky, G., et al.: Critical heart disease in the neonate: Presentation and outcome at a tertiary care center. *Pediatric Critical Care Medicine*, 9(3):1–10, 2008.

Dryzek, P., Goreczny, S., and Kopala, M.: Interventional treatment of critical coarctation of the aorta in an extremely low birth weight preterm neonate. *Cardiology in the Young*, 22(4):475–477, 2012.

Dutta, S. and Albanese, C.T.: Minimal access surgery in the neonate. *NeoReviews*, 7(8):e400–e409, 2006.

Evans, N. and Seri, I.: Cardiovascular compromise in the newborn infant. In H.W. Taeusch, R.A. Ballard, and C.A. Gleason (Eds.): *Avery's diseases of the newborn.* Philadelphia, 2005, Elsevier Saunders, pp. 398–437.

Fadel, B.M., Manlhiot, C., Al-Halees, Z., et al.: The fate of the neoaortic valve and root after the modified Ross-Konno procedure. *Journal of Thoracic and Cardiovascular Surgery*, 145(2):430–437, 2013.

Flanagan, M.F., Yeager, S.B., and Weindling, S.N.: Cardiac disease. In M.G. MacDonald, M.M.K. Seshia, and M.D. Mullett (Eds.): *Avery's neonatology: Pathophysiology and management of the newborn* (6th ed.). Philadelphia, 2005, Lippincott, Williams & Wilkins, pp. 633–709.

Fleiner, S.: Recognition and stabilization of neonates with congenital heart disease. *Newborn and Infant Nursing Reviews*, 6(3):137–150, 2006.

Forbes, T.J., Kim, D.W., Turner, D.R., et al.: Comparison of surgical, stent, and balloon angioplasty of native coarctation of the aorta: An observational study by the CCISC (Congenital Cardiovascular Interventional Study Consortium). *Journal of the American College of Cardiology*, 58(25):2664–2674, 2011.

Friedberg, M.K., Su, X., Tworetzky, W., et al.: Validation of 3D echocardiographic assessment of left ventricular volumes, mass, and ejection fractions in neonates and infants with congenital heart disease. *Imaging*, 3:735–742, 2010.

Frost, M.S., Fashaw, L., Hernandez, J.A., and Jones, M.D. Jr.: Neonatal nephrology. In S.L. Gardner, B.S. Carter, M.I. Enzman-Hines, and J.A. Hernandez (Eds.): *Merenstein & Gardner's handbook of neonatal intensive care* (7th ed.). St. Louis, 2011, Elsevier Mosby, pp. 717–747.

Gandhi, R., Almond, C., Singh, T.P., et al.: Factors associated with in-hospital mortality in infants undergoing heart transplantation in the United States. *Journal of Thoracic and Cardiovascular Surgery*, 141:531–536, 2011.

Ghanayem, N.S., Allen, K.R., Tabbutt, S., et al.: Interstage mortality after the Norwood procedure: Results of the multicenter Single Ventricle Reconstruction trial. *Journal of Thoracic and Cardiovascular Surgery*, 144:896–906, 2012.

Glickstein, J.S.: Cardiology. In R.A. Polin, and A.R. Spitzer (Eds.): *Fetal and neonatal secrets* Philadelphia, 2007, Elsevier Mosby, pp. 80–114.

Goff, D.A., Luan, X., Gerdes, M., et al.: Younger gestational age is associated with worse neurodevelopmental outcomes after cardiac surgery in infancy. *Journal of Thoracic and Cardiovascular Surgery*, 143:535–542, 2012.

Grant, B., Morgan, G.J., McCrossan, B.A., et al.: Remote diagnosis of congenital heart disease: The impact of telemedicine. *Archives of Disease in Childhood*, 95:276–280, 2010.

Habib, A., Jacobs, H.F., Mavroudis, J.P., et al.: Contemporary patterns of management of tetralogy of Fallot: Data from the Society of Thoracic Surgeons Database. *Annals of Thoracic Surgery*, 90(3):813–819, 2010.

Hartman, R.J., Rasmussen, S.A., Botto, L.D., et al.: The contribution of chromosomal abnormalities to congenital heart defects: a population-based study. *Pediatric Cardiology*, 32(8):1147–1157, 2011.

Hartman, D.M. and Medoff-Cooper, B.: Transition to home after neonatal surgery for congenital heart disease. *MCN: American Journal of Maternal Child Nursing*, 37(2):95–100, 2012.

Hay, W.W., Hayward, A.R., Levin, M.J. and Sondheimer, J.M.: Cardiovascular diseases. In S. Reinhardt, H. Lebowitz, and L.A. Sheinis (Eds.): *Current pediatric diagnosis and treatment* (16th ed.). New York, 2003, McGraw-Hill.

Hermes-DeSantis, E.R. and Aranda, J.V.: Clinical experience with intravenous ibuprofen lysine in the pharmacologic closure of patent ductus arteriosus. *Journal of Pediatric Pharmacology and Therapeutics*, 12 (3):171–182, 2007.

Hiremath, G., Natarajan, G., Math, D. and Aggarwal, S.: Impact of balloon atrial septostomy in neonates with transposition of the great arteries. *Journal of Perinatology*, 31(7):494–499, 2011.

Holzer, R.J., Gauvreau, K., Kreutzer, J., et al.: Safety and efficacy of balloon pulmonary valvuloplasty: A multicenter experience. *Catheterization & Cardiovascular Interventions*, 80(4):663–672, 2012.

Hraska, V., Sinzobahamvya, N., Haun, C., et al.: The long-term outcome of open valvotomy for critical aortic stenosis in neonates. *Annals of Thoracic Surgery*, 94 (5):1519–1526, 2012.

Jonas, J.M. and Demmer, L.A.: Genetic syndromes determined by alterations in genomic imprinting pathways. *NeoReviews*, 8(20):e120–e126, 2007.

Jones, K.J., Willis, M. and Uzark, K.: The blues of congenital heart disease. *Newborn and Infant Nursing Reviews*, 6(3):117–127, 2006.

Kanter, K.R., Kogon, B.E., Kirshbom, P.M. and Carlock, P.R.: Symptomatic neonatal tetralogy of Fallot: Repair or shunt? *Annals of Thoracic Surgery*, 89 (3):858–863, 2010.

Kaplan, J.H., Ades, A.M. and Rychik, J.: Effect of prenatal diagnosis on outcome in patient with congenital heart disease. *NeoReviews*, 6(7):e326–e331, 2005.

Karamichalis, J.M., Thiagarajan, R.R., Liu, H., et al.: Stage I Norwood: optimal technical performance improves outcomes irrespective of preoperative physiologic status or case complexity. *Journal of Thoracic and Cardiovascular Surgery*, 139(4):962–968, 2010.

Karlsen, K.A.: Transporting newborns the S.T.A.B.L.E. way. A manual for community hospital caregivers: Pre-transport stabilization of sick newborns. In *The S.T.A.B.L.E. program instructor manual.* Park City, UT, 2006, S.T.A.B.L.E. Program, pp. 130–149.

Karlsen, K.A. and Tani, L.Y.: *S.T.A.B.L.E. cardiac module.* Park City, UT, 2003, S.T.A.B.L.E. Program.

Kelle, A.M., Backer, C.L., Gossett, J.G., Kaushal, S. Mavroudis, C.: Total anomalous pulmonary venous connection: results of surgical repair of 100 patients at a single institution. *Journal of Thoracic and Cardiovascular Surgery*, 139(6):1387–1394, 2010.

Kemper, A.R., Mahle, W.T., Martin, G.R., et al.: Strategies for implementing screening for critical congenital heart disease. *Pediatrics*, 128:e1259–e1266, 2011.

Khairy, P., Clair, M., Fernandes, S.M., et al.: Cardiovascular outcomes after arterial switch operation for *d*-transposition of the great arteries. *Circulation*, 127:331–339, 2013.

Khoshnood, B., Lelong, N., Houyel, L., et al.: Prevalence, timing of diagnosis and mortality of newborns with congenital heart defects: A population-based study. *Heart*, 98:1667–1673, 2012.

Kipps, A. and Silverman, N.H.: Historical perspectives: The introduction of ultrasonography in neonatal cardiac diagnosis. *NeoReviews*, 6(7):e315–e325, 2005.

Kensey, P.M., Howser, D., Williams, L.C. and Iskersky, V.: Cardiovascular diseases and surgical interventions. In S.L. Gardner, B.S. Carter, M.I. Enzman-Hines, and J.A. Hernandez (Eds.): *Merenstein & Gardner's handbook of neonatal intensive care* (7th ed.). St. Louis, 2011, Elsevier Mosby, pp. 678–716.

Knowles, R.L., Bull, C., Wren, C. and Dezateux, C.: Mortality with congenital heart defects in England and Wales, 1959-2009: Exploring technological change through period and birth cohort analysis. *Archives of Disease in Childhood*, 97:861–865, 2012.

Koren, G. and Nordeng, H.: Antidepressant use during pregnancy: The benefit-risk ratio. *American Journal of Obstetrics & Gynecology*, 207(3):157–163, 2012.

Kunanithy, V.: An approach to neonatal cyanosis. *Learn Pediatrics.* 2011. Available at www.learnpediatrics.com; accessed March 12, 2013.

LaPar, D.J., Mery, C.M., Peeler, B.B., et al.: Short and long-term outcomes for bidirectional Glenn procedure performed with and without cardiopulmonary bypass. *Annals of Thoracic Surgery*, 94(1):164–170, 2012.

Lott, J.L.: Cardiovascular system. In C. Kenner, and J.W. Lott (Eds.): *Comprehensive neonatal care: An interdisciplinary approach* (5th ed.). St. Louis, 2014, Elsevier Saunders, pp. 152188.

Mahle, W.T., Newburger, J.W., Matherne, G.P., et al.: Role of pulse oximetry in examining newborns for congenital heart disease: A scientific statement from the American Heart Association and American Academy of Pediatrics. *Circulation*, 120: 447–458, 2009.

Marino, B.S., Lipkin, P.H., Newburger, J.W., et al.: Neurodevelopmental outcomes in children with congenital heart disease: Evaluation and management. A scientific statement from the American Heart Association. *Circulation*, 126:1143–1172, 2012.

Markham, M.: Patent ductus arteriosus in the premature infant: A clinical dilemma. *Newborn and Infant Nursing Reviews*, 6(3):151–157, 2006.

Massaro, A.N., Glass, P., Brown, J., et al.: Neurobehavioral abnormalities in newborns with congenital heart disease requiring open-heart surgery. *Journal of Pediatrics*, 158:678–681, 2011.

Mayo Clinic Staff: Coarctation of the aorta. 2006: Retrieved February 8, 2008, from www.mayoclinica.com.

McElhinney, D.B., Tworetzky, W. and Lock, J.E.: Current status of fetal cardiac intervention. *Circulation*, 121:1256–1263, 2010.

Mezu-Ndubuisi, O.J., Agarwal, G., Raghavan, A., et al.: Patent ductus arteriosus in premature neonates. *Drugs*, 72(7):907–916, 2012.

Miller, A., Riehle-Colarusso, T., Alverson, C.J., et al.: Congenital heart defects and major structural noncardiac anomalies, Atlanta, Georgia, 1968 to 2005. *Journal of Pediatrics*, 159:70–78, 2011.

Mo, X., Zuo, W., Ma, Z., et al.: Hybrid procedure with cardiopulmonary bypass for muscular ventricular septal defects in children. *European Journal of Cardio-Thoracic Surgery*, 40(5):1203–1206, 2011.

Moake, L. and Ramaciotti, C.: Atrial septal defect treatment options. *AACN Clinical Issues*, 16(2):252–266, 2005.

Newazhay, T., Chernogrivov, A., Biryukov, E., et al.: Arterial switch in the first hours of life: No need for Rashkind septostomy? *European Journal of Cardio-Thoracic Surgery*, 42(3):520–523, 2012.

Newburger, J.W., Sleeper, L.A., Bellinger, D.C., et al.: Early developmental outcome in children with hypoplastic left heart syndrome and related anomalies. *Circulation*, 125:2081–2091, 2012.

Nyrnes, S.A., Lovstakken, L., Skogvoll, E., et al.: Does a new ultrasound flow modality improve visualization of neonatal pulmonary veins? *Echocardiography*, 27 (9):1113–1119, 2010.

Oncel, M.Y., Yurttutan, S., Uras, N., et al.: An alternative drug (paracetamol) in the management of patent ductus arteriosus in ibuprofen-resistant or contraindicated preterm infants. *Archives of Disease in Childhood: Fetal and Neonatal Edition*, 98:F94, 2013.

Ofori-Amanfo, G. and Cheifetz, I.M.: Pediatric postoperative cardiac care. *Critical Care Clinics*, 29 (2):185–202, 2013.

Oster, M.E., Strickland, M.J. and Mahle, W.T.: Racial and ethnic disparities in post-operative mortality following congenital heart surgery. *Journal of Pediatrics*, 159:222–226, 2011.

Overmeire, B.V.: Common clinical and practical questions on the use of intravenous ibuprofen lysine for the treatment of patent ductus arteriosus. *Journal of Pediatric Pharmacology and Therapeutics*, 12 (3):194–206, 2007.

Oyen, N., Poulsen, G., Boyd, H., et al.: Recurrence of congenital heart defects in families. *Circulation*, 120:295–301, 2009.

Park, C.S., Kim, W.H., Kim, G.B., et al.: Symptomatic young infants with tetralogy of Fallot: one-stage versus staged repair. *Journal of Cardiac Surgery*, 25 (4):394–399, 2010.

Park, M.K.: *Pediatric cardiology for practitioners:* (5th ed.). St. Louis, 2008, Elsevier Mosby.

Parra, D.A. and Vera, K.: New imaging modalities to assess cardiac function: Not just pretty pictures. *Current Opinion in Pediatrics*, 24:557–564, 2012.

Pike, N.A. and Falco, D.A.: Postoperative care of the neonate/infant after cardiac surgery. In B.A. Reitz, and D.D. Yuh (Eds.): *Congenital cardiac surgery*, New York, 2002, McGraw-Hill, pp. 193–202

Prakash, A., Powell, A.J. and Geva, T.: Multimodality of noninvasive imaging for assessment of congenital heart disease. *Circulation and Cardiovascular Imaging*, 3:112–125, 2010.

Pridham, K., Harrison, T., Krolikowski, M., et al.: Internal working models of parenting: Motivations of parents of infants with a congenital heart defect. *Advances in Nursing Science*, 33(4):E1–E16, 2010.

Punukollo, M., Harnden, A., and Tulloh, R.: Coarctation of the aorta in the newborn. *BMJ*, 343:1–5, 2011.

Reade, C., Maziarz, D.M., and Koutlas, T.C.: Coarctation of the aorta and interrupted aortic arch: Surgical perspectives. *eMedicine*. 2006. Retrieved February 1, 2008, from www.emedicine.com/Ped/topic2824.htm, 2006.

Rossi, R.I., Manica, J.L., Petraco, R., et al.: Balloon aortic valvuloplasty for congenital aortic stenosis using the femoral and the carotid artery approach: A 16-year experience from a single center. *Catheterization & Cardiovascular Interventions*, 78(1):84–90, 2011.

Russell, H.M., Pasquali, S.K., Jacobs, J.P., et al.: Outcomes of repair of common arterial trunk with truncal valve surgery: A review of the Society of Thoracic Surgeons Congenital Heart Surgery Database. *Annals of Thoracic Surgery*, 93(1):164–169, 2012.

Sakurai, T., Stickley, J., Stumper, O., et al.: Repair of isolated aortic coarctation over two decades: Impact of surgical approach and associated arch hypoplasia. *Interactive Cardiovascular and Thoracic Surgery*, 15 (5):865–870, 2012.

Sansoucie, D.A. and Cavaliere, T.A.: Newborn and infant assessment. In C. Kenner and J.W. Lott (Eds.): *Comprehensive neonatal care: An interdisciplinary approach* (4th ed.). St. Louis, 2007, Elsevier Saunders, pp. 677–718.

Satou, G.M.: Pediatric congestive heart failure. *Medscape: Drugs, Diseases & Procedures*, Updated February 11, 2013. Retrieved April 2, 2013, from www.emedicine.medscape.com.

Sedmera, D.: Function and form in the developing cardiovascular system. *Cardiovascular Research*, 91 (2):252–259, 2011.

Seri, I. and Evans, J.: Controversies in the diagnosis and management of hypotension in the newborn infant. *Current Opinion in Pediatrics*, 13(2):116–123, 2001.

Smithells, R.W. and Newman, C.G.H.: Recognition of thalidomide defects. *Journal of Medical Genetics*, 29:716–723, 1992.

Spence, K.: Surgical considerations in the newborn and infant. In C. Kenner, and J.W. Lott (Eds.): *Comprehensive neonatal care: An interdisciplinary approach* (4th ed.). St. Louis, 2007, Elsevier Saunders, pp. 385–391.

Stein, P.: Total anomalous pulmonary venous connection. *AORN Journal*, 85(3):509–520, 2007.

Stone, D.H.: Long-term survival of children born with congenital anomalies. *Lancet*, 375:614–615, 2010.

Stumper, O.: Hypoplastic left heart syndrome. *Heart*, 96:231–236, 2010.

Tabbutt, S., Gaynor, J.W. and Newburger, J.W.: Neurodevelopmental outcomes after congenital heart surgery and strategies for improvement. *Current Opinion in Cardiology*, 27(2):82–91, 2012.

Takemoto, C.K., Hodding, J.H., and Kraus, D.M.: *Pediatric & neonatal dosage handbook* (18th ed.). Cleveland, OH, 2011, Lexi-Comp.

Tao, K., Lin, K., Shi, Y., et al.: Periventricular device closure of perimembranous ventricular septal defects in 61 young children: Early midterm follow-up results. *Journal of Thoracic and Cardiovascular Surgery*, 140:864–870, 2010.

Tararbit, K., Houyel, L., Bonnet, D., et al.: Risk of congenital heart defects associated with reproductive technologies: A population-based evaluation. *European Heart Journal*, 32:500–508, 2011.

Thammineni, K., Lohr, J., Trefz, M. and Sivanandam, S.: Perinatal/neonatal case presentation: Familial recurrence of congenital heart disease. *Journal of Perinatology*, 31:742–743, 2011.

Trivedi, B., Smith, P.B., Barker, P.C.A., et al.: Arrhythmias in patients with hypoplastic left heart syndrome. *American Heart Journal*, 161:138–144, 2011.

Tweddell, J.S., Sleeper, L.A., Ohye, R.G., et al.: Intermediate-term mortality and cardiac transplantation in infants with single ventricles: Risk factors and their interaction with shunt type. *Journal of Thoracic and Cardiovascular Surgery*, 144:152–159, 2012.

U.S. Food and Drug Administration: FDA approves mechanical cardiac assist device for children with heart failure. *FDA News Release*. Washington, DC, 2011, U.S. Food and Drug Administration.

Van de Berg, G. and Moorman, A.F.M.: Concepts of cardiac development in retrospect. *Pediatric Cardiology*, 30:580–587, 2009.

van der Born, T., Zomer, A.C., Zwinderman, A.H., et al.: The changing epidemiology of congenital heart disease. *Nature Reviews: Cardiology*, 8:50–60, 2011.

Vyas, H.V., Greenberg, S.B. and Krishnamurthy, R.: MR imaging and CT evaluation of congenital pulmonary vein abnormalities in neonates and infants. *Radiographics*, 32(1):87–98, 2012.

Webb, G.D., Smallhorn, J.F., Therrien, J., and Redington, A.N.: Congenital heart disease. In R.O. Bonow, D.L. Mann, D.P. Zipes, and P. Libby (Eds.): *Braunwald's heart disease: A textbook of cardiovascular medicine* (9th ed.). Philadelphia, 2011, Elsevier Saunders.

Wechsler, S.B. and Wernovsky, G.: Cardiac disorders. In J.P. Cloherty, E.C. Eichenwald, and A.R. Stark (Eds.): *Manual of neonatal care* (5th ed.). Philadelphia, 2004, Lippincott, Williams & Wilkins, pp. 407–460.

Wernovsky, G., Ades, A.M. and Spray, T.L.: Management of congenital heart disease in the low-birth-weight infant. In H.W. Taeusch, R.A. Ballard, and C.A. Gleason (Eds.): *Avery's diseases of the newborn* (8th ed.). Philadelphia, 2005, Elsevier Saunders, pp. 888–895.

Wernovsky, G. and Gruber, P.J.: Common congenital heart disease: Presentation, management, and outcomes. In H.W. Taeusch, R.A. Ballard, and C.A. Gleason (Eds.): *Avery's diseases of the newborn* (8th ed.). Philadelphia, 2005, Elsevier Saunders, pp. 827–871.

Young, T.E. and Mangum, B.: *Neofax:* (21st ed.). Montvale, NJ, 2008, Thomson Healthcare.

Zahorec, M., Hrubsova, Z., Skrak, P., et al.: A comparison of Blalock-Taussig shunts with and without closure of the ductus arteriosus in neonates with pulmonary atresia. *Annals of Thoracic Surgery*, 92 (2):653–658, 2011.

CHAPTER

# 29 Gastrointestinal Disorders

WANDA T. BRADSHAW

**OBJECTIVES**

1. Discuss normal and abnormal abdominal assessment findings.
2. Discuss common laboratory and diagnostic tests used to evaluate the gastrointestinal system.
3. Differentiate between omphalocele and gastroschisis.
4. Identify four common associations in infants with intestinal obstruction.
5. Identify the clinical presentation of a neonate with tracheoesophageal fistula.
6. Describe radiographic findings in an infant with duodenal atresia.
7. Identify one gastrointestinal disorder that is considered a surgical emergency.
8. Identify the gastrointestinal presentation of infants with cystic fibrosis.
9. Describe the defect in Hirschsprung's disease.
10. Identify the three mechanisms involved in the pathogenesis of necrotizing enterocolitis.
11. Describe the clinical presentation of an infant with biliary atresia.
12. Identify at least three management strategies for the infant with cholestasis.
13. Identify at least three management strategies for the infant with gastroesophageal reflux.
14. Identify the triad of anomalies occurring in prune-belly syndrome.
15. Describe the symptoms of diaphragmatic hernia.
16. Differentiate between unconjugated and conjugated bilirubin.
17. Compare and contrast physiologic and nonphysiologic jaundice.
18. Describe management of an infant receiving phototherapy.
19. Define "hydrops."

Unique embryologic features of the gastrointestinal (GI) tract, such as the obliteration and recanalization of the GI tract, midgut herniation into the umbilical cord, and rotation of the intestines, make the GI tract prone to a variety of congenital anomalies. Anomalies may affect any part of the GI tract, from the mouth to the anus. Atresias, stenoses, and functional obstructions account for the vast majority of congenital defects. As for acquired defects, necrotizing enterocolitis (NEC) is the most common serious GI illness in neonates. This chapter will review the more common GI anomalies and a variety of multisystem disorders that have significant GI involvement, such as prune-belly syndrome, congenital diaphragmatic hernia (CDH), hyperbilirubinemia, and hydrops.

## GASTROINTESTINAL EMBRYONIC DEVELOPMENT

A. **Week 3.** Tubular intestine begins to form; omphalomesenteric (yolk stalk) duct forms; mesentery is forming; major digestive (salivary, liver, pancreas, gallbladder) and endocrine (thyroid) gland formation is initiated.
B. **Week 4.** Intestine is present; esophagus and trachea separate and are distinct; stomach becomes obvious; liver is present.
C. **Week 5.** Esophagus, stomach, proximal duodenum present; intestine elongates into a loop and begins to rotate.

D. **Week 6.** Stomach rotates into adult position; distal duodenum, jejunum, ileum, cecum, ascending colon, and proximal two thirds of transverse colon present; rapidly developing midgut herniates into umbilical cord.
E. **Week 7.** Rapid endothelial proliferation results in temporary duodenal occlusion; intestinal loops herniate into umbilical cord, lengthen, and rotate; and urorectal septum fuses with cloacal membrane, separating rectum from the developing urinary bladder.
F. **Week 8.** Small intestine recanalizes; intestinal villi develop; diaphragm complete.
G. **Weeks 9 and 10.** Intestines begin to reenter abdominal cavity and continue counterclockwise rotation around the axis of the superior mesenteric artery.
H. **Week 12.** Muscular layers of intestine are present; active transport of amino acids begins; pancreatic islet cells appear; bile appears; lactase appears.
I. **Week 16.** Meconium is present; swallowing is observed.
J. **Week 24.** Ganglion cells are detected in the rectum.
K. **Week 26.** Random peristalsis begins.
L. **Weeks 34 to 36.** Sucking and swallowing become coordinated.
M. **Weeks 36 to 38.** Maturity of GI system completed.
N. **Weeks 5 to 40.** Intestine elongates approximately 100-fold (small intestine is 6 times the length of the colon).

## FUNCTIONS OF THE GASTROINTESTINAL TRACT

A. **Absorption and digestion of nutrients.**
B. **Elimination of waste products.**
C. **Maintenance of fluid and electrolyte balance.**
D. **Protection of host from toxins and pathogens.**

## ASSESSMENT OF THE GASTROINTESTINAL SYSTEM

A. **History.**
   1. Family: presence of GI disease.
   2. Presence of genetic syndrome: Major syndromes associated with GI defects include the following (Jones et al., 2013):
      a. Apert's syndrome: pyloric stenosis, tracheoesophageal fistula/esophageal atresia (TEF/EA), CDH.
      b. Beckwith–Wiedemann syndrome: umbilical defects, diastasis recti, posterior diaphragmatic eventration, pancreatic hyperplasia resulting in hypoglycemia.
      c. Fetal hydantoin syndrome: umbilical hernia, duodenal atresia.
      d. Meckel–Gruber syndrome: liver defects (bile duct proliferation, fibrosis, cysts), single umbilical artery, patent urachus, omphalocele, intestinal malrotation, imperforate anus.
      e. Sirenomelia: imperforate anus, anal agenesis.
      f. Trisomy 13: umbilical defects, intestinal malrotation, CDH.
      g. Trisomy 18: umbilical defects, pyloric stenosis, intestinal malrotation, TEF/EA, CDH, single umbilical artery.
      h. Trisomy 21: Hirschsprung's disease, pyloric stenosis, duodenal atresia, intestinal malrotation.
      i. VATERR association (*v*ertebral defects, imperforate *a*nus, *t*racheo*e*sophageal fistula and/or esophageal atresia, and *r*adial and *r*enal dysplasia). Additional: single umbilical artery.
      j. VACTERL association (*v*ertebral defects, *a*nal atresia, *c*ardiac abnormalities, *t*racheoesophageal fistula and/or esophageal atresia, *r*enal agenesis or dysplasia, and *l*imb defects).
   3. History of present illness.
      a. Fetal ultrasonography.
         (1) Abdomen can be seen by 10 weeks of gestation, stomach by 13 weeks.
         (2) Abdomen can be assessed for intactness of abdominal wall, umbilical cord insertion, stomach as fluid-filled chamber, bowel dilation, or indication of obstruction.

(3) Polyhydramnios (>2000 mL) may indicate interference with fetal swallowing or intestinal obstruction.
(4) Oligohydramnios (<500 mL) may indicate renal agenesis or dysgenesis.

**b.** Birth weight, weight loss/gain, reflux, gastric aspirates, vomiting (bilious vs. nonbilious, projectile), timing of passage of first meconium stool, stool color, presence of blood, diarrhea, constipation, abdominal distention or tenderness, jaundice (Seidel et al., 2010).

**B. Abdominal assessment (Goodwin, 2009; Seidel et al., 2010).**

**1.** Inspection.

**a.** Size, shape, and color.
(1) Normal: rounded, soft, symmetrical, pink.
(2) Abnormal: erythematous, dusky, mottled.
(3) Distended: intestinal obstruction, infection, organomegaly, ascites.
(4) Scaphoid: associated with CDH.
(5) Asymmetrical: mass, organomegaly, intestinal obstruction.

**b.** Muscular development.
(1) Flat, flabby, lumpy: prune-belly syndrome.
(2) Gap between rectus muscles: diastasis recti.
(3) Externalization of abdominal contents: omphalocele, gastroschisis, bladder exstrophy.
(4) Hernias: protrusions of an organ or tissue through an abnormal opening. Common in three areas:
(a) Umbilical: common in African Americans, low birth weight males, trisomy 21, hypothyroidism, and mucopolysaccharidosis.
(b) Inguinal.
(i) More common in males, especially very low birth weight.
(ii) Frequently bilateral.
(iii) May not be evident until second or third month of life.
(iv) Usually readily reducible.
(c) Femoral.
(i) Rare but more common in females.
(ii) Located just below inguinal ligament on anterior aspect of thigh.

**c.** Umbilicus/umbilical cord.
(1) Normally pearly white.
(2) Normally three vessels: two ventrally situated arteries, one dorsally situated vein.
(3) Usually dries and spontaneously detaches in 10 to 14 days.
(4) Green or yellow staining suggests in-utero meconium passage.
(5) Wet, foul-smelling cord, or periumbilical redness: omphalitis.
(6) Persistent clear drainage: patent urachus.
(7) Ileal fluid drainage: omphalomesenteric duct.
(8) Serous or serosanguineous drainage: granuloma.
(9) Abnormally thick: single herniated loop of intestine.
(10) Thick, gelatinous: large for gestational age.
(11) Thin, small: intrauterine growth restriction.

**d.** Bowel loops.
(1) Normally not visible.
(2) Presence: obstruction.

**e.** Movements.
(1) Should move in synchrony with respirations.
(2) Movements not in synchrony may represent respiratory distress, peritoneal irritation, or central nervous system (CNS) disease.
(3) Peristalsis: not normally seen.
(a) May be seen in premature infants with thin abdominal walls.
(b) Presence: associated with hypertrophic pyloric stenosis.

**f.** Veins.
(1) Superficial veins become more prominent with abdominal distention.
(2) Dilated veins: venous obstruction.

**g.** Perineum: inspected for patency of anus and presence of fistulas.

2. Auscultation.
   a. Done before palpation (to avoid altering sounds).
   b. Bowel sounds.
      (1) Become audible within 15 to 30 minutes after birth (Montrawl, 2014).
      (2) Should have a metallic clicking quality.
      (3) Hyperactive or hypoactive does not necessarily represent pathologic change. Other historical or clinical findings should be taken into consideration when interpreting bowel sounds.
      (4) Increased sounds.
         (a) Malrotation.
         (b) Hirschsprung's disease.
         (c) Diarrhea.
      (5) Decreased or absent sounds.
         (a) Ileus.
         (b) Starvation.
         (c) Medication administration: opiates, magnesium, anesthesia.
   c. Vascular sounds: bruit, similar to murmur. Caused by turbulent blood flow through an artery, especially if heard despite position change of infant. Bruits may indicate partial vascular obstruction.
   d. Friction rub: peritoneal inflammation, splenic involvement, hepatic tumor, abscess.
3. Percussion.
   a. Provides information regarding size and location of organs, presence of masses, fluids, gases. Not a significantly useful tool in the newborn infant.
   b. Two main sounds to listen for:
      (1) Tympanic: low-pitched, heard over gas-filled structures (stomach).
      (2) Dullness: high-pitched, short, heard over dense or solid organs (liver, spleen).
4. Palpation.
   a. Performed to assess:
      (1) Abdominal tone.
      (2) Organ position.
         (a) Liver should be 1 to 2 cm below right costal margin, midclavicular line.
         (b) Spleen rarely palpable. Tip should not be more than 1 cm below left costal margin.
         (c) Kidneys are about 4 to 5 cm in length. Right kidney is easier to palpate and is lower than left.
      (3) Organomegaly.
      (4) Masses.
      (5) Pulsations.
      (6) Fluid.
   b. Technique: start in lower quadrants and progress to upper quadrants using a bimanual approach. Place one hand under infant's back; using free hand, start with light palpation, then progress to deep palpation.
   c. Hints to relax infant.
      (1) Use warm hands.
      (2) Flex legs.
      (3) Use gentle circular motion.
      (4) Slowly increase depth of palpation.
      (5) Palpate any known areas of tenderness last.

**C. Diagnostic tests.**
1. Gastric tests.
   a. Gastric aspirate. Measure pH of gastric contents.
   b. Apt test.
      (1) Differentiates swallowed maternal blood from fetal blood. Fetal hemoglobin remains pink; adult hemoglobin turns yellow-brown.
      (2) Can be done on gastric fluid or stool.
2. Stool examination.
   a. Normal: initially meconium followed by soft, yellow stool after milk introduction.

b. Examined for color, consistency, odor, blood, mucus, pus, tissue fragments, bacteria, and parasites.
c. Color may be influenced by diet, dyes, drugs, pathology.
(1) Green: indomethacin, meconium.
(2) Greenish black: iron, meconium.
(3) Black: iron, swallowed blood, blood from high GI tract lesion.
(4) Pale: biliary atresia.
(5) White: antacids, barium.
(6) Red: bright red indicates blood from low GI tract lesion or anal fissure; currant jelly indicates intussusception.
d. Odor.
(1) Sweet, yeasty, or acidic in odor suggests carbohydrate (CHO) malabsorption typical of osmotic diarrhea of viral enteritis.
(2) Purulent odor suggests colitis.
e. CHO malabsorption.
(1) pH less than 5 in infants is suggestive.
(2) Reducing substance test (Clinitest Reagent Tablets, Bayer Corp., Diagnostic Division, Elkhart, Ind.) detects CHO malabsorption indicating impaired bowel mucosal integrity or dysfunction that may be seen with NEC (Pinheiro et al., 2003).
f. Guaiac.
(1) Detects occult blood.

3. pH probe test: 24-hour pH probe study to diagnose GI reflux. Detects acid reflux only; does not detect nonacid (milk) or gas reflux.
4. Radiologic studies.
a. Plain radiograph (see Chapter 14).
(1) Bowel gas pattern (Montrawl, 2014).
(a) At birth, GI tract is fluid-filled and gasless.
(b) Within 30 minutes, gas should be in stomach.
(c) By 3 to 4 hours, gas should be in small intestine.
(d) After 6 to 8 hours, gas should be in entire intestine.
(2) Absence of gas below pylorus: possible indication of obstruction.
b. Upper GI series: done to assess structure and function of esophagus and evaluate for pyloric stenosis, malrotation, and strictures.
(1) Contrast material such as barium or a water-soluble product is administered via a nasogastric tube and observed by fluoroscopy.
(2) Water-soluble products are preferred in cases of suspected perforation.
c. Lower GI series: may be used to detect presence of malrotation, Hirschsprung's disease, meconium ileus, and meconium plug syndrome. May be therapeutic in meconium ileus and meconium plug syndrome.
5. Ultrasonography: may be used to diagnose suspected cases of pyloric stenosis, duplications, gastroesophageal reflux (GER), or biliary atresia.
6. Scintigraphy (nuclear scan): used to evaluate gastric emptying, aspiration with swallowing, reflux with aspiration, and liver excretory function. Radionuclide-tagged formula is fed to the infant and recorded by a gamma camera.
7. Endoscopy: used to directly visualize the upper or lower GI mucosa. Endoscopic retrograde cholangiopancreatography (ERCP) visualizes the biliary pancreatic ducts.
8. Fecal fat: used to diagnosis malabsorption syndromes. Fecal fat content greater than 6 g/24 hours is associated with malabsorption syndrome.
9. Culture: helpful in differentiating bloody diarrhea caused by infection versus hypoxic insult to intestine.

**D. Laboratory tests (Table 29-1) (Kee, 2005).**
1. Albumin.
a. Synthesized in the liver; it is the most abundant plasma protein.
b. Decreased levels occur in hepatocellular injury; usually a late finding.
2. Alkaline phosphatase (ALP).

■ TABLE 29-1
■ ■ **Laboratory Tests Used to Evaluate the Gastrointestinal System**

| Test | Preterm | Term | Reference |
|---|---|---|---|
| Alanine aminotransferase (ALT) (units/L) | — | 10 to 33 | 1 |
| Aspartate aminotransferase (AST) (units/L) | | 24 to 81 | 1 |
| Alkaline phosphatase (ALP) (units/L) | $207 \pm 60$ to $320 \pm 142$ | $164 \pm 68$ | 1 |
| Albumin (g/dL) | — | 2.8 to 4.4 | 2 |
| Bile acids | ⅙ of adult value | ½ of adult value | 3 |
| Bilirubin, total (mg/dL) | | | 1 |
| Cord | <2.8 | <2.8 | |
| 24 hours | 1 to 6 | 2 to 6 | |
| 48 hours | 6 to 8 | 6 to 7 | |
| 3 to 5 days | 10 to 12 | 4 to 6 | |
| ≥1 month | <1.5 | <1.5 | |
| Bilirubin, direct (mg/dL) | <0.5 | <0.5 | |
| Ammonia (mcg/dL) | — | 90 to 150 | 1 |
| γ-Glutamyltransferase (GGT) (units/L) | — | 14 to 131 | 1 |
| 5′-Nucleotidase (5′N, 5′NT) (units/L) | — | 5 to 10 | 4 |
| Prothrombin time (PT) (seconds) | — | 13 to 18 | 2 |

Adapted from [1]Blackburn, S.T.: *Maternal, fetal, and neonatal physiology: A clinical perspective* (4th ed.). St. Louis, 2013, Elsevier Mosby; [2]Martin, R.J., Fanaroff, A.A., and Walsh, M.C. (Eds.): *Fanaroff and Martin's neonatal-perinatal medicine: Diseases of the fetus and infant* (8th ed.). Philadelphia, 2006, Elsevier Mosby; [3]Malarkey, L.M. and McMorrow, M.E.: *Saunders nursing guide to laboratory and diagnostic tests.* St. Louis, 2005, Elsevier Saunders; [4]Simone, S.: Gastrointestinal critical care problems. In M.C. Curley and P.A. Moloney-Harmon (Eds.): *Critical care nursing of infants and children* (2nd ed.). Philadelphia, 2001, Saunders, pp. 765-804.

- **a.** ALP is derived from the epithelium of the intrahepatic bile ducts and excreted into the bile. It is also found in the bone, kidney, and small intestine.
- **b.** Elevated levels occur in obstructive liver disease (e.g., biliary atresia) and hepatitis, as well as in bone disease.

**3.** Aminotransferase activity.
- **a.** Alanine aminotransferase (ALT) catabolizes the reversible transfer of the α-amino group of aspartic acid to the α-keto group of α-ketoglutaric acid, leading to the formation of pyruvic acid.
- **b.** Aspartate aminotransferase (AST) catabolizes the reversible transfer of the α-amino group of aspartic acid to the α-keto group of α-ketoglutaric acid, leading to the formation of oxaloacetic acid.
- **c.** ALT and AST are the most sensitive tests of hepatocyte necrosis. ALT is more specific than AST because it is not found in high concentrations in other tissues.
- **d.** High elevations occur in hepatocellular injury. Slight elevations occur in cholestasis. Serum ALT greater than 300 units coupled with jaundice signals a liver disorder and not a hemolytic disorder.
- **e.** ALT-to-AST ratio is often performed to help differentiate types of liver disease.

**4.** Ammonia.
- **a.** Produced from the deamination of amino acids during protein metabolism and is a by-product of colonic bacteria protein breakdown. Liver is responsible for metabolizing ammonia.
- **b.** Elevated in liver failure.
- **c.** Elevations occur in acute or chronic liver disease.

**5.** Bilirubin.
- **a.** By-product of heme breakdown.
- **b.** Increased indirect bilirubin occurs when liver function is reduced (prematurity, injury) or when there is an excessive load of unconjugated bilirubin (hemolysis).
- **c.** Increased direct bilirubin occurs when the liver cannot excrete conjugated bilirubin into the bile ducts or biliary tract (biliary atresia, cholestasis).

6. Prothrombin time (PT).
   a. Measures the time required for prothrombin (factor II) to be converted to thrombin.
   b. In cases of obstructive liver disease in which bile acids do not reach the intestine, fat-soluble vitamins are not absorbed (required for coagulation factors).
   c. Prolonged PT occurs in patients with hepatocellular injury and biliary obstruction.
7. International Normalized Ratio (INR): ratio of a patient sample PT to a normal PT.
8. Serum bile acids.
   a. In the absence of abnormalities of the ileum, normal serum values reflect functioning of the enterohepatic circulation.
   b. Elevations occur in acute and chronic liver disease.

## ABDOMINAL WALL DEFECTS (CHRISTISON-LAGAY ET AL., 2011; ISLAM, 2012; LEDBETTER, 2012)

**A. Omphalocele (exomphalos).**

1. Definition: central defect with herniation of the abdominal viscera into the umbilical cord covered by a thin, avascular membranous sac composed of amnion and peritoneum with a small amount of Wharton's jelly. Umbilical arteries and veins insert into the apex of the defect (Fig. 29-1).
2. Etiology: multifactorial, including environmental, chromosomal (recessive and dominant forms), and folding abnormality of the germ disc, with failure to close the ventral abdominal wall.
3. Incidence: 2.5 per 10,000 live births.
4. Associated conditions: many will have associated anomalies or be part of a syndrome.
   a. Prematurity; small for gestational age.
   b. Cardiac defects (50%).
   c. Intestinal malrotation and/or atresia.
   d. Pentalogy of Cantrell: upper abdominal omphalocele above the umbilical cord, diaphragmatic hernia, sternal cleft, pericardial defect, ectopia cardiac defect.
   e. Neurologic anomalies, neural tube (40%).
   f. Genitourinary anomalies.
   g. Skeletal anomalies.

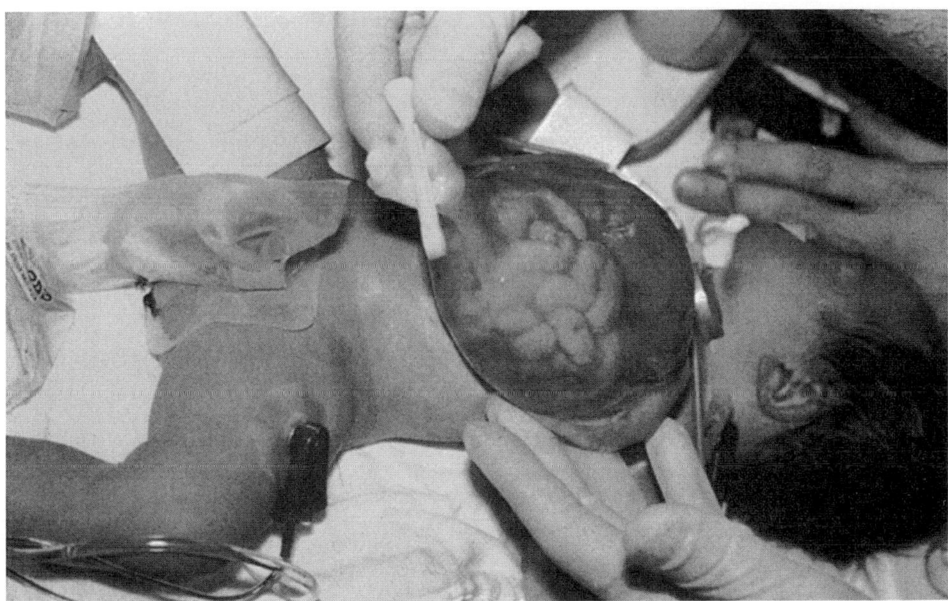

FIGURE 29-1 ■ Omphalocele.

h. Chromosomal anomalies (50% to 65%). Common anomalies include trisomy 13, 18, and 21, with 18 being the most frequent. Frequent in infants with Beckwith–Wiedemann syndrome (chromosome 11).

5. Diagnosis.
   a. Maternal serum markers: elevated serum α-fetoprotein to detect open defects.
   b. High-resolution prenatal ultrasound.
   c. Amniocentesis: chromosome analysis for associated defects; amniotic fluid α-fetoprotein and acetylcholinesterase levels to evaluate for defects associated with abnormal values.
   d. Inspection at birth.
      (1) Small defect: contains few loops of intestine, slightly enlarged umbilical ring. Any umbilical cord that is unusually fat should be inspected carefully before clamping to prevent intestinal trauma.
      (2) Large defect: may contain intestines, stomach, liver, spleen, bladder, uterus and ovaries, testicles; deficient upper musculature of umbilical ring.
      (3) The thin, avascular membranous sac may rupture before or at time of delivery; must be differentiated from gastroschisis because of the high rate of associated anomalies with omphalocele.
6. Prognosis.
   a. Mortality rate is related to size of defect and severity of associated anomalies.

**B. Gastroschisis (Sadler and Rasmussen, 2010).**

1. Definition: herniation of abdominal contents through an abdominal wall defect lateral to the umbilical ring; umbilical ring and cord are normal; right-sided predominance (Fig. 29-2). See Table 29-2 for a comparison of omphalocele and gastroschisis.
2. Etiology: unclear; theories include rupture of umbilical stalk, right periumbilical ischemia due to atrophy or persistence of the right umbilical vein, or a vascular accident of the right omphalomesenteric artery.
3. Incidence: overall 1 per 10,000 live births, with 7 per 10,000 in women less than 20 years old, of low socioeconomic status, and with exposure to vasoconstrictors (decongestants, nonsteroidal antiinflammatory drugs, cocaine).
4. Associated conditions.
   a. Prematurity.
   b. Intestinal malrotation (100%) and atresia (5% to 25%).
   c. Other anomalies are uncommon.

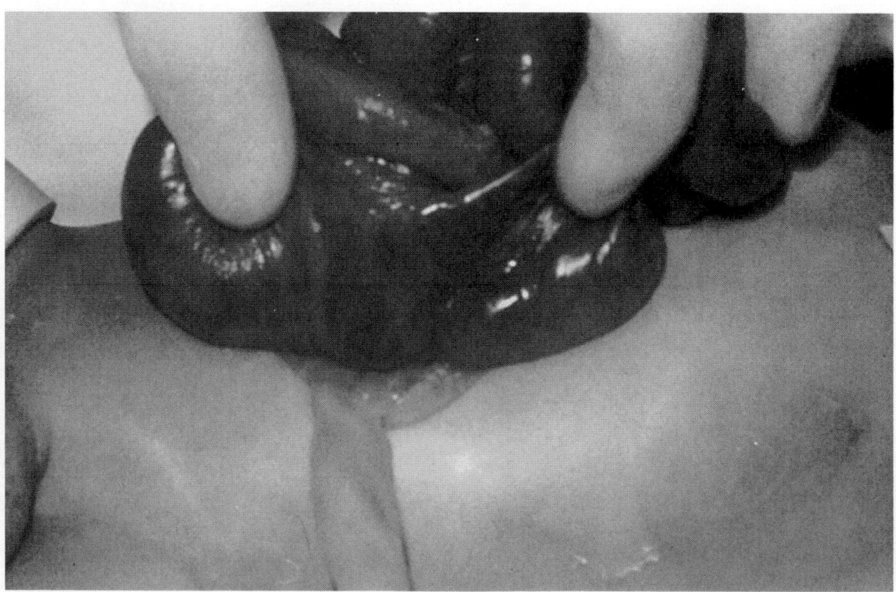

FIGURE 29-2 ■ Gastroschisis.

■ TABLE 29-2
■ ■ **Comparison of Omphalocele and Gastroschisis**

| | Omphalocele | Gastroschisis |
|---|---|---|
| Incidence | 1:5000 to 1:6000 | 1:30,000 to 1:50,000 |
| Covering | Present, may be ruptured | None |
| Site | Umbilical | Paraumbilical, usually to the right |
| Fascial defect | Small or large | Small |
| Herniated organs | Intestines; stomach, liver, spleen sometimes | Intestines; rarely liver |
| Appearance of herniated bowel | Normal, unless sac is ruptured | Often edematous, matted |
| Associated anomalies | 45% to 55% | 10% to 15% |
| IUGR | Less common | Common |

*IUGR*, Intrauterine growth restriction.

5. Diagnosis.
   a. Maternal serum markers: elevated serum α-fetoprotein to detect open defects.
   b. Prenatal ultrasonography, including a high-resolution method.
   c. Amniocentesis: chromosome analysis for associated defects; amniotic fluid α-fetoprotein and acetylcholinesterase levels to evaluate for defects associated with abnormal values.
   d. Inspection at birth.
      (1) Eviscerated abdominal organs without a thin, avascular membranous sac to protect the viscera.
      (2) Usually includes small and large intestines and rarely the liver.
      (3) Intestine may be thickened, edematous, and inflamed as a result of amniotic fluid exposure.
      (4) Fascial defect is smaller than with omphalocele.
      (5) Umbilical cord is intact.
      (6) Must be differentiated from ruptured omphalocele because of the high rate of associated anomalies with omphalocele.
6. Prognosis.
   a. Mortality rate is related to size of defect and severity of associated anomalies.
   b. Morbidity almost entirely related to intestinal dysfunction (impaired absorption, reduced enzymes, dysmotility) as a result of in-utero injury to eviscerated, unprotected bowel.

**C. Care of the neonate with an abdominal wall defect (omphalocele and gastroschisis).**

1. No research has demonstrated the efficacy of delivering infants with omphalocele or gastroschisis early.
2. Goals.
   a. Prevent hypothermia and hypovolemia (heat and evaporative fluid loss).
      (1) At the time of delivery, if there are exposed viscera, place infant in a sterile bowel bag from the feet to the axilla. Secure drawstring around torso at axilla. The bowel bag maintains a sterile environment for, and allows visualization of, the exposed viscera. If bowel bag is not available, cover the exposed defect and viscera with warm, sterile normal saline dressings. Then cover the dressing with plastic. Gauze dressings require rehydration to prevent drying, adherence to viscera, and tissue trauma when removed. Such dressings may contribute to hypothermia as the gauze cools over time. Close assessment for adequate perfusion is imperative.
      (2) Begin intravenous (IV) fluid as soon as possible. Add amino acids for injection and electrolytes as needed. IV fluid may need to be increased to approximately 150 mL/kg/day because of increased fluid loss through exposed bowel. Ideally, IV infusions should not be started in the lower extremities owing to postoperatively increased intra-abdominal pressure and venous stasis.

b. Nutrition: nothing by mouth (NPO).
c. Gastric decompression with a vented sump tube to low continuous suction until gastric output is minimal. To prevent dehydration, measure amount every 4 hours and replace milliliter for milliliter (mL for mL) with physiologic IV fluid. Bowel distention restricts normal intestinal blood flow and makes primary surgical repair more difficult.
d. Maintain perfusion to the viscera; prevent vascular compromise from torqued viscera.
   (1) Position infant side lying or support viscera with a small roll.
e. Prevent infection.
   (1) Maintain sterile environment. Minimize handling of viscera, wear sterile gloves.
   (2) Administer antibiotics.

3. Laboratory studies: complete blood count (CBC) with manual differential; electrolytes; acid–base and blood gas values; clotting studies; and blood type and cross-match.
4. Assess for associated anomalies, syndromes, or malformations.
5. Most newborn infants with abdominal wall defects require surgical repair. The types of repair include the following:
   a. Primary repair: All contents are returned to the abdominal cavity, and the fascia and skin are closed. The infant may require prolonged respiratory support because of increased intra-abdominal pressure. Preferred repair, but not possible in all cases.
   b. Staged repair: Not all the organs are returned to the abdominal cavity during the primary surgery.
      (1) The viscera remaining outside the cavity are managed three ways.
         (a) Placement in an extra-abdominal prosthetic compartment (typically a mesh-reinforced, Silastic-covered Marlex sac [silo]). The sac is either sutured to the edge of the defect or secured underneath the fascia, allowing gradual reduction of the intestines on a daily basis. The silo must be supported at a 90-degree angle to the infant to promote reduction by gravity and prevent vascular compromise. This technique is employed with infants with large defects and for those who cannot tolerate primary repair.
         (b) A variation of the silo technique is the insertion of a spring-loaded silo over the exposed viscera under the fascia, performed in the delivery room or in the NICU with subsequent closure on an elective basis. This latter technique is gaining in popularity and has been associated with fewer complications, fewer ventilator days, and shorter hospital stays.
         (c) The umbilical turban, where the defect is reduced and the umbilical cord is coiled over the defect and fixed into place with an adhesive dressing that epithelializes. This technique may result in umbilical hernia (Kunz et al., 2013).
      (2) Reduction minimizes the stress on the respiratory and vascular systems by allowing these systems to adjust slowly to the increased pressure of the organs as they are slowly returned to the abdominal cavity.
      (3) Reduction can usually be accomplished during a period of 10 days or less, after which infection becomes a major consideration.
      (4) Assess perfusion of herniated contents frequently. Compromise of mesenteric vasculature can occur within the silo.
      (5) The abdominal wall is closed after the reduction is completed.
   c. Skin flap closure. Only the skin is pulled over the exposed organs. This method is not a long-term solution and is used when the fascia cannot be initially repaired.
      (1) Definitive repair done at 6 to 12 months of age.
   d. Closure by porcine small intestinal submucosal graft using a biomaterial (collagen, proteins, and biomolecules) such as Alloderm (LifeCell Corp., Branchburg, N.J.), Surgisis ES (Cook, Bloomington, Ind.), or Permacol (Tissue Science Laboratories, Hampshire, U.K.). The graft is sewn to the fascia. Complete epithelialization and vascularization over the graft occurs, closing the abdomen (Beale et al., 2012).
   e. Nonsurgical repair. The omphalocele defect is painted with an escharotic agent such as silver nitrate or silver sulfadiazine and allowed to air dry and epithelialize.
      (1) This uncommon procedure is used only if the defect is large, if the infant cannot tolerate surgery or has uncorrectable congenital anomalies, or if the reduction fails.

(2) Systemic side effects are associated with most of the escharotic agents. The health care team should be aware of such effects and assess the infant for them.

6. Postoperative care.
   a. Pain management (see Chapter 16).
   b. Prevent infection: dressing changes are performed with aseptic technique; administer antibiotics.
   c. Oxygen saturation, urine output, and blood pressure are monitored continuously. Other parameters to watch closely include fluid and electrolyte balance, pH, and clotting times.
   d. Observe for complications: respiratory distress, sepsis, intestinal obstruction, abdominal compartment syndrome, skin necrosis over repaired defect, and venous stasis distal to the repair.
   e. When staged reduction is employed, the silo must be supported to prevent tilting or torsion of the enclosed viscera. Sterile gauze may be wrapped around the base of the silo for this purpose.
   f. Gastric suction is required postoperatively until the gastric output is minimal. Gastric losses should be replaced with physiologic IV solutions. To prevent dehydration, measure gastric suction drainage every 4 hours and replace this volume over the ensuing 4 hours with physiologic IV fluid.
   g. Establish long-term IV access: percutaneously inserted central line, subclavian catheter, central venous catheter. Total parenteral nutrition (TPN) is provided until the infant tolerates full enteral feedings.
   h. Bowel sounds are assessed to determine readiness to feed. A prolonged ileus is a common complication in gastroschisis, but relatively uncommon in omphalocele.
   i. Feeding is begun very slowly when gastric output is minimal and bowel sounds are active.
      (1) Low-osmolality feeding, such as half-strength formula, breast milk, or mineral–electrolyte solution (Pedialyte, Abbott, Abbott Park, IL), is usually preferred. Feedings are frequently stopped and started because of reduced intestinal function.
      (2) Soy-based and elemental formulas are used for infants who exhibit signs of feeding intolerance or malabsorption.
   j. Support parents through the often long recovery process (see Chapter 17).

## OBSTRUCTIONS OF THE GASTROINTESTINAL TRACT

**A. General considerations (Juang and Snyder, 2012; Vinocur et al., 2012).**

1. Obstructions may be either mechanical (in which there is a specific point of obstruction) or functional (usually related to motility) in nature and can be found anywhere from the esophagus to the anus.
2. Obstruction occurs because of an intrinsic or extrinsic blockage (Table 29-3).
3. Common associations in infants with intestinal obstruction.
   a. History of polyhydramnios.
      (1) Occurs more often in proximal obstructions.
      (2) Fifteen percent to 20% of polyhydramnios cases are associated with fetal GI obstructions.
   b. Failure to pass meconium within 24 to 48 hours: 95% of term infants pass meconium by 24 hours (Anderson et al., 2011).
   c. Abdominal distention: occurs more often in distal obstructions and tracheoesophageal fistula.
   d. Bilious vomiting: occurs when obstruction is distal to the ampulla of Vater, located in the duodenum.
4. General preoperative management.
   a. NPO.
   b. Gastric decompression with a vented sump tube to low continuous suction until gastric output is minimal. To prevent dehydration, measure amount every 4 hours and replace mL for mL with physiologic IV fluid.
   c. Correct fluid, electrolyte, and acid–base status (see Chapter 8).

■ TABLE 29-3
■ ■ **Causes of Intestinal Obstruction in the Newborn Infant**

| Mechanical | | |
|---|---|---|
| **Congenital** | **Acquired** | **Functional** |
| INTRINSIC | | |
| Atresias | Necrotizing enterocolitis | Hirschsprung disease |
| Stenoses | Intussusception | Meconium plug syndrome |
| Meconium ileus | Peritoneal adhesions | Ileus |
| Anorectal malformations | | Peritonitis |
| Enteric duplications | | |
| EXTRINSIC | | |
| Volvulus | | Intestinal pseudo-obstruction syndrome |
| Peritoneal bands | | |
| Annular pancreas | | |
| Cysts and tumors | | |
| Incarcerated hernias | | |

From Gleason, C.A., and Devaskar, S.U.: *Avery's diseases of the newborn* (9th ed.). Philadelphia, 2012, Saunders.

  - **d.** Maintenance IV therapy (may include TPN).
  - **e.** Antibiotics.

**B. Esophageal atresia and tracheoesophageal fistula (Juang and Snyder, 2012; Pinheiro et al., 2012; Vinocur et al., 2012).**

1. Definitions: EA, an interruption in the esophagus; TEF, an abnormal communication between the esophagus and trachea. EA and TEF may occur as separate defects or, more commonly, in association with each other.
   - **a.** Types of TEFs (Fig. 29-3).
     - (1) Esophageal atresia (blind proximal pouch) with distal esophageal communication with the trachea (85%).
     - (2) Isolated esophageal atresia (blind proximal pouch), no esophageal–tracheal communication (8%).
     - (3) H-type: communication between normal esophagus and normal trachea (5%).
     - (4) Esophageal atresia (blind proximal pouch) with proximal or proximal and distal communication with trachea (2%).
2. Etiology: hedgehog signaling abnormality and other genetic factors leading to incomplete elongation and separation of esophagus and trachea during the fourth week of gestation (Felix et al., 2009).
3. Incidence: approximately 1 per 1000 to 2500 live births.
4. Associated anomalies.

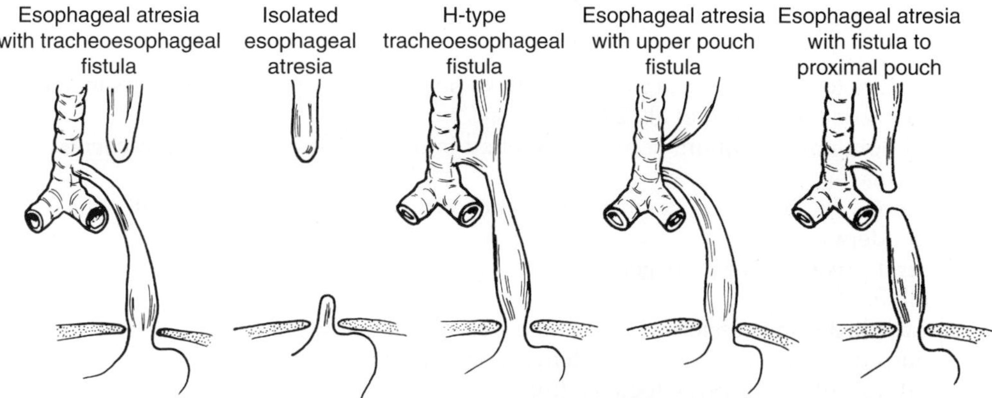


FIGURE 29-3 ■ Esophageal malformations.

a. Low birth weight is associated with other malformations and poor outcome.
b. Cardiac defects: primarily atrial septal defects and ventricular septal defects.
c. GI anomalies: pyloric stenosis, duodenal obstruction, and imperforate anus.
d. EA/TEF are components of both VATERR and VACTERL associations. Infants with EA/TEF should have a cardiac, renal, and skeletal evaluation.
e. Esophageal abnormalities are also seen in the CHARGE (*c*olobomata, *h*eart disease, choanal *a*tresia, mental *r*etardation, *g*enital hypoplasia, and *e*ar anomalies with deafness) association.

5. Diagnosis.
   a. Fetal ultrasound showing small or absent stomach.
   b. History of polyhydramnios.
   c. Clinical presentation.
      (1) Dependent on the type of tracheoesophageal anomaly.
      (2) Accumulation of oral secretions in mouth, drooling.
      (3) Coughing, choking, respiratory distress, or cyanosis.
      (4) Inability to pass gastric tube. Passage terminates in proximal esophageal pouch at approximately 10 cm. On radiographic examination, gastric tube appears coiled in the proximal esophageal pouch. In addition, air in the GI tract indicates the presence of a TEF. A gasless abdomen indicates an isolated EA (see Chapter 14).
      (5) Abdominal distention if fistula between distal esophagus and trachea.
      (6) Recurrent pneumonia (especially with communication between normal esophagus and normal trachea [H-type]).
      (7) Use of contrast studies is not recommended because of the risk of aspiration and subsequent chemical pneumonitis.
6. Prognosis: survival rate excellent for healthy term infants. Prognosis is dependent on birth weight; presence of other congenital anomalies, especially cardiac; and preoperative condition. Highest mortality occurs in infants less than 1500 g and those with associated cardiac or chromosomal abnormalities.
7. Preoperative care.
   a. See A. "General Considerations."
   b. Manage airway; prevent aspiration-induced lung injury.
      (1) EA/TEF: elevate head of bed 30 to 45 degrees to avoid reflux and aspiration of gastric secretions.
      (2) EA without TEF: normal positioning.
      (3) Evacuate EA pouch using a Replogle (Kendall, Covidien, Mansfield, MA) tube to low continuous suction. Replogle is the desired tube because evacuation holes are near the distal end. Assess and maintain patency of tube. If tube appears clogged, move tube slightly as it may have adhered to the esophageal mucosa or inject air only (to prevent aspiration) into the pigtail.
      (4) Use comfort measures to prevent crying, which leads to increased swallowed air, abdominal distention, and increased risk of gastric content reflux into the trachea.
      (5) Medications: gastric acid blockade and antibiotics.
      (6) For lung disease requiring ventilatory support: avoid nasal continuous positive airway pressure; for endotracheal ventilation, use low mean airway pressures or use high-frequency oscillation. These techniques minimize shunting of tidal volume from the trachea to the stomach, which results in inadequate ventilation and may result in a ruptured viscus.
   c. Perform complete evaluation for associated anomalies.
8. Surgical repair.
   a. Primary repair.
      (1) EA: end-to-end anastomosis of the esophagus.
      (2) TEF: ligation of the TEF.
   b. Staged repair is used with infants who are very premature, who have pneumonia or other coexisting life-threatening problems, or in whom the gap between the two esophageal segments is great (more than four vertebral bodies, with both segments in a neutral position).

(1) Initial surgery: ligation of TEF, placement of gastrostomy tube for gastric decompression, minimize risk of aspiration of gastric contents, and provide route for enteral feedings.
(2) Continue suction of proximal esophageal pouch until final surgery.
(3) Final surgery is usually delayed for 6 to 12 months.

c. When end-to-end anastomosis is impossible because the gap between the esophageal pouches is too great or a previous repair has failed, the upper segment may be elongated surgically.

9. Postoperative care.
   a. Provide pain management (see Chapter 16).
   b. Prevent aspiration: continue elevation of head of bed and gastric acid blockade.
   c. Prevent infection: administer antibiotics.
   d. Protect anastomosis site.
      (1) Ventilate using low mean airway pressure.
      (2) Suction length of endotracheal tube (ETT) only. Prevent suction catheter extrusion beyond the ETT.
      (3) Do not extubate until certain that reintubation will not be necessary.
      (4) If accidental extubation occurs, do not bag-and-mask ventilate; only experienced personnel should reintubate if needed.
      (5) Suction posterior pharynx using a premeasured catheter to limit the distance.
      (6) If the orogastric/nasogastric tube placed during surgery is dislodged, do not attempt to reinsert.
   e. Monitor: extrathoracic drain, gastric drainage. Note amount, color, and consistency.
   f. Gastrostomy tube care.
   g. Nutrition.
      (1) TPN is used until sufficient enteral intake is established.
      (2) Enteral nutrition is initiated when the anastomosis site has healed. Confirmation may be obtained by esophagram.
10. Postoperative complications.
   a. Aspiration.
   b. Infection, pneumonia.
   c. Anastomosis site complications.
      (1) Leak: delays feeding, may result in infection.
      (2) Stricture: suspect in infants exhibiting dysphagia, inability to handle secretions, or respiratory distress after the immediate postoperative period. Strictures require long-term periodic dilation.
   d. Dysmotility of lower esophageal segment. Most often a problem with long gap atresia and when oral intake is delayed for a prolonged period of time.
   e. Recurrent fistula, usually resulting from a leak.
   f. Unilateral diaphragmatic paralysis.
   g. Tracheomalacia. This complication is occasionally severe enough to require a tracheostomy. Caused by deformation and softening of tracheal cartilages from compression of posterior trachea by enlarged proximal esophageal pouch.
   h. TEF cough. Characterized by stridor, brassy cough, and bronchospastic airway symptoms.
   i. GER (common).

**C. Pyloric stenosis (Feenstra et al., 2012; Huether, 2010; Taylor et al., 2013).**

1. Definition: obstruction of pylorus caused by hypertrophy of the pyloric musculature.
2. Etiology: unknown but higher incidence in infants whose mothers had increased gastrin secretion in the third trimester of pregnancy or infants who received prostaglandin E administration. The pyloric muscle demonstrates both hypertrophy and hyperplasia.
3. Incidence: overall 3 per 1000 live births.
   a. Predominance: males 5 per 1000 live births; females 1 per 1000 live births.
   b. Prevalence: more common in infants who are white, full-term, and have trisomy 21.
   c. Occurs in approximately 20% of males and 10% of females who had affected mothers.
4. Associated conditions: uncommon. Three major malformations associated with pyloric stenosis are Apert's syndrome, trisomy 18, and trisomy 21 (Jones et al., 2013).

5. Diagnosis.
   a. Presence of signs and symptoms usually between 3 weeks and 5 months of age.
   b. Clinical presentation.
      (1) Nonbilious vomiting that becomes projectile over time.
      (2) Visible peristaltic waves in epigastrium.
      (3) Palpable pyloric "olive" in right upper quadrant (70% to 90%).
      (4) Dehydration, electrolyte imbalances, acid–base disturbance (hypochloremia, hypokalemia, metabolic alkalosis).
      (5) Chronic weight loss, malnutrition, and failure to thrive (late sign).
   c. Ultrasound (almost exclusively).
   d. Upper GI tract contrast study.
6. Prognosis: excellent. Generally, complete recovery with no residual effects; some continued vomiting possible in the first few days after surgery, followed by quick resolution.
7. Preoperative care.
   a. See A. "General Considerations."
   b. Prevent aspiration-induced lung injury: use gastric decompression.
8. Medical repair.
   a. Pyloric stenosis may resolve spontaneously before 1 year of life. Infant requires medical and nutritional support. Procedure is associated with slow improvement and higher mortality.
9. Surgical repair.
   a. Pyloromyotomy: pyloric muscles are split/separated either by laparotomy or laparoscopic techniques.
10. Postoperative care.
   a. Pain management (see Chapter 16).
   b. Routine wound care.
   c. Nutrition: initially NPO for a few hours, then rapid progression of enteral feeds leading to full volume and discharge 24 hours after surgery.
   d. Prevention of perforation of the mucosa at the pyloromyotomy site by avoiding placement of a gastric tube postoperatively.

**D. Duodenal atresia and stenosis (Burjonrappa et al., 2011; Shalkow et al., 2012).**

1. Definition: congenital obstruction of the duodenum. The defect usually occurs distal to the ampulla of Vater. The obstruction can be partial or complete and is further stratified as intrinsic or extrinsic. Duodenal atresia exhibits three forms: a membranous web causes obstruction in type I and is associated with common bile duct anomalies; a fibrous atretic cord connects two segments of duodenum in type II; and type III exhibits discontinuous segments of the duodenum.
2. Etiology: During early gestation, the duodenal epithelium proliferates rapidly and completely obliterates the bowel lumen. Obstruction is thought to be a failure of recanalization during weeks 8 to 10 of fetal life. With extrinsic obstruction, anomalies outside the duodenum affect patency. These anomalies include malrotation with Ladd's bands, annular pancreas, and supraduodenal portal vein.
3. Incidence: approximately 1 per 7000 live births.
4. Associated conditions.
   a. Trisomy 21 syndrome (approximately 30%).
   b. Congenital heart disease (approximately 30%).
   c. Intestinal malrotation (approximately 20%).
   d. Tracheoesophageal abnormalities (10% to 20%).
   e. Anorectal defects (10% to 20%).
5. Diagnosis.
   a. Fetal ultrasound showing classic "double bubble" echogenicity.
   b. History of polyhydramnios.
   c. Clinical presentation.
      (1) Abdominal distention.
      (2) Absence of stools.

(3) Bilious vomiting within the first 24 hours; nonbilious vomiting does not rule out duodenal atresia or obstruction.
(4) Jaundice.

**d.** Plain radiograph showing double bubble pattern (see Chapter 14).

**6.** Prognosis: excellent. Long-term outcome is primarily dependent on associated anomalies and malformations.

**7.** Preoperative care.

**a.** See A. "General Considerations."

**b.** Gastric decompression with a vented sump tube to low continuous suction until gastric output is minimal. To prevent dehydration, measure amount every 4 hours and replace mL for mL with physiologic IV fluid.

**c.** Perform complete evaluation for associated anomalies.

**8.** Surgical repair.

**a.** For intrinsic lesions, surgery is performed to excise the atretic or stenosed portions and perform primary reanastomoses. For extrinsic etiology, surgery removes or redirects the tissue causing duodenal blockage.

**b.** Surgery may be by open laparotomy or laparoscopy assisted.

**9.** Postoperative care.

**a.** Pain management (see Chapter 16).

**b.** Prevent infection.
(1) Routine wound care.
(2) Continue antibiotics.

**c.** Gastric decompression with a vented sump tube to low continuous suction until gastric output is minimal. To prevent dehydration, measure amount every 4 hours and replace mL for mL with physiologic IV fluid.

**d.** Gastrostomy tube care if placed (rare).

**e.** Nutrition: initially NPO for 3 to 10 days. Initiate enteral feeding and progress slowly as tolerated. Expect possible intolerance due to delayed gastric emptying and microcolon distal to repair site. Continue TPN until adequate enteral nutrition is established.

**E. Jejunal or ileal atresia (Best et al., 2012; Sadler and Rasmussen, 2010; Shalkow et al., 2012).**

**1.** Definition: congenital obstruction of the jejunum, ileum, or both. Type I: membranous web; type II: segments connected by fibrous cord; type IIIa: segments separated by V-shaped mesenteric defect; type IIIb: apple-peel defect, with distal small bowel corkscrewing around the ileocecal artery; type IV: multiple atresias (Fig. 29-4).

**2.** Etiology: two proposed etiologies: failure of recanalization during weeks 8 to 10 of fetal life or, second, and most supported hypothesis is a mesenteric vascular insult with subsequent necrosis and resorption of the affected segment or segments.

**3.** Incidence: 1 per 1000 live births. Males and females are equally affected. Anatomic distribution: jejunal (50%), ileum (50%).

**4.** Associated conditions.

**a.** Intestinal malrotation (10% to 18%).

**b.** Meconium peritonitis (12%).

**c.** Meconium ileus (10%).

**5.** Diagnosis.

**a.** Fetal ultrasound showing distended intestinal loops.

**b.** History of polyhydramnios.

**c.** Clinical presentation.
(1) Abdominal distention. The lower the obstruction, the greater the distention.
(2) Absence of stools.
(3) Bilious vomiting within the first 24 to 48 hours.
(4) Jaundice.

**d.** Radiologic studies.
(1) Plain radiograph showing dilated bowel loops and multiple air–fluid levels (see Chapter 14). With proximal jejunal atresia, classic "triple bubble" is noted. With in-utero bowel perforation, peritoneal calcifications may be visible.
(2) Barium enema reveals a microcolon.

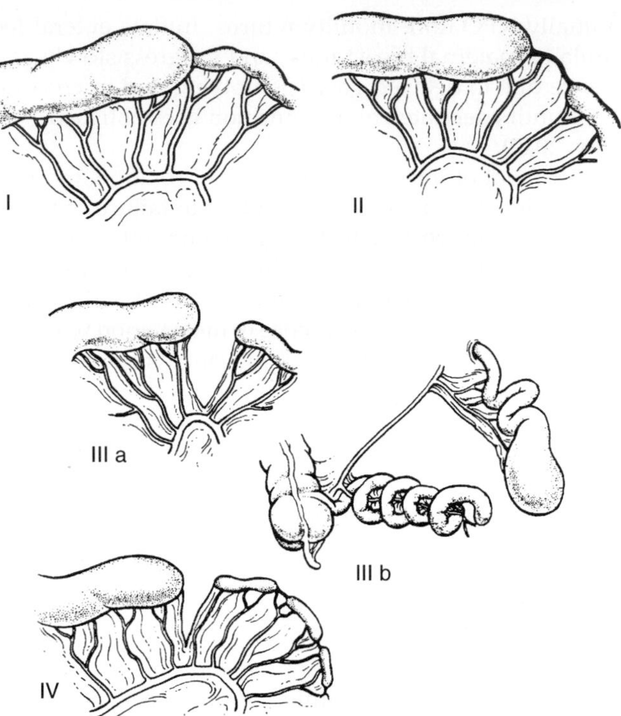


FIGURE 29-4 ■ Types of jejunal atresia. Type I—mucosal atresia with intact muscularis. Type II—atretic ends are separated by a fibrous band. Type IIIa—atretic ends are separated by a V-shaped gap defect. Type IIIb—apple-peel deformity of the distal atretic segment with retrograde blood supply from the ileocolic or right colic artery. Type IV—multiple atresias ("string-of-sausage" effect). (From Rowe, M.I., O'Neill, J.A., Grosfeld, J.L., et al.: *Essentials of pediatric surgery*. St. Louis, 1995, Mosby, p. 511.)

6. Prognosis: generally good, with return to normal bowel function within 10 days. Mortality is usually related to short-bowel syndrome and complex defects (types IIIb and IV). Morbidity includes ileus, peritonitis, and prolonged intestinal dysfunction.
7. Preoperative care.
   a. See A. "General Considerations."
   b. Gastric decompression with a vented sump tube to low continuous suction until gastric output is minimal. To prevent dehydration, measure amount every 4 hours and replace mL for mL with physiologic IV fluid.
   c. Perform complete evaluation for associated anomalies.
8. Surgical repair.
   a. Surgery may be by open laparotomy or laparoscopy assisted.
   b. Dependent on location of atresia and amount of intestinal involvement.
   c. Atretic intestinal portion is often resected proximally to the point of normal bowel dimensions and then connected to the distal segment using an end-to-oblique-side anastomosis.
   d. Occasionally, exteriorization of the proximal and even distal ends may be necessary with reanastomosis later.
9. Postoperative care.
   a. Pain management (see Chapter 16).
   b. Prevent infection.
   c. Routine wound care.
   d. Continue antibiotics.
   e. Gastric decompression with a vented sump tube to low continuous suction until gastric output is minimal. To prevent dehydration, measure amount every 4 hours and replace mL for mL with physiologic IV fluid.

f. Nutrition: initially NPO until motility returns. Initiate enteral feeding (often with elemental formula or maternal breast milk) and progress slowly as tolerated. Expect possible intolerance due to delayed gastric emptying and microcolon distal to repair site. Continue TPN until adequate enteral nutrition is established.

**F. Malrotation (Hatley, 2012).**

1. Definition: an assortment of intestinal anomalies of rotation and retroperitoneal fixation.
2. Etiology: hedgehog signaling abnormality leading to failure of the intestines to rotate and fixate appropriately during weeks 6 to 10 of gestation. Intestines may twist on themselves (midgut volvulus), occluding the intestinal lumen, or may twist around the superior mesenteric artery, occluding intestinal blood supply. Ischemia and bowel necrosis follow.
3. Incidence: 1 per 5000 live births. The incidence of malrotation without significant symptoms is much higher than cases with clinically significant symptoms. More males affected than females.
4. Associated anomalies.
   a. Intestinal atresia.
   b. Diaphragmatic hernia.
   c. Duodenal obstruction due to peritoneal (Ladd's) bands encircling the duodenum.
   d. Omphalocele.
   e. Gastroschisis.
5. Diagnosis.
   a. Presence of symptoms.
      (1) 80% of patients who become symptomatic do so within the first month of life, with the majority presenting within the first week. Approximately 90% of clinical symptoms appear in children in the first year of life.
      (2) Acute presentation.
         (a) Bilious vomiting, suggestive of malrotation with volvulus formation; needs immediate attention.
         (b) Abdominal distention.
         (c) Abdominal pain.
         (d) Signs of shock and sepsis.
         (e) Rectal bleeding.
      (3) Less acute presentation.
         (a) Intermittent bilious vomiting.
         (b) Abdominal tenderness.
         (c) Failure to thrive.
   b. Imaging studies.
      (1) Upper GI radiograph is the gold standard.
      (2) Plain radiographs. May appear normal in 20% of cases.
      (3) Ultrasound.
      (4) Classic early studies show distended stomach and proximal duodenum and scanty gas distributed throughout remainder of bowel. An airless abdomen is an ominous sign.
6. Prognosis: excellent if uncomplicated by infarction or associated anomalies. Mortality increases with intestinal necrosis, prematurity, or other abnormalities. Amount of intestinal resection is an important predicting factor in outcome. Major postoperative complication is short-bowel syndrome.
7. Preoperative care.
   a. See A. "General Considerations."
   b. Perform complete evaluation for associated anomalies.
   c. Assess general perfusion; consider volume resuscitation for shock state.
8. Surgical repair.
   a. Surgery is emergent and cannot be delayed. Degree of surgery is dependent on pathology and amount of intestinal involvement.
   b. Volvulus is detorsed, Ladd's bands are divided, incidental appendectomy, and nonrotational return of bowel to the abdomen with the small bowel to the right and large bowel to the left.

9. Postoperative care.
   a. Pain management (see Chapter 16).
   b. Prevent infection.
      (1) Routine wound care.
      (2) Continue antibiotics.
   c. Gastric decompression with a vented sump tube to low continuous suction until gastric output is minimal. To prevent dehydration, measure amount every 4 hours and replace mL for mL with physiologic IV fluid.
   d. Nutrition: initially NPO until motility returns. Initiate enteral feeding (often with elemental formula or maternal breast milk) and progress slowly as tolerated. Expect possible intolerance due to delayed gastric emptying and microcolon distal to repair site. Continue TPN until adequate enteral nutrition is established.

**G. Meconium ileus (Carlyle et al., 2012).**

1. Definition: mechanical obstruction of the distal ileum due to intraluminal accumulation of thick, inspissated meconium. Although meconium ileus has been reported in a few patients without cystic fibrosis (CF), it is the predominant cause of meconium ileus in infants.
   a. Types of meconium ileus.
      (1) Simple meconium ileus.
         (a) More common.
         (b) Distal segment of the small bowel is obstructed with thick, tar-like, tenacious meconium and the proximal segment of the small bowel is dilated.
         (c) Clinical presentation is usually within 48 hours.
      (2) Complicated meconium ileus.
         (a) Volvulus.
         (b) Intestinal necrosis and perforation.
         (c) Meconium peritonitis or pseudocyst formation.
         (d) Clinical presentation is usually within 24 hours.
2. Etiology: exact cause unknown. Two implicating factors are hyposecretion of pancreatic enzymes, which may play a part in some but not all cases of meconium ileus (as a result, meconium contains an abnormal amount of proteins and glycoproteins, making the meconium thick and viscid); or abnormal viscid secretions from the mucous glands of the small intestine.
3. Incidence: exact incidence unknown. CF occurs in 1 in 2000 live births of white infants; 10% to 15% of children with CF have meconium ileus.
4. Associated conditions.
   a. CF.
   b. Hepatobiliary disease.
5. Diagnosis.
   a. Abdominal distention at birth.
   b. Bilious vomiting.
   c. Failure to pass meconium within 12 to 24 hours.
   d. Palpable, rubbery loops of bowel. Small grapelike pellets of meconium may be palpated distally.
   e. Complicated form has earlier presentation, and these infants appear sicker, with signs of sepsis and respiratory distress.
   f. Family history of CF. Definitive diagnosis of CF based on sweat chloride iontophoresis (sodium and chloride concentrations >60 mEq/L), or chromosome analysis (defect located on chromosome 7).
   g. Radiologic studies.
      (1) Plain radiograph shows "soap bubble" or ground-glass appearance of distal intestine created by the mixture of air and meconium; distended bowel loops without air–fluid levels; scattered calcifications due to intrauterine intestinal perforations may be seen in complicated form.
      (2) Contrast radiograph may show microcolon.
6. Prognosis: dependent on number and degree of organs affected by CF as well as associated anomalies.

7. Pre–nonsurgical procedure and preoperatively.
   a. See A. "General Considerations."
   b. Perform complete evaluation for associated conditions; volvulus, atresia, perforation, and peritonitis must be ruled out.
   c. Evaluation by pediatric surgeon who remains in attendance during nonsurgical procedure.
   d. Patient should be prepared for surgery should complications occur during nonsurgical procedure.
8. Nonsurgical procedure.
   a. A hypertonic contrast water-soluble enema may be successful in dislodging the meconium by drawing fluid into the intestine and allowing for normal intestinal activity. Successful in up to 60% of patients. Usually meconium pellets are passed quickly, followed by liquid meconium for 24 hours after the procedure. A second enema may be required.
9. Surgical repair: uncomplicated meconium ileus.
   a. Used when nonsurgical procedure has failed.
   b. A T-tube (Fig. 29-5) is inserted into the ileum, which is irrigated postoperatively with *N*-acetylcysteine pancreatic enzymes.
10. Surgical repair: complicated meconium ileus.
    a. Always requires surgical intervention.
    b. Compromised intestine is resected.
    c. If the bowel is viable, end-to-end anastomosis is performed.
    d. In extreme cases in which bowel necrosis has occurred, all compromised intestine is resected and an ostomy is placed at the proximal and/or distal segments.
11. Postprocedural care.
    a. Fluids at one-and-one-half times maintenance. Hypovolemic shock can occur secondary to rapid fluid shift resulting from hypertonic solution used for enema. Careful monitoring of urine output, urine specific gravity or osmolality, blood urea nitrogen, creatinine, and serum osmolality.
    b. Physical assessment. Intestinal perforation may occur up to 48 hours after administration of enema. Risk of intestinal perforation increases with successive attempts at nonoperative techniques.
12. Postprocedural management and postoperative care.
    a. Pain management (see Chapter 16).
    b. Prevent infection: administer antibiotics; chest physiotherapy, aerosolized mucolytic agents (acetylcysteine sodium [Mucomyst]), and supplemental humidity to prevent atelectasis and pneumonia, which infants with CF are prone to develop.
    c. NPO.

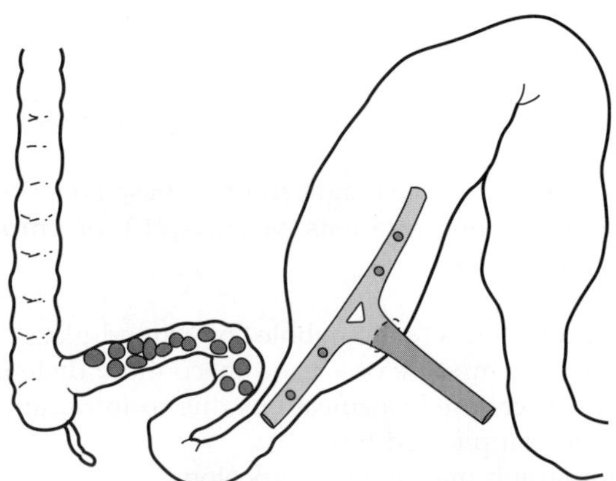

FIGURE 29-5 ■ T-tube. (From Mak, G.Z., Harberg, F.J., Hiatt, P., et al.: T-tube ileostomy for meconium ileus: Four decades of experience. *Journal of Pediatric Surgery*, 35[2]:349-352, 2000.)

d. Gastric decompression with a vented sump tube to low continuous suction until gastric output is minimal. To prevent dehydration, measure amount every 4 hours and replace mL for mL with physiologic IV fluid.
e. Irrigation of distal stoma or T-tube with *N*-acetylcysteine or pancreatic enzymes around postoperative day 3.
f. Nutrition.
(1) TPN is used until sufficient enteral intake is established.
(2) Enteral nutrition is initiated when the surgical site has healed.
(3) Begin feedings with elemental formula or breast milk, supplemented with pancreatic enzymes.
g. Parental education.
(1) Genetic counseling.
(2) Pulmonary hygiene, infection prevention, nutritional supplements.
h. Observe for postoperative complications.
(1) Volvulus.
(2) Gangrene.
(3) Perforation.

**H. Meconium plug syndrome (Cuenca et al., 2012).**

1. Definition: a mechanical obstruction, usually of the distal segment of the colon and the rectum, that occurs from thick, inspissated meconium in the absence of an abnormality of ganglion cells or enzymatic deficiency. Because the meconium plug is formed primarily by mucous and intestinal secretions, the plug appears yellowish white and is gelatinous.
2. Etiology: unclear; results from diminished colonic motility and meconium clearance. More common with:
a. Maternal diabetes, probably because of increased fetal glycogen production leading to decreased bowel motility.
b. Neonatal hypermagnesemia: usually occurs after mother has been treated with magnesium sulfate for pregnancy-induced hypertension or preterm labor; the decreased bowel motility is secondary to myoneural depression.
c. Prematurity.
d. Hypotonia in infant with CNS disease.
e. Sepsis.
3. Incidence: 1 in 100 newborns; 75% of newborns are able to expel the plug spontaneously, avoiding the complication of intestinal obstruction.
4. Associated conditions.
a. Hirschsprung's disease.
b. CF.
5. Diagnosis.
a. Clinical presentation.
(1) Abdominal distention. Multiple dilated loops of bowel.
(2) Failure to pass meconium by 48 hours of life.
(3) Hyperactive bowel sounds.
(4) Bilious vomiting (late sign).
b. Plain radiograph showing multiple distended loops of bowel (see Chapter 14).
c. Water-soluble contrast enema often outlines an intraluminal plug. Such an enema will commonly dislodge the plug, and no further interventions will be required.
6. Prognosis: generally excellent if no associated conditions exist.
7. Pre–nonsurgical procedure and preoperatively.
a. See A. "General Considerations."
b. Medications: generally not required.
c. Perform complete evaluation for associated conditions; volvulus, atresia, perforation, and peritonitis must be ruled out.
8. Interventions.
a. Rectal examination may expel plug in some circumstances.
b. Enemas of warm saline, meglumine diatrizoate, or acetylcysteine.

(1) Meglumine diatrizoate is hyperosmolar, drawing fluid into the bowel from interstitial space. Careful assessment and management of fluid status are important.

c. Surgery rarely necessary.

**I. Hirschsprung disease (congenital megacolon, aganglionic megacolon) (Arshad et al., 2012; Langer, 2013).**

1. Definition: a non-mendelian congenital genetic absence of parasympathetic innervation to the colon with partial penetrance and variable expressivity. The affected intestine is unable to relax, resulting in a functional obstruction.
   a. Length of bowel involvement is dependent on the time during which migration of neuroblasts ceased.
   b. Agangliosis commonly involves rectum or rectosigmoid portion of colon only.
   c. Agangliosis may extend to proximal colon. Total colon agangliosis is rare.
2. Etiology: failure of ganglion cells to migrate cephalocaudally before week 12 of gestation, resulting in partial or complete agangliosis of the submucosal and mesenteric plexuses of the colon. Eight genomes have been associated with Hirschsprung disease (HD). The lack of intestinal ganglion cells prevents the inhibitory relaxation normally regulated by parasympathetic nerves. The affected segment is unable to relax, and functional obstruction ensues. The normally innervated proximal colon becomes hypertrophied from its attempts to overcome the functional obstruction. The oral, facial, and cranial ganglia arise from the same craniocervical neural crest as the ganglionic plexus of the bowel, explaining associated conditions (Kenny et al., 2010).
3. Incidence: 1 in 5000 live births. Males are affected 4 times more often than females. More than one third of affected patients have a relative with HD.
4. Associated conditions:
   a. Sensorineural deafness with central alveolar hypoventilation and Shah–Waardenburg syndromes.
   b. Cardiovascular, skeletal, and limb anomalies seen with DiGeorge and X-linked aqueductal stenosis syndromes.
   c. Systemic anomalies seen with multiple endocrine neoplasia and Smith–Lemli–Opitz syndrome.
   d. Other: colonic atresia or imperforate anus; 3% to 10% of children with trisomy 21 have HD; ocular neuropathies.
5. Diagnosis.
   a. Clinical presentation.
      (1) Early symptom: failure to pass meconium within 24 to 48 hours after birth.
      (2) Bilious vomiting.
      (3) Progressive abdominal distention.
      (4) Poor feeding with failure to thrive.
      (5) Late symptom: inability to stool normally. Abnormal stooling since birth is a common symptom of HD. As the obstruction continues, enterocolitis may develop, with fever, abdominal distention, and diarrhea. The infant usually has symptoms in the first several weeks and then has diarrhea, abdominal distention, and/or vomiting. In advanced cases, urinary obstruction may occur secondary to mechanical compression of the ureters and bladder.
   b. Radiologic examination.
      (1) Plain radiograph demonstrating proximal bowel dilation with an absence of air in the rectum is suggestive.
      (2) Contrast studies showing a nondistensible rectal ampulla, with a dilated bowel above and a transition zone (an area between the normal and abnormal aganglionic intestine having a conical tapering appearance) is suggestive.
      (3) Retained barium in the rectum for more than 24 hours after the procedure is suggestive.
   c. Anal manometry is useful in very-short-segment agangliosis or in patients who have normal findings on contrast studies.
   d. Confirmation: rectal biopsy demonstrating absence of ganglion cells. Punch or suction biopsy may be done in the nursery. Full-thickness biopsy under general anesthesia is

rarely needed. Increased acetylcholinesterase content in rectal tissue is identified by histochemical staining.
e. Within the past 4 years, a monoclonal antibody (anti-MAP2 antibody neuronal marker, Abcam, Cambridge, MA) has been developed with exceptional specificity and sensitivity to detect ganglionic cells in rectal biopsy specimens.
6. Prognosis: excellent. Mortality rate increases when diagnosis is delayed and enterocolitis occurs as a result of bowel wall distention and ischemia followed by bacterial translocation into circulation, resulting in sepsis. Enterocolitis is the leading cause of death. Approximately 10% of patients with HD will have subsequent elimination problems, such as constipation and delayed toilet training.
7. Preoperative care.
   a. See A. "General Considerations."
   b. Perform complete evaluation for associated conditions; volvulus, atresia, perforation, and peritonitis must be ruled out.
   c. Rectal irrigation is routinely performed to allow repeated emptying of colon and prevent enterocolitis.
8. Surgical repair. Goal: bring the normal ganglionated bowel down to the anus. The transanal procedure eliminates an abdominal incision and results in a primary pull-through repair.
9. Postoperative care.
   a. Pain management (see Chapter 16).
   b. NPO.
   c. Gastric decompression with a vented sump tube to low continuous suction until gastric output is minimal. To prevent dehydration, measure amount every 4 hours and replace mL for mL with physiologic IV fluid.
   d. Nutrition.
      (1) TPN is used until sufficient enteral intake is established.
      (2) Enteral nutrition is initiated when the anastomosis site has healed.
   e. Careful monitoring of fluid and electrolyte balance.
   f. Close observation for shock and recurrent enterocolitis.
   g. Routine ostomy care if applicable. Complications include ostomy prolapse, intestinal obstruction, skin dehiscence and excoriation, and stomal ulceration and bleeding.
   h. Routine rectal irrigations with normal saline to decrease risk of postoperative enterocolitis.
   i. If frequent and liquid stools cause perineal irritation, loperamide may be administered to reduce stool frequency and kaolin–pectin suspension can solidify stools.
   j. Special diets may be necessary to improve stool consistency.
   k. Genetic counseling should be offered to the infant's family.
   l. A regimen of anal dilation begins approximately 2 weeks postoperatively in primary pull-through patients.
10. Complications.
   a. Fecal incontinence.
   b. Persistent constipation.
   c. Anastomotic leakage with subsequent stricture formation.
   d. Rectal stenosis.

**J. Imperforate anus (anorectal agenesis) (Rosen and Beals, 2012).**
1. Definition: a broad spectrum of anorectal malformations characterized by a stenotic or atretic anal canal. A fistula between the rectum and the perineum, vagina in females or urethra in males, may also occur.
2. Classified dependent on level of defect (i.e., above [high] or below [low] a line drawn from the symphysis pubis to the coccyx [pubococcygeal line]).
   a. High imperforate anus.
      (1) More common and generally more complex.
      (2) Male predominance.
      (3) Rectourinary and rectovaginal fistulas are common associations. Infants with a fistula are at risk for hyperchloremic acidosis as a result of colonic absorption of urine.

(4) High imperforate anus with sacral anomaly can be associated with lack of innervation of the bowel and/or bladder, resulting in incontinence.

b. Low imperforate anus.
   (1) Male/female ratio closer to 1:1.
   (2) Perineal fistula is common.

3. Etiology: failure of differentiation of the urogenital sinus and cloaca during embryologic development (Blackburn, 2013).
4. Incidence: 1 in 5000 live births.
5. Common associations: anomalies, including vertebral, genitourinary, cardiovascular, and GI malformations, in 20% to 75% of infants. Specific anomalies include cryptorchidism, congenital heart defects, esophageal atresia, spinal dysraphism.
6. Diagnosis.
   a. Physical examination. An infant with anal stenosis or imperforate anal membrane may have a normal-appearing rectum, with the condition detected only after the absence of stooling is noted.
   b. Imaging studies.
      (1) Plain and contrast radiographs. An inverted lateral radiograph may be obtained to determine the level of the air-filled rectal pouch in relation to the pubococcygeal line.
      (2) Ultrasonography.
7. Prognosis: level of defect significantly influences outcome regarding fecal continence (Fig. 29-6).
8. Outcome is generally excellent with low imperforate anus, although there is an association with constipation. High imperforate anus is associated with bowel incontinence.
9. Preoperative care.
   a. See A. "General Considerations."
10. Surgical repair.
    a. Surgical intervention is always necessary, with the procedure dependent on the level of the anorectal pouch. High and intermediate pouches are treated with a colostomy and a definitive pull-through procedure performed after the infant is approximately 8 months of age and weighs 18 pounds. A low pouch can usually be repaired by anoplasty with good results.
11. Postoperative care.
    a. Pain management (see Chapter 16).
    b. NPO.

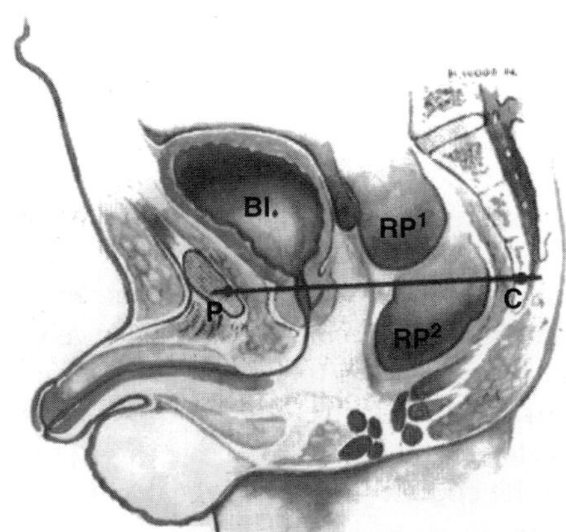


FIGURE 29-6 ■ Imperforate anus. Rectal pouch 1 ($RP^1$) sits above the pubococcygeal line (PC) and would be classified as a "high type" anomaly. Rectal pouch 2 ($RP^2$) sits below the PC line and represents a "low type" anomaly. The level of the rectal pouch is crucial in decisions of management. *Bl*, Bladder. (From Ross, A.J.: Intestinal obstruction in the newborn. *Pediatrics in Review*, 15[9]:338-347, 1994.)

c. Gastric decompression with a vented sump tube to low continuous suction until gastric output is minimal. To prevent dehydration, measure amount every 4 hours and replace mL for mL with physiologic IV fluid.
d. Nutrition.
   (1) TPN is used until sufficient enteral intake is established.
   (2) Enteral nutrition is initiated when the anastomosis site has healed.
e. Routine ostomy care if applicable. Complications include ostomy prolapse, intestinal obstruction, skin dehiscence and excoriation, and stomal ulceration and bleeding.
f. Anal dilation for approximately 2 weeks postoperatively in infants with anoplasty to prevent anal stenosis.

## NECROTIZING ENTEROCOLITIS (CILIEBORG ET AL., 2012; DOMINQUEZ AND MOSS, 2012; DOWNARD ET AL., 2012; NEU AND WALKER, 2011)

**A. General considerations.**

1. Definition: an acquired disease that affects the GI system, particularly that of premature infants. It is characterized by inflammation of the bowel wall followed by areas of necrosis, most commonly in the terminal ileum and proximal colon, but may affect any or all of both small and large intestine.
2. Etiology: unknown, thought to be multifactorial. Three mechanisms have been suggested:
   a. Intestinal ischemia (asphyxia/hypoxemia; redistribution of blood flow [hypotension, hypovolemia, polycythemia, patent ductus arteriosus, severe stress, hypothermia, umbilical catheter, blood transfusion, exchange transfusion]).
   b. Bacterial colonization of the initially sterile intestinal tract. The occurrence of NEC in clusters suggests a role for microorganism involvement. Organisms commonly associated with NEC include *Klebsiella*, *Escherichia coli*, *Clostridium* species.
   c. Enteral feedings. Majority of NEC cases preceded by enteral feeding (90% to 95%). Increased occurrence when hyperosmolar formulas and medications (aminophylline, vitamin E) are administered enterally, and when feeding volume increases exceed 20 mL/kg/day. Mechanism is unclear; formula may provide a substrate for bacterial proliferation; feeding and medications may increase intestinal oxygen demand during absorption, resulting in tissue hypoxia; fluid shifts into the intestine, resulting in decreased GI blood flow and intestinal ischemia. Breast milk may have a protective effect against development of NEC. Protective ingredients include secretory immunoglobulin A, lactobacilli (antistaphylococcal agents), complement components, lysozymes, lactoferrins, macrophages, and lymphocytes. However, NEC can occur in infants who have received breast milk.
   d. Prevention.
      (1) Emphasis is on minimizing the factors contributing to NEC.
      (2) Prevent/correct acid–base imbalance, hypoxemia, hypovolemia, hypotension.
      (3) Correct hyperviscosity.
      (4) Cautious initiation of enteral feedings in small premature infants and in infants who have had perinatal asphyxia.
      (5) Careful monitoring of feeding tolerance.
      (6) Oral administration of immunoglobulins and bifidobacterium may be beneficial (AlFaleh et al., 2011).
3. Focal intestinal perforation.
   a. Can occur in the absence of NEC.
   b. Factors distinguishing focal perforation from NEC:
      (1) Less hemodynamic instability.
      (2) Less metabolic acidosis.
      (3) Improved survival rate.
      (4) Use of umbilical artery catheter and administration of indomethacin or ibuprofen more common.

(5) Pathologic finding of coagulation necrosis found in NEC is absent in focal intestinal perforations.

**4.** Incidence: up to 10% of all admissions to the NICU; approximately 90% of cases occur in preterm infants. Occurs sporadically and in clusters. Occurs within first week of life to several weeks after birth.

**a.** Factors contributing to the preterm infant's susceptibility to NEC:

(1) Decreased immunologic factors in the intestinal tract.

(2) Increased gastric pH.

(3) Immature intestinal barrier.

(4) Decreased intestinal motility.

**5.** Associated conditions.

**a.** Prematurity.

**b.** Patent ductus arteriosus.

**c.** Infection.

**6.** Diagnosis.

**a.** Physical examination.

(1) Positive abdominal signs: distention, visible bowel loops, diminishing peristalsis, tenderness, discoloration.

**b.** Clinical presentation.

(1) Gastric residuals.

(2) Lethargy.

(3) Apnea and bradycardia.

(4) Blood in stools: occult or frank blood.

(5) Temperature instability.

(6) Diminished urinary output.

(7) Hypoperfusion.

(8) Hypotension due to third-space fluid loss from the intravascular space into the extracellular (third-space) compartment.

(9) Bilious vomiting.

**c.** Radiologic examination (plain film).

(1) Diffuse gaseous distention of intestines is an early but nonspecific sign.

(2) Asymmetric bowel gas pattern and a relative lack of gas in a certain area with dilation in another area.

(3) Persistently dilated loop of bowel usually represents advanced disease.

(4) Pneumatosis intestinalis (air within the wall of the intestine) is pathognomonic of NEC (see Chapter 14).

(5) Air in the portal venous system (see Chapter 14).

(6) Pneumoperitoneum: represents intestinal perforation (see Chapter 14). Absence of free air does not rule out intestinal perforation.

**d.** Laboratory studies.

(1) Abnormal CBC: leukocytosis or leukopenia, thrombocytopenia.

(2) Abnormal blood chemistry: metabolic acidosis, electrolyte imbalances.

(3) Abnormal blood gases: hypoxemia, hypercapnia.

(4) Abnormal clotting studies: disseminated intravascular coagulation (DIC).

(5) Presence of blood in stools.

(6) CHO malabsorption; may be an early sign of NEC.

**7.** Prognosis: survival rate varies between institutions and also depends on amount of bowel involvement and resection.

**B. Care of the infant with NEC.**

**1.** Medical management.

**a.** See A. "General Considerations."

**b.** NPO.

**c.** Gastric decompression with a vented sump tube to low continuous suction until gastric output is minimal. To prevent dehydration, measure amount every 4 hours and replace mL for mL with physiologic IV fluid.

**d.** Medications: antibiotics (both penicillin-based β-lactam and an aminoglycoside), 3 to 14 days, depending on clinical status.

e. Frequent CBCs and electrolytes to evaluate infant for thrombocytopenia and electrolyte imbalances.
f. Serial plain radiographs (usually every 6 to 8 hours).
g. Respiratory and ventilatory support as needed.
h. Circulatory support as needed to prevent hypotension. Fresh frozen plasma, vasopressors should be considered.
i. Platelet transfusions for thrombocytopenia.
j. Fresh frozen plasma for DIC; consider use of vitamin K.
k. Careful monitoring of intake and output. "Third spacing" of fluids is common and may lead to hypovolemia and hypotension.
l. Frequent serial abdominal girth measurements.
m. Frequent blood glucose measurements.

2. Surgical management.
   a. Preoperative care: continue medical management.
   b. Surgery is used if medical management is not possible or fails. Indications for surgery include:
      (1) Absolute indication.
         (a) Pneumoperitoneum.
      (2) Relative indications.
         (a) Intestinal gangrene.
         (b) Progressive clinical deterioration.
         (c) Portal venous gas.
         (d) Persistent fixed dilated loop of bowel.
         (e) Abdominal wall edema or erythema.
         (f) Progressive pneumatosis.
         (g) Progressive acidosis.
         (h) Progressive thrombocytopenia.
         (i) Leukopenia or leukocytosis.
   c. Surgical repair.
      (1) Principles of surgery for NEC are to decompress the bowel, resect necrotic bowel, and divert the proximal fecal stream. Actual procedures performed are dependent on condition and age of infant and amount of bowel necrosis.
      (2) In an infant who has isolated necrosis with remaining bowel appearing viable and no intestinal perforation, resection of necrotic bowel and primary anastomosis is appropriate.
      (3) When there is less than 25% viable bowel, options include simple closure of abdomen (always fatal), resection of all necrotic bowel and creation of stomas (frequently results in short-bowel syndrome), and proximal diversion without bowel resection (may allow healing of part of bowel). Subsequent operations are usually required to resect gangrenous bowel, but there may be enough remaining bowel for survival.
      (4) Placement of peritoneal drains without surgery has had some success with the initial management of critically ill, extremely low birth weight infants with perforated NEC or isolated intestinal perforation (Rao et al., 2011).
   d. Postoperative care.
      (1) Pain management (see Chapter 16).
      (2) NPO.
      (3) Gastric decompression with a vented sump tube to low continuous suction until gastric output is minimal. To prevent dehydration, measure amount every 4 hours and replace mL for mL with physiologic IV fluid.
      (4) Nutrition.
         (a) TPN is used until sufficient enteral intake is established.
         (b) Enteral nutrition is initiated when the operative site has healed. Initiate enteral feeding (often with elemental formula or maternal breast milk) and progress slowly as tolerated.
      (5) Routine ostomy care if applicable. Complications include ostomy prolapse, intestinal obstruction, skin dehiscence and excoriation, and stomal ulceration and bleeding.

(6) Maintenance of fluid and electrolyte balance.
(7) Medications: continue antibiotics.
(8) Observation of stomas for color and drainage.
(9) Observe for complications.
(a) Strictures occur in approximately a third of infants with resection. Signs of strictures include bloody stools, failure to thrive, feeding abnormalities, and diarrhea.
(b) Enteric fistulas and short-bowel syndrome (malabsorption and diarrhea).
(c) Recurrent NEC is not common but can occur.

## SHORT-BOWEL SYNDROME (AMIN ET AL., 2013; GOULET ET AL., 2013; LIGHTDALE ET AL., 2013)

**A. General considerations.**

1. Definition: syndrome of chronic malabsorption and malnutrition as a result of bowel shortening. Pathophysiology depends on length of intestine, segment of remaining intestine, and whether or not the ileocecal valve is intact. Following bowel resection, the remaining bowel has the ability to adapt to increase its digestive and absorptive capabilities. Villi and crypts elongate and epithelial hyperplasia occurs. Adaptive process is greater in the ileum than in the jejunum. Adaptation occurs over 1 to 2 years. Consequences of short-bowel syndrome are related to malabsorption due to decreased surface area and loss of specific functions of resected segments.
2. Etiology.
   a. Surgery requiring extensive resection of bowel.
      (1) NEC (most common, as high as 50%).
      (2) Jejunal or ileal atresia.
      (3) Midgut volvulus.
      (4) Extensive Hirschsprung's disease.
      (5) Omphalocele or gastroschisis.
3. Incidence: 2 per million per year.
4. Associated conditions.
   a. GI tract defects: atresia, malrotation, gastroschisis, omphalocele, Hirschsprung's disease.
5. Diagnosis.
   a. Substantial small intestine is removed during surgery.
   b. Clinical presentation: In general, infants experience malabsorption and diarrhea; specific problems are dependent on length of small bowel remaining, presence of ileocecal valve, and site of intestinal loss.
6. Prognosis.
   a. Both the length of intestine and site of intestinal loss influence survival of infants receiving enteral nutrition. Increasing length alone permits longer contact between the product of digestion and the mucosa. If enteral feeding is inadequate, TPN is required. Long-term TPN carries the risk of cholestasis and hepatic damage. Cholelithiasis may occur, owing to depletion of bile acids, resulting in a cholesterol–bile salt ratio abnormality.
   b. Loss of stomach is well tolerated if vitamin $B_{12}$ is periodically given parenterally to prevent anemia.
   c. Jejunum is the primary site of digestion and absorption; however, these functions can be performed in other areas of the intestine after adaptation occurs. Infants with loss of jejunum tend to do much better than those whose ileum is removed. Loss of jejunum can result in nutritional deficiencies, steatorrhea, and cholestasis.
   d. Ileum is responsible for absorption of fat-soluble vitamins, vitamin $B_{12}$, and bile salts. Loss of ileum has significant metabolic and nutritional consequences.
   e. Ileocecal valve delays intestinal transit time and prevents overgrowth of colonic bacteria in the small intestine. Loss of ileocecal valve results in small-bowel colonization with colonic bacteria and less time for digestion and absorption of nutrients in the small intestine.
   f. Loss of the colon may result in hypovolemia, dehydration, and electrolyte disturbances.

g. Overall survival has improved with new therapies.
h. With an intact ileocecal valve, infants with as little as 15 cm of small bowel can survive.
i. Without an intact ileocecal valve, infants require approximately 30 to 45 cm of small bowel for survival.

**B. Care of the infant with short-bowel syndrome.**

1. Medical management.
   a. Stabilize fluid and electrolytes and maintain normal profile.
   b. Nutrition.
      (1) TPN is used until sufficient enteral intake is established to sustain adequate growth. Cyclic administration of TPN is often used. Careful monitoring for associated complications is required.
      (2) Initiate enteral feeding (often with elemental formula or maternal breast milk) and progress very slowly as tolerated.
   c. Medications:
      (1) Gastric acid blockade (50% have a temporary increase in gastric acid postoperatively).
      (2) Cholestyramine for steatorrhea.
      (3) Antiperistaltic agents for persistent diarrhea. Somatostatin is used to suppress intestinal hormones, decrease gastric and pancreatic secretions, and decrease GI motility. Octreotide is a somatostatin mimetic.
      (4) Trimethoprim-sulfamethoxazole, metronidazole, or other nonabsorbable antibiotics for bacterial overgrowth.
      (5) Vitamin $B_{12}$ is required if the stomach or ileum is lost.
      (6) Vitamins A, D, E, and K are required if the ileum is lost.
   d. Provision of nonnutritive sucking.
   e. Prevention of skin breakdown due to diarrhea.
2. Surgical management.
   a. Any of a variety of surgical procedures to increase intestinal surface area or decrease intestinal motility.
   b. Small-bowel transplant. Successful for only a small number of infants; reserved for infants in whom medical and other surgical management has been unsuccessful or who have life-threatening complications of TPN. Contraindications: profound neurologic disabilities, life-threatening and other noncorrectable illnesses not directly related to the digestive system, severe congenital or acquired immunologic deficiencies, and insufficient vascular patency to guarantee easy central venous access for up to 6 months following transplantation.

## BILIARY ATRESIA (BRUMBAUGH AND MACK, 2012; DAVENPORT, 2012; WILDHABER, 2012)

**A. General considerations.**

1. Definition: obstruction of bile flow in the bile duct system. Two types:
   a. Intrahepatic. An embryonic form with failure of ductal formation. Associated with other congenital anomalies.
   b. Extrahepatic. Perinatal fibro-obliteration of ducts, which has three forms: type I with atresia of the common bile duct with patent proximal ducts; type II with atresia of the common hepatic duct with patent proximal ducts; and type III with atresia of the right and left hepatic ducts at the porta hepatis.
   c. With both intra- and extrahepatic forms of biliary atresia, bile fails to exit the liver, resulting in hepatic fibrosis and cirrhosis with progressive liver failure and portal hypertension. With liver failure, liver functions diminish (clotting factors, albumin, drug biotransformation, phagocytosis of foreign substances and bacteria, and excretion of waste material and toxins). Deficiencies of fat-soluble vitamins and vitamin K occur as a result of alterations in fat digestion and absorption.
2. Etiology: exact mechanism unknown. Suggested theories: alteration in embryologic development, immune or autoimmune response, and association with viral infections. Research points to a genetic causation in some cases.

3. Incidence: 1 in 8,000 to 18,000 live births, with a slight preponderance in females; 20% intrahepatic and 80% extrahepatic.
4. Associated anomalies: occurrence in 10% to 15% of infants; including cardiovascular disorders, polysplenia or asplenia with or without situs inversus, preduodenal or absent portal vein, malrotation, and intestinal atresias.
5. Diagnosis.
   a. Clinical presentation.
      (1) Normal appearance at birth, with gradual manifestation during first month of life.
      (2) Jaundice: usually becomes apparent between second and sixth weeks of life. Skin is not yellow but rather of green-bronze color because of conjugated hyperbilirubinemia, which is always pathologic.
      (3) Acholic stools (meconium is normal in color). Dark urine.
      (4) Portal hypertension. Seen in advanced liver disease when high pressure exists between portal vein and inferior vena cava.
         (a) Engorged veins: periumbilical, esophageal, and rectal.
         (b) Ascites: result of low albumin levels and increased hydrostatic pressure in abdominal vessels.
   b. Physical examination.
      (1) Abdominal distention.
      (2) Distended, tortuous abdominal veins.
      (3) Hepatosplenomegaly. Liver is hard.
   c. Imaging studies.
      (1) Ultrasound.
      (2) Hepatobiliary scintigraphy (hepatobiliary iminodiacetic acid [HIDA] scan).
      (3) Operative cholangiography.
      (4) ERCP. Recent development of a new side-view instrument makes ERCP now possible in infants.
   d. Laboratory studies.
      (1) Elevated serum levels of aminotransferase, alkaline phosphatase (ALP), $\gamma$-glutamyl transpeptidase, and 5′-nucleotidase and hyaluronic acid.
      (2) Late findings: abnormal clotting studies, hypoalbuminemia.
   e. Other.
      (1) Liver biopsy.
6. Prognosis.
   a. Without surgical treatment, most infants will die by 2 years of age.
   b. Less than 20% of patients who have a portoenterostomy survive to adulthood without a liver transplant.
   c. Survival is improved for patients who initially undergo a portoenterostomy, followed by liver transplantation.

**B. Care of the infant with biliary atresia.**

1. Preoperative care.
   a. Evaluation for additional anomalies.
2. Surgical procedures.
   a. Intrahepatic form requires liver transplantation. Lack of intrahepatic ducts precludes any drainage procedures.
   b. Extrahepatic form. Goal: reestablishment of bile drainage. Treatment is dependent on the type.
      (1) Resection of atretic segments and end-to-end anastomosis: possible in only a few cases.
      (2) Hepatoportoenterostomy (Kasai procedure). Intestinal conduit is created between the liver surface and small intestine. Typically performed by laparotomy, recently performed using robotic laparoscopic technique (Yamataka et al., 2012). This is most successful when performed by 2 months of age. The conduit is sometimes exteriorized temporarily to allow assessment of bile flow. Complications include the following:

(a) Cholangitis: most common complication; results from bile stasis and bacterial contamination of the intestinal conduit. Presents with fever, leukocytosis, increased serum bilirubin, and nonspecific signs of infection.
(b) Cessation of bile flow.
(c) Portal hypertension.
(3) Liver transplant.

**3.** Postoperative care.
**a.** Pain management (see Chapter 16).
**b.** NPO.
**c.** Gastric decompression with a vented sump tube to low continuous suction until gastric output is minimal. To prevent dehydration, measure amount every 4 hours and replace mL for mL with physiologic IV fluid.
**d.** Medications.
(1) Antibiotics to decrease risk of cholangitis.
(2) Fat-soluble vitamins (A, D, E, K).
(3) Choleretic agents such as ursodiol (Actigall) may be given to increase bile flow.
(4) Steroids are commonly given for a month, then tapered. Used for their choleretic effect and to decrease scarring at the site of anastomosis.
**e.** Nutrition.
(1) TPN is used until sufficient enteral intake is established.
(2) Enteral nutrition is initiated when the operative site has healed. Initiate enteral feeding containing medium-chain triglycerides and progress as tolerated.
**f.** Assessment of bile flow and replacement as appropriate (if exteriorized).
**g.** Monitor for hemorrhage secondary to portal hypertension and bleeding tendencies.

## CHOLESTASIS (BRUMBAUGH AND MACK, 2012; GOSSARD, 2013; HARTLEY ET AL., 2013)

**A. General considerations.**
**1.** Definition: marked impairment in bile flow.
**2.** Etiology: the main determinant of bile flow is the enterohepatic circulation, with the rate-limiting step being secretion of bile by the hepatocyte. The neonatal liver is prone to cholestasis because its bile acid pool size is diminished and hepatic uptake and excretion mechanisms are immature. In addition, new research points to a genetic causation in some cases. Causes of cholestasis by anatomic location:
**a.** Extrahepatic bile duct: biliary atresia, choledochal cyst, choledocholithiasis, and bile duct perforation.
**b.** Intrahepatic bile duct: syndromic paucity of bile ducts (Alagille syndrome [70% with abnormal chromosome 20p12]), nonsyndromic paucity of bile ducts, bile duct dysgenesis, CF, Langerhans cell histiocytosis, and hyper-immunoglobulin M syndrome.
**c.** Hepatocyte: bacterial and viral infection, progressive familial intrahepatic cholestasis syndrome, inborn errors of metabolism, neonatal hemochromatosis, and total parenteral nutrition–associated cholestasis (TPNAC).
**3.** Incidence: overall incidence is 1 in 2500. Incidence of cholestasis associated with TPN varies from 7% to 50%. Frequency increases with younger gestational age and longer duration of TPN. Most cases occur within 2 to 10 weeks after starting TPN; 90% of infants develop cholestasis within 13 weeks.
**4.** Associated conditions: see 2. Etiology, above.
**5.** Diagnosis: there is no one test for cholestasis. Once it is established that the infant has conjugated hyperbilirubinemia, the diagnostic evaluation should be individualized.
**a.** History.
**b.** Clinical presentation.
(1) Normal appearance at birth, with gradual manifestation during first month of life.
(2) Jaundice; usually becomes apparent between second and sixth weeks of life. Skin is not yellow but rather of green-bronze color due to conjugated hyperbilirubinemia.

(3) Acholic stools, malabsorption of fat (steatorrhea) and lipid-soluble vitamins, mineral and trace mineral deficiency, growth failure. Dark urine.
(4) Hepatomegaly due to hepatocellular damage. Portal hypertension if cholestasis is prolonged and liver failure occurs.
(5) Pruritus, xanthomas due to retention of bile acids and cholesterol.

**c.** Imaging studies.
(1) Ultrasound.
(2) Hepatobiliary scintigraphy (HIDA scan).
(3) Percutaneous or endoscopic cholangiography.
(4) ERCP.
(5) Radiographs of long bones and skull for congenital infections.

**d.** Laboratory studies.
(1) Urinalysis.
(2) Bacterial cultures of blood and urine.
(3) Serology for vital hepatitides, human immunodeficiency virus, and TORCH (*t*oxoplasmosis, *o*ther [congenital syphilis and viruses], *r*ubella, *c*ytomegalovirus, *h*erpes simplex).
(4) Bilirubin fractionation: Direct bilirubin greater than 2 mg/dL. Direct-to-total bilirubin ratio greater than 15%.
(5) Liver enzymes: Elevated aminotransferase concentrations (hepatocellular damage). Elevated ALP, 5′-nucleotidase or $\gamma$-glutamyl transpeptidase (biliary injury or obstruction).
(6) Assessment of synthetic liver function: serum albumin, glucose, ammonia, cholesterol, PT.
(7) Test for inborn errors of metabolism.
(8) Sweat chloride iontophoresis.

**e.** Other.
(1) Ophthalmologic examination.
(2) Liver biopsy.

**6.** Prognosis: related to underlying cause.

**B. Management of the infant with cholestasis: Management is specific to the etiology.** No specific therapy reverses cholestasis or prevents its progression. In cases of outflow obstruction, eliminate the obstruction (see Biliary Atresia). Chromosomal abnormalities cannot be reversed but may be palliated. With an infectious etiology, treat underlying infection. For TPNAC, minimize TPN concentration and duration and provide enteral nutrition if possible. Goals of therapy are to improve nutritional status, maximize growth, and minimize discomfort.

**1.** TPN management.
**a.** Decrease parenteral protein to 1 to 2 g/kg/day.
**b.** Decrease parenteral dextrose concentration to 10%.
**c.** Eliminate hepatic trace elements.

**2.** Enteral feeding management.
**a.** Increase enteral feedings as tolerated. Caloric intake should be 125% to 150% of recommended dietary additives.
**b.** Administer formulas with medium-chain triglycerides (e.g., Pregestimil, Alimentum).
**c.** Encourage breastfeeding as long as infant grows appropriately.

**3.** Medications.
**a.** Supplemental fat-soluble vitamins. TPGS-tocopherol (Liqui-E or Nutr-E-Sol) is the preferred vitamin E preparation, to be given with a multivitamin supplement (e.g., Poly-Vi-Sol) and vitamin K. These preparations should all be mixed together for administration.
**b.** Cholestyramine to increase fecal excretion of bile acids. The decrease in bile acids returning to the liver stimulates the production of new bile acids from cholesterol, resulting in the reduction of toxic bile acids in the liver and a decrease in cholesterol. May help decrease pruritus.
**c.** Ursodeoxycholic acid for pruritus and to increase intestinal excretion of bile acids.
**d.** Phenobarbital to decrease bile acid pool size.

## GASTROESOPHAGEAL REFLUX (AMERICAN ACADEMY OF PEDIATRICS, TASK FORCE ON SUDDEN INFANT DEATH SYNDROME, AND MOON, 2011; BLACKBURN, 2013; CZINN AND BLANCHARD, 2013; LIGHTDALE ET AL., 2013)

**A. General considerations.**

**1.** Definition: GER is the retrograde movement of gastric contents into the esophagus and above. With gastroesophageal reflux disease (GERD), there are symptoms of disease resulting from GER events. GERD has not been well defined in neonates. Regurgitation is a movement of gastric contents into the mouth. Regurgitation may be a sign of GER, but GER can occur without regurgitation.

**a.** Spectrum of GER.

(1) Reflux episodes occur to some extent in all individuals, especially after meals.

(2) Reflux is considered physiologic as long as the individual continues to thrive and has no complications.

(3) Complications generally do not occur as long as the frequency and duration of reflux are in the normal range.

(4) Infants who have regurgitation as their only sign of reflux are considered to have physiologic GER and are referred to as "happy spitters."

(5) Pathologic GER usually manifests as malnutrition, respiratory disorders, or esophagitis.

**2.** Etiology. Mechanisms for reflux in infants includes a transient relaxation of the lower esophageal segment (LES), delay in esophageal clearance of contents, air entry into stomach during swallowing, excessive swallowing, delayed gastric emptying, and decreased esophageal motility. A complete understanding of the pathophysiology of GER remains unclear.

**3.** Incidence: varied; 40% to 50% of infants regurgitate more than once a day. GER with symptoms has been noted in 3% to 10% of premature infants less than 1500 g.

**4.** Associated conditions.

**a.** Prematurity.

**b.** Birth asphyxia with neurodevelopmental delay. Infants treated with extracorporeal membrane oxygenation (ECMO) are at risk for GER because of the acute status requiring ECMO.

**c.** GI tract anomalies/conditions: EA/TEF, esophagitis, hiatal hernia, pyloric stenosis, gastroschisis/omphalocele, duodenal atresia, malrotation.

**d.** Diaphragmatic hernia/paralysis.

**e.** Chronic lung disease.

**f.** Medications: xanthines, β-mimetics, prostaglandin $E_1$, dopamine.

**5.** Diagnosis.

**a.** Clinical presentation.

(1) Feeding difficulties.

(a) Regurgitation; most common presentation in infants.

(b) Gagging.

(c) Feeding refusal.

(d) Aspiration.

(e) Failure to thrive.

(2) Fussiness, irritability, colic-like behavior, back arching with feeding.

(3) Respiratory difficulty.

(a) Apnea.

(i) Protective airway reflexes may respond to refluxed pharyngeal material, causing laryngospasm and obstructive apnea.

(ii) Reflux-related apnea most commonly occurs after a meal, with the infant supine or seated. The infant may not cough, choke, or gag prior to the apneic episode.

(b) Stridor.

**b.** Radiologic examination.

(1) Fluoroscopy or upper GI series (30% false positive).

(2) Scintigraphy.

c. Other studies.
   (1) Esophageal pH probe. Detects acid reflux only; does not detect nonacid (milk) or gas reflux.
   (2) Intraesophageal electrical impedance (pH independent).
   (3) Esophageal manometry.
   (4) Endoscopy.

6. Prognosis. Resolves in almost all infants by 12 to 18 months of age; 10% to 15% require prolonged medical management; 10% to 15% also require surgery. Success after fundoplication varies. Prognosis depends on complications: respiratory (worsening of chronic lung disease; bronchospasm and pneumonia), esophageal (esophagitis [occurs in 61% to 83% of infants with clinically significant reflux], bleeding, strictures), and hematologic (anemia from chronic bleeding).

**B. Management of the infant with GER.**

1. Conservative measures.
   a. Interventions to minimize simple regurgitation.
      (1) Thicken feedings with rice cereal or other commercially available thickeners. Thickening increases viscosity. It also increases caloric density, thus reducing the volume needed to supply adequate calories.
      (2) Feed slowly.
      (3) Frequent burping.
      (4) Small frequent feedings.
      (5) Position infant at a 45- to 60-degree angle during feeding.
      (6) Avoid pressure on abdomen during and immediately after feeding.
      (7) Avoid jiggling or bouncing the infant during feeding and for at least an hour afterward.
   b. Minimize/eliminate provoking and aggravating factors.
      (1) Provoking factors: frequent suctioning, chest physical therapy.
      (2) Aggravating factors: xanthine and β-mimetic agents (increase LES relaxation).
   c. Position.
      (1) Upright for 30 minutes after feeding (infant held upright by caregiver). Upright position in a car seat can makes reflux worse as typically the infant's lower body slides forward, increasing intraabdominal pressure and possibly compromising the airway by a chin-on-chest position.
      (2) Supine position. Preterm delivery and GER do not exempt an infant from supine position recommendations (American Academy of Pediatrics [AAP], Task Force on Sudden Infant Death Syndrome, and Moon, 2011).
      (3) The surface on which the infant is placed for sleep should be firm and without soft bedding or gas-trapping objects (AAP, Task Force on Sudden Infant Death Syndrome, and Moon, 2011).
2. Pharmacologic measures.
   a. Prokinetics. Used to increase gastric motility. Commonly used agents include bethanechol, metoclopramide, and erythromycin.
   b. Histamine$_2$-receptor antagonists or proton pump inhibitors. Reduce gastric acid when complications such as esophagitis occur. Commonly used agents include ranitidine, famotidine, and omeprazole.
   c. Acid-neutralizing agents (e.g., calcium- and aluminum-containing antacids). Facilitate healing of esophagitis but are infrequently given to neonates because of the side effect of constipation.
3. Surgical measures: initiated when conservative and medical management has failed and the infant has developed or is anticipated to develop sequelae and complications. Frequently performed using laparoscopic technique.
   a. Nissen fundoplication (Fig. 29-7). Stomach fundus is wrapped 360 degrees around the LES. Is the procedure most commonly performed.
   b. Variations of Nissen technique including the Thal (270-degree) procedure; the Mutaf gastric tube cardioplasty; posterior 180-degree procedure; anterior 180-degree procedure; and recently an anterior 90-degree procedure.

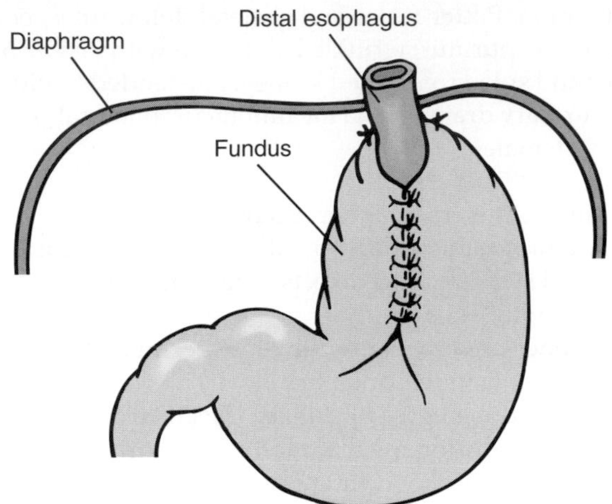


FIGURE 29-7 ■ Nissen fundoplication for repair of hiatal hernia. Fundus of stomach is wrapped around distal esophagus and sutured to itself. (From Lewis, S.L., Dirksen, S.R., Heitkemper, M.M., and Bucher, L.: *Medical-surgical nursing: Assessment and management of clinical problems* [9th ed.]. St. Louis, 2014, Elsevier Mosby.)

## MULTISYSTEM DISORDERS WITH GASTROINTESTINAL INVOLVEMENT (HASSETT ET AL., 2012; LESAVOY ET AL., 2012; WOODS AND BRANDON, 2007; ZUGOR ET AL., 2012)

**A. Eagle–Barrett syndrome (prune-belly syndrome; prune-belly association).**

1. Definition: triad of congenital anomalies consisting of absence of abdominal musculature, genitourinary tract abnormalities, and cryptorchidism (undescended testes). Most common genitourinary defects are as follows:
   a. Megaloureter.
   b. Cystic renal dysplasia.
   c. Urethral obstruction.
   d. Megacystitis.
2. Etiology: unclear, but may be the result of a generalized developmental defect of abdominal parietes and mesenchyma. The condition is rarely familial, and no cytogenic abnormality has been discovered, although recent genetic analyses point to several genes producing inconsistent phenotype (Woolf et al., 2013).
3. Incidence: 1 in 35,000 to 50,000 live births. Approximately 97% of affected infants are male. With familial cases, the incidence of affected males decreases to 72%. The incidence is also higher in twin gestations, African American infants, and cases of trisomy 21.
4. Associated conditions.
   a. Pulmonary conditions: hypoplasia.
   b. GI tract anomalies (30%): malrotation, volvulus, atresia or stenosis, imperforate anus, persistent cloaca.
   c. Cardiac anomalies (10%): patent ductus arteriosus, atrial and ventricular septal defects, tetralogy of Fallot.
   d. Genitourinary conditions: patent urachus, posterior urethral valves, bilateral hydroureter and hydronephrosis.
   e. Musculoskeletal anomalies: limb abnormalities (clubfoot and other positional deformations), scoliosis, congenital hip dysplasia, contractures.
5. Diagnosis.
   a. Prenatal ultrasonography, including high-resolution method. May show a dilated renal pelvis (>5 mm at 16 to 18 weeks of gestation), dilated ureters, and bladder distention.
   b. History of oligohydramnios: suggestive of renal pathologic changes.
   c. Inspection at birth: shapeless, flat abdomen with wrinkled skin; respiratory distress, compression deformities.

   d. Physical examination: Potter facies and skeletal deformities; bell-shaped chest, respiratory distress, cardiac murmur; wrinkled abdomen with visible bowel loops and possible margins of liver and spleen, enlarged kidneys, distended bladder (4 cm from symphysis by percussion), urinary drainage via the umbilicus; bilateral cryptorchidism, pseudohermaphroditism in females.
6. Imaging studies.
   a. Ultrasound: kidneys, ureters, bladder, urethra.
   b. Voiding cystourethrogram: controversial. Evaluates urethra, bladder, vesicoureteral reflux, and ureteral stenosis, and detects patent urachus.
   c. Computed tomography scan.
   d. Nuclear scan: technetium (Tc-99 m) dimethylsuccinic acid (DMSA) renal scan.
7. Other: karyotyping if sex is indeterminate.
8. Prognosis: directly related to degree of urinary tract dysfunction, especially renal. Approximately 20% of infants die during the first month of life from renal dysplasia or hypoplasia. Renal failure develops in childhood in approximately 30% of those who survive infancy. Treatment required includes dialysis or transplantation. Long-term considerations include difficulty voiding and the need for nephrostomy or ureterostomy; constipation is common; long-term antibiotic therapy may be necessary to prevent infection.

**B. Management of the infant with Eagle–Barrett syndrome.**

1. Medical management.
   a. Respiratory: support as needed; alert for pulmonary air leak.
   b. Correct fluid, electrolyte, and acid–base status. Sodium reabsorption is diminished or deficient; hyponatremia may rapidly result. Blood urea nitrogen and serum creatinine: rising values may indicate renal insufficiency.
   c. Nutrition. Low protein intake reduces renal workload.
   d. Antibiotics to prevent urinary tract infection due to urinary stasis and reflux, and invasive procedures.
2. Surgical procedures.
   a. Prenatal: shunting to preserve renal function by preventing bladder distention. Procedures include vesicoamniotic shunting, open fetal surgery, and fetoscopic surgery.
   b. Postnatal: Urinary diversion is essential to sustain renal function. Procedures include urethrotomy for urethral obstruction; cutaneous vesicostomy with the bladder brought to the abdominal surface; repair of posterior urethral valves; closure of patent urachus, although many spontaneously close; orchiopexy to prevent testicular malignancy; and abdominal wall reconstruction.

**C. Congenital diaphragmatic hernia (Benjamin et al., 2013; Greer, 2013; Hedrick, 2013).**

1. Definition: herniation of abdominal organs into the thoracic cavity through a defect in the diaphragm. About 85% occur on the left. Approximately 95% occur posteriorly (Bochdalek type), while 5% occur anteriorly (Morgagni type). The defect can vary from a small slit to the complete absence of the diaphragm on the affected side. Severity is related to timing and degree of prenatal herniation. Early herniation through a large defect is associated with bilateral pulmonary hypoplasia, pulmonary hypertension, and intrapulmonary shunt (V/Q mismatch). A right-to-left shunt occurs through the ductus arteriosus and/or foramen ovale, further compromising pulmonary blood flow and sending deoxygenated blood to the body.
2. Etiology: unknown; retinoid signaling and transcription factors are considered. May occur as isolated defect or part of a syndrome. Numerous genetic abnormalities are associated with CDH.
3. Incidence: 1 in 2200 to 3000 live births.
4. Associated conditions.
   a. Chromosomal abnormalities: most common are trisomies 13, 18, and 21, and 45,X.
   b. Associated anomalies are reported to be greater than 40% and include CNS, cardiovascular, skeletal, GI, and genitourinary defects. Intestinal malrotation is common.
5. Diagnosis.
   a. Prenatal ultrasonography, including the high-resolution method. Hallmark finding: fluid-filled stomach just behind the left atrium.

b. History of polyhydramnios.
c. Clinical presentation.
(1) Respiratory distress and cyanosis at birth or shortly after birth, typically followed by worsening presentation. Condition worsens rather than improves with bag-and-mask ventilation as intestines distend with air and further compromise lung function.
(2) Hypoperfusion and decreased oxygen saturation due to right-to-left shunting through the ductus arteriosus, foramen ovale, and intrapulmonary shunts.
d. Physical examination.
(1) Diminished breath sounds: decreased on ipsilateral side due to lung compression by abdominal organs; decreased on contralateral side due to mediastinal shift.
(2) Heart tones may be shifted from their normal point of maximal intensity.
(3) Barrel chest.
(4) Scaphoid abdomen.
e. Radiologic examination.
(1) Plain radiograph showing displaced gastric bubble and a bowel gas pattern in the thorax (see Chapter 14). A radiograph taken immediately after birth may not demonstrate bowel gas in the intestines, while later radiographs demonstrate it clearly.
f. Laboratory tests: blood gas analysis demonstrating hypoxemia, hypercapnia, and combined metabolic and respiratory acidosis.
6. Prognosis: survival varies depending on the size of the defect and amount of herniated viscera, early intervention (especially at a tertiary care center), pulmonary hypertension, and associated conditions. Despite current interventions and a shift from early surgical repair to supportive therapy and techniques to avoid lung injury, survival ranges from 70% to 92%. Although some institutions report higher survival rates, the reported survival rates do not include infants who expired prior to arrival at the respective institution. Structured follow-up care is required for infants with long-term sequelae (AAP, Section on Surgery and Committee on Fetus and Newborn, Lally, and Engle, 2008).

**D. Management of the infant with CDH.**
1. Prenatal treatment: the gravid mother must be transferred to a facility capable of management of the infant postpartum, including neonatal intensive care, inhaled nitric oxide (iNO), ECMO, pediatric surgery, and genetic evaluation.
2. Preoperative care: CDH is no longer considered a surgical emergency. Concerns immediately after birth include pulmonary hypoplasia and pulmonary hypertension. In addition, not rushing to surgery allows stabilization of the infant and evaluation for associated conditions that may preclude ECMO or surgery.
a. Respiratory.
(1) Intubate and support as needed. Avoid bag-mask ventilation to prevent GI distention. Remain alert for pulmonary air leak. Immediate treatment must be prompt and aggressive. Primary considerations are as follows:
(a) Establishment of adequate perfusion. Use of inotropes to increase systemic blood pressure and decreased right-to-left shunting.
(b) Correction of acid–base imbalances and provision of adequate oxygenation.
(c) May require high-frequency ventilation, administration of iNO. Prophylactic surfactant treatment at birth has no benefit in either preterm or term infants because surfactant maturation is unaffected in infants with CDH. Hyperventilation and hyperalkalinization to force alkalinization are no longer recommended because they cause ventilation-induced lung injury, complicate electrolyte management, and decrease cerebral blood flow.
b. ECMO is instituted if ventilation does not effectively stabilize the pulmonary status. ECMO may be used preoperatively to stabilize the patient for surgery, intraoperatively, and/or postoperatively to rest the lungs.
c. NPO.
d. Gastric decompression with a vented sump tube to low continuous suction until gastric output is minimal. To prevent dehydration, measure amount every 4 hours and replace mL for mL with physiologic IV fluid.

e. Complete examination for other anomalies.
3. Surgical procedures.
a. Prenatal surgery.
(1) Procedures to occlude the trachea have been used in fetuses but have not proven beneficial. Ongoing fetal lamb studies are evolving.
(2) In-utero repair of CDH does not improve survival over conventional postpartum care.
b. Postnatal surgery.
(1) Primary closure of the diaphragmatic defect is usually possible. With large defects or a totally absent diaphragm, a synthetic patch can be used to close the diaphragmatic defect.
c. Postoperative care.
(1) Pain management (see Chapter 16).
(2) Continue preoperative care.
(a) Respiratory support with oxygenation, ventilation, iNO, ECMO.
(b) NPO.
(c) Gastric decompression with a vented sump tube to low continuous suction until gastric output is minimal and peristalsis is normal. To prevent dehydration, measure amount every 4 hours and replace ml for ml with physiologic IV fluid.
(d) Inotropes: decrease right-to-left shunting.
(e) If placed during surgery, a chest tube for drainage should be placed on water seal (without suction) to prevent acute mediastinal shift.
(f) Coordinated long-term follow-up is required as some survivors demonstrate neurologic issues: abnormal muscle tone and delayed neurocognitive and language skills.

E. **Hyperbilirubinemia (AAP, Subcommittee on Hyperbilirubinemia, 2004; Bhutani et al., 2013; Kamath et al., 2011; National Association of Neonatal Nurses, Board of Directors, 2010).**
1. Definitions.
a. Hyperbilirubinemia: an elevated total serum bilirubin (TSB) level. Abnormal values differ by gestational age, days of life, and concomitant illness or conditions. A recognizable sign is jaundice. TSB is the combination of conjugated and unconjugated serum bilirubin levels (Fig. 29-8).
b. Jaundice (icterus): the yellowish coloration of the skin and sclera caused by the presence of bilirubin in elevated concentrations. Jaundice appears cephalad to caudal and regresses in the reverse order.
c. Conjugated: direct serum hyperbilirubinemia.
d. Unconjugated: indirect hyperbilirubinemia.
e. Acute bilirubin encephalopathy: acute bilirubin toxicity manifested by a direct correlation between lethargy and unconjugated serum bilirubin concentration, and abnormal brainstem auditory evoked response. Brain magnetic resonance images show focal changes. If not reversed, the process progresses to permanent neurologic impairment or death. Survivors demonstrate cerebral palsy and sensorineural hearing loss. Autopsy also reveals renal, intestinal, and pancreatic cell involvement. Calculation of a risk index score:
(1) Phase 1: poor sucking, hypotonia, depressed sensorium.
(2) Phase 2: fever, retrocollis, hypertonia, opisthotonos, high-pitched cry.
(3) Phase 3: shrill cry, hearing and visual derangements, no feeding, athetosis, apnea, seizures, deep stupor to coma, death.
f. Kernicterus: for consistency the AAP recommends this definition: irreversible, chronic sequelae of bilirubin toxicity (AAP, Subcommittee on Hyperbilirubinemia, 2004).
(1) During the first year of life, characteristic findings are hypotonia, active deep tendon reflexes, persistent tonic neck reflex, and delayed acquisition of motor skills.
(2) Characteristics of fully developed encephalopathy include hearing loss, choreoathetoid cerebral palsy, and gaze abnormalities, especially upward gaze. Intellectual deficits are common but usually not severe.
(3) Treatment: none.

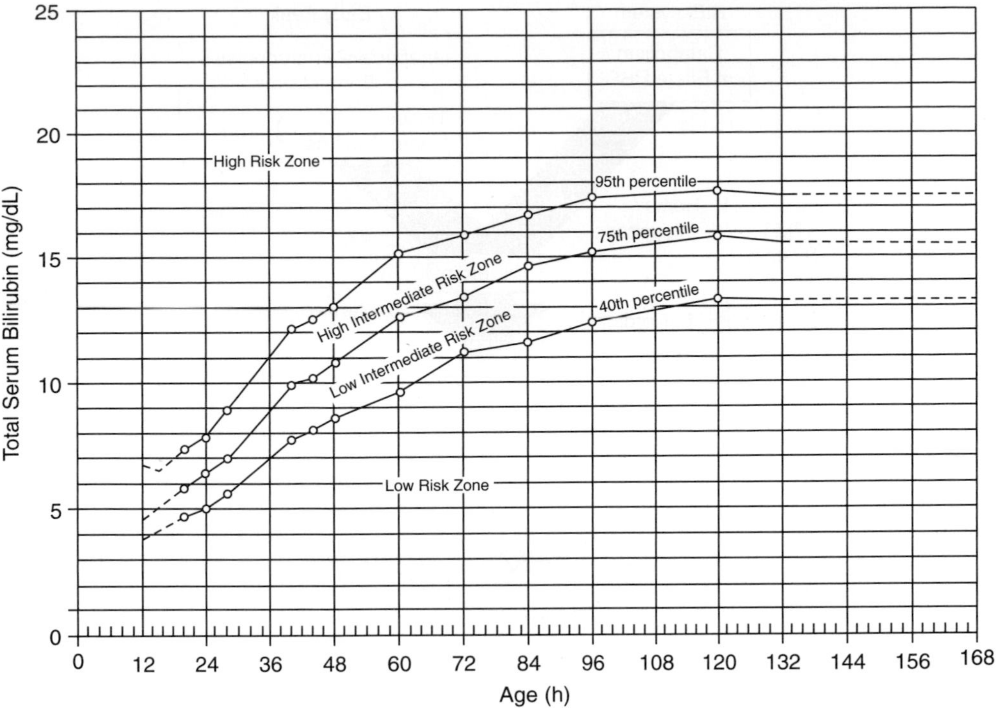


FIGURE 29-8 ■ Risk designation of term and near-term well newborns based on their hour-specific serum bilirubin values. The high-risk zone is designated by the 95th percentile track. The intermediate-risk zone is subdivided to upper- and lower-risk zones by the 75th percentile track. The low-risk zone has been electively and statistically defined by the 40th percentile track. (Dotted extensions are based on <300 total serum bilirubin [TSB] values/epoch.) (From Bhutani, V.K. and American Academy of Pediatrics, Committee on Fetus and Newborn: Phototherapy to prevent severe neonatal hyperbilirubinemia in the newborn infant 35 or more weeks of gestation. *Pediatrics*, 128[4]:e1046-e1052, 2011.)

2. Etiology.
   a. Bilirubin metabolism (Fig. 29-9).
      (1) Synthesis: bilirubin is primarily the metabolic end-product of erythrocyte (red blood cell [RBC]) breakdown. One gram of heme produces 34 mg of bilirubin; normal neonates produce 8 to 10 mg/kg/day.
      (2) Transport: heme reversibly binds to albumin (1 g of albumin can bind with approximately 8 mg of bilirubin) and is transported via the bloodstream to the liver as an unconjugated, fat-soluble product with a propensity for fatty tissues such as subcutaneous and brain tissue.
      (3) Metabolism: glucuronyl transferase converts bilirubin and glucuronic acid into water-soluble glucuronide.
      (4) Excretion: glucuronide is excreted into bile and enters the intestine, where bacteria convert it to urobilinogen. Urobilinogen is converted to stercobilin and excreted in feces, giving feces a brownish color.
      (5) Enterohepatic reabsorption of bilirubin: In the small intestine, the high concentration of β-glucuronidase in the brush border in newborn infants can convert conjugated bilirubin into the unconjugated form, which is easily absorbed from the small intestine into the portal circulation. In fetal life, this permits bilirubin to be transported across the placenta for maternal excretion. Increased amounts of bilirubin in the amniotic fluid may indicate hemolytic disease or fetal intestinal obstruction below the bile ducts.
   b. Nonpathologic unconjugated hyperbilirubinemia: a result of an elevated hematocrit level at birth, increased RBC destruction (neonatal RBCs have a 70- to 90-day life span), reduced hepatic uptake of unconjugated bilirubin, and enterohepatic reabsorption of

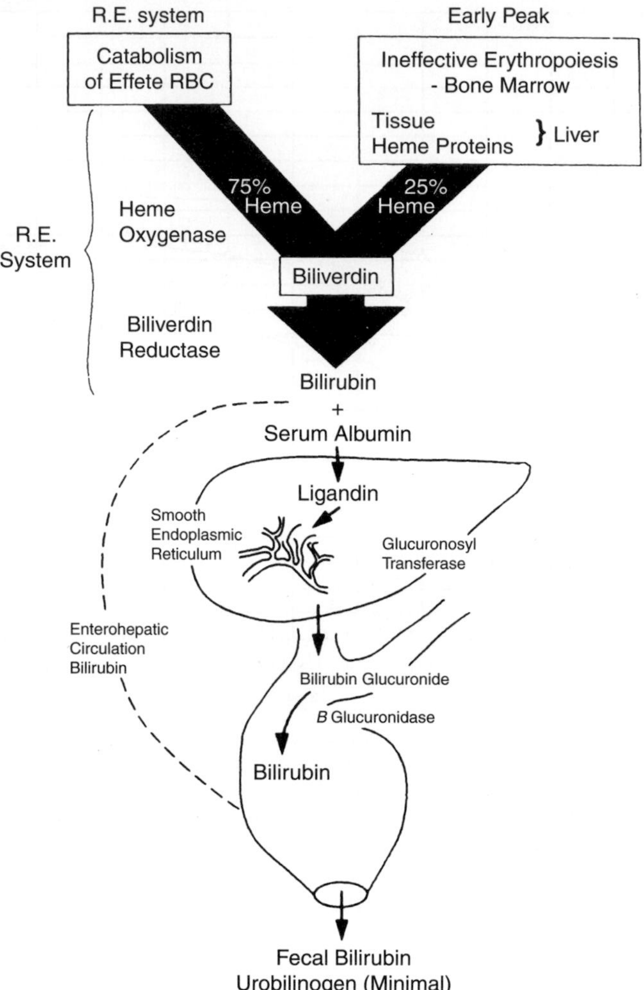


FIGURE 29-9 ■ Neonatal bile pigment metabolism. *RBC*, Red blood cells; *R.E.*, reticuloendothelial. (From Maisels, M.J.: Jaundice. In G.B. Avery, M.A. Fletcher, and M.G. MacDonald [Eds.]: *Neonatology: Pathophysiology and management of the newborn* [5th ed.]. Philadelphia, 1999, Lippincott, Williams & Wilkins, p. 767.)

bilirubin. TSB levels generally peak on day 3 of life in full-term infants and on days 5 to 6 in preterm infants. Factors that may further accentuate this normal process include:

(1) Hemolysis.
  (a) ABO/Rh incompatibilities.
  (b) Bacterial and viral infection (especially TORCH infections).
  (c) Inherited disorders of RBC metabolism.
    i. RBC membrane defects: spherocytosis, elliptocytosis.
    ii. RBC enzyme defects: glucose-6-phosphate dehydrogenase (G6PD) deficiency and pyruvate kinase deficiency.
  (d) Inherited disorders of bilirubin metabolism: Crigler–Najjar syndrome types I and II, Gilbert syndrome.
  (e) Medications that cause hemolysis or compete with albumin for binding sites, and free fatty acids from emulsified fats (Intralipid®).
(2) Extravasation of blood.
  (a) Cephalohematoma or bruising.
  (b) Pulmonary, cerebral, or retroperitoneal hemorrhage.
(3) Increased enterohepatic circulation.
  (a) Delayed feeding.
  (b) Intestinal obstructions.

(4) Decreased hepatic function and perfusion.
   (a) Metabolic derangements: hypoxia, acidosis, hypothermia, hypoglycemia, starvation.
   (b) Infection.
(5) Endocrine disorders.
   (a) Hypothyroidism.
   (b) Hypopituitarism.
(6) Inborn errors of metabolism (with both unconjugated and conjugated hyperbilirubinemia).
   (a) Galactosemia.
   (b) $\alpha_1$-Antitrypsin deficiency.
   (c) Tyrosinosis.
   (d) Hypermethioninemia.
   (e) CF.
(7) Globin synthesis defect: $\alpha$-thalassemia.

**c.** Pathologic unconjugated hyperbilirubinemia (for blood incompatibilities, see Chapter 31): When the nonpathologic unconjugated hyperbilirubinemia processes are exaggerated and when available albumin-binding sites are saturated, unconjugated bilirubin circulates as free bilirubin and can cross the blood–brain barrier (BBB). This BBB breach is accentuated with meningitis.
(1) Unconjugated hyperbilirubinemia is pathologic when
   (a) Jaundice appears in the first 24 hours of life,
   (b) TSB level increases by more than 5 mg/dL/day,
   (c) TSB level exceeds 12.9 mg/dL in a term infant or 15 mg/dL in a preterm infant,
   (d) TSB level is in the 95th percentile for age in hours or is "jumping the tracks" (see Fig. 29-8), or
   (e) Jaundice lasts for more than 1 week in a term infant or 2 weeks in a preterm infant.

**d.** Conjugated hyperbilirubinemia.
(1) Hepatic cell injury: TPN, infection (TORCH and viral hepatitis, and systemic bacterial), medications, metabolic derangements and inborn errors of metabolism.
(2) Biliary obstruction: see Biliary Atresia.
(3) Excessive bilirubin load.
(4) Maternal–fetal blood group incompatibility: ABO, Rh (see Chapter 31).

**e.** Breastfeeding jaundice: onset 2 to 4 days of life; related to low enteral intake. Self-limiting as milk supply increases.

**f.** Breast milk jaundice: onset 4 to 7 days of life; exaggerated physiologic jaundice related to substances in maternal breast milk that cause glucuronyl transferase inhibition. Occurs in 10% to 30% of breastfed newborns; TSB levels may reach 12 to 20 mg/dL and persist for up to 2 months.

**3.** Incidence: dependent on etiology.

**a.** Influenced by the following:
(1) Ethnicity (higher in infants of East Asian and Mediterranean descent).
(2) Elevated hematocrit level (delayed cord clamping, maternal diabetes).
(3) Extravasated blood (bruising, cephalohematoma, intracranial hemorrhage, swallowed blood).
(4) Maternal medications: oxytocin and bupivacaine. Mechanism is unclear but may involve hemolysis.
(5) Hepatic dysfunction: prematurity, asphyxia.
(6) Feeding: early enteral feeds promote peristalsis and passage of bilirubin-containing stool, and introduce bacteria into the gut (contributes to the conversion of bilirubin to urobilin, a substance that cannot be reabsorbed).

**b.** Nonpathologic unconjugated hyperbilirubinemia (physiologic jaundice): jaundice develops in more than 60% of term newborn infants and 80% of preterm infants; it is visible when the serum bilirubin concentration is greater than 6 to 7 mg/dL.

**c.** Conjugated hyperbilirubinemia: dependent on etiology.

d. Breastfeeding jaundice: 1 in 10 breastfed infants.
e. Breast milk jaundice: 1 in 200 breastfed infants.

4. Associated conditions.
   a. Prematurity.
   b. Infection.
   c. Dehydration.
5. Diagnosis.
   a. Nonpathologic unconjugated hyperbilirubinemia.
      (1) Clinical presentation: onset of jaundice around day 2 to 3 of life. No hepatosplenomegaly.
      (2) Laboratory tests: transcutaneous bilirubin meter helps establish a risk assessment but does not determine exact TSB levels. Usefulness in preterm infants, infants receiving phototherapy, and infants with TSB values above 15 mg/dL requires further study. Definitive bilirubin levels are obtained only by analysis of TSB levels.
   b. Pathologic unconjugated hyperbilirubinemia.
      (1) See nonpathologic unconjugated hyperbilirubinemia.
      (2) Clinical presentation: jaundice within 24 hours of birth. Signs of acute bilirubin encephalopathy.
      (3) Laboratory tests: TSB increase of 5 mg/dL or more in a 24-hour period or above the 95th percentile for age (hours).
   c. Conjugated hyperbilirubinemia.
      (1) See Biliary Atresia.
   d. Breastfeeding jaundice: Peaks around day 3 as enteral intake increases, then resolves.
   e. Breast milk jaundice: Prolonged appearance, no signs of bilirubin encephalopathy.
6. Prognosis: dependent on etiology and early detection and treatment, when necessary.

**F. Care of the infant with hyperbilirubinemia.**

1. **Management of nonpathologic unconjugated hyperbilirubinemia.**
   a. Frequent enteral feeding, including promotion and support of breastfeeding. This promotes removal of meconium from the intestines. Meconium contains 1 mg of bilirubin per 1 g of meconium. Delayed stooling promotes enterohepatic recirculation of bilirubin.
   b. Establish protocols to identify hyperbilirubinemia and measure bilirubin levels. Interpret results by infant's age—gestationally and hours of life. Follow-up care postdischarge is required for all infants discharged before 48 hours of age.
   c. At discharge, provide caregivers with verbal and written information about hyperbilirubinemia, need for follow-up monitoring, and how monitoring will be accomplished.
2. **Management of pathologic unconjugated hyperbilirubinemia.**
   a. Goal: prevent bilirubin toxic effects. Recognize that all infants are at risk. Risk is increased with decreasing gestational age, in infants less than 38 weeks of gestation who are breastfeeding, and in the ill neonate.
   b. Guidelines for treating hyperbilirubinemia in healthy term infants are listed in Table 29-4. Management of hyperbilirubinemia in low birth weight infants is determined by clinical status, age, weight, and history (Table 29-5).
   c. Jaundice before 24 hours of age and rising TSB levels exceeding 5 mg/dL per day requires investigation.
   d. Phototherapy: converts bilirubin to a water-soluble product at 0.5 to 1 mg percent per hour, and by 30% to 40% after 24 hours of treatment. Effectiveness influenced by the following:
      (1) Energy output of phototherapy unit. Bulbs require changing as energy output decreases. Light irradiance meters are used to determine bulb output.
      (2) Spectrum of light: special blue light labeled F20T12/BB (General Electric, Westinghouse, Sylvania) or TL52/20 W (Phillips, Eindhoven, The Netherlands) at 450 nm is most effective. Disadvantage: distortion of infant's color. White lamps, high-intensity gallium nitride light-emitting diodes, and fiberoptic blankets are effective alternatives.
      (3) Amount of infant's body surface area exposed to light. Turn infant frequently to allow all areas of the skin to be exposed.

■ TABLE 29-4
■ ■ **Management of Hyperbilirubinemia in Healthy Term Neonate***

| | TSB Level, mg/dL (mcmol/l) | | | |
|---|---|---|---|---|
| **Age (hours)** | **Consider Phototherapy*** | **Phototherapy** | **Exchange Transfusion If Intensive Phototherapy Fails†** | **Exchange Transfusion and Intensive Phototherapy** |
| ≤24‡ | | | | |
| 25 to 48 | ≥12 (170) | ≥15 (260) | ≥20 (340) | ≥25 (430) |
| 49 to 72 | ≥15 (260) | ≥18 (310) | ≥25 (430) | ≥30 (510) |
| >72 | ≥17 (290) | ≥20 (340) | ≥25 (430) | ≥30 (510) |

From American Academy of Pediatrics, Provisional Committee for Quality Improvement and Subcommittee on Hyperbilirubinemia: Practice parameter: Management of hyperbilirubinemia in the healthy term newborn. *Pediatrics*, 94(4 Pt. 1):558-565, 1994.
*TSB,* Total serum bilirubin.
*Phototherapy at these TSB levels is a clinical option, meaning that the intervention is available and may be used on the basis of individual clinical judgment.
†Intensive phototherapy should produce a decline of TSB of 1 to 2 mg/dL within 4 to 6 hours and the TSB level should continue to fall and remain below the threshold level for exchange transfusion. If this does not occur, it is considered a failure of phototherapy.
‡Term infants who are clinically jaundiced at ≤24 hours of age are not considered healthy and require further evaluation.

■ TABLE 29-5
■ ■ **Management of Hyperbilirubinemia in the Low-Birth-Weight Infant**

| | Total Serum Bilirubin Level, mg/dL | | | |
|---|---|---|---|---|
| | Healthy | | Sick | |
| **Gestational Age** | **Phototherapy** | **Exchange Transfusion** | **Phototherapy** | **Exchange Transfusion** |
| **Premature** | | | | |
| <1000 g | 5 to 7 | Variable | 4 to 6 | Variable |
| 1001 to 1500 g | 7 to 10 | Variable | 6 to 8 | Variable |
| 1501 to 2000 g | 10 to 12 | Variable | 8 to 10 | Variable |
| 2001 to 2500 g | 12 to 15 | Variable | 10 to 12 | Variable |

From Martin, R.J., Fanaroff, A.A., and Walsh, M.C.: *Fanaroff and Martin's neonatal-perinatal medicine: Diseases of the fetus and infant* (9th ed.). Philadelphia, 2011, Elsevier Mosby.

(4) Distance between light and infant. Follow equipment manufacturer's recommendations. Monitor infant's temperature. Fluorescent lights should be at a distance of 10 cm from the infant, who is placed naked in a bassinet. When bank lights are used, lamps should be covered with a clear acrylic shield to protect the infant from ultraviolet light.

**e.** Monitor fluid and electrolytes. Phototherapy increases insensible water loss and stooling. The AAP, Subcommittee on Hyperbilirubinemia (2004) recommends milk-based enteral feeding that inhibits enterohepatic reabsorption of bilirubin.

**f.** Monitor TSB during and after therapy. A rebound of 1 to 2 mg/dL can be expected.

**g.** Side effects: bronze skin if conjugated bilirubin is elevated; lethargy; skin rashes; risk of eye damage if eye patches are not secure; abdominal distention; hypocalcemia; lactose intolerance; and thrombocytopenia.

**h.** Home phototherapy: an option that decreases hospitalization time for an otherwise healthy infant.

**i.** Intensive phototherapy uses multiple phototherapy units above and below the completely naked infant. In addition, aluminum foil or a white cloth on the bassinet side is employed to reflect light onto the infant. All facilities providing care to infants should be capable of providing intensive phototherapy.

**j.** Exchange transfusion.

(1) Used when intensive phototherapy has been unsuccessful in controlling TSB, and at any time signs of acute bilirubin encephalopathy are present regardless of TSB level; used more often in hemolytic conditions.

(2) Hemolyzed and antibody-coated RBCs are removed over approximately 2 hours in small aliquots (3 to 5 mL/kg in preterm infants, 10 mL/kg in term infants) and replaced with donor blood. Double volume exchange (160 mL/kg) will reduce the TSB by 50%. Expect a rebound TSB of 60% to 70% of the preexchange transfusion level.

(3) IV gamma globulin (0.5 to 1 mg/kg over 2 hours) if phototherapy fails to control bilirubin levels or the TSB is approaching exchange transfusion level decreases isoimmune hemolysis.

(4) The administration of albumin prior to the exchange transfusion is not recommended.

(5) Stabilize infant prior to procedure: treat hypoglycemia, acid–base derangements, hypotension, and temperature abnormalities.

(6) Cytomegalovirus-negative blood less than 48 hours old should be used to minimize problems with elevated potassium that occurs in older blood.

(7) Procedure.

(a) Exchange transfusion is performed only by trained personnel in a NICU with monitoring and resuscitation capabilities.

(b) Secure infant on radiant warmer bed. Ensure oxygen, suction, and resuscitation equipment are immediately available. Observe neonate with a cardiorespiratory monitor and assess vital signs frequently.

(c) Ideally, an umbilical artery catheter and umbilical venous catheter are placed (see Chapter 15 for procedure).

(d) Laboratory studies.

(i) On initial blood removed: CBC, bilirubin and calcium levels, and blood cultures.

(ii) During procedure: calcium level (if signs of hypocalcemia present).

(iii) On final aliquot removed: CBC, bilirubin, and calcium.

(e) Accurate recording of blood volumes exchanged is essential during the procedure.

(f) Observe for hypocalcemia. Anticoagulant citrates (acid–citrate–dextrose and citrate–phosphate–dextrose negative [CPD−] adenosine) bind to calcium. Symptoms of hypocalcemia include irritability, tachycardia, and prolonged Q–T interval.

(g) Calcium gluconate is used to treat hypocalcemia. Normal dose is 1 to 2 mL/kg (100 to 200 mg/kg) per dose of 10% calcium solution.

(h) Evaluate medications. Medications whose levels are known to decrease significantly during an exchange transfusion should be administered after the exchange: ampicillin, gentamicin, digoxin, phenobarbital, vancomycin.

(8) Complications.

(a) Electrolyte and substrate abnormalities: hyperkalemia, hypocalcemia, hypomagnesemia, hypoglycemia, hyperglycemia.

(b) Clotting abnormalities: thrombocytopenia, embolization, thrombosis.

(c) Respiratory and cardiovascular events: apnea, bradycardia, cardiac dysrhythmias and arrest, cyanosis, vasospasm, heart failure, acidosis.

(d) NEC and infection.

(9) Postexchange care.

(a) Continue phototherapy.

(b) Laboratory studies: TSB every 4 hours. Rebound usually occurs within 1 hour after the exchange.

(c) Monitor blood glucose levels frequently. Dextrose in the blood preservative is equivalent to 300 mg of glucose per liter of blood. Rebound hypoglycemia can occur following an insulin response to the glucose.

(d) Monitor for complications.

3. **Management of conjugated hyperbilirubinemia.**
   a. Management is related to etiology.
   b. Eliminate or reduce causative factors; treat the remainder as appropriate (see Biliary Atresia, and Cholestasis).
   c. Evaluate liver function; evaluate for infection, including urinalysis and urine culture; check newborn screen for thyroid deficiency and galactosemia. Evaluate for G6PD deficiency.
4. **Management of breastfeeding jaundice.**
   a. Increase enteral intake by breastfeeding 8 to 12 times per day. The AAP does not encourage the interruption of breastfeeding (AAP, Subcommittee on Hyperbilirubinemia, 2004).
   b. No supplementation with water or glucose water in term, nondehydrated infants.
   c. Systematic assessment for hyperbilirubinemia risk, including maternal blood typing and neonatal direct antibody testing for incompatibility.
   d. Establish protocols for jaundice assessment and follow-up, including when the nurse can obtain a transcutaneous and serum bilirubin level (TSB) if jaundiced before 24 hours of age; follow-up required.
5. **Management of breast milk jaundice.**
   a. Obtain total and direct serum bilirubin to evaluate for cholestasis if jaundice is present at or beyond 3 weeks of age. Ensure normal thyroid and galactosemia screen.
6. **Alternative therapies.**
   a. Binding agents: agar and activated charcoal bind bilirubin in the gut and decrease the enterohepatic circulation.
   b. Phenobarbital: increases hepatic ligandin concentration and induces the cytochrome P-450 enzymatic system.
   c. Metalloporphyrins: inhibit heme oxygenase, the enzyme that catalyzes the conversion of heme to biliverdin, thereby decreasing bilirubin production. Tin mesoporphyrin and tin protoporphyrin are the two metalloporphyrins most commonly used; however, their use is not approved by the U.S. Food and Drug Administration and is still investigational.

G. **Hydrops (Hamdan, 2012; Hasnani-Samnani et al., 2013; Maheshwari and Carlo, 2011).**
1. Definition: a prenatal form of heart failure almost always caused by fetal anemia; characterized by generalized subcutaneous edema and fluid in two compartmental spaces.
2. Etiology: an imbalance of interstitial fluid production and lymphatic return.
   a. Immune hydrops (IH), also known as alloimmune or isoimmune hydrops: fetal RBCs enter maternal circulation, inducing maternal antibodies that cross the placenta and attack and destroy fetal RBCs. Seen in Rh and ABO disease.
   b. Nonimmune hydrops (NIH): disease or anomalies interfere with fetal fluid management. Most conditions associated with hydrops cause edema either through anemia with hypoxia and subsequent capillary leak or through cardiovascular anomalies with heart failure and subsequent tissue hypoxia, vascular permeability, and decreased lymphatic flow.
      (1) Cardiovascular (most frequent cause).
         (a) Dysrhythmias: supraventricular tachycardia, atrial flutter, complete heart block.
         (b) Cardiac malformation: left and right outflow tract obstructions; hypoplastic left heart syndrome and endocardial cushion defects are the most common.
         (c) Myocarditis.
      (2) Chromosomal: aneuploidy, including trisomies 13, 18, 21, triploidy, and 45,X (Turner's syndrome); achondroplasia.
      (3) Infection: TORCH, parvovirus B19, and congenital hepatitis.
      (4) Hematologic.
         (a) α-Thalassemia.
         (b) G6PD deficiency.
         (c) Chronic fetal-to-maternal or twin-to-twin transfusion.
         (d) Hemorrhage, including fetomaternal hemorrhage.
         (e) Bone marrow failure.
         (f) RBC enzyme deficiency.

(5) Renal.
(a) Nephrosis.
(b) Renal vein thrombosis.
(c) Renal hypoplasia.
(d) Urinary obstruction.
(6) Pulmonary.
(a) Pulmonary hypoplasia.
(b) Cystic adenomatoid malformations.
(c) Pulmonary lymphangiectasis.
(d) CDH.
(7) Gastrointestinal.
(a) In-utero volvulus.
(b) Meconium peritonitis.
(c) Prune-belly syndrome.
(8) Inborn errors of metabolism: lysosomal storage disease.
(9) Maternal.
(a) Toxemia.
(b) Diabetes.
(c) Systemic lupus erythematosus.
(10) Placenta and cord (uncommon).
(a) Chorioangioma.
(b) Umbilical vein thrombosis.
(c) Arteriovenous malformation.
(11) Idiopathic: approximately 25% of cases have no identifiable cause. Incidence of idiopathic NIH is dependent on the thoroughness of the diagnostic workup of the populations studied.

**3.** Incidence: Exact figure unknown, as some fetuses die or hydrops resolves in utero. Current estimates range from 1 in 600 to 1 in 4000 live births. Males affected more than females.
**a.** IH: Incidence has significantly decreased to approximately 10% to 20% of hydrops cases with the wide use of anti-D antibody prophylaxis using Rh immunoglobulin for Rh-negative mothers at 28 weeks of gestation (following suspected fetomaternal hemorrhage) and postpartum (following the delivery of an Rh-positive infant). In addition, in-utero fetal transfusion has lessened the incidence.
**b.** NIH: approximately 80% to 90% of hydrops cases.

**4.** Associated conditions.
**a.** Chromosomal abnormalities.
**b.** Congenital malformations: heart defects, especially outflow tract obstruction (both left and right).
**c.** Prematurity.
**d.** Inborn errors of metabolism.

**5.** Diagnosis.
**a.** Prenatal.
(1) Polyhydramnios.
(2) High-resolution ultrasound and fetal echocardiography: hepatosplenomegaly, cardiomegaly, cardiac defects, pleural effusion, pericardial effusion, ascites, generalized edema.
(3) Fetal blood sampling via cordocentesis.
(4) Amniocentesis: chromosome analysis for associated defects, bilirubin level.
(5) Serologic testing for isoimmunization and infection (TORCH; polymerase chain reaction for parvovirus B19).
(6) Kleihauer–Betke test for fetomaternal hemorrhage.
**b.** Postnatal.
(1) Clinical presentation.
(a) Physical examination: generalized edema; respiratory distress; cardiovascular abnormalities, including dysrhythmia, murmur, diminished perfusion; abdominal findings, including hepatosplenomegaly, distention.

(2) Imaging studies: skeletal radiographs, ultrasound.
(3) Laboratory studies.
(a) Hematology: CBC to evaluate anemia, thrombocytopenia, reticulocytosis; hemoglobin electrophoresis.
(b) Other: serum albumin, metabolic panel, chemistries, karyotype if not already done.

**6.** Prognosis. IH is associated with a survival rate of approximately 75%. Prognosis in NIH is very poor and is related to the underlying cause. Multiple anomalies and chromosomal abnormalities carry an extremely high mortality. Neurologic outcome in survivors is concerning.

**H. Care of the infant with hydrops.**

**1.** Prenatal: depends on etiology. The gravid mother must be transferred to a facility capable of management of the infant postpartum, including neonatal intensive care, ventilatory and inotropic support, and genetic evaluation.
**a.** Intrauterine transfusion to ameliorate anemia.
**b.** Amniocentesis to determine karyotype, follow bilirubin level, and reduce uterine volume to prevent premature delivery.
**c.** Thoracentesis or thoracoamniotic shunt placement.
**d.** Maternal medication administration to control fetal dysrhythmias.
**e.** Fetal medication administration.
**f.** Delivery.

**2.** Postnatal.
**a.** Resuscitation is frequently required, including intubation, bilateral thoracentesis (which may include bilateral tube thoracotomy), pericardiocentesis, and umbilical venous catheter placement (generalized edema prohibits successful peripheral IV placement). Umbilical artery catheter placement can be obtained once initial stabilization is accomplished.
**b.** Respiratory support as needed with acid–base determination and management. Paracentesis and additional thoracentesis or tube thoracotomy drainage may be required to enhance ventilation efforts. Frequent monitoring of breath sounds and chest movement and radiographs are essential.
**c.** Anticipate and treat metabolic abnormalities.
**d.** Exchange transfusion or partial exchange transfusion for severe anemia.
**e.** Cardiovascular support: inotropes to improve cardiac output; pericardiocentesis; diuretic therapy.
**f.** Fresh frozen plasma may be given for hypoalbuminemia.
**g.** Assess for associated anomalies, syndromes, or malformations. Determine etiology of hydrops if unknown.

## REFERENCES

AlFaleh, K., Anabrees, J., Bassler, D. and Al-Kharfi, T.: Probiotics for prevention of necrotizing enterocolitis in preterm infants. *Cochrane Database of Systematic Reviews*, (3): CD005496, 2011.

American Academy of Pediatrics, Section on Surgery and Committee on Fetus and Newborn, Lally, K.P., and Engle, W.: Post-discharge follow-up of infants with congenital diaphragmatic hernia. *Pediatrics*, 121(3):627–632, 2008.

American Academy of Pediatrics, Subcommittee on Hyperbilirubinemia: Management of hyperbilirubinemia in the newborn infant 35 or more weeks of gestation. *Pediatrics*, 114(1):297–316, 2004.

American Academy of Pediatrics, Task Force on Sudden Infant Death Syndrome and Moon, R.Y.: SIDS and other sleep-related infant deaths: Expansion of recommendations for a safe infant sleeping environment. *Pediatrics*, 128(5):1030–1039, 2011.

Amin, S.C., Pappas, C., Iyengar, H., and Maheshwari, A.: Short bowel syndrome in the NICU. *Clinics in Perinatology*, 40(1):53–68, 2013.

Anderson, M.S., Wood, L.E., Keller, J.A., and Hay, W.W.: Enteral nutrition. In S.L. Gardner, B.S. Carter, M. Enzman-Hines, and J.A. Hernandez (Eds.): *Merenstein & Gardner's handbook of neonatal intensive care* (17th ed). St. Louis, 2011, Elsevier Mosby, pp. 398–433.

Arshad, A., Powell, C., and Tighe, M.P.: Hirschsprung's disease. *BMJ*, 345:e5521–e5524, 2012.

Beale, E.W., Hoxworth, R.E., Livingston, E.H., and Trussler, A.P.: The role of biologic mesh in abdominal wall reconstruction: A systematic review of the current literature. *American Journal of Surgery*, 204 (4):510–517, 2012.

Benjamin, J.R., Gustafson, K.E., Smith, P.B., et al.: Perinatal factors associated with poor neurocognitive outcome in early school age congenital diaphragmatic hernia survivors. *Journal of Pediatric Surgery*, 48 (4):730–737, 2013.

Best, K.E., Tennant, P.W., Addor, M.C., et al.: Epidemiology of small intestinal atresia in Europe: A register-based study. *Archives of Disease in Childhood: Fetal and Neonatal Edition*, 97(5):F353–F358, 2012.

Bhutani, V.K.: American Academy of Pediatrics, Committee on Fetus and Newborn: Phototherapy to prevent severe neonatal hyperbilirubinemia in the newborn infant 35 or more weeks of gestation. *Pediatrics*, 128(4):e1046–e1052, 2011.

Bhutani, V.K., Stark, A.R., Lazzeroni, L.C., et al. for the Initial Clinical Testing Evaluation and Risk Assessment for Universal Screening for Hyperbilirubinemia Study Group: Predischarge screening for severe neonatal hyperbilirubinemia identifies infants who need phototherapy. *Journal of Pediatrics*, 162(3):477–482, 2013.

Blackburn, S.T.: *Maternal, fetal, and neonatal physiology: A clinical perspective* (4th ed.). St. Louis, 2013, Elsevier Saunders.

Brumbaugh, D. and Mack, C.: Conjugated hyperbilirubinemia in children. *Pediatrics in Review*, 33 (7):291–302, 2012.

Burjonrappa, S., Crete, E., and Bouchard, S.: Comparative outcomes in intestinal atresia: A clinical outcome and pathophysiology analysis. *Pediatric Surgery International*, 27(4):437–442, 2011.

Carlyle, B.E., Borowitz, D.S., and Glick, P.L.: A review of pathophysiology and management of fetuses and neonates with meconium ileus for the pediatric surgeon. *Journal of Pediatric Surgery*, 47(4):772–781, 2012.

Christison-Lagay, E.R., Kelleher, C.M., and Langer, J.C.: Neonatal abdominal wall defects. *Seminars in Fetal and Neonatal Medicine*, 16(3):164–172, 2011.

Cilieborg, M.S., Boye, M., and Sanqild, P.T.: Bacterial colonization and gut development in preterm neonates. *Early Human Development*, 88(Suppl. 1):S41–S49, 2012.

Cuenca, A.G., Ali, A.S., Kay, D.W., and Islam, S.: "Pulling the plug"—management of meconium plug syndrome in neonates. *Journal of Surgical Research*, 175(2): e43–e46, 2012.

Czinn, C.J. and Blanchard, S.: Gastroesophageal reflux disease in neonates and infants: When and how to treat. *Paediatric Drugs*, 15(1):19–27, 2013.

Davenport, M.: Biliary atresia: Clinical aspects. *Seminars in Pediatric Surgery*, 21(3):175–184, 2012.

Dominquez, K.M. and Moss, R.L.: Necrotizing enterocolitis. *Clinics in Perinatology*, 39(2):387–401, 2012.

Downard, C.D., Renaud, E., and St. Peter, S.D.: et al. for the 2012 American Pediatric Surgical Association Outcomes Clinical Trials Committee: Treatment of necrotizing enterocolitis: An American Pediatric Surgical Association Outcomes and Clinical Trials Committee systematic review. *Journal of Pediatric Surgery*, 47(11):2111–2122, 2012.

Feenstra, B., Geller, F., Krogh, C., et al.: Common variants near MBNL1 and NKX2-5 are associated with infantile hypertrophic pyloric stenosis. *Nature Genetics*, 44:334–337, 2012.

Felix, J.F., de Jong, E.M., Torfs, C.P., et al.: Genetic and environmental factors in the etiology of esophageal atresia and/or tracheoesophageal fistula: An overview of the current concepts. *Birth Defects Research Part A: Clinical and Molecular Teratology*, 85:747–754, 2009.

Goodwin, M.: Abdomen assessment. In E.P. Tappero and M.E. Honeyfield (Eds.): *Physical assessment of the newborn: A comprehensive approach to the art of physical examination* (4th ed.). Santa Rosa, CA, 2009, NICU Ink, pp. 105–114.

Gossard, A.A.: Care of the cholestatic patient. *Clinics in Liver Disease*, 17(2):331–344, 2013.

Goulet, O., Olieman, J., Ksiazyk, J., et al.: Neonatal short bowel syndrome as a model of intestinal failure: Physiological background for enteral feeding. *Clinics in Nutrition*, 32(2):162–171, 2013.

Greer, J.J.: Current concepts on the pathogenesis and etiology of congenital diaphragmatic hernia. *Respiratory Physiology & Neurobiology* 2013. Retrieved May 15, 2013, from http://www.sciencedirect.com/science/article/pii/S1569904813001201.

Hamdan, A.H.: Hydrops fetalis. *Medscape* 2012. Retrieved May 15, 2013, from http://emedicine.medscape.com/article/974571-overview.

Hartley, J.L., Gissen, P., and Kelly, D.A.: Alagille syndrome and other hereditary causes of cholestasis. *Clinics in Liver Disease*, 17(2):279–300, 2013.

Hasnani-Samnani, Z., Mahmoud, M.I., Farid, I., et al.: Non-immune hydrops: Qatar experience. *Journal of Maternal-Fetal & Neonatal Medicine*, 26(5):449–453, 2013.

Hassett, S., Smith, G.H.H., and Holland, A.J.A.: Prune belly syndrome. *Pediatric Surgery International*, 28 (3):219–228, 2012.

Hatley, R.: Intestinal malrotation. *Medscape* 2012. Retrieved May 15, 2013, fromhttp://emedicine.medscape.com/article/930313-overview.

Hedrick, H.L.: Management of prenatally diagnosed congenital diaphragmatic hernia. *Seminars in Pediatric Surgery*, 22(1):37–43, 2013.

Huether, K.L.: Alterations of digestive function in children. In K.L. McCance, and S.E. Huether (Eds.): *Pathophysiology: The biologic basis for disease in adults and children* (6th ed). St. Louis, 2010, Elsevier Mosby, pp. 1452–1515.

Islam, S.: Advances in surgery for abdominal wall defects: Gastroschisis and omphalocele. *Clinics in Perinatology*, 39(2):375–386, 2012.

Jones, K.L., Jones, M.C., and del Campo, M.: *Smith's recognizable patterns of human malformation* (7th ed.). Philadelphia, 2013, Elsevier Saunders.

Juang, D. and Snyder, C.L.: Neonatal bowel obstruction. *Surgical Clinics of North America*, 92(3):685–711, ix-x 2012.

Kamath, B.D., Thilo, E.H., and Hernandez, J.A.: Jaundice. In S.L. Gardner, B.S. Carter, M. Enzman-Hines, and J.A. Hernandez (Eds.): *Merenstein & Gardner's handbook of neonatal intensive care* (7th ed.). St. Louis, 2011, Mosby Elsevier, pp. 531–552.

Kee, J.L.: *Handbook of laboratory and diagnostic tests with nursing implications* (5th ed.). Upper Saddle River, NJ, 2005, Pearson Prentice Hall.

Kenny, S.E., Tam, P.H., Garcia-Barcelo, M., and Phil, M.: Hirschsprung's disease. *Seminars in Pediatric Surgery*, 19:194–200, 2010.

Kunz, S.N., Tiedel, J.S., Whitlock, K., et al.: Primary fascial closure versus staged closure with silo in patients with gastroschisis: A meta-analysis. *Journal of Pediatric Surgery*, 48(4):845–857, 2013.

Langer, J.C.: Hirschsprung disease. *Current Opinions in Pediatrics*, 25(3):368–374, 2013.

Ledbetter, D.J.: Congenital abdominal wall defects and reconstruction in pediatric surgery: Gastroschisis and omphalocele. *Surgical Clinics of North America*, 92 (3):713–727, 2012.

Lesavoy, M.A., Chang, E.I., Suliman, A., et al.: Long-term follow-up of total abdominal wall reconstruction for prune belly. *Plastic and Reconstructive Surgery*, 129(1):104e–109e, 2012.

Lightdale, J.R. and Gremse, D.A.: Section on Gastroenterology, Hepatology, and Nutrition: Gastroesophageal reflux: Management guidance for the pediatrician. *Pediatrics*, 131(5):e1684–e1685, 2013.

Maheshwari, A. and Carlo, W.A.: Hemolytic disease of the newborn (erythroblastosis fetalis). In R.M. Kliegman, B.F. Stanton, and J.W. St. Geme III, et al.: (Eds.): *Nelson textbook of pediatrics* (19th ed.). Philadelphia, 2011, Elsevier Saunders, pp. 615–619.

Montrawl, S.: Gastrointestinal system. In C. Kenner, and J.W. Lott (Eds.): *Comprehensive neonatal nursing: A physiologic perspective* (5th ed.). St. Louis, 2014, Saunders, pp. 189–228.

National Association of Neonatal Nurses, Board of Directors: Prevention of acute bilirubin encephalopathy and kernicterus in newborns: Position statement #3049. *Advances in Neonatal Care*, 11(5 Suppl.):S3–S9, 2010.

Neu, J. and Walker, W.A.: Necrotizing enterocolitis. *New England Journal of Medicine*, 364(3):255–264, 2011.

Pinheiro, J.M., Clark, D.A., and Benjamin, K.G.: A critical analysis of the routine testing of newborn stools for occult blood and reducing substances. *Advances in Neonatal Care*, 3(3):133–138, 2003.

Pinheiro, P.F.: Simoes e Silva, A.C., and Pereira, R.M.: Current knowledge on esophageal atresia. *World Journal of Gastroenterology*, 18(28):3662–3672, 2012.

Rao, S.C., Basani, L., Simmer, K., et al.: Peritoneal drainage versus laparotomy as initial surgical treatment for perforated necrotizing enterocolitis or spontaneous intestinal perforation in preterm low birth weight infants. *Cochrane Database of Systematic Reviews* (6): CD006182, 2011.

Rosen, N.G. and Beals, D.A.: Pediatric imperforate anus. *Medscape* 2012. Retrieved May 15, 2013, from http://emedicine.medscape.com/article/929904-overview.

Sadler, T.W. and Rasmussen, S.A.: Examining the evidence for vascular pathogenesis of selected birth defects. *American Journal of Medical Genetics Part A*, 152A(10):2426–2436, 2010.

Seidel, H.M., Ball, J.W., Dains, J.E., et al.: *Mosby's guide to physical examination*. (7th ed.). St. Louis, 2010, Elsevier Mosby.

Shalkow, J., Florens, A., Shorter, N.A., and Quiros, J.A.: Small intestinal atresia and stenosis. *Medscape* 2012. Retrieved May 15, 2013, from http://emedicine.medscape.com/article/939258-overview.

Taylor, N.D., Cass, D.T., and Holland, A.J.: Infantile hypertrophic pyloric stenosis: Has anything changed? *Journal of Paediatrics and Child Health*, 49:33–37, 2013.

Vinocur, D.N., Lee, E.Y., and Eisenberg, R.L.: Neonatal intestinal obstruction. *AJR: American Journal of Roentgenology*, 198(1):W1–W10, 2012.

Wildhaber, B.E.: Biliary atresia: 50 years after the first Kasai. International Scholarly Research Network. *ISRN Surgery*, 2012: Retrieved May 15, 2013, from 132089, 2012. http://www.ncbi.nlm.nih.gov/pmc/articles/PMC3523408/pdf/ISRN.SURGERY2012-132089.pdf.

Woods, A.G. and Brandon, D.H.: Prune belly syndrome: A focused physical assessment. *Advances in Neonatal Care*, 7(3):132–143, 2007.

Woolf, A.S., Stuart, H.M., and Newman, W.G.: Genetics of human congenital urinary bladder disease. *Pediatric Nephrology* 2013. Retrieved May 15, 2013, from http://link.springer.com/content/pdf/10.1007%2Fs00467-013-2472-1.pdf.

Yamataka, A., Lane, G.J., and Cazares, J.: Laparoscopic surgery for biliary atresia and choledochal cyst. *Seminars in Pediatric Surgery*, 21(3):201–210, 2012.

Zugor, V., Schott, G.E., and Labanaris, A.P.: The prune belly syndrome: Urological aspects and long-term outcomes of a rare disease. *Pediatric Reports*, 4(2): e20, 2012.

CHAPTER

# 30 Endocrine Disorders

LAURA STOKOWSKI

**OBJECTIVES**

1. Define the endocrine system.
2. Describe endocrine system regulation.
3. Identify and discuss endocrine disorders that manifest in the neonatal period, including disorders of the thyroid, pituitary, adrenal gland, pancreas, and genital development.
4. List effective ways to help parents cope with the birth of an infant with a disorder of sexual development.

Disorders of the endocrine system are relatively rare in neonates, but usually have lifelong consequences.

## THE ENDOCRINE SYSTEM

The classic endocrine system is a group of nine ductless glands (Table 30-1), but in reality it includes every organ and cell in the body that produces and responds to hormones. A system of communication between different cells of the body, the endocrine system is intricately linked with the neurologic and immune systems in a vast, interacting control network (Wilson, 2005). Coordination and regulation of metabolism and energy, the internal environment, growth and development, and sexual differentiation and reproduction are among the functions of this complex system.

**A. Hormones.**

1. Hormones are the molecular messengers of the endocrine system, allowing communication between organs, tissues, and cells throughout the body. In composition, hormones are steroids, proteins, glycoproteins, peptides, or amines.
2. Hormones bind to specific receptors on the surface of or within the cytoplasm or nucleus of target cells to produce physiologic actions. Sensitivity of a target cell to its hormones is critical to normal function.
3. Many hormones are secreted directly into the circulation for transport to various target tissues. Hormones can also act on cells in the immediate vicinity of their release (paracrine action) or on the cell that produced the hormone (autocrine or intracrine action).
4. Some hormones circulate partly in free form and partly bound to transport proteins. It is the free form that is available for receptor binding and that dictates regulatory influences on hormone release. Clinical states of hormone excess and deficiency correlate best with free hormone levels.
5. Most hormones are secreted in their biologically active form (such as insulin), but others (such as thyroxine) must be converted to their final active form in peripheral tissues.

**B. Endocrine system regulation (Fig. 30-1).**

1. Many hormones are regulated by a negative-feedback loop involving the hypothalamic–pituitary axis and target endocrine glands. Beginning with hormonal or neural input, the hypothalamus produces one of two substances: releasing hormones or inhibiting hormones. These are transported via the pituitary portal system to the anterior pituitary, the gland that controls the secretory activity of most target organs. The anterior pituitary releases trophic hormones that in turn stimulate release of target gland hormones. As blood concentrations of target hormones reach certain thresholds, a negative message to the anterior pituitary inhibits further release of trophic hormones. Examples of hormones regulated by negative feedback are thyroid hormone and cortisol. Negative feedback can be direct (at the level of the pituitary gland) or indirect (at the level of the hypothalamus).

■ TABLE 30-1
■ ■ **Major Glands and Hormones of the Endocrine System**

| Endocrine Gland | Hormones Produced |
|---|---|
| Hypothalamus | Corticotropin-releasing hormone (CRH) |
| | Thyrotropin-releasing hormone (TRH) |
| | Gonadotropin-releasing hormone (GnRH) |
| | Somatostatin |
| | Growth hormone–releasing hormone (GHRH) |
| | Prolactin-releasing factor (PRF) |
| | Prolactin release–inhibiting hormone (PIH; dopamine) |
| Anterior pituitary | Adrenocorticotropic hormone (ACTH) |
| | Thyroid-stimulating hormone (TSH; thyrotropin) |
| | Follicle-stimulating hormone (FSH) |
| | Growth hormone (GH) |
| | Luteinizing hormone (LH) |
| | Prolactin (PRL) |
| Posterior pituitary | Antidiuretic hormone (ADH; arginine vasopressin) |
| | Oxytocin (OCT) |
| Thyroid gland | Thyroxine ($T_4$) |
| | Triiodothyronine ($T_3$) |
| | Calcitonin |
| Parathyroid gland | Parathyroid hormone (PTH) |
| Adrenal medulla | Epinephrine (adrenaline) |
| | Norepinephrine (noradrenaline) |
| Adrenal cortex | Cortisol (hydrocortisone) |
| | Aldosterone |
| Pancreas | Insulin |
| | Glucagon |
| | Somatostatin |
| Pineal gland | Melatonin |

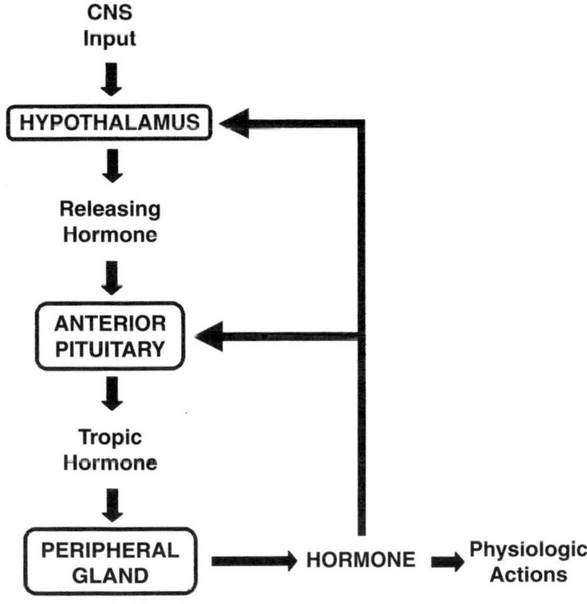


FIGURE 30-1 ■ Negative-feedback-loop control of endocrine gland function. Hypothalamic releasing hormones stimulate pituitary trophic hormones, which in turn act on peripheral glands to release hormones. Levels of circulating hormones then exert feedback control on the pituitary and hypothalamus, modulating further output by these glands. *CNS*, Central nervous system.

2. Other endocrine glands, such as the parathyroids and the pancreatic islets, are not part of the hypothalamic–pituitary axis but have "freestanding" control mechanisms. These glands release hormones that stimulate a target tissue to produce an effect, which in turn directly modifies the output of the gland.
3. The neuroendocrine system plays a key role in body homeostasis. Hormones act as neurotransmitters, and neurotransmitters are involved in regulating endocrine function. Endocrine glands such as the hypothalamus, the pituitary, and the adrenal cortex respond to neural stimulation. The neuroendocrine system is important in the smooth adaptation of the neonate to the stresses of extrauterine life.

C. **Endocrine disruptors.**
1. Endocrine disruptors are synthetic or naturally occurring compounds that can mimic or block the body's endogenous hormones and disrupt endocrine function. Estrogens, androgens, and thyroid hormones are particularly vulnerable to interference by endocrine disruptors.
2. Exposure to an endocrine disruptor during embryonic gonadal sex differentiation can alter male germline epigenetics, a mechanism that can transmit adult-onset diseases, such as spermatogenic defects, prostate disease, kidney disease, and cancer, to both current and future generations (Anway and Skinner, 2008).
3. Sources of these chemicals include pharmaceuticals, dioxin and dioxin-like compounds, polychlorinated biphenyls, dichlorodiphenyltrichloroethane (DDT) and other pesticides, and plasticizers such as bisphenol A.

D. **Fetal origins of adult disease.**
1. Fetal origin of adult disease is a newly recognized phenomenon, describing effects of the maternal intrauterine environment on growth and development that can persist into adult life.
2. Chronic stress may induce the "thrifty phenotype fetus" and permanently alter the fetal hypothalamic–pituitary axis. In response to stressors, the fetus generates glucocorticoids and catecholamines that program the fetal endocrine system. Fetal endocrine programming has been associated with endocrine, metabolic, and cardiovascular disease in the adult.

E. **Endocrine disorders in the neonate.**
1. Most endocrine disorders are caused by hormone overproduction or underproduction, altered receptor function, or altered tissue response to hormones. In addition to well-described neonatal endocrine disorders (hypothyroidism, congenital adrenal hyperplasia [CAH]), endocrine dysfunction can affect the preterm infant in a variety of ways as a function of maturation.

## PITUITARY GLAND DISORDERS

A. **Anatomy and physiology.**
1. The pituitary gland has two distinct structures—the anterior and posterior glands. Although these two structures with different origins form a single gland, they are functionally separate.
2. Anterior pituitary arises from the oral ectoderm and its cells to differentiate into specific hormone-producing cells. The release of trophic hormones—growth hormone (GH), adrenocorticotropic hormone (ACTH), follicle-stimulating hormone (FSH), thyroid-stimulating hormone (TSH), luteinizing hormone (LH), and prolactin (PRL)—is influenced by hypothalamic releasing/inhibiting hormones.
3. Posterior pituitary develops from neuroectoderm evaginating ventrally from the brain. The posterior pituitary produces oxytocin and antidiuretic hormone (ADH).

B. **Hypopituitarism.**
1. Although rare in the newborn, hypopituitarism can be congenital or acquired by infection, hypovolemic shock, precipitous delivery, or low Apgar scores. Congenital hypopituitarism can be caused by mutations in signaling molecules of transcription factors regulating pituitary gland development, or may be part of a syndrome such as optic nerve hypoplasia, and be associated with absent septum pellucidum (Garcia-Fillon and Borchert, 2013). Congenital hypopituitarism can overlap with hypogonadotropic hypogonadal disorders such as Kallmann syndrome (Bancalari et al., 2012).

2. Types of hypopituitarism include absence of pituitary gland (pituitary agenesis), panhypopituitarism (deficiency of all pituitary hormones), and an isolated hormone defect, such as GH deficiency. A primary hypothalamic disorder can also result in hypopituitarism.
3. Neonates with congenital hypopituitarism can initially be asymptomatic, with evidence of pituitary hormone deficiencies developing over time (Alatzoglou and Dattani, 2009). Neonates with hypopituitary syndromes can present with midline craniofacial defects such as cleft lip, cleft palate, bifid uvula, or micropenis in boys (a normally formed and proportioned penis with a stretched penile length more than 2 standard deviations below the mean for age) (Tuladhar et al., 1998). Hypoglycemia can be mild or severe and persistent.
4. Later in the neonatal period, infants may present with prolonged jaundice and direct hyperbilirubinemia, or evidence of other endocrinopathy, such as diabetes insipidus (high urine output, dehydration, hypernatremia).
5. Diagnosis is made by hormone testing (including GH, thyroid hormone, cortisol), ultrasound or magnetic resonance imaging (MRI) of anatomic structures, and genetic analyses. Tests of pituitary function include stimulation tests (ACTH, thyrotropin-releasing hormone [TRH], glucagon) to test the response of pituitary hormones. A pediatric endocrinologist usually coordinates the diagnostic testing and interpretation for these infants.
6. Management involves correcting hypoglycemia and replacing deficient hormones.

**C. Diabetes insipidus.**

1. Diabetes insipidus (DI) is a deficiency of ADH (vasopressin). DI can be associated with midline facial defects, central nervous system (CNS) injury, hypoxia, or neoplasm.
2. Up to 90% of neonates with inherited nephrogenic DI are boys with an X-linked form caused by mutations in the arginine vasopressin receptor 2 gene (*AVP2R*) (Copelovitch and Kaplan, 2012).
3. ADH secretion is normally triggered by changes in osmolality, increasing or decreasing to regulate urine output. In DI, ADH is deficient, resulting in free water loss.
4. Clinical manifestations are vigorous sucking followed by vomiting, polyuria (high urine output with low specific gravity), irritability, fever, and evidence of dehydration.
5. Diagnosis is made by reviewing serum electrolytes, osmolality, plasma ADH levels, genetic analysis, urine output, and urinalysis. MRI may be done to visualize the posterior pituitary.
6. DI is treated with cautious fluid management to correct dehydration without causing rapid shifts in serum sodium levels. Desmopressin (DDAVP) may be required to supplement ADH if the neonate is unable to concentrate urine.

**D. Syndrome of inappropriate ADH.**

1. Impairment of free water clearance caused by an uncontrolled release of ADH.
2. Causes include CNS infection, birth asphyxia, intracranial hemorrhage, and meningitis. The release of ADH is inappropriate to the level of osmolality in the serum, causing fluid retention, oliguria, hyponatremia, weight gain, and edema.
3. Diagnosis is made by finding an elevated circulating ADH level with low serum osmolality and hyponatremia.
4. Treatment involves fluid restriction and monitoring of electrolytes, glucose, intake, and output. If it is not possible to manage DI with fluids alone, the agent of choice for pharmacologic treatment is DDAVP, a long-acting synthetic analogue of pituitary ADH.

## THYROID GLAND DISORDERS

### The Thyroid Gland

**A. Anatomy.**

1. The thyroid gland comprises two lateral lobes connected by a band of tissue (isthmus) and contains densely packed colloid-rich follicular cells and parafollicular cells. Parafollicular cells (C cells) produce the calcium-lowering hormone calcitonin.

**B. Normal physiology.**

1. Functions of the thyroid gland.
   a. Concentrates and stores iodide, a trace element required for thyroid hormone synthesis.
   b. Synthesizes *thyroglobulin*, a thyroid hormone precursor.
   c. Synthesizes and releases the thyroid hormones *thyroxine* ($T_4$) and *triiodothyronine* ($T_3$), catalyzed by the enzyme thyroid peroxidase (TPO).

2. Thyroid hormone metabolism.
   a. The thyroid gland produces $T_4$ and a small amount of $T_3$. Most of the plasma $T_3$ (the more potent hormone) is derived from peripheral metabolism (deiodination) of $T_4$.
   b. $T_4$ enters the cell and is converted to $T_3$ by enzymes.
   c. Deiodination of the outer ring of $T_4$ produces $T_3$. Deiodination of the inner ring of $T_4$ produces reverse $T_3$ ($rT_3$), a biologically inactive product.
3. Thyroid hormone transport.
   a. Thyroid hormones circulate in the blood bound to *thyroid-binding globulin* (TBG) and other albumins. Only a tiny fraction is in equilibrium as free hormone, but it is this free fraction that is responsible for hormonal action.
   b. TBG, synthesized in the liver, has a high affinity for $T_3$ and $T_4$, carrying 70% of circulating hormone. When TBG is deficient, total thyroid hormone concentrations may be lower but free hormone levels are normal.
4. Mechanisms of thyroid gland regulation.
   a. Hypothalamic–pituitary–thyroid (HPT) axis. Hypothalamic TRH is secreted in response to neural input, such as cooling of the skin. TRH stimulates synthesis and release of TSH (thyrotropin) by the anterior pituitary. TSH secretion is inhibited by dopamine, somatostatin, and high doses of corticosteroids. TSH binds to receptors on thyroid cell membranes and stimulates production of thyroid hormones. As thyroid hormone levels rise, TSH and TRH secretion is inhibited.
   b. Deiodinase enzymes in the anterior pituitary, brain, heart, liver, and other tissues regulate intracellular $T_3$ availability.
   c. Autoregulation of hormone synthesis by the thyroid gland itself in relationship to its iodine supply.
   d. Stimulation or inhibition of thyroid function by TSH receptor antibodies.
5. Physiologic effects of thyroid hormones.
   a. Metabolic processes such as oxygen consumption, thermogenesis, cardiac output, erythropoiesis, respiratory drive, gut motility, and metabolism of carbohydrates, proteins, and lipids.
   b. Growth and differentiation of organs and tissues, including the bones, lungs, and CNS. Thyroid hormones induce differentiation and maturation of neural circuits during critical periods of brain development. Absence of thyroid hormones delays critical events by interrupting intercellular communication (Brook and Dattani, 2012).

**C. Fetal thyroid development.**

1. The thyroid is the first endocrine gland to develop in the fetus, originating at 3 to 4 weeks of gestation (Forghani and Aye, 2008).
2. At about 10 to 12 weeks of gestation, the hypothalamus begins synthesizing TRH, the pituitary gland begins secreting TSH, and TBG is detectable in fetal serum.
3. The HPT axis begins to function at midgestation (weeks 18 to 20), when iodide uptake increases and the fetal thyroid gland begins to release $T_4$. Total and free $T_4$, TSH, and TBG increase steadily until term. The $T_3$ level remains low until 30 weeks of gestation, rising only in the last 10 weeks as mechanisms for deiodination of $T_4$ in fetal tissues mature.
4. Before 20 weeks of gestation, transplacental passage of maternal $T_4$ largely provides for fetal thyroidal needs, and is critical for normal development. Maternal hypothyroidism during early gestation can impair CNS development in the fetus. By the start of the second trimester, however, the fetal contribution to circulating thyroid hormones is significant.
5. The fetus is also dependent on the maternal–placental system for adequate supply of iodide, a critical substrate for fetal thyroid hormone synthesis. Autoregulation of iodide uptake is not yet mature, so the fetal thyroid is susceptible to inhibitory effects of both iodide deficiency and iodide excess.
6. Cord blood TSH and $T_4$ are directly proportional to birth weight and gestational age. At birth, 30% of thyroid hormone circulating in the infant is of maternal origin (Forghani and Aye, 2008).

**D. Neonatal thyroid physiology.**

1. At birth in term and late preterm neonates, the cooling of the skin and a surge of circulating catecholamines stimulate a sharp rise in the serum TSH level. TSH peaks in the 70 to

100 mU/l range at 30 minutes of age and then falls to a normal (<20 mU/l) level during the first 3 days of life.

2. The TSH surge stimulates an abrupt rise in thyroid hormone levels. $T_4$ and $T_3$ both increase in response to TSH, peaking at 24 to 36 hours after birth. This physiologic hyperthyroid state is temporary, and occurs in response to sudden exposure to a cold environment. $T_4$ increases in most infants to a level of 6.5 mcg/dL or higher. The rise in $T_4$ causes the TSH to decline to 20 mU/l or less (the cutoff used in most screening programs for congenital hypothyroidism) because of feedback inhibition.
3. Postnatal changes in TSH, $T_4$, and $T_3$ occur in less mature infants as well but are quantitatively lower. The extremely preterm infant exhibits a dramatic fall in $T_4$ over the first 1 to 2 weeks of life.

## Hypothyroidism

Hypothyroidism in the neonate can be considered either permanent (lifelong therapy required) or transient (spontaneously resolving in weeks or months; treatment is temporary or not required at all). Hypothyroidism can also be termed congenital (existing at birth) or acquired. Other labels indicate the origin of the hypothyroidism:

1. Primary hypothyroidism. A disorder involving the thyroid gland or some aspect of thyroid hormone synthesis, metabolism, or transport.
2. Central (also called secondary/tertiary). Deficient thyroid hormone secretion due to a disorder affecting pituitary control (TSH production) or hypothalamic control (TRH production).

**A. Etiologies of permanent congenital hypothyroidism (CH).**

1. Thyroid abnormalities.
   - a. Thyroid dysgenesis: absent (agenesis/athyreosis), hypoplastic, and/or ectopic (usually sublingual) gland. Ectopic gland is the most common etiology of CH. Familial thyroid dysgenesis is primarily caused by mutations in the thyrotropin receptor gene *TSHR* (Cangul et al., 2012).
   - b. Familial dyshormonogenesis: inborn errors of thyroid hormone biosynthesis, transport, or metabolism. About 10% to 20% of infants with CH have inherited defects of thyroid hormone metabolism, the most common of which is an organification defect related to deficient activity of the TPO enzyme.
2. Extrathyroid abnormalities.
   - a. Defects of the pituitary gland (e.g., hypopituitarism) or the hypothalamus.
   - b. TBG deficiency: X-linked disorder; more common in males.
   - c. Thyroid hormone resistance. Resistance to the actions of endogenous and exogenous $T_4$ and $T_3$, a form of "peripheral hypothyroidism," is becoming more common. All serum thyroid hormone levels are elevated, and many patients have goiter.

**B. Etiologies of transient hypothyroid states.**

1. Prenatally acquired:
   - a. Maternal autoimmune thyroid disorders characterized by transplacental passage of TSH receptor–blocking antibodies, which inhibit the binding of TSH to the thyroid cell.
   - b. Drugs given to the mother that cross the placenta and affect fetal thyroid production (propylthiouracil, methimazole, lithium, phenytoin, amiodarone, and radioiodine.)
   - c. Ingestion of excess iodine (Connelly et al., 2012) or severe dietary iodine deficiency (Zimmermann, 2012).
2. Postnatally acquired: transiently impaired thyroid hormone production from exposure to iodine-containing topical disinfectants, ointments, drugs such as amiodarone, or intravenously administered contrast media. Preterm infants can absorb and excrete large amounts of iodine; thus, exposure to iodinated products should be minimized.

**C. The preterm infant:** In addition to the same incidence of permanent CH as full term infants, several transient hypothyroid states have been described in preterm infants. Because two or more transient conditions can coexist, it is not always possible to determine the precise cause of low thyroid hormone levels in preterm infants.

1. *Hypothyroxinemia of prematurity*. Serum levels of thyroid hormones in preterm neonates are significantly lower and more variable than those of term neonates and correlate with gestational age and birth weight (Fisher, 2007). $T_4$ levels of most preterms reach a nadir at 7 to 14 days of age and then climb to normal within 4 to 8 weeks.
2. Sicker preterm infants demonstrate more variability in their $T_4$ values than healthy preterms of the same gestational age. Preterm infants do have an initial TSH surge after birth, but it is blunted in comparison to more mature neonates (Clemente et al., 2007). The TSH of preterm infants with hypothyroxinemia is not consistently elevated, suggesting relative lack of hypothalamic response to the lower $T_4$ level. This condition is believed to be a developmental phenomenon caused by one or more of the following:
   - **a.** Immaturity of thyroid hormone metabolism and the HPT axis.
   - **b.** Loss of maternal contributions to the thyroid hormone pool at birth.
   - **c.** Low TBG levels.
   - **d.** Increased use of $T_4$ to meet the demands of extrauterine life.
   - **e.** Insufficient enteral or parenteral iodine intake.
3. *Nonthyroidal illness syndrome*. In some ill preterm infants, $T_4$ is preferentially converted to $rT_3$ instead of $T_3$, possibly as an adaptive response to lower the metabolic rate during times of severe illness. The outcome is low serum concentrations of both $T_4$ and $T_3$. $rT_3$ is elevated and TSH is normal. This condition, also known as "low $T_3$ syndrome" or "euthyroid sick syndrome," occurs in infants who have immature lungs or infections, because the cytokines produced in response to illness or inflammation are believed to inhibit thyroid function, metabolism, or action (van Wassenaer and Kok, 2004). The low $T_4$ from nonthyroidal illness reverses spontaneously when the infant's condition improves without treatment. Similar effects are seen in infants who are receiving dopamine or glucocorticoids, both of which can lower serum $T_4$ concentrations.

**D. Clinical presentation and assessment.**

1. Few neonates are diagnosed with CH solely on clinical grounds. Signs and symptoms of CH can be slow to develop owing to persistence of maternal thyroid hormone and are subtle and nonspecific; thus they are not immediately linked with hypothyroidism. Early diagnosis is critical to ensure prompt treatment that will reduce the risk for cognitive impairment.
2. The signs and symptoms of hypothyroidism in the neonate reflect the wide-ranging actions of thyroid hormones on metabolism, intestinal motility, cardiac function, temperature regulation, neurologic function, and skeletal maturation (Box 30-1). The possibility of CH must be considered in infants presenting with birth weight in excess of the 90th percentile, prolonged jaundice, hypothermia and cold mottled skin, an enlarged (>1 cm) posterior fontanelle, umbilical hernia, and failure to feed well (Rastogi and LaFranchi, 2010).

**BOX 30-1**

**EARLY SIGNS AND SYMPTOMS OF CONGENITAL HYPOTHYROIDISM**

Large, open posterior fontanelle (>1 cm)
Birth weight greater than 4 kg; gestation longer than 42 weeks
Coarse features
Delayed bone age (identified on knee x-rays)
Umbilical hernia
Goiter
Thick skin
Poor perfusion (mottling, peripheral cyanosis)
Hypothermia
Abdominal distention
Poor feeding; sleepy and placid
Prolonged hyperbilirubinemia
Hoarse cry
Edema
Cardiomegaly, bradycardia

3. Other features traditionally associated with hypothyroidism (macroglossia, dry skin, lethargy, hypotonia, hoarse cry, coarse hair, and constipation) evolve over the first weeks of life. A palpable, enlarged thyroid gland (also called a goiter) can be associated with impaired thyroid hormone synthesis and hypothyroidism. Hyperplasia of the thyroid gland results from hypersecretion of TSH in response to low $T_3$ and $T_4$ levels. Infants with suspected central hypothyroidism may present with midline or cranial defects or other signs of pituitary deficiency. Central hypothyroidism should be suspected in infants presenting with optic nerve hypoplasia, hypoglycemia, micropenis, or cleft lip/palate.

E. **Diagnostic studies in hypothyroidism (Table 30-2):** Unless the infant is born to a mother with a history of thyroid dysfunction or has obvious clinical signs of hypothyroidism at birth, the diagnosis is usually made after the infant is identified by neonatal screening.

■ TABLE 30-2
■ ■ **Summary of Low Thyroid States in the Newborn Infant**

| Screening Results | Possible Conditions | Further Diagnostic Tests | Treatment |
|---|---|---|---|
| $T_4$ low,* TSH elevated† | Congenital hypothyroidism (thyroid agenesis, ectopia dyshormonogenesis) | Serum TFTs‡, Tg§ level; thyroid scan; ultrasonography; bone age radiography | Thyroid replacement |
| | Transient hypothyroidism | TSI, TBA | Monitoring |
| | Maternal (autoimmune, drugs) iodine exposure | Urinary iodine level | Monitoring |
| $T_4$ low, TSH normal or low-normal, TSH slightly elevated (borderline) | Congenital hypothyroidism | Repeat screen, other tests as for congenital hypothyroidism (above) | Thyroid replacement |
| | Early specimen collection (<24 hours) or false-positive | Repeat screen | |
| $T_4$ low, TSH normal | Hypothyroxinemia of prematurity | Serum TFTs or repeat screen to detect delayed TSH rise | Monitoring |
| | TBG deficiency | Serum TFTs; TBG level; $T_3$, resin uptake level‖{ParaMarks} | None |
| | Early specimen collection (<24 hours) or false-positive | Repeat screen | |
| $T_4$ low, delayed TSH rise | Atypical hypothyroidism Some VLBW infants (nonthyroidal illness?) | Serum TFTs | Close monitoring; possible treatment |
| | Congenital hypothyroidism (some functional thyroid; ectopic or hypoplastic) | Serum TFTs and other tests as for congenital hypothyroidism (above) | Thyroid replacement |
| $T_4$ low, TSH low | Central hypothyroidism (hypothalamic–pituitary) | Serum TFTs; TRH stimulation test¶; other tests of pituitary function (cortisol, growth hormone) | Thyroid replacement; other hormonal therapy |

*$T_3$*, Triiodothyronine; *$T_4$*, thyroxine; *TBA*, thyroid-blocking antibodies; *TBG*, thyroid-binding globulin; *TFTs*, thyroid function tests; *TSH*, thyroid-stimulating hormone; *TSI*, thyroid-stimulating immunoglobulins; *VLBW*, very low birth weight.

*$T_4$ low: less than 6 mcg/dL.

†TSH elevated: greater than 40 mU/l; TSH normal: less than 10 mU/l; TSH borderline: 20 to 40 mU/l. Note that a slightly elevated TSH level may be normal in the first 2 days of life.

‡TFTs: May include assays of total and free $T_4$ and $T_3$ along with TSH.

§Tg: Thyroglobulin, a thyroid hormone precursor produced by the thyroid gland. A low level suggests thyroid agenesis.

{ParaMarks}$T_3$, resin uptake level: an indirect measure of protein binding. A high level suggests low binding capacity, as in TBG deficiency.

¶TRH stimulation is a test of hypothalamic or pituitary control of thyroid function. A dose of thyrotropin-releasing hormone (TRH) is administered and TSH is measured serially. A subnormal TSH response suggests a deficient pituitary gland, and a delayed response suggests hypothalamic congenital hypothyroidism.

1. Newborn screening for hypothyroidism.
   a. Screening for CH uses either a two-tiered $T_4$-TSH testing approach or primary TSH testing. In the two-tiered system, TSH is measured only if the $T_4$ level is low.
   b. Owing to the physiologic surge in TSH in the first hours of life, the specimen must be collected when the infant is at least 24 hours of age, and preferably between 2 and 4 days of age. If collected earlier, particularly in the first 3 hours of life, a false-positive result can occur. In those instances, a repeat specimen must be collected within the first 7 days of life, regardless of first test results.
   c. The incidence of CH, as detected through newborn screening, is approximately 1 per 3000 to 4000. An elevated TSH level (>40 mU/l) is presumed to be CH until further testing proves otherwise. Rapid confirmation is essential.
   d. Screening errors caused by improper specimen collection, storage, or transport can result in a false-negative test. Thyroid medications taken by the mother during pregnancy can also produce false-negative results.
   e. Approximately 10% of infants with CH are missed on initial screening; they are detected only through routine second screening in states where this is required or on clinical grounds. Some of these infants have compensated hypothyroidism or delayed rise in the TSH level; most seem to have milder forms of hypothyroidism but still require treatment.
   f. Infants at risk of a missed or delayed diagnosis are those born at home, those who were extremely ill in the neonatal period, and those who were transferred to another hospital at an early age.
2. Thyroid function tests.
   a. A serum $T_4$ less than 6 mcg/dL and a serum TSH greater than 50 mU/L strongly suggest CH. A normal $T_4$ (e.g., >10 mcg/dL) with elevated TSH suggests enough functional thyroid tissue to respond to excess TSH stimulation (seen in compensated or subclinical hypothyroidism). Free $T_4$ and $T_3$ levels may also be measured, along with other tests, as needed, to determine the cause of abnormal screening results (see Table 30-2).
   b. Age-related reference norms, for both gestational age and hours of age, should be used when interpreting all thyroid test results.
   c. If maternal antibody-mediated hypothyroidism is suspected, maternal antithyroid antibody (TRBAb) testing is done. Other thyroid autoantibodies that can produce hypothyroidism include thyroglobulin antibodies (TGAb) and thyroid peroxidase antibodies (TPOAb).
   d. TBG levels can be measured to rule out TBG deficiency. Thyroglobulin levels in infants with possible CH can help to differentiate between thyroid agenesis and dyshormonogenesis, as an adjunct to thyroid imaging.
3. Imaging studies: Further evaluation for the cause of a CH blood profile includes Doppler ultrasonography of the neck, thyroid radionuclide imaging (to identify normal or ectopic thyroid tissue), and bone age radiography of the knee or foot (delayed bone ossification suggests long-standing thyroid deprivation).

**F. Management.**

1. CH.
   a. Early, adequate treatment of CH is critical for optimal neurologic development. The goal of hormone replacement therapy is to rapidly normalize the infant's serum $T_4$ level, and maintain it in the upper half of the normal range, which should result in a TSH of 0.5 to 4 mU/l (Bollepalli and Rose, 2012). The agent of choice is sodium levothyroxine because it is substantially converted to $T_3$ within the brain.
   b. Infants receiving thyroid replacement therapy must be monitored closely for adequacy of treatment and evidence of thyrotoxicosis (irritability, tachycardia, poor weight gain). Serum $T_4$ should normalize in 1 to 2 weeks; serum TSH can take longer to normalize.
      (1) Overtreatment can lead to advanced bone age, craniosynostosis, and thyrotoxicosis (tachycardia, irritability, hyperactivity, poor weight gain, and loose stools).
      (2) Undertreatment leads to clinical hypothyroidism, delayed bone maturation, and neurologic damage.
2. Transient hypothyroidism.
   a. Hypothyroxinemia of prematurity is associated with higher mortality and neurodevelopmental deficits, yet cumulative evidence to date has not been able to demonstrate

clear benefits of routinely supplementing these infants with thyroxine during early life (La Gamma and Paneth, 2012). A Cochrane Database review did not support the use of prophylactic thyroid hormones in preterm infants to reduce neonatal mortality or morbidity or improve neurodevelopmental outcomes (Osborn and Hunt, 2007). The exception is the infant with an elevated TSH level; these infants require treatment. Thyroid function tests should be followed carefully in preterm infants at risk for hypothyroxinemia, and treatment should be instituted promptly if indicated by elevated TSH.

**b.** Transient hypothyroidism caused by maternal antithyroid medication will resolve spontaneously when the drug is cleared from the infant's circulation, usually within a day or two after birth. The infant's serum $T_4$ and TSH should be monitored to ensure that they return to normal. Supplementation with levothyroxine is not usually necessary.

**c.** Transplacentally acquired TRBAb can be slow to degrade completely; therefore, most infants will require supplementation for several months.

**d.** TRBAb levels in the infant can be monitored to determine when to discontinue therapy. Breastfeeding is not contraindicated in neonates whose mothers continue their antithyroid medication in the postpartum period, as very little passes into the breast milk.

**G. Outcome.**

1. CH.

**a.** CH is one of the most preventable causes of mental retardation. Most infants with early diagnosis and early and adequate treatment will have normal IQs. A delay in treatment after birth can lower IQ by several points per week (Fisher, 2000).

**b.** Lifelong thyroid replacement therapy is necessary for normal growth and development.

**c.** Infants who are taking levothyroxine should not ingest soy-based products, including soy formula, because soy interferes with the absorption of levothyroxine, and the infant can remain hypothyroid (Fruzza et al., 2012).

2. Transient hypothyroidism.

**a.** Hypothyroxinemia of prematurity is transient, correcting spontaneously over 6 to 10 weeks as the infant matures.

**b.** More research is needed to determine whether hypothyroxinemia of prematurity is a benign physiologic phenomenon or a cause of psychomotor and neurodevelopmental sequelae in the preterm population.

## Hyperthyroidism

**A. Etiologies.**

1. Maternal Graves' disease (either active or inactive) causes neonatal Graves' disease in 1 of 70 affected pregnancies. Most babies born to mothers with Graves' disease have normal thyroid function.
2. Rare causes of neonatal hyperthyroidism include McCune–Albright syndrome and activating mutations in the TSH receptor.

**B. Pathophysiology of Graves' disease.**

1. The transient condition, neonatal Graves' disease, occurs in infants born to mothers with Graves' disease, to those who have undergone thyroidectomy or radioiodine ablation of the thyroid gland, and to women taking antithyroid drugs.
2. Maternal TSH receptor–stimulating antibodies (TRSAb) cross the placenta readily and stimulate the fetal thyroid gland, causing an overproduction of thyroid hormone and in some cases, development of a goiter. Usually the higher the TRSAb level in the mother, the more severely affected the infant.
3. Hyperthyroidism in the neonate is typically transient, lasting approximately 3 to 12 weeks. The clinical course varies depending on characteristics of the mother's disease and treatment. The onset of hyperthyroidism may be delayed for a week or longer in neonates whose mothers produce not only TRSAb but TRBAb as well.
4. Similarly, if the mother took antithyroid medication during pregnancy, the neonate might not exhibit evidence of hyperthyroidism for several days until the drugs are metabolized (and might even be hypothyroid during that time).

5. Occasionally, the hyperthyroidism persists beyond the expected recovery period and becomes true, permanent Graves' disease.

C. **Clinical presentation and assessment.**
1. Neonates may be born preterm, often with evidence of intrauterine growth restriction. Common clinical signs of thyrotoxicosis include tachycardia, arrhythmias, hypertension, tachypnea, poor feeding, vomiting, sweating, hyperthermia, flushing, diarrhea, restlessness, tremors, irritability, and hyperalertness.
2. In severe cases of untreated maternal Graves' disease, advanced bone age, craniosynostosis, and microcephaly are evident in both the fetus and newborn.
3. The infant should be examined for a goiter, which can be very small or large enough to compress the trachea and cause respiratory distress in the newborn. A goiter is a symmetrical, smooth enlargement of the gland and can be recognized as a swelling in the anterior neck of the neonate. To examine the neonate for goiter, place the infant supine and elevate the trunk while allowing the head to fall back gently (LynShue and Witchel, 2007).

D. **Diagnostic studies.**
1. Serum $T_4$, free $T_4$, and $T_3$ are elevated, and serum TSH is low, all relative to age-appropriate norms.
2. A TRSAb titer in the neonate will give an indication of the expected severity of the disease course. Infants at risk (e.g., high maternal titer of TRSAb) for severe thyrotoxicosis require frequent monitoring of free $T_4$ and TSH.
3. A thorough maternal history is essential (e.g., history of radioablation therapy, antithyroid drugs taken during pregnancy and when they were taken, and maternal symptoms, if any).

E. **Management.**
1. The mainstays of treatment of hyperthyroidism in the neonate are iodine, antithyroid medication, sedation, and β-adrenergic blockers, if needed. Treatment is tailored to the severity of the infant's symptoms. Lugol's iodine solution (potassium iodide), given in a single drop 3 times daily, acutely inhibits the release of thyroxine from the thyroid gland. Other preparations include iodine-based contrast agents (ipodate), propylthiouracil, and methimazole.
2. Propranolol can be used to manage cardiovascular symptoms. The infant's serum $T_4$ must be followed closely during treatment for possible iatrogenic hypothyroidism. TRSAb levels are also followed to monitor the infant's recovery and aid in determining the appropriate time for weaning antithyroid medication.
3. In cases of maternal thyrotoxicosis, thyrotoxicosis should be anticipated in the neonate so diagnosis and treatment can be instituted without delay.

F. **Complications.**
1. More severe manifestations of thyrotoxicosis, such as congestive heart failure, hepatosplenomegaly, thrombocytopenia, and hyperviscosity syndrome, may occur.

G. **Outcome.**
1. Neonatal hyperthyroidism is almost always transient.
2. The mortality rate of 12% to 16% is related to cardiovascular compromise, arrhythmia, tachycardia, and heart failure (Peters and Hindmarsh, 2007).
3. Survivors of severe, prolonged thyrotoxicosis often have permanent neurologic impairment from premature craniosynostosis and the direct effects of excess thyroid hormones on the brain.

# ADRENAL GLAND DISORDERS

## The Adrenal Gland

A. **Anatomy and physiology.**
1. The adrenal glands are located at the superior poles of the kidneys. Each highly vascular gland is composed of two endocrine organs: the inner adrenal medulla and the outer adrenal cortex.
2. The adrenal medulla produces and stores catecholamines (epinephrine, norepinephrine, dopamine) and is linked to the sympathetic nervous system.
3. All adrenocortical hormones (steroids) are synthesized from cholesterol. Three classes of steroids are produced by the adrenal cortex: glucocorticoids, mineralocorticoids, and androgens.

**B. Adrenocortical hormones.**

1. Cortisol, the primary glucocorticoid, has a major role in glucose homeostasis and key regulatory roles in development, growth, inflammatory responses, cardiovascular function, and response to stress.
2. Cortisol is closely regulated by ACTH and the hypothalamic–pituitary–adrenal axis via an acute or chronic negative-feedback loop. Increased plasma cortisol inhibits secretion of corticotropin-releasing hormone and ACTH, whereas decreased plasma cortisol permits their release. Cortisol is also released in response to stress, hypoglycemia, surgery, extreme heat or cold, decreased oxygen concentration, infection, or injury.
3. Aldosterone, the most important mineralocorticoid, regulates renal sodium ($Na^+$) and water retention and potassium ($K^+$) excretion, thus affecting not only electrolyte balance but also blood pressure and intravascular volume. Aldosterone is regulated by the plasma renin–angiotensin system and by plasma $K^+$ concentrations. A drop in intravascular volume or the $Na^+$ concentration or a rise in the $K^+$ level stimulates the renin–angiotensin system, which in turn stimulates production of aldosterone.
4. Adrenal androgens include dehydroepiandrosterone (DHEA), DHEA sulfate, and androstenedione and are regulated by ACTH. These steroids have minimal androgenic activity but are converted in the peripheral tissues to two more potent androgens: testosterone and dihydrotestosterone.

**C. Fetal adrenocortical development.**

1. Early in gestation, the fetal adrenal cortex begins to differentiate into distinct zones: a large, unique fetal zone and an outer definitive ("adult") zone. The fetal zone is responsible for most of the steroids produced during fetal life. Fetal adrenal growth is rapid; at term, the gland is twice the size of the adult's, but shrinks in size after birth as the fetal zone involutes.
2. The fetal adrenal gland and the placenta are an integrated endocrine organ known as the fetoplacental unit. The fetal zone, deficient in a critical enzyme for cortisol synthesis, produces mostly DHEA and DHEA sulfate. These are the precursors for placental estrogen, which is vital to maintenance of the pregnancy and fetal well-being. In turn, the placenta provides substrates for fetal cortisol production.
3. Until about 30 weeks of gestation, fetal cortisol comes from both the fetal gland and transplacental transfer. In the placenta, 80% of maternal cortisol is rapidly metabolized to inactive cortisone to protect the fetus from very high cortisol levels. Near term, maturation of fetal enzyme systems allows greater conversion of cortisone back to cortisol and synthesis of cortisol from cholesterol. Increases in circulating cortisol during the last 10 weeks of gestation (the prenatal cortisol surge) induce critical physiologic changes that prepare the fetus for extrauterine life, including maturation of pulmonary surfactant.
4. Aldosterone production increases throughout pregnancy, preparing the fetus to assume control of salt and water balance after birth.

**D. Neonatal adrenocortical function.**

1. Plasma cortisol levels are high at the time of birth but begin to fall in the first few days of life. In term infants, a nadir is seen on day 4. Likewise, levels of a cortisol precursor, 17-hydroxyprogesterone (17-OHP), are high at birth but decline to normal neonatal levels by 12 to 24 hours of age.
2. A diurnal pattern of cortisol secretion is evident at about 2 to 3 months of age in most infants, influenced more by environmental factors than genetic factors (Custodio et al., 2007). Cortisol in the newborn plays a key role in response to stress and illness, and is important in the maintenance of blood pressure (Ng, 2011).
3. Aldosterone concentration and plasma renin activity (PRA) are elevated compared with values for older infants, allowing for positive $Na^+$ balance until the kidneys fully mature. The hyponatremia and urinary $Na^+$ loss often seen in preterm infants during the early postnatal weeks are due to a relative mineralocorticoid deficiency as a consequence of immaturity of both the kidneys and the adrenal glands.

## Adrenal Disorders in the Neonate

A. **Transient adrenocortical insufficiency of prematurity.**
   1. A limited ability of the adrenal glands to maintain cortisol homeostasis in the early days of life has been observed in some preterm newborns.
   2. Manifestations are a low serum cortisol, normal or exaggerated pituitary response, and good recovery of adrenal function by day 14 of life (Ng, 2011).
   3. Some very low birth weight infants with inotrope and volume-resistant hypotension show an inadequate adrenal response to stress in the immediate postnatal period (Ng, 2011).
   4. Whether a relative adrenal insufficiency contributes to hemodynamic instability and hypotension in critically ill infants is still under debate (Nimkarn and New, 2012).

B. **Adrenal hemorrhage.**
   1. Adrenal hemorrhage in the neonate can be precipitated by traumatic delivery, breech presentation, macrosomia, or disseminated intravascular coagulation. The large size and vascularity of the fetal adrenal gland predisposes the gland to injury and rupture during the birth process.
   2. Although often asymptomatic, classic findings include jaundice, pallor, and a flank mass on either side (although hemorrhage is more common on the right) with discoloration and purpura of the overlying skin and discoloration of the scrotum (Mutlu et al., 2011). In severe cases, the infant may exhibit signs of adrenal insufficiency. Small hemorrhages can be initially undetected, but eventually manifest in anemia and persistent jaundice (Janjua and Batisky, 2012).
   3. Adrenal hemorrhage can be visualized on ultrasound, and usually resolves in 4 to 16 weeks (Mutlu et al., 2011).

## Congenital Adrenal Hyperplasia

A. **Definition:** A group of autosomal recessive genetic disorders resulting from deficient activity of one of the enzymes required to synthesize cortisol from cholesterol in the adrenal cortex. Each enzyme is encoded by its own gene. Mutation of the 21-hydroxylase (21-OHD) gene, *CYP21*, accounts for 95% of disorders, and is the most common cause of ambiguous genitalia in the neonate. Currently there are 127 known different mutations of CYP2A12 that range from having absolutely no enzyme activity to partial enzyme function. The worldwide incidence of classic 21-OHD is approximately 1 in 5000 to 1 in 15,000 live births (Witchel and Azziz, 2011; Stokowski, 2014).

B. **Pathophysiology (Fig. 30-2):**
   1. Because the overwhelming majority of CAH cases are the result of 21-OHD deficiency, the remainder of the discussion will pertain to this form of CAH.
   2. Lack of fetal 21-OHD prevents conversion of progesterone to its two end products: cortisol and aldosterone.
   3. By reduced negative-feedback regulation, the absence of cortisol causes oversecretion of ACTH, which chronically stimulates the adrenal cortex, resulting in hyperplasia.
   4. The cortisol precursor 17-OHP accumulates in the blood because its conversion to cortisol is blocked.
   5. The excess 17-OHP enters the unblocked androgen metabolic pathway, which results in an overproduction of androgens. At a critical stage in fetal development, androgens cause virilization of the external genitalia in female fetuses. Also important may be the effects of this androgen exposure on the developing CNS.

C. **Clinical presentation.**
   1. Infants with CAH are usually identified at birth by their abnormal genitalia, a key feature in CAH (Stokowski, 2014).
   2. Neonates with CAH may present with a range of findings, including clitoromegaly and posterior fusion of the labia majora with rugae. A single urogenital orifice, where the vagina joins the urethra above the perineum, may also be noted instead of separate urethral and vaginal openings (Witchel and Azziz, 2011; Stokowski, 2014).

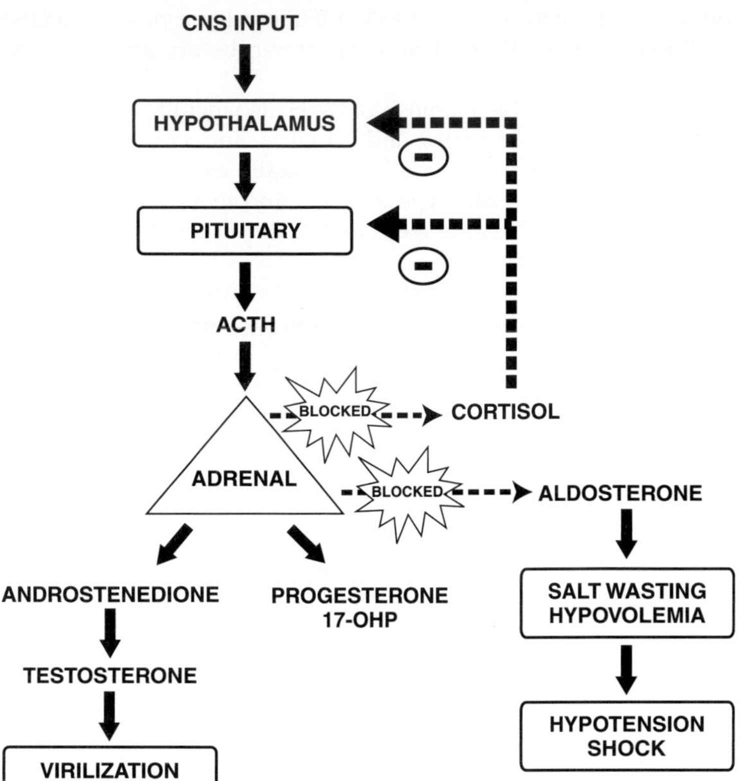


FIGURE 30-2 ■ Pathophysiology of congenital adrenal hyperplasia caused by 21-hydroxylase deficiency. In the absence of cortisol, adrenocorticotropic hormone (ACTH) stimulates the adrenal cortex to produce virilizing androgens. Diminished production of aldosterone leads to salt wasting and hypovolemia. *CNS*, Central nervous system; *17-OHP*, 17-hydroxyprogesterone. (Adapted from Martin, R.J., Fanaroff, A.A., and Walsh, M.C.: *Fanaroff and Martin's neonatal-perinatal medicine: Diseases of the fetus and infant* [9th ed.]. Philadelphia, 2011, Elsevier Mosby.)

3. In severe cases, clitoral hypertrophy is so marked that it resembles a penile urethra. These infants can be mistaken for boys with bilateral cryptorchidism and hypospadias.
4. There may also be hyperpigmentation of the genital skin resulting from excessive pituitary ACTH secretion.
5. Male infants with 21-OHD are phenotypically normal and may not be identified in the immediate neonatal period, because the onset of adrenal symptoms is delayed until 7 to 14 days of life.
6. Undetected infants may present to the emergency room with signs and symptoms of impending adrenal collapse: vomiting, weight loss, lethargy, dehydration, hyponatremia, hyperkalemia, hypoglycemia, hypovolemia, and shock.
7. Infants of either gender who are untreated will undergo rapid postnatal growth and sexual precocity; those with severe enzyme deficiencies can develop salt loss and die (Speiser et al., 2010).

**D. Diagnosis.**

1. Genital ambiguity can be lifesaving in females because it alerts the health care team to the possible diagnosis of CAH before a salt-losing crisis ensues. With neonatal screening, the diagnosis of CAH before the advent of a salt-losing state has become more common.
2. Diagnostic tests and findings in 21-OHD CAH are as follows:
   a. 17-OHP level is markedly elevated and is hyperresponsive to ACTH stimulation; levels of testosterone and its precursors are also increased. Random 17-OHP levels in affected infants can reach 10,000 ng/dL (normal is <100 ng/dL). However, such high 17-OHP levels may not be reached until the second or third day of life, so a specimen drawn too early could lead to false reassurance that the infant does not have CAH. Prenatal

or postnatal steroids can suppress the 17-OHP level and produce a false-negative result as well. Blood for 17-OHP level must be drawn before any hormone replacement is administered.

b. Biochemical support for the diagnosis of CAH also includes elevated serum DHEA and androstenedione levels in males and females, and elevated serum testosterone in females. Molecular genetic analysis is not usually essential for the diagnosis but may be helpful to confirm the exact type of defect and to aid in genetic counseling.

c. Serum aldosterone and PRA are measured to detect salt-losing states. The aldosterone level is low and PRA is high.

d. Serum and urine electrolytes and steroid profiles are determined. Positive findings are hyponatremia, hyperkalemia, and high urine $Na^+$ excretion. Other metabolic disturbances include hypoglycemia and metabolic acidosis.

e. Karyotype testing. It may be difficult for parents to accept that their severely virilized newborn is a genetic female without this testing. If genetic testing for *CYP21B* (gene for 21-OHD) is to be done, blood samples should be taken from both the infant and the parents (Ogilvy-Stuart and Midgley, 2006).

f. Ultrasonography and/or MRI of the pelvis and abdomen are done to visualize the uterus and adrenal glands.

3. Neonatal screening for CAH is currently required in all 50 states and the District of Columbia (National Newborn Screening and Genetics Resource Center, 2013). In Canada, 7 of 15 provinces and territories currently screen for CAH (Canadian Organization for Rare Disorders, 2012).

   a. The goals of screening are the presymptomatic identification of infants at risk for life-threatening adrenal crisis and prevention of incorrect sex assignment of affected females.

   b. The basis of screening for CAH is measurement of 17-OHP, which is markedly elevated in neonates with the disorder. False-positives occur in about 1% of all tests, and can also occur in preterm infants or sick infants, both of whom have higher levels of 17-OHP (Speiser et al., 2010).

E. **Management of CAH.**

1. Restore physiologic level of cortisol, suppress ACTH and androgen overproduction, and maintain fluid and electrolyte homeostasis, especially any salt deficit that is present.
2. Administer hydrocortisone (glucocorticoid) and 9-$\alpha$-fludrocortisone (mineralocorticoid). Further clinical management is guided by daily weights, adrenal steroid concentrations, PRA, electrolytes, blood glucose, and other data. PRA should be compared against age-specific norms, because basal PRA is higher in the newborn than in older infants.
3. Dietary sodium supplementation to prevent hyponatremia, if needed. Fludrocortisone is not effective without salt supplementation.
4. Additional measures. In a salt-losing state/adrenal crisis, these may include intravenous administration of fluids (glucose and sodium to correct dehydration and metabolic imbalances), treatment of shock, and correction of acidosis.
5. Genetic counseling.
   a. Prenatal diagnosis for subsequent pregnancies using direct molecular genetic analysis of the fetal DNA (Nimkarn and New, 2006).
   b. Intrauterine treatment can prevent some or all of the virilization of female fetuses. Dexamethasone given to the mother crosses the placenta and suppresses fetal ACTH. Treatment must begin before 8 weeks of gestation and continue to term in affected female fetuses.
6. Parent education. Parents need to understand that there is no cure for CAH, but it can be managed with medications and close monitoring. Their baby should receive care from a pediatric endocrinologist. Advise parents about immediate and long-term management of the disorder, the importance of compliance with therapy, and the need for follow-up of growth and development. Parents need to be aware of the requirement for double or even triple doses of steroids during illness and fever. Do not use the term *ambiguous genitalia* in discussions with parents as this term is disturbing to parents (Ogilvy-Stuart and Midgley, 2006).

F. **Management of virilized female neonates with CAH.** Two issues that might be raised regarding the neonate with virilizing CAH are gender of rearing and the type of surgery that will be needed, if any, and the timing of that surgery.
  1. Gender of rearing. Most 46,XX individuals with CAH develop a female gender identity, regardless of the degree of genital virilization present at birth (Houk and Lee, 2012). Therefore, even in cases in which babies are initially "misassigned" as boys, it is still generally recommended that these genetic females with CAH be raised as females, although some experts maintain that, in extensively virilized infants, a male sex assignment should be considered (Houk and Lee, 2012). Hypertrophy of the clitoris will gradually abate with medical therapy; however, severe virilization will not be reversed.
  2. Surgery. Parents of virilized female infants may have many questions about possible genital surgery. Although such surgery is not usually performed until the infant is 2 to 6 months of age, it is helpful for the parents to meet with the pediatric endocrinologist and pediatric urologic surgeon to discuss available options, one of which is to delay surgery performed for cosmetic purposes until the child is old enough to participate in the decision (Auchus et al., 2010; Intersex Society of North America, 2006). The goals of genital surgery for virilized girls with CAH are to achieve genital appearance compatible with gender, unobstructed urinary emptying without incontinence or infections, and good adult sexual and reproductive function.
  3. After discharge, infants with CAH must be closely followed by a pediatric endocrinologist for assessments of hormone levels, blood sugar, blood pressure, growth, skeletal maturation, and other parameters necessary to guard against over- or undertreatment.

G. **Complications of CAH.**
  1. Adrenal crisis can occur with sudden signs of cortisol insufficiency (shock, hypotension, acidosis, hypoglycemia, seizures) plus sodium depletion. This can be triggered by episodes of illness or stress (such as systemic infection or surgery) in the neonatal period. Stress therapy to prevent this complication requires 2 or 3 times the usual dosage of hydrocortisone.
  2. Consequences of poorly controlled CAH:
     a. Failure to suppress ACTH and androgen production can result in signs of virilization and accelerated growth or bone maturation.
     b. Overtreatment, resulting in hypertension, pulmonary edema, congestive heart failure, growth failure, adrenal atrophy, and lowered resistance to infection.

H. **Outcome.**
  1. Lifelong hormonal replacement is usually necessary to improve chances for normal growth, pubertal development, and fertility.
  2. Missed or delayed diagnosis can result in sudden deterioration or death in infants with undiagnosed CAH.

## SEXUAL DEVELOPMENT

Sexual development is a sequential process with three stages: (1) fertilization (determination of chromosomal sex), (2) gonadal differentiation, and (3) differentiation of phenotypic sex (internal ductal system and external genitalia) (Lin-Su and New, 2012). At the time of conception, the sex chromosome complement of the fertilizing sperm determines the chromosomal sex.

The next events are directed by genes. All embryos have bipotential gonads and structures for both male and female internal and external genitalia. Male-specific development requires the expression of the testis-determining gene (*SRY*) located on the short arm of the Y chromosome. This directs the gonad to differentiate to a testis, the key event in sex determination, by downstream regulation of sex-determining factors (Ocal, 2011). A large number of regulatory genes (including *SRY, SOX9, FGF9, FOXL2, WNT4,* and *GATA4*) acting in networks drives the process of embryonic gonadal development, and single mutations in some of these genes are known to cause disorders of sexual development (DSDs) (Ono and Harley, 2013). Because most genes related to gonadal development are expressed in other organs as well, mutations can cause syndromes of gonadal dysgenesis, such as Denys–Drash syndrome and camptomelic dysplasia.

A. **Internal genitalia:** The next events in sexual development are hormonally mediated, predicated on the established gonadal gender (Lin-Su and New, 2012).

1. By 7 weeks of gestation, the fetus has two sets of primitive ducts that will become the internal reproductive tracts: the müllerian (female) and wolffian (male). In the XY fetus, the testis differentiates by the end of week 7.
2. The embryonic testis develops two types of hormone-producing cells: the Sertoli and the Leydig cells. The Sertoli cells begin secreting müllerian-inhibiting factor (MIF), causing the müllerian ducts to regress. By the ninth week, testicular Leydig cells are secreting the androgens necessary for further virilization of the male fetus.
3. Testosterone, the major androgen produced by the testes, acts locally in high concentrations to induce development of the wolffian ducts into the epididymis, vas deferens, and seminal vesicles.
4. In the absence of testosterone, the wolffian ducts regress at 11 weeks of gestation. Müllerian ducts require no ovarian hormonal inducement to develop into fallopian tubes, uterus, and upper vagina. This occurs in fetuses with a normal ovary or on any side lacking a gonad.

B. **External genitalia.**

1. The primitive external genitalia are identical in both sexes (Fig. 30-3). At this indifferent stage, a genital tubercle forms and elongates to form a phallus and urogenital sinus, surrounded by inner urogenital folds and labioscrotal swellings.
2. Between the 8th and 14th weeks of gestation, male differentiation of the external genitalia takes place. Central to this development is availability of dihydrotestosterone (DHT), a potent metabolite produced from testosterone by the enzyme 5α-reductase-2 (5-ARD-2). With 10 times the binding affinity of testosterone, DHT binds to androgen receptors in the genital tissues, stimulating fusion of the urethral folds to form the penile shaft, and the labioscrotal swellings to form the scrotum. The urogenital sinus becomes the urethra.
3. Penile growth continues throughout gestation, and migration of the testes from the abdominal cavity to the scrotum is a late event, at 25 to 35 weeks of gestation. Androgen exposure after about 14 weeks contributes to further phallic enlargement (Lin-Su and New, 2012).
4. In the absence of DHT, feminization of the external genitalia occurs. The phallus becomes a clitoris, and the labioscrotal swellings remain unfused to form the labia majora and minora. The urogenital sinus develops into the lower vagina and urethra. Feminine external genital development is complete by 11 weeks of gestation. Androgen exposure after this critical period can promote growth of the clitoris but does not cause labial fusion or the development of a penile urethra (Lin-Su and New, 2012).

## DISORDERS OF SEXUAL DEVELOPMENT

A DSD is an incongruence between molecular, gonadal, and phenotypic sex (Houk and Lee, 2012). Many people still refer to DSDs as "ambiguous genitalia" but this is a feature of some DSDs, rather than a diagnosis. Most DSDs result from either a failure in one of the steps of the male sexual developmental pathway, or the exposure of an XX fetus to androgens during a sensitive period of development. Less frequent are DSDs resulting from gonadal differentiation, chromosomal disorders, and syndromes associated with ambiguous genitalia (Lin-Su and New, 2012).

## 46,XX DSD

The most frequently encountered DSD in the neonate is the virilized female, or the 46,XX infant with virilized external genitalia and normal female internal structures. By far, the most common etiology is 21-OHD deficiency CAH (Fig. 30-4). This enzyme deficiency results in an overproduction of androgens at a critical stage of development, causing masculinization of the external, but not the internal (ovaries, uterus, fallopian tubes), genitalia. In severe cases, the excess androgens also prevent the vagina from fully descending into the perineum, leaving a common urogenital canal. Rarer causes of virilization of external genitalia in the 46,XX infant are placental aromatase deficiency, maternal androgen-producing or adrenal tumors, and maternal medications with androgenic action taken during pregnancy.

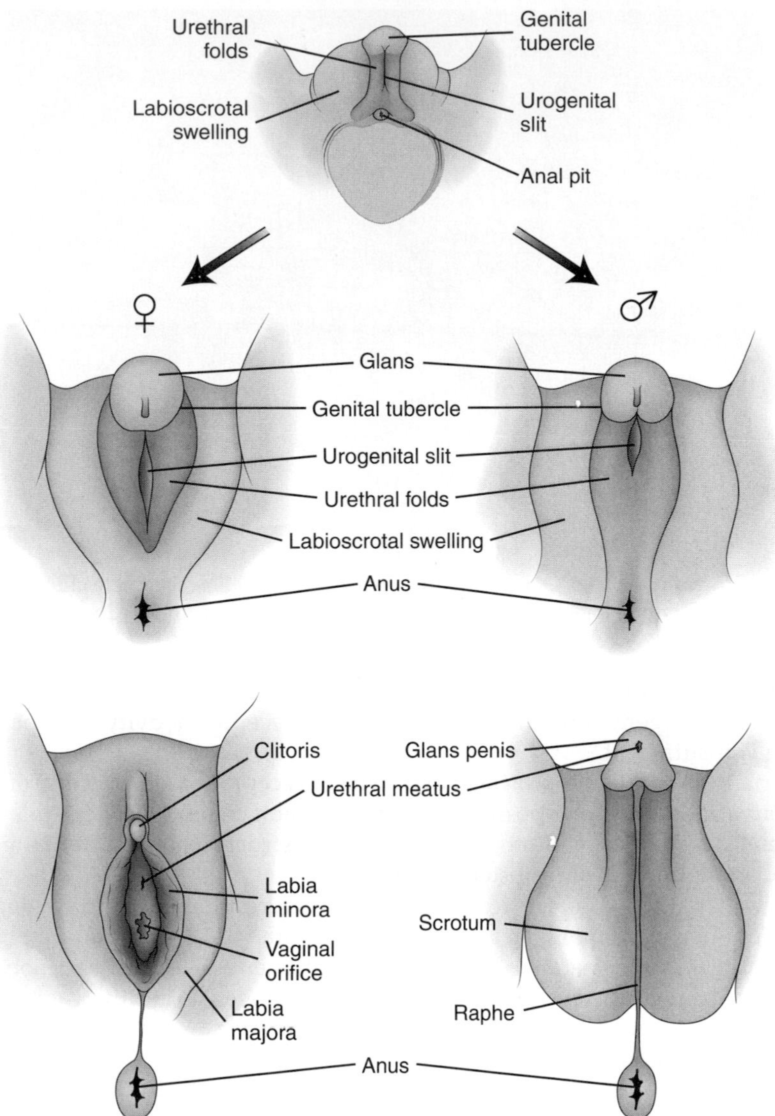


FIGURE 30-3 ■ Development and differentiation of male and female external genitalia. (Adapted from Spaulding, M.H.: The development of the external genitalia in the human embryo. *Contributions to Embryology of the Carnegie Institute*, 13:69-88, 1921; Kronenberg, H.M., Melmed, S., Polonsky, K.S., and Larsen, P.R. [Eds.]: *Williams textbook of endocrinology* [11th ed.]. Philadelphia, 2008, Elsevier Saunders.)

## 46,XY DSD

The combination of a 46,XY karyotype with ambiguous genitalia results from a failure in one of the steps involved in the synthesis of or response to testosterone during sexual differentiation and penile growth. These infants have bilateral testicular development, but incomplete virilization of the internal or external genitalia. This results in an external phenotype ranging from completely female to isolated hypospadias or cryptorchidism. Another condition associated with incomplete virilization in the XY male is cloacal exstrophy, a defect of embryogenesis involving exstrophy of the bladder. Although not a DSD, significant ambiguity of external genitalia may be present.

### Androgen Insensitivity Syndrome (AIS)

**A. Pathophysiology.**

1. AIS is caused by a loss-of-function mutation in the androgen receptor gene located on the long arm of the X chromosome.

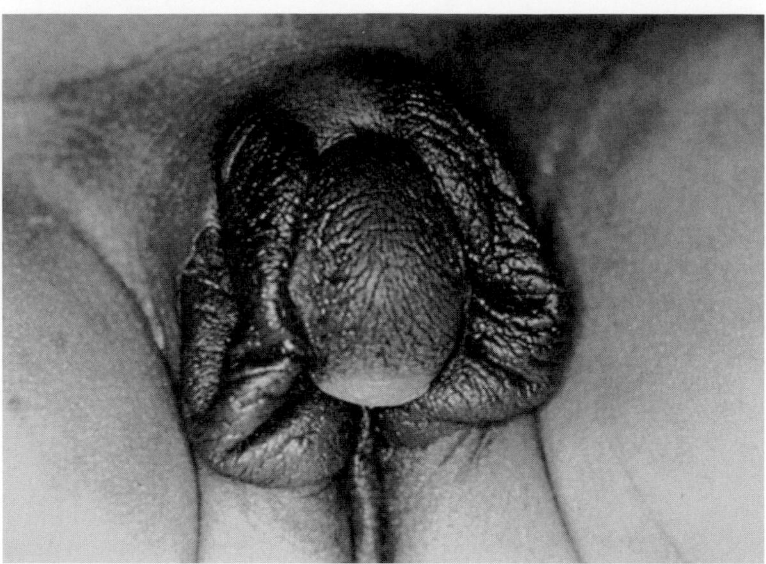

FIGURE 30-4 ■ Virilization in a 46,XX infant with 21-hydroxylase deficiency. Note clitoral hypertrophy and hyperpigmented and rugated labiosacral folds, resembling an empty scrotum. (Courtesy Michael S. Kappy, M.D., Ph.D.)

2. Both testosterone and its target tissue metabolite, DHT, must bind to androgen receptors to masculinize the genital tissues. When androgen receptor activity is impaired, androgen binding is insufficient.
3. One variant of AIS is receptor negative: cytosol receptors are incapable of binding DHT. Another variant is receptor positive: receptors are able to bind DHT but this does not result in normal differentiation. Both internal wolffian structures and external genitalia fail to respond to high levels of testosterone and DHT.
4. There are partial and complete forms of the disorder, resulting in different degrees of undervirilization. In partial androgen insensitivity syndrome (PAIS), the clinical phenotype varies considerably and often parallels the severity of androgen resistance, but genotype–phenotype correlations have not been found. A mild form of androgen insensitivity is not detected in the newborn because genitals are those of a typical male.

**B. Clinical manifestations.**

1. Infants with PAIS have undervirilization ranging from simple hypospadias to microphallus with a labia majora–like bifid scrotum, undescended testes, and a urogenital sinus. No visible features distinguish PAIS from other causes of incomplete masculinization.
2. Infants with complete androgen insensitivity syndrome (CAIS) are born with apparently female genitalia. However, these neonates may have palpable inguinal or labial masses, which further testing will reveal to be testes. Some may also have a short, blind-ending vagina.

**C. Diagnosis.**

1. The diagnosis of CAIS is missed in the newborn period unless the infant presents with bilateral masses in the labia or inguinal canals or a boy was expected based on a prenatal karyotype. CAIS might also be discovered at the time of inguinal hernia repair, or there may be a history of similarly affected family members.
2. Investigations include a karyotype and levels of testosterone, DHT, and LH. In PAIS, the ratio of androstenedione to testosterone is normal. Testosterone, estradiol, and LH are normal or high; FSH is usually normal.
3. Molecular genetic testing for mutations in the *AR* gene, and/or androgen binding assays.
4. Imaging studies reveal the absence of female internal reproductive structures (uterus, fallopian tubes). Two normal testes are present.

**D. Management.**

1. Infants with CAIS have unambiguously female external anatomy and are raised as girls. Testes are removed (usually after puberty) to prevent later malignancy.

2. The gender assignment of infants with PAIS can be more complex and is often based on the severity of the phenotype. When the phenotype is predominantly male, a male sex of rearing is recommended. However, no consensus exists for the management of infants with severe perineoscrotal hypospadias and microphallus. The detection of somatic mutations in AIS is of importance for correct gender assignment because the presence of a functional wild-type AR receptor can induce virilization at puberty (Kohler et al., 2005).
3. When a male sex of rearing is contemplated, a therapeutic trial with pharmacologic doses of androgen is often used to predict potential androgen responsiveness at puberty. If the phallus does not grow in response to testosterone, some experts would recommend consideration of a female gender assignment. However, many experts now believe that, given the putative influence of prenatal androgen exposure on the developing CNS and the possibility that the child will develop a male gender identity, it is more prudent to raise these infants as boys.

## Testosterone Biosynthetic Defects

**A. Pathophysiology.**

1. Defects in the chain of steroidogenic enzymes involved in the testosterone biosynthesis pathway result in insufficient androgen concentrations during fetal development.
2. Disorders include congenital lipoid adrenal hyperplasia (CLAH), 3β-hydroxysteroid dehydrogenase (3β-HSD) deficiency, 17α-hydroxylase/17,20-lyase deficiency, and 17β-hydroxysteroid dehydrogenase (17β-HSD) deficiency. CLAH is caused by a defect in the steroidogenic acute regulatory (StAR) protein, responsible for transporting cholesterol to the inner membrane of the mitochondria.
3. Insufficient testosterone in affected males leads to underdeveloped wolffian duct structures and external male anatomy. Müllerian structures are absent because there is normal testicular MIF production.

**B. Clinical manifestations.**

1. Male infants with CLAH present with complete adrenal insufficiency: vomiting, weight loss, and hypotension. Genital appearance is primarily female.
2. Infants with 3β-HSD can present with varying degrees of genital ambiguity and evidence of salt-losing crisis.
3. Infants with 17α-hydroxylase/17,20-lyase deficiency have genital ambiguity.
4. Patients with primary 17α-hydroxylase deficiency also have hypertension.
5. Infants with 17β-HSD present with what appear to be external female genitalia that may include mild clitoral enlargement. An inguinal hernia may be present, possibly the only finding that will bring the infant to medical attention.

**C. Diagnosis.**

1. Laboratory investigations in suspected testosterone biosynthetic defects include chromosomes; baseline levels of testosterone, androgen precursors, and DHT; and levels of steroids and steroid precursors.
2. A human chorionic gonadotropin (hCG) stimulation test can be performed to measure the ratio of androstenedione to testosterone; an elevated ratio suggests 17β-HSD deficiency.
3. In CLAH, ultrasound, computed tomography, or MRI may show enlarged, lipid-laden adrenal glands (Lin-Su and New, 2012).

**D. Management.**

1. Acute management of these disorders requires full steroid replacement with both glucocorticoids and mineralocorticoids.
2. In CLAH and 3β-HSD, general supportive measures may be necessary, because severe adrenal insufficiency can cause rapid metabolic decompensation if the disorder is not recognized at birth.
3. Genetic XY infants with CLAH are raised as girls. Children with 17β-HSD often virilize significantly at puberty owing to increased peripheral conversion of androstenedione to testosterone by 17β-HSD isoenzymes, making gender assignment of those diagnosed as neonates a less straightforward decision.

## 5α-Reductase-2 Deficiency

**A. Pathophysiology.**

1. 5-ARD-2 deficiency is an autosomal recessive disorder caused by more than 20 different mutations of the 5-ARD gene. 5-ARD-2 is an enzyme found in the genital skin and fibroblasts of the developing fetus, without which testosterone is not converted to DHT, and fetal external genitalia do not virilize.
2. Development of the internal structures is unaffected because DHT is not required, so the wolffian ducts differentiate normally in response to testosterone and the müllerian ducts regress. At puberty, the external genitalia become virilized and fertility is possible.

**B. Clinical manifestations (Fig. 30-5).**

1. The spectrum of findings ranges from mild (isolated micropenis or hypospadias) to severe (a female phenotype with clitoromegaly, mild rugation, or pigmentation) undervirilization.
2. Testes are intact and are found in the inguinal canals or labioscrotal folds, or are retained in the abdomen. The uterus and fallopian tubes regress because of normal secretion of MIF.
3. Wolffian duct differentiation is not affected because DHT is not required. Male internal ducts terminate either in a blind pseudovaginal pouch or on the perineum.

**C. Diagnosis.**

1. Diagnosis is made by assessing the ratio of testosterone to DHT following an hCG stimulation test. A normal testosterone/DHT ratio is less than 4:1. In 5-ARD-2 deficiency, this ratio is elevated, to higher than 14:1 (Lin-Su and New, 2012). The hCG stimulation test also rules out other causes of undervirilization, such as Leydig cell hypoplasia and testosterone biosynthetic defects.
2. Analysis of 5-ARD-2 activity in genital skin fibroblasts provides a definitive diagnosis.

**D. Management.**

1. Boys with 5-ARD-2 respond to endogenous testosterone and undergo virilization and penile growth at puberty. The mechanism behind this late virilization may be extraglandular DHT formation due to peripheral conversion of testicular testosterone by unaffected isoenzymes.
2. For this reason, it is recommended that when the diagnosis is made in the newborn period, a male gender assignment is made.

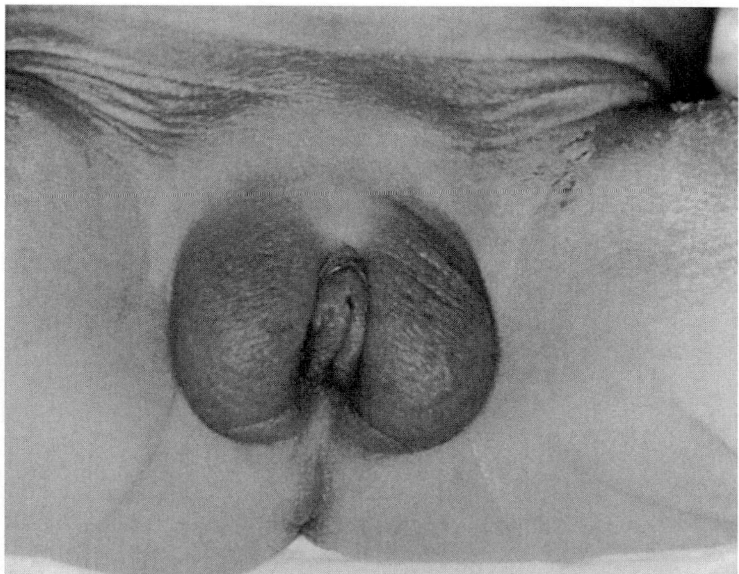

FIGURE 30-5 ■ Infant with 46,XY karyotype and ambiguous genitalia caused by 5-α-reductase deficiency. Note absence of a penis and lack of fusion of labiosacral folds, indicating incomplete virilization. (Courtesy Michael S. Kappy, M.D., Ph.D.)

## Gonadal Dysgenesis

This group of disorders is usually associated with chromosomal anomalies or mutations, or deletions of genes responsible for sexual differentiation. Karyotypes producing gonadal dysgenesis include 46,XY, 46,XX, 46,XY/46,X, and mosaic forms including the Y chromosome. Gonadal dysgenesis can occur as an isolated condition or as part of a complex syndrome such as Fraser syndrome, Denys–Drash syndrome, or camptomelic dysplasia.

**A. Pathophysiology.**

1. A dysgenetic testis either fails to produce testosterone at all or produces insufficient testosterone, resulting in varying degrees of undervirilization of the fetus.
2. Gonadal dysgenesis is considered partial or incomplete when the testes are dysgenetic or incompletely formed, and complete when the gonads are streaks containing only stromal tissue.
3. Mixed gonadal dysgenesis occurs when one gonad is a streak and the other is a well-formed testis. The internal ducts correlate with the ipsilateral gonad. On the side of a streak gonad, a fallopian tube and a hemiuterus will develop, and on the side of a normal testis, the vas deferens and epididymis will form.

**B. Clinical manifestations.**

1. The external genitalia are highly variable depending on how much testosterone is produced. In mixed gonadal dysgenesis, the external genitalia are asymmetrical, appearing male on one side and female on the other. A vagina and uterine cavity may be present.
2. Complete (or pure) gonadal dysgenesis is a form of sex reversal that results in unambiguously female genitalia with features of Turner's syndrome. These infants might not be identified in the newborn period unless a discrepancy is noted between a prenatal karyotype (46,XY) and appearance of the genitals.

**C. Diagnosis.**

1. Karyotyping.
2. Imaging studies are used to define the internal anatomy.
3. Gonadal histologic analysis is necessary to differentiate gonadal dysgenesis from ovotesticular DSD, a condition wherein elements of both testes and ovaries are present in the same individual.

**D. Management.**

1. Determining the sex of rearing for the infant with partial or mixed gonadal dysgenesis can be a difficult decision, one that is typically based on the degree of virilization and details of the internal anatomy.
2. When a uterus is present, the female gender assignment may be preferred. Most infants with complete gonadal dysgenesis are raised as females.

## Ovotesticular DSD

In ovotesticular DSDs, both ovarian and testicular components are present in the same individual. Possible combinations include an ovary on one side and a testis on the other, an ovary or testis with an ovotestis, or two ovotestes. More than half of affected babies will have an XX karyotype. This condition was formerly known as true hermaphroditism.

**A. Pathophysiology.**

1. The amount of testosterone produced by the testicular tissue determines the degree of differentiation of wolffian ducts, regression of müllerian ducts, and virilization of external genitalia.
2. The internal ducts usually parallel the ipsilateral gonadal histology. Ovarian tissue can be normal.

**B. Clinical manifestations.**

1. Asymmetry of the external genitalia is a hallmark of ovotesticular DSD. Genital ambiguity ranges from a female phenotype with slight clitoromegaly to a mildly undervirilized male phenotype.
2. The most common presentation is marked genital ambiguity: microphallus with penoscrotal or perineoscrotal hypospadias, fusion of labioscrotal folds, and cryptorchidism.

**C. Diagnosis.**

1. Karyotyping.
2. Imaging studies are used to define the internal anatomy. To diagnose ovotesticular dysgenesis, the presence of functional ovarian tissue containing follicles and testicular tissue with distinct seminiferous tubules must be established.
3. Laparoscopy with gonadal biopsy is necessary at some point to confirm the diagnosis.

**D. Management.** Principles of management for infants with true ovotesticular DSD are similar to those for gonadal dysgenesis.

## General Principles of Management of DSDs

**A. Delivery room management.**

1. Not being told immediately whether the newborn baby is a boy or a girl is one of the most incomprehensible things that can happen to parents in the delivery room. This situation requires a high degree of sensitivity and tact.
2. Many infants are identified prenatally following ultrasound recognition of genital ambiguity or a karyotype/phenotype discordance, and these families will be prepared, to some degree, for the experience of having a baby of uncertain sex. Others will be taken completely by surprise.
3. In spite of the family's desire for a quick answer, no attempt should be made by the health care team at the time of birth to guess the sex of the baby (Ogilvy-Stuart and Brain, 2004). The extreme phenotypic heterogeneity seen in DSDs makes it impossible to accurately predict either the diagnosis or the karyotype from a brief genital examination (Houk and Lee, 2005).
4. Neonates who do not have health concerns requiring intensive care monitoring or treatment should not be transferred to the neonatal intensive care unit, because this only heightens the parents' anxiety unnecessarily and impairs parent–infant bonding.
5. The Lawson Wilkins Pediatric Society and the European Society for Paediatric Endocrinology published a consensus statement on management of DSDs (Lee et al., 2006). That document represents the first agreed-upon set of guiding principles for approaching and managing the newborn with a DSD.

**B. Clinical manifestations.**

1. Obtain a detailed family history. Any of the following might suggest a congenital or inherited DSD: maternal virilization or ingestion of hormones or oral contraceptives during pregnancy; consanguinity; history of urologic abnormalities, infertility, or genital ambiguity in other family members; or previous neonatal deaths that might suggest an undiagnosed adrenal crisis. Dysmorphic features suggest the possibility of a syndrome.
2. Conduct a detailed assessment of the genitalia. All examinations should respect the privacy of the infant and the family as much as possible, avoiding overexposure of the infant even for educational purposes (Auchus et al., 2010). Because of considerable overlap in the genital anatomy among DSDs, the physical assessment alone does not permit a firm diagnosis (Lin-Su and New, 2012). However, some assessment findings can provide clues to the underlying pathophysiology, and guide the diagnostic process in one direction or another.
3. A precise description of the anatomy is more useful than simple staging classifications. If preferred, however, the degree of virilization can be documented by Prader staging (Fig. 30-6) from a phenotypic female with mild clitoromegaly (Prader stage II) to phenotypic male with glandular hypospadias (Prader stage III).
   a. Gonads. Determine whether gonads are palpable. Presence or absence of palpable gonads helps to differentiate the major categories of DSDs. An apparent male infant with bilateral or a single impalpable testis with hypospadias should be considered as having a potential DSD until proven otherwise. A palpable gonad excludes the diagnosis of virilized genetic female (46,XX) with CAH. A gonad palpated below the external inguinal ring is presumed to contain testicular tissue. Because ovaries are rarely palpable, a unilateral gonad is usually a testis or occasionally an ovotestis. To palpate testes, place finger flat from internal ring, and milk down into the labioscrotal folds. Gonads may be situated high in the inguinal canal, requiring a careful examination. Unilateral or bilateral absence of the testes is known as cryptorchidism.

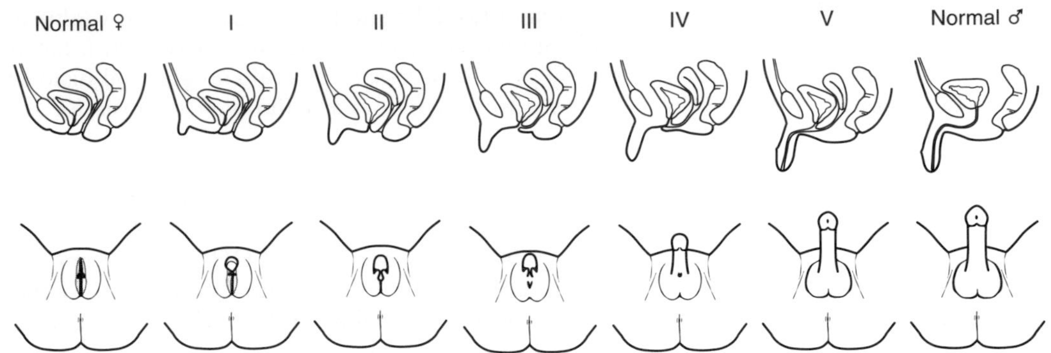


FIGURE 30-6 ■ Degrees of genital virilization based on the stages of Prader. The upper panel illustrates the sagittal view; the lower panel illustrates the perineal view. (From Scriver, C.R.: *The metabolic and molecular basis of inherited diseases* [7th ed.]. New York, 1995, McGraw-Hill Companies.)

b. Phallus. Phallic size should be measured with a straight-edge ruler, depressing the fat pad and measuring the stretched length from pubic tubercle to tip of penis, not including the foreskin. Both length and midshaft diameter of the penis should be noted. Chordee, ventral curvature of the penis caused by residual urethral tissue that tethers the phallus to the perineum, should be noted because it can reduce the apparent length of the penis (Lin-Su and New, 2012). The actual position of the urethral meatus and the severity of hypospadias, if present, should be determined.

c. Clitoral size should also be measured when clitoromegaly is present. Clitoral length greater than 9 mm in term infants is considered excessive. Clitoral size often appears large in preterm infants because breadth remains constant from 27 weeks onward. A prominent, but not truly enlarged, clitoris, or a normally sized penis concealed by an abundance of prepubic fat, are normal assessment findings.

d. Labioscrotal folds. Labial fullness, a benign finding, is another feature occasionally mistaken for genital ambiguity. The labioscrotal folds are examined for fusion, which starts posteriorly and moves anteriorly, increasing the anogenital distance. The perineum is inspected by gently separating the labia and using an examination light to confirm the presence of separate urethral and vaginal openings or a single urogenital orifice (an opening connected to both urinary and genital systems). Visualization of voiding is helpful. If skin tags with slightly bluish hue are seen, a hymen and vagina are present. Note rugosity or hyperpigmentation of the labioscrotal fold, signifying hypersecretion of ACTH associated with CAH. Other variations include a bifid scrotum (a deep midline cleft) or a shawl scrotum (scrotum surrounds the penis like a shawl).

**C. Diagnostic studies.**

1. DSDs are diagnosed with a combination of biochemical, hormonal, imaging, and molecular testing. A molecular diagnosis is possible for about 20% of DSDs (Ono and Harley, 2013).
2. The aim of the initial investigation is to rule out a life-threatening illness such as CAH, which can precipitate an adrenal crisis. Such testing includes serum 17-OHP level (after 24 to 48 hours of age), electrolytes, glucose, and baseline levels of testosterone, DHT, and other steroid precursors (progesterone, DHEA, Δ4-androstenedione, and 17α-hydroxypregnenolone). A karyotype with X- and Y-specific probe detection is obtained from all infants, even if a prenatal karyotype is available (Allen, 2009).
3. A urinary steroid profile is helpful in the diagnosis of disorders of steroid biosynthesis. Other investigations that may be warranted include ACTH stimulation test, PRA, and serum MIF, LH, and FSH. An hCG stimulation test is undertaken to delineate a block in testosterone biosynthesis from androstenedione (17β-HSD deficiency) or conversion of testosterone to DHT (5α-reductase deficiency). An hCG test involves measuring baseline levels of testosterone and its precursors DHEA or DHEA sulfate and androstenedione and its metabolite DHT.
4. Imaging studies include abdomino-pelvic ultrasound (to determine presence or absence of a uterus, to visualize the presence or absence of gonads in the inguinal region, and to assess

the müllerian anatomy), genitourethrogram (to delineate the anatomy of the vagina and urethra, and where the vagina opens into the urogenital sinus), and pelvic MRI. Laparoscopic exploration with gonadal biopsy may be necessary to evaluate gonadal histology. Finally, molecular analysis may be required to arrive at a definitive diagnosis for some disorders.

D. **Interpretation of findings:** It can be difficult even for health care professionals to understand that only a minority of patients will receive a definitive diagnosis and prognosis in the neonatal period (Ono and Harley, 2013).
   1. The most common cause of genital ambiguity in the newborn is 21-OHD CAH, responsible for more than 90% of cases of ambiguous genitalia. It presents with a virilized XX (female) infant, and should be suspected in the presence of a virilized infant with a uterus and no palpable gonads (Ocal, 2011).
   2. Among the remainder of cases of ambiguous genitalia, the most common diagnoses are gonadal dysgenesis, followed by PAIS and testosterone biosynthetic disorders. Symmetrical external genitalia, with or without palpable gonads, and no uterus suggest an undervirilized male (Ocal, 2011). A micropenis should prompt investigation for hypopituitarism or GH deficiency, particularly in the presence of hypoglycemia (Lin-Su and New, 2012).
   3. It is not always possible to reach a diagnosis in the undervirilized male infant. In a study of 67 XY infants with external sexual ambiguity, testicular tissue, and/or an XY karyotype, in 52% of cases no diagnosis could be reached, despite an exhaustive clinical and laboratory workup, including sequencing of the androgen receptor (Morel et al., 2002).

E. **Talking with families.**
   1. Optimal care of the infant with a DSD involves a well-coordinated team, comprising at minimum the attending neonatologist, neonatal nurse, endocrinologist, pediatric surgeon/pediatric urologic surgeon, social worker, counselor or other mental health professional, and in some instances, geneticist (Romao et al., 2012), where the team is experienced in the management of DSDs (Ono and Harley, 2013).
   2. The initial contact with parents of a newborn with a DSD is extremely important. This interaction should emphasize that a DSD is not a shameful condition and does not preclude the child from becoming a well-adjusted, functional adult, who can be expected to lead a fulfilling life (Houk and Lee, 2012).
   3. A single person should communicate diagnostic findings and plans with the family. When discussing possible diagnoses with the family, language must be carefully chosen. Words such as "hermaphrodite," "pseudohermaphrodite," "ambiguous genitalia," "intersex," and "sex reversal" are outdated, confusing, and perceived as distasteful by many (Ono and Harley, 2013). Use accurate, informative terms that describe the infant's diagnosis.
   4. A clear explanation of sexual development in the fetus will help parents understand how an infant can be born with atypical genitalia, an important component of parental coping (Houk and Lee, 2005). Parents may find comfort in knowing that the appearance of the external genitalia is the result of prenatal androgen exposure and not caused by the molecular sex (Witchel and Azziz, 2011; Stokowski, 2014).
   5. It is the parents who have the responsibility to make or defer decisions about care for their infant with a DSD, including gender-of-rearing (Houk and Lee, 2005). The role of the health care team is to provide information, to share and explain all diagnostic findings, to inform parents of all available options, and to support the parents in the decision-making process.
   6. The approach should be family-centered as well as culturally sensitive. Family concerns must be respected and addressed in strict confidence. A relationship of trust requires open and honest communication and full disclosure of available information, including candid discussion of the controversies and dilemmas concerning gender assignment and early genital surgery.
   7. Parental acceptance of the child with a DSD is a key determinant of a favorable outcome (Houk and Lee, 2012). Health care professionals must also recognize and respect the cultural and psychosocial influences on parents' decisions about care for their infant.

F. **Gender assignment.**
   1. Parents are naturally anxious to find out their baby's gender so that they can name the baby and announce the birth to family and friends. Nevertheless, it must be sensitively

communicated that, although their distress is acknowledged, when gender is in doubt, a gender-of-rearing decision is one with lifelong implications and cannot be made in haste. Gender assignment must be deferred until expert evaluation of the newborn takes place and sufficient data are available for a fully informed decision (Lee et al., 2006; Lin-Su and New, 2012).

2. Unfortunately, some tests required for evaluation of a DSD must be sent out to referral laboratories, and the long wait for results can be frustrating for the parents. It is helpful if an experienced mental health professional can meet very early with the parents to help them decide what to tell family and friends while awaiting a final diagnosis (Ogilvy-Stuart and Brain, 2004).

## PANCREAS

A. **The pancreas is both an exocrine and endocrine gland.** The endocrine pancreas is responsible for hormonal regulation of blood glucose levels. The endocrine functions are performed by clusters of cells called islets of Langerhans that include alpha, beta, and delta cells. Hormones secreted by the endocrine pancreas include glucagon, insulin, amylin, and somatostatin.

B. **Fetal insulin, present by 8 to 10 weeks of gestation, is secreted in response to both glucose and amino acids.** The fetus is critically dependent for growth on its own supply of insulin, which does not cross the placenta. Insulin stimulates uptake of glucose by muscle and adipose tissue. The fetal pancreas becomes progressively more responsive to glucose late in gestation and beta cell mass increases markedly.

C. **At birth, when maternal glucose supply ceases, the neonate's blood glucose and insulin levels decline.** A concomitant surge in counterregulatory hormones epinephrine and glucagon sets in motion the production of glucose that will sustain the neonate until milk feeding is established.

D. **The exocrine portion of the pancreas constitutes 80% of the total gland.** Acinar cells secrete digestive enzymes, including trypsin, lipase, and amylase, into the duodenum.

### Disorders of the Pancreas

Rare pancreatic disorders in the newborn include congenital conditions such as pancreatic agenesis, pancreatic hypoplasia, and annular pancreas. Disorders of the endocrine pancreas include neonatal diabetes mellitus and hyperinsulinism, as well as the developmental disorder of the pancreas seen in the infant of the diabetic mother. The most common newborn disorder of the exocrine pancreas is cystic fibrosis (CF).

**Infant of a Diabetic Mother (see Chapter 9).** Diabetes in pregnancy is on the rise, paralleling the marked increase in people with type 2 diabetes and prediabetes (Homko, 2010). This has led to more newborns being at risk for the problems associated with glucose intolerance and abnormal glucose regulation during pregnancy.

**Neonatal Diabetes Mellitus (NDM).** NDM is a rare disorder manifested by persistent, insulin-sensitive hyperglycemia occurring as early as the first week of life and lasting more than 2 weeks. About half of all cases of NDM are of the transient form (TNDM), and half the permanent form (PNDM). The frequency of NDM is 1 in 100,000 live births (Grulich-Henn et al., 2010).

A. **Pathophysiology.**
   1. The fundamental problem in NDM is a failure of the pancreas to release sufficient insulin in response to high blood glucose levels.
   2. NDM is unrelated to the presence of anti-insulin or anti–islet cell antibodies. In TNDM, diabetes develops within days of birth and resolves again within weeks or months, before recurring, in a milder form, in late childhood.
   3. PNDM develop shortly after birth and persists throughout life. Most cases of PNDM are caused by transcription factors involved in beta cell development and in insulin secretion, the glucose-sensing enzyme glucokinase, and a gene-regulating immune response.

B. **Clinical manifestations.**
   1. A common feature of NDM is intrauterine growth restriction, a result of insufficient insulin secretion and subsequent failure to thrive in utero.

2. In addition to being small for gestational age, infants with NDM exhibit hyperglycemia, glycosuria, osmotic polyuria, dehydration, and ketoacidosis.

C. **Diagnosis.**

1. The diagnosis is made by demonstrating hyperglycemia with low levels of insulin, insulin-like growth factor-1, and C-peptide. The hyperglycemia responds to insulin infusion. Antibodies to insulin or islet cells are absent.
2. If there are signs and symptoms of malabsorption, pancreatic agenesis should be ruled out by abdominal ultrasound.
3. TNDM and PNDM cannot be differentiated, based on clinical course, in the neonatal period; genetic testing for chromosome 6 anomalies is required. If the neonate is shown to have a mutation of the $K_{ATP}$ channel, treatment with oral sulfonylureas, rather than insulin, is possible.

D. **Management.**

1. Insulin therapy is necessary in some affected infants to manage hyperglycemia and achieve adequate growth, initially by continuous drip and transitioning to subcutaneous injection of an intermediate-acting insulin preparation when condition permits. A high caloric intake can be difficult to maintain.
2. In some infants, insulin therapy can be withdrawn after a period of time when it is observed that exogenous insulin induces hypoglycemia.
3. The course of disease in NDM is highly variable. Some infants with TNDM will have spontaneous recovery with no further disease recurrence, whereas others will have apparent remission with recurrence of permanent disease in late childhood. Infants with PNDM have no remission of their disease.
4. The opportunity for parents to speak with the pediatric endocrinologist and geneticist should be provided, if possible, for information and guidance about both the cause of NDM and the plans for continuing care for their infant. Close follow-up is essential even if the diabetes has resolved because of the high rate of recurrence later in childhood.

**Congenital Hyperinsulinism.** Congenital hyperinsulinism is not a single disorder, but a group of disorders with the common feature of hyperinsulinemic hypoglycemia, secondary to inappropriate secretion of insulin (Arnoux et al., 2011). It is the most frequent cause of severe, persistent hypoglycemia in the newborn, with an incidence of 1 in 30,000 to 50,000 live births (Jain et al., 2012). Several different genetic forms have been described. Between 10% and 15% of congenital hyperinsulinism is transient and will spontaneously resolve at 1 month of age. Beckwith–Wiedemann syndrome is a congenital overgrowth syndrome with hyperinsulinism caused by beta cell hyperplasia.

A. **Pathophysiology.**

1. Hyperinsulinism is due to unregulated insulin release either from the entire pancreas (diffuse beta cell hyperfunction) or from confined areas of the pancreas (focal adenomatous islet-cell hyperplasia).
2. Insulin lowers circulating glucose, suppressing lipolysis and ketogenesis and decreasing the availability of free fatty acids and ketone bodies. Because these are alternative energy substrates for the brain during hypoglycemia, hyperinsulinemia places the infant at risk for severe neurologic dysfunction and seizures as consequences of neuroglycopenia.

B. **Clinical manifestations.**

1. Most infants with congenital hyperinsulinism present shortly after birth. Generally they are born at term and are normal or large for gestational age.
2. Many are macrosomic with a characteristic facial appearance.
3. Neonates with Beckwith–Wiedemann syndrome present with a constellation of findings including macroglossia, abdominal wall defects, Wilms' tumors, renal abnormalities, and facial nevus.

C. **Diagnosis.**

1. Severe hypoglycemia with an insulin level that is inappropriate to the level of blood glucose (e.g., an insulin level >5 mU/ml with a plasma glucose level <50 mg/dL) suggests the diagnosis.
2. Other diagnostic criteria are a high glucose requirement (>6 to 8 mg/kg/min) needed to maintain normoglycemia, low serum blood glucose by laboratory analysis, measurable insulin, elevated C-peptide, low free fatty acids, and low ketone body concentrations.

3. Blood sampling must take place during hypoglycemia to be of diagnostic value (Jain et al., 2012).

D. **Management.**

1. Management involves a high caloric intake and pharmacologic therapy to inhibit insulin secretion by the pancreas. A central venous catheter is required for reliable and safe administration of high glucose infusates. Glucose infusion rates of 10 to 15 mg/kg/min or higher may be required, and the rate of glucose necessary to maintain normoglycemia (fasting blood glucose > 70 mg/dL) is an indicator of the severity of the disease (Arnoux et al., 2011).
2. Drugs include diazoxide, which inhibits insulin secretion by blocking the sulfonylurea receptor of the beta cell, and octreotide, a somatostatin analogue. Diazoxide must be used with caution in the presence of hyperbilirubinemia because it is highly protein bound and will displace bilirubin from albumin-binding sites. Glucagon to mobilize hepatic glucose can be added if needed as a short-term adjunct to therapy (Arnoux et al., 2011).
3. The response to these agents is inconsistent and variable. Infants who do not show an adequate and immediate response may require pancreatectomy to prevent recurrent neuroglycopenia. Preoperative localization procedures and intraoperative biopsies will determine the exact nature of the lesion and how much of the pancreas must be removed. Focal disease may require only a partial pancreatectomy, but a near-total (>95%) removal of the pancreas is indicated for diffuse congenital hyperinsulinism. Loss of the pancreas can pose additional risks such as pancreatic insufficiency and diabetes mellitus.

**Cystic Fibrosis.** CF is an autosomal recessive disorder caused by mutations in the gene encoding for the cystic fibrosis transmembrane conductance regulator (CFTR) protein, of which more than 1500 have been identified (O'Sullivan and Freedman, 2009). Data from newborn screening programs in the United States reveal that CF occurs in 1 in 3000 whites and 1 in 15,000 to 20,000 blacks (Walters and Mehta, 2007).

A. **Pathophysiology.**

1. Mutations in the CFTR gene affect the cyclic adenosine-5′-monophosphate (AMP)–mediated signals that stimulate chloride conductance in the epithelial cells of the exocrine ducts. Deficient chloride transport and the associated water-transport abnormalities result in the production of abnormally viscid mucus.
2. Nearly all organs and systems of the body are affected, including the lungs and upper respiratory tract, gastrointestinal tract, pancreas, liver, sweat glands, and genitourinary tract. Hyperviscous secretions in the intestines and a deficiency of pancreatic enzymes combine to create a sticky plug of meconium, a condition known as meconium ileus (see Chapter 29). The meconium has a higher protein and lower carbohydrate concentration, making it more viscid than normal meconium.

B. **Clinical manifestations.**

1. Without a family history or prenatal screening, CF is not recognized at the time of birth in most affected neonates unless a meconium ileus is present, typically identified by 24 to 48 hours of age.
3. Although not always present in the neonatal period, most patients with CF have pancreatic enzyme insufficiency and present with digestive symptoms or failure to thrive early in life.
4. Other neonatal signs and symptoms include intestinal atresia, prolonged jaundice, and abdominal or scrotal calcifications (O'Sullivan and Freedman, 2009).

C. **Diagnosis.**

1. The possibility of CF is raised in the neonate with meconium ileus, and can be confirmed with DNA testing. A sweat test can also be performed after the first 48 hours of life. A sweat test uses electrical–chemical stimulation of the skin to induce sweat, which is collected and analyzed for chloride content.
2. Newborn screening for CF is accomplished by measuring immunoreactive trypsinogen in dried blood samples. Screening for CF is conducted in all 50 states and the District of Columbia (Wagener et al., 2012).

D. **Management.**

1. A meconium ileus requires prompt attention to prevent complications such as volvulus, sepsis, bowel necrosis, or intestinal perforation.

2. CF is also managed with a diet high in energy and fat to compensate for malabsorption and the increased energy demand of chronic inflammation. In addition to vitamin and mineral supplementation, a hydrolyzed protein formula containing medium-chain triglycerides is used, because they do not require digestion by pancreatic enzymes for absorption.
3. Pancreatic enzyme supplements are also needed to improve fat absorption. Meticulous care of the perianal area must be taken because these enzymes can cause severe perianal dermatitis.
4. Breastfeeding has been shown to be beneficial for infants with CF, although growth might be slightly slower, and should be encouraged (Wagener et al., 2012).
5. Infants can also develop early pulmonary infections with *Staphylococcus aureus* followed often by *Pseudomonas aeruginosa* (Wagener et al., 2012).

## REFERENCES


Alatzoglou, K.S. and Dattani, M.T.: Genetic forms of hypopituitarism and their manifestation in the neonatal period. *Early Human Development*, 85(11):705–712, 2009.

Allen, L.: Disorders of sexual development. *Obstetrics and Gynecology Clinics of North America*, 36:25–45, 2009.

Anway, M.D. and Skinner, M.K.: Epigenetic programming of the germ line: Effects of endocrine disruptors on the development of transgenerational disease. *Reproductive Biomedicine Online*, 16(1):23–25, 2008.

Arnoux, J.B., Verkarre, V., Saint-Martin, C., et al.: Congenital hyperinsulinism: Current trends in diagnosis and therapy. *Orphanet Journal of Rare Diseases*, 3:63, 2011.

Auchus, R.H., Witchel, S.F., Leight, K.R., et al.: Guidelines for the development of comprehensive care centers for congenital adrenal hyperplasia: Guidance from the CARES Foundation Initiative. *International Journal of Pediatric Endocrinology*, 2010:275213, 2010.

Bancalari, R.E., Gregory, L.C., McCabe, M.J. and Dattani, M.T.: Pituitary gland development: an update. *Endocrine Development*, 23:1–15, 2012.

Bollepalli, S. and Rose, S.R.: Disorders of the thyroid gland. In C.A. Gleason, and S.U. Devaskar (Eds.): *Avery's diseases of the newborn* (9th ed.). Philadelphia, 2012, Elsevier Saunders, pp. 1307–1319.

Brook, C.G.D. and Dattani, M.T.: Handbook of clinical pediatric endocrinology. Hoboken NJ, 2012, Wiley-Blackwell.

Canadian Organization for Rare Disorders: *Newborn screening status report*, 2012. Retrieved May 18, 2013, from http://raredisorders.ca/documents/CanadaNBSstatusupdatedMay52012.pdf.

Cangul, H., Aycan, Z., Saglam, H., et al.: TSHR is the main causative locus in autosomal recessively inherited thyroid dysgenesis. *Journal of Pediatric Endocrinology and Metabolism*, 25(5–6):419–426, 2012.

Clemente, M., Ruiz-Cuevas, P., Carrascosa, A., et al.: Thyroid function in preterm infants 27-29 weeks of gestational age during the first four months of life: Results from a prospective study comprising 80 preterm infants. *Journal of Pediatric Endocrinology and Metabolism*, 20(12):1269–1280, 2007.

Connelly, K.J., Boston, B.A., Pearce, E.N., et al.: Congenital hypothyroidism caused by excess prenatal maternal iodine ingestion. *Journal of Pediatrics*, 161 (4):760–762, 2012.

Copelovitch, L. and Kaplan, B.S.: Glomerulonephropathies and disorders of tubular function. In C.A. Gleason, and S.U. Devaskar (Eds.): *Avery's diseases of the newborn* (9th ed.). Philadelphia, 2012, Elsevier Saunders, pp. 1222–1227.

Custodio, R.J., Junior, C.E., Milani, S.L., et al.: The emergence of the cortisol circadian rhythm in monozygotic and dizygotic twin infants: The twin-pair synchrony. *Clinical Endocrinology (Oxford)*, 66(2):192–197, 2007.

Fisher, D.A.: Thyroid function and dysfunction in premature infants. *Pediatric Endocrinology Reviews*, 4 (4):317–328, 2007.

Fisher, D.A.: The importance of early management in optimizing IQ in infants with congenital hypothyroidism. *Journal of Pediatrics*, 136(3):273–274, 2000.

Forghani, N. and Aye, T.: Hypothyroxinemia and prematurity. *NeoReviews*, 9(2):e66–e71, 2008.

Fruzza, A.G., Demeterco-Berggren, C. and Jones, K.L.: Unawareness of the effects of soy intake on the management of congenital hypothyroidism. *Pediatrics*, 130 (3):e699–e702, 2012.

Garcia-Fillon, P. and Borchert, M.: Optic nerve hypoplasia syndrome: A review of the epidemiology and clinical associations. *Current Treatment Options in Neurology*, 15(1):78–89, 2013.

Grulich-Henn, J., Wagner, V., Thon, A., et al.: Entities and frequency of neonatal diabetes: Data from the Diabetes Documentation and Quality Management System (DVP). *Diabetic Medicine*, 27:709–712, 2010.

Homko, C.J.: Gestational diabetes mellitus: can we reach consensus? *Current Diabetes Reports*, 10:252–254, 2010.

Houk, C.P. and Lee, P.A.: Update on disorders of sex development. *Current Opinion in Endocrinology, Diabetes, and Obesity*, 19:28–32, 2012.

Houk, C.P. and Lee, P.A.: Intersexed states: Diagnosis and management. *Endocrinology and Metabolism Clinics of North America*, 34(3):791–810, 2005.

Intersex Society of North America: What does the ISNA recommend for children with intersex? 2006. Retrieved February 28, 2008, from www.isna.org.

Jain, V., Chen, M. and Menon, R.K.: Disorders of carbohydrate metabolism. In C.A. Gleason, and S.U. Devaskar (Eds.): *Avery's diseases of the newborn* (9th ed.). Philadelphia, 2012, Elsevier Saunders.

Janjua, H.S. and Batisky, D.L.: Renal vascular disease in the newborn. In C.A. Gleason, and S.U. Devaskar

(Eds.): *Avery's diseases of the newborn* (9th ed.). Philadelphia, 2012, Elsevier Saunders.

Kohler, B., Lumbroso, S., Leger, J., et al.: Androgen insensitivity syndrome: Somatic mosaicism of the androgen receptor in seven families and consequences for sex assignment and genetic counseling. *Journal of Clinical Endocrinology and Metabolism*, 90:106–111, 2005.

La Gamma, E.F. and Paneth, N.: Clinical importance of hypothyroxinemia in the preterm infant and a discussion of treatment concerns. *Current Opinion in Pediatrics*, 24(2):172–180, 2012.

Lee, P.A., Houk, C.P., Ahmed, S.F., et al.: Consensus statement on management of intersex disorders. International consensus conference on Intersex. *Pediatrics*, 118(2):e488–e500, 2006.

Lin-Su, K. and New, M.I.: Ambiguous genitalia in the newborn. In C.A. Gleason, and S.U. Devaskar (Eds.): *Avery's diseases of the newborn* (9th ed.). Philadelphia, 2012, Elsevier Saunders.

LynShue, K.A. and Witchel, S.F.: Endocrinology. In B.J. Zitelli, and H.W. Davis (Eds.): *Atlas of pediatric physical diagnosis* Philadelphia, 2007, Elsevier Saunders.

Morel, Y., Rey, R., Teinturier, C., et al.: Aetiological diagnosis of male sex ambiguity: A collaborative study. *European Journal of Pediatrics*, 161:49–59, 2002.

Mutlu, M., Karaguzel, G., Aslan, Y., et al.: Adrenal hemorrhage in newborns: A retrospective study. *World Journal of Pediatrics*, 7:355–357, 2011.

National Newborn Screening and Genetics Resource Center: National newborn screening status report, January, 2013. Retrieved from http://genes-r-us.uthscsa.edu/sites/genes-r-us/files/nbsdisorders.pdf.

Ng, P.C.: Effect of stress on the hypothalamic-pituitary-adrenal axis in the fetus and newborn. *Journal of Pediatrics*, 158(2 Suppl.):e41–e43, 2011.

Nimkarn, S. and New, M.I.: Disorders of the adrenal gland. In C.A. Gleason, and S.U. Devaskar (Eds.): *Avery's diseases of the newborn* (9th ed.). Philadelphia, 2012, Elsevier Saunders.

Nimkarn, S. and New, M.I.: Prenatal diagnosis and treatment of congenital adrenal hyperplasia. *Pediatric Endocrinology Reviews*, 4(2):99–105, 2006.

Ocal, G.: Current concepts in disorders of sexual development. *Journal of Clinical Research in Pediatric Endocrinology*, 3:105–114, 2011.

Ogilvy-Stuart, A.L. and Brain, C.E.: Early assessment of ambiguous genitalia. *Archives of Diseases in Childhood*, 89(5):401–407, 2004.

Ogilvy-Stuart, A.L. and Midgley, P.: *Practical neonatal endocrinology*. Cambridge, MA, 2006, Cambridge University Press.

Ono, M. and Harley, V.R.: Disorders of sex development: New genes, new concepts. *Nature Reviews Endocrinology*, 9(2):79–91, 2013.

Osborn, D.A. and Hunt, R.W.: Postnatal prophylactic thyroid hormones for prevention of morbidity and mortality in preterm infants. *Cochrane Database of Systematic Reviews* (1): CD005948, 2007.

O'Sullivan, B.P. and Freedman, S.D.: Cystic fibrosis. *Lancet*, 373:1891–1904, 2009.

Peters, C.J. and Hindmarsh, P.C.: Management of neonatal endocrinopathies—best practice guidelines. *Early Human Development*, 83:553–561, 2007.

Rastogi, M.V. and LaFranchi, S.H.: Congenital hypothyroidism. *Orphanet Journal of Rare Diseases*, 5:17, 2010.

Romao, R.L., Salle, J.L. and Wherrett, D.K.: Update on the management of disorders of sex development. *Pediatric Clinics of North America*, 59(4):853–869, 2012.

Speiser, P.W., Azziz, R., Baskin, L.S., et al.: Congenital adrenal hyperplasia due to steroid 21-hydroxylase deficiency: An Endocrine Society Clinical Practice Guideline. *Journal of Clinical Endocrinology and Metabolism*, 95:4133–4160, 2010.

Stokowski, L.A.: Endocrine system. In C. Kenner, and J.W. Lott (Eds.): *Comprehensive Neonatal Nursing Care* (5th ed.). New York, 2014, Springer Publishing.

Tuladhar, R., Davis, P.G., Batch, J. and Doyle, L.W.: Establishment of a normal range of penile length in preterm infants. *Journal of Paediatric and Child Health*, 34:471–473, 1998.

van Wassenaer, A.G. and Kok, J.H.: Hypothyroxinaemia and thyroid function after preterm birth. *Seminars in Neonatology*, 9:3–11, 2004.

Wagener, J.S., Zemanick, E.T. and Sontag, M.K.: Newborn screening for cystic fibrosis. *Current Opinion in Pediatrics*, 24(3):329–335, 2012.

Walters, S. and Mehta, A.: Epidemiology of cystic fibrosis. In M. Hodson, D.M. Geddes, and A. Bush (Eds.): *Cystic fibrosis* (3rd ed.). London, 2007, Edward Arnold Ltd., pp. 21–45.

Wilson, J.D.: The evolution of endocrinology. *Clinical Endocrinology*, 62(4):389–396, 2005.

Witchel, S.F. and Azziz, R.: Congenital adrenal hyperplasia. *Journal of Pediatric and Adolescent Gynecology*, 24(3):116–126.

Zimmermann, M.B.: The effects of iodine deficiency in pregnancy and infancy. *Paediatric and Perinatal Epidemiology*, 26(Suppl. 1):108–117, 2012.

CHAPTER

# 31 Hematologic Disorders

WILLIAM DIEHL-JONES AND DEBBIE FRASER

**OBJECTIVES**

1. Understand the processes of hematopoiesis and erythropoiesis.
2. Recall erythrocyte and leukocyte development from pluripotent stem cells.
3. Relate the consequences of anemia to the management of the infant.
4. Evaluate the clinical presentation of disseminated intravascular coagulation in relation to the coagulation consumption and fibrinolysis.
5. Describe the etiologic factors of hemorrhagic disease of the newborn.
6. Describe key indicators for nursing assessment of the thrombocytopenic infant.
7. Evaluate the neonatal consequences of maternal immune thrombocytopenic purpura.
8. Discuss the role of partial exchange transfusion in the treatment of neonatal polycythemia.
9. Describe current recommendations for use of blood components.
10. Analyze the components of the complete blood cell count and describe the usefulness of each in the determination of neonatal sepsis.

To meet the objectives, this chapter presents an overview of blood cell development and coagulation factors, and includes normal birth values and common diagnostic tests. Blood products and transfusion therapies are discussed with current recommendations for use. Common hematologic problems and therapies affecting the newborn infant are outlined. An evaluation of the red blood cell (RBC) indices, useful for diagnosis of hematologic disorders, is included.

## DEVELOPMENT OF BLOOD CELLS

A. **Hematopoiesis:** formation, production, and maintenance of blood cells (Blackburn, 2013; Blanchette et al., 2005; Brugnara and Platt, 2009; Luchtman-Jones and Wilson, 2011; Ohls, 2011).
B. **Fetal hematopoiesis:** occurs in three distinct phases, mesoblastic, hepatic, and myeloid.
   1. RBCs arising from embryonic connective tissues or mesenchyme can be seen by the 14th day of gestation.
   2. Primitive erythroblasts arising from megaloblasts are detectable in circulating blood between 21 and 35 days of gestation.
   3. Extravascular liver hematopoiesis begins with migration of pluripotent stem cells from the yolk sac, well established by week 5 or 6 of gestation.
   4. Liver hematopoiesis peaks at 3 to 6 months of gestation and then slowly regresses as medullary (bone marrow) hematopoiesis predominates from 22 weeks of gestation.
   5. Sites of extramedullary hematopoiesis (spleen, lymph nodes, thymus, kidneys) aid production of cells during fetal life when long bones are small.
   6. Pluripotent cells develop into either colony-forming unit–granulocyte, erythrocyte, monocyte, macrophage (CFU-GEMM), colony-forming unit–erythroid (CFU-E), or colony-forming unit–granulocyte-macrophage (CFU-GM) cell lines, which evolve into specific cell lines (Fig. 31-1).
   7. Hypoxia, bacterial infection, and other forms of physiologic stress can influence the rate of differentiation of pluripotent cells.
   8. Hematopoietic factors include interleukins (ILs; e.g., IL-1 through IL-4, IL-6 through IL-8, and IL-10 through IL-12), growth and differentiation factors such as granulocyte

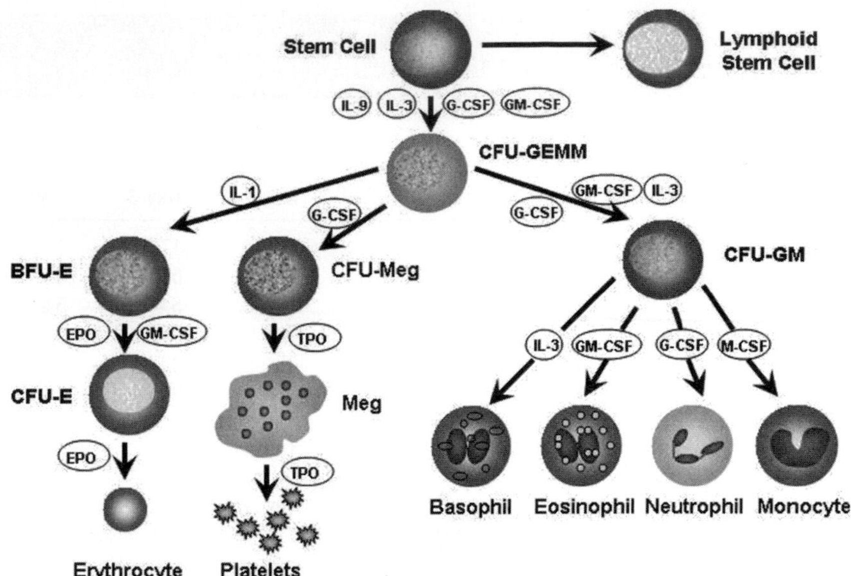


FIGURE 31-1 ■ Hematopoiesis and selected growth factors. *BFU-E*, Burst-forming unit, erythroid; *CFU-E*, colony-forming unit–erythroid; *CFU-GEMM*, colony-forming unit–granulocyte, erythrocyte, monocyte, macrophage; *CFU-GM*, colony-forming unit–granulocyte-macrophage; *CFU-Meg*, colony-forming unit–megakaryocyte; *EPO*, erythropoietin; *G-CSF*, granulocyte colony-stimulating factor; *GM-CSF*, granulocyte–macrophage colony-stimulating factor; *IL-1*, interleukin-1; *IL-3*, interleukin-3; *IL-9*, interleukin-9; *M-CSF*, macrophage colony-stimulating factor; *Meg*, megakaryocyte; *TPO*, thrombopoietin. (Adapted from Israels, L.G. and Israels, S.J.: *Mechanisms in hematology* [3rd ed.]. Toronto, 2002, Core Health Sciences, Inc., p. 402.)

colony-stimulating factor (G-CSF), macrophage colony-stimulating factor (M-CSF), granulocyte–macrophage colony-stimulating factor (GM-CSF), thrombopoietin, and erythropoietin.

C. **Erythropoiesis:** production of erythrocytes (RBCs).
   1. The erythrocyte precursor or burst-forming unit, erythroid (BFU-E) develops from a myeloid stem cell (CFU-GEMM), which also differentiates to produce a megakaryocyte precursor (CFU-Meg).
   2. Erythropoiesis and synthesis of hemoglobin are regulated by a hormone, erythropoietin, which is in turn regulated by hypoxia-sensing mechanisms in the fetal liver and kidney.
   3. Erythropoietin is produced postnatally in the kidneys, but during fetal life extrarenal sites (liver, submandibular glands) predominate.
   4. Erythropoietin levels are increased in response to anemia and low oxygen availability to tissues and are decreased in response to hypertransfusion.
   5. Erythropoietin levels are also elevated in infants with Down syndrome or intrauterine growth restriction, and those born to women with diabetes or pregnancy-induced hypertension.

D. **Hemoglobin:** major iron-containing component of the RBCs.
   1. Hemoglobin carries oxygen from the lungs to the tissue cells through the circulation
   2. Hemoglobin synthesis begins around 14 days of embryonic life.
   3. Transition from predominant production of fetal hemoglobin (HbF) to production of adult hemoglobin (HbA) begins at the end of fetal life. RBCs contain 70% to 90% HbF at birth. The switch to production of HbA is delayed in cases of maternal hypoxia or fetal growth restriction, and in infants of diabetic mothers.
   4. Hemoglobin binds with 2,3-diphosphoglycerate (2,3-DPG), releasing an oxygen molecule.
      a. HbF has far less affinity for 2,3-DPG than does HbA, resulting in a greater affinity for oxygen.
      b. Levels of 2,3-DPG are directly proportional to gestational age.
   5. Normal birth values (Table 31-1).
      a. Values depend on gestational age, volume of placental transfusion (timing of cord clamping, infant position), and blood sampling site; hemoglobin in capillary samples may be significantly higher than in venous samples.

■ TABLE 31-1
■ ■ **Normal Blood Values in Premature and Term Infants**

| Value | Gestational Age (weeks) 28 | 34 | Term Cord Blood | Day 1 | Day 3 | Day 7 | Day 14 |
|---|---|---|---|---|---|---|---|
| Hb (g/dl) | 14.5 | 15 | 16.8 | 18.4 | 17.8 | 17 | 16.8 |
| Hematocrit (%) | 45 | 47 | 53 | 58 | 55 | 54 | 52 |
| Red cells ($mm^3$) | 4 | 4.4 | 5.25 | 5.8 | 5.6 | 5.2 | 5.1 |
| MCV ($\mu^3$) | 120 | 118 | 107 | 108 | 99 | 98 | 96 |
| MCH (pg) | 40 | 38 | 34 | 35 | 33 | 32.5 | 31.5 |
| MCHC (%) | 31 | 32 | 31.7 | 32.5 | 33 | 33 | 33 |
| Reticulocytes (%) | 5 to 10 | 3 to 10 | 3 to 7 | 3 to 7 | 1 to 3 | 0 to 1 | 0 to 1 |
| Platelets (1000 s/$mm^3$) | | | 290 | 192 | 213 | 248 | 252 |

From Klaus, M.H. and Fanaroff, A.A.: *Care of the high-risk neonate* (5th ed.). Philadelphia, 2001, W.B. Saunders.
*Hb*, Hemoglobin; *MCH*, mean corpuscular hemoglobin; *MCHC*, mean corpuscular hemoglobin concentration; *MCV*, mean corpuscular volume.

**b.** Peripheral vasoconstriction and stasis yield higher values from capillary samples.
**c.** Hemoglobin levels are higher in newborns, and decrease by the end of the first week of life to values similar to cord blood.
**d.** Increased $Pa_{O_2}$ following delivery and increase in HbA causes a decrease in erythropoietin, leading to a gradual decline in hemoglobin (Luchtman-Jones and Wilson, 2011).

**E. Hematocrit:** percentage of RBCs in a unit volume of blood.
1. Values rise immediately after birth and then decline to cord levels in the first week.
2. Normal birth values (see Table 31-1).
   **a.** Values depend on gestational age and volume of placental transfusion (timing of cord clamping, infant position).
   **b.** Peripheral vasoconstriction and stasis yield higher values from capillary samples.

**F. RBCs.**
1. The erythrocyte BFU-E differentiates, under hormonal control, to form a CFU-E, which loses its nucleus as it forms erythrocytes (see Fig. 31-1).
2. The CFU-Es (or reticulocytes), in the absence of physiologic stress, mature 1 to 2 days in the bone marrow and then another day in the circulation before maturing to erythrocytes.
   **a.** Reticulocyte count is inversely proportional to gestational age at birth (see Table 31-1) but falls rapidly to less than 2% by 7 days.
   **b.** Persistent reticulocytosis may indicate chronic blood loss or hemolysis.
3. RBC function.
   **a.** Oxygen transport via oxyhemoglobin.
   **b.** Carbon dioxide transport via carboxyhemoglobin.
   **c.** Carbon dioxide reacts with water to form carbonic acid; reaction catalyzed by carbonic anhydrase in the cytoplasm of RBCs.
   **d.** Carbonic acid dissociation to form bicarbonate ions.
   **e.** Buffering of protons via binding with hemoglobin to form acid hemoglobin and by reaction with bicarbonate ions.
4. RBC count.
   **a.** Number of circulating mature RBCs per cubic millimeter (see Table 31-1).
   **b.** Count equals production versus destruction or loss.
   **c.** RBC life span proportional to gestational age.
      (1) Adult: 100 to 120 days.
      (2) Term infant: 60 to 70 days.
      (3) Premature infant: 35 to 50 days.
   **d.** Nucleated RBCs are circulating immature (prereticulocyte) RBCs.
      (1) Number is inversely proportional to gestational age and declines rapidly in the first week.

(2) Increase may indicate hemolysis, acute blood loss, hypoxemia, congenital heart disease, or infection.

5. RBC indices: measure of RBC size and hemoglobin content used for designation of anemias (see Table 31-1).
   a. Mean corpuscular volume (MCV): average size and volume of a single RBC.
      (1) MCV decreases as gestation progresses and continues to decrease after birth to adult size by 4 to 5 years.
      (2) Increased MCV: RBCs referred to as macrocytes.
      (3) Decreased MCV: RBCs referred to as microcytes.
   b. Mean corpuscular hemoglobin (MCH): average amount (by weight) of hemoglobin in each RBC.
      (1) A decrease in MCH parallels a decrease in MCV.
      (2) Increased MCH: RBCs appear hyperchromic.
      (3) Decreased MCH: RBCs appear hypochromic.
   c. Mean corpuscular hemoglobin concentration (MCHC): average concentration of hemoglobin per single RBC, calculated from the amount of hemoglobin per deciliter of cells.
      (1) Adult values for MCHC reached by 6 months.
      (2) Increased MCHC: RBCs appear hyperchromic.
      (3) Decreased MCHC: RBCs appear hypochromic.
   d. Erythrocyte mass: total mass of erythrocytes.
      (1) Best measure of anemia.
      (2) Direct correlation between erythrocyte mass and hemoglobin concentration.
      (3) Gold standard is use of chromium-labeled erythrocytes.

**G. White blood cells (WBCs).**

1. Leukocyte precursors mature in the bone marrow and lymphatic tissues, in the absence of physiologic stress, through the CFU-GEMM and CFU-GM stages (see Fig. 31-1).
2. WBCs can leave the circulation to enter the extravascular tissues, where they function as an important part of the immunologic system in reaction to foreign protein.
3. Granulocytes, lymphocytes, and monocytes are types of WBCs.
   a. Granulocytes: include basophils, eosinophils, and neutrophils.
      (1) Basophils.
         (a) Important in allergic and inflammatory responses.
         (b) Least numerous of the granulocytes: 0.5% to 1% of total WBC count.
      (2) Eosinophils.
         (a) Perform similar functions as neutrophils but are less effective in response.
         (b) Unlike neutrophils, can survive for prolonged periods in extravascular space.
         (c) Important in allergic and anaphylactic responses and most effective granulocyte for parasitic destruction.
         (d) Benign eosinophilia of prematurity, inversely proportional to gestational age, may reflect immaturity of barrier mechanisms in the gastrointestinal and/or respiratory tract (Blanchette et al., 2005).
         (e) Normally comprise 1% to 3% of total WBC count.
      (3) Neutrophils.
         (a) Neutrophils function as phagocytes that ingest and destroy small particles such as bacteria, protozoa, cells and cellular debris, and colloids.
         (b) Physiologic stress can increase production and bone marrow release of immature forms.
         (c) Neutrophils are increased at birth but decrease during the first week to reach percentages approximately equal to those of lymphocytes.
   b. Lymphocytes.
      (1) Thymus-derived (T) lymphocytes: important in graft-versus-host disease and delayed hypersensitivity reactions.
      (2) Bone marrow–derived (B) lymphocytes: important in the production and secretion of immunoglobulins and antibodies.
   c. Monocytes.
      (1) Circulating immature macrophages.

■ TABLE 31-2
■ ■ **Normal Leukocyte Values in Premature and Term Infants**

| Age (hours) | Total White Cell Count | Neutrophils | Bands/Metas | Lymphocytes | Monocytes | Eosinophils |
|---|---|---|---|---|---|---|
| **TERM INFANTS** | | | | | | |
| 0 | 10.0 to 26.0 | 5.0 to 13.0 | 0.4 to 1.8 | 3.5 to 8.5 | 0.7 to 1.5 | 0.2 to 2.0 |
| 12 | 13.5 to 31.0 | 9.0 to 18.0 | 0.4 to 2.0 | 3.0 to 7.0 | 1.0 to 2.0 | 0.2 to 2.0 |
| 72 | 5.0 to 14.5 | 2.0 to 7.0 | 0.2 to 0.4 | 2.0 to 5.0 | 0.5 to 1.0 | 0.2 to 1.0 |
| 144 | 6.0 to 14.5 | 2.0 to 6.0 | 0.2 to 0.5 | 3.0 to 6.0 | 0.7 to 1.2 | 0.2 to 0.8 |
| **PREMATURE INFANTS** | | | | | | |
| 0 | 5.0 to 19.0 | 2.0 to 9.0 | 0.2 to 2.4 | 2.5 to 6.0 | 0.3 to 1.0 | 0.1 to 0.7 |
| 12 | 5.0 to 21.0 | 3.0 to 11.0 | 0.2 to 2.4 | 1.5 to 5.0 | 0.3 to 1.3 | 0.1 to 1.1 |
| 72 | 5.0 to 14.0 | 3.0 to 7.0 | 0.2 to 0.6 | 1.5 to 4.0 | 0.3 to 1.2 | 0.2 to 1.1 |
| 144 | 5.5 to 17.5 | 2.0 to 7.0 | 0.2 to 0.5 | 2.5 to 7.5 | 0.5 to 1.5 | 0.3 to 1.2 |

From Oski, F.A. and Naiman, J.L.: *Hematologic problems in the newborn* (3rd ed.). Philadelphia, 1982, W.B. Saunders.

(2) Transformed into macrophages in tissues (i.e., lung—alveolar macrophages; liver—Kupffer cell macrophages).

(3) Responsible for clearance of old blood cells, cellular debris, opsonized bacteria, antigen–antibody complexes, and activated clotting factors from the circulation.

**4.** WBC count.

**a.** WBC count is the number of circulating WBCs per cubic millimeter (Table 31-2).

**b.** WBC count is proportional to gestational age, with the total counts of premature infants approximately 30% to 50% lower than those of term infants.

**H. Platelets.**

**1.** Small, nonnucleated, disk-shaped cells aid in hemostasis, coagulation, and thrombus formation.

**a.** Platelets are derived from megakaryocytes in the bone marrow.

**b.** Disrupted endothelium stimulates platelet plug formation and initiates hemostasis.

**2.** After release into the bloodstream, platelets will circulate 7 to 10 days before removal by the spleen. In the absence of injury, they circulate freely, without wall adhesion or aggregation with other platelets.

**3.** Normal range is 150,000 to 400,000/$mm^3$ in the term infant. Premature infants have a lower platelet count with a broader range of normal (100,000 to 450,000) (Nguyen-Vermillion and Juul, 2012). Counts are 20% to 25% lower in infants who are small for gestational age.

**4.** Neonatal platelets are hypoactive in the first few days after birth; this property protects against thrombosis but may increase risk of bleeding and coagulopathy.

**I. Blood volume.**

**1.** Volume of blood is measured in milliliters per kilogram of body weight.

**2.** Factors affecting blood volume are as follows:

**a.** Gestational age.

(1) Term infant: approximately 80 to 100 mL/kg.

(2) Preterm infant: approximately 90 to 105 mL/kg.

**b.** Placental transfusion.

(1) Timing of cord clamping.

(2) Position of infant relative to placenta (above or below) before cord clamping.

(3) Timing and strength of uterine contractions.

(4) Onset of respiration and decrease in pulmonary vascular resistance.

(5) Cord compression.

**c.** Maternal–fetal or fetal–maternal transfusion.

**d.** Twin-to-twin transfusion.

e. Placenta previa or abruptio placentae.
f. Nuchal cord.
g. Iatrogenic loss.

## COAGULATION

Hemostasis is accomplished by biochemical and physiologic events initiated to stop the flow of blood when vessel injury occurs (Young, 2012).

A. **Deficiencies in newborn clotting mechanisms.**
   1. Transient diminished platelet function.
   2. Transient deficiency of clotting factors II, VII, IX, X, XI, and XII. Neonatal levels are approximately 50% of adult levels in the early weeks after birth (Blackburn, 2013).
      a. Immaturity of hepatic enzymes responsible for production.
      b. Transient deficiency of vitamin K, needed for synthesis of factors II, VII, IX, and X.
      c. Factor concentrations: proportional to gestational age.

B. **Hemostatic mechanisms.**
   1. Vascular: damaged vessel contracts, minimizing blood loss.
   2. Intravascular: platelet plug formation. Platelet function is stimulated by exposure to damaged endothelial lining. Platelets:
      a. Swell and develop thornlike projections.
      b. Adhere to subendothelial fibers.
      c. Secrete adenosine diphosphate to trigger swelling and adhesiveness in nearby platelets.
      d. Aggregate and form platelet plug.
   3. Extravascular.
      a. Compression by surrounding tissue.
      b. Release of tissue thromboplastin by injured tissue.

C. **Coagulation process.**
   1. Cascade of events, requiring both cellular and plasma components (Fig. 31-2).
   2. Culminates in the formation of fibrin-based clots, and requires serial activation of precursor zymogens.
   3. Calcium, iron, and phospholipids are key components of the coagulation cascade.
      a. Extrinsic system triggered by tissue injury and exposure of cell membrane tissue factor.
      b. Intrinsic system triggered by vascular endothelial injury; amplifies factor X activation, which is a cofactor common to intrinsic and extrinsic pathways.
      c. Factor X activation begins the process of prothrombin-to-thrombin conversion. Conversion hydrolyzes fibrinogen (soluble protein in plasma) to fibrin (insoluble, threadlike polymer) and activates factor XIII, stabilizing fibrin threads into a meshwork to trap platelets and other cells to form the clot.
   4. Intravascular clotting is balanced by concurrent fibrinolysis.
      a. Inactive plasminogen synthesized by the liver is converted to plasmin, an active enzyme, when a fibrin clot is present.
      b. Plasmin begins fibrin clot dissolution, releasing fibrin degradation products (FDPs), also called fibrin split products (FSPs), into the circulation.
      c. FDPs exert an anticoagulant effect by interfering with clot formation and the function of platelets, thrombin, and fibrinogen.

D. **Coagulation tests (Kenet et al., 2010) (Table 31-3).**
   1. Platelet count is used to assess platelet number.
   2. Prothrombin time (PT) is used to assess extrinsic and common portions of the coagulation cascade. In neonates, a prolonged PT reflects decreased vitamin K–dependent clotting factors.
   3. Partial thromboplastin time (PTT) is used to assess intrinsic and common portions of the coagulation cascade. A prolonged PTT in a neonate reflects a decrease in both vitamin K–dependent factors and contact factors (XI, XII, prekallikrein).
   4. Fibrinogen level is used to assess the circulating level of this protein substrate, required for clot formation. The presence of fetal fibrinogen may result in falsely elevated fibrinogen levels in the newborn.

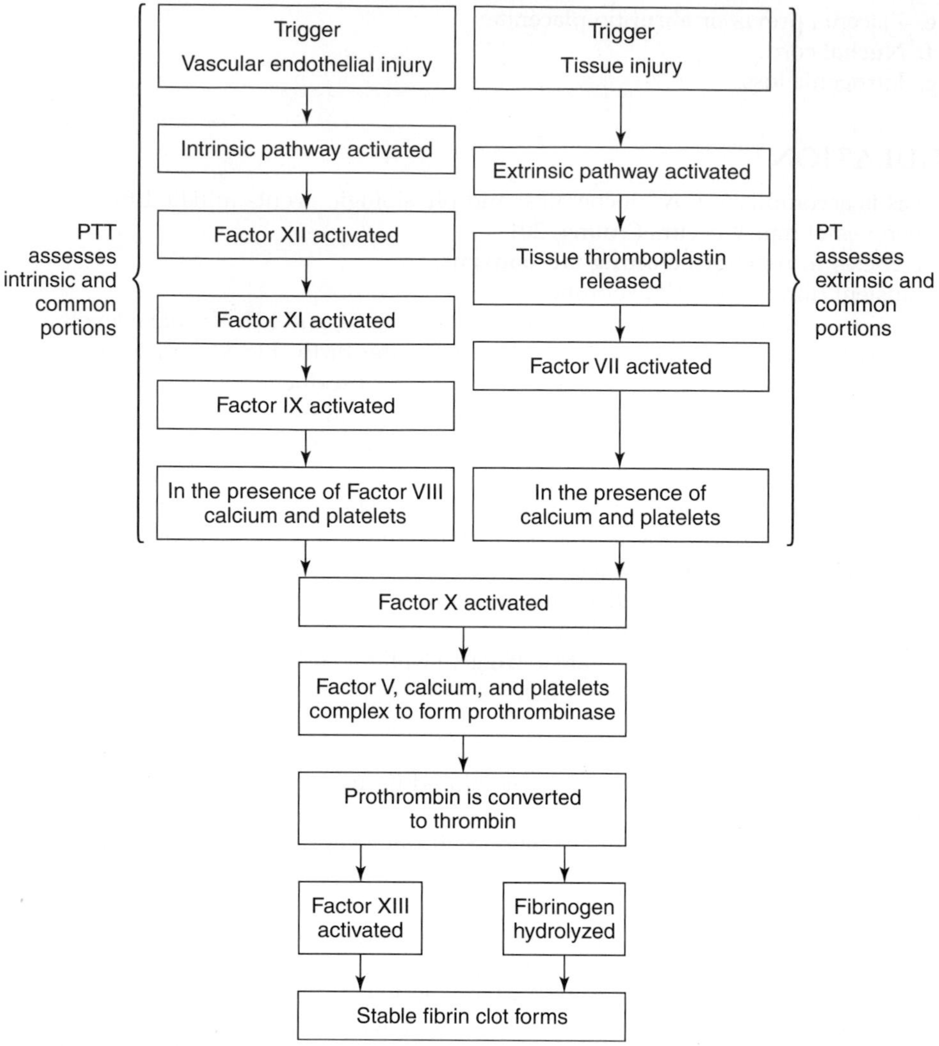


FIGURE 31-2 ■ Fibrin clot formation through activation of intrinsic or extrinsic pathways of coagulation process.

5. FDP/FSP level is used to assess fibrinolytic activity.
6. Individual clotting factors may be assayed, depending on results of the tests cited above.

E. **Physiologic anemia of infancy (Aher et al., 2008; Kates and Kates, 2007).**
   1. Hemoglobin levels decline after birth, reaching a physiologic nadir at 8 to 12 weeks. Hemoglobin levels at this time are typically 9 to 11 g/dL (90 to 110 g/L).

## ANEMIA

Low hemoglobin concentration and/or decreased number of RBCs diminishes the oxygen-carrying capacity of the blood and the level of oxygen available to the tissues. Anemia at birth can be classified into three major causes: (1) the result of blood loss (hemorrhage); (2) shortened RBC survival, including hemolysis; or (3) underproduction of erythrocytes (Manco-Johnson et al., 2011).

A. **Etiologic factors.**
   1. Hemorrhage: accounts for 5% to 10% of severe neonatal anemia (Aher et al., 2008).
      a. Fetal–maternal. Occurs in 50% to 75% of all pregnancies. May be acute or chronic. In 1% of pregnancies, the exchange of blood exceeds 30 mL.
         (1) Spontaneous.
         (2) Traumatic amniocentesis.
         (3) External cephalic version.

■ TABLE 31-3
■ ■ **Normal Values for Tests of Hemostasis**

| Parameter | Fetuses (Weeks of Gestation) 19 to 23 ($n$=20) | 24 to 29 ($n$=22) | 30 to 38 ($n$=22) | Newborns ($n$=60) | Adults ($n$=40) |
|---|---|---|---|---|---|
| PT (s) | 32.5 (19 to 45) | 32.2 (19 to 44)† | 22.6 (16 to 30)† | 16.7 (12.0 to 23.5)* | 13.5 (11.4 to 14) |
| PT (INR) | 6.4 (1.7 to 11.1) | 6.2 (2.1 to 10.6)† | 3 (1.5 to 5)* | 1.7 (0.9 to 2.7)* | 1.1 (0.8 to 1.2) |
| APTT (s) | 168.8 (83 to 250) | 154 (87 to 210)† | 104.8 (76 to 128)† | 44.3 (35 to 52)* | 33 (25 to 39) |
| TCT (s) | 34.2 (24 to 44)* | 26.2 (24 to 28)* | 21.4 (17 to 23.3) | 20.4 (15.2 to 25)† | 14 (12 to 16) |
| Factor | | | | | |
| I (g/l, Von Clauss) | 0.85 (0.57 to 1.50) | 1.12 (0.65 to 1.65) | 1.35 (1.25 to 1.65) | 1.68 (0.95 to 2.45)† | 3 (1.78 to 4.50) |
| I Ag (g/l) | 1.08 (0.75 to 1.50) | 1.93 (1.56 to 2.40) | 1.94 (1.30 to 2.40) | 2.65 (1.68 to 3.60)† | 3.5 (2.50 to 5.20) |
| IIc (%) | 16.9 (10 to 24) | 19.9 (11 to 30)* | 27.9 (15 to 50)† | 43.5 (27 to 64)† | 98.7 (70 to 125) |
| VIIc (%) | 27.4 (17 to 37) | 33.8 (18 to 48)* | 45.9 (31 to 62) | 52.5 (28 to 78)† | 101.3 (68 to 130) |
| IXc (%) | 10.1 (6 to 14) | 9.9 (5 to 15) | 12.3 (5 to 24)† | 31.8 (15 to 50)† | 104.8 (70 to 142) |
| Xc (%) | 20.5 (14 to 29) | 24.9 (16 to 35) | 28 (16 to 36)† | 39.6 (21 to 65)† | 99.2 (75 to 125) |
| Vc (%) | 32.1 (21 to 44) | 36.8 (25 to 50) | 48.9 (23 to 70)† | 89.9 (50 to 140) | 99.8 (65 to 140) |
| VIIIc (%) | 34.5 (18 to 50) | 35.5 (20 to 52) | 50.1 (27 to 78)† | 94.3 (38 to 150) | 101.8 (55 to 170) |
| XIc (%) | 13.2 (8 to 19) | 12.1 (6 to 22) | 14.8 (6 to 26)† | 37.2 (13 to 62)† | 100.2 (70 to 135) |
| XIIc (%) | 14.9 (6 to 25) | 22.7 (6 to 40) | 25.8 (11 to 50)† | 69.8 (25 to 105)† | 101.4 (65 to 144) |
| PK (%) | 12.8 (8 to 19) | 15.4 (8 to 26) | 18.1 (8 to 28)† | 35.4 (21 to 53)† | 99.8 (65 to 135) |
| HMWK (%) | 15.4 (10 to 22) | 19.3 (10 to 26) | 23.6 (12 to 34)† | 38.9 (28 to 53)† | 98.8 (68 to 135) |

From Nathan, D.G., Orkin, S.H., Ginsberg D., and Look, A.T. (Eds.): *Nathan and Oski's hematology of infancy and childhood* (6th ed.). Philadelphia, 2003, W.B. Saunders, p. 1855.
*Ag*, Antigenic value; *APTT*, activated partial thromboplastin time; *c*, coagulant activity; *HMWK*, high-molecular-weight kininogen; *INR*, International Normalized Ratio; *PK*, protein kinase; *PT*, prothrombin time; *TCT*, thrombin clotting time.
Values are the mean, followed in parentheses by the lower and upper boundaries including 95% of the population.
*$P$=0.05.
†$P$=0.01.

b. Twin-to-twin: 15% to 30% of monochorionic twins (Manco-Johnson et al., 2011).
   (1) Monozygotic, monochorionic (single) placenta.
   (2) Hemoglobin difference between twins greater than 5 g/dL (50 g/L).
c. Placental/cord.
   (1) Umbilical cord rupture.
   (2) Cord or placental hematoma.
   (3) Anomalous cord insertion.
   (4) Rupture of anomalous vessels of cord or placenta.
   (5) Accidental incision of cord or placenta.
   (6) Placenta previa or abruptio placentae.
d. Internal.
   (1) Intracranial (subdural, subarachnoid, intraventricular), subgaleal.
   (2) Organ rupture (liver, spleen, adrenal, kidney).
   (3) Pulmonary.
e. External.
   (1) Phlebotomy.
   (2) Iatrogenic (e.g., catheter losses).

2. Hemolysis.
   a. Blood group incompatibilities.
      (1) Rh incompatibility: erythroblastosis fetalis (Liley, 2009; Manco-Johnson et al., 2011).
         (a) Sequence of events: Fetal blood cells containing Rh antigen (Rh positive) enter the maternal circulation; maternal RBCs have no antigen (Rh negative); maternal immune system produces antibodies against the foreign fetal antigens; in

subsequent pregnancies maternal antibodies enter fetal circulation and destroy fetal RBCs.

(b) Predisposing factors.
 (i) Previous pregnancy or abortion.
 (ii) Fetal–maternal hemorrhage during pregnancy.
 (iii) Delivery (vaginal, breech, cesarean).
 (iv) Amniocentesis, chorionic villus sampling.
 (v) External version.
 (vi) Manual removal of placenta.

(c) Infant presentation.
 (i) Anemia (caused by hemolysis, resulting in increased production of very immature RBCs).
 (ii) Tissue hypoxia, acidosis (decreased RBC count and decreased oxygen-carrying capacity of immature cells).
 (iii) Congestive heart failure and hydrops fetalis (fetus attempts to expand blood volume and cardiac output, resulting in generalized edema).
 (iv) Ascites, pleural effusion (fluid collecting in large cavities).
 (v) Hepatosplenomegaly (increased extramedullary hematopoiesis).
 (vi) Petechiae (thrombocytopenia accompanying severe anemia).
 (vii) Hypoglycemia (increased RBC destruction stimulates insulin secretion, resulting in hyperplasia of pancreatic islets and hyperinsulinemia).
 (viii) Positive direct Coombs' test result.

(d) Prophylactic therapy: anti-D immune globulin.
 (i) Anti-D antibodies injected into maternal circulation (one dose accommodates approximately 15 mL of fetal whole blood or approximately 30 mL of RBCs).
 (ii) Destruction of fetal RBCs in maternal circulation, blocking maternal antibody production.
 (iii) Ninety percent effective in prevention of sensitization.
 (iv) Recommended administration at 28 weeks of gestation, within 72 hours after delivery, and after amniocentesis, chorionic villus sampling, percutaneous umbilical blood sampling, or evidence or possibility of fetal–maternal hemorrhage.

(2) ABO incompatibility (Manco-Johnson et al., 2011; Matthews and Glader, 2012).
 (a) More frequently occurring but less severe hemolytic disease than with Rh incompatibility.
 (b) Most often seen in mothers with O blood type (absence of antigen) carrying fetus with A or B blood type (see Table 31-4 for other potential incompatibilities).
 (c) Maternal exposure to naturally occurring A and B antigens in food, bacteria, and pollen initiates maternal production of anti-A, anti-B antibodies and accounts for occurrence of disease with first pregnancy.
 (d) ABO incompatibility protects against fetal Rh disease because of rapid destruction of fetal A/B cells, preventing Rh antigen exposure and maternal antibody production.
 (e) Infant presentation includes the following:
 (i) Mild hemolysis, anemia, reticulocytosis.
 (ii) Hyperbilirubinemia (occasionally requiring exchange).

■ TABLE 31-4
■ ■ **Potential Maternal–Fetal ABO Incompatibilities**

| Maternal Blood Group | Incompatible Fetal Blood Group |
|---|---|
| O | A or B |
| B | A or AB |
| A | B or AB |

b. Enzymatic defect: glucose-6-phosphate dehydrogenase (G6PD) deficiency (see also Chapter 29).
   (1) Most common inherited disorder of RBCs (sex-linked disease affecting mainly male offspring, occasionally female carriers).
   (2) Interaction of intracellular abnormality (deficiency of RBC enzyme) and extracellular factor (exposure to oxidant stress: drugs, infection), causing hemolysis and shortened erythrocyte life.
   (3) Most common occurrence in African American infants (10% to 15%) and in infants of Mediterranean, African, and Asian descent.
c. Hemoglobin disorders (Matthews and Glader, 2012; Steiner and Gallagher, 2007).
   (1) α-Thalassemia.
      (a) Deletion of one or more of the four α-globin genes.
      (b) Severity of expression is related to the number of globin genes missing.
         (i) Silent carrier—single gene deletion, asymptomatic.
         (ii) α-Thalassemia trait—deletion or dysfunction of two genes resulting in mild microcytic anemia.
         (iii) Hemoglobin H disease—absence or nonfunction of three globin genes. Mild to moderate hemolytic anemia exacerbated by oxidant stresses.
         (iv) α-Thalassemia (homozygous)—deletion of all four globin genes results in hydrops fetalis and, often, fetal death as a result of severe intrauterine hemolytic anemia.
      (c) Most common in infants of Southeast Asian, Middle Eastern, and Mediterranean descent.
   (2) β-Thalassemia.
      (a) Occurs as a result of deletion of β-globin gene.
      (b) Also most common in infants of Southeast Asian, African, or Mediterranean descent.
      (c) Neonates occasionally present with hemolytic anemia.
      (d) Does not usually present before 2 months of age because of the presence of HbF.
d. Infection. Intrauterine (viral, protozoan, spirochetal) and postnatal (bacterial) infection may cause neonatal hemolysis, anemia, thrombocytopenia, and disseminated intravascular coagulation (DIC).

3. Anemia of prematurity.
   a. Hemoglobin concentration at birth varies only slightly in relation to gestational age.
   b. During the first 2 to 3 months, hemoglobin concentration falls to the lowest value that occurs at any developmental period.
   c. Anemia of prematurity is considered physiologic because it is characteristic of healthy infants.
   d. Associated factors.
      (1) Rates of decline and nadir are inversely proportional to gestational age.
      (2) Iron concentration is low because of decreased blood volume and decreased concentration of circulating hemoglobin iron.
      (3) Improved extrauterine oxygen delivery causes a temporarily inactive stage of erythropoiesis.
      (4) Erythropoietin production in response to anemia is diminished.
      (5) Shortened RBC life span decreases RBC mass.
      (6) Growth causes dilutional anemia as a result of decreased hemoglobin concentration with expanding blood volume.
      (7) Despite rapid hemoglobin fall, tissue oxygenation is maintained by events responsible for right shift of the hemoglobin–oxygen dissociation curve.
   e. Some infants do manifest symptoms of hypoxemia (poor feeding and weight gain, dyspnea, tachypnea, tachycardia, diminished activity, pallor) in the absence of other problems and require transfusion.
4. Iatrogenic postnatal phlebotomy. Critically ill infants who require frequent monitoring may have excessive amounts of blood removed for diagnostic studies, thereby inducing anemia. Removal of greater than 20% of the blood volume over 24 to 48 hours can produce anemia; in a 1500-g infant this represents approximately 25 mL (Blanchette et al., 2005).

**B. Clinical presentation: varies with the volume of hemorrhage and the time period over which the blood is lost.**

1. Acute blood loss.
   a. Pallor initially, and then cyanosis and desaturation.
   b. Shallow, rapid, irregular respirations.
   c. Tachycardia.
   d. Weak or absent peripheral pulses.
   e. Low or absent blood pressure, low venous pressure.
   f. Hemoglobin concentration may be normal initially, with rapid decline over 4 to 12 hours with hemodilution.
2. Chronic blood loss.
   a. Pallor without signs of acute distress.
   b. Possible signs of congestive heart failure with hepatomegaly.
   c. Normal blood pressure, normal or elevated venous pressure.
   d. Low hemoglobin concentration.

**C. Clinical assessment.**

1. Family history.
   a. Bleeding, anemia, splenectomy.
   b. Consanguinity.
   c. Ethnic and geographic origins.
   d. Blood group incompatibilities.
   e. Previous child with anemia or jaundice.
2. Maternal history.
   a. Blood type.
   b. Late third-trimester bleeding.

**D. Physical examination.**

1. Signs of acute or chronic blood loss, as above.
2. Jaundice.
3. Cephalohematoma.
4. Abdominal distention or mass: liver, spleen, adrenal, kidney rupture.
5. Petechiae, purpura.
6. Cardiovascular abnormalities: tachycardia, murmur, gallop rhythm.
7. Hydropic changes.

**E. Diagnostic studies.**

1. Hemoglobin concentration: Normal hemoglobin values are dependent on gestational age, site of sampling, and timing of sampling (Brugnara and Platt, 2009). Values vary according to birth weight and postnatal age (Table 31-5).
2. Reticulocyte count: This reflects new erythroid activity and is persistently elevated with ongoing RBC destruction.
3. Peripheral blood smear.
   a. Test evaluates alterations in size, shape, and structure of RBCs that might enhance destruction because of decreased deformability.

■ TABLE 31-5
■ ■ **Serial Hemoglobin Values in Low Birth Weight Infants**

| | Hemoglobin Concentration (g/dL) by Age | | | | |
|---|---|---|---|---|---|
| **Birth Weight (g)** | **2 weeks** | **4 weeks** | **6 weeks** | **8 weeks** | **10 weeks** |
| 800 to 1000 | 16±0.6 | 10.2±3.2 | 8.7±1.5 | 8±0.9 | 8±1.1 |
| 1001 to 1200 | 16.4±2.3 | 12.8±2.5 | 10.5±1.8 | 9.1±1.3 | 8.5±1.5 |
| 1201 to 1400 | 16.2±1.3 | 13.4±2.8 | 10.9±1.2 | 9.9±1.9 | — |
| 1401 to 1500 | 15.6±2.2 | 11.7±1 | 10.5±0.7 | 9.8±1.4 | — |

From Oski, F.A.: Hematologic problems. In G.B. Avery (Ed.): *Neonatology: Pathophysiology and management of the newborn* (4th ed.). Philadelphia, 1994, Lippincott.

b. Fragmentation of RBCs can be identified.
4. Blood type to identify common blood group antigens: A, B, O, and Rh.
5. Coombs' test.
a. Positive result on direct Coombs' test indicates presence of maternal immunoglobulin G (IgG) antibodies on the surface of infant's RBCs.
b. Positive result on indirect Coombs' test means that antibodies against the infant's RBCs are present in the maternal serum.
6. Kleihauer–Betke test.
a. Test identifies fetal hemoglobin in maternal blood.
b. Calculations indicate volume of fetal–maternal hemorrhage and dose of anti-D immune globulin (Rhogam) required to prevent sensitization.

F. **Differential diagnosis: diseases that diminish oxygen delivery to the tissues** (e.g., pulmonary, cardiac).

G. **Complications.**
1. Inadequate tissue oxygenation, poor growth.
2. Transfusion.
a. Transfusion reaction.
b. Overhydration with pulmonary congestion.

H. **Patient care management** (see Transfusion Therapies).
1. Emergency treatment for acute blood loss resulting in hypovolemia.
a. Whole blood or packed RBCs (PRBCs).
(1) Type: group O, Rh negative.
(2) Amount: 10 to 20 mL/kg.
b. Saline solution if blood is unavailable.
(1) Amount: 10 to 15 mL/kg.
2. Nonemergency replacement transfusion: clinical decision based on adequacy of tissue oxygenation in the individual infant.
a. Advantages of transfusion must be weighed against risks, including infection, hypothermia, graft-versus-host disease, and other complications.
b. Consider gestational and postnatal age, intravascular volume, and coexisting cardiac, pulmonary, or vascular conditions.
3. Exchange transfusion.
a. Treatment of jaundice caused by blood group incompatibility.
b. Partial exchange if necessary to treat severe anemia of hydrops without increasing intravascular volume.

I. **Outcome.**
1. Improved tissue oxygenation and resolution of symptoms with replacement transfusion.
2. Long-term outcome varies with degree of anemia and underlying cause.

## HEMORRHAGIC DISEASE OF THE NEWBORN

Hemorrhagic disease of the newborn (HDN) is a hemorrhagic tendency caused by vitamin K deficiency and decreased activity of factors II, VII, IX, and X. Previously referred to as "hemorrhagic disease of the newborn," the newer term "vitamin K–dependent bleeding (VKDB)" is thought to describe more accurately the link between vitamin K deficiency and spontaneous hemorrhage and to exclude newborn infants with bleeding from other causes (Blackburn, 2013; Johnson, 2013; Pipe and Goldenberg, 2009).

A. **Etiologic factors: primary vitamin K deficiency.**
1. Required for activation of clotting factors II, VII, IX, and X and of proteins C and S after liver synthesis.
a. Vitamin K is important in the formation of calcium binding sites, which are necessary for functional activation of clotting factors.
b. In the absence of vitamin K, circulating proteins are decarboxylated; levels of protein induced by vitamin K absence (PIVKA) can be used as an indirect measure of bleeding risk.

2. Limited vitamin K availability.
   a. Inadequate placental transfer.
   b. Deficient hepatic stores.
   c. Limited postnatal dietary intake.
      (1) Human milk contains 1 to 5 mcg/L of vitamin K.
      (2) Recommended daily intake of vitamin K is 1 mcg/kg (Pichler and Pichler, 2008).
3. Three forms of vitamin K deficiency are recognized.
   a. Early—within 24 hours in neonates born to women taking certain anticonvulsants, antitubercular medications, and vitamin K antagonists such as warfarin (Coumadin).
   b. Classic or VKDB—seen at 2 to 6 days.
      (1) Incidence is 0.25 to 1.7 per 100 live births if no vitamin K is given (Johnson, 2013).
   c. Late onset—occurs at 2 to 12 weeks in infants not receiving vitamin K at birth or receiving an inadequate oral dose and breastfeeding or in infants with hepatobiliary disease. Intracranial bleeding is more common in late-onset disease.

B. **Clinical presentation of VKDB:** bleeding.
   1. Begins at 24 to 72 hours of age.
   2. May be localized or diffuse.
   3. Rarely life threatening.
   4. Late-onset bleeding possible at approximately 2 to 3 weeks of age.

C. **Clinical assessment:** oozing.
   1. Localized: frequently gastrointestinal (hematemesis, melena).
   2. Diffuse: umbilical cord, circumcision, puncture sites.

D. **Physical examination.**
   1. Diffuse ecchymosis, petechiae.
   2. Oozing puncture sites.
   3. Abdominal distention.
   4. Jaundice.

E. **Diagnostic studies.**
   1. Response to vitamin K administration establishes the diagnosis.
   2. PT and PTT are prolonged.
   3. Levels of vitamin K–dependent clotting factors are low.
   4. PIVKA levels are elevated.

F. **Differential diagnosis.**
   1. Decreased absorption of vitamin K.
      a. Biliary atresia.
      b. Cystic fibrosis.
      c. Cholestasis.
   2. Pharmacologic antagonism of vitamin K (Abbott et al., 2006).
      a. Anticonvulsants (hydantoin, phenobarbital, carbamazepine, diazepam), anticoagulants (coumarin, warfarin), and antibiotics (cephalosporins, isoniazid, quinolones, and rifampin).
         (1) Induce hepatic enzymes and increase vitamin K degradation.
         (2) Inhibit vitamin K transport across the placenta.
         (3) Depress vitamin K–dependent coagulation factors.
      b. Coumarol derivatives: replace with heparin during pregnancy.
      c. Maternal supplementation with oral vitamin K from 36 weeks of gestation to delivery might prevent neonatal hemorrhage associated with anticonvulsant therapy; extra vitamin K given to the mother to increase vitamin K available to the fetus.

G. **Complications.**
   1. Anemia.
   2. Intraventricular/intracranial hemorrhage.

H. **Patient care management.**
   1. Prophylactic vitamin K at the time of delivery.
      a. Phytonadione (naturally occurring vitamin K), 1 mg intramuscular (IM) administration for term infant, 0.5 mg for premature infants (American Academy of Pediatrics [AAP], 2009).

b. The Canadian Paediatric Society (Canadian Paediatric Society, Fetus and Newborn Committee, 2012) and the AAP (2009) recommend the use of only IM vitamin K at birth, because of the history of prevention of life-threatening HDN with the parenteral preparation, the unproven risks of cancer, and the need for further research on the efficacy, safety, and bioavailability of oral preparations.

c. Late HDN occurs primarily in breastfed infants who have not received adequate vitamin K prophylaxis.

(1) Parental concern with IM administration of vitamin K might stem from the following:

(a) Need for injection.

(b) Reports linking an earlier formulation of vitamin K to childhood cancer (Clarke and Shearer, 2007).

d. Commercial formulas contain vitamin K supplement.

e. Intestinal flora of breastfed infant may produce less vitamin K than that of formula-fed infant.

2. Significant bleeding (hemoglobin concentration <12 g/dL). PRBC infusion may be indicated.

3. Persistent bleeding in premature infant.

a. Fresh frozen plasma (FFP) infusion may be indicated to replace clotting factors.

b. Repeated doses of vitamin K are needed.

I. **Outcome.** Prophylactic treatment has virtually eliminated the disease.

## DISSEMINATED INTRAVASCULAR COAGULATION

DIC is an acquired hemorrhagic disorder associated with an underlying disease manifested as uncontrolled activation of coagulation and fibrinolysis. Consumption of clotting factors is thought to be initiated by release of thromboplastic material from damaged or diseased tissue into the circulation. In DIC, fibrinogen converts to fibrin to form microthrombi. Neonates are at increased risk of DIC because of inherent imbalances between fibrinolytic, anticoagulant, and procoagulant factors, particularly decreased levels of antithrombin and protein C (Blackburn, 2013; Luchtman-Jones and Wilson, 2011; Manco-Johnson et al., 2011; Pipe and Goldenberg, 2009).

A. **Common precipitating factors.**

1. Maternal.

a. Preeclampsia, eclampsia, placental abruption.

b. Placental abnormalities.

2. Intrapartal.

a. Fetal distress with hypoxia and acidosis.

b. Dead twin fetus.

c. Traumatic delivery.

3. Neonatal.

a. Infection (bacterial, viral, fungal).

b. Conditions causing hypoxia, acidosis, and shock.

c. Severe Rh incompatibility.

d. Thrombocytopenia.

e. Tissue injury (birth trauma, breech crush injury, necrotizing enterocolitis [NEC]).

B. **Clinical presentation (Fig. 31-3).**

1. Hemorrhage: predominant symptom.

a. Clotting factors and platelets are depleted.

b. Fibrinolysis is stimulated.

c. Endogenous thrombin and plasmin are formed.

2. Organ and tissue ischemia. Microvascular thrombosis (occlusion) by fibrin thrombi causes potential ischemia and necrosis of any organ, particularly the kidneys.

3. Anemia.

a. Blood loss.

b. RBC fragmentation by fibrin strands.

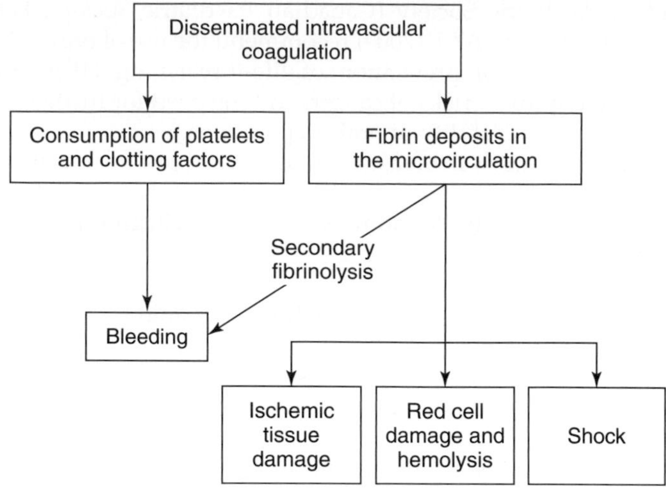


FIGURE 31-3 ■ Sequence of events in pathologic changes of disseminated intravascular coagulation (DIC).

C. **Clinical assessment.**
   1. Review the history for precipitating factors.
   2. Concurrent evidence of coagulation and fibrinolysis.

D. **Physical examination.**
   1. Variable signs, depending on underlying disease process.
   2. Prolonged oozing from puncture sites or umbilicus.
   3. Petechiae, purpura, ecchymosis.
   4. Hemorrhage (pulmonary, gastrointestinal, cerebral).
   5. Localized necrosis and gangrene resulting from microvascular thrombosis of peripheral vessels.

E. **Diagnostic studies.**
   1. Variable diagnostic studies are performed for delineation of the underlying disease process.
   2. Platelet count is low.
   3. PT and PTT may be normal in early DIC, then become significantly prolonged (Parker, 2005).
   4. Peripheral blood smear identifies microangiopathic hemolytic anemia, abnormalities of RBC shape, cell fragmentation, and decreased number of platelets.
   5. Fibrinogen level is low.
   6. Fibrinogen degradation products are significantly increased but are not specific markers of DIC.
   7. D-Dimer is a sensitive marker for endogenous thrombin/plasmin production and can detect much milder forms of DIC.
   8. Additional factors and levels might be evaluated: factors VIII and II are decreased, as well as protein C, protein S, and antithrombin III.

F. **Differential diagnosis.**
   1. Parenchymal liver disease.
   2. Vitamin K deficiency.
   3. Microangiopathic disease.
   4. Primary fibrinogenolysis.

G. **Complications.**
   1. Microvascular thrombosis.
   2. Organ failure resulting from ischemia and necrosis, especially renal.
   3. Intraventricular and parenchymal hemorrhage.

H. **Patient care management.**
   1. Aggressive treatment of the underlying disease.
   2. Supportive care.

a. Replacement transfusion with significant bleeding.
   (1) Whole blood for hypovolemia and shock.
   (2) PRBCs for isovolemic anemia.
   (3) Platelets for consumption.
b. Maintenance of blood pressure.

3. Measures to control DIC.
   a. Replacement of clotting factors.
      (1) FFP (replaces all factors, coagulation proteins, and coagulation inhibitors; small amount of fibrinogen).
      (2) Platelet concentrates.
      (3) Cryoprecipitate (replaces fibrinogen, factor VIII).
      (4) Antithrombin III (inhibits coagulation, controls fibrinolysis). High doses (120 to 250 units/kg/day) might attenuate organ failure and reverse coagulopathy in DIC without heparin therapy.
   b. Heparin therapy remains controversial; use if treatment of underlying disease and replacement of clotting factors fail to reverse the process or with evidence of significant large-vessel thrombosis.
      (1) Goals are to interrupt fibrin deposition and to achieve normal fibrinogen levels and platelet counts.
      (2) Continuous infusion is more physiologic and is safer because intermittent doses may aggravate existing hemorrhage.
      (3) Dosage is adjusted to maintain PTT within 60 to 70 seconds (once achieved, lower-dose heparin therapy may control ongoing consumption).

**I. Outcome: related to the prognosis of the underlying disease and the severity of the DIC.**

## THROMBOCYTOPENIA

Thrombocytopenia is an acquired disease in which there is a significant decrease in the platelet count (<150,000/mm$^3$) of the term or premature infant (Blanchette et al., 2005; Blickstein and Friedman, 2011). Thrombocytopenia occurs in 1% to 2% of healthy term neonates and in up to 35% of critically ill neonates (Holzhauer and Zieger, 2011).

**A. Etiologic factors.**

1. Platelet destruction.
   a. Maternal autoantibodies (autoimmune): idiopathic thrombocytopenic purpura, systemic lupus erythematosus.
      (1) Maternal autoantibodies bind to platelet surface antigens, making them susceptible to premature destruction.
      (2) IgG antibodies cross the placenta and destroy fetal platelets.
         (a) Approximately 10% to 15% have cord platelet counts of less than 100,000/mm$^3$ (half of these have counts <50,000/mm$^3$).
         (b) Nadir usually occurs on the second day.
         (c) Counts can be depressed for 2 to 4 months (as long as maternal IgG antibodies remain in circulation).
      (3) Maternal platelet count is low.
   b. Neonatal conditions.
      (1) Neonatal alloimmune thrombocytopenia—most common cause of significant, early-onset thrombocytopenia in a healthy neonate (Holzhauer and Zieger, 2011; Murphy and Bussel, 2007).
         (a) Analogous to Rh incompatibility.
            (i) Fetal platelets contain an antigen lacking in the mother.
            (ii) Fetal platelets enter maternal circulation, resulting in maternal production of antibodies against foreign platelets.
            (iii) Maternal antibodies cross into fetal circulation and coat fetal platelets, which are then destroyed.
         (b) Fetal thrombocytopenia can occur as early as 20 weeks of gestation.
         (c) Nadir occurs in the first few days; counts normalize by the end of the first month.

(d) About 15% to 25% have intracranial hemorrhage (approximately 10% occur in utero).
(e) Maternal platelet count remains normal.
(f) Workup includes both neonatal and parental blood screening for human platelet antigens (HPAs).
(g) Treatment includes platelet transfusion, preferably with matched platelets. IVIG may be used but its use is controversial (Bussel and Sola-Visner, 2009; Holzhauer and Zieger, 2011).

(2) Infection: bacterial (especially gram-negative sepsis) or congenitally acquired (rubella, cytomegalovirus, herpes, enterovirus, or human immunodeficiency virus).
(a) Megakaryocyte degeneration in bone marrow.
(b) Can cause DIC (platelet consumption).
(c) Activates reticuloendothelial system (increased platelet sequestration).
(d) Platelets may form antigen–antibody complexes with infectious agent.

(3) Thrombotic disorders.
(a) Large-vessel disease (renal vein thrombosis).
(b) Microvascular disease (NEC, respiratory distress syndrome, persistent pulmonary hypertension of the newborn).
(c) DIC (platelet consumption).

(4) Birth asphyxia. Fetal megakaryocytes may have increased sensitivity to hypoxic injury.

(5) Giant hemangiomas.
(a) Kasabach–Merritt syndrome. Vascular malformation results in platelet and fibrinogen consumption.
(b) Mechanical destruction and sequestration.

(6) Exchange transfusion: shortened survival of transfused platelets.

**2.** Impaired platelet production (rare, <5%) associated with congenital malformations.
**a.** Trisomy syndromes (13, 18). Bone marrow hypoplasia affects megakaryocyte production.
**b.** Thrombocytopenia with absent radii syndrome.
(1) Defective megakaryocyte progenitor cell.
(2) Presentation at birth, improvement thereafter.
(3) Anomalies of the radius but not the thumb.
**c.** Fanconi's anemia.
(1) Thumb, skeletal, renal, and central nervous system (CNS) anomalies; café-au-lait spots.
(2) Thrombocytopenia: presentation rare in the neonatal period; worsens with time.
**d.** Other rare syndromes associated with unusually small or giant platelets.

**3.** Platelet interference: maternal drug ingestion.
**a.** Interference with platelet aggregation.
**b.** Meperidine (Demerol), promethazine (Phenergan), acetylsalicylic acid, sulfonamides, quinidine, quinine, thiazides.

**B. Clinical presentation:** platelet-type bleeding.
**1.** Petechiae, purpura, epistaxis.
**2.** Ecchymosis over presenting part.
**3.** Cephalohematoma.
**4.** Bleeding (mucous membranes, gastrointestinal tract, genitourinary system, umbilical cord, puncture sites, superficial cuts, or abrasions).

**C. Clinical assessment.**
**1.** Family history: bleeding complications in previous children, other family members.
**2.** Maternal history.
**a.** History of bruising or bleeding, infections, collagen vascular disease, splenectomy.
**b.** Platelet count (low or normal).
**c.** Peripheral blood smear (may show low platelet count, increased immature forms).
**d.** Medication history.

3. Birth history.
   a. Hypoxia.
   b. Infection risk.

D. **Physical examination.**
   1. Signs of clinical presentation.
   2. Jaundice.
   3. Intrauterine growth restriction, microcephaly, hepatosplenomegaly with infectious cause (absent with immune etiology).
   4. Congenital anomalies consistent with syndromes.

E. **Diagnostic studies.**
   1. Platelet count is low.
   2. Peripheral blood smear shows low platelet count and increased immature forms; may show abnormal size.
   3. PT and PTT are normal for age.
   4. Bleeding time is prolonged.
   5. Maternal blood can be tested for HPA type and for the presence of platelet-specific antibody (up to 2 weeks postpartum).
   6. In severe cases, platelet typing of mother, father, and infant might be indicated.

F. **Differential diagnosis: DIC, vitamin K deficiency.**

G. **Complications.**
   1. Cranial hemorrhage with neurologic sequelae in alloimmune disease.
      a. Associated with approximately 12% mortality rate.
      b. Increased incidence in infants weighing less than 1500 g.
   2. Entrapped hemorrhage.
   3. Anemia.
   4. Hyperbilirubinemia.

H. **Infant management (see Table 31-5).**
   1. Supportive care and treatment of underlying disease. Majority of neonatal thrombocytopenias are secondary to other disease processes.
   2. Cesarean delivery.
      a. Autoimmune.
         (1) Rarely of benefit for infant.
         (2) Consider if:
            (a) Maternal disease is severe, with high antibody levels, or
            (b) Prior infant was severely affected.
      b. Alloimmune: maternal HPA typing not routinely done; infants identified postnatally.
   3. Platelet transfusion.
      a. Recommended goal: keep platelet count greater than 30,000/mm$^3$ in the first 48 hours, and greater than 50,000/mm$^3$ if surgery is necessary or infant is premature and at risk for intraventricular hemorrhage. The need for multiple platelet transfusions has been shown to be a predictor of higher mortality rates (Baer et al., 2007).
      b. Autoimmune.
         (1) Rarely needed; platelet counts greater than 20,000/mm$^3$, usually benign course.
         (2) Consider cranial ultrasonography if platelet counts less than 50,000/mm$^3$.
         (3) Consider transfusion if platelet counts less than 20,000/mm$^3$ (Del Vecchio and Motta, 2011).
      c. Alloimmune.
         (1) Serial transfusions may be necessary.
         (2) Obtain HPA type for infant before transfusion.
         (3) Transfusion of random donor platelets rarely results in sustained increase because of antibody destruction.
         (4) Transfuse maternal platelets (in absence of HPA) that have been washed and resuspended in AB-negative plasma.
      d. Production defects: repeated transfusions usually necessary.
   4. Steroids.
      a. May be used in infants with platelet counts less than 25,000/mm$^3$ and clinical bleeding.
      b. May be used for initial treatment of thrombocytopenia resulting from hemangioma.

I. **Outcome.**
   1. Varies with underlying disease, presence of congenital malformations.
   2. Autoimmune etiology: usually causes only mild, transient problems, with full recovery of platelet count in 8 to 12 weeks.
   3. Isoimmune etiology: causes mild to moderate problems with full recovery of platelet count in 6 to 8 weeks.

## POLYCYTHEMIA

Polycythemia is a condition in which infants demonstrate an excess in circulating RBC mass. The venous hemoglobin concentration is 2 standard deviations above the mean for gestational and postdelivery age (Sarkar and Rosenkrantz, 2008). Blood viscosity increases with hematocrits greater than 65% or when venous hemoglobin is greater than 22 g/dL (220 g/L) and leads to a reduction of blood flow to the organs. Occurs in 0.4% to 12% of healthy term newborns (Morag et al., 2011).

A. **Etiologic factors (Sarkar and Rosenkrantz, 2008).**
   1. Intrauterine hypoxia, placental insufficiency. Hypoxia stimulates erythropoiesis, increasing the fetal RBC mass.
      a. Maternal preeclampsia/eclampsia.
      b. Postmaturity syndrome, intrauterine growth restriction.
      c. Maternal smoking.
   2. Maternal–fetal and twin-to-twin transfusion.
   3. Placental hypertransfusion.
   4. Maternal diabetes: possibly resulting from abnormal fetal erythrocyte deformability.
   5. Congenital syndrome resulting in increased RBC mass.
   6. Perinatal hypoxia.

B. **Clinical presentation.**
   1. Many infants are asymptomatic.
   2. Plethora.
   3. Cyanosis.
   4. CNS abnormalities (lethargy, jitteriness, seizures).
   5. Respiratory distress (tachypnea, pulmonary edema, pulmonary hemorrhage).
   6. Tachycardia, congestive heart failure.
   7. Hypoglycemia.
   8. Poor feeding behaviors (poor nippling, regurgitation).

C. **Clinical assessment: history and physical examination usually identify cause.**

D. **Physical examination.**
   1. Findings may be normal except for plethora and occasionally cyanosis.
   2. Symptoms of clinical presentation cannot be attributed to other disease.

E. **Diagnostic studies.** Venous hemoglobin concentration and hematocrit are elevated. Computed tomography scan if stroke suspected.

F. **Complications.**
   1. Hyperbilirubinemia.
   2. Hypoglycemia—mechanism unknown.
   3. Hyperviscosity syndrome: elevated whole blood viscosity associated with reduced blood flow, vascular thrombosis (renal, cerebral, mesenteric), neurologic sequelae, fine motor abnormalities, speech delays up to 2 years of age (Drew et al., 1997).

G. **Patient care management.**
   1. Administration of a normal saline bolus. For asymptomatic infants with a hematocrit greater than 70% or those with symptoms and a hematocrit between 65% and 70%, a bolus of 10 mL/kg of normal saline may be adequate. Partial exchange is recommended if the postbolus hematocrit remains high (Morag et al., 2011).
   2. Partial exchange transfusion.
      a. Controversial in asymptomatic infants. Has not been shown to decrease neurologic morbidity (Ozek et al., 2010).
      b. Desired reduction of hematocrit to less than 60% (blood viscosity is thought to be relatively normal at this level).

c. Crystalloid shown to be as effective as colloid for reduction exchange at less cost and with fewer risks related to blood product exposure (Mimouni et al., 2011).
d. Gastrointestinal symptoms: possibility of bleeding, poor feeding tolerance, and NEC after partial exchange transfusion (Morag et al., 2011).
3. Supportive treatment of persistent symptoms.

**H. Outcome (Morag et al., 2011; Murray and Roberts, 2004).**
1. Neonates with proven hyperviscosity (less than 50% of neonates exhibit hyperviscosity even when packed cell volumes >70%) are at risk of an adverse neurologic outcome.
2. Adverse neurologic outcome may be independently related to underlying risk factors and race rather than polycythemia alone (Morag et al., 2011; Pappas and Delaney-Black, 2004).

## INHERITED BLEEDING DISORDERS

Although inherited bleeding disorders were recognized as early as AD 600, the specific clotting abnormalities have been delineated only in this century, with the last (deficiency of factor XIII) documented in 1963. While the overall incidence of these gene disorders is rare, and phenotypic expression is extremely variable it is estimated that 15% to 33% of infants with an inherited bleeding disorder will present with symptoms in the newborn period (Chalmers, 2004).

**A. Etiologic factors.**
1. Hemophilia.
   a. Ninety percent of infants with hemophilia will have either classic hemophilia (hemophilia A, factor VIII deficiency) or Christmas disease (hemophilia B, factor IX deficiency).
      (1) Incidence of hemophilia A is 1 per 10,000 live births (Parker, 2005).
      (2) Incidence of hemophilia B is 1 per 100,000 live births (Parker, 2005).
   b. X-linked recessive inheritance (Chalmers et al., 2011).
      (1) Gene is located on the X chromosome.
      (2) Females are carriers; disease is present in male infants because they have only one X chromosome, which carries the abnormal gene (no normal X chromosome as counterbalance).
      (3) Each pregnancy carries a 25% chance of occurrence (50% of the male offspring will be affected).
      (4) Seventy-five percent have a family history of a male with a bleeding disorder.
2. von Willebrand's disease.
   a. Autosomal dominant inheritance.
      (1) Males and females are equally affected.
      (2) Each pregnancy carries a 50% chance of occurrence.
      (3) Transmission is vertical (disease is seen in successive generations).
   b. Gene expression markedly variable (family history may be absent despite dominant inheritance).
3. Factor XIII deficiency: autosomal recessive inheritance.
   a. Both parents are phenotypically normal carriers.
   b. Males and females are equally affected.
   c. In each pregnancy, 25% of the offspring will be affected, 50% will be carriers, and 25% will be normal.
   d. Expression is horizontal (deficiency is seen in siblings; skips a generation).

**B. Clinical presentation (Kenet et al., 2010).**
1. Rare newborn presentation except for factor XIII deficiency.
2. Usually well infant with delayed bleeding.
3. Clotting screening results usually normal.

**C. Clinical assessment.**
1. Late bleeding.
   a. Delayed umbilical cord bleeding (>80% with factor XIII).
   b. Circumcision oozing: most common site of bleeding (45%) (significant hemorrhage is rare).
   c. Intracranial hemorrhage (17%).
2. Family history.

D. **Diagnostic studies.**
   1. PT, PTT, platelet count, fibrinogen level (usually normal).
   2. Specific factor assays (identification by factor levels and DNA analysis).
      a. Factor VIII levels should be comparable to normal adult levels in the newborn period.
      b. Factor IX levels are normally low in the neonatal period; however, infants with bleeding presentation will be severely affected, with less than 2% activity (clearly abnormal level).
E. **Patient care management.**
   1. Optimal mode of delivery for infants at risk of hemophilia is controversial (Chalmers et al., 2011).
   2. Initial correction is with FFP (contains adequate amounts of all clotting factors except factor VIII).
   3. Cryoprecipitate can be used if bleeding persists after use of FFP (enriched with approximately 20 units of factor VIII per milliliter).
   4. Diagnosis allows replacement of specific factor.
      a. Recombinant factor VIII is available for classic hemophilia.
      b. Purified (monoclonal antibody) factor IX is available for Christmas disease.
      c. Prothrombin concentrates are not recommended for neonatal use because of thrombogenicity.
   5. Use precautions to prevent bleeding.
      a. Immunizations should be given subcutaneously, with an ice pack applied to the site postinjection.
F. **Outcome: episodic bleeding requiring lifelong replacement.**

## TRANSFUSION THERAPIES

A. **Recommendations for use of blood components (Blanchette et al., 2005; Christensen et al., 2012; Canadian Paediatric Society, Fetus and Newborn Committee, 2012; Wong and Luban, 2005).**
   1. Develop and document criteria indicating need.
   2. Use only the blood components required for therapy.
   3. Use crystalloid or nonblood colloid whenever possible.
   4. Use Universal Precautions when handling blood products.
B. **Written, informed consent has been recommended since 1986 to ensure that families understand risks and explore alternatives.**
   1. Ethical or religious basis: autonomy—the right of choice.
   2. Legal basis: failure to inform adequately and to obtain consent constitutes negligence.
   3. Time-consuming: start a few days in advance of need (i.e., include in discussion on the first day of life of sick preterm infants).
C. **Informed consent includes discussion of the following:**
   1. Risks (American Cancer Society, 2011; American Red Cross, 2013; Galel and Fontaine, 2006).
      a. Infection.
         (1) Blood is screened for human immunodeficiency viruses types 1 and 2 (HIV-1, HIV-2), hepatitis B virus (HBV), hepatitis C virus (HCV), Chagas' disease (*Trypanosoma cruzi*), human T-lymphotropic virus, West Nile virus, and *Treponema pallidum* (syphilis).
         (2) Cytomegalovirus transmission can be prevented by using cytomegalovirus-seronegative blood or leukocyte-depleted, irradiated products.
         (3) Major risks for transmission via transfusion (Fasano and Luban, 2011; Zou et al., 2012).
            (a) HIV infection incidence is 1 per 2.3 million using nucleic acid testing.
            (b) HBV (hepatitis B surface antigen) infection incidence is 1:300,000.
            (c) HCV infection incidence is 1 in 1.8 million.
         (4) Predonation questions foster self-elimination of prospective donors with high-risk behaviors.
         (5) Confidential unit exclusion allows donors to designate the elimination of their donation if they recognize risk but want to avoid the embarrassment of refusing to donate.

**b.** Transfusion reactions (rare in neonates).
 (1) Febrile reactions (most common in adults but rare in neonates) (Fasano and Luban, 2011).
  (a) Probably caused by transfused (passenger) WBCs and/or their cytokine products (RBC and platelet transfusions).
  (b) Leukocyte reduction might prevent reaction.
   (i) Expensive and time-consuming.
   (ii) One unit of PRBCs can contain 1 billion WBCs.
   (iii) WBCs can be removed by centrifugation, or by filtering at donation (prestorage leukocyte depletion), or at transfusion (bedside filtration).
 (2) Allergic reactions.
  (a) Urticaria, angioedema, asthma.
  (b) Higher incidence with multiple transfusions.
 (3) Hemolytic reactions.
  (a) Usually ABO incompatibilities.
  (b) Possible acute or delayed hemolysis.
  (c) Most reactions can be eliminated by typing, screening, and cross-matching.
 (4) Transfusion-related acute lung injury (TRALI) (Fanaro, 2011).
  (a) Pulmonary edema occurring within 6 hours following a transfusion.
  (b) Probably under-recognized in preterm infants because of preexisting lung disease.

**c.** Graft-versus-host disease: rare in neonates (Wu and Stack, 2007).
 (1) Risk factors include neonates with congenital immunodeficiency syndromes, those receiving intrauterine or exchange transfusions, and low birth weight infants.
 (2) Immature immune system may not reject foreign lymphocytes (present in erythrocyte and platelet products); donor lymphocytes proliferate and damage the host (infection and neutropenia).
 (3) Clinical symptoms (within 100 days of transfusion) include rash, diarrhea, hepatic dysfunction, and bone marrow suppression with generalized reduction in all cell lines (pancytopenia).
 (4) Gamma irradiation of blood products will prevent lymphocyte proliferation.
  (a) Mature erythrocytes and platelets are resistant to radiation damage.
  (b) Enhances efflux of potassium ion from RBCs (store <28 days, wash to remove excess potassium before transfusion).

**d.** Hemodynamic complications
 (1) Fluid overload: Volumes should not exceed 20 mL/kg.
 (2) Hypoglycemia, metabolic acidosis, hyperkalemia, and hypocalcemia.

**e.** NEC, also referred to as transfusion-related acute gut injury (TRAGI) (La Gamma and Blau, 2012).
 (1) Emerging evidence suggests a relationship between RBC transfusions and late-onset NEC in low birth weight infants (Amin et al., 2012).

**2.** Expected benefits.

**a.** Whole blood (increases hematocrit approximately 35%).
 (1) Replacement of blood volume.
 (2) Treatment (massive hemorrhage, exchange transfusion).

**b.** PRBCs: 10 to 15 mL increases hemoglobin by 2 to 3 g/L (Wu and Stack, 2007).
 (1) Improved oxygen-carrying capacity and tissue oxygenation.
 (2) Relief of symptoms of anemia (tachypnea, apnea, periodic breathing, tachycardia, poor weight gain).
 (3) Treatment (active bleeding, hemolytic disease, extracorporeal membrane oxygenation).
 (4) Minimal fluid administration (approximate RBC mass of a whole unit of blood in one-half fluid volume).

**c.** Platelets.
 (1) Improved coagulation.
 (2) Treatment (hemorrhage caused by thrombocytopenia or platelet dysfunction).

d. FFP: replacement of clotting factor deficiency.
e. Albumin.
(1) Volume expansion; improved oncotic pressure.
(2) Treatment (for hypovolemia, third-space losses).

3. Alternatives.
a. Directed donation.
(1) Family and friends with compatible blood type can donate for infant.
(2) Blood must be irradiated to prevent graft-versus-host disease.
(3) There is no evidence of overall increased safety in comparison with anonymous volunteer donations.
(a) Donors might be more truthful (i.e., regarding acceptability for donation) because they know the recipient.
(b) Donors might be less truthful because they feel pressure to donate.
(4) Parental donation.
(a) Maternal plasma is unacceptable for transfusion to neonates because of the possible presence of antibodies directed against inherited paternal antigens on infant's cells.
(b) Maternal platelets and RBCs can be used if washed before transfusion.
(c) Paternal donation might be problematic if infant has circulating maternal antibodies produced by stimulation of inherited paternal antigens.
(5) All blood products from directed donors should be irradiated. Potential antigen similarities between close family members may impede recognition and destruction of foreign lymphocytes.

b. Delayed cord clamping has been shown to decrease the need for transfusions among very low birth weight infants (Christensen et al., 2012; Mercer and Erickson-Owens, 2012).

c. Erythropoietin (EPO) (Aher and Ohlsson, 2012; Bishara and Ohls, 2009; Juul, 2012).
(1) Recombinant human EPO (r-HuEPO) might be used to treat symptomatic anemia caused by physiologic decline in hematocrit or by blood loss from phlebotomy, or it might be used as a prophylactic therapy to minimize blood product exposure in preterm or sick neonates.
(2) Plasma EPO levels are lower in anemic preterm infants, suggesting responsibility for hematocrit decline.
(a) The liver, the initial site of EPO production at early gestation, is less responsive than the kidneys to tissue hypoxia caused by anemia.
(b) EPO pharmacokinetics differ in preterm infants: faster rate of clearance, larger volume of distribution, shorter elimination and mean residence times.
(c) Clearance increases with duration of r-HuEPO therapy, suggesting the need for progressively higher doses.
(3) Variable results and small sample sizes hamper clinical trials testing different doses and treatment schedules.
(a) Therapy with r-HuEPO and iron stimulates erythropoiesis and increases reticulocyte counts.
(b) Increase in reticulocyte count is dose dependent.
(c) Oral iron supplement, adequate to support enhanced erythropoiesis, may not be tolerated. Intravenous iron therapy has not yet been adequately studied to ensure absence of oxidant injury and toxic metabolites; however, preterm infants appear to need a supplement of 4 to 4.5 mg/kg of dietary iron to prevent late anemia (Canadian Paediatric Society, Fetus and Newborn Committee, 2012).
(d) The combination of r-HuEPO and iron stimulates erythropoiesis in infants of ≤1250 g birth weight; however, support for the use of EPO in neonates has been mixed. In a Cochrane Review done in 2012, Aher and Ohlsson concluded that the lack of impact on transfusion requirements combined with an increased risk of retinopathy of prematurity does not support routine use of r-HuEPO. Others have suggested that later administration of r-HuEPO combined with adequate nutritional support results in a decreased need for RBC transfusions in low birth weight infants (Bishara and Ohls, 2009; Juul, 2012; Strauss, 2010).

d. Thrombopoietin. Recombinant human thrombopoietin is currently under development and testing for use as a megakaryocyte enhancer.
e. G-CSF: currently under investigation; stimulates growth of neutrophil colonies and induces maturation of promyelocytes to mature neutrophils.

**D. Transfusion volumes.**

1. Transfusions with PRBCs: For prevention of overhydration, replacement is usually given in increments of 15 mL/kg.
2. Partial exchange transfusions.
   a. With normal saline solution: treatment of polycythemia (to reduce hematocrit without reducing blood volume).
   b. With PRBCs: treatment of hydrops fetalis (to correct anemia without increasing blood volume).
   c. Calculations for total exchange volume:
      (1) Volume of normal saline solution to exchange =

$$\frac{\text{Blood volume} \times (\text{Measured hematocrit} - \text{Desired hematocrit})}{\text{Measured hematocrit}}$$

      (2) PRBC volume to exchange =

$$\frac{\text{Blood volume} \times (\text{Desired hematocrit} - \text{Measured hematocrit})}{\text{PRBC hematocrit} - \text{Measured hematocrit}}$$

3. Exchange transfusions.
   a. Single unit of blood (approximately 250 mL) will usually exchange twice the blood volume and remove 85% of the initial RBCs and 25% to 45% of the available intravascular bilirubin (Fasano and Luban, 2011).
   b. For treatment of hyperbilirubinemia.
   c. Because preservatives provide a significant glucose load, rebound hypoglycemia may occur.
   d. Preservatives contain citrate, which binds calcium and magnesium; hypocalcemia and hypomagnesemia may occur.
   e. Potassium level rises as blood ages; blood should be less than 5 days old. Washed RBCs may reduce the level of extracellular potassium and prevent hyperkalemia (Wu and Stack, 2007).
4. Platelets.
   a. One unit (approximately 40 mL) provides approximately $5 \times 10^{10}$ platelets; transfusion of 10 to 15 mL/kg of platelets should increase the platelet count by 50,000 to 100,000/$mm^3$ (Fasano and Luban, 2011).
   b. Routine volume reduction (platelet concentration) before transfusion is not indicated in infants.
   c. Platelets are separated from single units of whole blood within 6 hours of collection and suspended in small amounts of plasma, or they are obtained by apheresis (single-donor platelets).
5. FFP.
   a. FFP is usually transfused in increments of 10 mL/kg to minimize overhydration.
   b. Transfusion of 15 to 20 mL/kg replaces all coagulation proteins present in adult concentrations.
   c. Plasma is obtained from a unit of whole blood and frozen within 6 hours of collection.
6. Cryoprecipitate.
   a. Transfusion volume is usually 1 unit/kg (approximate volume, 15 mL).
   b. One unit contains approximately 100 to 250 mg of factor I (fibrinogen), approximately 80 to 100 units of factor VIII (von Willebrand's factor), and 50 to 75 units of factor XIII.
7. Albumin.
   a. For volume expansion, 5% albumin is usually administered in increments of 10 mL/kg; for improvement of oncotic pressure, 25% albumin might be used in increments of 1 g/kg (4 mL/kg).

b. Albumin is a major contributor to oncotic pressure because of molecular size and weight.

8. Granulocytes.
   a. Collected by leukapheresis and selectively harvested from whole blood.
   b. Granulocyte transfusions are rarely used due to the difficulty in isolation and the efficacy of G-CSF in elevating neutrophil counts (Blanchette et al., 2005).

## EVALUATION BY COMPLETE BLOOD CELL COUNT

The complete blood cell count is used in evaluating RBCs, WBCs, and platelets. The WBC indices are reviewed in Chapter 32.

**A. Evaluation of RBC indices.**

1. Identification of diseases affecting synthesis of hemoglobin.
2. RBC morphology.
   a. Anisocytosis: abnormal variation in size of erythrocytes (severe anemia).
   b. Macrocytosis: diameter greater than 9 mcm (increased cell volume: vitamin $B_{12}$ and folic acid deficiencies).
   c. Microcytosis: diameter less than 9 mcm (decreased cell volume: iron deficiency, spherocytic and hemolytic anemias).
   d. Poikilocytosis: variation in shape (severe anemia).
   e. Spherocytosis: increased thickness and rounding (decreased deformability and greater susceptibility to destruction; seen in congenital spherocytosis, hemolytic anemias, after transfusion of stored blood).
   f. Target cells: thin, with large diameter, dark center and periphery, and a clear ring between the periphery and the center (hemoglobinopathies, sickle cell/thalassemia, liver disease).
   g. Burr cells: crenations; long spinous processes (hemolytic anemias, DIC, liver disease).
   h. Howell–Jolly bodies: spherical blue bodies in or on erythrocytes; nuclear debris (in asplenia, pernicious anemia).
   i. Nucleated RBCs: immature RBCs with nuclei still present (in chronic blood loss, significant hemolysis, chronic hypoxia, infection).

## REFERENCES


Abbott, M.B., Levin, R.H., and Wu, S.: Medication potpourri. *Pediatrics in Review*, 27(8):283–288, 2006.

Aher, S., Malwatkar, K., and Kadam, S.: Neonatal anemia. *Seminars in Fetal and Neonatal Medicine*, 13 (4):239–247, 2008.

Aher, S.M., and Ohlsson, A.: Early versus late erythropoietin for preventing red blood cell transfusion in preterm and/or low birth weight infants. *Cochrane Database of Systematic Reviews*, (10): CD004865, 2012.

American Academy of Pediatrics: Policy statement: AAP publications reaffirmed. *Pediatrics*, 124:845, 2009.

American Cancer Society: Risks of blood product transfusion. 2011. Retrieved January 24, 2013, from http://www.cancer.org/treatment/treatmentsandsideeffects/treatmenttypes/bloodproductdonationandtransfusion/blood-product-donation-and-transfusion-possible-transfusion-risks.

American Red Cross: Blood testing. 2013. Retrieved March 16, 2013, from http://www.redcrossblood.org/learn-about-blood/what-happens-donated-blood/blood-testing.

Amin, S.C., Remon, J.I., Subbarao, G.C., and Maheshwari, A.: Association between red cell transfusions and necrotizing enterocolitis. *Journal of Maternal-Fetal & Neonatal Medicine*, 25(Suppl. 5):85–89, 2012.

Baer, V.L., Lambert, D.K., Henry, E., et al.: Do platelet transfusions in the NICU adversely affect survival? Analysis of 1600 thrombocytopenic neonates in a multihospital healthcare system. *Journal of Perinatology*, 27(12):790–796, 2007.

Bishara, N., and Ohls, R.K.: Current controversies in the management of the anemia of prematurity. *Seminars in Perinatology*, 33(1):29–34, 2009.

Blackburn, S.T.: *Maternal, fetal, and neonatal physiology: A clinical perspective* (4th ed.). St. Louis, 2013, Elsevier Saunders.

Blanchette, V., Dror, Y., and Chan, A.: Hematology. In M. G. MacDonald, M.D. Mullett, and M.M.K. Seshia (Eds.): *Avery's neonatology: Pathophysiology and management of the newborn* Philadelphia, 2005, Lippincott Williams & Wilkins, pp. 1169–1234.

Blickstein, I., and Friedman, S.: Fetal effects of autoimmune disease. In R.J. Martin, A.A. Fanaroff, and M.C. Walsh (Eds.): *Fanaroff and Martin's neonatal-perinatal medicine: Diseases of the fetus and newborn* St. Louis, 2011, Elsevier Mosby, pp. 335–342.

Brugnara, C., and Platt, O.S.: The neonatal erythrocyte and its disorders. In S.H. Orkin, D.G. Nathan, and D. Ginsberg et al, (Eds.): *Nathan and Oski's hematology of infancy and childhood* (7th ed.). Philadelphia, 2009, Elsevier Saunders, pp. 21–66.

Bussel, J.B., and Sola-Visner, M.: Current approaches to the evaluation and management of the fetus and neonate with immune thrombocytopenia. *Seminars in Perinatology*, 33:35–42, 2009.

Canadian Paediatric Society, Fetus and Newborn Committee: Routine administration of vitamin K to newborns. *Pediatrics & Child Health*, 2(6):429–432, 1997. Reaffirmed 2012.

Chalmers, E., Williams, M., Brennand, J., et al.: for the Paediatric Working Party of United Kingdom Haemophilia Doctors' Organization: Guideline on the management of haemophilia in the fetus and neonate. *British Journal of Haematology*, 154(2):208–215, 2011.

Chalmers, E.A.: Neonatal coagulation problems. *Archives of Disease in Childhood: Fetal and Neonatal Edition*, 89:F475–F478, 2004.

Christensen, R.D., Del Vecchio, A., and Ilstrup, S.J.: More clearly defining the risks of erythrocyte transfusion in the NICU. *Journal of Maternal-Fetal & Neonatal Medicine*, 25(Suppl. 5):90–92, 2012.

Clarke, P., and Shearer, M.J.: Vitamin K deficiency bleeding: The readiness is all. *Archives of Disease in Childhood*, 92(9):741–743, 2007.

Del Vecchio, A., and Motta, M.: Evidence-based platelet transfusion recommendations in neonates. *Journal of Maternal-Fetal & Neonatal Medicine*, 24(Suppl. 1):38–40, 2011.

Drew, J.H., Guaran, R.L., Cichello, M., and Hobbs, J.B.: Neonatal whole blood hyperviscosity: The important factor influencing later neurologic function is the viscosity and not the polycythemia. *Clinical Hemorheology and Microcirculation*, 17(1):67–72, 1997.

Fanaro, S.: Blood transfusion in infants: Techniques and adverse events. *Journal of Maternal-Fetal & Neonatal Medicine*, 24(Suppl. 1):47–49, 2011.

Fasano, R., and Luban, L.C.: Blood component therapy for the neonate. In R.J. Martin, A.A. Fanaroff, and M. C. Walsh (Eds.): *Fanaroff and Martin's neonatal-perinatal medicine: Diseases of the fetus and newborn.* St. Louis, 2011, Elsevier Mosby, pp. 1360–1373.

Galel, S.A., and Fontaine, M.J.: Hazards of neonatal blood transfusion. *NeoReviews*, 7(2):e69, 2006.

Holzhauer, S., and Zieger, B.: Diagnosis and management of neonatal thrombocytopenia. *Seminars in Fetal and Neonatal Medicine*, 16(6):305–310, 2011.

Israels, L.G., and Israels, S.J.: *Mechanisms in hematology* (3rd ed.). Toronto, 2002, Core Health Sciences, Inc., p. 402.

Johnson, P.J.: Vitamin K prophylaxis in the newborn: Indications and controversies. *Neonatal Network*, 32 (3):193–199, 2013.

Juul, S.: Erythropoiesis and the approach to anemia in premature infants. *Journal of Maternal-Fetal & Neonatal Medicine*, 25(Suppl. 5):97–99, 2012.

Kates, E.H., and Kates, J.S.: Anemia and polycythemia in the newborn. *Pediatrics in Review*, 28:33–34, 2007.

Kenet, G., Chan, A.K., Soucie, J.M., and Kulkarni, R.: Bleeding disorders in neonates. *Haemophilia*, 16 (Suppl. 5):168–175, 2010.

La Gamma, E.F., and Blau, J.: Transfusion-related acute gut injury: Feeding, flora, flow, and barrier defense. *Seminars in Perinatology*, 36(4):294–305, 2012.

Liley, H.G.: Immune hemolytic disease. In S.H. Orkin, D.G. Nathan, and D. Ginsberg et al, (Eds.): *Nathan and Oski's hematology of infancy and childhood* (7th ed.). Philadelphia, 2009, Elsevier Saunders, pp. 67–101.

Luchtman-Jones, L., and Wilson, D.B.: The blood and hematopoietic system. In R.J. Martin, A.A. Fanaroff, and M.C. Walsh (Eds.): *Fanaroff and Martin's neonatal-perinatal medicine: Diseases of the fetus and newborn.* St. Louis, 2011, Elsevier Mosby, pp. 1303–1373.

Manco-Johnson, M., Rodden, D.J., and Hays, T.: Newborn hematology. In S.L. Garner, B.S. Carter, M. Enzman-Hines, and J.A. Hernandez (Eds.): *Merenstein & Gardner's handbook of neonatal intensive care* (7th ed.). St. Louis, 2011, Elsevier Mosby, pp. 503–530.

Matthews, D.C., and Glader, B.: Erythrocyte disorders in infancy. In C.A. Gleason, and S.U. Devaskar (Eds.): *Avery's diseases of the newborn* (9th ed.). Philadelphia, 2012, Elsevier Saunders, pp. 1080–1107.

Mercer, J.S., and Erickson-Owens, D.A.: Rethinking placental transfusion and cord clamping issues. *Journal of Perinatal & Neonatal Nursing*, 26(3):202–207, 2012.

Mimouni, F.B., Merlob, P., Dollberg, S., and Mandel, D.: for the Israeli Neonatology Association: Neonatal polycythaemia: Critical review and a consensus statement of the Israeli Neonatology Association. *Acta Paediatrica*, 100(10):1290–1296, 2011.

Morag, I., Strauss, T., Lubin, D., et al.: Restrictive management of neonatal polycythemia. *American Journal of Perinatology*, 28(9):677–682, 2011.

Murphy, M.F. and Bussel, J.B.: Advances in the management of alloimmune thrombocytopenia. *British Journal of Haematology*, 136(3):366–378, 2007.

Murray, N.A. and Roberts, I.A.: Neonatal transfusion practice. *Archives of Disease in Childhood: Fetal and Neonatal Edition*, 89(2):F101–F107, 2004.

Nguyen-Vermillion, A., and Juul, S.E.: Hematologic system and disorders of bilirubin metabolism. In C.A. Gleason, and S.U. Devaskar (Eds.): *Avery's diseases of the newborn* (9th ed.). Philadelphia, 2012, Elsevier Saunders, pp. 1047–1055.

Ohls, R.K.: Developmental erythropoiesis. In R.A. Polin, W.W. Fox, and S.H. Abman (Eds.): *Fetal and neonatal physiology* (4th ed.). Philadelphia, 2011, Elsevier Saunders, pp. 1495–1520.

Ozek, E., Soll, R., and Schimmel, M.S.: Partial exchange transfusion to prevent neurodevelopmental disability in infants with polycythemia. *Cochrane Database of Systematic Reviews*, (1): CD005089, 2010.

Pappas, A., and Delaney-Black, V.: Differential diagnosis and management of polycythemia. *Pediatric Clinics of North America*, 51(4):1063–1086, 2004.

Parker, R.I.: Neonatal thrombosis, hemostasis, and platelet disorders. In A.R. Spitzer (Ed.): *Intensive care of the fetus and newborn* (2nd ed.). Philadelphia, 2005, Mosby, pp. 1295–1312.

Pichler, E., and Pichler, L.: The neonatal coagulation system and vitamin K deficiency bleeding—a mini review. *Wiener Medizinische Wochenschrift*, 158 (13–14):285–395, 2008.

Pipe, S.W., and Goldenberg, N.A.: Acquired disorders of hemostasis. In S.H. Orkin, D.G. Nathan, and D.

Ginsberg et al, (Eds.): *Nathan and Oski's hematology of infancy and childhood* (7th ed.). Philadelphia, 2009, Elsevier Saunders, pp. 1591–1620.

Sarkar, S., and Rosenkrantz, T.S.: Neonatal polycythemia and hyperviscosity. *Seminars in Fetal and Neonatal Medicine*, 13(4):248–255, 2008.

Steiner, L.A., and Gallagher, P.G.: Erythrocyte disorders in the perinatal period. *Seminars in Perinatology*, 31:254–261, 2007.

Strauss, R.G.: Anaemia of prematurity: Pathophysiology and treatment. *Blood Reviews*, 24(6):221–225, 2010.

Wong, E.C., and Luban, N.L.: Intrauterine, neonatal, and pediatric transfusion. In P.D. Mintz (Ed.): *Transfusion therapy: Clinical principles and practice* (2nd ed.). Bethesda, MD, 2005, AABB Press, pp. 159–201.

Wu, Y., and Stack, G.: Blood product replacement in the perinatal period. *Seminars in Perinatology*, 31:262–271, 2007.

Young, G.: Hemostatic disorders of the newborn. In C.A. Gleason, and S.U. Devaskar (Eds.): *Avery's diseases of the newborn* Philadelphia, 2012, Elsevier Saunders, pp. 1056–1107.

Zou, S., Stramer, S.L., and Dodd, R.Y.: Donor testing and risk: Current prevalence, incidence, and residual risk of transfusion-transmissible agents in US allogeneic donations. *Transfusion Medicine Reviews*, 26(2):119–128, 2012.

CHAPTER

# 32 Infectious Diseases in the Neonate

DIANA J. WILSON AND CAROL INGALS TYNER

**OBJECTIVES**

1. Differentiate the methods of acquisition of neonatal infection.
2. Identify risk factors for infection associated with term and preterm infants.
3. Describe clinical signs and symptoms of infection and septic shock.
4. Calculate the absolute neutrophil count and immature/total neutrophil ratio from a complete blood cell count and differential cell count.
5. Identify the common gram-positive and gram-negative organisms responsible for bacterial infections in the neonatal period.
6. Name common broad-spectrum antimicrobial agents used to treat neonatal sepsis and discuss indications for and risks of their use.
7. Differentiate between mucocutaneous, systemic, and cutaneous candidiasis.
8. Identify clinical symptoms and therapies associated with ToRCHES CLAP spectrum infections.
9. List prevention strategies for hospital-acquired infections.

The immature immune system of a neonate is characterized by immature activation and function of immune responses that make newborns more susceptible to infections with a frequency and an intensity greater than at any other period of life. In the first month of life, the risk of sepsis is the highest and remains the major cause of death. Up to 40% of the survivors will have some neurologic sequelae.

Greater than 1 million newborns globally die each year from sepsis. In the United States, as many as 1 to 5 infants per 1000 live births will have early-onset sepsis (EOS) and as many as 250 infants per 1000 live births will acquire late-onset sepsis (LOS) (Weston et al., 2011; Wynn and Wong, 2010). The incidence of septicemia increases substantially in very low birth weight (VLBW) and extremely low birth weight (ELBW) premature infants and results in 50% to 61% mortality. *Neonatal sepsis* is a general term used to define actual or potential infection in the neonatal and newborn period and is defined on a continuum. The diagnosis of sepsis remains one of the most difficult diagnostic tasks. Early detection and implementation of therapy are critical. Failure to identify early signs of sepsis contributes to morbidity, mortality, and increased health care costs. This chapter provides a comprehensive review of common neonatal infections, treatment modalities, and the latest recommendations for reducing hospital-acquired infections.

## TRANSMISSION OF INFECTIOUS ORGANISMS IN THE NEONATE

A. **Vertical transmission:** mother to infant.
   1. Intrauterine acquisition with intact membranes—organism most commonly crosses transplacentally from maternal bloodstream through the placenta to the fetus, but may be a direct extension of an infected uterus, ascend from the genital tract, or descend through the fallopian tubes.
      a. May result in death and embryo reabsorption, abortion, stillbirth, premature delivery, low birth weight (LBW), congenital anomalies, sepsis, or congenital disease.
   2. Intrapartum acquisition after rupture of membranes: organism may ascend through genital tract with prolonged rupture of membranes. Infection may also result from aspiration of

infected amniotic fluid or occur by colonization during passage of the fetus through the birth canal. Infection has also been demonstrated to occur through skin abrasions such as scalp electrodes during labor.

3. Postpartum acquisition: transmission through maternal breast milk to infant of several viruses, including HIV, hepatitis B virus, and cytomegalovirus.

B. **Horizontal transmission:** transmission to the infant from nursery personnel, family members and visitors, contaminated hospital equipment, invasive procedures and devices, and blood products; also known as a nosocomial infection or hospital-acquired infection (HAI).

## RISK FACTORS

### Identification of Predisposing Risk Factors for Neonatal Infection

A. **Maternal.**

1. Antepartum risk factors include: inadequate prenatal care, inadequate nutrition, low socioeconomic status, recurrent abortion, substance abuse, history of maternal sexually transmitted diseases, maternal urinary tract infection (UTI), and premature rupture of membranes.
2. Intrapartum risk factors include: prolonged rupture of membranes (>12 to 18 hours), vaginal GBS colonization, chorioamnionitis, uterine tenderness, purulent amniotic fluid, foul-smelling amniotic fluid, maternal fever greater than 38° C/101° F, prolonged or difficult labor, premature labor, maternal UTI, invasive intrapartum procedures (i.e., internal fetal monitoring), elevated maternal heart rate (>100 beats per minute [bpm]), and elevated fetal heart rate (>180 bpm).

B. **Neonatal.**

1. Neonatal risk factors include: prematurity, LBW, difficult delivery, birth asphyxia, meconium staining, resuscitation, low Apgar score (<6 at 5 minutes), congenital anomalies (i.e., abdominal wall and spinal defects), breach of skin integrity, and multiple-order births.

C. **Environmental.**

1. Environmental risk factors include: hospital admission, length of stay, invasive procedures (i.e., peripheral intravenous [IV] punctures, endotracheal tubes, umbilical catheters, central and peripherally inserted venous lines, thoracostomy tubes, and other surgical interventions), common use of broad-spectrum antibiotics, use of humidification systems in ventilation, and incubator care.

## DIAGNOSIS AND TREATMENT

### Recognition of Clinical Manifestations of Neonatal Infection

A. **Variable nonspecific presentation of sepsis:** appearance of infant "just not right," accompanied by subtle changes in feeding and activity. Culture-proven sepsis is difficult in the newborn infant; most are symptomatic without correlation of positive cultures.

B. **Specific manifestations of sepsis by systems:**

1. Thermoregulatory instability: temperature instability, fever, and hypothermia.
2. Neurologic: lethargy, jitteriness, irritability, seizures, hypotonia or hypertonia, bulging fontanelles, high-pitched or abnormal cry.
3. Respiratory distress (most common clinical sign): tachypnea, grunting, nasal flaring, retractions, cyanosis, apnea, respiratory acidosis, respiratory insufficiency, and radiologic evidence of pneumonia or pleural effusion.
4. Cardiovascular: tachycardia or bradycardia; arrhythmias; hypotension or hypertension; cold, clammy, or mottled skin; decreased peripheral perfusion or vasoconstriction; poor peripheral pulses; delayed capillary refill (>3 seconds); cardiomegaly; and poor cardiac function.
5. Gastrointestinal: poor feeding, vomiting, diarrhea, abdominal distention, feeding intolerance, hypoactive bowel sounds, and radiologic evidence of ileus, portal venous gas, pneumatosis, or free air.
6. Integumentary: rash, pustules or vesicles, jaundice, pallor, and petechiae.
7. Internal organ: hepatomegaly and splenomegaly.
8. Metabolic: hyperglycemia, hypoglycemia, or glucose instability, and metabolic acidosis.

C. **Septic/distributive shock:** profound sepsis resulting in insufficient perfusion, oxygenation, and delivery of nutrients to satisfy tissue requirements, resulting in cellular dysfunction and ultimately cell destruction. Rapid identification and treatment is paramount to preventing impending death (Agrawal, 2012) (see also Chapter 28).
  1. Clinical presentation of septic shock:
     a. Tachycardia or bradycardia.
     b. Increased work of breathing, tachypnea, retractions, apnea, progressing to respiratory insufficiency and failure.
     c. Persistent pulmonary hypertension with resulting decreased oxygenation.
     d. Poor perfusion with pallor, mottling, delayed capillary refill (>3 seconds), weak pulses, cool extremities, wide pulse pressures.
     e. Hypotension, decreased urinary output, organ dysfunction, ileus.
     f. Metabolic acidosis and other electrolyte disorders.
     g. Coagulopathy, oozing or bleeding, may progress to disseminated intravascular coagulation.
     h. Edema from capillary leak.
     i. Myocardial dysfunction, arrhythmias, impending cardiac arrest.

## Hematologic Evaluation

A. **Complete blood cell count (CBC).**
  1. White blood cell (WBC) count: interpretation is often difficult because of the wide range of normal values in the neonate (5000 to 30,000 cells/mm$^3$) (Oski and Naiman, 1966). WBC count is an unreliable indicator of infection as leukocyte counts are normal in greater than 30% of infants with proven bacteremia, and leukopenia (<5000 cells/mm$^3$) or leukocytosis (>20,000 cells/mm$^3$) may be present when greater than 50% of culture results are negative (Weinberg and D'Angio, 2011). This suggests leukocytosis can be a normal finding in the newborn infant. Leukopenia less than 1750 cells/mm$^3$ is generally considered an abnormal finding and may be due to sepsis, but may also be associated with maternal hypertension, asphyxia, or hemolytic disease.
  2. Differential cell count (Fig. 32-1).
     a. Neutrophil count.
        (1) Absolute neutrophil count (ANC) is calculated as:

$$ANC = WBCs \times (\%\ Immature\ neutrophils + \%\ Mature\ neutrophils) \times 0.01.$$

           (a) Manroe and colleagues (1979) developed a reference range for the ANC in term infants (Fig. 32-2).

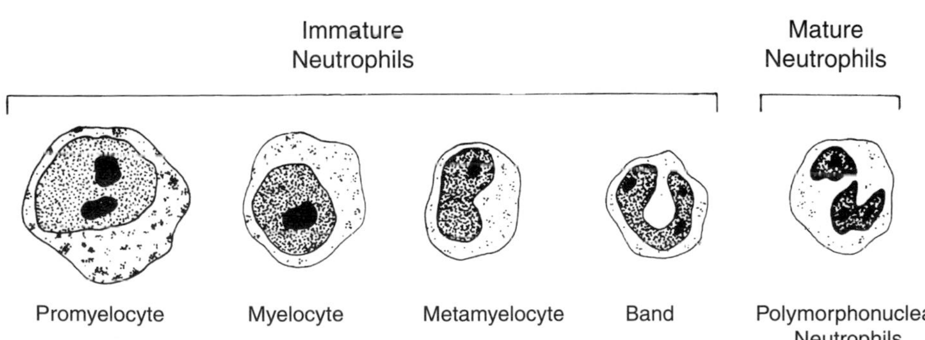


FIGURE 32-1 ■ Neutrophils represent a percentage of the total white blood cell count and are reported as the differential on a complete blood cell count.

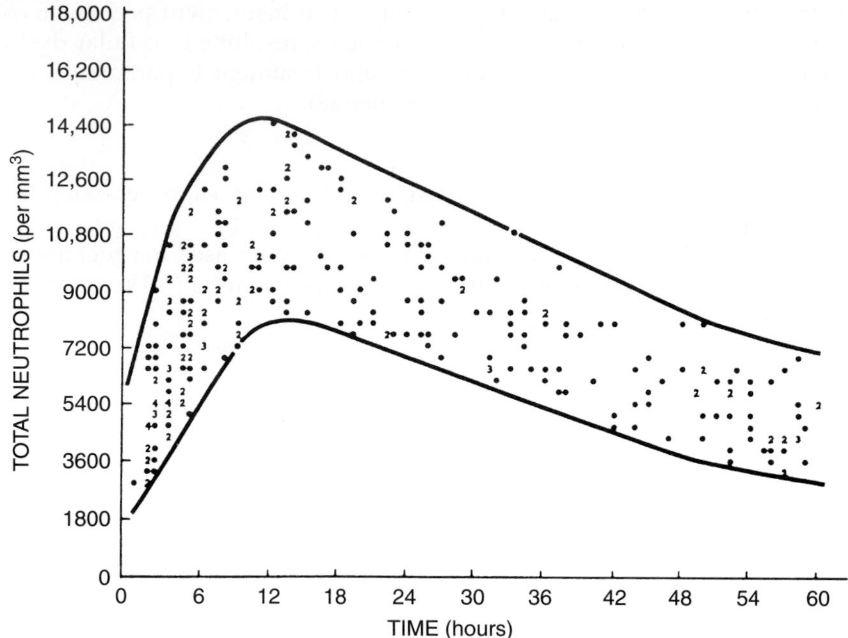


FIGURE 32-2 ■ Absolute neutrophil count reference range in the first 60 hours of life. (From Manroe, B.L., Weinberg, A.G., Rosenfeld, C.R., et al.: The neonatal blood count in health and disease. *Journal of Pediatrics*, 95[1]:89-98, 1979.)

(2) Neutropenia: less than 1800 cells/mm$^3$ (Manroe et al., 1979). Affects 6% to 8% of all NICU patients, or as many as 48,000 infants in the United States annually (Maheshwari and Black, 2012). Incidence is highest in premature infants and LBW infants, with 6% to 58% occurrence.

(a) Relationship between neutropenia and risk of infection is not well established in neonates, and infants with greater than 1000 cells/mm$^3$ may not be at increased risk (Maheshwari and Black, 2012).

(b) Decision to treat should not be based upon neutropenia alone.

(3) Neutrophilia.

(a) Inconsistent response to infection, often normal with serious infection.

(b) May be elevated at birth (as high as 26,000 cells/mm$^3$) because of birth stress, maternal fever, ≥6 hours of oxytocin, asphyxia, meconium aspiration, pneumothorax with uncomplicated hyaline membrane disease, seizures, prolonged crying (≥4 minutes), hypoglycemia less than 30 mg/dL, hemolytic disease, surgery, and high altitude (Weinberg and D'Angio, 2011).

**b.** Immature/total neutrophil (I/T) ratio.

(1) Increase in the I/T ratio is known as a left shift; reflects an increase in immature neutrophils.

(2) Not a consistent correlation with presence of serious infection. Low immature band counts may be due to depleted bone marrow reserves producing misleading low I/T ratios.

(3) Best used for negative predictor value. If I/T ratio is normal, likelihood infection is absent with 99% predictive value (Weinberg and D'Angio, 2011).

(4) I/T ratio greater than 0.2 to 0.25 is suggestive of infection (Fig. 32-3).

(5) Calculation of I/T ratio:

$$\frac{\%\ \text{Bands} + \%\ \text{Immature}\ \textit{forms}}{\%\ \text{Mature} + \%\ \text{Bands} + \%\ \text{Immature forms}}$$

**3.** Platelet count.

**a.** Normal count: 100,000 to 400,000/mm$^3$ in the first 10 days of life, greater than 150,000/mm$^3$ during the next 3 weeks of life.

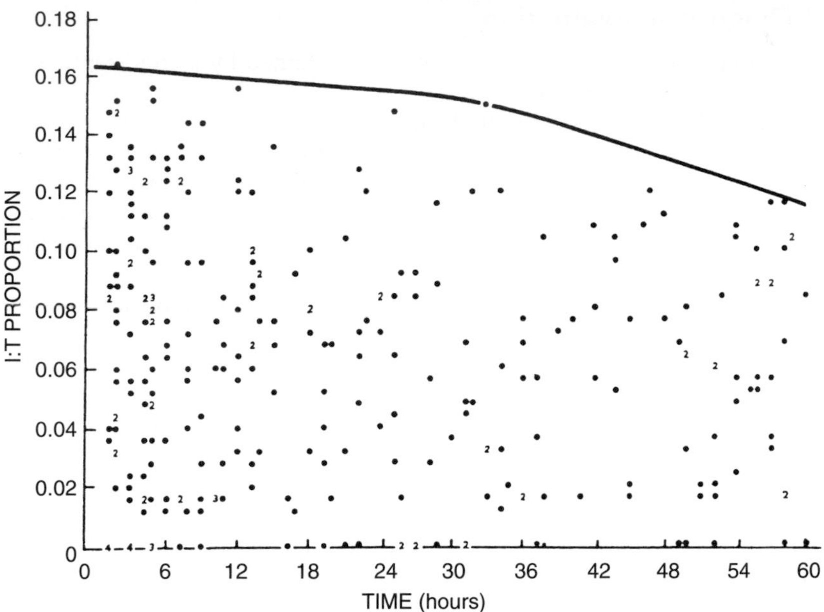


FIGURE 32-3 ■ I/T ratio. Reference range for the proportion of immature to total neutrophils in the first 60 hours of life. (From Manroe, B.L., Weinberg, A.G., Rosenfeld, C.R., et al.: The neonatal blood count in health and disease. *Journal of Pediatrics*, 95[1]:89-98, 1979.)

b. Thrombocytopenia (<100,000/mm$^3$): possible association with bacterial sepsis or viral infection, but usual onset does not occur until 1 to 3 days after infection onset (late indicator). May also occur with maternal HELLP syndrome (*h*emolysis, *e*levated *l*iver function test results, and *l*ow *p*latelet count), pregnancy-induced hypertension, and intrauterine growth restriction, as well as some syndromes such as trisomies 13, 18, and 21, Turner's syndrome, and hemolytic disease.

c. Severe and early-onset thrombocytopenia (<50,000/mm$^3$) is often an indicator of bacterial infection (Saxonhouse and Sola-Visner, 2012). With a clinically well infant without proven infection, neonatal alloimmune thrombocytopenia must be considered.

**B. C-Reactive protein (CRP).**

1. Nonspecific acute-phase reactant globulin that appears in the blood during an acute inflammatory process and is closely associated with tissue injury.
2. May act as a carrier protein facilitating removal of foreign or altered materials from invading microorganisms or damaged tissues. Role remains unclear in activation of immune system pathways (Weinberg and D'Angio, 2011).
3. Elevated cord blood CRP levels are associated with chorioamnionitis with prolonged rupture of membranes.
4. Elevated CRP is also associated with noninfectious conditions that cause tissue damage or inflammation, including: asphyxia, respiratory distress syndrome, intracerebral hemorrhage, surgery, gastroschisis, meconium aspiration, and recent immunizations. This reduces the positive predictive value of the CRP level and its usefulness as a diagnostic tool.
5. Serial CRP levels are helpful in exclusion of serious infection. CRP levels increase rapidly and are elevated within 1 day of bacterial infection, peak at 2 to 3 days, and remain elevated until infection and associated inflammatory process are resolved. CRP levels then return to normal within 5 to 10 days in most infants. For infants undergoing sepsis evaluation, normal CRP levels 1 to 3 days after initiation of evaluation may have a negative predictive value of 99%, allowing the discontinuation of antibiotic therapy in light of negative cultures.

## Additional Diagnostic Evaluation

A. **Culture:** isolation of a pathogen in a blood culture obtained by using aseptic technique is the "gold standard" for diagnosing infection.
   1. A minimum of 1 mL of blood should be obtained to improve chances for detection of bacteremia. Collection of only 0.5 mL has been shown to be unreliable in detection of pathogens (Nizet and Klein, 2011). Many clinicians suggest cultures from two sites are preferable in order to substantiate a positive culture. Adequate blood sample volume is associated with 90% sensitivity for bacterial detection and is twice as likely to yield a noncontaminant positive result (Piantino et al., 2013).
      a. May be falsely negative if mother received antibiotics in labor or if the infant has been exposed to multiple courses of antibiotics.
      b. Bacterial growth is evident within 48 hours for most cultures. Culture results are followed at 24-hour intervals, with a final report at 5 to 7 days.
      c. About 92% of positive blood cultures will be positive by 24 hours (Byington et al., 2003).
      d. False-positives can occur with contaminated specimens. Differentiating true sepsis from contamination can be challenging. Indicators of possible contamination include: increased time (>2 to 3 days) until culture became positive, only a single culture is positive, infant is clinically well, organism is part of normal skin flora, multiple organisms grow in one culture bottle, or different organisms grow in separate cultures. If the infant has clinical deterioration, bacteremia must be presumed rather than a contaminant.
      e. In light of positive cultures, appropriate therapy should be continued and daily cultures drawn until a minimum of two consecutive cultures are negative.

B. **Cerebrospinal fluid (CSF) culture and polymerase chain reaction (PCR).**
   1. Routine use of lumbar puncture remains controversial in early sepsis evaluation. Up to 15% of infants with sepsis develop meningitis, and may not have any accompanying clinical symptoms to indicate meningitis. Bacterial meningitis occurs in less than 1 case per 1000 infants, but risk increases with LBW and prematurity (Nizet and Klein, 2011).
   2. Lumbar puncture may be reserved for infants with clinical symptoms of central nervous system (CNS) involvement or proven bacteremia, or delayed for several days in an unstable infant until stabilization is achieved. The CSF culture results may be sterile after several days on antibiotic therapy, but abnormal CSF assays will still identify the presence of pleocytosis and an inflammatory reaction.
   3. Interpreting CSF findings.
      a. Cell counts vary widely in the first few weeks of life, making interpretation difficult. Additionally, blood in the CSF complicates interpretation.
      b. Polymorphonuclear leukocytes are often present in newborns.
      c. Elevated protein concentration occurs in newborns and is higher in premature and VLBW than term infants. By the third month of life, protein levels reach the normal values for older infants in term babies (<40 mg/dL), but may take longer in premature infants.
      d. CSF glucose concentrations are lower in neonates than in older infants, and may be as low as 30 mg/dL in term infants or 20 mg/dL in premature infants (Nizet and Klein, 2011).
      e. Gram stain smear of CSF can detect organisms in up to 78% of gram-negative meningitis, and up to 83% of group beta streptococci (GBS) meningitis. Gram-positive bacteria can be detected for up to 36 hours of antimicrobial therapy, and some gram-negative organisms can be seen for several days (Nizet and Klein, 2011).
      f. CSF culture.
         (1) Positive culture may reflect bacteremia from a bloody tap.
         (2) Repeat the CSF tap every 24 to 36 hours until culture is sterile.
         (3) Duration of antibiotic therapy is based on when the first negative culture is documented.
         (4) There is a direct correlation between adverse neonatal outcomes and persistence of bacteria in the CSF.

C. **Urine culture.**
   1. Incidence of UTI is low in EOS (1% to 2%), yield is significantly higher in LOS (7% to 8%) (Nizet and Klein, 2011).
   2. Contamination with urine obtained by an external collection bag is high. Urine sample should be obtained by sterile catheterization to avoid contamination and false-positive results.
      a. If urine is obtained by urethral catheterization, a bacterial count greater than 50,000 to 100,000 organisms per milliliter suggests infection.

D. **Repeat studies.**
   1. If a positive culture result has been obtained from blood, CSF, or urine specimen, a follow-up culture specimen should be obtained to document sterilization.
   2. Persistent bacteremia may be caused by resistance to antibiotics, incorrect administration of antibiotics, an occult site of infection that may require surgical intervention (e.g., abscess), or presence of invasive devices left in place during treatment for bacteremia.

## Systemic Inflammatory Response Syndrome (SIRS)

A. The neonatal SIRS is considered a state of physiologic dysregulation that is associated with deviations in laboratory values and vital signs, and despite scientific advances, remains poorly understood. In the neonatal population, SIRS is generally *presumed* to be caused by infection. SIRS, however, has many more noninfectious etiologies that produce symptoms mimicking sepsis, and prolonged treatment of presumed occult infection with negative cultures may cloud the timely identification and treatment of the causes of SIRS.

B. Definitions of and guidelines for SIRS have been modified from adult literature to fit the neonatal population by the International Pediatric Sepsis Consensus Conference, and published in 2005, (Goldstein, et al., 2005) but have limitations due to significant variations in normal vital sign values in premature and term infants alike (Piantino et al., 2013). Based on the guidelines, a neonate must have the presence of two of the following criteria, one of which must be an abnormal temperature or leukocyte count:
   1. Core temperature of greater than 38.5° C/101.3° F or less than 36° C/96.8° F.
   2. Tachycardia, defined as a mean heart rate greater than 2 standard deviations above normal for age in the absence of external stimulus, painful stimulus, or chronic medications. Otherwise, persistent unexplained elevation over a half-hour to 4-hour time frame.
   3. Bradycardia with heart rate less than 10th percentile for age in the absence of external vagal stimulus, β-blocker medications, or heart disease. Otherwise, persistent unexplained bradycardia over a half-hour to 4-hour time frame.
   4. Mean respiratory rate greater than 2 standard deviations above normal for age, mechanical ventilation related to acute deterioration, not due to neuromuscular disease or general anesthesia.
   5. Elevated or depressed leukocyte count for gestation, or greater than 10% immature neutrophils.
   6. Proven or suspected sepsis caused by any pathogen, or a clinical syndrome associated with high likelihood of infection. Positive evidence of infection, including derangements in examination, imaging, or laboratory tests, such as WBCs in normally sterile body fluid, perforated viscus, chest x-ray with pneumonia, petechial or purpuric rash, or purpura fulminans.
   7. SIRS in the presence of or as a result of proven or suspected infection.

C. Practitioners have the difficult task of deciding to discontinue empirical antibiotics with negative cultures.
   1. Differential etiologies for SIRS with negative cultures include: viral infections, cardiopulmonary diseases (structural heart lesions, patent ductus arteriosus, pulmonary hypertension, pulmonary hypoplasia, surfactant protein deficiency, and bronchopulmonary dysplasia), intraventricular hemorrhage, seizures, subgaleal and intracranial hemorrhage, opiate withdrawal, NEC, malrotation, bowel obstruction (meconium plug syndrome, meconium ileus, Hirschsprung's disease), metabolic disorders, and inborn errors (galactosemia, urea cycle disorders, organic acidemias, adrenal hyperplasia, hypoglycemia, autoinflammatory diseases) (Piantino et al., 2013).

## Therapy

A. **Antimicrobial therapy.**
   1. Appropriate antibiotic choice depends on prevalent organisms, age of onset of symptoms, and environmental setting. Additional factors include pharmacokinetics, efficacy, and potential toxicity of antimicrobial agents used.
      a. Treatment for suspected EOS must include antibiotics effective against gram-positive cocci (especially GBS), streptococci species, *Listeria monocytogenes*, and gram-negative enteric bacilli.
      b. Treatment for suspected LOS must include coverage for prevalent HAIs such as coagulase-negative staphylococci (CoNS) and *Staphylococcus aureus*, or organisms with increased incidences specific to the individual nursery.
   2. Ampicillin is commonly used in combination with an aminoglycoside such as gentamicin or tobramycin for synergy for initial broad-spectrum treatment of suspected or confirmed bacterial EOS.
      a. If GBS is identified in EOS, antibiotic coverage is changed to penicillin for the remainder of therapy. Additional aminoglycoside coverage is not necessary for synergy.
   3. If meningitis is suspected with EOS, ampicillin and cefotaxime are the antibiotics of choice until a specific organism has been identified.
      a. Third-generation cephalosporins, including cefotaxime and ceftazidime, have increased antimicrobial activity against gram-negative bacilli and enhanced penetration across the blood–brain barrier over gentamicin.
      b. Third-generation cephalosporins may lead to rapid emergence of drug-resistant bacteria when used extensively for presumptive therapy and therefore should be limited to infants with evidence of meningitis or gram-negative sepsis.
   4. Vancomycin and an aminoglycoside for synergy are used for initial treatment of suspected bacterial LOS due to penicillin G and ampicillin resistance of the majority of *S. aureus* organisms.
      a. Currently all staphylococcal strains in neonates have been susceptible to vancomycin, but vancomycin-resistant *S. aureus* has been identified in older populations (Nizet and Klein, 2011). Judicious use of vancomycin may help prevent further development of resistance in neonates.
   5. Duration of antibiotic therapy is a minimum of 10 to 14 days for proven sepsis with minimal or absent focal infection, and a minimum of 21 days for meningitis.
   6. If culture results are negative, antimicrobial agents may be discontinued after 48 to 72 hours, though antibiotics are often continued for 5 to 7 days of treatment in symptomatic infants or infants with deteriorating clinical condition despite negative culture results.
   7. If the mother was treated before delivery, the antimicrobial course may be extended in the face of negative culture results, or if multiple courses of antibiotics have presumably induced low bacterial load (i.e., recent course within 4 days of new-onset infection).

## Treatment of Septic Shock

A. **Treatment goals of septic shock** includes timely management of airway, breathing, and circulation to rapidly restore adequate tissue perfusion and improve patient outcomes (Adcock, 2012; Agrawal, 2012).
   1. Provide adequate ventilatory support and secure appropriate airway.
   2. Treat hypovolemia with isotonic crystalloid (normal saline, lactated Ringer's solution) for acute volume expansion.
   3. Transfuse with packed red blood cells (RBCs), platelets, fresh frozen plasma, or cryoprecipitate for anemia, blood loss for disseminated intravascular coagulation.
   4. Correct metabolic and electrolyte derangements, provide adequate nutrition, and avoid hypoglycemia due to increased energy demands and to avoid catabolism.
   5. Treat hypotension with inotropic agents and consider cortisol.
      a. Dopamine—positive inotropic and chronotropic effects that increase myocardial contractility, dependent on myocardial norepinephrine stores.

b. **Epinephrine**—potent inotropic and chronotropic effects, frequently used in infants non-responsive to dopamine.
c. **Hydrocortisone**—cortisol therapy in premature neonates is often used as a third-line treatment of refractory hypotension due to suspected adrenal insufficiency and may result in improved myocardial contractility, stroke volume, and cardiac output. It has been shown to increase blood pressure, decrease heart rate, and reduce the need for other vasoactive medications in neonates (Wang et al., 2010).

6. Treat underlying infection.
7. Evaluate cardiac function and arrhythmias with echocardiogram and electrocardiogram.
8. Extracorporeal membrane oxygenation for infants greater than 34 weeks of gestation if non-responsive to other interventions.

## Treatment Goals and Prevention Strategies

A. **Differential Diagnosis.** Because the findings are so nonspecific, it is often difficult to differentiate neonatal sepsis from other disease. The differential diagnosis for neonatal sepsis in the term or near-term infant generally includes the following systemic infections. Appropriate culture and/or serology distinguish these infections from neonatal sepsis.

1. Viral infections such as enteroviruses, herpes simplex virus (HSV), cytomegalovirus, influenza viruses, respiratory syncytial virus.
2. Spirochete infections—syphilis.
3. Parasitic infections—congenital malaria, toxoplasmosis.
4. Fungal infection—candidiasis.
5. Other bacterial infections include UTIs, osteomyelitis or septic arthritis, pneumonia, and tuberculosis.
6. Other diagnoses that may present with similar nonspecific findings include neonatal hypoxia, inborn errors of metabolism, cyanotic congenital heart disease, and neonatal respiratory distress.

## NEONATAL SEPTICEMIA

A. **Neonatal Sepsis and Incidence.** Neonatal sepsis is a clinical syndrome in an infant 28 days of life or younger. It is manifested by systemic signs of infection and/or isolation of a bacterial pathogen from the bloodstream. Most commonly presents as bacteremia and/or meningitis.

1. The overall incidence of neonatal sepsis in the United States in the last 10 years is between 1 and 5 per 1000 live births. Term infants have a reported rate of 1 to 2 per 1000 live births. The late preterm rate was 4 to 6 per 1000 live births (Cohen-Wolkowiez et al., 2009).
2. Defined by the age at which onset occurs.
   a. EOS is infection presenting at less than 72 hours to 7 days of life, caused by maternal intrapartum transmission of invasive organism.
   b. LOS is infection presenting at greater than 72 hours or ≥7 days of age and is attributed to pathogens acquired postnatally.
   c. Late-late-onset sepsis is defined as occurring in infants born at ≤28 weeks and infection presenting after 3 months of age.
3. Recent database results from the NICHD Neonatal Research Network in infants born from 2006 to 2009 estimated the overall incidence of EOS to be 0.98/1000 live births, with increasing rates in premature infants. Mortality was 7% (CDC, Active Bacterial Core Surveillance, Emerging Infections Program Network, 2011; Stoll et al., 2011).
   a. In VLBW infants (<1500 g birth weight) the incidence was 11 in 1000 live births. Mortality was 18%.
   b. Rates of LOS are most common in preterm LBW infants, with rates from 1.87% to 5.42%, with decreasing rates as birth weight increases.
   c. African American preterm neonates account for 5.14 cases per 1000 births, with a case fatality rate of 24.4%.

**B. Responsible Organisms.**

1. Currently, GBS accounts for 43% followed by *E. coli* with 29%. Combined they account for 70% of EOS and LOS cases.
2. In VLBW infants with birth weights of less than 2500 g, rates of GBS were 2.1 in 1000 births, *E. coli* infection rate was 5.1 in 1000 births.
   a. Other bacterial agents associated with early onset are *L. monocytogenes, Haemophilus influenzae, Enterobacter* spp., *Streptococcus pyogenes*, and *Streptococcus pneumoniae.*
3. Cases with LOS are most commonly associated with CoNS (rate of 48%), *S. aureus* (rate of 8%), *Klebsiella pneumoniae, Pseudomonas aeruginosa, Enterobacter* spp., *Citrobacter* spp., and *Candida*. Gram-negative LOS is less common but has the greater mortality of 19% to 36%. Fungal infections account for roughly 12% of LOS in VLBW infants, although the incidence among centers varies widely (Edwards, 2012; Stoll et al., 2011).

## Common Focal Sites and Pathogens

Following are brief descriptions of common focal sites and pathogens that contribute to the overall septicemia seen in neonates.

**A. Meningitis.** Any isolation of a pathogen from CSF culture is generally considered evidence of meningitis, regardless of the CSF cell count or chemistries.

1. Incidence of meningitis has remained stable since the 1970s. Depending upon the inclusion criteria, the incidence is between 0.25 and 0.32 per 1000 live births. Occurs in as many as 15% of neonates with bacteremia. In a study done between 2006 and 2009 in the United States, 72% of infants who had sepsis or meningitis and who presented within 72 hours of birth had infection caused by GBS or *E. coli* (Stoll, et al., 2011).
2. EOS infections acquired in the first 2 to 6 days after birth reflect vertical transmission from maternal genital tract flora. Those infections acquired after the first week of life suggest vertical transmission with neonatal colonization from maternal flora or horizontal transmission through contact with colonized household or community caregivers.
3. Of neonates who present with early-onset GBS bacteremia, 5% to 10% will develop meningitis. Of those with late-onset GBS infection, 25% will have meningitis (Heath et al., 2003, Stoll et al., 2011).
   a. Other gram-positive organisms that contribute to 4% of cases overall are *Enterococcus*, coagulase-negative staphylococci, *S. aureus, L. monocytogenes*, and α-hemolytic streptococci. Mortality with gram-positive meningitis is approximately 10%.
4. Gram-negative bacillus is responsible for 3.6% of cases in which neonates present with meningitis. It is the fifth most common cause of meningitis in infants. Gram-negative bacilli seed the CSF secondary to bacteremia, trauma, and surgery. Subsequent meningitis can develop as a result of bacterial multiplication and induction of inflammation in the subarachnoid and ventricular space; this is followed by a progression of inflammation and development of neuronal damage.
   a. *E. coli* and *Klebsiella pneumoniae* account for the majority of cases; other less frequent pathogens include *Pseudomonas aeruginosa, Acinetobacter, Enterobacter*, and *Serratia*. Gram-negative bacillary meningitis is commonly accompanied by bacteremia. Mortality range in children has ranged from 40% to 80%.
5. Chronic complications of neonatal meningitis include (Libster et al., 2012):
   a. Hydrocephalus, multicystic encephalomalacia, porencephaly, and white matter atrophy. The clinical manifestations of these complications include:
      (1) Developmental delay in approximately 25%.
      (2) Late-onset seizures in approximately 25%.
      (3) Cerebral palsy in approximately 20%.
      (4) Hearing loss in approximately 10%.
      (5) Cortical blindness in less than 10%.
   b. Term infants, after GBS meningitis, had mild to moderate neurologic impairment in 25% of cases, and 19% had severe neurologic impairment (Libster, et al., 2012).
6. The clinical presentation of neonatal meningitis typically is indistinguishable from that of neonatal sepsis without meningitis. The most commonly reported clinical signs are:

a. Temperature instability: presents in approximately 60% of neonates with bacterial meningitis. Term infants are more likely to have fever, whereas preterm infants are more likely to have hypothermia.
b. Neurologic signs of neonatal meningitis (Nizet and Klein, 2011; Pong and Bradley, 1999):
   (1) Irritability is present in up to 60% of infants.
   (2) Seizures have been reported as a presenting feature in 20% to 50%. Meningitis resulting from gram-negative pathogens presents with seizures, usually focal rather than generalized, more often than gram-positive pathogens.
   (3) Bulging fontanelle is present in approximately 25% of infants, and nuchal rigidity in approximately 15%. Findings of a full, but not bulging, fontanelle and normal neck flexion at the time of initial presentation are more the rule than the exception.
c. Other findings reported are:
   (1) Poor feeding/vomiting in approximately 50%.
   (2) Respiratory distress in 33% to 50%.
   (3) Apnea in 10% to 30%.
   (4) Diarrhea in 20%.

7. Diagnostic features that are characteristic of neonatal bacterial meningitis include:
   a. Isolation of a bacterial pathogen from the CSF by culture and/or by visualization by Gram stain. CSF result may be positive even though blood culture result is negative.
      (1) When the CSF culture is positive, a repeat culture should be done in 24 to 36 hours after initiation of treatment to ensure adequate therapy and document sterilization of the CSF.
      (2) Neonates in whom a traumatic lumbar puncture occurred should be treated for presumed sepsis and meningitis, pending results of CSF culture.
   b. Increased white blood cell counts in CSF of greater than 1000 WBCs/mcl with predominately neutrophils.
   c. Decreased CSF glucose of less than 30 mg/dL in term and less than 20 mg/dL in preterm infants.
   d. Elevated CSF protein of greater than 100 mg/dL in term and greater than 150 mg/dL in preterm infants.
   e. Neuroimaging is indicated to assist in defining the potential complications of neonatal meningitis. It is suggested that a neuroimaging study be done 48 to 72 hours before the anticipated end of therapy.
      (1) Cranial ultrasound can be performed at the bedside, and when completed early in the course of infection is most helpful for assessing ventricular size and the presence of intraventricular hemorrhage. It can also demonstrate ventriculitis and extracerebral fluid collections.
      (2) Computed tomography or magnetic resonance imaging can demonstrate the degree of cerebral edema, obstruction of CSF flow, infarction, abscess, and subdural fluid collections.

8. Antibiotic therapy. Prompt initiation is crucial for optimal outcome, and antibiotics may be administered before results of CSF specimen are obtained.
   a. In EOS, appropriate broad-spectrum antimicrobial therapy for suspected bacterial meningitis within the first 3 to 6 days of age is ampicillin and an aminoglycoside, usually gentamicin.
   b. When meningitis resulting from a gram-negative organism is strongly suspected or CSF Gram stain reveals gram-negative bacilli, the empirical regimen of ampicillin and an aminoglycoside should be expanded to include cefotaxime for CSF penetration.
      (1) Duration of therapy is dependent on recovered pathogens and clinical response, generally 14 to 21 days.
   c. Antibiotic choice in the neonate who presents with LOS bacterial meningitis depends on the preliminary CSF findings.
      (1) LOS without meningitis in neonates need to be treated with vancomycin and an aminoglycoside, if the lumbar puncture suggests meningitis. Cefotaxime should be added to provide an extended spectrum for gram-negative enterics and for optimal activity in the CSF against pneumococci.

(2) Once the causative pathogen and susceptibility pattern are known, the antimicrobial therapy should be altered accordingly.

d. GBS is uniformly susceptible to penicillin and ampicillin, and a combination of either with an aminoglycoside is recommended. The aminoglycoside is to improve synergy.

e. Gram-negative enteric bacteria: *E. coli*—ampicillin is the antimicrobial of choice.

f. Ampicillin-resistant *E. coli* and other gram-negative organisms usually are treated with cefotaxime in combination with gentamicin.

(1) Once sterility of the CSF is documented, the combination is continued for 7 to 14 days.

g. Coagulase-negative staphylococci—vancomycin is the antibiotic of choice.

9. Management.

a. Lumbar puncture should be repeated routinely at 24 to 48 hours after initiation of antimicrobial therapy to document CSF sterilization.

b. Gram-positive bacteria usually clear from the CSF within 24 to 48 hours after initiation of appropriate therapy. Gram-negative pathogens may persist for several days in severe cases.

c. Failure to respond to clinically and bacteriologically appropriate antimicrobial therapy can lead to significant neurologic sequelae such as hydrocephalus, multicystic encephalomalacia, porencephaly, and cerebral cortical and/or white matter atrophy.

d. Infants with suspected bacterial meningitis need to be in the NICU setting and monitored for signs of increased intracranial pressure, such as bradycardia, hypertension, respiratory distress, bulging fontanelle, accelerated head growth, separation of the cranial sutures, hemiparesis, and focal seizures and/or new-onset seizures.

(1) Development of these complications may necessitate additional evaluation and neurologic consultation.

(2) Evaluation and management with infectious disease experts to ensure adequate duration of antimicrobial therapy.

e. Long-term follow-up for survivors of neonatal meningitis includes monitoring of hearing, visual acuity, and development status.

(1) Hearing should be evaluated by evoked-response audiometry within 4 to 6 weeks of completion of therapy (Estripeaut and Saez-Llorens, 2009).

f. Survivors are also at risk for developmental delay and may be eligible to receive early intervention services in the United States (eligibility criteria vary by state).

g. Appropriate referrals should be made as indicated, and developmental surveillance should continue throughout childhood.

**B. Pneumonia**

1. In developed countries, the estimated incidence of pneumonia in full-term infants is less than 1% and increases to 10% in preterm infants. Early-onset pneumonia is generally within 3 days of birth and is acquired by vertical transmission from the mother to the infant by one of three routes:

a. Transplacental transmission of organisms from the mother to the fetus through the placental circulation.

b. Intrauterine aspiration of contaminated amniotic fluid.

c. Aspiration of infected amniotic fluid during or after birth. The neonate can aspirate vaginal organisms that are colonizing the maternal genital area, leading to respiratory colonization.

2. Late-onset pneumonia usually occurs after 3 days of life, and generally arises from colonized organisms present in the hospitalized newborn. Horizontal transmission, or nosocomial infection, is acquired from infected caregivers, family members, or contaminated equipment. Microorganisms can invade through injured tracheal or bronchial mucosa or through the bloodstream.

3. The pathologic changes vary with the type of organism, either bacterial or viral.

a. Bacterial pneumonia is characterized by inflammation of the pleura, infiltration or destruction of bronchopulmonary tissue, and leukocyte and fibrinous exudate within alveoli and the bronchi/bronchioles. Bacteria often reside within the interstitial spaces, alveoli, and bronchi.

b. Viruses typically cause an interstitial pneumonia. The extensive inflammation occasionally occurs with hyaline membrane formation, followed by varying degrees of interstitial fibrosis and scarring.
c. In the United States, GBS is the most common early-onset pathogen. Injury from GBS in the lungs increases the permeability that contributes to the development of alveolar edema and hemorrhage and possibly the mechanism that is responsible for bloodstream extension.

4. Pathogens responsible for EOS with pneumonia include: *E. coli* > GBS > *Klebsiella* > *S. aureus* > *S. pneumoniae* (Duke, 2005).
   a. Other less common bacterial pathogens include *L. monocytogenes* and *Mycobacterium tuberculosis*, both of which can be transmitted transplacentally.
   b. Viral—Of the viral infections, HSV is the most common viral agent to cause early-onset pneumonia. HSV pneumonia occurs in 33% to 54% of disseminated HSV infections and usually is fatal in spite of treatment (Speer, 2012).
   c. Fungal—Approximately 25% of VLBW infants are colonized by *Candida* in the gastrointestinal and respiratory tracts, presumably during labor and delivery.
      (1) Pneumonia occurs in 70% of infants with systemic candidiasis (Baley et al., 1986).
5. Late-onset pneumonia occurs usually in those infants who have prolonged hospitalization that results in deviations to normal flora. There is a predominance of gram-positive organisms, including *S. pyogenes*, *S. aureus*, and *S. pneumoniae*.
   a. *S. aureus* and *K. pneumoniae* cause extensive tissue damage, abscess formation, and empyema.
   b. *E. coli*, *Serratia marcescens*, *Enterobacter cloacae*, *S. pneumoniae*, and *P. aeruginosa* may cause pneumatoceles.
   c. *Citrobacter diversus* is frequently associated with brain abscess and can also cause lung abscess.
   d. *Chlamydia trachomatis* has a long incubation period and typically is associated with pneumonia occurring between 2 and 4 weeks of age. Occurs where untreated sexually transmitted disease is present.
6. Risks: Patients who require assisted ventilation are at highest risk for late-onset pneumonia.
7. Clinical manifestations:
   a. Early-onset pneumonia commonly presents with respiratory distress beginning at or soon after birth. Infants may have associated lethargy, apnea, tachycardia, and poor perfusion. It can progress to septic shock.
   b. Some infants develop pulmonary hypertension.
   c. Ventilatory-dependent infants may have increased oxygen and ventilator requirements or purulent tracheal secretions.
8. Diagnosis: Because signs of pneumonia are nonspecific, any newborn infant with sudden onset of respiratory distress or other signs of illness should be evaluated for pneumonia and/or sepsis.
   a. Cultures of blood and CSF should be obtained.
   b. If viral or other nonbacterial infection is suspected, specific studies should be obtained, including PCR.
   c. Gram stain and culture of tracheal aspirates may identify the causative organism.
   d. Chest x-ray examination.
      (1) Bilateral alveolar densities with air bronchograms are characteristic, but irregular patchy infiltrates can occur.
         (a) Pneumonia caused by GBS or other pathogens is difficult to distinguish from respiratory distress syndrome (RDS) in premature infants.
         (b) Pleural effusions occur in up to 67% of infants with pneumonia, but are rarely found in RDS. However, pleural effusions can also be seen in infants with transient tachypnea of the newborn, congenital heart disease, and hydrops fetalis.
9. Therapy: The choice of empirical regimens is based upon whether the infection is early- or late-onset.

a. In early-onset pneumonia, a frequently used initial regimen for empirical coverage is ampicillin and gentamicin. Ampicillin is effective against GBS and most other strains of streptococci.
   (1) Third-generation cephalosporins should not be used for suspected sepsis or pneumonia.
   (2) Gram-negative bacilli can rapidly develop resistance to cephalosporins.
b. For late-onset pneumonia, antibiotic choice depends on the prevalence sensitivity of bacteria in both the community and the hospital. The choice for term infants is vancomycin plus gentamicin.
c. The usual treatment course for uncomplicated pneumonia is 10 to 14 days.

C. **Urinary tract infections.** UTIs in newborns frequently are associated with bacteremia and may result in long-term complications. Newborns with UTI should be evaluated for associated systemic infection and anatomic or functional abnormalities of the urinary tract.

1. Incidence: In term newborns, the incidence of bacteriuria was 0.1% to 1%, and in preterm infants, the incidence is 2% to 6%. UTI occurs in males 1.5 to 5 times more than females. The incidence decreases in boys and increases in girls during the first 6 months after birth. Approximately one third of newborns with UTI have an accompanying bacteremia, and 1% will have meningitis.
2. *E. coli* is the most common organism found, accounting for 80% of cases responsible for UTIs.
   a. Other organisms found were *Klebsiella* > *Enterobacter* > *Citrobacter*.
   b. Most common gram-positive organisms were *Staphylococcus* and *Enterococcus* species, but they occur less frequently than do gram-negative pathogens.
3. Most UTIs in newborns represent upper tract infection (pyelonephritis). Pathogenesis includes either hematogenous spread secondary to bacteremia or ascending infections, especially in infants with urinary tract abnormalities. Approximately 30% to 50% of term newborns with a UTI have urinary tract abnormalities, of which vesicoureteric reflux is the most common. Other lesions found in infants with UTI include obstructive abnormalities such as posterior urethral valves, malformations such as ectopic ureter, and renal conditions such as polycystic diseases.
4. Clinical manifestations: General signs are often nonspecific and may include temperature instability, poor weight gain, poor feeding, cyanosis, abdominal distention, hyperglycemia, hematuria, and proteinuria. Localized signs consist of a weak urinary stream and/or bladder distention.
5. Diagnosis: A urine specimen should be obtained by sterile catheterization.
   a. Diagnosis of UTI is based on culture of an organism from the urine.
   b. Because of the associated risk of bacteremia, blood cultures should be obtained.
6. Therapy: antimicrobial agents. Treatment with parenteral IV broad-spectrum antibiotics as soon as cultures of urine, blood, and CSF (if indicated) have been obtained.
   a. Ampicillin and gentamicin provide coverage for the most common bacterial pathogens. Changes in antibiotic therapy are based on culture results, including antimicrobial susceptibilities. Usual duration for therapy is 10 to 14 days.
7. Management: Repeat urine culture should be sterile within 36 to 48 hours after initiation of antimicrobial therapy.
   a. If a UTI has been documented in an infant, voiding cystourethrogram should be performed to evaluate the possibility of any congenital abnormalities of the urinary tract.

## INFECTION WITH SPECIFIC PATHOGENS

### Group B Streptococcus

A. ***Streptococcus agalactiae* is a gram-positive diplococcus encapsulated bacterium that has been the principal GBS pathogen in the neonate for over 50 years.** GBS accounts for more than 95% of EOS and more than 90% of LOS in neonates in the United States today. The reported fatality rate among preterm neonates with birth weights greater than 1500 g was 20%, nearly an eight-fold increase compared to term infants (Phares et al., 2008).

1. There are 10 GBS serotypes, with serotypes Ia, Ib, II, III, and V recognized as the most common organisms colonizing the gastrointestinal and genital tracts of 15% to 40% of pregnant women and as the primary risk factor for GBS infection in neonates from 0 to 90 days of age.
2. GBS infection in neonates is classified by age at onset into early-onset GBS, occurring within 24 hours of birth up to day 7 of life; late-onset GBS, which has a broader range from 7 to 89 days; and late, late-onset GBS, which occurs in infants older than 3 months of age.
   a. Nearly 50% of infants who pass through a colonized birth canal become colonized. However, only 1% to 2% will develop invasive disease, dependent on the presence or absence of additional risk factors.
3. Risk factors include:
   a. Delivery at less than 37 weeks of gestation.
   b. Premature rupture of membranes.
   c. Rupture of membranes ≥18 hours before delivery.
   d. Clinical signs of chorioamnionitis, maternal temperature ≥100.4° F or (38° C) during labor.
   e. Maternal GBS bacteriuria during the current pregnancy.
   f. Prior delivery of an infant with GBS disease.
   g. Heavy maternal colonization inoculum (>$10^5$ colony-forming units/mL) vaginally.
4. Since the implementation of universal screening of pregnant women at 35 to 37 weeks of gestation and recommendations for providing intrauterine antibiotic prophylaxis (IAP) in 2002, surveillance data by the CDC from 2010 demonstrate a decline from 1.7 cases per 1000 live births (1993) to 0.28 cases per 1000 live births (2008) in the United States.
   a. Racial disparities remain, with approximately twice the incidence occurring among African Americans than non–African Americans for all age groups.
   b. Despite highly effective prevention efforts, an estimated 1100 infants still become infected each year in the United States. Early-onset GBS accounts for 80% to 85% of cases. Late-onset GBS accounts for 50% of cases that present usually at 5 to 6 weeks after birth (American Academy of Pediatrics, Committee on Infectious Diseases, 2012; CDC, 2010; Remington et al., 2011).
   c. Late-onset GBS usually occurs at 4 or 5 weeks of age. Up to 50% of LOS is thought to be attributable to vertical transmission at birth and horizontally in household and community settings.
   d. Late, late-onset GBS occurs in infants older than 3 months of age. The infants who most commonly develop late, late-onset GBS are infants who were born before 28 weeks of gestation or those with a history of immunodeficiency.
5. Early-onset GBS infection most commonly manifests as:
   a. Generalized sepsis.
   b. Pneumonia.
   c. Meningitis.
   d. Infants whose mothers receive IAP are less likely to have sepsis, need assisted ventilation, or have documented GBS bacteremia (Feng-Ying, et al., 2011).
6. Sepsis without a focus of infections occurs in 80% to 85% of cases of early-onset GBS. The signs and symptoms are nonspecific. Late-onset GBS disease most often presents as bacteremia without a focus in about 65% of cases. Meningitis remains the most common presentation of late-onset GBS and occurs in approximately 25% to 30% of cases.
   a. Refer to sections on neonatal sepsis, pneumonia, and meningitis discussed earlier for clinical manifestations, diagnostics, therapy, management, and prevention.
   b. Penicillin remains the preferred agent, with ampicillin an acceptable alternative.
7. Other less common (2% to 3%) but well-described late-onset GBS focal infections are:
   a. Bacteremic cellulitis.
   b. Osteoarthritis.
8. Guidance with empirical therapy for early- or late-onset GBS can be reviewed online at http://www.cdc.gov/groupbstrep/guidelines/index.html. New in the 2010 guidelines:
   a. There are expanded options for laboratory detection of GBS, including use of pigmented media and PCR assays.

b. There is a revised colony count threshold for laboratories to report GBS in the urine of pregnant women.
c. There are revised algorithms for GBS screening and use of IAP for women with threatened preterm delivery, including one algorithm for preterm labor and one for preterm premature rupture of membranes.
d. Recommendations for IAP agents are presented in an algorithm format in an effort to promote use of the most appropriate antibiotic for penicillin-allergic women.
e. A minor change has been made to penicillin dosing to facilitate implementation in facilities with different prepackaged penicillin products.
f. The neonatal management algorithm's scope was expanded to apply to all newborns.
g. It provides management recommendations that depend upon clinical appearance of the neonate and other risk factors such as maternal chorioamnionitis, adequacy of IAP if indicated for the mother, gestational age, and duration of membrane rupture.
h. Changes were made to the algorithm to reduce unnecessary evaluations in well-appearing newborns at relatively low risk for early-onset GBS disease.

## Fungal Infection: Candidiasis

**A. Candidiasis is caused by *Candida*, budding yeasts that form long chains called pseudohyphae.**

1. Species causing most infections is *Candida albicans*, though *Candida parapsilosis* and *Candida glabrata* are also responsible for candidiasis in increasing numbers over the last 10 years in VLBW neonates (Remington et al., 2011).
2. *Candida* species are found on the skin and in the mouth, intestinal tract, and vagina. Transmission to neonate can occur in utero, intrapartum, or postnatally through breastfeeding. Risk factors include infants less than 1500 g, intubation, abdominal or cardiac surgery, NEC, spontaneous intestinal perforation, neutropenia, use of corticosteroids and histamine$_2$ ($H_2$) blockers, long-term use of broad-spectrum antibiotics, use of total parenteral nutrition and lipids, hyperglycemia, and invasive central catheters. Of VLBW infants less than 1000 grams, 5% to 20% develop disseminated or invasive candidiasis and approximately 75% have prolonged hospitalization, neurodevelopmental impairment (AAP, Committee on Infectious Diseases, 2012), and up to 30% mortality even with appropriate therapy (Remington et al., 2011).
3. Mucocutaneous candidiasis results in oral–pharyngeal (thrush) or vaginal and cervical candidiasis (lesions of gluteal folds, buttocks, groin, neck, and axillae).
   a. Most common form of candidiasis in the newborn infant.
   b. Mucosal lesions appear as white plaques on oral mucosa.
   c. Diaper dermatitis presents with intense erythema and satellite lesions.
4. Congenital candidiasis presents with widespread erythematous maculopapular rash, and preterm infants may present with pneumonia.
5. Disseminated candidiasis may involve any organ or anatomic site and may present with acute respiratory deterioration, acidosis, feeding intolerance, hypotension, skin abscesses, temperature instability, and/or erythematous rash.
   a. Common sites of lesions include the brain, kidneys, liver, spleen, lungs, and retinas but lesions typically do not appear until late in the course of the disease (AAP, Committee on Infectious Diseases, 2012).
6. Mucocutaneous candidiasis is usually diagnosed clinically with the visualization of lesions. Disseminated candidiasis is confirmed through isolation of the organism from blood, CSF, or urine cultures. Focal lesions are diagnosed with ophthalmologic examination, ultrasonography, computed tomography, and magnetic resonance imaging.
7. Treatment: Guidelines for management were updated in 2009 by the Infectious Diseases Society of America and contain recommendations for neonates (available at: http://cid.oxfordjournals.org/content/48/5/503.1.full#sec-6) (Pappas, et al., 2009).
   a. Mucocutaneous candidiasis is treated with oral nystatin suspension and topical nystatin cream or powder. Fluconazole is also used for oral therapy and may be more effective

than nystatin. IV fluconazole or amphotericin B can be used for chronic, severe, or refractory cases.

b. Invasive disease is treated by prompt removal of infected invasive catheters, and IV amphotericin B remains the drug of first choice for neonates.
   (1) Fluconazole has limited data for treatment of meningitis and can be considered if UTI and meningitis are excluded.
   (2) Echinocandins are reserved for drug-resistant species and should be used with caution as safety and dosing have not been established in neonates.
   (3) Most *Candida* species are susceptible to amphotericin B, though lipid preparations of amphotericin B may not penetrate into the kidney parenchyma.

c. Fungal prophylaxis of VLBW infants less than 1000 or less than 1500 g has demonstrated significant reduction in *Candida* colonization, invasive disease, and related mortality in four prospective randomized controlled trials and 10 retrospective cohort studies. Based on these studies, fluconazole has been shown to be safe and effective as prophylaxis in this population and is recommended for NICUs with moderate (5% to 10%) or high ($\geq$10%) incidence of invasive disease (AAP, Committee on Infectious Diseases, 2012; Remington et al., 2011). Routine prophylaxis is not recommended for all NICUs due to the potential development of drug resistance, which has been documented in adult populations.

8. Isolation procedures: Standard Precautions.

## ToRCHES CLAP Infections

**A. Classification of ToRCHES CLAP organisms.**

1. Common congenital infections were traditionally classified as TORCH infections for ease of identification and management. Some professionals have expanded the "O" (other infections) category beyond the original syphilis to include other well-described pathogens (Johnson et al., 2013). A new acronym—ToRCHES CLAP—has been suggested to be more inclusive of other well-described pathogens acquired congenitally and in the neonatal period (Remington et al., 2011) and is utilized here with the addition of respiratory syncytial virus (RSV) under the "R" and hepatitis B virus (HBV) under the "H" due to their prevalence as causes of neonatal infection.
   a. To—*To*xoplasmosis (*Toxoplasma gondii*)
   b. R—*R*ubella virus and *R*espiratory syncytial virus
   c. C—*C*ytomegalovirus
   d. H—*H*erpes simplex virus and *H*epatitis B virus
   e. E—*E*nteroviruses
   f. S—*S*yphilis (*Treponema pallidum*)
   g. C—*C*hickenpox (varicella-zoster virus)
   h. L—*L*yme disease (*Borrelia burgdorferi*)
   i. A—*A*cquired immunodeficiency syndrome/human immunodeficiency virus
   j. P—*P*arvovirus B19

**B. ToRCHES CLAP organisms.**

1. To—*To*xoplasmosis.
   a. Caused by intracellular protozoan parasite, *Toxoplasma gondii.*
   b. Maternally acquired from consumption of poorly cooked meat or by exposure to infected cat feces. Highest risk to fetus is primary acute maternal infection during pregnancy, but can occur with subsequent infections in immunocompromised women. Risk of transmission increases with increasing gestational age, but severity of the disease decreases. Estimated incidence of congenital toxoplasmosis ranges from 1 in 1000 live births in some areas of Latin America to 0.1 in 1000 live births in the United States (Guerina et al., 2013a).
   c. Most infants are asymptomatic and without apparent abnormalities at birth. Some may present with fever, maculopapular rash, petechiae, purpura, hepatosplenomegaly, jaundice, pneumonitis, microcephaly, meningoencephalitis, hydrocephalus, intracranial calcifications, seizures, thrombocytopenia, lymphadenopathy, myocarditis,

chorioretinitis, cataracts, optic atrophy, and bone lesions (Johnson et al., 2013; Remington et al., 2011).

(1) Classic triad of associated morbidities includes chorioretinitis, hydrocephalus, and intracranial calcifications, but triad occurs in less than 10% of cases (Guerina et al., 2013a).

(2) The most common late finding is chorioretinitis, which can result in vision loss, retinal detachment, cataracts, glaucoma, and blindness. Additional sequelae include mental retardation, seizures, deafness, spasticity, and learning disabilities.

**d.** Diagnosis may be made by a number of methods: isolation or histologic demonstration of the organism by PCR of amniotic fluid, CSF, urine, blood, or cord blood; observation of parasites (detection of *Toxoplasma* cysts) in tissues and body fluids or placenta; detection of parasites from blood or body fluids by mouse inoculation or tissue culture; and other serologic tests.

**e.** Treatment consists of an antiparasitic regimen for a year, including pyrimethamine plus sulfadiazine, and folinic acid to aid in prevention of bone marrow suppression. Glucocorticoids (prednisone) are added when chorioretinitis threatens vision. Clindamycin may be used for infants who develop an allergy to sulfadiazine (Guerina et al., 2013b).

**f.** Isolation procedures: Standard Precautions.

**2.** R—*R*ubella virus and *R*espiratory syncytial virus.

**a.** Congenital rubella syndrome (CRS).

(1) *Rubivirus*: enveloped, positive-stranded ribonucleic acid (RNA) virus from the family Togaviridae.

(2) Virus found in nasopharyngeal secretions and is transmitted through direct or droplet contact. Most prevalent in winter and early spring. About 25% to 50% of infected individuals are asymptomatic. Outbreaks now occur in those born outside the United States or underimmunized people (AAP, Committee on Infectious Diseases, 2012). Acquiring rubella during pregnancy can result in a wide range of complications, including miscarriage, fetal death, and a group of anomalies described as CRS. Up to 85% of infants will have congenital defects if maternal infection occurs in the first trimester, and 25% to 50% with second-trimester infection (AAP, Committee on Infectious Diseases, 2012).

(3) Mild forms of CRS may have few or no apparent clinical symptoms at birth. Associated symptoms of CRS include: cataracts, glaucoma, retinopathy, microphthalmos, myocarditis, patent ductus arteriosus, peripheral pulmonary artery stenosis, hearing impairment, meningoencephalitis, microcephaly, hydrocephalus, behavioral disorders, mental retardation, intrauterine growth restriction, pneumonitis, hepatosplenomegaly, jaundice, thrombocytopenia, bone disease, "blueberry muffin" purpura, and petechiae.

(4) Diagnosis is made by detection of specific rubella immunoglobulin M (IgM) antibody. Most congenital cases are IgM positive at birth to 3 months of age, and postnatal cases are positive by 5 days after symptom onset. Congenital infection is also confirmed by stable or rising rubella immunoglobulin G (IgG) titers in serial sera obtained for the first 7 to 11 months. Virus is isolated primarily from throat or nasal secretions, and less consistently from urine, blood, and cataract specimens, with inoculation of appropriate cell culture. Special cell cultures are required for cultivation of rubella virus.

(5) Treatment is supportive, and prevention measures are as follows:

(a) Pregnant women should be screened for immunity whether or not they have received prior rubella immunization. Susceptible pregnant women should avoid exposure to infected persons. Pregnant women are not given the vaccine because of the small risk of transmission of virus to the fetus (1.3%, of whom 2% had subclinical infection and none had congenital defects) (AAP, Committee on Infectious Diseases, 2012).

(b) Seronegative women should be vaccinated postpartum, before discharge from the hospital. Vaccine virus is excreted in breast milk, but breastfeeding is not a contraindication to vaccination.

(c) Vaccination in the United States is a live-virus subcutaneous injection combined with measles and mumps vaccines (MMR) or MMR plus varicella (MMRV), recommended at 12 to 15 months of age, and repeated at 4 to 6 years of age. Routine vaccination should be administered to all infants with few exceptions for immunocompromised children and those who have recently received immune globulin (AAP, Committee on Infectious Diseases, 2012).

(6) Isolation procedures: Droplet precautions for 7 days after onset of rash, and Contact Precautions in addition to Standard Precautions. Contact Isolation is recommended from birth until ≥1 year of age for proven or suspected congenital rubella unless two separate negative cultures 1 month apart after 3 months of age are obtained.

**b.** RSV.

(1) Enveloped, nonsegmented, negative-stranded RNA virus of the Paramyxoviridae family. Only one identified serotype, but multiple strain variations may affect virulence and susceptibility to infection.

(2) Virus is found in oral, nasal, and respiratory secretions. Transmission is by exposure to large-particle droplets or contaminated surfaces. RSV can survive for several hours on environmental surfaces. Incubation period is most commonly 4 to 6 days, but ranges from 2 to 8, and may last as long as 3 to 4 weeks in immunosuppressed people. RSV is one of the most common diseases of early childhood. Most infants are infected in the first year of life, and almost all children have had RSV by age 2. Approximately 20% to 30% of infants develop lower respiratory tract disease and 1% to 3% of infants under 1 year old require hospitalization for bronchiolitis and pneumonia (AAP, Committee on Infectious Diseases, 2012). One in 1000 infants die as a result of RSV infection (Remington et al., 2011).

(a) Infection is most prevalent during winter and early spring (November through March, but varies year to year) in temperate climates.

(b) Severe and often fatal in high-risk populations, including premature infants, infants with chronic lung disease or congenital heart disease, or immunocompromised infants.

(3) Symptoms may be nonspecific and include poor feeding, lethargy, apnea, and irritability. Symptoms of bronchiolitis may include cough, wheezing, tachypnea, rales, rhonchi, increased work of breathing (retractions, nasal flaring, and use of accessory muscles), pneumonia, cyanosis, and pulmonary infiltrates.

(a) May result in respiratory failure.

(4) Diagnosis is most commonly made by rapid viral antigen detection isolated from nasopharyngeal aspirate. Molecular testing using reverse transcriptase PCR assays is now commercially available and detects RSV at significantly higher rates than antigen or viral culture, but will detect viral RNA for weeks after the infectious period.

(5) Treatment of infants with RSV is primarily supportive care and includes oxygen, clearing airway secretions as indicated, hydration, and isolation. High-risk infants may progress to assisted ventilation because of hypoxemia and hypercapnia.

(a) Aerosolized ribavirin has been associated with increased oxygen saturation during the acute phase of infection, but is not recommended for routine use due to potential toxic effects of exposed health care personnel and clinical trials with conflicting efficacy results. May be considered for select cases of potentially life-threatening RSV (AAP, Committee on Infectious Diseases, 2012; Remington et al., 2011).

(b) Prophylaxis of RSV is indicated for high-risk infants less than 24 months old with a history of preterm birth (<35 weeks of gestation), and infants with chronic lung disease or significant congenital heart disease (AAP, Committee on Infectious Diseases, 2012). Number of doses to be received is determined by clinical status and associated risk factors such as attending day care or having one or more siblings under 5 years of age.

(i) Palivizumab (Synagis), a humanized mouse monoclonal antibody, is administered intramuscularly once every 30 days during RSV season, and reduces associated hospitalization rates by 39% to 82% (AAP, Committee on Infectious Diseases, 2012).

(6) Isolation procedures: Contact Precautions in addition to Standard Precautions. Cohort infected infants to prevent widespread nursery infection.

3. C—Cytomegalovirus (CMV).
   a. Viral genome double-stranded DNA, of the herpesvirus family Herpesviridae.
   b. Virus is found in saliva, urine, blood, breast milk, and seminal and cervical fluids. Transmission occurs horizontally from person to person with contaminated secretions, vertically from mother to infant in utero, perinatally or postnatally, and via transfusion or transplantation from infected donors. CMV is the most common congenital viral infection, with approximately 1% of all live-born infants infected in utero and excreting CMV at birth (AAP, Committee on Infectious Diseases, 2012). Severe sequelae are most commonly associated with primary maternal infection in the first trimester, though sequelae can occur regardless of trimester or reinfection. Intrapartum or postpartum infection in term infants is not usually associated with clinical illness, but in preterm or immunocompromised infants, infection after delivery can cause systemic infections.
   c. Asymptomatic infections are most common in children, but vary with age and immunocompetence of the individual. Congenital infection is usually not evident at birth, with approximately 10% of infected newborn infants presenting with clinical manifestations of the disease (AAP, Committee on Infectious Diseases, 2012). Symptoms of congenital infection include: intrauterine growth restriction, hepatosplenomegaly, jaundice, purpura, pneumonitis, microcephaly, hydrocephalus, intracerebral calcifications, hearing loss, chorioretinitis, and optic atrophy. Prognosis is poor, with one third dying in infancy and up to 90% of survivors having severe neurologic sequelae. Progressive and late-onset sensorineural hearing loss is the most common sequela of congenital CMV. Twenty-one percent of all hearing loss at birth and 25% of all hearing loss at 4 years of age are attributable to CMV. Perinatal and postnatal infections of preterm or immunocompromised infants include lower respiratory tract disease, interstitial pneumonia, prolonged fever, thrombocytopenia, and hepatitis.
   d. Diagnosis of congenital CMV is made by viral isolation in cell culture from the infant's urine or saliva, or by a high anti-CMV IgM titer in the first 2 to 4 weeks of life.
   e. Infants with symptomatic congenital CMV involving the CNS may benefit from treatment with antiviral ganciclovir IV or oral valganciclovir for 6 weeks. Data suggest this therapy is protective against hearing deterioration and possibly decreases developmental delays. Due to possible toxicities, including neutropenia, antiviral therapies are not recommended for all neonates, just those with CNS involvement who are able to start therapy within the first month of life. Current clinical trials involving these antivirals and investigative vaccines are ongoing.
   f. CMV transmission from blood products can be eliminated by use of CMV antibody—negative donors, by freezing red blood cells in glycerol before administration, or by filtration processes. Breastfeeding is not contraindicated due to low incidence of developing clinical illness and transfer of maternal antibodies. Donor breast milk should be pasteurized, and freezing may also decrease the likelihood of transmission.
   g. Isolation procedures: Standard Precautions.
4. H—*H*erpes simplex virus and *H*epatitis B virus.
   a. HSV.

      (1) Enveloped, double-strand DNA viruses, two distinct types: HSV-1 and HSV-2.

         (a) HSV-1 usually involves the face and skin above the waist, but can cause genital HSV.

         (b) HSV-2 usually involves the genital area and skin below the waist in the sexually active, but also can be found above the waist. Causes approximately 75% of neonatal disease (AAP, Committee on Infectious Diseases, 2012).

         (c) Both viruses establish latency following primary infection and have periodic reactivation that causes recurrent symptomatic disease or viral shedding without symptoms.

(2) Transmission to fetus may be by ascending infection through ruptured membranes, but is more common during birth through an infected genital tract, and occurs occasionally postnatally through a nongenital infection such as hands or mouth of a care provider, or from breast lesions during breastfeeding. Causes serious disease in fetus and neonate, with incidence estimated at 1 in 3000 to 1 in 20,000 births (AAP, Committee on Infectious Diseases, 2012). Primary maternal genital infection during pregnancy near the time of delivery accounts for as much as 25% to 60% of neonatal infection. Risk to the neonate of reinfection during the first half of pregnancy is less than 2%. More than 75% of infants who acquire neonatal HSV infection have been born to women who had no history or clinical findings suggestive of active HSV infection during pregnancy (AAP, Committee on Infectious Diseases, 2012).

(3) Symptoms of HSV infection include: skin vesicles or scarring, microcephaly, meningoencephalitis, keratoconjunctivitis, and liver failure.
   (a) Disseminated disease (25% of cases) involving multiple organs, with up to 75% having CNS involvement, and approximately 67% have lesions that may not be initially present.
      (i) Typically presents at 7 to 14 days of life.
      (ii) Severe liver dysfunction, abnormal CSF findings, seizures, profound sepsis, septic shock, high morbidity and mortality.
   (b) Localized CNS disease (30% of cases), may have skin involvement.
      (i) Typically presents at 14 to 21 days of life.
   (c) Localized skin, eyes, and mouth (SEM) disease (45% of cases); 80% of SEM cases have skin lesions; remainder are localized to eyes and oral mucosal lesions only.
      (i) Typically presents at 7 to 14 days of life.

(4) Diagnosis: Positive culture result with specimen obtained from vesicular fluid, blood, or CSF results in a diagnosis. The diagnostic yield of CSF culture for neonates with CNS disease is less than 50%. The PCR test has a much higher yield in CSF and should be performed if available. Other rapid identification tests include direct fluorescent antibody staining of vesicle scrapings and enzyme immunoassay antigen detection in vesicles or body fluids.
   (a) Surface cultures from mouth, nasopharynx, conjunctivae, and anus greater than 12 to 24 hours after delivery and initial bath (to ascertain viral replication versus intrapartum exposure).
   (b) Skin swabs of vesicles.
   (c) Blood and CSF for HSV culture and HSV PCR, serum alanine aminotransferase (ALT)

(5) Treatment of choice is acyclovir intravenously for 10 days for asymptomatic infants born to mothers with suspected or proven primary infection with active lesions at delivery, 14 days for SEM infection, or 21 days minimum for disseminated infection or CNS infections.
   (a) Repeat CSF HSV PCR near end of 21-day course and continue for additional 7 days or more if CSF remains positive.
   (b) Acyclovir suppressive therapy for 6 months following acute phase improves neurodevelopmental outcomes and helps to suppress skin recurrences.
   (c) For infants with ocular involvement, a topical ophthalmic drug such as 3% vidarabine, 1% trifluridine, or 0.1% iododeoxyuridine is used in addition to parenteral antiviral therapy. An ophthalmology consultation should be obtained.

(6) **Active maternal lesions at birth:** For asymptomatic infants born to women with *recurrent* HSV genital lesions at birth, surface cultures and HSV blood PCR should be obtained at approximately 24 hours of life. If infant remains asymptomatic, acyclovir is not indicated at this time. Parents should be educated on signs and symptoms and infant followed closely. Full evaluation and treatment should occur if any culture results become positive or infant becomes symptomatic. If active *primary* maternal HSV infection is proven or suspected, CSF for cell count, chemistries, HSV PCR, and a serum ALT should be sent in addition to surface cultures and

HSV blood PCR. Acyclovir is then initiated. If infant remains asymptomatic with negative cultures and non-indicative CSF and normal ALT, treatment is continued for 10 days. If maternal type-specific serology for HSV-1 and HSV-2 antibodies testing is available and infection proves to be recurrent, treatment can be discontinued at 48 to 72 hours (AAP, Committee on Infectious Diseases and Committee on Fetus and Newborn, 2013).

(7) Isolation procedures: Contact Precautions in addition to Standard Precautions.
  (a) Mothers with HSV infections need to use strict handwashing techniques before touching their infant.
  (b) Mothers with active lesions may wear clean covering gown to provide care, and a surgical mask should be worn for oral/cold sore lesions. Breastfeeding is permissible if there are no breast lesions and other lesions are covered.

**b.** HBV.
  (1) DNA double-shelled virus.
  (2) Virus is found in any bodily secretion, including human milk. Transmission to fetus is vertical. There is no added risk to the infant of acquiring HBV infection while breast-feeding if appropriate immunoprophylaxis recommendations are followed. Two billion people worldwide are estimated to have acquired HBV, and more than 350 million are chronically infected (Remington et al., 2011; Tovo et al., 2012). In the United States, over 1 million people have HBV (CDC, Advisory Committee on Immunization Practices, 2013).
  (3) Infants are usually asymptomatic at birth. Elevated liver enzymes or acute fulminating hepatitis is occasionally present. Infants infected at delivery or after birth may become hepatitis B surface antigen (HBsAg) positive 4 to 12 weeks after birth and are lifelong carriers; the time of onset of symptoms after exposure ranges from 6 weeks to 6 months. Infants who become chronically infected are at risk of having chronic hepatitis, cirrhosis, or hepatocellular carcinoma later in life (Venkatesh et al., 2011). Mortality rate of fulminating hepatitis is around 67%, and many survivors require liver transplantation (Tovo et al., 2012).
  (4) Routine screening is used for all pregnant women with each pregnancy, and universal screening for all exposed infants should occur at 9 to 18 months of age or 1 to 2 months following primary immunization series. Routine neonatal immunization is with hepatitis B vaccine:
    (a) Term infant is immunized at discharge and again at 1 to 2 months, and at 6 to 18 months of age (AAP, Committee on Infectious Diseases and Committee on Fetus and Newborn, 2013; CDC, Advisory Committee on Immunization Practices, 2013).
    (b) Preterm infant is immunized at discharge if weight is $\geq$2 kg or at 2 months of age.
  (5) Treatment of the infant born to an HBsAg-positive mother is 85% to 90% effective in preventing the development of the hepatitis B carrier state and should include:
    (a) Administration of hepatitis B immune globulin, in addition to a hepatitis B vaccine $\leq$12 hours after birth (AAP, Committee on Infectious Diseases and Committee on Fetus and Newborn, 2013, CDC, Advisory Committee on Immunization Practices, 2013).
  (6) Isolation procedures: Standard Precautions.

**5.** E—*E*nteroviruses.

**a.** RNA virus of the family Picornaviridae; grouped together with Parechoviruses due to shared physical properties and symptoms that they cause.
  (1) More than 100 serotypes identified as pathogenic in neonates, including polioviruses, coxsackieviruses, and echoviruses.

**b.** *Enterovirus* infections occur worldwide and are a common cause of neonatal infection, but clear data are unavailable regarding the incidence of symptomatic congenital and neonatal infections. Infections are most prevalent in the summer and fall in temperate climates, but occur all year in tropical settings. The virus is spread by fecal–oral and respiratory routes and from mother to infant in utero and peripartum, and may also be transmitted by breastfeeding. Polio vaccines have virtually eliminated poliomyelitis in the United States, but it remains endemic in parts of the world.

c. Clinical manifestations of *Enterovirus* infection include but are not limited to: nonspecific febrile illness, respiratory symptoms (including bronchiolitis and pneumonia), pulmonary edema and hemorrhage, hand-foot-and-mouth disease, meningitis, encephalitis, paralysis, vomiting, diarrhea, hepatitis, acute hemorrhagic conjunctivitis, myocarditis, sepsis, and coagulopathy. Neonates present with more severe clinical disease and have increased incidence of long-term morbidities than do older children (Remington et al., 2011).

d. Diagnosis of *Enterovirus* infection is made by PCR assay and cultures from stool, rectal, throat, and conjunctival swabs, as well as tracheal aspirates, urine, blood, CSF, and tissue biopsy.

e. No specific treatment other than supportive care. The antiviral drug pleconaril is currently being studied for neonatal enteroviral sepsis by the National Institute of Allergy and Infectious Disease Collaborative Antiviral Study Group.

f. Isolation procedures: Standard Precautions, Contact Precautions, and cohorting are used for controlling nursery outbreaks.

6. S—*Syphilis*.

a. Caused by *T. pallidum*, a thin, motile spirochete.

b. Maternally acquired through sexual contact. Vertical transmission across placenta, or via direct contact with active lesion at birth. Congenital infection can occur at any gestation but frequency increases with advancing gestation. Maternal untreated primary or secondary syphilis causes highest risk to fetus, with 60% to 100% transmission (Remington et al., 2011) and up to 30% to 40% spontaneous abortion occurring with early untreated syphilis. Incidence of congenital syphilis is about 0.2 per 1000 live births in the United States and affects an estimated 1 million pregnancies per year worldwide (Dobson, 2013).

c. Presentation at birth varies with timing of intrauterine infection. Up to two thirds of infected neonates are asymptomatic at birth. Manifestations may include an edematous "barber's pole" umbilical cord with stripes of red, light blue, and chalky white; hepatomegaly; splenomegaly; jaundice; nasal rhinitis ("snuffles"); lymphadenopathy; fever; edema; rash; fissures and condylomata lata (wart-like lesions) around mucous membranes of mouth, nares, and anus; long bone abnormalities; pneumonia alba; anemia; thrombocytopenia; and CNS involvement.

(1) Skin lesions: initially red or pink-colored maculopapular rash that is most prominent on the back, buttocks, posterior thighs, and soles, usually appears 1 to 2 weeks after rhinitis. Subsequent desquamation and crusting, lesions become copper-colored. Lesions present at birth may be bullous, ulcerative, and widely disseminated.

(2) CNS involvement may be asymptomatic but occurs in approximately 40% of symptomatic infants. Symptoms include progressive hydrocephalus, cranial nerve palsies, optic atrophy, seizures, and neurodevelopmental delay.

(3) Periostitis of long bones, with guarding of extremities, or "pseudoparalysis of Parrot" (lack of movement associated with pain from bone lesion).

d. Diagnosis is made by serologic testing of maternal blood with Venereal Disease Research Laboratory (VDRL) or rapid plasma reagin (RPR) test early in pregnancy and at the time of delivery.

(1) Diagnosis of active disease in the neonate includes:

(a) High VDRL titer ($\geq$4 times higher than maternal titer).

(b) Reactive RPR.

(c) Serum IgM level greater than 20 mg/dL.

(d) Confirmation with a positive result on darkfield microscopic examination or direct fluorescent antibody staining of suspicious lesions, body fluids, placenta, or umbilical cord.

(2) Uninfected infants possess maternally acquired antibodies at concentrations similar to those of infected infants. It may be difficult to interpret neonatal laboratory data;

therefore, it is important to determine adequacy of maternal treatment, possibility of reexposure, and family compliance with follow-up.

**e.** Treatment.

(1) Treatment recommendation for infants with proven or highly probable congenital syphilis is 10 to 14 days of parenteral penicillin (aqueous penicillin G intravenously or procaine penicillin G intramuscularly).

(2) Treatment of at-risk neonates who are asymptomatic and have nonreactive VDRL or RPR or values less than four-fold the maternal titer varies depending on maternal history and treatment (Dobson, 2012; Remington et al., 2011).

(a) Treat with full 10- to 14-day course if mother was not treated, was inadequately treated, or has evidence of reinfection ($\geq$four-fold increase in titers after treatment).

(b) May treat with single dose of benzathine penicillin G intramuscularly if mother had adequate treatment.

(3) No treatment necessary if all of the following are true: mother adequately treated with appropriate response in titers (decrease four-fold after therapy; VDRL $\leq$1:2 or RPR $\leq$1:4) and levels remained stable and low, maternal treatment occurred more than 4 weeks prior to delivery, and mother has no evidence of relapse or infection.

**f.** Isolation procedures: Standard Precautions.

**7.** C—Chickenpox.

**a.** Varicella-zoster virus (*Varicellovirus*) is a member of the Herpesviridae family that also includes HSV-1 and HSV-2, CMV, Epstein-Barr virus, and other herpesviruses.

**b.** Remains one of the most communicable human diseases. Transmission occurs through person-to-person contact of individuals with vesicular lesions, and may occur through infected respiratory tract secretions. Transplacental transmission occurs with maternal infection. Congenital varicella syndrome occurs in approximately 1% to 2% of infants with maternal infection before 20 weeks of gestation. Incubation period may be as short at 2 to 16 days after birth for infants born to actively infected mothers at the time of delivery (AAP, Committee on Infectious Diseases, 2012). Infected individuals are contagious 1 to 2 days before onset of lesions and until all lesions are crusted.

**c.** Infection during the first or second trimester can result in fetal death, limb hypoplasia, cutaneous scarring, eye abnormalities, and CNS derangements. If maternal infection occurs 5 days before to 2 days after delivery, subsequent infant mortality is higher due to the immature immune system of the infant and insufficient maternal antibody transfer. Additional symptoms of chickenpox are a generalized pruritic, vesicular rash, low-grade fever, potential superinfection of skin lesions, pneumonia, thrombocytopenia, and rarely glomerulonephritis, hepatitis, and arthritis. Latent infection can occur, as well as infection after vaccination.

**d.** Diagnosis is made by PCR assay of vesicular fluid or scab, or saliva and buccal swabs, or by tissue culture of vesicles, CSF, or biopsy.

**e.** Acyclovir is commonly used to treat neonatal HSV, but few data are available for its use in treating progressive varicella, and it is not recommended unless the infant has active zoster (Remington et al., 2011). Passive immunization using varicella-zoster immune globulin (VZIG or VariZIG) is recommended for infants born to women who developed active infection 5 days or fewer prior to delivery to 2 days after delivery, given as soon as possible after birth. Additional therapy of the neonate is supportive.

**f.** Isolation procedures: Standard, airborne, and Contact Precautions for hospitalized neonates, continued 21 to 28 days if treated with VZIG. Infants with embryopathy without active lesions do not require isolation.

**8.** L—*Lyme disease.*

**a.** Spirochete of the species *B. burgdorferi*; common vector-borne illness transmitted by ticks.

**b.** Lyme disease occurs throughout the world, and in the United States most cases occur in endemic areas, including New York, New Jersey, Pennsylvania, Minnesota, and Wisconsin. Disease progression can cause severe sequelae, including meningitis and encephalitis, and carditis. Concern regarding transplacental transmission in humans exists due to known transmission and congenital infection of other spirochetes of the *Borrelia* genus, but documentation of congenital disease or complications of pregnancy due to Lyme disease have not been reported (AAP, Committee on Infectious Diseases, 2012). *B. burgdorferi* has not been isolated in breast milk. Studies have isolated transplacental transmission in animals with reproductive failure and severe fetal infection (Remington et al., 2011), but studies in humans have shown no adverse effect to the fetus from maternal Lyme disease.

**c.** No diagnostic studies or treatment of the neonate are indicated with confirmed maternal Lyme disease. Parents should be assured there is no evidence suggesting increased risk to the infant.

**9.** A—*A*cquired immunodeficiency syndrome/human immunodeficiency virus.

**a.** HIV is a cytopathic lentivirus of the family Retroviridae; human RNA retrovirus.

(1) HIV type 1 (HIV-1) prevalent in the United States; HIV type 2 (HIV-2) predominantly found in West Africa, few cases have been reported in the United States.

(a) HIV-2 milder disease course with longer time to develop.

(2) HIV-1 requires reverse transcriptase enzyme to convert RNA to DNA, then becomes integrated in the host cell genome as a provirus.

(3) Suppression of T-helper lymphocytes. This results in B-cell and suppressor T-cell dysfunction, with subsequent defects in cell-mediated immunity and development of opportunistic infections.

**b.** Virus is found in blood, semen, cervicovaginal secretions, and breast milk. Most infants are infected perinatally, accounting for 91% of cases (Remington et al., 2011), though intrauterine transmission may occur. Infants with a positive HIV peripheral blood test within the first 48 hours of life are considered to be infected in utero and tend to have early onset of symptoms. Intrapartum transmission during exposure to maternal blood or genital tract secretions is presumed. The risk of mother-to-child transmission without interventions is 12% to 40%, with an average of 25% to 30% in the United States. The CDC estimates 215 to 370 infants with HIV infection are born each year in the United States (AAP, Committee on Infectious Diseases, 2012; Remington et al., 2011).

**c.** Infants are asymptomatic at birth and are classified as exposed, infected, or seroreverted according to their immunologic status. Disease progression is more rapid in children than in adults, and infected infants may become seriously ill within 2 to 4 weeks of life. Ten percent to 20% of untreated infants die before 4 years of age, with a median age at death of 11 months. Symptoms of infection include:

(1) Failure to thrive.

(2) Generalized lymphadenopathy, hepatomegaly, and splenomegaly.

(3) Recurrent oral and diaper candidiasis.

(4) Systemic bacterial infections.

(5) Lymphoid interstitial pneumonitis.

(6) Hyperreflexia, hypertonia, floppiness, developmental delay.

(7) Parotitis, hepatitis, nephropathy, and cardiomyopathy.

(8) Recurrent diarrhea.

(9) Opportunistic infections (viral and bacterial).

(10) Unexplained fevers.

(11) Malignancies.

**d.** The preferred diagnostic test for neonatal HIV-1 is DNA PCR (AAP, Committee on Infectious Diseases and Committee on Fetus and Newborn, 2013).

(1) May detect proviral DNA before 48 hours of life with a sensitivity of 55% (Schwarzwald, 2012); considered in-utero transmission if positive.

(2) Test is 93% positive by 2 weeks of life, 96% to 99% by 1 month of age, with 97% specificity (AAP, Committee on Infectious Diseases, 2012; Remington et al., 2011).

(a) Western blot; confirmatory test, but unreliable for HIV-2.

(3) Plasma viral RNA assesses viral load and can aid in monitoring disease progression and therapy efficacy, but is unreliable for diagnosis in the first 2 weeks of life.

(4) Viral culture; expensive and long time for results, not recommended.

(5) Timing of initial testing varies from less than 48 hours of life to 14 days, and should be repeated at 1 to 2 months of age and again at 4 to 6 months of age. An infant is considered infected with two positive test samples by DNA or RNA PCR (AAP, Committee on Infectious Diseases and Committee on Fetus and Newborn, 2013).

**e.** Initiation of early antiretroviral (ARV) therapy reduces maternal–child transmission, morbidity, and mortality. Maternal therapy should include a combination ARV therapy that includes oral zidovudine (ZDU) beginning at 14 to 34 weeks of gestation and continuing throughout pregnancy. During labor, IV ZDU is recommended, and delivery via cesarean section prior to rupture of membranes is recommended for women with unknown plasma viral loads or greater than 1000 copies/mL (http://aidsinfo.nih.gov/Guidelines). Infants should receive ARV therapy from birth regardless of clinical symptoms, viral load, or immune status.

(1) Bathe as soon as possible after birth.
(2) Initiate oral ZDU from birth through 6 weeks of life.
(3) An additional one- to two-drug regimen is used for infants born to HIV-infected mothers who did not receive any ARVs prior to onset of labor or for infants proven to be infected while on ZDU prophylaxis. Additional medications include lamivudine, nelfinavir, didanosine, stavudine, nevirapine, or lopinavir–ritonavir, but not all may be paired due to adverse reactions. Standards are still evolving, and collaboration with an HIV treatment center is recommended.
(4) In the United States, where formula is readily available and safe, breastfeeding is not recommended (John-Stewart, 2013).
(5) Follow-up at 2 to 4 weeks is recommended to assure drug regimen compliance and to monitor for ZDU-associated anemia.
(6) Long-term follow-up and prompt intervention during bacterial and treatable opportunistic infections.
(7) Routine immunization schedule and doses for all inactivated vaccines, with MMR considered for children not severely immunosuppressed as they are at high risk for complications associated with varicella-zoster and measles (Tovo et al., 2012).

**f.** Isolation procedures: Standard Precautions should be strictly followed.

**10.** P—*Parvovirus* B19.

**a.** Single-stranded, nonenveloped DNA virus of the family Parvoviridae.

**b.** Common cause of infection worldwide. Transmitted through respiratory secretions and blood, and vertical transmission from mother to fetus. Intrauterine transmission rates range from 25% to 50%, with adverse fetal outcomes less than 10%; highest risk associated with initial infection before 20 weeks of gestation, though may cause fetal demise in all trimesters (Remington et al., 2011).

**c.** Neonatal morbidities associated with primary maternal infection during pregnancy include nonimmune hydrops fetalis, myocarditis, pericardial effusions, meconium ileus, peritonitis, hyperechoic bowel, anemia, and fetal demise, but also has been associated with asymptomatic neonatal infections and normal deliveries. Maternal symptoms include malaise, arthralgia, rash, coryza, or fever.

**d.** Mothers and fetuses with symptoms should be considered high risk and tested for serum IgG and IgM antibodies to parvovirus B19. Presence of IgG but not IgM indicates prior infection as IgG is present for life. Serum PCR assay also can detect low levels of the virus up to 9 months after acute infection.

**e.** Some cases of associated hydrops fetalis have successfully been treated with intrauterine blood transfusions. Other therapy is supportive.

**f.** Isolation precautions: Standard Precautions and droplet precautions for infants with unresolved hydrops fetalis associated with parvovirus B19 at the time of delivery.

## INFECTION CONTROL

**A. Hospital-acquired infections** (HAIs) are a major cause of morbidity and mortality in infants and children. The CDC estimates approximately 5% to 10% of hospitalized patients in the United States develop HAIs, and the estimated cost for each central line–associated infection is $16,550 (The Joint Commission, 2012). In the NICU, HAIs are primarily acquired from the neonate's own flora, but the NICU environment and hands of health care workers play an important role in transmission. Risk factors are confounded by multiple factors, including birth weight and the immature immune system. LBW remains one of the strongest risk factors, although the presence of indwelling intravascular or transmucosal medical devices has also been identified as one of the greatest risk factors of HAIs. Hand hygiene remains the single most important prevention of HAIs (AAP, Committee on Infectious Diseases, 2012).

1. The CDC has published guidelines and recommendations for the prevention of HAIs, including isolation precautions, guidelines for protecting health care workers, and guidelines for the prevention of postoperative and device-related infections. These guidelines can be found on the CDC website (http://www.cdc.gov/HAI/prevent/prevention.html). Additional resources are available through the Society for Healthcare Epidemiology, the Association for Professionals in Infection Control and Epidemiology, and The Joint Commission.
2. Standard Precautions should be strictly adhered to for all patients regardless of diagnosis, gestational age, or presence of infection. Transmission-Based Precautions should be utilized in addition to Standard Precautions for patients who are infected or colonized with pathogens that are transmitted by airborne, droplet, or direct contact. All health care providers are responsible for following infection control practices and staying informed and educated on the latest guidelines and practices to help prevent HAIs.
3. Central line–associated bloodstream infections (CLABSIs) remain a prominent concern in NICU settings. VLBW infants less than 750 g are at highest risk, with an associated rate of 3.4 per 1000 catheter days, and those less than 1500 g who develop late-onset CLABSI have 3 times higher mortality than those who do not (The Joint Commission, 2012). CDC guidelines for prevention of CLABSIs were established in 2011 (available at: www.cdc.gov/HAI/pdfs/bsi/checklist-for-CLABSI.pdf) and include:
   - **a.** Prompt removal of unnecessary central lines with daily audits of necessity.
   - **b.** Proper insertion practices.
     - (1) Proper hand hygiene.
     - (2) Strict aseptic technique with maximal sterile barrier precautions, including gown, mask, cap, sterile gloves, and full-body drape.
     - (3) Appropriate skin cleansing.
     - (4) Choose best insertion site to minimize infection and complications.
     - (5) Maintain intact sterile transparent, semipermeable dressings.
   - **c.** Maintain central lines appropriately.
     - (1) Proper hand hygiene.
     - (2) Scrub access port or hub immediately prior to use with antiseptic (e.g., chlorhexidine, povidone–iodine, an iodophor, or 70% alcohol).
     - (3) Access with sterile devices only.
     - (4) Replace soiled, nonocclusive dressings.
     - (5) Dressing changes under aseptic technique using clean or sterile gloves.
   - **d.** Empower staff to monitor proper procedures.
   - **e.** Bundle supplies for ease of accessibility.
   - **f.** Provide checklists for providers to ensure compliance with proper practices.
   - **g.** Provide adequate access to hand hygiene and monitor adherence to procedure.
   - **h.** Provide education to all staff regarding insertion, usage, and maintenance.
4. Prevention of ventilator-associated pneumonia (VAP). VAP is the second most common HAI in NICU patients. VAP is associated with increased hospitalization and health care costs. Rates of VAP range from 1 to 4 cases per 1000 ventilator days, but rates greater than 10 cases per 1000 ventilator days have been reported in some neonatal and surgical populations (Coffin et al., 2008).
   - **a.** Associated with aspiration of secretions, colonization or use of contaminated equipment.
   - **b.** Risk factors include prematurity, LBW, sedation, paralytic agents, intubation, mechanical ventilation, orogastric/nasogastric tube placement, and use of medications that increase bacterial colonization (e.g., broad-spectrum antibiotics, antacids, or $H_2$ blockers), (Remington et al., 2011).

c. Prevention strategies are based upon adult studies (Coffin et al., 2008; Remington et al., 2011) and include:
   (1) Active surveillance for VAP.
   (2) Minimize use of mechanical ventilation using weaning protocols and promote use of noninvasive ventilation when possible.
   (3) Educate providers who work with ventilated patients regarding VAP.
   (4) Disinfect, sterilize, maintain respiratory equipment; remove condensation from circuit, and change circuit when visibly soiled.
   (5) Perform regular oral care.
   (6) Maintain semirecumbent position (30- to 45-degree head-of-bed elevation) unless medically contraindicated.
   (7) Avoid unplanned extubations.
   (8) Avoid gastric overdistention.
   (9) Avoid $H_2$ blockers.
   (10) Use in-line suctioning devices.

5. Optimal staffing-to-patient ratios have not been established for NICUs, but low nurse–to–high patient ratios have been correlated with increased rates of nosocomial infections. Understaffing has also been correlated with periods of decreased hand hygiene compliance, leading to further infection rates (Remington et al., 2011).

**B. Vaccination remains a critical component to preventing and controlling the spread of infection nationally and globally.**

1. The four major strategies for protecting neonates are:
   a. Maternal immunization during pregnancy.
   b. Passive immunization with antibodies or immune globulins.
   c. Active immunization of neonates.
   d. Immunization of contacts to prevent transmission (herd immunity).
2. Recommendations and schedules for vaccination use are constantly changing. Health care providers must review current guidelines from regulatory and advisory bodies for current practice standards.
   a. Guidelines and recommendations are available from the Advisory Committee on Immunization Practices (ACIP) of the CDC and can be found at: http://www.cdc.gov/vaccines/pubs/acip-list.htm.
   b. The Recommended Immunization Schedules for Persons Aged 0 Through 18 Years are updated annually and approved by the ACIP, the AAP, the American Academy of Family Physicians, and the American College of Obstetricians and Gynecologists. The 2013 schedule is available at: http://www.cdc.gov/vaccines/schedules/hcp/child-adolescent.html.

## REFERENCES


Adcock, L.: Etiology, clinical manifestations, and evaluation of neonatal shock. *Up To Date*. Wolters Kluwer Health, updated October 2013. Available at: www.uptodate.com/contents/etiology-clinical-manifestations-and-evaluation-of-neonatal-shock.

Agrawal, P.: Shock. In J.P. Cloherty, E.C. Eichenwald, and A.R. Stark (Eds.): *Manual of neonatal care* (7th ed.). Philadelphia, 2012, Lippincott, Williams & Wilkins.

American Academy of Pediatrics, Committee on Infectious Diseases: *2012 Red book: Report of the Committee on Infectious Diseases* (29th ed.). Elk Grove Village, IL, 2012, American Academy of Pediatrics.

American Academy of Pediatrics, Committee on Infectious Diseases and Committee on Fetus and Newborn: Guidance on management of asymptomatic neonates born to women with active genital herpes lesions. *Pediatrics*, 131:e635, 2013.

Baley, J.E., Kliegman, R.M., Boxerbaum, B., and Fanaroff, A.A.: Fungal colonization in the very low birth weight infant. *Pediatrics*, 78:225, 1986.

Byington, C.L., Rittichier, K.K., Bassett, K.E., et al.: Serious bacterial infections in febrile infants younger than 90 days of age: The importance of ampicillin-resistant pathogens. *Pediatrics*, 111(5 Pt. 1):964–968, 2003.

Carr, R., Modi, N., and Doré, C.: G-CSF and GM-CSF for treating or preventing neonatal infections. *Cochrane Database of Systematic Reviews*, (3), CD003066, 2003.

Centers for Disease Control and Prevention: Prevention of perinatal group B streptococcal disease in newborns. *MMWR Recommendations and Reports*, 59(RR-10):1–32, 2010.

Centers for Disease Control and Prevention, Active Bacterial Core Surveillance, Emerging Infections Program Network: ABCs report: Group B *Streptococcus*, 2011. Available at: http://www.cdc.gov/abcs/reports-findings/survreports/gbs11.pdf; accessed June 29, 2013.

Centers for Disease Control and Prevention Advisory Committee on Immunization Practices: The Recommended Immunization Schedules for Persons Aged 0 Through 18 Years—United States, 2013. *MMWR Morbidity and Mortality Weekly Report*, 62(Suppl. 1): 1–19, 2013.

Coffin, S., Klompas, M., Classen, D., et al.: Strategies to prevent ventilator-associated pneumonia in acute care hospitals. *Infection Control and Hospital Epidemiology*, 29(Suppl. 1):S31–S40, 2008. Available at: http://www.jstor.org/stable/10.1086/591062.

Cohen-Wolkowiez, M., Moran, C., Benjamin, D.K., et al.: Early and late onset sepsis in late preterm infants. *Pediatric Infectious Disease Journal*, 28:1052, 2009.

Dobson, S.: Congenital syphilis: Clinical features and diagnosis. *Up To Date*. Wolters Kluwer Health, updated January 2013. Available at: www.uptodate.com/contents/congenital-syphilis-clinical-features-and-diagnosis

Dobson, S.: Congenital syphilis: Evaluation, management, and prevention. *UpToDate*. Wolters Kluwer Health, updated December 2012. Available at: www.uptodate.com/contents/congenital-syphilis-evaluation-management-and-prevention.

Duke, T.: Neonatal pneumonia in developing countries. *Archives of Disease in Childhood: Fetal and Neonatal Edition*, 90(3):F211, 2005.

Edwards, S.: Treatment and outcome of sepsis in term and late preterm infants. *UpToDate*. Wolters Kluwer Health Updated December 2012. Available at: www.uptodate.com/contents/treatment-and-outcome-of-sepsis-in-term-and-late-preterm-infants.

Estripeaut, D., and Saez-Llorens, X.: Perinatal bacterial diseases. In R.D. Feigin, J.D. Cherry, G.J. Demmler-Harrison, and S.L. Kaplan (Eds.): *Textbook of pediatric infectious diseases* (6th ed.). Philadelphia, 2009, Elsevier Saunders, p. 979.

Feng-Ying, C.L., Weisman, L.E., and Robbins, J.B.: Assessment of intrapartum antibiotic prophylaxis for the prevention of early-onset group B streptococcal disease. *Pediatric Infectious Disease Journal*, 30 (9):759–763, 2011.

Goldstein, B., Giroir, B. and Randolph, A.: International consensus conference on pediatric sepsis. *Pediatric Critical Care Medicine*, 6(1):2–8, 2005.

Guerina, N., Lee, J., Lynfield, R., et al.: Congenital toxoplasmosis: Clinical features and diagnosis. *Up To Date*. Wolters Kluwer Health, 2013a. Available at: www.uptodate.com/contents/congenital-toxoplasmosis-clinical-features-and-diagnosis.

Guerina, N., Lee, J., Lynfield, R., et al.: Congenital toxoplasmosis: Treatment, outcome, and prevention. *Up To Date*. Wolters Kluwer Health, 2013b. Available at: www.uptodate.com/contents/congenital-toxoplasmosis-treatment-outcome-and-prevention.

Heath, P.T., Nik Yusoff, N.K., and Baker, C.J.: Neonatal meningitis. *Archives of Disease in Childhood: Fetal and Neonatal Edition*, 88:F173, 2003.

Johnson, K.: Overview of TORCH infections. *UpToDate*. Wolters Kluwer Health, 2013. Updated May 2013. Available at: www.uptodate.com/contents/overview-of-torch-infections.

John-Stewart, G.: Prevention of HIV transmission during breastfeeding in resource limited settings. *UpToDate*. Wolters Kluwer Health, 2013. Updated September 2013. Available at: www.uptodate.com/contents/prevention-of-hiv-transmission-during-breastfeeding-in-resource-limited-settings.

The Joint Commission: Preventing central line–associated bloodstream infections: A global challenge, a global perspective. 2012: Oak Brook, IL, 2012, Joint Commission Resources. Available at: http://www.PreventingCLABSIs.pdf.

Libster, R., Edwards, K.M., Levent, F., et al.: Long-term outcomes of group B streptococcal meningitis. *Pediatrics*, 130:e8, 2012.

Maheshwari, A. and Black, L.V.: A practical approach to the neutropenic neonate. In R.K. Ohls and A. Maheshwari, (Eds.): *Hematology, immunology and infectious disease: neonatology questions and controversies* (2nd ed.). Philadelphia, 2012, Elsevier Saunders.

Manroe, B.L., Weinberg, A.G., Rosenfeld, C.R., et al.: The neonatal blood count in health and disease. *Pediatrics*, 95:89–98, 1979.

Nizet, V. and Klein, J.O.: Bacterial sepsis and meningitis. In J.S. Remington, J.O. Klein, C.B. Wilson, et al. (Eds.): *Infectious diseases of the fetus and newborn infant* (7th ed.). Philadelphia, 2011, Elsevier Saunders.

Oski, F. and Naiman, J.: *Hematologic problems in the newborn*. Philadelphia, 1966, W.B. Saunders.

Pappas, P.G., Kauffman, C.A., Andes, D., et al.: Clinical practice guidelines for the management of candidiasis: 2009 update by the Infectious Diseases Society of America. *Clinical Infectious Diseases*, 48(5):503–535, 2009.

Phares, C.R., Lynfield, R., Farley, M.M., et al.: for the Active Bacterial Core Surveillance/Emerging Infections Program Network: Epidemiology of invasive group B streptococcal disease in the United States, 1999-2005. *JAMA*, 299:2056, 2008.

Piantino, J.H., Schreiber, M.D., Alexander, K., and Hageman, J.: Culture negative sepsis and systemic inflammatory response syndrome in neonates. *NeoReviews*, 14:e294, 2013.

Pong, A. and Bradley, J.S.: Bacterial meningitis and the newborn infant. *Infectious Disease Clinics of North America*, 13:711, 1999.

Remington, J.S., Klein, J.O., Wilson, C.B. et al. (Eds.): *Infectious diseases of the fetus and newborn infant* (7th ed.). Philadelphia, 2011, Elsevier Saunders.

Saxonhouse, M.A. and Sola-Visner, M.C.: Current issues in the pathogenesis, diagnosis, and treatment of neonatal thrombocytopenia. In R.K. Ohls and A. Maheshwari (Eds.): *Hematology, immunology and infectious disease: Neonatology questions and controversies* (2nd ed.). Philadelphia, 2012, Elsevier Saunders.

Schwarzwald, H.: Diagnostic testing for HIV infection in infants and children younger than 18 months. *UpToDate*. Wolters Kluwer Health, 2012. Updated December 2012. Available: www.uptodate.com/contents/diagnostic-testing-for-hiv-infection-in-infants-and-children-younger-than-18-months.

Speer, M.: Neonatal pneumonia. *Up To Date*. Wolters Kluwer Health, updated October 2012. Available at: www.uptodate.com/contents/neonatal-pneumonia.

Stoll, B.J., Hansen, N.I., Sánchez, P.J., et al.: Early onset neonatal sepsis: The burden of group B streptococcal and E. coli disease continues. *Pediatrics*, 127:817, 2011.

Tovo, P., Bezzio, S., and Gabiano, C.: Fetal infections: Rubella, HIV, HCV, HBV, and human parvovirus B19. In G. Buonocore, R. Bracci, and M. Weindling (Eds.): *Neonatology: A practical approach to neonatal diseases*. 2012, Springer-Verlag Italia.

Venkatesh, M., Adams, K., and Weisman, L.: Infection in the neonate. In S.L. Gardner, B.S. Carter, M. Enzman-Hines, and J.A. Hernandez (Eds.): *Merenstein & Gardner's handbook of neonatal intensive care* (7th ed.). St. Louis, 2011, Elsevier Mosby, pp. 553–579.

Wang, H., Tang, J., Xiong, Y., et al.: Neonatal community-acquired pneumonia: pathogens and treatment. *Journal of Paediatric and Child Health*, 46(11):668–672, 2010.

Weinberg, G.A. and D'Angio, C.T.: Laboratory aids for diagnosis of neonatal sepsis. In J.S., Remington, J.O., Klein, C.B., Wilson, et al. (Eds.): *Infectious diseases of the fetus and newborn infant* (7th ed.). Philadelphia, 2011, Elsevier Saunders.

Weston, E.J., Pondo, T., Lewis, M.M., et al.: The burden of invasive early-onset neonatal sepsis in the United States, 2005-2008. *Pediatric Infectious Disease Journal*, 30(11):937–941, 2011.

Wynn, J.L. and Wong, H.R.: Pathophysiology and treatment of septic shock in neonates. *Clinical Perinatology*, 37(2):439–479, 2010.

CHAPTER

# 33 Renal and Genitourinary Disorders

JAN SHERMAN

**OBJECTIVES**

1. Relate congenital renal/genitourinary disorders to embryologic development.
2. Apply knowledge of normal renal anatomy and physiology to renal pathophysiology that presents in the neonatal period.
3. Explain the etiology of selected neonatal renal/genitourinary disorders.
4. Describe clinical manifestations and complications that may be associated with selected neonatal renal/genitourinary disorders.
5. Determine the appropriate management of each disorder discussed.
6. Formulate an appropriate plan of care for each disorder discussed.

## OVERVIEW

Homeostasis of the newborn is dependent on a functional renal system. In utero, the placenta is the organ responsible for fluid and electrolyte homeostasis. After birth, the kidney must assume its role as the regulator. An understanding of basic principles in renal developmental physiology is essential for successful clinical management of sick preterm and term neonates. This chapter presents information on the anatomy and physiology of the kidney as a base from which to discuss selected renal/genitourinary disorders. Fetal renal function is closely linked to both the developmental stage of the kidney and the intrauterine or extrauterine environment of the fetus. Maternal exposure to a variety of drugs not only may alter function of the fetal kidney but also may cause permanent impairment of renal development and function. The Barker hypothesis, as well as the theory of the developmental origins of disease, contend that adverse events in utero induce compensatory responses in the fetus, such as altered kidney development. These changes in organ structure may persist permanently and have long-term consequences for renal functions, such as the future development of hypertension. These considerations underscore the lifetime importance of optimal prenatal and neonatal care.

## FETAL DEVELOPMENT OF THE KIDNEY

A. **General concepts.**
   1. The fetal kidney develops from three successive structures: the pronephros, the mesonephros, and the metanephros.
   2. Nephrogenesis is the formation of new nephron units.
   3. Embryologic development of the urinary system begins within the first weeks after conception and progresses through three stages.
   4. Both the urinary and the genital systems develop from the same germ layer of the embryo.

B. **Pronephros.**
   1. Pronephros is a primitive and nonfunctional kidney that appears early in the fourth week of gestation, then disappears by the fifth week (Moore et al., 2013).
   2. Pronephroi degenerate but the ducts and tubes persist, which are then used by the mesonephroi (Moore et al., 2013).

C. **Mesonephros.**
   1. This intermediate kidney appears from 5 to 12 weeks' gestation and consists of glomeruli and tubules (Moore et al., 2013).
   2. The pronephric tube extends into the cell lining of the mesonephros to form the wolffian duct. An outbranch of the Wolffian duct called the ureteric bud aids in the development of the metanephros (Guignard and Sulyok, 2012).
   3. The mesonephroi function as the intermediate kidney, then undergo involution through apoptosis (programmed cell death) in preparation for the next stage of development (Guignard and Sulyok, 2012).

D. **Metanephros.**
   1. Differentiation of the metanephros—a primitive form of the permanent kidney—starts around 5 weeks' gestation, and the first nephrons are formed by week 8 (Moore et al., 2013).
   2. This primitive kidney is functional at around the ninth week of gestation and begins the formation of urine (Moore et al., 2013).
   3. Interactions between the ureteric bud and the metanephric mesenchyme result in the formation of both the collecting duct system and the nephrons of the permanent kidney. The stalk of the ureteric bud becomes the ureter and the cranial part of the bud branches to form the collecting tubules. This branching morphogenesis leads to the formation of the renal collecting system, with the first generations of the collecting tubules enlarging to form the major calices while subsequent generations form the minor calices (Guignard and Sulyok, 2012; Moore et al., 2013).
   4. Nephrogenesis is complete at 34 weeks of gestation, when each kidney contains its definitive complement of approximately 800,000 to 1.2 million nephrons (Vogt and Dell, 2011).

E. **Positional changes of the fetal kidney (Moore et al., 2013).**
   1. Initially the fetal kidneys are closely approximated and located down in the pelvis in the area of the sacrum. As the abdomen and the pelvis grow, the kidneys move upward and apart from each other. The kidneys attain their adult location in the ninth week of gestation.
   2. Early in development, the hilum of the kidney (area where the veins, arteries, and ureters enter the kidney) faces ventrally (toward the abdomen). As the kidneys ascend upward, they also rotate medially, and by the ninth week of gestation the hilum is directed anteromedially. Eventually the kidneys are located on the posterior abdominal wall.
   3. The kidneys become fixed once they come into contact with the suprarenal (adrenal) glands in the ninth week of gestation.

F. **Changes in blood supply of the fetal kidney (Moore et al., 2013).**
   1. As the fetal kidneys change location, they obtain their blood supply from local blood vessels. Initially the renal arteries are branches of the common iliac arteries. Future blood is supplied from the distal aorta; then, as the kidneys rise upward, new branches to the aorta develop. Normally the old vessels involute and disappear.
   2. The permanent renal arteries develop from branches of the abdominal aorta. The right renal artery is longer and often more superior.

## DEVELOPMENT OF THE BLADDER AND URETHRA (VOGT AND DELL, 2011)

A. **The bladder and urethra are formed during the second and third months of gestation.**
   1. During the fourth to seventh week of development, the cloaca begins to divide and develop. As the cloaca develops, portions of the mesonephric ducts are absorbed into the bladder wall.
   2. Caudal portions of the ureters, which originate from the mesonephric ducts, enter the bladder.
   3. During these processes, the ureteral orifices move cranially and the mesonephric ducts move closer together to enter the prostatic urethra, forming the trigone of the bladder.

## RENAL FUNCTION

A. **During intrauterine life, the kidneys play only a minor role in regulating fetal salt and water balance because this function is maintained primarily by the placenta.** The most important functions of the prenatal kidneys are the formation and excretion of urine to maintain an adequate amount of amniotic fluid (Chevalier and Norwood, 2011).
B. **Renal blood flow is low during fetal life, only 2% to 4% of the total cardiac output.** This proportion increases after birth, from a value of 5% in the first 12 hours of life to 10% at the end of the first week (Guignard and Sulyok, 2012).

## RENAL ANATOMY

A. **Gross anatomy.**
   1. Cortex: outermost portion of the kidney, which contains the glomeruli, proximal and distal convoluted tubules, and collecting ducts of the nephron.
   2. Medulla: middle section of the kidney, which contains the renal pyramids, straight portions of tubules, loops of Henle, vasa recta, and terminal collecting ducts.
   3. Renal sinus and pelvis: innermost portion of the kidney. The renal sinus contains the uppermost part of the renal pelvis and calyces, surrounded by some fat in which branches of the renal vessels and nerves are embedded.
   4. Ureter: excretory duct of the kidney, which transports urine from the kidney to the bladder.
B. **Microscopic renal anatomy: the nephron (Hall, 2011).**
   1. The nephron is the functional unit of the kidney and produces urine. Each kidney contains about 800,000 to 1 million nephrons.
   2. Each nephron contains a tuft of glomerular capillaries called the glomerulus, through which large amounts of fluid are filtered from the blood, and a long tubule in which the filtered fluid is converted into urine on its way to the pelvis of the kidney.
   3. The glomerulus contains a network of glomerular capillaries that is encased in Bowman's capsule. Fluid filtered from the glomerular capillaries flows into Bowman's capsule and then into the proximal tubule, which lies in the cortex of the kidney.
   4. From the proximal tubule, fluid flows into the loop of Henle, which dips into the renal medulla. Each loop consists of a descending and an ascending limb.
   5. Collecting ducts empty into the renal pelvis of the kidney. Urine flows from the collecting ducts into the renal calyces, then into the ureters. Peristaltic contractions force urine down the ureters into the bladder.

## REGULATION OF POSTNATAL RENAL HEMODYNAMICS (SOLHAUG AND JOSE, 2011)

A. **The postnatal regulation of renal hemodynamics is a combination of related cardiac output, perfusion pressure, and renal vascular resistance.** The low renal blood flow is the result of several factors such as decreased number of glomeruli, lower systemic pressure, and higher renal vascular resistance.
B. **Cardiac output:** The proportion of cardiac output distributed to the kidneys is 4% to 6% in the first 12 hours of life and increases to 8% to 10% in the first week of life. In comparison, 25% of cardiac output is distributed to the kidneys in the normal adult.
C. **Systemic vascular resistance:** Systemic vascular resistance increases markedly after birth, which may cause a redistribution of blood flow to organs other than the kidneys, which may immediately contribute to the low neonatal renal blood flow.
D. **Contribution of structural changes:** New vascular channels from nephrogenesis, as well as the continued formation of new glomeruli and vascular remodeling, may influence renal hemodynamics postnatally.
E. **Vasoactive factors that regulate renal blood flow:** Several vasoactive agents participate in the regulation of renal blood flow in the postnatal maturing kidney:

1. **Renin–angiotensin system** is a powerful system to control blood pressure. Renin is a protein enzyme released by the kidneys when the arterial pressure is low. Renin acts on another plasma protein, angiotensinogen, to release an amino peptide, angiotensin I.
2. **Angiotensin I** rapidly converts to angiotensin II predominantly in the lungs, although other tissues such as the kidneys and blood vessels contain converting enzyme and can form angiotensin II.
3. **Angiotensin II** is an extremely powerful vasoconstrictor but is rapidly inactivated in the blood after 1 to 2 minutes. A second effect is to decrease excretion of sodium and water, which slowly increases the extracellular fluid volume (Hall, 2011).
4. **Natriuretic peptides:** atrial natriuretic peptide (ANP), brain natriuretic peptide (BNP), and C-type natriuretic peptide (CNP). ANP and BNP are produced in the atria and ventricles, whereas CNP is found mainly in the brain, pituitary gland, vascular endothelium, and kidneys. The primary effects of ANP are: (1) vasodilation and decrease in mean blood pressure; (2) increase in renal blood flow, glomerular filtration rate (GFR), and filtration fraction; (3) inhibition of sodium and water reabsorption in both proximal and distal tubules; and (4) decreased concentrating ability.
5. **Nitric oxide** synthesized endogenously is an important regulator of renal hemodynamics in the immature kidney. Nitric oxide can function as a vasodilator to counterbalance vasoconstrictors such as angiotensin II (Solhaug et al., 1996).
6. **Prostaglandins,** which are endogenously produced, can cause vasodilation. Renal prostaglandin production is increased during the perinatal period, and the urinary excretion of prostaglandin E is 5 times that noted at term (Peruzzi et al., 1999).

**F. Glomerular filtration (Vogt and Dell, 2011).**

1. As blood passes through the capillaries, plasma is filtered through the glomerular capillary walls. Filtrate is collected in Bowman's space and enters the tubules, where composition is modified until it is excreted as urine.
2. GFR.
   a. Factors that may contribute to decreased GFR at birth include:
      (1) Small glomerular capillary area available for filtration.
      (2) Structural immaturity of glomerular capillary, which is associated with decreased water permeability.
      (3) Decreased blood pressure.
      (4) Increased hematocrit.
      (5) Renal vasoconstriction, which results in decreased glomerular plasma flow.
   b. Neonates born at less than 34 weeks' gestation have low GFR (0.5 mL/min) until nephrogenesis is completed.
3. Three primary factors determine GFR:
   a. Glomerular capillary hydrostatic pressure.
   b. Hydrostatic pressure in Bowman's capsule.
   c. Capillary colloid osmotic pressure.
4. Glomerular capillary hydrostatic pressure is the major controller of GFR.
5. Additional factors that affect GFR are:
   a. Capillary surface area.
   b. Permeability of capillary basement membrane.
   c. Rate of renal plasma flow.
   d. Changes in renal blood flow.
   e. Changes in blood pressure.
   f. Vasoactive changes in afferent or efferent arterioles.
   g. Ureteral obstruction.
   h. Edema of kidney.
   i. Changes in the concentration of plasma proteins:
      (1) Dehydration.
      (2) Hypoproteinemia.
   j. Increased permeability of the glomerular filter.
   k. Decrease in total area of glomerular capillary bed.

G. **Tubular function (Vogt and Dell, 2011).**
1. Components of the tubular system include the proximal tubule, loop of Henle, distal tubule, and collecting ducts.
2. Tubules modify the glomerular ultrafiltrate, leading to production of urine, which is accomplished by the process of tubular reabsorption and secretion.
   a. Tubular reabsorption is the movement of substances into the peritubular capillary plasma from the tubular epithelium, which occurs by diffusion and active transport. The proximal tubule is the major site of reabsorption.
   b. Tubular secretion is the movement of substances into the tubular epithelium from the peritubular capillary plasma. Tubular secretion is necessary for regulation of fluid and electrolyte balance, along with other renal processes.
3. Regulation of fluids and electrolytes is an important tubular function.
4. Tubular function is altered in the neonate as a result of decreased renal blood flow and GFR.
5. Tubular portions of the neonatal nephron are smaller and less functionally mature, resulting in an altered ability to transport sodium, urea, chloride, and glucose, with decrease renal thresholds for many substances.
6. Rapid maturation of proximal tubular cells occurs between 32 and 35 weeks of gestation.

H. **Concentration and dilution mechanism (Vogt and Dell, 2011).**
1. Maintenance of osmolality. The preterm and term neonate's ability to dilute urine is well developed, but concentrating ability is limited. A major function of the kidney is to maintain osmolality of extracellular fluid within the narrow range compatible with optimal cellular function.
2. Sites of urinary concentration and dilution:
   a. Loop of Henle.
   b. Collecting duct.
3. Factors responsible for the limited ability of the neonatal kidney to concentrate urine:
   a. Anatomic immaturity of the renal medulla.
   b. Decreased medullary concentration of sodium chloride and urea.
   c. Diminished responsiveness of the collecting ducts to arginine vasopressin.
4. Normal range of neonatal specific gravity is 1.002 to 1.010.
5. Maximum concentrating ability:
   a. Term neonate: 700 mOsm of water/kg.
   b. Preterm neonate: 600 to 700 mOsm of water/kg.
6. Capacity for urine dilution:
   a. Thirty to 50 mOsm of water/kg.
   b. Ability of neonate to excrete a hypotonic load is limited, presumably because of the low GFR.

I. **Renal regulation of acid–base balance (Hall, 2011).**
1. The kidneys are one of the most powerful acid–base regulatory systems.
   a. Molecules containing hydrogen atoms that can release hydrogen ions ($H^+$) in solutions are referred to as acids. The body produces acids mainly from the metabolism of proteins. These acids are called nonvolatile since they cannot be excreted by the lungs; they must be excreted by the kidneys.
   b. The term *alkalosis* refers to excess removal of $H^+$ from the body fluids, in contrast to the excess addition of $H^+$, which is referred to as *acidosis*.
   c. Excreting acidic urine reduces the amount of acid in extracellular fluid, while excreting alkaline urine removes base from the extracellular fluid.
2. The kidneys regulate extracellular $H^+$ concentration through three processes: (1) secretion of $H^+$, (2) reabsorption of filtered bicarbonate, and (3) production of new bicarbonate.
   a. Glucocorticoids can accelerate the renal processes of acidification (Guignard and Sulyok, 2012).

J. **Renal regulation of potassium (Benchimol and Satlin, 2011).**
1. Some 98% of potassium in the body is intracellular. Potassium is required for cell growth and division, DNA and protein synthesis, conservation of cell volume and pH, and optimal enzyme function.

2. The kidney is the major excretory organ for potassium.
3. Acidosis is associated with intracellular potassium release resulting in an increase in plasma potassium. Alkalosis results in a shift of potassium into cells and a consequent decrease in plasma potassium.
4. Acute metabolic acidosis causes the urine pH and potassium excretion to decrease. Acute respiratory alkalosis and metabolic alkalosis result in increases in urine pH and potassium excretion.
5. Potassium uptake into cells is stimulated by insulin, β-adrenergic agonists (e.g., albuterol and terbutaline), and alkalosis.

## CLINICAL EVALUATION OF RENAL AND URINARY TRACT DISEASE (VOGT AND DELL [2011])

A. **Renal anomalies may be diagnosed prenatally.** The kidneys may be visualized at 10 weeks' gestation, but accurate determination of renal anatomy is usually not possible until 16 weeks (Stamilio and Morgan, 1998).
B. **The antenatal history should be reviewed thoroughly, with particular attention devoted to medications, toxins, and unusual environmental exposures during the pregnancy.**
C. **A review of the medical history of the family is important, including any prior fetal or neonatal deaths.** While there is no established genetic basis for many congenital renal anomalies, certain disorders such as renal hypoplasia/dysplasia, multicystic dysplastic kidney, and vesicoureteral reflux may be familial. Certain diseases such as polycystic kidney disease and congenital nephrotic syndrome do have a clear genetic basis.

### Prenatal Diagnosis of Renal Disorders (Bates and Schwaderer, 2012)

A. **Prenatal findings that suggest renal or urinary tract disease** include hydronephrosis, renal cysts, hyperechoic kidneys, renal mass, oligohydramnios, and polyhydramnios. Hydronephrosis (dilation of the renal pelvis) is the most common identified renal anomaly (Dicke et al., 2006).
B. **Hydronephrosis may indicate upper urinary tract obstruction (ureteropelvic junction obstruction) and lower urinary tract obstruction (posterior urethral valves and prune-belly syndrome).**
C. **Prenatal renal cysts can be seen with autosomal dominant polycystic kidney disease, multicystic dysplastic kidneys, and cystic renal dysplasia.**
D. **Hyperechoic kidneys can result from tubular dilations (autosomal recessive polycystic kidney disease), dysplasia, or multiple microscopic cysts (Meckel–Gruber syndrome and nephrotic syndrome).**
E. **Oligohydramnios is not limited to renal disorders.** However, it can indicate renal agenesis, renal dysplasia, and lower urinary tract obstruction.
F. **Polyhydramnios is generally caused by gastrointestinal anomalies but may have a renal etiology in a small percentage of cases.** Renal dysplasia, nephrotic syndrome, or inherited renal tubular defects may present with polyhydramnios.
G. **Congenital renal tumors are rare.** The most common tumor is a mesoblastic nephroma, which appears as a unilateral, single, solid mass on prenatal ultrasound.

### Postnatal Evaluation of Renal and Urinary Tract Disease (Bates and Schwaderer, 2012)

A. **A family history of renal agenesis in parents or siblings, polycystic kidney disease, increases the risks of congenital kidney disease.**
B. **Hypertension in the newborn period is suggestive of renal disease and should be evaluated. Hypotension usually results from hypovolemia, hemorrhage, or sepsis, which may lead to acute kidney injury.**
C. **Delayed voiding greater than 12 hours may be seen after stressful deliveries but nearly all neonates will produce urine within 24 hours of birth. Prolonged anuria should be evaluated.**

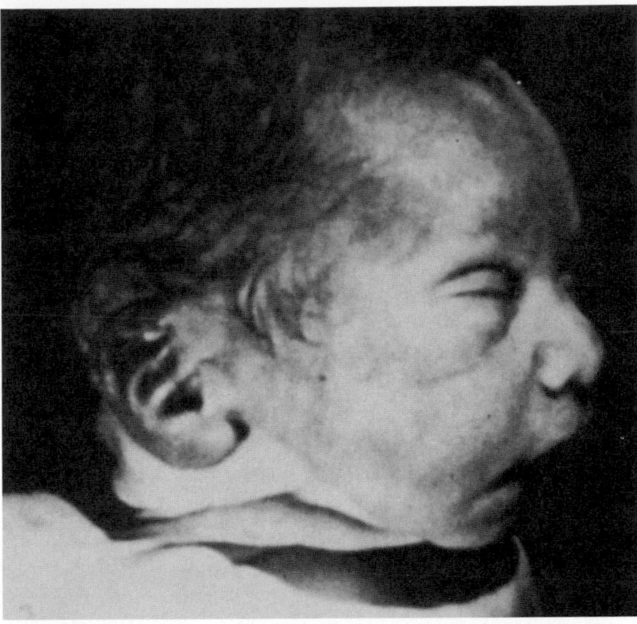

FIGURE 33-1 ■ Potter facies. Note epicanthal folds, hypertelorism, low-set ears, crease below lower lip, and receding chin. (From Martin, R.J., Fanaroff, A.A., and Walsh, M.C.: *Fanaroff and Martin's neonatal-perinatal medicine: Diseases of the fetus and infant* [9th ed.]. St. Louis, 2011, Elsevier Mosby.)

D. **Palpable abdominal masses, in particular flank masses, most often originate from the urinary tract and must be evaluated.**

E. **Edema occurs when there is an imbalance between capillary hydrostatic and interstitial oncotic forces.** The major renal causes include fluid overload secondary to a decrease in GFR from acute or chronic renal injury. Low intravascular oncotic pressure from urinary protein losses (congenital nephrotic syndrome) may also cause edema.

F. **Ascites can arise as an imbalance between hydrostatic and oncotic pressures, but it can also occur secondary to decreased lymphatic drainage.** The most common renal cause is urinary ascites from perforation of the ureter, renal pelvis, or bladder from obstruction (e.g., posterior urethral valves). Congenital nephrotic syndrome and renal vein thrombosis may also cause ascites.

G. **Other anomalies such as abnormal ears, microcephaly, meningomyelocele, pectus excavatum, abnormal genitalia, cryptorchidism, imperforate anus, and limb deformities may be associated with underlying renal defects.**

H. **Oligohydramnios (Potter) sequence may be seen in infants with bilateral renal agenesis.** The absence of fetal renal function results in anhydramnios, which causes fetal deformation from compression by the uterine wall. Features generally include wide-set eyes, depressed nasal bridge, beaked nose, receding chin, and posteriorly rotated, low-set ears. Other anomalies include a small, compressed chest wall and arthrogryposis. The condition is uniformly fatal. "Potter-like" features may be seen in infants with significant renal impairment and oligohydramnios. Such patients often have pulmonary hypoplasia and require careful respiratory management (Vogt and Dell, 2011) (Fig. 33-1).

I. **A single umbilical artery raises the suspicion of renal disease.** Bourke et al. (1993) found that 7% of otherwise normal infants with a single umbilical artery had significant renal anomalies.

## LABORATORY EVALUATION OF RENAL FUNCTION

A. **Serum creatinine level is the simplest and most commonly used indicator of neonatal kidney function.** The serum creatinine concentration immediately after birth reflects the maternal creatinine concentration, neonatal muscle mass, and GFR at the time of delivery.

1. In term infants, the serum creatinine level gradually decreases from 1.1 mg/dL to a mean value of 0.4 mg/dL within the first 2 weeks of life.
2. However, in preterm infants, the plasma creatinine level does not fall steadily from birth but instead rises in the first 48 hours before beginning to fall to equilibrium levels (Vogt and Dell, 2011).

B. **Failure of the serum creatinine level to fall or a persistent increase in serum creatinine suggests impairment of renal function.** In general, each doubling of the serum creatinine level represents an approximately 50% reduction in GFR; for example, a rise in serum creatinine from 0.4 to 0. 8 mg/dL represents a 50% reduction in GFR (Vogt and Dell, 2011).

C. **Blood urea nitrogen (BUN) is used as an indirect measure of kidney function.** The BUN may be elevated as a result of increased production of urea nitrogen in catabolic states, sequestered blood, tissue breakdown, or increased protein intake. Renal insufficiency is suspected if the BUN is greater than 20 mg/dL or if it rises at a rate of 5 mg/dL/day or higher (Bates and Schwaderer, 2012; Kim and Herrin, 2008) (Table 33-1).

TABLE 33-1

**Urine Evaluation of Renal Function**

| Evaluation | Discussion |
|---|---|
| Urine output | Anuria is absence of urine output.<br>Oliguria is less than 0.5 mL/kg/hr.<br>Ideally, urine output should be $\geq$2 mL/kg/hr. |
| Urine source | A clean-catch sample may be used for a urinalysis. If a culture is desired, a sterile sample must be obtained by a sterile catheterization. |
| Urine color and visual inspection | Cloudiness may represent a urinary tract infection or the presence of crystals.<br>Yellow-brown to deep olive green color may represent large amounts of conjugated bilirubin.<br>Porphyrins, certain drugs such as phenytoin, bacteria, and urate crystals may stain the diaper pink and be confused with bleeding.<br>Brown urine suggests bleeding from the upper urinary tract, hemoglobinuria, or myoglobinuria. Hemoglobinuria occurs secondary to intravascular hemolysis, of which the most common etiology is ABO blood group incompatibility.<br>In infants with myoglobinuria and hemoglobinuria, the urine may look red or brown and test dipstick-positive for blood, *but red blood cells are not present on microscopic examination of the urine.* |
| Specific gravity | Normal: 1.002 to 1.010.<br>May be falsely elevated by high-molecular-weight solutes such as contrast agents, glucose or other reducing substances, or large amounts of protein.<br>Urinary osmolality may be a more reliable measurement of the concentrating and diluting capacity of the kidney. |
| Hematuria | Defined as 5 or greater red blood cells per high-powered field on microscopic evaluation. Causes include renal vein thrombosis, polycystic kidney disease, obstructive nephropathy, tumor, congenital malformations, urinary tract infection, and acute kidney injury. |
| Proteinuria | Any form of renal injury, glomerular or tubular, will increase urinary protein excretion. |
| Glycosuria | Occurs when the serum glucose concentration exceeds the renal threshold.<br>Isolated glycosuria with a normal serum glucose concentration is defined as renal glycosuria, a benign condition caused by an abnormality in the transport of proximal tubular glucose. |
| Microscopic analysis | May detect the presence of red blood cells, casts, white blood cells, bacteria, or crystals. |

Data from Bates, C.M. and Schwaderer, A.L.: Clinical evaluation of renal and urinary tract disease. In C.A. Gleason and S.U. Devaskar (Eds.): *Avery's diseases of the newborn* (9th ed.). Philadelphia, 2012, Elsevier Saunders, pp. 1176-1181; Gomella, T.A.: *Neonatology: Management, procedures, on-call problems, diseases, and drugs* (6th ed.). New York, 2009, McGraw-Hill Medical; and Vogt, B.A. and Dell, K.M.: The kidney and urinary tract. In R.J. Martin, A.A. Fanaroff, and M.C. Walsh (Eds.): *Fanaroff and Martin's neonatal-perinatal medicine* (9th ed.). St. Louis, 2011, Elsevier Mosby, pp. 1681-1704.

## RADIOGRAPHIC EVALUATION (VOGT AND DELL, 2011)

A. **Ultrasonography has become the most common method of imaging the neonatal urinary tract.** It offers a noninvasive evaluation without exposure to contrast agents or radiation. A Doppler-flow study of the renal arteries and aorta may be helpful in the evaluation of thrombosis, suspected renovascular hypertension, or acute kidney injury.
B. **A voiding cystourethrogram (VCUG) is utilized to evaluate for lower urinary tract obstruction and vesicoureteral reflux.** Films of the urethra during voiding and of the bladder and ureters toward the end of voiding are essential.
C. **Radioisotopic renal scanning may be used to locate anomalous kidneys, determine kidney size, and identify obstruction or renal scarring.** Radioisotopic scans may also provide information about the relative blood flow to each kidney and the contribution of each kidney to overall renal function.
D. **Abdominal computed tomography (CT) is useful in the diagnosis of renal tumors, renal abscesses, and nephrolithiasis.** There has been recent concern related to the amount of radiation received with a CT scan.
E. **Fetal magnetic resonance imaging (MRI) provides detailed anatomy.** The typical indication for fetal urinary tract MRI evaluation is a second- or third-trimester pregnancy with oligohydramnios and an inconclusive prenatal renal ultrasound examination (Poutamo et al., 2000).

## ACUTE KIDNEY INJURY

A. **Previously referred to as acute renal failure, acute kidney injury is characterized by a deterioration in kidney function leading to an inability to excrete waste products and maintain fluid and electrolyte homeostasis.** This condition is defined as a serum creatinine of more than 1.5 mg/dL (Vogt and Dell, 2011).
B. **Oliguric acute kidney injury is characterized by a urine flow rate of less than 1 mL/kg/hr. With nonoliguric acute kidney injury, the urine flow rate is greater than 1 mL/kg/hr.**
C. **The risk factors for developing acute kidney injury** include very low birth weight (<1500 g), low 5-minute Apgar score, maternal drug administration (nonsteroidal antiinflammatory drugs and antibiotics), respiratory distress syndrome, patent ductus arteriosus, phototherapy, and neonatal medication administration (nonsteroidal antiinflammatory drugs, antibiotics, diuretics).
D. **Signs of acute kidney injury** may include elevated serum creatinine and BUN, hyperkalemia, metabolic acidosis, and evidence of fluid overload or dehydration.
E. **Half-life for medications excreted by the kidney (e.g., aminoglycosides, vancomycin) may also be prolonged.**
F. **The causes of acute kidney injury are multiple and can be divided into three categories: prerenal, renal, and postrenal (Table 33-2).**

### Evaluation of Acute Kidney Injury (Vogt and Dell, 2011)

A. **A careful review of the history should focus on prenatal ultrasound abnormalities, perinatal asphyxia, the prenatal or postnatal administration of potentially nephrotoxic drugs, and a family history of renal disease.**
B. **The physical examination should focus on signs of dehydration or volume overload, the abdomen, genitalia, and a search for congenital anomalies.**
C. **Electrolytes, BUN, creatinine, calcium, and phosphorus should be monitored frequently.**
D. **Urine should be sent for urinalysis, urine culture, and urine sodium and creatinine determination.**
E. **The fractional excretion of sodium and other diagnostic indices may be useful in differentiating prerenal from intrinsic acute kidney injury (Table 33-3).**
F. **Renal ultrasound is helpful in the identification of congenital renal disease and urinary tract obstruction.**

■ TABLE 33-2
■ ■ **Categories and Etiologies of Acute Kidney Injury**

| Category of AKI | Cause | Discussion |
|---|---|---|
| Prerenal | **1.** Respiratory distress syndrome<br>**2.** Hemorrhage<br>**3.** Sepsis<br>**4.** Necrotizing enterocolitis<br>**5.** Hypoxia<br>**6.** Congestive heart failure<br>**7.** Dehydration<br>**8.** Drugs that reduce renal blood flow: angiotensin-converting enzyme inhibitors, indomethacin, ibuprofen, amphotericin, tolazoline | Most common type. Often called prerenal azotemia.<br>Characterized by inadequate renal perfusion.<br>Prompt treatment is followed by improvements in renal function and urine output. |
| Renal (intrinsic) | **1.** Acute tubular necrosis (ATN)<br>**2.** Congenital anomalies<br>**a.** Renal dysplasia/agenesis<br>**b.** Polycystic kidney disease<br>**3.** Thromboembolic disease<br>**a.** Renal artery/vein thrombosis<br>**b.** Disseminated intravascular coagulation<br>**4.** Infection/inflammatory disease<br>**a.** Acute pyelonephritis<br>**b.** Congenital syphilis and toxoplasmosis | ATN is the most common cause and appears to involve renal tubular cellular injury.<br>The causes of ATN include perinatal asphyxia, sepsis, cardiac surgery, a prolonged prerenal state, and nephrotoxic drug administration. |
| Postrenal (obstructive) | **1.** Posterior urethral valves<br>**2.** Bilateral ureteropelvic junction obstruction<br>**3.** Bilateral ureterovesical junction obstruction<br>**4.** Neurogenic bladder<br>**5.** Obstructive nephrolithiasis | Caused by urinary tract obstruction and can usually be reversed by relief of the obstruction.<br>Compression of the ureters or bladder by a tumor or obstruction by renal calculi or fungus balls may also occur. |

Data from Vogt, B.A. and Dell, K.M.: The kidney and urinary tract. In R.J. Martin, A.A. Fanaroff, and M.C. Walsh (Eds.): *Fanaroff and Martin's neonatal-perinatal medicine* (9th ed.). St. Louis, 2011, Elsevier Mosby, pp. 1681-1704.

■ TABLE 33-3
■ ■ **Diagnostic Indices Related to Acute Kidney Injury (AKI)**

| Test | Prerenal AKI | Renal (Intrinsic) AKI |
|---|---|---|
| BUN/Cr ratio (mg/mg) | >30 | <20 |
| $FE_{Na}$ (%)* | ≤2.5 | ≥3.0 |
| Urinary Na (mEq/L) | ≤20 | ≥50 |
| Urinary Osm (mOsm/kg) | ≥350 | ≤300 |
| Urinary specific gravity | >1.012 | <1.014 |
| Ultrasonography | Normal | May be abnormal |
| Response to volume challenge | UO >2 mL/kg/hr | No increase in UO |

From Vogt, B.A. and Dell, K.M.: The kidney and urinary tract. In R.J. Martin, A.A. Fanaroff, and M.C. Walsh (Eds.): *Fanaroff and Martin's neonatal-perinatal medicine* (9th ed.). St. Louis, 2011, Elsevier Mosby, pp. 1681-1704.

*BUN*, Blood urea nitrogen; *Cr*, creatinine; *$FE_{Na}$*, fractional excretion of sodium; *Na*, sodium; *Osm*, osmolality; *UO*, urinary output.

*Fractional excretion of sodium $(FE_{Na}) = (U_{Na} \times P_{Cr})/(P_{Na} \times U_{Cr}) \times 100$, where $U_{Na}$ = urine sodium; $P_{Cr}$ = serum creatinine; $P_{Na}$ = serum sodium; $U_{Cr}$ = urine creatinine.

## Medical Management of Acute Kidney Injury (Vogt and Dell, 2011)

A. **The prevention of acute kidney injury requires maintenance of an adequate circulatory volume, careful fluid and electrolyte management, prompt diagnosis and treatment of hemodynamic or respiratory abnormalities, and close monitoring of potentially nephrotoxic medications.**
B. **The goal of medical management is to provide supportive care until there is spontaneous improvement in renal function.**
C. **With persistent oliguria, a urinary catheter should be placed to exclude lower urinary tract obstruction.** If there is no improvement in urine output after bladder drainage is established, a fluid challenge of 10 to 20 mL/kg should be administered over 1 to 2 hours to exclude prerenal acute kidney injury. A lack of improvement in urine output and increased serum creatinine suggests intrinsic acute kidney injury.
D. **Fluids are generally restricted.**
E. **Daily weights and careful intake and output measurements are necessary to follow volume status.**
F. **Nephrotoxic medication troughs should be monitored closely to reduce the risk of additional renal injury.**
G. **Potassium and phosphorus should be restricted in those neonates with hyperkalemia or hyperphosphatemia.**
H. **Metabolic acidosis may require treatment.**

## RENAL TUBULAR ACIDOSIS

A. **Renal tubular acidosis (RTA) is defined as metabolic acidosis resulting from the inability of the kidney to excrete $H^+$ or to reabsorb bicarbonate.** It may be a primary disorder or secondary to acquired renal injury. Poor growth may result from RTA (Kim and Herrin, 2008).
B. **Generally RTA is secondary to tubular damage from medications or obstructive uropathy (Dell, 2011).**
C. **Maternal toluene abuse from paint or glue sniffing during pregnancy causes severe renal tubular acidosis in the mother and neonate (Lindemann, 1991).**
D. **There are three main forms of RTA:** type I (distal), type II (proximal), and type IV (hyperkalemic) (Table 33-4).

## DEVELOPMENTAL RENAL ABNORMALITIES

Many of the disorders of the kidney and urinary tract that present in infancy are the result of congenital malformations or inherited disorders.

A. **Unilateral renal agenesis (Moore et al., 2013).**
    1. Unilateral renal agenesis, or the congenital absence of the kidney, occurs in 1 in 500 to 3200 live births. Bilateral renal agenesis occurs in 1 in 4000 to 10,000 live births.
    2. Males are affected more often than females, and the left kidney is usually the one that is absent.
    3. Unilateral renal agenesis often causes no symptoms and is usually not discovered during infancy because the other kidney usually undergoes compensatory hypertrophy and performs the function of the missing kidney.
B. **Bilateral renal agenesis (Moore et al., 2013).**
    1. Renal agenesis results when the ureteric buds do not develop or the primordia (stalks of buds) of the ureters degenerate.
    2. Bilateral renal agenesis is associated with oligohydramnios because little or no urine is excreted into the amniotic cavity.
        a. This condition occurs in approximately 1 in 3000 births, and is incompatible with postnatal life.
C. **Horseshoe kidney (Moore et al., 2013).**
    1. The poles of the kidneys are fused. The large U-shaped kidney usually lies in the pubic region, anterior to the inferior lumbar vertebrae.

■ TABLE 33-4
■ ■ **Three Types of Renal Tubular Acidosis**

| Type of RTA | Etiology | Presentation | Diagnosis | Treatment |
|---|---|---|---|---|
| Type I (distal or classic)<br>Primary—genetic defect<br><br>Secondary—tubular injury | Defect in the secretion of $H^+$ in the distal tubule<br>Primary may be autosomal recessive with associated nerve deafness<br>Secondary due to tubular injury, nephrocalcinosis, or medications | 1. Hypotonia<br>2. Persistently low serum bicarbonate<br>3. Elevated serum chloride<br>4. Urine cannot be acidified less than 6 pH | Urine pH that is greater than 6.5 in the presence of a non–anion gap metabolic acidosis<br>This diagnosis may be made erroneously in patients with diarrhea who develop a hyperchloremic metabolic acidosis and have an inappropriate urine pH (>6) | Alkali supplementation, either as bicarbonate or citrate to maintain normal serum bicarbonate concentration |
| Type II (proximal) | Defect in the proximal tubule with reduced reabsorption results in bicarbonate wastage<br>May be seen with Fanconi syndrome | | | Alkali supplementation |
| Type IV (hyperkalemic) | Combined impaired ability of the distal tubule to excrete hydrogen ions and potassium<br>May be associated with aldosterone deficiency<br>May be induced with angiotensin-converting enzyme inhibitors or spironolactone | 1. Non–anion gap metabolic acidosis<br>2. Hyperkalemia<br>3. Elevated urine sodium<br>4. Decreased urine potassium | | Alkali supplementation<br>Mineralocorticoid supplementation in conditions characterized by a deficiency of aldosterone<br>Treatment of hyperkalemia may reverse many of the abnormalities |

Data from Vogt, B.A. and Dell, K.M.: The kidney and urinary tract. In R.J. Martin, A.A. Fanaroff, and M.C. Walsh (Eds.): *Fanaroff and Martin's neonatal-perinatal medicine* (9th ed.). St. Louis, 2011, Elsevier Mosby, pp.1681-1704; and Guignard, J.P. and Sulyok, E.: Renal morphogenesis and development of renal function. In C.A. Gleason and S.U. Devaskar (Eds.): *Avery's diseases of the newborn* (9th ed.). Philadelphia, 2012, Elsevier Saunders, pp. 1165-1175.

2. Normal ascent of the fused kidneys is prevented because they are held down by the root of the inferior mesenteric artery.
3. A horseshoe kidney usually produces no symptoms because its collecting system develops normally and the ureters enter the bladder.
4. Approximately 7% of persons with Turner's syndrome have horseshoe kidney.

D. **Autosomal recessive polycystic kidney disease (Moore et al., 2013).**
1. Both kidneys contain many small cysts, which results in renal insufficiency.
2. Death of the infant usually occurs shortly after birth; however, an increasing number of these infants are surviving because of postnatal dialysis and kidney transplantation.

E. **Multicystic dysplastic kidney (MCDK).**
1. MCDK is a nonfunctional kidney, composed of multiple large cysts that resemble a cluster of grapes.

2. A possible etiology is failure of the ureteric bud to integrate and branch appropriately into the metanephros.
3. The majority of MCDKs undergo partial or complete spontaneous involution over time. The contralateral kidney, if normal, generally grows larger because of compensatory hypertrophy, allowing the child to maintain normal renal function.
4. MCDK does pose a risk of hypertension and malignancy. Surgical removal is reserved for children in whom the MCDK fails to involute or grows larger over time (Vogt and Dell, 2011).

**F. Ureteropelvic junction obstruction (Vogt and Dell, 2011).**
1. The most common cause of moderate to severe congenital hydronephrosis.
2. Ureteropelvic junction obstruction is more common in males and may be associated with other congenital anomalies, syndromes, or other genitourinary malformations.
3. Many clinicians advocate antibiotic prophylaxis to prevent urinary tract infection, although this practice remains somewhat controversial.
4. Surgical repair is the treatment.

**G. Posterior urethral valves.**
1. Represent the most common cause of lower urinary tract obstruction, with an incidence of 1 in 5000 to 8000 live male births.
2. A posterior urethral valve is composed of a congenital membrane that obstructs or partially obstructs the posterior urethra.
3. At birth, the infant may present with a palpable, distended bladder and a poor urinary stream.
4. The VCUG is diagnostic for posterior urethral valves.
5. The initial treatment is placement of a urinary catheter and later primary ablation of the valves (Vogt and Dell, 2011).

**H. Eagle–Barrett syndrome (prune-belly syndrome).**
1. Infants generally present with a distinct, flabby abdomen that is indicative of absent or deficient abdominal musculature.
2. Characterized by a triad of findings:
   a. Dilated, unobstructed urinary tract.
   b. Deficiency of abdominal wall musculature.
   c. Bilateral cryptorchidism.
3. The estimated incidence is 1 in 35,000 to 50,000 live births, with more than 95% of the cases occurring in males.
4. The two theories of pathogenesis are in-utero urinary tract obstruction and a specific mesodermal injury between the 4th and 10th weeks of gestation (Vogt and Dell, 2011).
5. Cardiac, pulmonary, gastrointestinal, and orthopedic anomalies may also be present.
   a. Treatment in the neonatal period involves the optimization of urinary tract drainage, the management of renal insufficiency, and antibiotic prophylaxis (Vogt and Dell, 2011).

## DISORDERS OF THE GENITALIA

**A. Undescended testes—cryptorchidism (Zderic and Lambert, 2012).**
1. Three percent of full-term males have an undescended testicle. Up to 30% of patients with undescended testes present with bilateral undescended testes.
2. Bilateral impalpable undescended testes in a newborn male warrants a genetic and endocrine evaluation for a disorder of sexual differentiation.
   a. Failure to appreciate the significance of bilateral and impalpable undescended testes in the NICU could result in missed diagnosis of congenital adrenal hyperplasia in a virilized female neonate.
   b. The neonate with a unilateral undescended testis and a normal phallus may be referred for a urologic follow-up evaluation at 3 to 6 months of age. If at 6 months of age the testis remains out of position, surgical intervention should be undertaken to reposition the testis within the scrotum.
   c. Long-term issues associated with cryptorchidism include an increased risk of infertility and testicular malignancy.

**B. Testicular torsion.**

1. The newborn who presents in the delivery room with a painful, blue, and edematous hemiscrotum will likely have had an antenatal torsion.
2. If the infant was born with a normal scrotal examination but subsequently develops scrotal swelling and erythema, the infant should undergo a Doppler ultrasound and surgical exploration if blood flow cannot be confirmed (Guerra et al., 2008).

**C. Hypospadius.**

1. The diagnosis of hypospadias is established when the urethral meatus is not present in the normal glanular position; the meatus may be present anywhere along the ventral penile surface from the glans to the perineum.
2. In addition, there is an asymmetrical or dorsally hooded foreskin, and the penis may be tethered, creating a significant bend (chordee).
3. There are four main types (Moore et al., 2013):
   a. Glanular hypospadias, the most common type.
   b. Penile hypospadias.
   c. Penoscrotal hypospadias.
   d. Perineal hypospadias.
4. Although the etiology remains unclear, hypospadias is thought to result from inadequate production of androgens by the fetal testes and/or inadequate receptor sites for the hormones (Moore et al., 2013). A family history is reported in 5% to 10% of cases.
5. The infant must not undergo circumcision; the foreskin is crucial for use in the urethral reconstruction and correction of the chordee. However, up to 10% of patients with a hypospadias may have an intact foreskin, and the diagnosis is determined only after circumcision.
   a. Congenital adrenal hyperplasia in a female neonate may be misdiagnosed as hypospadias with undescended testis.
   b. For an infant with hypospadias and bilaterally descended testes, an outpatient urologic evaluation should be arranged within 2 to 6 months of age (Zderic and Lambert, 2012).

---

## REFERENCES


Bates, C.M. and Schwaderer, A.L.: Clinical evaluation of renal and urinary tract disease. In C.A. Gleason, and S.U. Devaskar (Eds.): *Avery's diseases of the newborn* (9th ed.). Philadelphia, 2012, Elsevier Saunders.

Benchimol, C. and Satlin, L.M.: Potassium homeostasis in the fetus and neonate. In R.A. Polin, W.W. Fox, and S.H. Abman (Eds.): *Fetal and neonatal physiology* (4th ed.). Philadelphia, 2011, Elsevier Saunders.

Bourke, W.G., Clarke, T.A., Mathews, T.G., et al.: Isolated single umbilical artery—the case for routine renal screening. *Archives of Disease in Childhood*, 68:600, 1993.

Chevalier, R.L. and Norwood, V.F.: Functional development of the kidney in utero. In R.A. Polin, W.W. Fox, and S.H. Abman (Eds.): *Fetal and neonatal physiology* (4th ed.). Philadelphia, 2011, Elsevier Saunders.

Dell, K.M.: The kidney and urinary tract. In R.J. Martin, A.A. Fanaroff, and M.C. Walsh (Eds.): *Fanaroff and Martin's neonatal-perinatal medicine* (9th ed.). St. Louis, 2011, Elsevier Mosby.

Dicke, J.M., Blanco, V.M., Yan, Y. and Coplen, D.E.: The type and frequency of fetal renal disorders and management of renal pelvis dilatation. *Journal of Ultrasound in Medicine*, 25:973–977, 2006.

Gomella, T.A.: *Neonatology: Management, procedures, on-call problems, diseases, and drugs:* (6th ed.). New York, 2009, McGraw-Hill Medical.

Guerra, L.A., Wiesenthal, J. and Pike, J.: Management of neonatal testicular torsion: Which way to turn? *Canadian Urological Association Journal*, 2:376–379, 2008.

Guignard, J.P. and Sulyok, E.: Renal morphogenesis and development of renal function. In C.A. Gleason, and S.U. Devaskar (Eds.): *Avery's diseases of the newborn* (9th ed.). Philadelphia, 2012, Elsevier Saunders.

Hall, J.E.: *Guyton and Hall textbook of medical physiology: Guyton and Hall textbook of medical physiology (Guyton and Hall textbook of medical physiology*, (12th ed.). Philadelphia, 2011, Elsevier Health Sciences. Enhanced E-book (Guyton Physiology), Kindle Edition.

Kim, M.S. and Herrin, J.T.: Renal conditions. In J.P. Cloherty, E.C. Eicherwald, and A.R. Stark (Eds.): *Manual of neonatal care* (6th ed.). Philadelphia, 2008, Lippincott, Williams & Wilkins.

Lindemann, R.: Congenital renal tubular dysfunction associated with maternal sniffing of organic solvents. *Acta Paediatric Scandinavia*, 80(8–9):882–884, 1991.

Moore, K.L., Persaud, T.B.N. and Torchia, M.G.: *The developing human: Clinically oriented embryology:* (9th ed.). Philadelphia, 2013, Elsevier Saunders.

Peruzzi, L., Gianoglio, B., Porcellini, M.G. and Coppo, R.: Neonatal end-stage renal failure associated with maternal ingestion of cyclo-oxygenase-type-1 selective inhibitor nimesulide as tocolytic. *Lancet*, 354:1615, 1999.

Poutamo, J., Vanninen, R., Partanen, K. and Kirkinen, P.: Diagnosing fetal urinary tract abnormalities: Benefits of MRI compared to ultrasonography. *Acta Obstetricia et Gynecologica Scandinavica*, 79:65, 2000.

Solhaug, M.J. and Jose, P.A.: Postnatal maturation of renal blood flow. In R.A. Polin, W.W. Fox, and S.H. Abman (Eds.): *Fetal and neonatal physiology* (4th ed.). Philadelphia, 2011, Elsevier Saunders.

Solhaug, M.J., Wallace, M.R. and Granger, J.P.: Nitric oxide and angiotensin II regulation of renal hemodynamics in the developing piglet. *Pediatric Research*, 39:527, 1996.

Stamilio, D.M. and Morgan, M.A.: Diagnosis of fetal renal anomalies. *Obstetrics and Gynecology Clinics of North America*, 25:527–552, 1998.

Vogt, B.A. and Dell, K.M.: The kidney and urinary tract. In R.J. Martin, A.A. Fanaroff, and M.C. Walsh (Eds.): *Fanaroff and Martin's neonatal-perinatal medicine* (9th ed.). St. Louis, 2011, Elsevier Mosby.

Zderic, S.A. and Lambert, S.M.: Developmental abnormalities of the genitourinary system. In C.A. Gleason, and S.U. Devaskar (Eds.): *Avery's diseases of the newborn* (9th ed.). Philadelphia, 2012, Elsevier Saunders.

CHAPTER

# 34 Neurologic Disorders

M. TERESE VERKLAN

**OBJECTIVES**

1. Identify the six primary stages of neurodevelopment and the congenital anomalies that result from defective development at each stage.
2. Define autoregulation.
3. Review a complete neurologic examination.
4. Examine birth injuries and patient care management.
5. Differentiate between the different types of intracranial hemorrhages and their origins, clinical presentation, and outcomes.
6. Recognize neonatal seizures, their distinguishing characteristics, and issues in patient care management.
7. Describe hypoxic–ischemic encephalopathy.
8. Describe the clinical implications of periventricular leukomalacia.
9. Distinguish pathophysiologic factors, clinical presentation, and patient care management of early- and late-onset meningitis.

The human brain is an intricate, fragile organ requiring precise development from the moment of conception. Several crucial developmental landmarks pinpoint major events in the development of the human brain. If the process is interrupted, difficulties ranging from simple, easily treatable conditions to major neurologic malformations may occur. Neurologic problems account for a significant number of admissions into the neonatal intensive care unit each year. This chapter provides a comprehensive review of neurodevelopment, neurophysiology, and neuromalformations.

## ANATOMY OF THE NEUROLOGIC SYSTEM (MOORE ET AL. 2012; VOLPE, 2008)

A. **Embryologic development (Table 34-1).**
   1. Primary neurulation (dorsal induction).
      a. Occurs within the first month of life, ending between 24 and 28 days of gestation.
      b. Induction events of dorsal aspect of embryo.
      c. Neural tube is formed by the invagination and curling of the distal neural plate.
      d. Closure of the neural tube gives rise to the central nervous system (CNS), including the cranial nerves.
      e. This evolution results in the formation of the skull and vertebrae.
      f. Inaccuracies of primary neurulation result in craniorachischisis totalis, anencephaly, myeloschisis, encephalocele, myelomeningocele with Arnold–Chiari type II malformation.
   2. Prosencephalic development.
      a. Peak development is in the second and third months of gestation.
      b. Inductive interactive events that occur primarily at the rostral end on the ventral aspect of the embryo.
      c. This influences the formation of the face, forebrain, corpus callosum and septum pellucidum, optic nerves/chiasm, the hypothalamic structures (thalamus and hypothalamus [diencephalon]), and the cerebral hemispheres (telencephalon).
      d. Absence of olfactory bulbs and tracts is not uncommon.
      e. Disturbance in prosencephalic development causes facial and forebrain alterations.
         (1) Holoprosencephaly (abnormal formation of telencephalon and diencephalon).

■ TABLE 34-1
■ ■ **Major Events in Human Brain Development and Peak Times of Occurrence**

| Major Developmental Event | Peak Time of Occurrence |
|---|---|
| Primary neurulation | 3 to 4 weeks of gestation |
| Prosencephalic development | 2 to 3 months of gestation |
| Neuronal proliferation | 3 to 4 months of gestation |
| Neuronal migration | 3 to 5 months of gestation |
| Organization | 5 months of gestation to years postnatal |
| Myelination | Birth to years postnatal |

From Volpe, J.J.: *Neurology of the newborn* (5th ed.). Philadelphia, 2008, Elsevier Saunders.

(2) Midline and midfacial defects.
(a) Hypotelorism (less common: hypertelorism).
(b) Cyclopia.
(c) Cleft lip with or without cleft palate.
(3) Agenesis of corpus callosum, corpus pellucidum.
**f.** Most common karyotype is normal (chromosomal disorder is possible).

**3.** Neuronal proliferation.
**a.** Occurs initially at 2 months, with peak between 3 and 4 months of gestation.
**b.** Toxins and inherited diseases can significantly alter the number of neurons.
**c.** Chemical and environmental substances can reduce the number of neurons, causing microcephaly vera.
**d.** Insufficient neurons in absence of apoptotic events are primary micrencephaly; excess neurons can produce macrencephaly.
**e.** Disorders of proliferation of small veins cause Sturge–Weber syndrome (6% unilateral, 24% bilateral facial lesions).

**4.** Neuronal migration.
**a.** Can occur as early as 2 months; peaks between 3 and 5 months.
**b.** By 6 months of gestation, the neurons have migrated to their final, permanent place in the cortex.
**c.** Neurons follow glial paths outward.
**d.** Cells migrate and differentiate into six cortical layers.
**e.** Migration is critical for development of the cerebral cortex and the deeper nuclear structures.
(1) Basal ganglia.
(2) Hypothalamus.
(3) Thalamus.
(4) Brainstem.
(5) Cerebellum.
(6) Spinal cord.
**f.** Dysfunction at this stage results in cortical malformation with abnormalities of neurologic function.
**g.** Seizures may be the first clinical manifestation in the early postnatal period.
**h.** Defects associated with abnormal migration range in severity and may be associated with other neurologic development.
**i.** Abnormal development of gyrus denotes a neuronal migration disorder.
**j.** Disorders include lissencephaly ("smooth brain"), pachygyria, agenesis of the corpus callosum, and schizencephaly (clefts found in the cerebral wall).

**5.** Neuronal organization.
**a.** Peaks at 5 months of gestation to several years after birth.
**b.** Provides the basis for brain function and its complex circuitry.
**c.** Includes cell differentiation, cell death, synaptic development, neurotransmitters, and myelination.

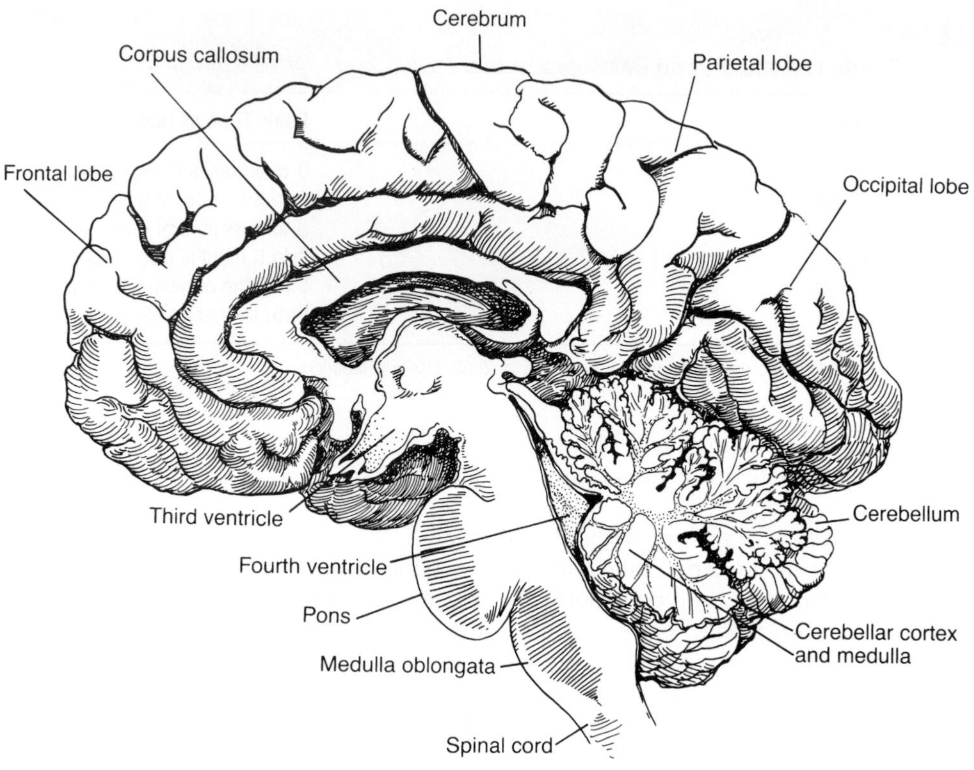


FIGURE 34-1 ■ Anatomy of the brain.

  - **d.** Achieves stabilization of cell connections.
  - **e.** Disorders due to organizational deficits and detrimental retardation (as with Down syndrome, fragile X syndrome, and mild Duchenne's muscular dystrophy).
- **6.** Myelination.
  - **a.** Begins in the second trimester and continues into adult life.
  - **b.** Involves myelin deposition around axons.
  - **c.** Myelin, a fatty covering, insulates the circuitry; prevents leakage of current and enables rapid, efficient transmission of nerve impulses.
  - **d.** Enhances intercellular communication.
  - **e.** Deficiencies occur in some acquired and inherited diseases.

**B. Brain anatomy (Fig. 34-1) (Moore et al., 2012; Volpe, 2008).**

- **1.** Cerebellum.
  - **a.** Promotes integrative muscle function.
  - **b.** Maintains balance.
  - **c.** Enables smooth, purposeful movements.
- **2.** Cerebrum: main components of cerebral hemisphere.
  - **a.** Contains four lobes: frontal, parietal, occipital, and temporal.
    - (1) Frontal lobes make up command center; concerned with decision making and other "executive" tasks.
    - (2) Parietal lobes are responsible for hearing, understanding speech, and forming an integrated sense of self.
    - (3) Occipital lobes process vision.
    - (4) Temporal lobes are centers for smell with associative areas for memory and learning.
  - **b.** Corpus callosum: fiber bundles connecting the cerebral hemispheres.
  - **c.** Cerebral cortex.
    - (1) Encompasses the mind, the intellect.
    - (2) Gray matter.
  - **d.** Lateral ventricles.

e. Third ventricle: fluid-filled space.
f. Thalamus: integrates sensory input.
g. Hypothalamus: regulates body temperature.

3. Brainstem.
   a. Relays input and output signals between higher brain centers and the spinal cord.
   b. Three main components.
      (1) Medulla oblongata.
         (a) Gives origin to cranial nerves VIII, IX, X, XI, and XII.
         (b) Controls areas of the abdomen, thorax, throat, and mouth.
      (2) Pons: carries information between the brainstem and the cerebellum.
      (3) Midbrain: involved in eye movements.

## PHYSIOLOGY OF THE NEUROLOGIC SYSTEM (McLEAN ET AL., 2012; VOLPE, 2008; YAGER, 2012).

**A. Glucose metabolism.**

1. Cerebral metabolism is influenced by the availability of glucose and oxygen.
2. Glucose is transported from blood to brain by a glucose transporter found in capillaries.
3. Serum glucose provides the brain with a glucose pool.
4. The neonatal brain is glucose dependent. The CNS is quickly and significantly affected by hypoglycemia.
5. Glycogen stores are minimal or nonexistent in the premature baby.
6. The brain depends on adequate circulation to supply both oxygen and glucose to create enough energy for normal growth and metabolism.
7. Anaerobic metabolism causes lactic acid buildup.
8. Anaerobic metabolism produces significantly smaller amounts of energy.
9. Newborn blood glucose levels less than 30 mg/dL are associated with significant increases in cerebral blood flow.
10. Defining the lower limit of the neonatal blood glucose level is difficult because the infant's ability to present overt symptoms of hypoglycemia is not developed.

**B. Cerebral blood flow.**

1. Cerebral blood flow is affected by pH (controlled by hydrogen ions and carbon dioxide levels), potassium, hypoxemia, osmolarity, and calcium ion concentrations.
   a. The brain increases cerebral blood flow to spare itself inadequacies.
   b. As pH decreases, cerebral blood flow increases.
   c. As potassium levels increase, cerebral blood flow increases.
   d. Hypoxemia causes an increase in cerebral blood flow to provide adequate oxygenated blood to the brain.
   e. Increased osmolarity causes increased cerebral blood flow.
   f. An increase in calcium ions causes a decrease in cerebral blood flow.
   g. Cerebral blood flow increases when blood glucose levels fall to less than 30 mg/dL; the hypoglycemic brain recruits previously unperfused capillaries to maintain glucose levels. Degree and duration of hypoglycemia are significant.
   h. Studies have shown that neonatal neurologic signs can be minimal or absent with subsequent abnormal cognitive development.
2. Autoregulation.
   a. Maintains steady-state cerebral blood flow over a broad range of perfusion pressures.
   b. Important vasoactive factors in the brain: hydrogen ions, potassium ions, adenosine, prostaglandins, osmolarity, calcium.
   c. Cerebral blood flow increases with advancing gestational age and concomitant cerebral metabolic demands.
   d. Normal arterial blood pressure in the preterm neonate is thought to be near or at the lower autoregulatory limit. This suggests an increased vulnerability to ischemic brain injury with modest hypotension, especially with decreasing gestational age.

e. Cerebral vasculature vasodilates maximally in response to hypoxemia, hypercapnia, and acidosis.
   (1) Hypotension leads to ischemia.
      (a) Ischemia damages blood vessels and surrounding elements supporting the blood vessels.
      (b) Blood flow to cerebral white matter is restored only after reperfusion of other brain regions.
      (c) Once adequate blood supply resumes, hemorrhage can occur into ischemic areas.
   (2) Hypertension leads to hemorrhage.

## NEUROLOGIC ASSESSMENT (RENNIE AND HUERTAS-CEBALLOS, 2012; VOLPE, 2008)

A. **History.**
B. **Observation.**
   1. Determine behavioral state.
   2. Note posture.
      a. Gestational age determines posture.
         (1) Premature infants: open, extended position reflecting diminished tone.
         (2) Term infants: flexed position reflecting adequate tone.
      b. Sequelae of intrauterine position may be evident.
      c. Abnormal findings are as follows:
         (1) Hyperextension.
         (2) Asymmetry.
         (3) Flaccidity.
   3. Note movements.
      a. Symmetrical or asymmetrical body movements.
      b. Note movement quality (jitteriness, seizures, tremors, and clonus).
      c. Quantity (absent or pronounced).
   4. Note respiratory activity.
      a. Signs of distress.
      b. Hypoventilation (apnea).
      c. Quality of cry.
         (1) High pitched (consider meningitis, drug withdrawal, neurologic abnormalities).
         (2) Stridor (consider vocal cord damage or paralysis).
   5. Observe skin.
      a. Lesions (note number, size, shape, color, and texture).
         (1) Café-au-lait spots (six or more lesions of $\geq$1.5 cm; may indicate neurofibromatosis).
         (2) Port-wine facial hemangioma (consider Sturge–Weber syndrome).
         (3) Areas of depigmentation.
      b. Abrasions, lacerations, bruises, and forceps marks (consider intracranial bleeding, injury).
C. **Physical examination (Fenichel, 2007; Scher, 2013; Volpe, 2008).**
   1. Check the skull size, shape, symmetry, hair whorls, fontanelles, and sutures.
   2. Measure frontal–occipital circumference (FOC).
      a. Document less than 10th percentile (symmetrical vs. asymmetrical compared with total body growth; may indicate microcephaly).
      b. Document greater than 90th percentile (symmetrical vs. asymmetrical compared with total body growth; may indicate macrocephaly).
   3. Examine the face for abnormalities in structure.
      a. Placement of ears.
      b. Neck skinfolds.
   4. Spine (intact, openings, masses).
   5. Cranial nerve function.
      a. Refer to Table 34-2.
      b. May be difficult to assess in the preterm newborn.

■ TABLE 34-2
■ ■ **Cranial Nerves**

| Number | Name | Type of Nerve | Function | Bedside Testing Mechanism | Expected Results and Comments |
|---|---|---|---|---|---|
| I | Olfactory | Sensory | Smell | Soak cotton pledget in strong odor and place under nares | Startle |
| II | Optic | Sensory | Conveys visual information from retina to brain | Check PERL; funduscopic examination | PERL intact; presence of red reflex |
| III | Oculomotor | Motor | Motor fibers to eyelid (lid elevation), some eye muscles, pupil (constriction and accommodation), and light reflex | Check EOM, PERL | PERL intact; EOM full and conjugate |
| IV | Trochlear | Motor | Movement of superior oblique muscles of eye, uvula movement | Check EOM | EOM full and conjugate |
| V | Trigeminal | Mixed | Sensation of face, scalp, and cornea; motor of jaw (mastication) | Touch cheek | Turns cheek toward stimulus |
| VI | Abducens | Motor | Lateral gaze; abducts eyeball | Rotate infant | Movement of eyes in direction of travel |
| VII | Facial | Mixed | Facial muscle movement, lid closure, taste | Elicit cry and observe facial movement | Symmetrical facial movements |
| VIII | Auditory | Sensory | Hearing | Talk softly to baby or clap loudly near baby's ear | Quiets to voice; blinks to clap |
| IX | Glossopharyngeal | Mixed | Taste, swallow, gag | Elicit gag response | Strong gag response |
| X | Vagus | Mixed | Most extensive innervation of any cranial nerve; motor, sensory, and autonomic innervation of neck, thorax, abdomen; swallow and gag | Elicit cry | Strong, lusty cry |
| XI | Accessory | Motor | Movement of head and neck | Turn supine infant's head to side | Attempts to bring head to midline; full range of shoulder and neck |
| XII | Hypoglossal | Motor | Tongue movement and symmetry | Insert gloved finger into baby's mouth while sucking | Suck should be strong and steady without fasciculations, tongue symmetry |

Adapted from Scanlon, J.W., Nelson, T., Grylack, L.J., and Smith, Y.F.: *A system of newborn physical examination.* Baltimore, 1979, University Park Press; Hockenberry, M.J. and Wilson, D.: *Wong's nursing care of infants and children* (9th ed.). St. Louis, 2011, Elsevier Mosby; Fletcher, M.A.: *Physical diagnosis in neonatology.* Philadelphia, 1997, Lippincott, Williams & Wilkins; http://library.med.utah.edu/pedineurologicexam/html/newborn_n.html#02; and http://www.fpnotebook.com/Nicu/Exam/NwbrnNrlgcExm.htm.
*EOM*, Extraocular movements; *PERL*, pupils equal and reactive to light.

c. Blink reflex requires intact cranial nerves III and VII.
d. Corneal reflex requires intact cranial nerves V and VII.
   (1) Generally elicited only if one suspects brain damage.
   (2) Consider testing integrity of reflex in the presence of eye damage.
e. Cranial nerves IX, X, and XII regulate the tongue, swallow, gag, and cry.
f. Rooting reflex starts at 28 weeks, with a complete response established by 32 weeks.

g. Sucking reflex present at 28 to 30 weeks but slow, weak, and unsustainable; mature and robust by 34 to 36 weeks of gestation.
h. Rooting and sucking reflexes test partial function of cranial nerves V, VII, and XII.
i. Swallowing tests cranial nerves IX and X.
6. Muscle tone.
a. Evaluate head lag, ventral suspension, clonus, and recoil from extension.
b. Check symmetry; briskness versus flaccidity.
7. Reflexes.
a. Check primitive reflexes (automatisms).
(1) Blinking: An infant will close his or her eyes in response to bright lights.
(2) Palmar and plantar grasp (bilaterally): An infant's fingers or toes will curl around a finger placed in the area.
(3) Babinski: As the infant's foot is stroked, the toes will extend upward and fan outward.
(4) Moro: A quick change in the infant's position will cause the infant to throw back his or her head, extend his or her arms outward, and open the hands.
(5) Startle: A loud noise will cause the infant to extend and flex the arms, while the hands remain in a fist.
b. Evaluate symmetry and strength of response of all primitive reflexes.
c. Consider clavicular or humeral fractures or brachial plexus injury in the presence of an abnormal Moro reflex.
d. Grasp varies with gestational age; if grasp is absent, consider nerve damage.

## NEURAL TUBE DEFECTS (NTDs)

As the neural tube develops, developmental processes can be altered by intrinsic or extrinsic factors, resulting in defective closure or a reopening of the neural tube. Defects range from anencephaly to open or skin lesions of the spinal cord.

**A. Incidence and etiology. (Back and Plawner, 2012)**
1. Neural tube defects are among the most commonly occurring congenital malformation of the CNS.
a. Incidence of NTDs in the United States is estimated as 1 per 1000 live births (Moore et al., 2012).
2. Risks for recurrence are significantly higher if a previous pregnancy has resulted in a child with an NTD. The risk may actually be nearly triple for subsequent pregnancies.
3. The etiology of NTDs is multifactorial. This complex interaction of genetic and environmental factors operates independently to determine individual and population risk. The majority of defects occur sporadically.
a. Environmental risk factors most commonly identified with development of an NTD include: maternal febrile illness, maternal heat exposure in the first trimester, hyperglycemia secondary to maternal diabetes, lower socioeconomic status, dietary factors, and prenatal exposure to drugs.
4. The defects result from a failure in closure of the neural groove to form an intact neural tube. The type and severity of the defect is dependent on the location and extent of failure.

## Anencephaly (Volpe, 2008)

**A. Incidence and etiology.**
1. Anencephaly is the most common and severe of disorders of anterior neural tube closure, comprising over half of the NTDs (Back and Plawner, 2012). It is a primary defect in anterior neural tube closure. Presentation of the anomaly is variable, may extend from the level of the lamina terminalis to the foramen magnum.
a. About 75% of infants are stillborn; of the infants who do survive into the neonatal period, it is uniformly lethal within the first months of life. The onset of the defect is estimated to occur no later than 24 days of gestation.
2. Incidence is 1.0 to 10.0 per 1000 live births (Back and Plawner, 2012). Recurrence risk for parents who have had one affected child is 1.9% (Jones et al., 2013).

3. Genetic and environmental influences appear to be important in the development of the defect.

B. **Clinical presentation.**
   1. General: no documented growth deficiency.
   2. Craniofacial: commonly involves the forebrain and upper brainstem, resulting in absence of the calvaria; cerebral hemispheres are missing. The lower brainstem is present, with rudimentary function. Hypothalamus and cerebellum are frequently malformed. Varied facial features, cleft palate and/or lip, altered auricular development, and cervical abnormalities are also common. (Back and Plawner, 2012).
   3. Musculoskeletal: malformation of the ribs, thoracic cage, abdominal wall, anterior spina bifida, and short neck.

C. **Associated findings.**
   1. Polyhydramnios.
   2. Diaphragmatic defects with or without herniation, hypoplastic lung.

D. **Diagnosis.**
   1. Fetal ultrasound or radiographs in the second trimester to detect absence of vital structures.
   2. Maternal serum screening at 16 to 18 weeks identifies infants at risk. AFP is a major serum protein in the early embryo and is fetus specific. Leakage of fetal serum through an open NTD directly into the amniotic fluid results in elevation of AFP levels. These increases are detected by maternal serum and amniocentesis evaluation (Back and Plawner, 2012).

E. **Treatment/prevention.**
   1. U.S. Public Health Service recommends that women of childbearing age consume 0.4 mg of folic acid daily to decrease their risk for conceiving a child with an NTD. Periconceptional use of vitamins and folate have resulted in a 60% to 70% reduction in the recurrence of these malformations when given to women who had previously given birth to an infant with a neural tube disorder (Back and Plawner, 2012). In the United States, cereals and bread products are enriched with folate.
   2. As most anencephalic infants are stillborn or die within a few days of delivery, the parents must prepare for the death of their infant at a time when they would be anticipating the birth. Support for the family must take into account their individual preferences and needs.
   3. The opportunity for these infants to serve as organ donors is complex. Ethical and legal concerns over the diagnosis of brain death and persistent clinical signs of brainstem function have limited the donation of organs from anencephalic infants.

## Encephalocele

Defects are secondary to restricted failure of the anterior neuropore to close at approximately day 26 of gestation, resulting in extension of the brain tissue through a defect in the skull.

A. **Incidence and etiology (Back and Plawner, 2012).**
   1. The defect occurs in 1 per 10,000 live births. In 70% to 80% of babies the lesion is found in the occipital region (Volpe, 2008).
   2. Precise mechanism for development is unclear.
   3. Genetic factors may be causative, autosomal recessive patterns of inheritance have been reported. Meckel's syndrome and Walker–Warburg syndrome are the most commonly associated syndromes.
   4. Environmental factors, including maternal teratogens, have been linked to development of encephalocele.
      a. Maternal febrile illness resulting in temperatures of 38.9° C (102.2° F) or greater within the first one third to one half of gestation have been found to be teratogenic (Jones et al., 2013).

B. **Clinical presentation.**
   1. Craniofacial: cranial defect through which brain protrudes. Defects are commonly occipital (80%), with frontal, temporal, and parietal composing the remainder. Lesions generally are covered by skin or membrane.

C. **Associated findings (Back and Plawner, 2012).**
   1. Approximately 50% of infants presenting with an encephalocele have other major anomalies. Microcephaly, arrhinencephaly, cleft lip/palate, craniosynostosis, and hydrocephalus

occur in approximately one half of the affected children. Agenesis of the corpus callosum occurs in two thirds of affected infants (Volpe, 2008).
2. Though normal intelligence is reported in approximately 50% of cases, intellectual deficiencies occur.
3. Hypotonia and associated motor defects.

D. **Diagnosis.**
1. Evaluation of these defects is supported through the use of radiographs of the skull, transillumination of the defect, cranial ultrasound, and CT or MRI imaging.
2. Chromosomal studies should be undertaken if suspicion of a genetic syndrome is present.
3. Careful history of maternal exposure to teratogens or adverse environmental events may provide clues to etiology.

E. **Treatment.**
1. Based on the individual position and extent of the lesion.
   a. Neurosurgical relief is indicated for most lesions, especially if cerebrospinal fluid is leaking from the lesion. Mortality and morbidity are dependent on the individual lesion. Of those children surviving initial repair, a significant number will have neurologic defects, paralysis, seizures, and deficits in muscular coordination.
2. For those families who experience a child with an encephalocele, genetic counseling is essential as recurrence risk is estimated at 3% to 5%, depending on the etiology of the defect.

## Spina Bifida

These spinal cord malformations include myelomeningocele and meningoceles and result from restricted failure of the posterior neuropore to close at approximately 26 days of gestation.

A. **Incidence and etiology (Volpe, 2008).**
1. Overall incidence is 2 in 10,000 live births (Back and Plawner, 2012).
2. The etiology of these defects include: multifactorial inheritance, single mutant genes, chromosomal anomalies, and specific teratogens.
   a. Females are more commonly affected than males.
   b. The level of the myelomeningocele in the first affected infant has a direct effect on risk for subsequent infants. Recurrence risk for infants whose sibling had a lesion at T11 is 7.8%. If the index lesion was below T11, the subsequent risk was 0.7%.

B. **Clinical presentation (Volpe, 2008).**
1. Defects are divided into two categories:
   a. Spina bifida occulta: Mildest form of the defect presenting with skin covering the opening in the spinal column. This developmental anomaly involves a separation of overlying ectoderm from the neural tube. Impairment of the mesoderm to develop between ectoderm and neural tube results in disturbance of vertebrae and mesodermal tissue.
      (1) These lesions occur most commonly in the caudal region. Overt lesions include ectodermal abnormalities, dermal tracts and sinuses. Vertebral defects are present in 85% to 95% of lesions.
      (2) Approximately 80% of affected infants will exhibit a dermal lesion in the lumbosacral region. These defects include cutaneous dimples, cutaneous abnormalities or masses, and abnormal collections of hair.
      (3) Neurologic deficits are unusual in the newborn; sensory abnormalities in legs, feet or sphincter abnormalities may occasionally be present.
   b. Spina bifida manifesta: Spinal dysraphic conditions result from defects in caudal neural tube formation.
      (1) Meningocele: restricted herniation of meninges at the site of defect. Defect is uniformly localized to the lumbar region, is closed defect with intact dermal covering (Back and Plawner, 2012).
      (2) Myelomeningocele: characterized by herniation of meninges and spinal cord at the site of the defect. Lesions may or may not have vertebral or dermal covering. These defects are 4 times more common than meningoceles (Back and Plawner, 2012).
         (a) Rarely occurs as an isolated malformation, commonly associated with CNS abnormalities (Back and Plawner, 2012).

**C. Associated findings.**
1. Hydrocephalus is a common associated development either at birth or shortly after.
   a. Development correlates with the site of the lesion: 60% in patients with occipital, cervical, or thoracic lesions; 90% in infants with thoracolumbar, lumbar, or lumbosacral lesions (Back and Plawner, 2012).
2. Infants with myelomeningocele experience serious urinary tract complications. These urinary issues are a major cause of death after the first year of life (Volpe, 2008).
3. Kyphosis at birth; scoliosis later in childhood.
4. Clubfeet secondary to neurologic and orthopedic abnormalities.
5. Dislocation of hips, delay in walking, asymmetry of legs.
6. Arnold–Chiari malformation occurs in 95% of patients with a lumbar lesion (Back and Plawner, 2012). Downward displacement of the medulla and the fourth ventricle through the foramen magnum into the upper cervical canal sets in motion a chain of events that are potentially lethal secondary to brainstem dysfunction and hydrocephalus. Development of a hoarse weak cry may indicate vocal cord paralysis and is a sign of herniation.
7. Tethered cord.
8. Seizure activity secondary to cortical dysgenesis occurs in 20% to 25% of infants with myelomeningocele (Volpe, 2008).

**D. Diagnosis.**
1. AFP elevation in maternal serum at 16 to 18 weeks.
2. Amniotic fluid acetylcholinesterase and amniotic AFP at 14 to 16 weeks.
3. Fetal ultrasound.
4. Radiographs, CT, cranial ultrasonography, and MRI are done to provide visual record of anomalies.

**E. Treatment.**
1. Scheduled delivery by cesarean section before onset of labor should be considered for the fetus with known meningomyelocele.
2. Clinical management is individualized to the type and position of the lesion.
   a. Early surgical repair is advocated for most infants to preserve cognitive function, improve prognosis for ambulation, and decrease mortality.
   b. Assessment of function at the level of the lesion allows for estimates of potential capabilities; motor, sensory, and sphincter function.
   c. Examine lesion and measure size.
   d. Culture specimen from lesion if sac is open. Wrap lesion with sterile gauze moistened with warm sterile saline solution; place a sterile feeding tube within the gauze mesh for intermittent infusion of warm saline solution. Maintain the infant in a prone kneeling position, and protect the knees from skin breakdown. Place a drape over the buttocks below the lesion; utilize the drape's adhesive backing to secure the drape to the body.
   e. Obtain immediate consultation:
      (1) Neurosurgery
      (2) Urology: evaluation must be undertaken to demonstrate deformity and determine the type and frequency of follow-up management needed.
3. Secondary to the extensive associated finding for these defects, parents must be made aware of the need for continuing care and support. Often a team approach is needed to ensure that complications are minimized.

## NEUROLOGIC DISORDERS

**A. Microcephaly (Back and Plawner, 2012; Volpe, 2008).**
1. Definition.
   a. FOC $\geq$2 standard deviations below the mean for age and gender.
   b. Small brain implies neurologic impairment.
2. Risk factors.
   a. Maternal:
      (1) Viral infections under the TORCH spectrum (*t*oxoplasmosis, *o*ther [syphilis], *r*ubella, *c*ytomegalovirus, or *h*erpes).

(2) Exposure to radiation.
(3) Metabolic conditions such as diabetes or phenylketonuria.
(4) Use of prescription and/or street drugs, especially in the first trimester.
(5) Genetic foundation may be autosomal recessive, autosomal dominant, or X-linked.
(6) Malnutrition is the most common etiology worldwide.

**b.** Fetal:
(1) Prenatal/perinatal insult: inflammation; hypoxia; birth trauma.

**c.** Neonatal:
(1) Very low birth weight infant.
(2) Hypoxic–ischemic encephalopathy (HIE).
(3) Nutrition: most common worldwide cause.

**3.** Pathophysiology.
- **a.** Neuronal proliferation defect.
- **b.** Occurs between 3 and 4 months of gestational age.
- **c.** Destructive microcephaly occurs when the normal brain suffers prenatal/perinatal insult.

**4.** Clinical presentation.
- **a.** Small head, backward sloping of the forehead, small cranial volume.
- **b.** Neurologic deficits rarely evident at birth.

**5.** Diagnostic evaluation.
- **a.** Perform a complete physical examination, including neurologic assessment.
- **b.** Elicit a thorough maternal history.
- **c.** Use tests to confirm or rule out etiologic factors aligned with maternal history.
- **d.** Computed tomography (CT) or magnetic resonance imaging (MRI) is performed.

**6.** Patient care management.
- **a.** Record accurate measurement of FOC, length, and weight weekly.
- **b.** Note percentiles and alert physician to abnormalities.
- **c.** Document clearly any deviations from normal.
- **d.** Obtain tests as ordered; note dates to follow up results.
- **e.** Ensure that the family is informed.
- **f.** Obtain consultations as needed: genetics, infectious diseases.

**7.** Outcome.
- **a.** Dependent on severity.
- **b.** May be associated with developmental delays.

**B. Hydrocephalus (Prabhu et al., 2012; Verklan and Lopez, 2011; Volpe, 2008).**

**1.** Definition: excess cerebrospinal fluid (CSF) in the ventricles of the brain due to a decrease in reabsorption or overproduction.
- **a.** CSF is in balance between formation and absorption.
- **b.** CSF is produced at a rate of 0.35 mL/min from brain parenchyma, cerebral ventricles, areas along the spinal cord, and the choroid plexus (70% is from the choroid plexus).

**2.** Pathophysiology.
- **a.** Excessive CSF production (rare).
- **b.** Inadequate CSF absorption secondary to abnormal circulation.
- **c.** Excess ventricular CSF secondary to aqueductal outflow obstruction causes obstructive, noncommunicating hydrocephalus (refer to Fig. 34-2 for a simplified diagram of the brain).
  (1) The condition is most common in newborn infants.
  (2) Obstructive hydrocephalus may progress rapidly.
- **d.** Excess ventricular CSF with flow between the lateral ventricles and the subarachnoid space results in communicating, nonobstructive hydrocephalus.

**3.** Congenital hydrocephalus.
- **a.** Risk factors.
  (1) Aqueductal stenosis.
  (2) Dandy–Walker cyst (cystic transformation of fourth ventricle).
  (3) Myelomeningocele with Arnold–Chiari malformation (herniation of the hindbrain, usually causing obstructive hydrocephalus).

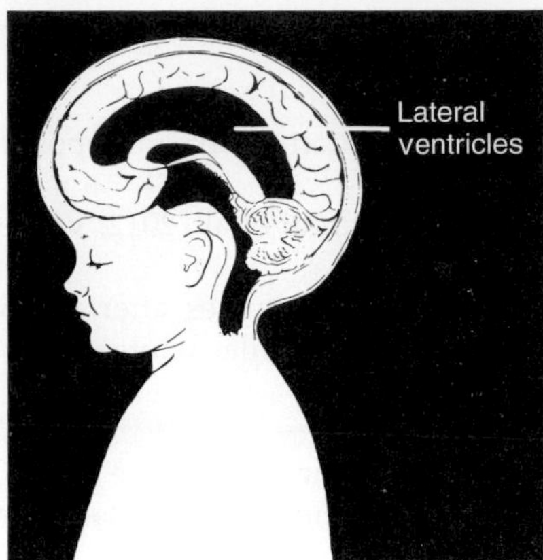


FIGURE 34-2 ■ Hydrocephalus. (From Ross Laboratories: *New perspectives on intraventricular hemorrhage.* Columbus, OH, 1988, Ross Laboratories.)

(4) Congenital masses and tumors.
(5) Congenital infection (toxoplasmosis, cytomegalovirus infection).

**b.** Associated etiologies and/or congenital defects.
(1) Spina bifida.
(2) Encephalocele.
(3) Holoprosencephaly.

**c.** Clinical presentation.
(1) Large head.
(2) Widened sutures.
(3) Full (bulging) and tense fontanelles.
(4) Increasing FOC.
(5) "Setting-sun" eyes (may signify brain tissue damage).
(6) Vomiting, lethargy, irritability.
(7) Visible scalp veins.

**d.** Diagnostic evaluation.
(1) Serial intracranial ultrasonography.
(2) Neuroimaging techniques: CT, MRI, and cranial ultrasonography.

**e.** Patient care management.
(1) Intrauterine diagnosis affords the family more options and allows time for preparation and anticipation.
(2) Perform a thorough physical examination, assessing for further anomalies.
(3) Obtain neurosurgery and genetics consultations.
(4) Confirm diagnosis and cause.
(5) Consider the possible need for reservoir placement versus ventriculoperitoneal (VP) shunt placement.
(6) Support the infant by decreasing noxious stimuli (dim lights, minimal handling).
(7) Position the head carefully.
(8) Provide normal infant care as much as possible.
(9) Involve parents in infant's care as soon as family is ready.
(10) Allow parents to view an infant with a VP shunt or review pictured handouts.
(11) Review VP shunt with parents preoperatively and postoperatively.
(12) Prevent skin breakdown by not allowing the infant to put his or her head on the shunt side postoperatively.
(13) Relieve the infant's probable stiff neck by holding the child's neck on the shunt side during feedings.
(14) Review signs of infection or blocked shunt with the family.
(a) Irritability.
(b) Vomiting.
(c) Increasing head size.

(d) Lethargy.
(e) Changes in feeding patterns.
(f) Bulging fontanelle.

(15) If incision site reddens, position infant on opposite side to relieve pressure from this area.

**4.** Posthemorrhagic hydrocephalus (Prabhu et al., 2012; Volpe, 2008).

**a.** Etiology.

(1) Progressive dilatation of the ventricles after intraventricular hemorrhage (IVH) caused by injury to the periventricular white matter.

(2) Two types: acute and chronic.

(a) Acute.

(i) Rapidly appears—within days of the initial hemorrhage.

(ii) Probably occurs secondary to malabsorption of CSF secondary to a blood clot.

(b) Subacute, chronic.

(i) Inhibition of CSF flow.

(ii) Blood from IVH.

**b.** Incidence.

(1) Approximately 45% of infants with IVH have no evidence of hydrocephalus (Volpe, 2008).

(2) Acute ventricular dilatation develops in approximately 50% of surviving infants with hemorrhage; in the majority, it resolves spontaneously or remains static (Papile, 2006).

**c.** Clinical presentation.

(1) Insidious following mild ventricular dilatation.

(2) May be profound following severe ventricular dilatation.

(a) Rapid increase in head size (begins days to weeks after ventricular dilatation present).
(b) Episodic apnea and bradycardia.
(c) Lethargy.
(d) Increased intracranial pressure.
(e) Tense, bulging anterior fontanelle.
(f) Cranial sutures separating.
(g) Ocular movement abnormalities.

**d.** Diagnostic evaluation.

(1) Graph of weekly FOC measurements.
(2) CT scan.
(3) Cranial ultrasonography.
(4) MRI.

**e.** Patient care management (Verklan, 2012; Verklan and Lopez, 2011; Volpe, 2008).

(1) Obtain daily FOC measurements.
(2) Serial cranial ultrasonography.
(3) Neurosurgical consultation.
(4) Interventions to maintain lumbar or ventricular pressure at approximately 5 cm $H_2O$ while evaluating for shunt placement.

(a) Serial lumbar punctures or direct ventricular access may be helpful.
(b) Administer medications that diminish CSF production rates:

(i) Furosemide (Lasix): 1 mg/kg/day.
(ii) Acetazolamide (Diamox): up to 100 mg/kg/day.

(5) Consideration given to placing a reservoir or VP shunt.
(6) Observe the infant for signs of increasing intracranial hemorrhage and hydrocephalus.
(7) Support the family: neonate is very susceptible to shunt infections and shunt malfunction.

**f.** Outcome (Prabhu et al., 2012; Verklan, 2012; Volpe, 2008).

(1) Poor outcomes are likely when cerebral decompression does not occur after VP shunt placement.

(2) Initial IVH severity is the major determining factor in posthemorrhagic hydrocephalus development.
(3) In slightly more than 50% of the cases, severe hemorrhage results in progressive ventricular dilatation.
(4) Without therapy, a considerable number of infants exhibit halted progression, with or without resolution.
(5) Deficits are motor and/or cognitive.

**C. Craniosynostosis (Evans et al., 2012).**

1. Definition.
   - **a.** Premature closure of cranial sutures.
   - **b.** Occurs along one or more suture lines (see Fig. 34-3 for names and placement of cranial sutures).
2. Risk factors. Usually sporadic and without associated anomalies.
3. Pathophysiology.
   - **a.** Cause unclear. May be a defect in the mesenchymal layer of the ossification center within the skull.
   - **b.** Etiology includes developmental, mechanical, metabolic, and genetic factors that influence skull growth.
4. Incidence.
   - **a.** Reported as 1 in 2000 to 2500 births.
   - **b.** Sagittal craniosynostosis most common.

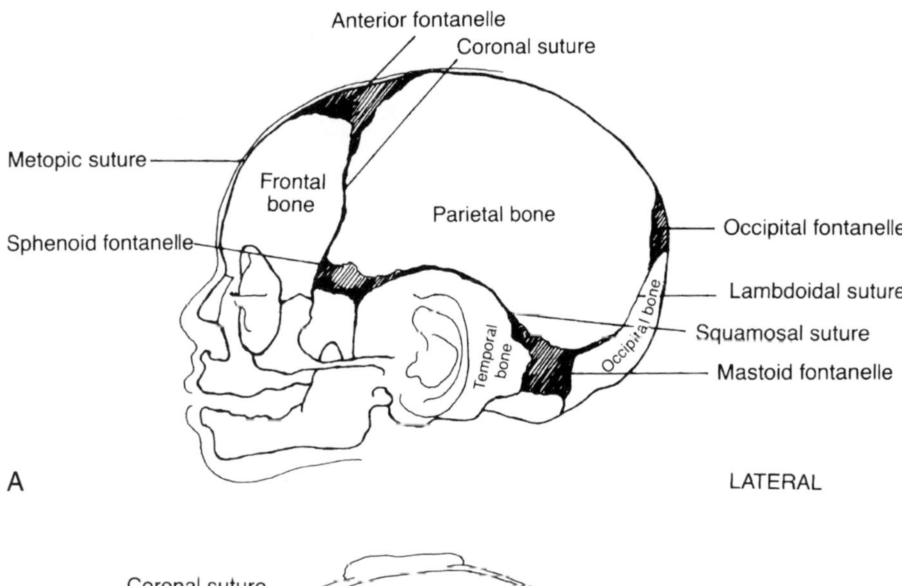


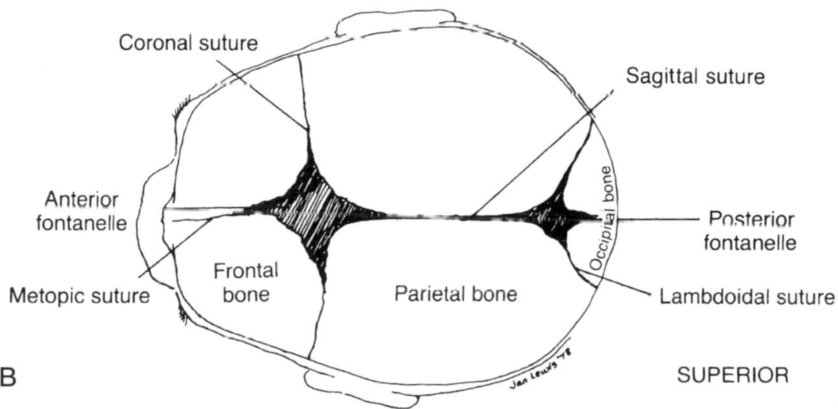


FIGURE 34-3 ■ **A** and **B**, Two views of neonatal skull, showing clinically important fontanelles and sutures. (From Scanlon, J.W., Nelson, T., Grylack, L., and Smith, Y.F.: *A system of newborn physical examinations*. Baltimore, 1979, University Park Press, p. 47.)

5. **Clinical presentation.**
   a. Asymptomatic.
   b. Cranial suture line reveals bony prominence; even and smooth bilaterally.
   c. Inability to move the suture.
   d. Abnormal cranial shape.
   e. Later signs:
      (1) Increased intracranial pressure.
      (2) Increased irritability.
      (3) Possible separation of other sutures.
6. Diagnostic evaluation.
   a. Skull x-ray examination.
   b. High-resolution three-dimensional CT reconstruction scanning to determine the extent of premature bone fusion.
   c. Weekly graph of FOCs.
7. Patient care management.
   a. Thorough physical examination.
   b. Obtain neurosurgery consultation.
   c. Educate and support the family.
   d. Observe for signs of increased intracranial pressure.
      (1) Irritability.
      (2) Lethargy.
      (3) Vomiting.
      (4) Bulging fontanelle.
   e. Early surgical treatment is recommended.
8. Outcome.
   a. Surgically correctable.
   b. Good outcome; possible absence of sequelae.
   c. Cosmetically pleasing outcome.
   d. Multiple craniosynostoses associated with numerous syndromes.

**D. Cleft lip and cleft palate (Evans et al., 2012).**

1. Development of orofacial structures occur before the seventh week of gestation. Cleft lip and palate result in medial and lateral nasal processes failing to fuse with maxillary process, producing cleft lip with or without cleft palate.

**E. Etiology and incidence.**

1. Orofacial clefts of the primary and secondary palate represent one of the most common structural defects; overall frequency is approximately 1 in 500 to 550.
2. Cleft lip and palate are the most common defect, followed by isolated cleft lip, and then cleft palate only.
3. Racial predilection exists, with Native American, white, and Hispanic populations experiencing increased incidence.
4. Sixty percent to 80% of infants affected with cleft lip are male. Cleft palate is more common in females than males (Moore et al., 2012).
5. The causes of most orofacial clefts are unknown and are nonsyndromic. The etiology of these defects are multifactorial, likely secondary to the interaction between environmental and genetic factors. Most cases represent sporadic events, but recurrence within families has been documented.
6. Seventy percent to 75% of cleft lip with cleft palate defects are nonsyndromic.
7. Recurrence risk is dependent on specific syndrome and genetic diagnosis. For families with one child affected with cleft lip and palate, risk is 2% to 5%, increasing to 10% to 15% if other family members have clefts. Risk for cleft lip only is less as cleft lip with or without cleft palate is genetically distinct from cleft palate.

**F. Clinical presentation.**

1. Presentation of the defect is variable, affecting the primary palate and/or the posterior palate.
   a. Unilateral cleft lip most commonly occurs on the left side.
   b. Bilateral cleft lip is usually accompanied by a cleft palate.

2. Defect may occur as a part of a syndrome of anomalies. Over 400 syndromes have been associated with orofacial clefting.
3. True median cleft is the rarest type of cleft and is commonly associated with serious risk for underlying CNS abnormalities, growth hormone deficiencies, adrenal hypoplasia, thyroid deficiency, and diabetes insipidus.

**G. Associated findings.**
1. Hypodontia in the area of the cleft, natal teeth.
2. Disruption of facial growth resulting in reduced facial height, flat facial profile, increased nasopharyngeal width, and a shortened mandible.
3. Feeding difficulties, failure to thrive.
4. Speech deficits and language delay.
5. Eustachian tube dysfunction, recurrent otitis media, and acquired conductive hearing loss.
6. Airway obstruction issues, especially if Pierre Robin sequence is associated.

**H. Diagnosis.**
1. Ultrasound evaluation with close attention to the oral and facial areas may provide a clue to the presence of the defect prenatally.
2. Careful physical examination following delivery as 25% of infants with cleft lip and/or palate have associated syndromes.

**I. Treatment.**
1. Secondary potential effects of these defects on respiratory, auditory, language, growth, and feeding; multidisciplinary team is important in long-term management.
2. Degree of defect may markedly alter the ability for the infant to breast- or bottle-feed effectively. A variety of feeding systems and nipples are available, and trial of many types may be needed to find the appropriate system.
3. Breastfeeding may be difficult as an open palate will not assist in generating negative pressure needed for sucking. Expressed breast milk should be offered.
4. Growth velocity must be followed closely as these infants are at higher nutritional risk.
   a. Dental appliances can be helpful to provide a palatal surface.
   b. Dentition patterns should be monitored closely, timing interventions with surgical intervention.
5. Auditory evaluations utilizing otoacoustic emissions or brainstem auditory evoked response are necessary if initial hearing screens are abnormal. As hearing loss may be responsible for speech distortion, development of speech must be closely monitored and therapy provided as an ongoing portion of care.
6. Though site specific, surgical correction of the lip and nasal deformities occurs first—usually within the first 3 to 6 months of life. Palatal repair occurs later at 9 to 12 months of age.
7. Airway management is a primary concern. Those infants with associated micrognathia and glossoptosis may require protective positioning and possible tracheostomy.
8. Genetic counseling is needed to assign potential risk and to exclude chromosomal disorder and single-gene defects.

**J. Birth injuries.**
1. Definition.
   a. Any injury that occurs during the entire phase of the birth process, comprising labor and delivery.
   b. Classification of the injury is anatomic or etiologic.
2. Risk factors.
   a. Abnormal labor time (long or short).
   b. Large size for gestational age.
   c. Cephalopelvic disproportion.
   d. Prematurity.
   e. Birth dystocia.
   f. Abnormal presentation (transverse, breech, face, and brow).
   g. Instrument-assisted extraction (vacuum or forceps).
3. Pathophysiology (see specific injury).
4. Specific injuries.

**a.** Cephalhematoma (Bonifacio et al., 2012).
   (1) Pathophysiology.
      (a) Subperiosteal hemorrhage.
      (b) Does not extend across the cranial suture lines.
      (c) Usually unilateral.
   (2) Incidence approximates 1.5% to 2.5% of deliveries and is seen twice as often in males.
   (3) Clinical presentation.
      (a) Enlarges during the first few days after birth.
      (b) Feels firm.
      (c) Does not transilluminate.
      (d) Presents bilaterally in 15% of patients.
      (e) Linear fractures found in 5% of unilateral lesions and 18% of bilateral lesions.
   (4) Diagnostic evaluation for presence of cranial fractures.
   (5) Patient care management (Verklan and Lopez, 2011).
      (a) Provide supportive care to the family and their baby.
      (b) Observe for hyperbilirubinemia.
      (c) If sudden enlargement occurs, question infection.
      (d) Educate the family.
      (e) Assess neurologic status.
   (6) Outcome.
      (a) Bony calcified ring may develop; usually disappears within 6 months.
      (b) Usually takes 2 weeks to 3 months for resolution.
      (c) Essentially all cases resolve.

**b.** Caput succedaneum.
   (1) Pathophysiology.
      (a) Hemorrhagic edema crossing cranial suture lines.
      (b) Commonly seen after vaginal delivery.
   (2) Clinical presentation.
      (a) Evident at birth.
      (b) Hemorrhagic scalp edema, causing discoloration at the site.
      (c) Does not grow in size after birth.
   (3) Diagnostic evaluation as per physical examination.
   (4) Patient care management.
      (a) No treatment is given.
      (b) Educate and counsel the family.
   (5) Outcome: resolution occurs during first few days of life.

**c.** Subgaleal hemorrhage (Bonifacio et al., 2012; Waller et al., 2012).
   (1) Pathophysiology.
      (a) Hemorrhage beneath the scalp into the loose connective tissue below the aponeurotic membrane.
      (b) Possible entry of blood into the subcutaneous tissue of the neck.
      (c) Hematoma may cross suture lines in sufficient quantities to lead to exsanguination of the infant.
   (2) Incidence.
      (a) Approximately 1.54 per 10,000 births.
      (b) Occurs much less often than caput succedaneum.
      (c) Associated with vacuum extraction.
   (3) Clinical presentation.
      (a) Often a fluctuant mass of the scalp.
      (b) May increase in size postnatally.
      (c) Hypotonia, pallor, lethargy, seizures.
      (d) Falling hematocrit levels.
   (4) Diagnostic evaluation.
      (a) Palpate: hemorrhage crosses suture lines, is firm but fluctuant to palpation.
      (b) Vital signs: monitor for symptoms of shock.

(c) Serial hematocrit levels.
(d) Monitor bilirubin levels during recovery.
(5) Patient care management.
(a) Rapid diagnosis and blood replacement is key to management.
(i) Observe for signs/symptoms of shock/hypovolemia.
(ii) Monitor blood pressure, heart rate, and serial complete blood cell counts.
(iii) Management for supporting organs, such as kidney, if shock occurs.
(b) Infant may need blood transfusion on an emergent basis.
(c) Ensure that infant receives vitamin K promptly.
(d) Observe for hyperbilirubinemia.
(6) Outcome: once the infant has survived the acute phase, recovery occurs in 2 to 3 weeks (Volpe, 2008).

**d.** Skull fractures.
(1) Pathophysiology.
(a) Linear fracture can occur.
(b) Depressed fractures occur secondary to excessive force used with forceps and extreme molding.
(2) Incidence.
(a) Unknown.
(b) Linear fracture fairly common finding.
(c) Depressed fracture much less common than linear.
(3) Clinical presentation.
(a) Linear fracture: asymptomatic.
(b) Depressed fracture.
(i) Presents with depressed surface of skull; indented, without craniotabes.
(ii) Does not cross the suture lines.
(iii) Possible marked separation of adjacent sutures.
(iv) Most often occurs in right parietal bone.
(4) Diagnostic evaluation.
(a) X-ray examination.
(b) CT scan.
(5) Patient care management.
(a) Obtain neurosurgery consultation.
(b) Assess closely for neurologic deficits.
(c) If lesion is less than 2 cm and patient is without neurologic deficits, follow clin ically; spontaneous resolution expected within a few weeks.
(6) Outcome.
(a) Linear fractures usually heal completely within 3 months.
(b) Depressed fracture outcome is dependent on degree of cerebral injury and success of therapy.

**e.** Brachial nerve plexus injuries (Bonifacio et al., 2012; Verklan and Lopez, 2011).
(1) Pathophysiology.
(a) Excessive stretching of brachial plexus during delivery.
(b) Erb's palsy, involving cervical nerves V and VI. Denervation of the deltoid, supraspinatus, biceps, and brachioradialis leads to upper arm paralysis.
(c) Klumpke's paralysis, involving cervical nerve VI to thoracic nerve I. Denervation of the intrinsics of the hand, flexors of the wrist, fingers, and sympathetics (Horner's syndrome) leads to lower arm paralysis.
(d) Combination of Erb–Duchenne paralysis and Klumpke's paralysis, involving the entire arm from cervical nerve V to thoracic nerve I (entire arm paralyzed). Paralysis of the diaphragm will occur if injury involves cervical nerve IV.
(2) Incidence: 0.5 to 2 per 1000 live births.
(3) Risk factors.
(a) Multiparous mother.
(b) Prolonged labor.

(c) Large size for gestational age.
(d) Shoulder dystocia.

(4) Clinical presentation.
(a) Erb's palsy.
(i) Affected arm is abducted and internally rotated.
(ii) The elbow is extended, with arm pronation and wrist flexion ("waiter's tip" position).
(iii) Asymmetrical Moro reflex (absent in the affected arm), with a normal grasp.
(b) Klumpke's paralysis.
(i) Swelling in shoulder and supraclavicular fossa; clavicle may be fractured.
(ii) Involves intrinsic muscles of the hand, with a clawhand deformity.
(iii) No grasp in the affected hand.
(c) Erb–Duchenne–Klumpke paralysis.
(i) A combination of the above.
(ii) Occurs more often than isolated Klumpke's paralysis.
(iii) Entire affected arm is flaccid.
(iv) Moro and grasp reflexes are absent.

(5) Diagnostic evaluation.
(a) Obtain x-ray examination of affected arm and shoulder.
(b) Obtain serial electromyographic studies.
(c) Rule out fracture of the clavicle or humerus.
(d) Rule out shoulder dislocation.
(e) Rule out cerebral injury.

(6) Patient care management.
(a) Obtain neurology consultation.
(b) Obtain serial electromyographic examinations to note improvements.
(c) Primary goal: avoid contractures of involved joints.
(i) Begin passive range-of-motion exercise, beginning after the swelling and inflammation subside.
(ii) Exercise the arm with every diaper change.
(iii) Request a physical therapy consultation (infant may be able to benefit from splints at some point).
(iv) Educate the family about the importance of maintaining normal joint function.
1. Reinnervated musculature needs supple joints.
2. Will have wider choice of reconstructive procedures in the absence of contractures in the event there is no recovery.

(7) Outcome.
(a) Generally spontaneous recovery occurs.
(b) About 88% fully recover by 4 months, and 92% fully recover by 12 months (Volpe, 2008).
(c) If no appreciable recovery is noted by 3 months, surgical exploration may be warranted (Volpe, 2008).

**f.** Phrenic nerve paralysis (Volpe, 2008).

(1) Pathophysiology.
(a) Diaphragmatic paralysis involving overstretching of cervical nerves III, IV, and V.
(b) Results from torn nerve sheaths with edema and hemorrhage.
(c) Eighty percent to 90% occur in association with brachial plexus injury, but it may also occur in isolation.

(2) Clinical presentation.
(a) History of traumatic delivery, especially difficult breech delivery.
(b) First hours after birth.
(i) Respiratory distress with cyanosis, tachypnea, hypoxemia, hypercapnia, and acidosis.

(ii) Diagnosis may be missed as the elevated hemidiaphragm may not be present early in the course, especially with use of positive pressure ventilation.

(c) Next several days.

(i) Improvement with oxygen and ventilatory support.

(3) Diagnostic evaluation.

(a) Chest x-ray examination may not be useful, especially if positive pressure ventilation is in use.

(b) Ultrasonographic or fluoroscopic examination will show elevated hemidiaphragm and the paradoxical movement of the affected side with breathing.

(c) Serial ultrasonography to evaluate diaphragmatic function.

(4) Patient care management.

(a) Administer oxygen and ventilatory support as needed.

(b) Place the infant affected side down (splint the affected side).

(c) Follow physical examination closely to note improvements.

(d) Family education and support because prolonged ventilatory support may be required.

(5) Outcome.

(a) Mortality rate 10% to 15%.

(b) Majority recover within the first 6 to 12 months.

(c) Prolonged ventilatory support associated with 50% mortality rate.

**g.** Traumatic facial nerve palsy (Bonifacio et al., 2012; Verklan and Lopez, 2011; Volpe, 2008).

(1) Pathophysiology.

(a) Trauma causes hemorrhage and edema into the nerve sheath, rather than a true disruption of the nerve fiber.

(b) Site of the lesion typically at or near the exit of the nerve from the stylomastoid foramen.

(c) Weakness of the facial muscles results.

(2) Incidence: approximately 0.75% of term infants.

(3) Clinical presentation.

(a) Varies with the degree of nerve involvement.

(b) Usually presents the first 2 days after birth.

(c) Persistently open eye on the affected side.

(d) Suck with drooling.

(e) Mouth drawn to normal side during crying.

(f) Corner of mouth does not pull down on affected side.

(g) Eyeball may roll up behind open eyelid.

(h) Usually does not increase in severity.

(4) Patient care management.

(a) Artificial tears for the open eye.

(b) Possible need to tape or patch affected eye to protect cornea.

(c) Support of parents.

(d) Necessary to watch for signs of improvement.

(5) Outcome.

(a) High rate of spontaneous recovery by 7 to 10 days, especially between 1 and 3 weeks of age.

(b) Detectable deficits rarely evident after several months.

(c) For persistence beyond a few weeks, pediatric neurology should be consulted.

## INTRACRANIAL HEMORRHAGES

**A. Subdural hemorrhage.**

**1.** Definition (Bonifacio et al., 2012).

**a.** Due to laceration of the major veins and sinuses, usually associated with a tear of the dura overlying the cerebral hemispheres or cerebellum.

**b.** Occurrence with or without laceration of the dura.

2. Risk factors (Bonifacio et al., 2012; Volpe, 2008).
   a. Macrosomia.
   b. Cephalopelvic disproportion.
   c. Forceps delivery.
   d. Vaginal breech delivery.
   e. Premature delivery.
   f. Malpresentation (breech, face, brow, foot).
   g. Skull is unusually compliant and/or pelvic structures unusually rigid.
   h. Labor is either very short (not enough time for dilation) or too long (head subjected to prolonged compression/molding).
   i. Forceps, vacuum extraction, or rotational maneuvers required to effect delivery.
3. Pathophysiology (Volpe, 2008).
   a. Excessive vertical molding and frontal–occipital elongation, or oblique expansion of the head, results in stretching of the falx and tentorium.
   b. Venous sinuses are stretched, with possible rupture of the vein of Galen or cerebellar bridging veins.
   c. Tear of the dura, including the falx or tentorium, may also occur.
4. Incidence.
   a. Uncommon occurrence, accounts for less than 10% of intracranial hemorrhages.
5. Clinical presentation.
   a. Decreased level of consciousness.
   b. Seizure activity.
   c. Asymmetry of motor function.
   d. Determined by the extent of associated HIE injury.
   e. Often minimal to no clinical symptoms for first 24 hours because of slowly enlarging hematoma.
   f. On day 2 or 3: signs of increasing intracranial pressure due to block in CSF flow in posterior fossa.
      (1) Full fontanelle, irritability, lethargy.
   g. Signs of brainstem disturbance:
      (1) Dilated, poorly reactive pupil on same side as the hemorrhage.
      (2) Respiratory abnormalities, facial paralysis.
      (3) Doll's eye reflex: normal to abnormal.
   h. Chronic subdural effusion: present within the first 6 months of life with enlarging FOC.
6. Diagnostic evaluation.
   a. CT scan.
   b. MRI scan more effective if hemorrhage is in the posterior fossa.
   c. Skull radiographs demonstrate skull fractures.
7. Outcome.
   a. Major laceration of tentorium and falx with massive hemorrhage has poor prognosis.
   b. Mortality rate approximately 45%.
   c. Survivors develop hydrocephalus and other sequelae.
   d. Concomitant hypoxic–ischemic injury critical factor in determining outcome.

**B. Primary subarachnoid hemorrhage (Bonifacio et al., 2012; Volpe, 2008).**

1. Definition: an intracranial hemorrhage into the CSF-filled space between the arachnoid and pial membranes on the surface of the brain.
2. Pathophysiology.
   a. Bleeding of venous origin in the subarachnoid space as a result of rupture of small vessels in the leptomeningeal plexus or bridging veins in the subarachnoid space.
   b. Bleeding is not secondary to an extension of subdural hemorrhage, intraventricular hemorrhage, or cerebellar hemorrhage.
   c. Self-limited.
   d. May be precipitated by trauma (term infant) or hypoxia (preterm infant).
3. Incidence: common type of neonatal intracranial hemorrhage.
4. Clinical presentation.
   a. Most commonly no symptoms develop.

b. Seizure activity may begin on day 2 of life, especially in the term infant.
c. Infant looks healthy between seizures: "well baby with seizures" (Volpe, 2008).
d. Recurrent apnea (more common in preterm infants).

5. Diagnostic evaluation.
a. Diagnosis of exclusion. Other forms of intracranial bleeding are eliminated by CT scan.
b. Lumbar puncture demonstrates uniformly blood-stained CSF.

6. Outcome.
a. Sequelae very uncommon.
b. Ninety percent of term infants who exhibited seizures have normal follow-up.

C. **Intracerebellar hemorrhage.**

1. Definition: hemorrhage(s) within the cerebellum resulting from primary bleeding or extension of intraventricular or subarachnoid hemorrhage into the cerebellum.
2. Risk factors: association exists with respiratory distress, hypoxic events, prematurity, and traumatic delivery.
3. Pathophysiology.
a. Intravascular, vascular, and extravascular factors (Volpe, 2008).
(1) Breech presentation and difficult forceps delivery secondary to a compliant skull, with external pressure causing occipital pressure.
(2) Vitamin K deficiency, thrombocytopenia.
(3) Vulnerable cerebral capillaries exposed to rapid colloid infusion, causing hypertensive spikes.
(4) Richly vascularized subpial and subependymal locations.
(5) Poor vascular support for subependymal and subpial germinal matrices.
(6) Extension of blood into the cerebellum associated with:
(a) Large volume of blood present with IVH,
(b) Increased intracranial pressure, and
(c) Incomplete myelination of the cerebellum.
4. Incidence (Volpe, 2008).
a. About 5% to 10% of neonatal deaths studied by autopsy.
b. Higher in preterm infants than in term.
c. Occurrence of 15% to 25% in premature infants born at less than 32 weeks of gestation or weighing less than 1.5 kg at birth.
5. Clinical presentation (Hill, 2005).
a. May have a history of hypoxic–ischemic insult.
b. Catastrophic deterioration with apnea, bradycardia, decreasing hematocrit values, and bloody CSF may occur.
c. Signs appear within the first 3 weeks, most commonly within the first 2 days of life.
d. Term infants may have a history of difficult breech delivery.
6. Diagnostic evaluation.
a. Cranial ultrasonography (lack of symmetrical echogenicity may be important).
b. CT scan necessary to define the hemorrhage.
c. MRI provides definitive diagnostic information.
7. Outcome.
a. More favorable in term infant than in premature infant.
b. Poor outcome in premature infant.
c. Probable neurologic deficits.

D. **Periventricular–intraventricular hemorrhage (Blackburn, 2013; Bonifacio et al., 2012; Verklan and Lopez, 2011; Volpe, 2008).**

1. Definition.
a. Occurs once subependymal germinal matrix hemorrhage extends into lateral ventricles.
b. Most extensive periventricular–intraventricular hemorrhage is a parenchymal intracerebral hemorrhage.
(1) Involves bleeding into the periventricular (i.e., intracerebellar) white matter and may also precipitate cerebral infarction.
(2) With time, on follow-up scans, may see formation of porencephalic cyst at the original hemorrhage site.

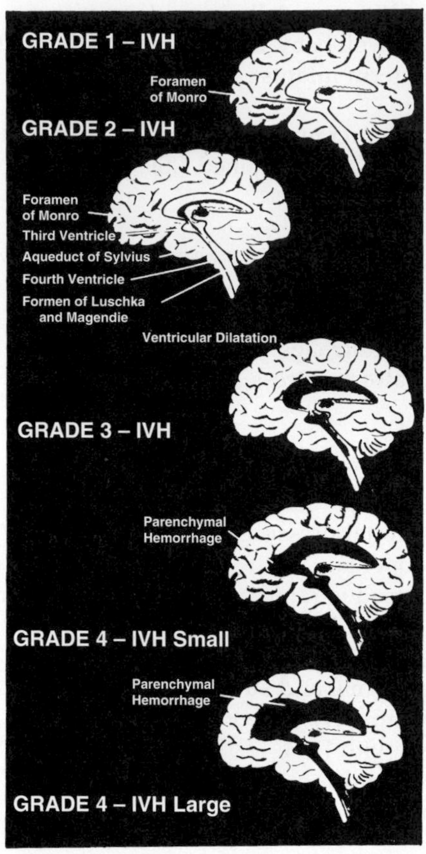


**Grade 1 IVH:** Subependymal hemorrhage in the periventricular germinal matrix. Often localized at the foramen of Monro.

**Grade 2 IVH:** Partial filling of lateral ventricles without ventricular dilatation.

**Grade 3 IVH:** Intraventricular hemorrhage with ventricular dilatation.

**Grade 4 IVH** (small and large): Parenchymal involvement or extension of blood into the cerebral tissue itself. Can be present to a lesser degree.

Correlation between the severity or extent of involvement and subsequent impairment is not absolute. Because outcomes are so varied, assessment of early symptoms and the practice of purposeful interventions are extremely important.

FIGURE 34-4 ■ Quantification of extent of intraventricular hemorrhage (IVH). Four grades of hemorrhagic involvement categorized IVH, as differentiated by Papile and Burstein. (From Ross Laboratories: *New perspectives on intraventricular hemorrhage*. Columbus, OH, 1988, Ross Laboratories.)

**c.** See Figure 34-4 for description and grading system (Papile, 2006).
   (1) Small hemorrhage: grade 1 or 2.
   (2) Moderate hemorrhage: grade 3.
   (3) Severe hemorrhage: grade 4.

**2.** Risk factors.
   **a.** Prematurity: birth at less than 34 weeks of gestation; respiratory failure requiring mechanical ventilation.
   **b.** Associated with increasing arterial blood pressure and perinatal asphyxia.
   **c.** Associated clinical factors.
      (1) Low 5-minute Apgar score.
      (2) Asphyxia or birth trauma.
      (3) Very low birth weight.
      (4) Acidosis.
      (5) Hypotension or hypertension.
      (6) Low hematocrit.
      (7) Respiratory distress requiring mechanical ventilation.
      (8) Rapid administration of sodium bicarbonate.
      (9) Rapid volume expansion.
      (10) Infusion of hyperosmolar solution.
      (11) Coagulopathy.
      (12) Pneumothorax.
      (13) Ligation of patent ductus arteriosus.
      (14) Transport.

3. Pathophysiology.
   a. Occurs once subependymal germinal matrix hemorrhage extends into lateral ventricles.
   b. Most extensive periventricular–intraventricular hemorrhage is a parenchymal intracerebral hemorrhage.
      (1) Involves bleeding into the periventricular (i.e., intracerebellar white matter) and may also precipitate cerebral infarction.
      (2) Only 10% to 15% of infants with hemorrhages.
      (3) With time, on follow-up scans, may see formation of porencephalic cysts at the original hemorrhage site.
4. Incidence.
   a. Incidence: 40% to 60% of very low birth weight neonates.
   b. Infants born at less than 28 weeks of gestation have a 3 times higher risk than infants born at 28 to 31 weeks of gestation.
      (1) Primary site of bleeding is the germinal matrix in the subependymal area next to the caudate nucleus.
   c. Approximately 3.5 to 4.6% of term infants have a periventricular–intraventricular hemorrhage.
      (1) More than half of these hemorrhages originated at the choroid plexus of the lateral ventricles.
      (2) Timing of onset.
         (a) About 50% occur by 24 hours of age.
         (b) About 80% occur by 48 hours of age.
         (c) About 90% occur by 72 hours of age.
         (d) By 7 days of age, 99.5% have occurred.
         (e) Twenty percent to 40% exhibit progression of the hemorrhage over 3 to 5 days.
5. Clinical presentation.
   a. Presentation ranges from unnoticeable to dramatic.
      (1) Sudden deterioration.
      (2) Oxygen desaturation.
      (3) Bradycardia.
      (4) Metabolic acidosis.
      (5) Significant decrease in hematocrit.
      (6) Hypotonia.
      (7) Shock.
      (8) Hyperglycemia.
      (9) Tense anterior fontanelle.
   b. Symptoms of worsening hemorrhage.
      (1) Full, tense fontanelles.
      (2) Increased ventilatory support.
      (3) Seizure activity.
      (4) Apnea.
      (5) Decrease in level of consciousness and/or activity.
6. Diagnostic evaluation.
   a. Optimal time to screen: 7 days of age because greater than 90% of all hemorrhages have occurred.
      (1) If test result is normal, there is no need to recheck.
      (2) If test result is positive for periventricular–intraventricular hemorrhage, repeat test in 2 weeks.
   b. Serial cranial ultrasonography has replaced CT as the principle diagnostic technique.
   c. Lumbar puncture (CSF studies show elevated red blood cells, increased protein concentration, xanthochromia, and decreased glucose concentration).
   d. Rule out septic shock or meningitis.
7. Patient care management.
   a. Prevent preterm birth, perinatal asphyxia, and birth trauma.
   b. Promote in-utero transport.
   c. Promote nonstressful intrapartum course.

- **d.** Provide efficient, expedient intubation.
- **e.** Appropriate handling; minimal stimulation with clustering of care activities as tolerated.
- **f.** Minimize noxious stimuli (dim the lights, quiet the environment).
- **g.** Avoid noxious procedures when possible.
- **h.** Avoid events associated with wide swings in arterial and venous pressures.
  - (1) Seizures.
  - (2) Excess motor activity.
  - (3) Apnea.
  - (4) Crying.
  - (5) Pneumothorax.
- **i.** Avoid administration of hyperosmolar solutions.
- **j.** Prevent blood pressure swings: give volume replacement slowly.
- **k.** Avoid overventilation leading to pneumothorax.
- **l.** Use two people for endotracheal suctioning.
- **m.** Use noninvasive monitoring of oxygen and carbon dioxide levels (maintain within normal limits).
- **n.** Monitor and maintain normal pH.

**8.** Correct abnormal clotting.
- **a.** Be alert to signs of a hemorrhage.
- **b.** Educate and support the parents.

**9.** Outcome.
- **a.** Grade 1 and grade 2 hemorrhage typically have resolution.
- **b.** Grade 3 hemorrhage evolves over 1 to 3 weeks. There may be destruction of the subarachnoid space leading to ventricular dilatation and hydrocephalus.
- **c.** Mortality rate is 50% with severe hemorrhage, 10% with moderate hemorrhage, and 5% with small hemorrhage.
- **d.** These hemorrhages are an important cause of morbidity and death in low birth weight infants.
- **e.** Hemorrhage alone does not account for all neurologic deficits.
- **f.** Approximately 50% of premature infants are free of neurologic symptoms.
- **g.** Approximately 25% to 30% of very low birth weight infants discharged from a level III neonatal intensive care unit have a periventricular–intraventricular hemorrhage without major neurodevelopmental sequelae.
- **h.** Outcome depends on degree of severity of hemorrhage.
  - (1) Small hemorrhage.
    - (a) Neurodevelopmental disability similar to that in premature infants without hemorrhage.
    - (b) Major neurodevelopmental disability in 10%.
  - (2) Moderate hemorrhage.
    - (a) Major neurodevelopmental disability in 40% during infancy.
    - (b) Mortality rate 10%, with progressive hydrocephalus in less than 20%.
  - (3) Severe hemorrhage.
    - (a) Major neurodevelopmental disability in 80%.
    - (b) Mortality rate 50% with hydrocephalus common in survivors.

## SEIZURES (SCHER, 2012, 2013; VERKLAN AND LOPEZ, 2011).

**A. Definition:** symptom of neurologic dysfunction (not a disease).

**B. Risk factors.**

**1.** Metabolic encephalopathies.
- **a.** Decreased production of adenosine triphosphate.

**2.** Ischemia.

**3.** Hypoxemia.

**4.** Hypoglycemia.
- **a.** Hyponatremia or hypernatremia.

   b. Hypocalcemia, hypomagnesemia.
   c. Inborn errors of metabolism.
   d. Pyridoxine dependency.
   e. Hyperammonemia.
5. Structural.
   a. IVH.
   b. Intrapartum trauma.
   c. Cerebral cortical dysgenesis: result of abnormal neuronal migration.
   d. HIE, the most common diagnosis of neonatal seizures.
6. Intracerebral meningitis.
   a. Bacterial infection.
      (1) Group B β-hemolytic streptococci and *Escherichia coli* may account for up to 65% of cases.
      (2) Many other bacterial organisms may be implicated and include but are not limited to other streptococcus and staphylococcus species, such as group D streptococci, *Staphylococcus epidermidis, Staphylococcus aureus, Listeria monocytogenes, Haemophilus influenzae, Neisseria meningitidis,* and *Streptococcus pneumoniae.*
   b. Nonbacterial infection: TORCH.
7. Withdrawal from maternal drugs.
   a. Uncommon cause of seizures (may cause jitteriness).
   b. Onset during first 3 days of life.
   c. Drugs.
      (1) Narcotic analgesics.
      (2) Sedative–hypnotics.
      (3) Alcohol.
8. Familial (genetic).
   a. Onset in second and third days of life.
   b. Infant appears well between seizures.
   c. Self-limiting: within 1 to 6 months, seizures stop.
   d. Autosomal dominant inheritance.

C. **Pathophysiology:** seizures result from excessive simultaneous electrical discharge or depolarization of neurons.

D. **Incidence.**
1. 57.5 per 1000 infants less than 1500 grams.
2. 2.8 per 1000 infants weighing 2500 to 3999 grams.

E. **Clinical presentation.**
1. Subtle.
   a. Most frequent of neonatal seizures.
   b. Present in most term and premature newborn infants having seizures.
   c. Often unrecognized.
   d. Presentation varies.
      (1) Horizontal deviation of the eyes.
      (2) Pedaling movements.
      (3) Rowing, stepping movements.
      (4) Eye blinking or fluttering.
      (5) Nonnutritive sucking.
      (6) Smacking of lips.
      (7) Drooling.
      (8) Apnea (convulsive apnea usually does not occur by itself).
2. Tonic.
   a. Characteristic in premature infants weighing $\leq$500 g.
   b. Often seen with severe IVH.
   c. Generalized tonic extension of all extremities or flexion of upper limbs with extension of lower extremities.
   d. Often mimics decorticate posturing.

3. Multifocal clonic.
   a. Characteristic in term infants with HIE.
   b. Clonic movements migrating from one limb to another without a specific pattern.
4. Focal clonic.
   a. Uncommon.
   b. Presents as localized clonic jerking.
5. Myoclonic.
   a. Very rare in neonatal period.
   b. Multiple jerks of upper or lower limb flexion.

**F. Diagnostic evaluation.**

1. Perform physical examination.
   a. Rule out jitteriness.
      (1) Characterized by trembling of hands and feet.
      (2) No involvement of eye movements.
      (3) Stopped by gentle, passive flexion of affected extremity.
   b. Note infant's history, which may provide a predisposed underlying etiology.
2. Laboratory work.
   a. Serum glucose level.
   b. Electrolyte levels (sodium, potassium, chloride, calcium, magnesium).
   c. Arterial blood gas analysis.
   d. Urea, ammonia.
3. Diagnostic study for sepsis.
   a. Lumbar puncture.
   b. Culture of blood, urine, and CSF specimens; bacterial and viral.
   c. Complete blood cell count and platelet count.
4. Electroencephalography (EEG), CT scan, cranial ultrasonography, MRI.
5. Skull films if etiology is trauma.
6. Twelve-lead electrocardiography.
7. Consideration of following laboratory tests:
   a. Blood pyruvate.
   b. Lactate.
   c. TORCH.
   d. Urinary drug screen.
8. Neurology consultation.

**G. Patient care management.**

1. Determine underlying etiology.
2. Resuscitate as necessary.
3. Obtain diagnostic studies as ordered.
4. Provide pharmaceutical therapy.
   a. Phenobarbital.
      (1) Loading dosage: 20 mg/kg slow intravenous (IV) push for 10 to 15 minutes. Additional 5 mg/kg may be given 1 hour later for refractory seizures, to a maximum of 40 mg/kg.
      (2) Closely monitor respiratory status.
      (3) Maintenance dosage: 3 to 4 mg/kg/day, beginning 12 to 24 hours after the loading dose.
      (4) Therapeutic range: 15 to 40 mcg/mL.
      (5) Excretion.
         (a) Metabolized by liver: 50% to 70%.
         (b) Unchanged in urine: 20% to 30%.
      (6) Consider as the drug of choice.
   b. Fosphenytoin (Cerebyx).
      (1) Loading dosage: 15 to 20 mg PE/kg IV over 10 minutes. Normal saline should be flushed before and after the dosing. [Fosphenytoin dose expressed in phenytoin equivalents (PE). Fosphenytoin 1 mg PE = 1 mg phenytoin.]
      (2) May be given intramuscularly (IM).
      (3) Maintenance dosage: 4 to 8 mg PE/kg/day slow IV push or IM 24 hours after loading dose.

(a) Term neonates greater than 7 days of age may require up to 8 mg PE/kg/dose every 8 to 12 hours.

(4) Therapeutic range: 10 to 20 mcg/mL. Serum trough level of phenytoin measured (not fosphenytoin) 48 hours after the IV loading dose.

(a) Peak plasma concentrations: about the time that the IV infusion is complete; half-life is 4 to 10 minutes.

(b) Rapidly converted by the body to generate therapeutic levels of phenytoin.

(5) Excretion.

(a) Protein bound (approximately 90%).

(b) Displaced by bilirubin, increasing free drug levels. Caution with hyperbilirubinemia.

**c.** Phenytoin.

(1) Loading dosage: 15 to 20 mg/kg IV over at least 30 minutes. Flush with normal saline prior to and after dosing. Never given IM and never give in central lines.

(a) Is very irritating to veins; extravasation may result in tissue necrosis.

(2) Maintenance.

(a) Dosage: 4 to 8 mg/kg/day slow IV push or per os (PO). *Caution:* Absorption is erratic with PO route.

(b) Therapeutic range: trough level of 6 to 15 mcg/mL 48 hours after loading dose; and 10 to 20 mcg/mL after 2 weeks.

**d.** Lorazepam.

(1) Administer: 0.05 to 0.1 mg/kg slow IV push (for status epilepticus).

(2) Repeat dose based on clinical response.

(3) Note routes of excretion.

(a) By kidneys.

(b) Lipid soluble.

(4) Lorazepam produces anticonvulsant effect in minutes after administration.

(5) Monitor oxygenation and vital signs.

(6) Document precisely.

**H. Outcome.**

**1.** Related to underlying etiology.

## HYPOXIC–ISCHEMIC ENCEPHALOPATHY (BONIFACIO ET AL., 2012; LAPTOOK, 2012; SCHER 2013; VERKLAN AND LOPEZ, 2011)

**A. Definition of HIE.**

**1.** Hypoxemia and anoxia (diminished oxygen in blood supply; partial or complete). Moderate to severe hypoxia leads to metabolic acidosis.

**2.** Ischemia (diminished blood supply perfusing the brain).

**a.** Systemic hypotension.

**b.** Occlusive vascular disease.

**3.** Hypoxia and ischemia, which lead to neurologic dysfunction.

**4.** Asphyxia.

**a.** Impairment of gas exchange of respiratory gases—oxygen and carbon dioxide.

**b.** Mixed respiratory and metabolic acidosis.

**c.** Failure of systemic multiorgan systems, including heart, lungs, liver, and kidneys.

**B. Diagnosis.**

**1.** History and risk factors.

**a.** Antepartum risk factors: socioeconomic status, maternal thyroid disease, severe pregnancy-induced hypertension, fetal growth restriction, postdatism.

**b.** Intrapartum risk factors: maternal pyrexia; persistent occiput posterior fetal position; acute intrapartum events, such as cord accident, uterine rupture, abruption; evidence of intrapartum hypoxia defined by composite of abnormal fetal heart rate, fresh meconium, and low Apgar scores.

**2.** EEG.

**C. Incidence of HIE.**
  **1.** Approximately 1.5 per 1000 live births. About 0.3 per 1000 live births will have significant neurologic sequelae.
  **2.** About 2% to 4% of term infants.
  **3.** Approximately 60% of very low birth weight infants.
  **4.** Timing of insult occurrence (Volpe, 2008).
    **a.** Antepartum occurrence: 20%.
    **b.** Intrapartum occurrence: 30%.
    **c.** Antepartum–intrapartum occurrence: 35%.
    **d.** Postpartum occurrence: 10%.

**D. Clinical presentation and staging using Sarnat criteria.**
  **1.** Stage I (mild encephalopathy): characteristic features.
    **a.** Hyperalert state.
    **b.** Normal muscle tone, active suck, strong Moro reflex, normal/strong grasp, and normal doll's eye reflex.
    **c.** Increased tendon reflexes.
    **d.** Myoclonus present.
    **e.** Hyperresponsiveness to stimulation.
    **f.** Tachycardia possible.
    **g.** Dilation of pupils, reactive.
    **h.** Sparse secretions.
    **i.** No convulsions (unless due to hypoglycemia or preexisting conditions that predisposed the infant to perinatal distress).
    **j.** Electroencephalographic findings: within normal limits.
  **2.** Stage II (moderate encephalopathy).
    **a.** Characteristic features.
      (1) Lethargy.
      (2) Hypotonia.
      (3) Increased tendon reflexes.
      (4) Myoclonus.
      (5) Seizure activity frequent.
      (6) Weak suck.
      (7) Incomplete Moro reflex.
      (8) Strong grasp.
      (9) Overactive doll's eye reflex.
      (10) Pupils constrictive and reactive.
      (11) Respirations variable in rate and depth; respirations may be periodic.
    **b.** Critical period: infant's condition either improves or deteriorates.
    **c.** Indications of deterioration.
      (1) No signs of improvement.
      (2) Development of any of the following:
        (a) Seizures.
        (b) Cerebral edema.
        (c) Lethargy.
        (d) Abnormalities on electroencephalogram.
    **d.** Recovery.
      (1) No further seizure activity.
      (2) Electroencephalographic findings return to normal.
      (3) Transient jitteriness.
      (4) Improvement in level of consciousness.
  **3.** Stage III (severe encephalopathy).
    **a.** Clinical course.
      (1) Level of consciousness deteriorates from obtunded to stuporous to comatose.
      (2) Mechanical ventilation is required to sustain life.
    **b.** Clinical features.
      (1) Apnea/bradycardia.

(2) Seizures appearing within the first 12 postnatal hours; 50% to 60% of patients who do ultimately seize do so within the first 6 to 12 hours. Premature infants present with generalized seizures. Term infants demonstrate multifocal clonic seizures. All these infants display subtle seizures (Volpe, 2008).
(3) Severe hypotonia and flaccidity; suck, Moro, and grasp reflexes absent.
(4) Stuporous to comatose.
(5) Absent or depressed reflexes.
(6) Doll's eye reflex weak or absent.
(7) Pupils often unequal; variable reactivity and poor light reflex.

**c.** Deterioration.
(1) Deterioration occurs within 24 to 72 hours.
(2) Severely affected infants often worsen, sinking into deep stupor or coma.
(3) Death may ensue.

**d.** Survivors.
(1) Infants who survive to this point often improve in the next several days to months.
(2) Feeding difficulties often develop secondary to abnormalities of suck and swallow. This is due to the poor muscle tone connected to involvement of cranial nerves for these functions.
(3) Generalized hypotonia is common; hypertonia is uncommon.
(4) Severe neurologic disabilities may ensue.

**E. Diagnostic studies.**

**1.** Valuable in assessing the nature of the brain insult and the extent of the brain injury.

**2.** Used to track the evolution of HIE.

**a.** Precise history.

**b.** Complete neurologic examination.

**c.** EEG.
(1) Confirm or deny clinical diagnosis of seizures.
(2) Provide prognostic information regarding severity of permanent brain damage.
(3) Two common types of EEG: conventional EEG (cEEG) or amplitude EEG (aEEG).
(a) cEEG: used to measure impact of neurologic insult and detect presence of seizure activity.
(i) Twelve to 16 sensors applied by specialist technician. Sensors are usually invasive.
(ii) Usually recorded for 40 to 60 minutes.
(iii) Provides information about entire cerebral cortex.
(iv) Logistically challenging to schedule technician to interpret and neurologist to interpret study.
(b) aEEG: measures, filters, and time-compresses raw EEG signal to create simplified pattern easy to interpret by nonneurologist.
(i) May be single (2 sensors) channel to monitor single parietal channel or dual (4 sensors) channels in parietal and central positions.
(ii) Usually recorded continuously.
(iii) Provides hemispheric information of the cerebral cortex.
(iv) No technician needed for sensor application, and nonneurologist can interpret study.
(v) Abnormal aEEG is more specific (89% vs. 78%), has a greater positive predictive value (73% vs. 58%), and has a similar sensitivity (79% vs. 78%) as well as negative predictive value (90% vs. 91%) compared with abnormal neurologic examination by Sarnat criteria alone.

**d.** Evoked potentials.

**e.** Creatinine kinase and other biochemical/enzyme markers.

**f.** Lumbar puncture, CSF analysis.

**g.** CT scan.

**h.** Cranial ultrasonography.

**i.** Technetium scan.

j. MRI.
k. Intracranial pressure monitoring.

F. **Patient care management.**
1. Prevent perinatal hypoxia, ischemia, and asphyxia (anticipation of risk factors, appropriate intervention).
2. Perform prompt, efficient resuscitation by trained staff.
3. Maintain physiologic oxygenation and acid–base balance.
4. Correct fluid, electrolyte, and caloric abnormalities.
5. Monitor blood volume; avoid blood pressure swings and hypotension.
6. Maintain optimal perfusion.
7. Treat seizures.
8. Consider cerebral hypothermia.
   a. Total body cooling.
   b. Selective head cooling.
   c. Goal of hypothermia: maintain brain energy phosphorylated metabolites, improve coupling between blood flow and oxidative metabolism, decrease release of excitatory transmitters that lead to seizures, reduce nitric oxide production, and decrease apoptosis.
   d. See Table 34-3 for comparison between total body and selective cooling.
9. Perform a thorough neurologic examination.
10. Monitor and manage disturbances of other body organs.
   a. Pulmonary.
   b. Cardiac.
   c. Hepatic.
   d. Renal.
11. Educate and support the family.
12. Obtain neurology consultation.

G. **Outcome.**
1. Based on severity of brain insult; selective neuronal necrosis.
2. Death within newborn period in 20% to 50% of asphyxiated infants who exhibit HIE.
3. Overall neurologic sequelae with HIE at 3{1/2} years of age: approximately 17%. With more follow-up data, the rate may change as cooling strategies have become widely used.

■ TABLE 34-3
■ ■ **Comparison of Brain Cooling Trials**

| Parameter | CoolCap | Body Cooling |
|---|---|---|
| Mode of cooling | Head and systemic | Systemic only |
| Equipment | Cooling cap and radiant warmer | Cincinnati Sub-Zero Hyper-Hypothermia System |
| Target core: temperature | 34° to 35°C | 33.5°C |
| Target core: site | Rectum | Esophagus |
| Temperature control method at core site | Servo control of abdominal skin temperature 36.8° to 37.2°C; manual control of CoolCap to achieve target core temperature at rectum | Servo control of esophagus |
| Age at therapy initiation | <6 hours | <6 hours |
| Time to achieve target core temperature | 2 hours | Approximately 1.5 hours |
| Duration of cooling therapy | 72 hours | 72 hours |
| Rate of rewarming after therapy cessation | 0.5°C/hour | 0.5°C/hour |

From Laptook, A.R.: Brain cooling for neonatal encephalopathy: Potential indications for use. In J.M. Perlman (Ed.): *Neurology: Neonatal questions and controversies*. Philadelphia, 2008, Elsevier Saunders, pp. 66-78.

4. Factors associated with poor outcome.
   a. Apgar score.
      (1) If score is 0 to 3 for 20 minutes or more, approximately 60% die.
      (2) If score is less than 3 at 1 minute and less than 5 at 5 minutes, with abnormal neurologic signs (feeding difficulties, apnea, hypotonia, seizures):
         (a) About 20% die.
         (b) About 40% are normal.
         (c) About 40% have neurologic sequelae.
   b. Encephalopathy.
      (1) Mild: no subsequent deficits.
      (2) Severe: 75% die, 25% have sequelae.
      (3) Term infants: 60% normal, 30% abnormal, and 10% die.
      (4) Premature infants: 50% normal, 20% abnormal, and 30% die.
      (5) Duration of abnormal neurologic signs: good indicator of severity of HIE injury.
      (6) Disappearance of abnormal neurologic signs by 1 to 2 weeks: good chance of being normal (possibility of learning disabilities not ruled out).
5. Seizures early (first 12 hours of life) and/or difficult to control: associated with poorer prognosis.
6. Hyperactivity and attention difficulties: in infants with less severe encephalopathy.
7. Rapid initial improvement indicative of better outcomes.
8. Long-term sequelae based on:
   a. Site,
   b. Extent of cerebral injury, and
   c. Duration of abnormal clinical presentation.

## PERIVENTRICULAR LEUKOMALACIA (SCHER, 2013).

**A. Definition of periventricular leukomalacia (PVL).**
1. Ischemic, necrotic periventricular white matter.
2. Principally ischemic lesion of arterial origin.
3. Multicystic encephalomalacia with or without secondary hemorrhage into ischemic area.

**B. Pathophysiology.**
1. Predisposition.
   a. Systemic hypotension severe enough to impair cerebral blood flow.
   b. Occurrence of focal cerebral infarction and cerebral ischemia.
   c. Major systemic hypotension.
   d. Episodes of apnea and bradycardia.
2. Occurrence secondary to inadequate cerebral perfusion.
3. Manifestation of HIE in premature infants.

**C. Incidence (Volpe, 2008).**
1. Unknown.
2. Approximately 3% to 10% of those with bilateral cystic leukomalacia.
3. Increases to approximately 26% if noncystic PVL is included.

**D. Clinical presentation (Volpe, 2008).**
1. Acute phase: hypotension and lethargy.
2. Six to 10 weeks later, characteristic picture:
   a. Irritable, hypertonic, increased flexion of arms and extension of legs.
   b. Frequent tremors and startles.
   c. Moro reflex may be abnormal.

**E. Diagnostic evaluation (Scher, 2013).**
1. Cranial ultrasonography.
2. CT scan.
3. MRI.

**F. Outcome (Scher, 2013; Volpe, 2008).**

1. Spastic diplegia (major motor deficit common in premature infants with PVL).
2. Motor deficits in premature infants; possible spontaneous resolution in first several years of life.
3. Significant upper arm involvement associated with intellectual deficits.
4. Visual impairment.
5. Lower limb weakness.
6. Outcome based on:
   a. Location, and
   b. Extent of injury.

## MENINGITIS (SEE CHAPTER 32).

## REFERENCES


Back, S.A., and Plawner, L.L.: Congenital malformations of the central nervous system. In C.A. Gleason, and S.U. Devaskar (Eds.): *Avery's diseases of the newborn* (9th ed.). Philadelphia, 2012, Elsevier Saunders, pp. 844–868.

Blackburn, S.T.: *Maternal, fetal, and neonatal physiology: A clinical perspective:* (4th ed.). St. Louis, 2013, Elsevier Saunders.

Bonifacio, S.L., Gonzalez, F., and Ferriero, D.M.: Central nervous system injury and neuroprotection. In C.A. Gleason, and S.U. Devaskar (Eds.): *Avery's diseases of the newborn* (9th ed.). Philadelphia, 2012, Elsevier Saunders, pp. 869–891.

Evans, K., Hing, A.V., and Cunningham, M.: Craniofacial malformations. In C.A. Gleason, and S.U. Devaskar (Eds.): *Avery's diseases of the newborn* (9th ed.). Philadelphia, 2012, Elsevier Saunders, pp. 1331–1350.

Fenichel, G.M.: *Neonatal neurology:* (4th ed.). Philadelphia, 2007, Churchill Livingstone, pp. 1–18.

Hill, A.: Neurological and neuromuscular disorders. In M.G. MacDonald, M.D. Mullett, and M.M.K. Seshia (Eds.): *Neonatology: Pathophysiology and management of the newborn* (5th ed.). Philadelphia, 2005, Lippincott Williams & Wilkins, pp. 1384–1409.

Jones, K.L., Jones, M.C., and Casanelles, M.D.C.: *Smith's recognizable patterns of human malformation:* (7th ed.). Philadelphia, 2013, Elsevier Saunders.

Laptook, A.R.: The use of hypothermia to provide neuroprotection for neonatal hypoxic-ischemic brain injury. In J.M. Perlman (Ed.): *Neurology: Neonatal questions and controversies* (2nd ed.). Philadelphia, 2012, Elsevier Saunders, pp. 77–90.

McLean, C.W., Noori, S., Cayabyab, R.G., and Seri, I.: Cerebral circulation and hypotension in the premature infant: Diagnosis and treatment. In J.M. Perlman (Ed.): *Neurology: Neonatology questions and controversies* (2nd ed.). Philadelphia, 2012, Elsevier Saunders, pp. 3–36.

Moore, K.L., Persaud, T.V.N., and Torchia, M.G.: Nervous system. In K.L. Moore, T.V.N. Persaud, and M.G. Torchia (Eds.): *Before we are born: Essentials of embryology and birth defects* (8th ed.). Philadelphia, 2012, Elsevier Saunders, pp. 247–270.

Papile, L.: Intracranial hemorrhage and vascular lesions. In A.A. Fanaroff, R.J. Martin, and M.C. Walsh (Eds.): *Fanaroff and Martin's neonatal-perinatal medicine: Diseases of the fetus and infant* (8th ed.). Philadelphia, 2006, Elsevier Mosby, pp. 891–899.

Prabhu, S.P., Grant, P.E., Robertson, R.L., and Taylor, G. A.: Neonatal neuroimaging. In C.A. Gleason, and S.U. Devaskar (Eds.): *Avery's diseases of the newborn* (9th ed.). Philadelphia, 2012, Elsevier Saunders, pp. 816–843.

Rennie, J.M., and Huertas-Ceballos, A.: Examination of the nervous system. In J.M. Rennie, and N.R.C. Roberton (Eds.): *Rennie and Roberton's textbook of neonatology* (5th ed.). Edinburgh, 2012, Churchill Livingstone, pp. 1067–1079.

Scher, M.S.: Brain disorders of the fetus and neonate. In A.A. Fanaroff, and J.M. Fanaroff (Eds.): *Klaus & Fanaroff's care of the high-risk neonate* (6th ed.). Philadelphia, 2013, Elsevier Saunders, pp. 476–524.

Scher, M.S.: Neonatal seizures. In C.A. Gleason, and S. U. Devaskar (Eds.): *Avery's diseases of the newborn* (9th ed.). Philadelphia, 2012, Elsevier Saunders, pp. 901–919.

Verklan, M.T.: Hemolytic disorders and congenital anomalies. In D.L. Lowdermilk, S.E. Perry, K. Cashion, and K. R. Alden (Eds.): *Maternity & women's health care* (10th ed.). St. Louis, 2012, Elsevier Mosby, pp. 867–893.

Verklan, M.T., and Lopez, S.M.: Neurologic disorders. In S.L. Gardner, B.S. Carter, M. Enzman-Hines, and J.A. Hernandez (Eds.): *Merenstein & Gardner's handbook of neonatal intensive care* (7th ed.). St. Louis, 2011, Elsevier Mosby, pp. 748–786.

Volpe, J.J.: *Neurology of the newborn:* (5th ed.). Philadelphia, 2008, Elsevier Saunders.

Waller, S.A., Gopalani, S., and Benedetti, T.J.: Complicated deliveries: Overview. In C.A. Gleason, and S. U. Devaskar (Eds.): *Avery's diseases of the newborn* (9th ed.). Philadelphia, 2012, Elsevier Saunders, pp. 146–158.

Yager, J.Y.: Glucose and perinatal brain injury: Questions and controversies. In J.M. Perlman (Ed.): *Neurology: Neonatology questions and controversies* (2nd ed.). Philadelphia, 2012, Elsevier Saunders, pp. 153–171.

CHAPTER

# 35 Congenital Anomalies

LEANN STERK

**OBJECTIVES**

1. Describe assessment strategies for diagnosis of infants experiencing a congenital defect.
2. Identify methods of initial management and care for individual congenital anomalies.
3. List possible causative factors that result in common congenital abnormalities.
4. Verbalize the importance of parental involvement in the development of infants affected with congenital anomalies.

In North America, congenital malformations account for more than 20% of infant deaths (Moore and Persaud, 2013). In the United States, nearly 1 in 120 live-born infants will experience a chromosomal abnormality (Moore and Persaud, 2013). These statistics represent a significant challenge to health care providers and pose life-changing challenges for the families of these infants.

A congenital anomaly is defined as a physical, metabolic, anatomic, or behavioral deviation from the normal pattern of development (Moore and Persaud, 2013) (Box 35-1). This chapter presents information concerning the incidence, etiology, clinical presentation, and treatment modalities for some common abnormalities. The reader is directed to Chapter 20 for a foundation on genetics.

A. **Incidence.**
   1. The frequency of medically significant malformations diagnosed in the newborn period is documented as 2% of all live births (Parikh and Wiesner, 2011). These defects present as single or multiple defects, all with varying clinical significance.
      a. By 1 year of age, the incidence of congenital anomalies requiring surgery or interfering with normal functioning ranges from 4% to 7% (Lashley, 2005).
      b. Minor single anomaly rates are estimated to be as high as 14% (Moore and Persaud, 2013). Infants experiencing three or more minor abnormalities commonly have one or more major defects.
      c. The identification of neonates with a major malformation is vital as these infants have a five-fold increase in morbidity (Parikh and Wiesner, 2011).
   2. Birth defects are a significant cause of miscarriage and fetal death.
      a. Of recognized conceptions, 10% to 20% will end in spontaneous abortion secondary to abnormal genetic development.
      b. Fifty percent to 60% of all infants spontaneously aborted will have a detectable chromosomal abnormality (Lashley, 2005). Of those infants, trisomic abnormalities account for 50% of pregnancy losses (Parikh and Weisner, 2011).

B. **Etiology.** The etiology of 50% to 60% of congenital anomalies is unknown (Moore and Persaud, 2013). Congenital malformations may have more than one cause, are often associated with multiple anomalies of major or minor significance, and have variable recurrence risks. Congenital anomalies may result from chromosomal disorders, single-gene defects, infective agents, teratogens, combinations of genetic and environmental factors, maternal metabolic factors, and mechanical constraints on the uterus (Lashley, 2005).
   1. Genetic factors.
      a. Genetic factors are numerically the most frequent cause of congenital anomalies and are responsible for approximately 0.5% to 0.7% of all anomalies (Matthews and Robin, 2011). Chromosomal disorders account for 10% of all of the major malformations (Parikh and Wiesner, 2011). Of anomalies with known causes, 85% are due to genetic factors (Moore and Persaud, 2013).

**BOX 35-1**
**TERMINOLOGY**

Consistent language, definitions, and accurate presentation of dysmorphology are vital to understanding congenital anomalies.

1. Malformation: a primary morphologic defect of an organ or body part that results from an intrinsic abnormal developmental process (Lashley, 2005) (e.g., neural tube defect).
2. Deformation: alteration of a previously normal body part by unusual forces on normal tissue (*Dorland's Illustrated Medical Dictionary*, 2007). Timing of event usually occurs in the fetal period as a secondary alteration, often involving cartilage, joints, and bones (Lashley, 2005) (e.g., clubfoot).
3. Disruption: extrinsic breakdown or interruption of a normal developmental process resulting in a defect of an organ or larger body system (e.g., amniotic banding sequence).
4. Dysplasia: abnormal organization of cells in tissue.
5. Syndrome: a recognized pattern of multiple anomalies derived from a single anomaly or mechanical factor (*Dorland's Illustrated Medical Dictionary*, 2007) (e.g., Down syndrome).
6. Sequence: a pattern of multiple anomalies related to a single prior anomaly (Lashley, 2005) (e.g., Pierre Robin sequence).

**b.** Chromosomal errors are produced in the germline of either parent, secondary to errors in fertilization, meiosis, or mitosis (commonly nondisjunction and anaphase lag), and chromosome breakage and reunion (Lashley, 2005).

**c.** Embryos resulting from these unions display missing or extra chromosomes (numeric abnormality) or rearranged segments (structural abnormalities). Chromosomal aberrations result in defective zygotes, blastocysts, and early embryos.

**d.** Both sex chromosomes and/or autosomes may be affected.

**e.** Categories of genetic factors:

(1) Numeric abnormalities commonly result from nondisjunction of genetic material. This error in cell division occurs during mitosis or meiosis when a chromosomal pair or two chromatids of a chromosome fail to disjoin (Moore and Persaud, 2013). The end result is the loss or gain of one or more chromosomes (Matthews and Robin, 2011).

(a) Trisomy: fertilization of an aneuploid gamete by a normal gamete resulting in a zygote with an extra chromosome.

(b) Monosomy: zygote develops missing a specific chromosome.

(c) Mosaicism: Results secondary to nondisjunction in early cleavage division of a single zygote. The result is an embryo having two or more cell lines with different cell numbers (Moore and Persaud, 2013). Symptoms are generally less severe than if all cells are affected.

**f.** Numeric chromosomal abnormalities are frequently associated with intrauterine growth retardation, dysmorphic features, mental retardation, and physical malformations (Matthews and Robin, 2011).

**g.** Structural abnormalities frequently result from chromosome breakage that results in a loss or rearrangement of the broken segment to a different location on the chromosome or to a different chromosome. The resulting change in structure is dependent on the final disposition of the broken pieces. Chromosome breakage may be caused by radiation, drugs, chemicals, and viruses (Moore and Persaud, 2013).

(1) Deletions are chromosome breaks that result in the loss of part of the chromosome. Breakage can occur at either end, resulting in a ring chromosome, or in the body of the chromosome. Microdeletions are submicroscopic chromosomal abnormalities that involve specific minute portions of chromosomes. Loss of chromosomal material is associated with serious malformation.

(2) Duplication anomalies result as a duplication of genetic material within, attached to, or as a separate fragment of the chromosome (Moore and Persaud, 2013). Though there is no loss of genetic material, individuals commonly experience mental retardation or other birth defects.

(3) Inversion defects result when a chromosome segment is reversed. Risk for abnormality is dependent on the portion of the chromosome involved.

h. Single-gene or Mendelian disorders are responsible for 4% of major malformations (Parikh and Wiesner, 2011). The mode of Mendelian inheritance for many major malformations is autosomal dominant (Parikh and Wiesner, 2011). Autosomal recessive, or less frequently X-linked, inheritance accounts for a minority of major malformations. The mechanism for development of abnormality is related to dysfunction of the gene or disturbance of the developmental pathway.

i. Multifactorial disorders result secondary to interaction of genes and additive environmental influences. In order for an abnormality to be expressed, a threshold of traits must be exceeded.

j. Disorders are familial, but lack the inheritance traits of single-gene defects.

k. Most isolated single malformations, such as congenital heart defects, neural tube defects, and cleft lip and palate, develop secondary to multifactorial inheritance patterns (Matthews and Robin, 2011).

l. Recurrence rates are higher for first-degree relatives, are greater if a larger number of family members are affected, and are increased if the malformation is severe (Matthews and Robin, 2011).

2. Disorders resulting from exposure to teratogens that affect the developing fetus.

a. A teratogen is defined as any organism, substance, deficiency state, or physical agent capable of inducing abnormal structure or function (Blackburn, 2013).

b. Environmental factors are causative for 7% to 10% of congenital anomalies (Moore and Persaud, 2013). The exact mechanism resulting in a disruption of embryonic development and induction of anomalies remains unclear, but environmental factors do not appear to exert effect until cellular differentiation begins.

c. The majority of teratogenic agents exert their effect by interfering with cellular metabolic activity. The end result is failure of cellular replication, cell migration, cellular fusion, and death. Moore and Persaud (2013) define the most critical periods of development as the time when cell division, cell differentiation, and morphogenesis are at their peak.

d. The ability of a particular agent to exert a teratogenic effect is determined by the timing of the exposure (critical time once cellular differentiation has begun), dosage of the teratogen (higher the dose, greater the effect), the individual properties of the teratogen, and the genetic susceptibility of the mother and fetus (Matthews and Robin, 2011).

e. The range of teratogenic agents is large and continues to increase. McLean (2005) describes classifications of teratogens as infectious agents, drugs and chemical agents, radiation, and maternal factors, as well as mechanical forces upon the fetus.

f. Exposure of the fetus to alcohol carries significant risk throughout pregnancy and is considered to be the most common teratogen (Parikh and Wiesner, 2011). Fetal alcohol spectrum disorder is estimated to affect as much as 1% of the general population (Moore and Persaud, 2013).

C. **Evaluation.** When a newborn is identified as having one or more malformations, a detailed history and physical examination is needed to aid in accurate diagnosis.

1. Family history should include the past three generations, with health information about all relatives—parents, siblings, grandparents, uncles and aunts, as well as cousins.

2. A pedigree analysis should be developed.

a. Reproductive losses and infertility.

b. Relatives with mental retardation or known malformations.

c. Infants within the family with malformations or birth defects.

d. Neonatal deaths, childhood deaths, stillbirths.

e. Familial disorders or physical features common to the family.

f. Consanguinity in parents.

g. Ethnic background.

3. Prenatal and perinatal history should detail information about maternal and fetal well-being.

a. Maternal age, parity, and health—including maternal illness and medications.

b. Pregnancy mode (natural or assisted), complications.

c. Teratogenic exposures, including alcohol, drugs, herbal preparations, medications, bacterial infections, viral infections, and parasitic infections.
d. Duration of pregnancy, intrapartum course, prenatal testing, and duration.
e. Fetal growth and behavior in utero—patterns of movement throughout pregnancy.
f. Delivery mode, complications, condition of infant at delivery.
g. Birth weight, length, and head circumference and whether measurements are appropriate for gestation.

4. Detailed physical examination is undertaken with attention to physical variations and malformations. It is essential to determine if an anomaly is isolated or part of a pattern of malformation. Clinical photographs should be obtained. Photographs of unusual features provide a permanent record that allows initial diagnosis and later consultation (Lashley, 2005).
   a. Growth parameters: weight, length, head circumference—assessment of proportionality and symmetry. Specific measurements of features for abnormality in shape, size, or symmetry should be undertaken. Measurements should be compared against gestational norms. Variation may reflect degree of prenatal insult.
   b. Estimation of gestational age.
   c. General appearance: posture, tone, and position.
   d. Systematic examination of all body surfaces.
      (1) Head: size measured as occipital–frontal circumference, shape (assess for dolichocephaly, premature fusion of cranial sutures, frontal bossing), size of anterior fontanelles (Haldeman-Englert et al., 2012a).
      (2) Scalp: hair patterns, including placement of whorls, hairline, texture, pigmented areas, eyebrow length and pattern, eyelash length, widow's peaks, or alterations in pigmentation.
      (3) Face: configuration, elfin, coarse, flat, triangular, round, birdlike, expressionless.
      (4) Eyes: spacing of eyes, interpupillary distances, epicanthal folds, palpebral fissures (length and degree of slanting), iris color, colobomas, ptosis.
      (5) Nose: appearance—beaked, pinched, upturned, flattened bridge, position on face, number and patency of nares, length of the columella.
      (6) Mouth: shape of palate and uvula, presence of cleft lip or palate, size of tongue or deformities, natal teeth, deformities of frenulum, shape of mouth, philtrum, and vermilion border.
      (7) Ears: location, position, rotation, unilateral/bilateral defect, protruding/prominent shape, patency of auditory meatus, preauricular and postauricular pits and tags.
      (8) Neck: length, webbed/redundant skinfolds, posterior hairline, torticollis, small or receding chin, bony abnormalities of the neck.
      (9) Chest: shape, size, symmetry; location, spacing, and number of nipples, internipple distance.
      (10) Cardiovascular: murmurs, pulses, blood pressure.
      (11) Lungs: equality, character of breath sounds.
      (12) Abdomen: integrity of abdominal wall, location and appearance of umbilicus, presence of masses, organomegaly, hypoplasia of musculature, omphalocele, gastroschisis. Umbilicus should be examined for number of vessels, hernias (Haldeman-Englert et al., 2012a).
      (13) Genitalia: presence of ambiguity, size, appearance.
      (14) Anus: location and patency.
      (15) Spine: neural tube defects, unusual pigmentary lesions, hair tufts, dimples, sinuses.
      (16) Extremities: proportions, appearance, range of motion, number and placement of hands, feet, digits. Epidural ridges, creases, absence deformities, polydactyly, syndactyly, contracture deformities, clinodactyly, camptodactyly (Parikh and Wiesner, 2011).
      (17) Skin: pigmentation, lesions, texture; hair distribution, patterns—whorls, widow's peaks.

5. Diagnostic evaluation of a congenital abnormality.
   a. Radiographs, computed tomography (CT), ultrasound, and magnetic resonance imaging (MRI) are used to rule out structural abnormalities. These tests are also performed to investigate dysmorphic features that may be part of a syndrome or sequence.

b. Cytogenic, molecular, and biochemical examination are useful in determining etiology of congenital anomalies.
c. Chromosome analysis should be obtained for all infants having two or more major malformations, infants with growth restriction in association with anomalies, infants having multiple minor abnormalities, and infants with ambiguous genitalia.
   (1) Karyotype analysis is performed on cells undergoing mitosis (Haldeman-Englert et al., 2012a). As chromosomes condense, they are stained and a representation of chromosome number results. Normal karyotype consists of 46 chromosomes—22 pairs of autosomes and one set of sex chromosomes.
d. Microarray technology allows for detection and analysis of thousands of genes at the same time. Assay provides information about patterns of gene expression and interaction (Haldeman-Englert et al., 2012a). The focus of microarray-based techniques is centered on examination of chromosome number changes. Diagnostic confirmation of microdeletion error is possible. Comparative genomic hybridization, single-nucleotide polymorphism or oligonucleotide arrays, and molecular analysis are being utilized in greater frequency to determine etiology of abnormalities (Haldeman-Englert et al., 2012a).
   (1) Fluorescent in-situ hybridization (FISH) utilizes segments of fluorescently labeled DNA probes that attach to a specific segment of the chromosome and appear fluorescent under microscopic evaluation. Where material is missing from the segment, the probe is unable to attach to the chromosome, resulting in identification of microdeletion (Murray, 2012).
e. Biochemical studies are performed on ill neonates who have a condition that may be secondary to an inborn error of metabolism, or for whom a specific diagnosis cannot be made. Laboratory studies should be obtained before treatment is begun. Presenting symptoms guide the specific tests to be ordered. Newborn screening using tandem mass spectrometry allows for a single drop of blood to effectively screen for 40 inborn errors of metabolism.
f. Ophthalmologic examination may be useful as abnormalities are often associated with neurologic or brain malformations.

**D. Genetic counseling.**

1. The diagnosis of a congenital anomaly places the family in a crisis. Genetic counseling should be available to all parents of children with a major malformation or multiple anomalies.
   a. Genetic counseling is offered to prospective parents to help them evaluate risks for hereditary or genetic conditions based on the individual family pedigree (Parikh and Wiesner, 2011).
   b. Goals of counseling are centered around provision of information concerning diagnosis, needed care, impact of the illness, prediction for recurrence, and future support. Counseling is aimed toward assisting parents to make informed decisions.
   c. Counseling can be offered by family physicians, neonatologists, or genetic specialists. Counseling is provided in a quiet location with all family members desired by the family present.
   d. Principles of genetic counseling.
      (1) Supportive, nonjudgmental attitude.
      (2) Respectful of family privacy, confidentiality.
      (3) Sensitive to ethnic, cultural, and language differences.
      (4) Supportive of family's movement through the grieving process.
      (5) Content of counseling should take into account medical issues, mechanisms causing the abnormality, a realistic prognosis, and a plan for treatment and support resources.
      (6) Risk for recurrence and reproductive options.
      (7) Assistance with family adjustment and social services as needed.

## SPECIFIC DISORDERS

See Figure 35-1 for the division of congenital anomalies.

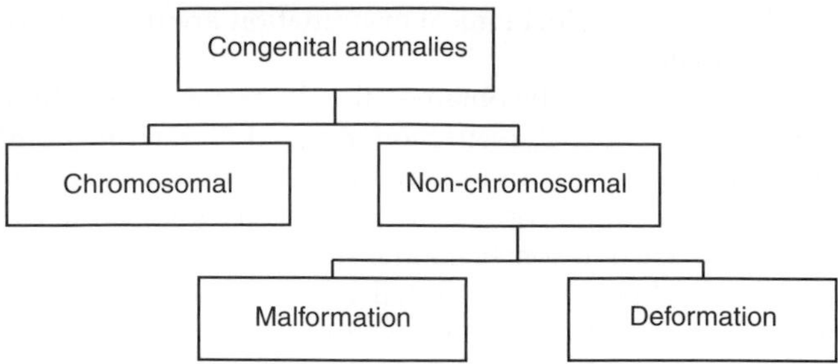


FIGURE 35-1 ■ Division of anomalies.

## Abnormalities of Chromosomes

### Trisomy 21 (Down Syndrome)

A. **Incidence and etiology.**
   1. Most common autosomal chromosomal abnormality in live-born infants; occurring in 1 in 800 infants (Haldeman-Englert et al., 2012b).
   2. Full trisomy 21 occurs in 94% of cases (all or large part of the chromosome). Affected individuals have 47 chromosomes (three of chromosome 21) (Fig. 35-2).
   3. Greater than 90% of trisomy 21 cases result secondary to meiotic disjunction. Maternal age exerts a significant effect. Three percent to 5% of cases are de novo or caused by a balanced translocation that becomes unbalanced (Haldeman-Englert et al., 2012b).
   4. Mosaic or mitotic nondisjunction Down syndrome, presenting with variable phenotypic expression, is demonstrated in 3% of affected infants (Haldeman-Englert et al., 2012b).
   5. Greater than 50% of trisomy 21 fetuses abort early in pregnancy.

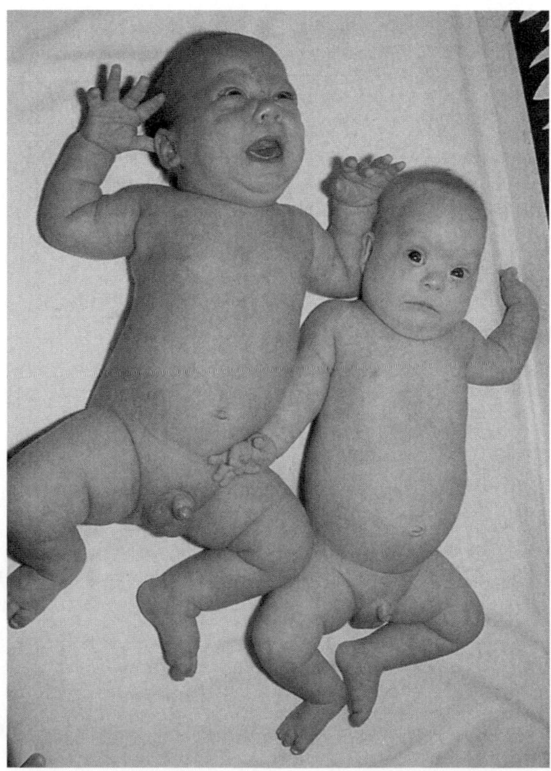

FIGURE 35-2 ■ Anterior view of dizygotic (fraternal) male twins discordant for Down syndrome (trisomy 21). The twin at right is smaller and hypotonic compared with the unaffected twin. The twin at right developed from a zygote that contained an extra 21 chromosome. (Courtesy Dr. A.E. Chudley, Department of Pediatrics and Child Health, University of Manitoba, Children's Hospital, Winnipeg, Manitoba, Canada.)

6. Recurrence risk approximately 1% overall. For those parents who are known translocation carriers, the risk is substantially higher. Risk for carrier parent is dependent on the type of translocation and the sex of the parent (Jones et al., 2013).
7. Incidence of Down syndrome related to maternal age is as follows (Moore and Persaud, 2013):
   a. 20 to 24 years—1 in 1400.
   b. 25 to 29 years—1 in 1100.
   c. 30 to 34 years—1 in 700.
   d. 35 years—1 in 350.
   e. 37 years—1 in 225.
   f. 41 years—1 in 85.
   g. 43 years—1 in 50.
   h. Over 45 years—1 in 25.

**B. Clinical presentation.**

1. Craniofacial.
   a. Brachycephaly with flattened occiput, presence of third fontanelle.
   b. Upslanting palpebral fissures, iris speckled with Brushfield's spots, colobomatous cataracts, and glaucoma.
   c. Prominent epicanthal folds.
   d. Flattened facial profile, micrognathia, flattened nasal bridge.
   e. Small, posteriorly rotated, rounded ears; low-set and malformed ears (overfolding of superior helices), hearing loss.
   f. Prominent, protruding tongue; high-arched palate with tendency to keep mouth open (Jones et al., 2013).
2. Musculoskeletal.
   a. Hypotonia: generalized—poor Moro reflex present in 80% of infants. Suck may be weak.
   b. Hyperflexibility of joints, dysplasia of pelvis: narrow acetabular angle.
   c. Clinodactyly of fifth digits, single or bilateral transverse simian crease—present in 50% of cases. Brachydactyly.
   d. Prenatal growth restriction, short stature, often 10% to 25% of affected children.
   e. Wide spacing between first and second toes (Matthews and Robin, 2011).
3. Skin.
   a. Short neck with excess nuchal skin.

**C. Associated findings.**

1. Prematurity.
2. Mental retardation: present in all cases, variable degree, mild to moderate impairment (Lashley, 2005).
3. Hematologic: bone marrow dyscrasias, including neonatal thrombocytopenia and transient self-resolving myeloproliferative disorders, have been described within the first year of life (Haldeman-Englert et al., 2012b). Thirty percent of infants with Down syndrome and transient myeloproliferative disease develop acute megakaryoblastic leukemia within the first 4 years of life (Luchtman-Jones et al., 2011).
4. Gastrointestinal: duodenal atresia/stenosis—occur in 2% to 5% of cases; esophageal atresia, imperforate anus, fistulas, webs.
5. Cardiac anomalies in approximately 50% of infants: endocardial cushion defect, ventral septal defect, patent ductus arteriosus, atrial septal defect, tetralogy of Fallot (Haldeman-Englert et al., 2012b).
6. Otitis media, hearing impairment.

**D. Diagnosis.**

1. Chorionic villus sampling at 9 to 12 weeks of gestation.
2. Amniocentesis at 16 weeks.
3. Maternal serum screening for low values of α-fetoprotein (AFP).
4. Ultrasound targeting growth, polyhydramnios, heart defects.
5. Standard chromosome banding techniques provide confirmation of trisomy 21 and differentiate those infants having nondisjunctional trisomy from a translocation. In those infants with confirmed translocation, each parent should have karyotype analysis done to rule out carrier status as recurrence risk is significantly increased (Lewanda et al., 2006).
6. FISH: region on chromosome affected is q22.2.

**E. Treatment.**

1. Initial treatment geared to expressed symptoms.
2. Parent education and support are essential for treatment of continuing health issues.
3. Ophthalmologic evaluation should be undertaken as children with Down syndrome have greater incidence of cataracts, strabismus, myopia, and glaucoma (Haldeman-Englert et al., 2012b).
4. Monitor cerebral spine for spinal cord compression.
5. Monitor growth as velocity often decreases—weight and head circumference.
6. Screen for hypothyroidism.
7. Upper respiratory infections and ear infections are common.
8. Cardiac sequelae, including congestive heart failure.
9. Aimed at optimizing potential for intellectual and social growth.
10. Developmental delays—muscle tone increases with age, rate of developmental progress slows with age (Jones et al., 2013). Early developmental enrichment programs seem to be of the most value.
11. Social performance is usually above the expected level. Emotional problems are apparent in many affected individuals. Parents must be provided with resources for emotional and medical support.
12. Following correction of associated congenital malformations, less than 50% of individuals with Down syndrome survive to age 60. Less than 15% survive to age 68 (Haldeman-Englert et al., 2012b).

### Trisomy 18

**A. Incidence and etiology.**

1. Affected infants have 47 chromosomes (three of chromosome 18) (Fig. 35-3).
2. Occurs in 1 in 600 births; females more often than males (3:1) (Jones et al., 2013). Trisomy 18 is the third most common autosomal disorder. Associated with a high rate of intrauterine demise—5% of affected cases will survive to birth (Haldeman-Englert et al., 2012b).
3. Eighty percent of cases are caused by chromosomal nondisjunction (Lewanda et al., 2006); 95% of infants have three copies of entire chromosome 18, and 5% have either partial trisomy or mosaicism of most of the long arm of 18 (Haldeman-Englert et al., 2012b).
4. Occurs more frequently as maternal age advances: mean maternal age is 32 (Jones et al., 2013).
5. Three patterns of presentation have been described:
   a. Severe: most body cells display abnormality. Handicaps are severe, with a short life expectancy.
   b. Mosaic form: some cells have the normal complement of genetic material, the remaining cells having the typical pattern for trisomy 18. Infants are less severely affected and have a longer life expectancy.
   c. Partial: dependent on the portion of the chromosome affected. Infants with trisomy of the short arm of the chromosome have minimal handicaps and few abnormalities are expressed. Infants with trisomy involving the entire long arm of the chromosome display the full spectrum of the syndrome. Infants with trisomy of the distal one third of the chromosome demonstrate a partial syndrome with less profound mental deficit and longer survival (Jones et al., 2013).
6. Estimate for risk of recurrence for future pregnancies is 1% over the maternal age-specific risk for any viable autosomal trisomy (Haldeman-Englert et al., 2012b). Infants whose defect is secondary to a structural arrangement warrant parental karyotype analysis.

**B. Clinical presentation.**

1. General: growth deficiency, hypoplasia of skeletal muscle, subcutaneous and adipose tissue (Haldeman-Englert et al., 2012b).
2. Craniofacial: small narrow cranium, prominent occiput, low-set malformed auricles, atresia of auditory canals, narrow palpebral fissures, microphthalmia, corneal opacities, colobomas, micrognathia, microstomia and high-arched palate, cleft palate (Lewanda et al., 2006).
3. Musculoskeletal: clenched hand, with index finger overlapping the third finger and the fifth finger overlapping the fourth, abnormal creases, low-arch dermal ridge pattern on six or

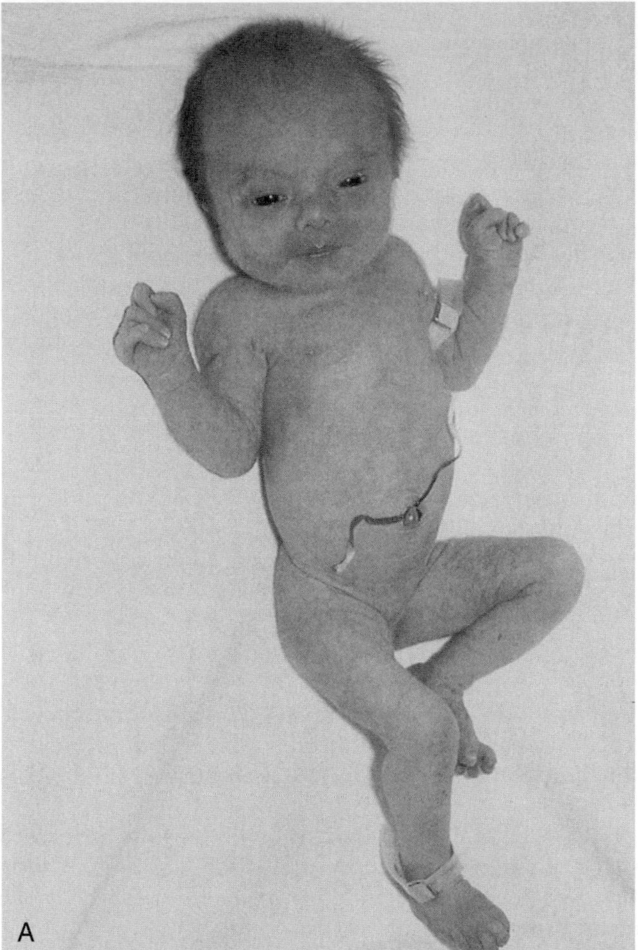

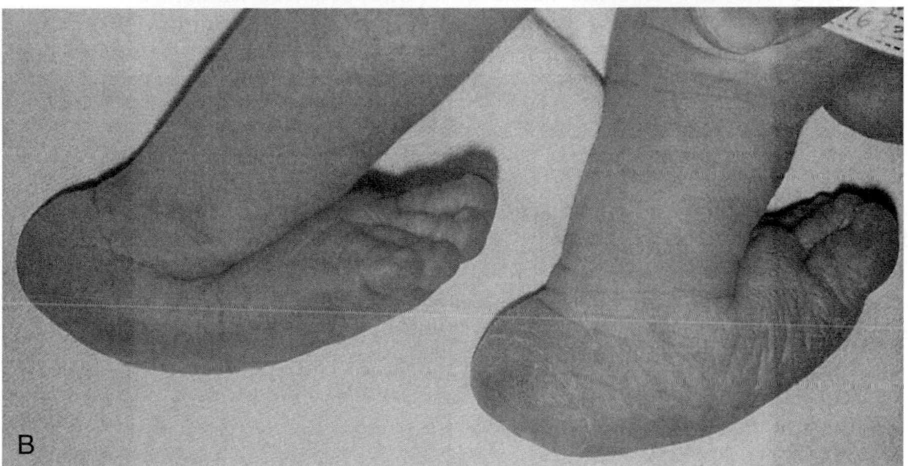

FIGURE 35-3 ■ **A**, Female neonate with trisomy 18. Note growth retardation, clenched fists with characteristic positioning of fingers (second and fifth digits overlap third and fourth digits). **B**, Feet of another trisomy 18 infant showing characteristic rocker-bottom appearance as a result of vertical position of tali (ankle bones). Also observe prominent calcanei (heel bones). (Courtesy Dr. A.E. Chudley, Department of Pediatrics and Child Health, University of Manitoba, Children's Hospital, Winnipeg, Manitoba, Canada.)

more fingertips, hypoplasia of nails, short sternum, narrow pelvis with hip dislocation, rocker-bottom appearance to feet, hammer toes, clubfeet, and syndactyly between toes 2 and 3 (Jones et al., 2013).
4. Skin: redundant skin, mild hirsutism of back and forehead.

C. **Associated findings.**
1. Cardiac anomalies: varied. Occur in 95% of cases (Lashley, 2005). Ventricular septal defects and patent ductus arteriosus, atrial septal defects, pulmonic stenosis, coarctation of the aorta are most common (Haldeman-Englert et al., 2012b).
2. Renal anomalies: horseshoe kidneys, ectopic kidneys, double ureters, and cystic kidneys.
3. Genital abnormalities: cryptorchidism in males. Hypoplasia of labia and prominent clitoris in females.
4. Umbilical hernias.
5. Severe psychomotor retardation.

D. **Diagnosis.**
1. Chorionic villus sampling at 9 to 12 weeks of gestation.
2. Amniocentesis at 16 weeks.
3. Maternal serum triple screening revealing low levels of AFP, unconjugated estradiol, and total human chorionic gonadotropin. Fifty percent to 60% of trisomy 18 cases can be detected with second-trimester screening utilizing the triple screen (Blackburn, 2013).
4. Ultrasound targeting growth retardation, oligohydramnios and polyhydramnios, heart defects, myelomeningocele, and limb abnormalities.
5. Following delivery, standard chromosome banding assay or FISH.

E. **Treatment.**
1. Infants with full trisomy 18 are usually fragile, with a history of feeble fetal activity (Jones et al., 2013). Prognosis for infants with this disorder is poor. More than 90% of infants will succumb in the first 6 months of life, 5% will survive to 1 year (Haldeman-Englert et al., 2012b).
2. Children who survive the first year of life deal with feeding issues secondary to hypotonia, growth issues, and significant developmental disability. These children generally do not walk unsupported or develop expressive language, but can be capable of limited verbal communication and some social interaction.
3. Once a diagnosis has been confirmed, decisions about extraordinary medical means for prolongation of life present nearly overwhelming challenges for families. Individual circumstances for each family must be considered (Jones et al., 2013). Most deaths result secondary to congestive heart disease, infection, and central apnea (Haldeman-Englert et al., 2012b).
4. For those infants surviving the immediate newborn period, care is supportive and individualized to the infant's needs.
5. Parents should be offered genetic counseling and provided with resources for support.

### Trisomy 13

A. **Incidence and etiology.**
1. Affected infants are born with 47 chromosomes instead of the usual 46, with the extra genetic material located on chromosome 13. This abnormality is the rarest of the trisomies, severe external malformations are common, and only 2% to 3% survive to term (Lashley, 2005).
2. Defect occurs in 1 in 12,500 to 1 in 21,000 live births (Haldeman-Englert et al., 2012b), making it the fourth most common autosomal dominant disorder.
   a. Older mothers are more likely to have an infant with this aneuploidy defect.
   b. Slightly more boys than girls are affected (Jones et al., 2013).
3. Seventy-five percent of cases result from chromosomal nondisjunction (Lewanda et al., 2006).
4. The etiology for this disorder is trisomy of all or part of chromosome 13.
   a. Eighty percent of affected infants have three complete copies of chromosome 13.
   b. Mosaicism accounts for 5% of cases, with these infants demonstrating a wide range of expression from near normal to severe full pattern malformation.
      (1) Survival for infants with mosaicism is usually longer.

(2) Degree of mental deficit is variable (Jones et al., 2013).

c. Partial trisomy of the proximal segment is characterized by infants with severe mental deficiency and an overall pattern of full trisomy 13.

d. Partial trisomy of the distal segment results in severe mental deficiency and characteristic phenotype (Jones et al., 2013).

**B. Clinical presentation.**

1. General: growth deficiency.
2. Craniofacial: cebocephaly, microcephaly, microphthalmia, colobomata, glaucoma, midline scalp defects, retinal dysplasia, cleft lip and/or palate (60% to 80%) (Jones et al., 2013), malformed ears, atresia of external auditory canals, deafness, prominent nasal bridge, short neck with excessive skin.
   a. Aplasia cutis congenita is a congenital localized absence of skin often involving the scalp along the midline. Lesions have sharp margins and may present as ulcers, bullae, or scars (Tran and Cohen, 2012). Lesions are frequently noted on the scalp near the parietal hair whorl (Graham, 2007). Most defects are small and superficial; 20% involve absence of the skull, exposing the infant to hemorrhage and infection.
3. Musculoskeletal: polydactyly, single palmar crease, overlapping of fingers, flexion deformities of hands and wrists, prominent heel resulting in rocker-bottom feet, thin posterior ribs with or without missing rib, and hypoplasia of pelvis with shallow acetabular angle.
4. Genital abnormalities: males—cryptorchidism, abnormal scrotum; females—bicornuate uterus.
5. Central nervous system (CNS): holoprosencephaly found in 50% of patients with incomplete development of the forebrain and olfactory and auditory nerves, seizure activity, apnea in early infancy, and severe mental deficiency (Haldeman-Englert et al., 2012b).
6. Capillary hemangiomas, localized scalp defects—cutis aplasia.

**C. Associated findings.**

1. Cardiac anomalies occur in approximately 80% of infants: ventral septal defects, dextrocardia, patent ductus arteriosus, atrial septal defects.
2. Renal abnormalities: polycystic kidneys.
3. Inguinal or umbilical hernias, single umbilical artery.

**D. Diagnosis.**

1. Chorionic villus sampling between 9 and 12 weeks of pregnancy.
2. Amniocentesis at 16 weeks.
3. Ultrasound targeting growth parameters, abnormalities of heart, kidneys, and brain.
4. Following delivery, standard chromosome banding assay, FISH.

**E. Treatment.**

1. The presence of holoprosencephaly is the single most important finding predicting survival.
2. Prognosis is extremely poor—80% mortality in the newborn period has been documented (Haldeman-Englert et al., 2012b). Survivors frequently have seizures, severe mental retardation, and failure to thrive.
3. Feeding issues are related to the smallness of the lower jaw and poor muscle tone.
4. For those infants with cleft lip and/or palate, feeding issues present additional challenges.
5. The high rate of early mortality for this syndrome requires the parents to prepare for the infant's death as well as plan for supportive care. The desires of the parents must be taken into account as care is designed for each patient.

**22q11.2 Deletion Syndrome.** This syndrome has been referred to as DiGeorge syndrome, Sprintzen syndrome, or velocardiofacial syndrome. It is the most commonly occurring microdeletion syndrome in humans (Haldeman-Englert et al., 2012b).

**A. Incidence and etiology.**

1. Occurs in 1 in 3000 infants (Haldeman-Englert et al., 2012b). This syndrome is extremely variable in expression and varies from patient to patient.
2. Inherited as an autosomal dominant pattern.
3. Individuals have an interstitial deletion of 22q11.2; 80% to 90% of patients have the same large deletion (Haldeman-Englert et al., 2012b).
4. Most 22q11 deletions occur as de novo lesions—less than 10% are inherited from an affected parent. Both parents must be tested to determine carrier status (Jones et al., 2013).

B. **Clinical presentation.**
   1. Growth: postnatal onset of short stature (Jones et al., 2013).
   2. Craniofacial: microcephaly, velopharyngeal insufficiency, palatal anomalies, small or absent adenoids, prominent nose with bulbous tip, narrow palpebral fissures, long face, retruded mandible with chin deficiency, small mouth—associated with swallowing abnormalities, hooded eyelids, hypertelorism, hearing deficits, and minor auricular abnormalities.
   3. Musculoskeletal: limbs are slender, hypotonic; hands and fingers are hyperextensible (Jones et al., 2013).

C. **Associated findings.**
   1. Cardiac defects are present and usually significant in 85% of patients. Most common defects include ventral septal defects, right interrupted aortic arch, tetralogy of Fallot, and truncus arteriosus (Jones et al., 2013).
   2. Atresia or hypoplasia of the thymus and parathyroid glands (Haldeman-Englert et al., 2012b).
   3. Functional T-cell abnormalities.
   4. Hypocalcemia: occurs as a transient finding in neonates (60%). Seizures can occur—usually as a result of hypocalcemia.
   5. Learning disabilities: 62% of patients will have normal or mild learning issues, with severe or moderate learning difficulties in 18% (Jones et al., 2013). Developmental delays in language and speech are common (Haldeman-Englert et al., 2012b).
   6. IQ range variable. One third of patients function within normal range.
   7. Psychiatric disorders—schizophrenia.
   8. Speech and language are often delayed. Speech pattern is frequently nasal secondary to poor pharyngeal musculature.

D. **Diagnosis.**
   1. Defect is detected by FISH.

E. **Treatment.**
   1. Death primarily secondary to cardiac defects—occurs in approximately 8% of infants (Jones et al., 2013).
   2. Hypotonia is common, resulting in developmental delays. Early intervention, physical and speech therapy are helpful, especially with feeding issues.
   3. Infants may require surgical intervention for palatal abnormalities to improve speech.
   4. Infants frequently demonstrate greater socialization skills than intellectual skills.
   5. Onset of psychiatric symptoms is usually between 10 and 21 years of age—schizophrenia and depression are the most common conditions. Ongoing assessment and support are essential (Jones et al., 2013).

## Sex Chromosome Abnormalities

### Turner's Syndrome

A. **Incidence and etiology.**
   1. Affected individuals have monosomy—loss of all or part of one copy of the X chromosome in a female. Most 45,X conceptuses die early—0.1% survive to term, the majority are spontaneously aborted (Haldeman-Englert et al., 2012b).
      a. Loss of the entire chromosome occurs in approximately 50% of cases (Lewanda et al., 2006).
   2. Occurs in approximately 1 in 2500 live-born phenotypic females (Haldeman-Englert et al., 2012b).
   3. In 70% to 80%, the paternal X chromosome is missing (Lashley, 2005).
   4. Mosaicism is associated with complex karyotypes, ring chromosomes, and deletions.
   5. Disorder generally occurs as a sporadic event in a family (Jones et al., 2013).

B. **Clinical presentation.**
   1. Growth: short stature.
   2. Craniofacial: narrow palate, low-set ears with anomalous auricles, hearing loss, ptosis of eyelids, epicanthal folds, broad nasal bridge, low posterior hairline with appearance of a webbed neck.

3. Musculoskeletal: broad chest with wide-spaced nipples, pectus excavatum, short fourth metacarpal/metatarsal, marked lymphedema of extremities, bone dysplasia, dislocation of the hip, knee abnormalities (Lewanda et al., 2006).
4. Skin: excessively pigmented nevi, loose skin—especially posterior folds of neck.
5. Lymphatic: Impaired lymph drainage leads to distention of lymphatics, and peripheral lymphedema, particularly of dorsa of hands and feet (Kalhan and Devaskar, 2011).

**C. Associated anomalies.**

1. Cardiac defects: bicuspid aortic valve, coarctation of aorta, valvular aortic stenosis, and mitral valve prolapse (Haldeman-Englert et al., 2012b).
2. Renal: horseshoe kidney, unilateral renal agenesis.
3. Gonads: ovarian dysgenesis with hypoplasia owing to lack of germinal elements (Jones et al., 2013).
4. Performance issues: delayed motor skills, poor coordination, clumsiness, problems with nonverbal problem solving, depression and poor self-esteem in young adults (Jones et al., 2013).

**D. Diagnosis.**

1. Ultrasound for short stature, monitoring of growth throughout gestation.
2. Standard chromosome banding assay or FISH.

**E. Treatment.**

1. Growth issues persist throughout childhood and adolescence. Growth is commonly normal within the first 3 years of life, decreasing during school-age years, more dramatically during teenage years when these girls do not get their usual growth spurt at puberty. Growth hormone therapy is generally begun at around 4 to 5 years of age. Significant improvement in final height has been achieved (Haldeman-Englert et al., 2012b).
2. Congenital lymphedema requires symptomatic treatment initially, presenting with edema of hands and feet secondary to faulty lymph drainage.
3. Ovarian function is affected, with primary ovarian failure occurring secondary to gonadal dysplasia. The result can be delay in development of secondary sex characteristics and primary amenorrhea. Treatment options include cyclic estrogen replacement therapy for hypogonadotropic girls beginning at ages 13 to 14 (Haldeman-Englert et al., 2012b).
4. Ongoing evaluation of congenital heart defects is necessary secondary to the increased risk for dissection of the aorta. Coarctation of aorta must be surgically repaired.
5. With increasing age, greater incidences of osteoporosis, autoimmune thyroid disease, and chronic liver disease have been reported (Jones et al., 2013). Close monitoring for these conditions is needed.
6. For those infants for whom their physical appearance would be aided by plastic surgery, concerns for the formation of keloid scars must be considered.
7. School performance may be affected primarily in word comprehension, perceptual thinking, and presentation (Haldeman-Englert et al., 2012b). Intelligence is usually normal.

### Klinefelter's Syndrome

**A. Incidence and etiology.**

1. Affects approximately 1 in 1000 males, making it the most common single cause of hypogonadism and infertility in males (Moore and Persaud, 2013).
2. Chromosomal analysis reveals a 47,XXY karyotype.
   a. Parental nondisjunction errors account for one half of the affected infants; maternal meiosis errors accounting for the majority of remaining cases (Lewanda et al., 2006).
   b. Advanced maternal age is related to an increased incidence for those whose defect is secondary to maternal factors.
   c. According to Jones et al. (2013), older fathers are at higher risk for producing a higher number of XY sperm, resulting in a higher risk of having an infant with Klinefelter's syndrome.
3. Infants with XXY/XY mosaicism may have a greater potential for testicular function.
4. Infants carrying XXYY karyotype are more often developmentally delayed.

**B. Clinical presentation.**

1. General: affected males frequently have long limbs, reduced upper- to lower-segment ratio (Moore and Persaud, 2013). Tall and slim stature.
2. Musculoskeletal: elbow dysplasia, fifth finger clinodactyly.
3. Genital: hypogonadism, cryptorchidism, hypospadias, gynecomastia.

C. **Associated findings.**
   1. Cancers: teratoma, leukemia, breast most common.
   2. Scoliosis during adolescent years (Jones et al., 2013).
   3. School performance and behavioral issues: delayed speech and language development, difficulties with auditory processing and auditory memory. Aggressive behavior is observed (Moore and Persaud, 2013).

D. **Diagnosis.**
   1. Prepubertal males have no significant dysmorphism. Condition may not be diagnoses until puberty, with incomplete development of secondary sex characteristics and infertility (Lashley, 2005). Minor abnormalities are helpful in providing clues for diagnosis: penile size, skeletal defects (Lewanda et al., 2006).
   2. Chromosomal testing, FISH to determine XXY or XXYY or XXXY status.

E. **Treatment.**
   1. As adolescence progresses, screening for scoliosis is needed.
   2. Deficient testosterone and elevated gonadotropin levels signal the need for hormone replacement. Boys must be monitored for prospective testosterone replacement as they near ages 10 to 12. As some males have incomplete or inadequate puberty, replacement will assist in development of a more masculine physique, increase pubic and facial hair, and improve bone density and muscle mass (Jones et al., 2013). Delays in treatment can increase risk for osteoporosis.
   3. The incidence of breast cancer for affected infants is 20 times higher than the general population, but only 1 in 5000 affected men. Routine mammography is not required (Jones et al., 2013). Incidence of mediastinal teratomas is 34 to 40 times that of nonaffected populations. Ongoing assessment of these individuals is needed.
   4. IQ range for affected individuals is variable, from well below to well above average. Assistance in school is commonly required, especially in the areas of reading and spelling.
   5. Emotional and behavioral problems persist and may increase throughout childhood. Formation of peer relationships may be difficult secondary to insecurity, shyness, and poor judgment activity. Support with psychological adjustment is needed.

## NONCHROMOSOMAL ABNORMALITIES

### Malformation Disorders

Malformation sequences occur with a single, localized, poor formation of tissue that initiates a chain of subsequent defects (Jones et al., 2013). Expressed manifestations range from nearly normal to severe and carry a variable recurrence risk.

**Osteogenesis Imperfecta.** Clinically and genetically heterogeneous hereditary disease involving connective tissue disorders and skeletal dysplasia.

A. **Incidence and etiology.**
   1. Disorder is caused by mutations of *COL1A1* and *COL1A2* genes on chromosomes 17q21 and 17q22.1. The result of the mutation is an abnormality of type I collagen (Rimoin and Tiller, 2012). Overall incidence is 3 to 4 per 100,000.
   2. Six clinical types are identified:
      a. Type I: autosomal dominant, resulting from mutations of *COL1A1* gene on chromosome 17q21 (Jones et al., 2013). Most common form found in most populations. Characterized by bone fragility with onset of fractures following birth.
      b. Type II: autosomal dominant, inheritance pattern occurring secondary to a sporadic, dominant mutation in one of the two collagen genes (Jones et al., 2013).
         (1) Frequency 1 in 20,000 to 60,000 (Rimoin and Tiller, 2012). Lethal in the perinatal period—either as stillborn or secondary to respiratory failure; 80% die within the first month of life. Recurrence risk is described as 6%.
      c. Type III: primarily an autosomal dominant inheritance pattern, although rare autosomal recessive pattern has been identified (Jones et al., 2013). Progressive and deforming; if not present at birth, fractures and deformations develop in first and second years of life (Rimoin and Tiller, 2012).
      d. Type IV: autosomal dominant pattern resulting from mutations of the two collagen genes. Significant bone deformities are common.

e. Type V: autosomal dominant inheritance pattern that is not associated with collagen type I mutations (Jones et al., 2013). Moderate tendencies to fracture long bones.
f. Type VI: pattern of inheritance is unknown. Results from a mineralization defect; fractures occurring later between 4 and 18 months.

**B. Clinical presentation.**
1. Type I.
   a. Growth: near-normal or normal growth pattern.
   b. Craniofacial: macrocephaly, triangular appearing facies, hearing impairment, altered dentition with hypoplasia of dentin and pulp (Jones et al., 2013).
   c. Musculoskeletal: postnatal onset of mild limb problems; bowing of femur, tibia, scoliosis, hyperextensibility of joints, and osteopenia.
   d. Skin: translucent, easy bruising, blue sclerae secondary to partial visualization of the choroid.
2. Type II.
   a. Growth: short-limbed growth deficiency with prenatal onset, low birth weight.
   b. Craniofacial: head is soft and boggy, with minimal calvarial bone palpable, large fontanelles, deep blue sclerae, shallow orbits; head assumes a triangular shape (Rimoin and Tiller, 2012).
   c. Musculoskeletal: shortened and bowed limbs with extra skin, flexed and abducted hips, flattened vertebrae (Jones et al., 2013).
3. Type III.
   a. Growth: prenatal onset of growth deficiency, extremely short stature.
   b. Craniofacial: macrocephaly, triangular facies, deep blue sclera, hearing loss, dentinogenesis imperfecta.
   c. Musculoskeletal: kyphoscoliosis, which may lead to respiratory distress (Jones et al., 2013), multiple fractures, and deformations of limbs at birth.
4. Types IV to VI.
   a. Presentation less severe for these forms. Stature and growth may be mildly affected; fractures, if they occur, present later. Sclerae may be mildly affected or absent. Dentition is less commonly affected.

**C. Associated findings.**
1. Conductive hearing loss secondary to deformity of the small bones of the ear.
2. Platelet function is decreased due to defects in adhesion and clot retraction.
3. Corneal clouding and keratoconus, megalocornea (Jones et al., 2013).
4. Cardiac: floppy mitral valve.
5. Scoliosis developing later, progressing during puberty, sometimes resulting in severe deformity in adulthood. Loss of height may occur secondary to progressive spinal osteoporosis in adults.

**D. Diagnosis.**
1. Prenatal diagnosis is possible with ultrasonography and mutation analysis.
2. Radiographs: entire skeleton, including skull, hands, feet, and lateral spine.
   a. Type I: femurs are short, broad, or crumpled. Fibulas may be thin.
   b. Type II: femurs are short and deformed, but not crumpled. The long bones appear thin with bowing and deformations. Cranial bones are undermineralized, with wormian bones.
3. Ultrasound of brain, heart, and kidneys.
4. Detailed family history, including measurements of family members.
5. Chromosomal study confirming genetic mutation on 17q21 and 17q22.1.

**E. Treatment.**
1. Depending on the type of osteogenesis, treatment will vary extensively. Type I patients may require little or no treatment, whereas type II patients may die before any treatment is begun. Types III and IV are the most complex, requiring intensive support. Treatment is centered around minimizing pain and prevention of future fractures.
   a. Initial treatment of fractures is aimed toward alignment of bones to avoid deformity, comfort measures, prevention of further deformity, optimizing function following healing, and prevention of further fractures.

b. Laxity of ligaments and previous fracture abnormalities complicate the healing process.
c. Lightweight splints or braces provide the first-line treatment; depending on previous bone damage, surgical procedures may be necessary to provide strengthening and support.
d. Administration of bisphosphonates to increase bone density and decrease fracture has been suggested (Rimoin and Tiller, 2012).

2. Early intervention for hearing loss is essential for development of language and later learning.
3. Dentition may be difficult or delayed; these children are more prone to cavities. Ongoing examination and treatment is vital.
4. Scoliosis may progress quickly for those nearing puberty—bracing is often ineffective. Early surgical fusion may provide the best option for treatment.
5. If a diagnosis has been made prenatally, operative delivery to avoid fractures and intracranial bleeding is recommended.

### Achondroplasia

**A. Incidence and etiology.**

1. Achondroplasia occurs with a frequency of 1 in 25,000 live births (Rimoin and Tiller, 2012).
   a. Most common skeletal dysplasia in humans (Lewanda et al., 2006).
2. Defect has an autosomal dominant inheritance pattern. Eighty percent are sporadic occurrences of *FGFR3* (fibroblast growth factor receptor 3), representing a new mutation on chromosome 4p16.3 (Rimoin and Tiller, 2012).
   a. New mutations occur in the father's sperm and are associated with advanced paternal age (Lewanda et al., 2006).
   b. Transmitted as a fully penetrant autosomal dominant trait; each person who inherits the mutant gene will show the condition (Rimoin and Tiller, 2012).

**B. Clinical presentation.**

1. General: small stature. Small at birth, with increasingly apparent growth deficiency secondary to failure of endochondral ossification.
2. Craniofacial: megalocephaly, small foramen magnum, low nasal bridge, flat midface, short flat nose with broad tip, anteverted nares, long philtrum, hypotelorism (Jones et al., 2013).
3. Musculoskeletal: short limbs, lumbar lordosis, mild thoracolumbar kyphosis, short tubular bones, vertebral anomalies, short trident hand, hyperextensible joints, shortened upper limbs, and flexion contractures at elbows.

**C. Associated findings.**

1. Mild hypotonia, especially in the trunk and extremities, with delayed milestones.
2. Bowing of the legs after ambulation has started.
3. Orthodontic problems related to maxillary hypoplasia.
4. Stenosis of the magnum and spine leading to compression of the upper cord and resultant symptoms of apnea, growth delays, hydrocephalus, quadriparesis, and sudden death.
5. Upper airway is often small, leading to obstructive apnea, snoring, and serous otitis media (Rimoin and Tiller, 2012).

**D. Diagnosis.**

1. Chromosomal studies to confirm mutation on 4p16.3 chromosome.
2. Diagnosis is confirmed for achondroplasia through radiographic survey: iliac bones are short and round, lumbar vertebrae have short pedicles and scalloping, long bones have mildly flared metaphyses and are shortened.

**E. Treatment.**

1. Infants with known achondroplasia must be closely monitored for developmental delay, hypotonia, and abnormal growth patterns.
2. Unsupported sitting is associated with development of kyphosis. Infants should not be allowed to be carried in flexed positions before trunk muscle strength is adequate (Rimoin and Tiller, 2012). Most infants lose kyphosis and develop lumbar lordosis when ambulation begins.
3. Hydrocephalus may develop within the first 2 years of life. Radiologic imaging of the skull as a baseline is recommended for monitoring; monthly head circumference should be obtained and plotted to determine abnormal growth.

4. Obstructive apnea may represent a serious threat. Treatment may consist of tonsillectomy or adenoidectomy. Evaluation for foramen magnum stenosis should be done.
5. Treatment for severe bowing of the legs is often deferred until full growth has occurred. Osteotomies provide needed corrections (Jones et al., 2013).
6. Close monitoring of auditory performance is needed as shortened eustachian tubes may lead to middle ear infections and resultant hearing loss. Many infants require placement of tympanic membrane tubes.
7. Dental crowding is frequently encountered, requiring removal of one or more teeth.
8. Obesity develops toward late childhood and should be monitored closely.

## Specific Neural Tube Defects

See Chapter 34.

## Developmental Dysplasia of the Hip

A wide spectrum of abnormalities that affect the femoral head and acetabulum.

**A. Incidence and etiology.**

1. Defect occurs in 11.5 per 1000 live births, frank dislocations occurring in 1 to 2 per 1000 (White and Goldberg, 2012). Dislocations are described as syndromic or typical.
2. Syndromic dislocations are associated with neuromuscular or dysmorphic conditions. These defects occur in either week 12 or 18 of gestation, and are associated with arthrogryposis and myelodysplasia (White and Goldberg, 2012).
3. Typical dislocations present in healthy infants in prenatal or perinatal period.
4. Risk factors include female gender (19 per 1000), positive family history, and breech presentation.
5. In 60% of infants the left hip is affected, in 20% the right hip is affected, and in 20% both hips (White and Goldberg, 2012).
6. Frank breech positioning with hips flexed and knees bent increases risk of dislocation.
7. Etiology is multifactorial; interaction of genetic and environmental factors is considered to be causative.
8. Ligamentous laxity secondary to circulating maternal hormone (relaxin) exerts an effect, resulting in hip dislocation. Familial ligamentous laxity has also been described.

**B. Clinical presentation.**

1. The defect is considered a deformation anomaly. A full range of severity from a lax dislocatable hip to a nonreducible dislocation (Lashley, 2005).
2. Not all dislocated hips are present at birth.
3. Not all dislocated hips present at birth are present in the newborn period.
4. Despite newborn screening, 1 in 50,000 children will have a dislocated hip detected at 18 months or greater of age (White and Goldberg, 2012).
5. Anatomic changes are minimal in the neonate. As the hip becomes permanently dislocated, pathologic changes of the acetabulum, femoral head, hip capsule joints, and ligaments can occur. End result is degenerative changes in femoral head and acetabulum.
6. Physical examination will demonstrate limitations in adduction, apparent shortening of the affected femur, and extra skinfolds.

**C. Associated findings.**

1. Associated with other postural adductus deformities such as torticollis, talipes equino varus, and metatarsus deformities.
2. A strong correlation with Larsen's syndrome (multiple joint dislocations) exists (Jones et al., 2013).
3. Unilateral defects often have secondary problems with limb-length inequality, ipsilateral knee deformity, scoliosis, and disturbances in gait.

**D. Diagnosis.**

1. Physical tests are aimed at determining if the femoral head is fixed in the acetabulum. Tests should be repeated at intervals within the first year of life as a dislocation may not be demonstrated for several months following delivery.
   a. Barlow's test: attempts to dislocate or subluxate a located, but unstable hip.
   b. Ortolani test: determines if femoral head is dislocated laterally.

c. If the dislocation is a fixed type of lesion, Barlow's and Ortolani tests are not helpful as the femoral head is locked outside of the acetabulum. Diagnosis is made by palpation of the femoral head posteriorly (Smith, 2012).
d. Galeazzi sign: presence of asymmetrical thigh and/or buttock folds.

2. Radiographs are helpful but are difficult to interpret before 4 to 5 months of age secondary to the high percentage of cartilage in newborn infants.
   a. Ultrasound screening of the cartilaginous femoral head and acetabulum has become common, with sensitivity for detection of over 90% (Lashley, 2005).

**E. Treatment.**

1. Following delivery, unstable hips must be monitored closely. A percentage of unstable hips will stabilize, whereas others progress to subluxation or dislocation. The outcome of hip stability cannot be predicted: all newborns with clinical hip instability should be treated.
2. Initial goal of treatment is reduction of the displaced femoral head and support of acetabular and femoral head growth. Reduction and stability of the femoral head are needed for normal growth and development of the hip joint.
3. For children 0 to 6 months of age, infants with reducible hip abnormalities are treated with the Pavlik harness (Fig. 35-4). The Pavlik harness is the most commonly used device to prevent adduction while allowing flexion and abduction. Length of treatment is dependent on the age of presentation. The harness encourages deepening and stability of the acetabulum. Progress is judged by serial physical examinations and ultrasonography. Treatment is successful in 90% of patients (White and Goldberg, 2012).
4. For those infants for whom harnessing is not effective or the lesion is fixed, surgical intervention with subsequent spica casting.
5. Ongoing developmental assessment of these infants is needed to monitor for secondary deformities.
6. Parents play a pivotal part in the success in management of harnessing therapy. It is vital for parents to have a clear understanding of the deformity and plan for care.

## Talipes Equinovarus

Developmental deformity of the hindfoot, resulting from an arrest in embryonic development in weeks 6 to 8 of gestation.

**A. Incidence and etiology.**

1. Defect occurs in 1 per 1000 live births (Cooperman and Thompson, 2011).
2. Clubfoot is bilateral in 50% of cases, with males affected twice as often as females.
3. Classified as congenital, teratogenic, or positional (Cooperman and Thompson, 2011).
4. The cause of congenital clubfoot is unknown.

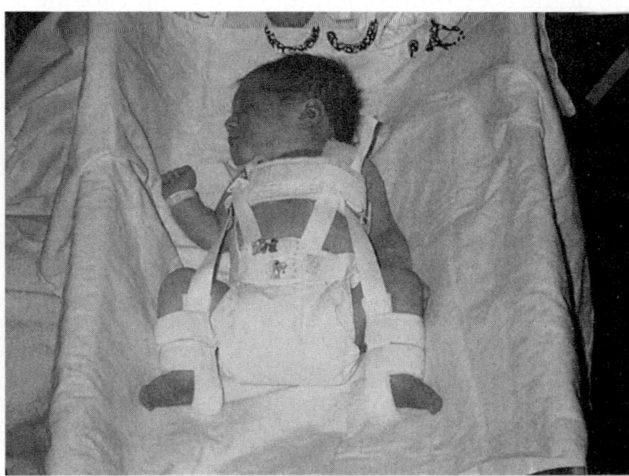

FIGURE 35-4 ■ Infant with dislocated hips in a Pavlik harness. (Courtesy Jane Deacon, RNC, MS, NNP, The Children's Hospital, Denver, Colorado.)

a. Causative factors are thought to be multifactorial, with strong influence from single autosomal dominant gene (Cooperman and Thompson, 2011).
b. Extrinsic causes: related to changes within the uterine environment, uterine abnormalities, oligohydramnios, and effects of uterine pressure during critical periods of development.
c. Neural origin: neuromuscular pathologic conditions, resulting in muscle fibrosis, shortening of muscles, and development of contractures.

5. Within affected families, recurrence rates are 3% for subsequent siblings and 20% to 30% for offspring of affected parents (Cooperman and Thompson, 2011).

**B. Clinical presentation.**

1. Classic deformity presents with numerous anatomic deformities. Clinically, the foot has a medial crease, with toes pointing toward midline; the sole of the foot is angulated medially; and the hindfoot is plantar flexed (White and Goldberg, 2012) (Fig. 35-5).
   a. The calf and foot of the clubfoot are smaller than the contralateral side.
   b. Infants may demonstrate dysplasia of bones, muscles, tendons, cartilage, skin, and neurovascular tissues distal to the knee of the affected extremity (White and Goldberg, 2012).
   c. Weight bearing is not possible secondary to position of the foot.
   d. Postural clubfoot presents without deep medial creasing and minimal to no calf atrophy.

**C. Associated anomalies.**

1. Deformity is associated with Smith–Lemli–Opitz, Larsen's, Freeman–Sheldon, and Poland's syndromes. These arthrogrypotic or neuromuscular defects result in rigid deformity with absence of skin creases, suggesting early in-utero involvement. These defects fail to improve without operative strategies.
2. Congenital hip dysplasia, neural tube defects, particularly myelomeningocele.

**D. Diagnosis.**

1. Physical examination and manipulation of the foot through range of motion.
2. Anteroposterior and lateral radiographs are helpful, assist with diagnosis of other bony abnormalities.

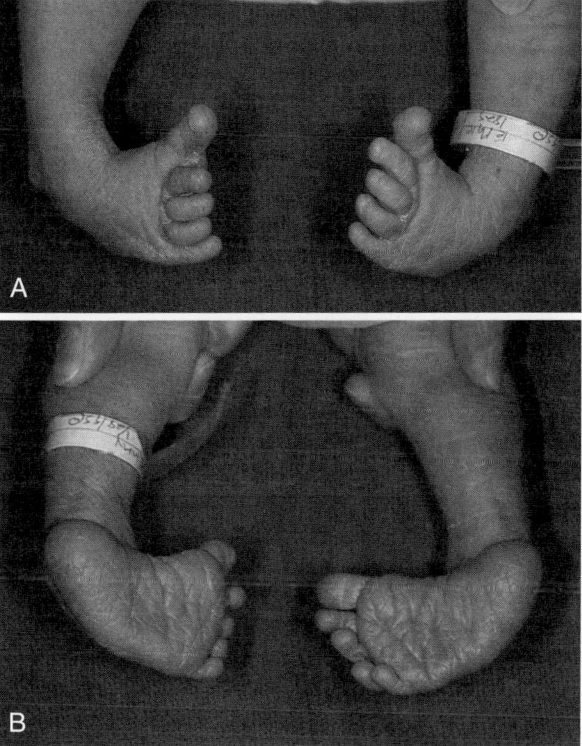


FIGURE 35-5 ■ Bilateral talipes equinovarus. Note structural deformity of hind part of foot. (Courtesy Jane Deacon, RNC, MS, NNP, The Children's Hospital, Denver, Colo.)

**E. Treatment.**

1. All clubfoot deformities should be evaluated by a pediatric orthopedist.
2. Depending on the lesion, operative and nonoperative methods are used to treat clubfoot deformities. Initial treatment for all congenital clubfoot is nonoperative; early treatment is more successful secondary to pliability of tissues and resilience to immobilization.
   a. Manipulation, serial casting, and taping are first-line treatment, lasting for 3 to 6 months. Failure to achieve clinical and radiographic correction by 3 months of age may indicate the need for surgical correction (Cooperman and Thompson, 2011).
   b. Untreated clubfoot results in development of degenerative changes in foot joints. Long-term results of early surgical correction have yielded poor results with recurrence rate approaching 15% (White and Goldberg, 2012).
   c. Nonoperative treatment consisting of casting, augmented with percutaneous tenontotomy and occasionally tendon transfer, appears to provide some success. Recurrences of the deformity are common and require further casting or bracing (White and Goldberg, 2012).
3. Parents must be educated as to the importance of their role in ongoing treatment as adherence to prescribed therapy is mandatory for a positive outcome.

## Polydactyl

**A. Incidence and etiology.**

1. Inherited as an autosomal dominant trait. Occurs in 2 per 1000 live births (Cooperman and Thompson, 2011). Approximately 30% of affected infants will have a positive family history.
2. Incidence is common: anomaly results from a duplication error in which a stimulus induces excessive limb bud formation.

**B. Clinical findings.**

1. Commonly involves the ulnar aspect of the hand; affected digits are often incomplete and lack muscular development. Defects are often bilateral (Fig. 35-6).
2. Abnormalities are divided into three classifications: soft tissue mass connected by a tissue pedicle; partial duplication involving the phalanges; and complete duplication of the digit with bony formation (Moore and Persaud, 2013).

**C. Associated findings.**

1. The anatomic placement of the digit varies and is associated with genetic syndromes.
   a. Preaxial or duplicate thumbs occur most commonly as an isolated lesion. Defect has been associated with Holt–Oram, Fanconi, and Ellis–van Creveld syndromes.
   b. Triphalangeal thumb; also referred to as a thumbless, five-fingered hand. Defect is associated with trisomies 13 and 15, and Blackfan–Diamond and Fanconi syndromes.

**D. Diagnosis.**

1. Physical examination.
2. Radiologic examination to identify bony defects.

**E. Treatment.**

1. Treatment is dependent on defect.
2. Therapy is aimed toward preservation of function and motion, as well as provision of cosmetic remedy.
3. Education of parents as to the risks for recurrence and associated syndromes is essential.

# DEFORMATION ABNORMALITIES

## Amniotic Band Syndrome

**A. Incidence and etiology.**

1. Amniotic band sequence occurs in 1 in 1200 live-born infants (Moore and Persaud, 2013).
2. Etiology is primarily idiopathic, generally a sporadic event in an otherwise normal family, with little risk of recurrence. Exceptions are presumed to occur secondary to trauma. Secondary to amnion rupture, strands of amnion encircle developing structures (Jones et al., 2013).

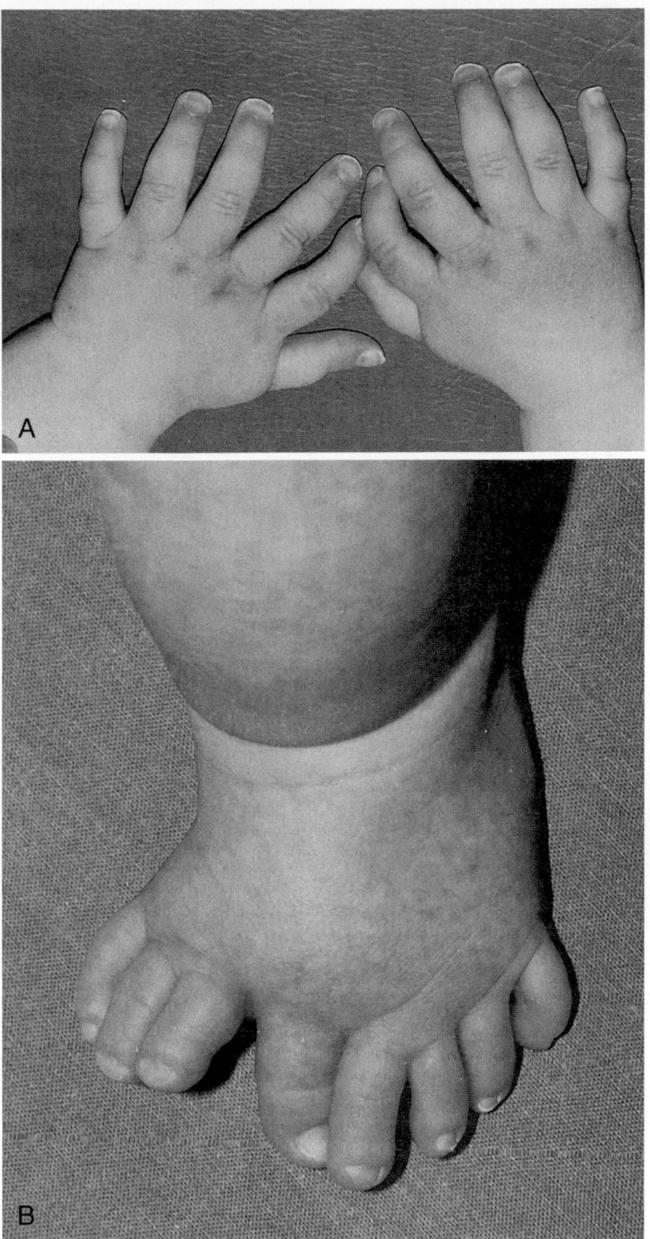


FIGURE 35-6 ■ Polydactyly of hands (**A**) and feet (**B**). This condition results from formation of one or more extra digital rays during the embryonic period. (Courtesy Dr. A.E. Chudley, Department of Pediatrics and Child Health, University of Manitoba, Children's Hospital, Winnipeg, Manitoba, Canada.)

**a.** Defects are dependent on the degree of entanglement, timing of insult, and the body part affected.

**B. Clinical findings.**

**1.** Constriction bands commonly involve the distal portion of limbs, resulting in annular constrictions, pseudosyndactyly, intrauterine amputations, and umbilical cord constriction (Jones et al., 2013) (Fig. 35-7).

**a.** Deformational defects result secondary to the primary insult.

(1) Loss of fetal movement can occur following tethering of a limb, resulting in foot or hand abnormalities.

(2) Constraint deformities result from a lack of amniotic fluid.

(3) Neurologic defects distal to the defect may occur.

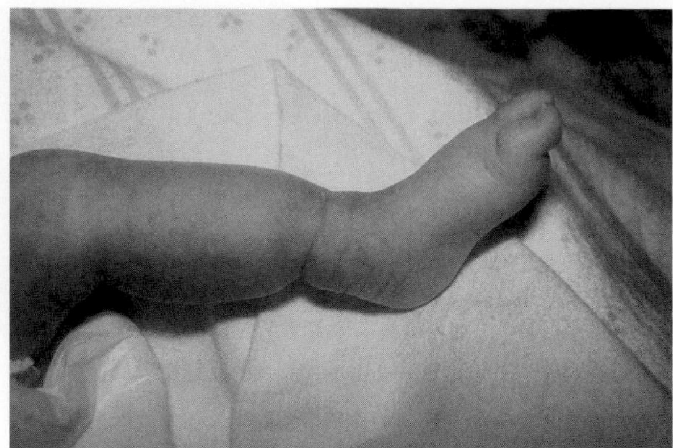

FIGURE 35-7 ■ Amniotic band constriction of lower leg. (Courtesy Jane Deacon, RNC, MS, NNP, The Children's Hospital, Denver, Colo.)

(4) Defect may involve veins, arteries, and nerves, compromising circulation and growth of affected extremities.

C. **Associated findings.**
1. Clubfeet occurs in 12% to 56% of affected infants. Treatment may be difficult owing to the rigid position and paralysis secondary to nerve damage.
2. Angular deformity, bone dysplasia, pseudarthrosis, and anterolateral bowing of the tibia may occur secondary to deep constriction bands in extremities.
3. Syndactyly, brachydactyly.
4. Cranial vault defects.
5. If amniotic fluid has been leaking, features of oligohydramnios deformation may occur (Jones et al., 2013).

D. **Diagnosis.**
1. No one feature consistently occurs as this is a disruption sequence abnormality. No two infants will present with exactly the same defect.
   a. Physical examination, including vascular supply, joint function.
   b. Examination of the placenta for aberrant bands or strands of amnion, or rolled-up remnants of amnion at the placental base of the umbilical cord (Jones et al., 2013).
2. Radiographs assist with definition and classification of defect.

E. **Treatment.**
1. Dependent on anatomic position, associated abnormalities.
   a. If constriction is severe, early surgical relief is needed to preserve vascular, lymph, and nerve integrity.
   b. Deformities that pose no emergent threat are best repaired at ages 1 to 2 years. Repair may require a staged approach; repair is seldom completed in one surgery.
2. Genetic counseling is necessary to educate parents as to the rare likelihood of recurrence. The appearance of some defects is significantly severe as to discourage further pregnancies, and accurate diagnosis of these defects is essential.
3. Life expectancy is normal unless brain malformation or deep facial clefts are present.

## Talipes Calcaneovalgus

A. **Incidence and etiology.**
1. Thought to be a postural defect secondary to intrauterine positioning, characterized by marked dorsiflexion of the entire foot at the ankle joint (White and Goldberg, 2012).
2. Incidence of defect is estimated at 0.4 to 1 per 1000 births (White and Goldberg, 2012).
   a. More common following breech deliveries.
   b. Girls are affected more often than boys.

**B. Clinical findings.**
1. Dorsum of the foot is, or is easily, positioned directly apposed to the anterior aspect of the leg.
   a. Soft tissues of the dorsal and lateral aspects of the foot are often contracted, limiting plantar flexion and inversion (White and Goldberg, 2012).

**C. Associated findings.**
1. Increased association with hip dysplasia (White and Goldberg, 2012).
2. May occur with external rotation of the tibia, and posteromedial bowing of the tibia.

**D. Diagnosis.**
1. Physical examination provides the diagnosis for this condition.
   a. Reveals free mobility of the foot to passive manipulation.
   b. Hindfoot is in the dorsiflexed position so that the plantar aspect of the forefront is in line. Plantar flexion of the foot is limited.
2. Defect must be differentiated from congenital vertical talus, posteromedial bowing of the tibia, and neuromuscular abnormalities (Cooperman and Thompson, 2011).

**E. Treatment.**
1. Evaluation for hip dysplasia is essential; repeated examinations are needed.
2. Gentle stretching exercises, done with diaper changes, will usually resolve this positional deformity within 3 to 6 months (White and Goldberg, 2012).
3. Infrequently, serial casting may be required; rarely ankle–foot orthoses are needed.
4. Parents provide an active part in resolution of this condition and must be aware of the need for ongoing treatment and follow-up examinations.

## CONGENITAL METABOLIC PROBLEMS

The process by which the body converts food into energy is complex. Disturbances in these processes result in a wide array of medical problems. The following section reviews some of the more common inborn biochemical disorders that affect the newborn.

### Inborn Errors of Metabolism

**A. Incidence and etiology.**
1. Inborn errors of metabolism are genetic biochemical disorders in which the function of a protein is compromised, resulting in alteration of the structure or amount of the protein synthesized.
2. Gene mutations produce deficiencies in enzymes, cofactors, transport proteins, and cellular processes. Interruptions of any of the steps in the formation of the coenzyme can lead to disease (Cederbaum, 2012).
3. In newborns, the majority of conditions are inherited as autosomal recessive traits (Rezvani and Rezvani, 2011). The majority of mutations are inconsequential, but some mutations produce disease states that range from minor to severe.
   a. The majority of conditions are inherited as autosomal recessive traits (Rezvani and Rezvani, 2011).
4. Newborn metabolic diseases can be classified into three groups:
   a. Defects involving complex molecules: lysosomal storage diseases. Result from defective function of a catabolic hydrolase responsible for breaking down complex glycosaminoglycans and sphingolipids. These compounds accumulate intracellularly, and are not removed by maternal circulation. Symptoms are not generally evident at birth as pathologic metabolites accumulate slowly (Cederbaum, 2012).
   b. Disorders of fatty acid metabolism: defects concerning the intermediary metabolism of small molecules—glucose, lactate, amino acids, organic acids, and ammonia.
   c. Metabolic disorders in which there is insufficient generation of energy by mitochondrial machinery. This complex process involves problems in the manufacture of substrates, failure of delivery of substrates to the site of oxidation, the inability to break down fatty acids, or deficient function of mitochondrial respiratory pathway and energy-generating systems (Cederbaum, 2012).

**B. Clinical presentation.**

1. The fetus is afforded protection as the placenta effectively removes circulating toxins. The newborn appears normal at birth but may quickly present with life-threatening symptoms as the underlying metabolic defect is manifested.
2. Symptoms of inborn errors commonly include the following:
   - a. Metabolic encephalopathy: lethargy, changes in muscle tone, seizures, irritability, weak suck, and apnea.
   - b. Respiratory: tachypnea and apnea secondary to underlying metabolic acidosis and metabolic encephalopathy.
   - c. Gastrointestinal symptoms: vomiting secondary to protein intolerance, failure to gain weight despite adequate intake and formula changes.
   - d. Cardiac symptoms: cardiomyopathy, arrhythmias.
   - e. Hepatic symptoms: appear within the first 2 weeks of life. Jaundice: usually direct reacting associated with vomiting, diarrhea, poor weight gain, hepatomegaly, cataract formation, and hypoglycemia.
   - f. Unusual body or urinary odor. In phenylketonuria (PKU), infant's urine has a musty odor, whereas the urine of infants with maple syrup urine disease has a sweet odor secondary to isovaleric acidemia.
   - g. Ocular findings: cataracts, glaucoma, corneal clouding, and dislocated lenses.

**C. Diagnosis.**

1. The newborn presenting with deterioration represents an emergency state. Septic evaluation should be undertaken to rule out infectious etiology. Metabolic workup is undertaken when the newborn's symptoms no longer fits the expected pattern for sepsis. The goals of treatment are rapid identification, treatment, and prevention of major sequelae.
   - a. Mandatory screening of newborns: tandem mass spectrometry enables a single spot of blood to test for more than 40 inborn errors of metabolism. The only acutely presenting disorders not tested by expanded newborn screen include hyperammonemias and lactic acidosis (Cederbaum, 2012).
     - (1) All states require screening for PKU, hypothyroidism, and galactosemia.
     - (2) Expanded newborn screening is mandated by individual states.
     - (3) Collection of samples must be undertaken early (before 7 days of age) and repeated at prescribed intervals.

# DISORDERS OF METABOLISM

## Errors of Amino Acid Metabolism

### Phenylketonuria

**A. Incidence and etiology.**

1. PKU is the most common inborn error of amino acid metabolism that may result in mental retardation (Haldeman-Englert et al., 2012b).
   - a. Occurs in more frequently in whites, 1 per 10,000 live births (Thomas and Van Hove, 2012).
   - b. Gene location: chromosome 12q22-q24.1. Inherited as an autosomal recessive trait.
   - c. Results from a deficiency of the liver enzyme phenylalanine hydrolase to convert phenylalanine to tyrosine. It is the deficiency of this liver enzyme that is responsible for the development of brain disease.

**B. Clinical findings.**

1. Following birth, the infant ingesting breast milk or formula will experience a gradual and persistent increase in plasma phenylalanine levels. Early symptoms include vomiting, poor feedings, hyperactivity, and irritability. Untreated PKU will result in severe mental retardation, hyperactivity, and seizures.
2. After 6 months of age, developmental delays are evident; seizures, infantile spasms, and musty-smelling urine (Cederbaum and Berry, 2012b). Untreated, the infant will demonstrate postnatal microcephaly.

**C. Diagnosis.**

1. Standard newborn screening is done with the infant receiving a regular diet.

2. DNA sequencing and mutational analysis are used to identify carriers in families, and assist with family genetic counseling (Cederbaum and Berry, 2012b).

D. **Treatment.**

1. Therapy consists of a low-protein diet and use of special amino acid–containing formula that does not have phenylalanine.
2. Parents must be counseled to understand the importance of continued dietary restrictions. A phenylalanine exchange system that allows for normal daily utilization of foods containing phenylalanine while maintaining safe plasma phenylalanine levels is essential.

**Maple Syrup Urine Disease**

A. **Incidence and etiology.**

1. Maple syrup urine disease (MSUD) is a rare inborn error in 1 of 200,000 live births that is caused by a disturbance in the metabolism of leucine, isoleucine, and valine. The end result of this failure is an elevation of branched-chain amino acids (BCAAs) (Cederbaum and Berry, 2012a).
   a. Exception: Pennsylvania Mennonites, in whom frequency is 1 in 358 (Cederbaum and Berry, 2012a).
2. Inherited as an autosomal recessive trait. Males and females equally affected.

B. **Clinical findings.**

1. Infants are usually well at the time of delivery, but after 2 to 3 days of feedings, infants demonstrate poor feeding and lethargy. The infant worsens, with high-pitched cry and hypotonia, eventually becoming obtunded and lapsing into a coma and death unless medical intervention is provided.
2. Odor of maple syrup is evident on breath, in urine and feces, and in saliva.

C. **Diagnosis.**

1. Laboratory findings include metabolic acidosis, ketonuria. Elevation of plasma BCAAs leucine, isoleucine, and valine (Cederbaum and Berry, 2012b).
2. Standard metabolic screening.
3. Molecular diagnosis may be useful in target populations.

D. **Treatment.**

1. Initial therapy in the acute crisis includes parenteral nutrition modified to be BCAA-free and insulin therapy to manage catabolic stress. Peritoneal dialysis has also been utilized to decrease circulating plasma BCAAs.
   a. For those infants treated within 7 days of life, incidence of mental retardation is diminished. Delays beyond this time result in significant IQ deficiencies, with spastic diplegia or quadriplegia (Cederbaum and Berry, 2012a).
2. Long-term management requires a special formula devoid of BCAAs. The intake of formula must be carefully monitored. Supplemental isoleucine and valine may be needed.
3. The long-term management of these infants requires that parents are vigilant in the provision of the diet and the need for follow-up.

## Errors of Carbohydrate Metabolism

**Galactosemia.** Defects in the enzyme involved with the metabolism of galactose may result in the development of galactosemia.

A. **Incidence and etiology.**

1. The condition is caused by a nearly total deficiency of galactose 1-phosphate uridyltransferase (GALT).
2. Enzymes involved in the galactose metabolic pathway are responsible for the conversion of galactose to glucose in the liver. The most common enzymatic deficiency is GALT (Cederbaum and Berry, 2012b).
   a. Lactose is a disaccharide composed of galactose and glucose—deficiency of GALT enzyme blocks conversion, so infants are unable to metabolize lactose.
3. Incidence is 1 in 40,000 live births (Thomas and Van Hove, 2012).
4. Inherited as an autosomal recessive condition (Cederbaum and Berry, 2012b).

**B. Clinical findings.**

1. Infant appears normal at birth; once milk feeding begins, galactose and other metabolites accumulate in blood and urine. Symptoms occur quickly—vomiting, diarrhea, jaundice, failure to thrive, hepatomegaly, hypoglycemia.
2. Jaundice; presenting in the first weeks of life, persisting.
3. Later signs: multiorgan toxicity, with liver disease that progresses to cirrhosis, portal hypertension, splenomegaly, ascites, sometimes progressing to renal Fanconi syndrome.
   a. *Escherichia coli* sepsis occurs as a complication in 50% of the affected infants (Thomas and Van Hove, 2012).

**C. Associated findings.**

1. Speech defects—especially expressive speech, delayed speech, language and learning disabilities.
2. Behavioral disorders, short attention span.
3. Infertility: ovarian failure and amenorrhea and hypogonadism.
4. Cataracts developing within 2 months of birth, reverse with treatment.

**D. Diagnosis.**

1. Newborn screening demonstrating absence of the enzyme necessary for breakdown and metabolism of galactose.
2. Laboratory: serum blood galactose levels, red blood cell galactose 1-phosphate levels, and elevated urine galactitol. Albuminuria, hyperbilirubinemia, elevated alanine transaminase (ALT) and aspartate transaminase (AST) levels, elevated prothrombin time.
   a. Positive reducing substances in urine are present in severe hypergalactosemia.

**E. Treatment.**

1. Initiation of a lactose-free diet is essential. This reflects a lifelong change; parents must receive appropriate counseling to ensure long-term success. Galactose 1-phosphate levels in red blood cells are monitored.
2. With treatment, intellectual development may be normal or near normal. But even for infants who receive treatment, rates of mental retardation remain higher.
3. Communication problems continue throughout life despite speech therapy.

## Errors of Fatty Acid Oxidation

### Medium-Chain Acyl-Coenzyme A Dehydrogenase Deficiency

**A. Incidence and etiology.**

1. Defect involves an abnormality in the enzyme that encourages mitochondrial beta oxidation of fatty acids.
   a. Fatty acid oxidation provides energy during periods of caloric deprivation. When normal metabolism is disrupted, the quickly depleted glycogen stores lead to hypoglycemia.
2. Medium-chain acyl-coenzyme A dehydrogenase (MCAD) deficiency is the most commonly occurring fatty acid oxidation disorder, occurring in 1 in 20,000 infants (Cederbaum and Berry, 2012b).
   a. MCAD gene has been cloned and sequenced, several mutations have been isolated.
   b. A single mutation accounts for more than 90% of mutant alleles (Lashley, 2005). Inherited as an autosomal recessive trait.

**B. Clinical findings.**

1. Though severe enzyme deficiencies may manifest within the first days of life, presentation of symptoms is frequently in later infancy: following an infection, the infant experiences anorexia, vomiting, dehydration, lethargy, and hypoglycemia associated with seizures.
   a. High mortality rates are common with initial episodes. Thought to be causative in sudden infant death syndrome in 25% to 30% of cases (Cederbaum and Berry, 2012b).
2. Symptoms may mimic Reye's syndrome, death occurring from brain edema.

**C. Associated findings.**

1. Carnitine deficiency develops as a result of excess excretion of acylcarnitine.
2. In infants who die suddenly and have fat accumulation in the liver, suggests a disorder of fatty acid oxidation.

**D. Diagnosis.**

1. Chorionic villus sampling, amniocentesis, DNA analysis.
2. Newborn screening.
3. Laboratory studies: hypoglycemia, absence of moderate to large ketones in urine. Plasma ammonium values may be increased, AST and ALT may also be elevated.
4. MCAD enzyme may be assayed in cultured skin fibroblasts (Cederbaum and Berry, 2012a).

**E. Treatment.**

1. Symptomatic hypoglycemia is treated aggressively. Intravenous glucose and caloric support must be provided quickly.
2. Prevention of hypoglycemia is the cornerstone of therapy; avoid free fatty acid mobilization during times of catabolic stress and relative insulin deficiency.
3. Limiting fasting to no more than 12 hours, particularly if infant is experiencing an associated illness.
4. Diagnosis and treatment of associated carnitine deficiency.
5. Infants having MCAD often have a sibling who has died of sudden infant death syndrome. Accurate diagnosis and genetic counseling are essential.

## REFERENCES


Cederbaum, S.: Introduction to metabolic and biochemical genetic disease. In C.A. Gleason and S.U. Devaskar (Eds.): *Avery's diseases of the newborn* (9th ed.). Philadelphia, 2012, Elsevier Saunders, pp. 209–257.

Cederbaum, S. and Berry, G.T.: Inborn errors of carbohydrate, ammonia, amino acid, and organic acid metabolism. In C.A. Gleason and S.U. Devaskar (Eds.): *Avery's diseases of the newborn* (9th ed.). Philadelphia, 2012a, Elsevier Saunders, pp. 215–238.

Cederbaum, S. and Berry, B.: Lysosomal storage, peroxisomal, and glycosylation disorders and Smith-Lemli-Opitz syndrome in the neonate. In C.A. Gleason and S.U. Devaskar (Eds.): *Avery's diseases of the newborn* (9th ed.). Philadelphia, 2012b, Elsevier Saunders, pp. 239–257.

Cooperman, D. and Thompson, G.: Neonatal orthopedics. In R.J. Martin, A.A. Fanaroff, and M.C. Walsh (Eds.): *Fanaroff and Martin's neonatal-perinatal medicine: Diseases of the fetus and newborn* (9th ed.). St. Louis, 2011, Elsevier Mosby, pp. 1771–1797.

*Dorland's illustrated medical dictionary* (31st ed.). Philadelphia, 2007, Elsevier Saunders.

Graham, J: Aplasia cutis congenita. In J. Graham (Ed.): *Smith's recognizable patterns of human deformation* (3rd ed.). Philadelphia, 2007, Elsevier Saunders, pp. 235–239.

Haldeman-Englert, C., Saitta, S., and Zackai, E.: Evaluation of the dysmorphic infant. In C.A. Gleason and S.U. Devaskar (Eds.): *Avery's diseases of the newborn* (9th ed.). Philadelphia, 2012a, Elsevier Saunders, pp. 186–195.

Haldeman-Englert, C., Saitta, S., and Zackai, E.: Specific chromosome disorders in newborns. In C.A. Gleason and S.U. Devaskar (Eds.): *Avery's diseases of the newborn* (9th ed.). Philadelphia, 2012b, Elsevier Saunders, pp. 196–208.

Jones, K.L., Jones, M.C., and Casanelles, M.D.C.: *Smith's recognizable patterns of human malformation* (7th ed.). Philadelphia, 2013, Elsevier Saunders.

Kalhan, S. and Devaskar, S.: Metabolic and endocrine disorders. In R.J. Martin, A.A. Fanaroff, and M.C. Walsh (Eds.): *Fanaroff and Martin's neonatal-perinatal medicine: Diseases of the fetus and newborn* (9th ed.). St. Louis, 2011, Elsevier Mosby, pp. 1598–1599.

Lashley, F.: Birth defects and congenital anomalies. In *Clinical genetics in nursing practice* (3rd ed.). New York, 2005, Springer Verlag, pp. 103, 107, 111, 115, 147–160.

Lewanda, A., Boyadjiev, S., and Jabs, E.: Dysmorphology: Genetic syndromes and associations. In J. McMillan, R. Feigin, C. DeAngelis, and M. Jones (Eds.): *Oski's pediatrics* (4th ed.). Philadelphia, 2006, Lippincott, Williams & Wilkins, pp. 2629–2669.

Matthews, A. and Robin, N.: Genetic disorders and malformations and inborn errors of metabolism. In S.L. Gardner, B.S. Carter, M. Enzman-Hines, and J.A. Hernandez (Eds.): *Merenstein and Gardner's Handbook of neonatal intensive care* (7th ed.). St. Louis, 2011, Elsevier Mosby, pp. 787–811.

McLean, S.D.: Congenital anomalies. In M.G. MacDonald, M.M.K. Seshia, and M.D. Mullett (Eds.) *Avery's neonatology: Pathophysiology and management of the newborn* (6th ed.). Philadelphia, 2005, Lippincott, Williams & Wilkins, pp. 892–913.

Moore, K. and Persaud, T.: Human birth defects. In K. Moore, T. Persaud, and M.G. Torchia (Eds.): *The developing human: Clinically oriented embryology* (9th ed.). Philadelphia, 2013, Elsevier Saunders, pp. 471–500.

Murray, J.: Impact of the Human Genome Project on neonatal care. In C.A. Gleason and S.U. Devaskar (Eds.): *Avery's diseases of the newborn* (9th ed.). Philadelphia, 2012, Elsevier Saunders, pp. 173–179.

Parikh, A. and Wiesner, G.: Congenital anomalies. In R.J. Martin, A.A. Fanaroff, and M.C. Walsh (Eds.): *Fanaroff and Martin's neonatal-perinatal medicine: Diseases of the fetus and newborn* (9th ed.). St. Louis, 2011, Elsevier Mosby, pp. 531–550.

Rimoin, D. and Tiller, G.: Skeletal dysplasias and connective tissue disorders. In C.A. Gleason and S.U. Devaskar (Eds.): *Avery's diseases of the newborn* (9th ed.). Philadelphia, 2012, Elsevier Saunders, pp. 258–276.

Rezvani, I. and Rezvani, G.: An approach to inborn errors of metabolism. In R. Kliegman, B. Stanton, J. St. Gemell, et al. (Eds.): *Nelson textbook of pediatrics* (19th ed.). Philadelphia, 2011, Elsevier Saunders, pp. 416–418.

Smith, J.B.: Initial evaluation: History and physical examination of the newborn. In H.W. Taeusch, R.A. Ballard, and C.A. Gleason (Eds.): *Avery's diseases of the newborn* (9th ed.). Philadelphia, 2012, Elsevier Saunders, pp. 277–299.

Thomas, J. and Van Hove, J.: Inborn errors of metabolism. In W. Hay, M. Levin, R. Deterding, et al. (Eds.): *Current diagnosis & treatment: pediatrics* (21st ed.). New York, 2012, McGraw-Hill, pp. 1068–1069.

Tran, M. and Cohen, B.: Congenital and hereditary disorders of the skin. In C.A. Gleason and S.U. Devaskar (Eds.): *Avery's diseases of the newborn* (9th ed.). Philadelphia, 2012, Elsevier Saunders, pp. 1380–1381.

Blackburn, S.T.: *Maternal, fetal, and neonatal physiology:* (4th ed.). St. Louis, 2013, Elsevier Saunders.

White, K. and Goldberg, M.: Common neonatal orthopedic ailments. In C.A. Gleason and S.U. Devaskar (Eds.): *Avery's diseases of the newborn* (9th ed.). Philadelphia, 2012, Elsevier Saunders, pp. 1351–1361.

CHAPTER

# 36 Neonatal Dermatology

CATHERINE L. WITT

**OBJECTIVES**

1. Name three functions of the skin.
2. Describe two ways in which the skin of a newborn or preterm infant differs from that of an adult.
3. Identify three factors that affect the appearance of the neonate's skin.
4. Identify two nursing interventions that provide protection for the preterm infant's skin.
5. Recognize three common skin lesions that are normal variations in the newborn infant. Describe their appearance and treatment, if any.
6. Describe three common vascular lesions in the neonate, their appearance, and appropriate treatment.
7. Identify two syndromes associated with vascular lesions.
8. Evaluate two pigmented lesions occurring in the newborn infant and list implications associated with each.
9. Name two types of infectious skin lesions and select the appropriate treatment.

Careful assessment of the skin is an important element of the neonatal physical examination. The appearance of the skin gives the nurse important clues regarding gestational age, nutritional status, function of organs such as the heart and liver, and the presence of cutaneous or systemic disease. It is important for the clinician to be familiar with normal variances in the skin of the newborn infant as well as those variances that signify disease.

Proper care of the neonate's skin can directly affect mortality and morbidity, especially in the preterm infant. The skin is the first line of defense against infection. Proper skin care can protect the integrity of the skin and prevent breakdown.

## ANATOMY AND PHYSIOLOGY OF THE SKIN

**A. Anatomy of the skin—three main layers (Fig. 36-1).**

1. Epidermis: outermost layer, which functions as a barrier against outside penetration. The epidermis is subdivided into the following:
   a. Stratum corneum: outermost layer, consisting of closely packed dead cells that are consistently brushed off and replaced by lower levels of the epidermis. These cells are flatter and have thicker walls than other cells. The cells are held together by intracellular lipids, which aid in forming the protective barrier of the skin.
   b. Lower layers of epidermis: contain keratin-forming cells that create the outer layer of skin as well as melanocytes, which produce melanin, or pigment. Despite racial differences in pigmentation, the number of melanocytes in a given surface area of skin is the same (Paller and Mancini, 2011; Weston et al., 2007).
2. Dermis: directly under epidermis; 2 to 4 mm thick at birth. The dermis is composed of:
   a. Collagen and elastic fibers that connect the epidermis and dermis and provide the skin with the ability to stretch and then to return to normal shape.
   b. Blood vessels and nerves that carry sensations of heat, touch, pain, and pressure from the skin to the brain and provide protection against injury, infections, or other invasions.
   c. Sweat glands, sebaceous glands, and hair shafts.
3. Subcutaneous layer: fatty tissue functions as insulation, protection of internal organs, and calorie storage.

**B. Functions of the skin.**

1. Physical protection.
   a. Mechanical.

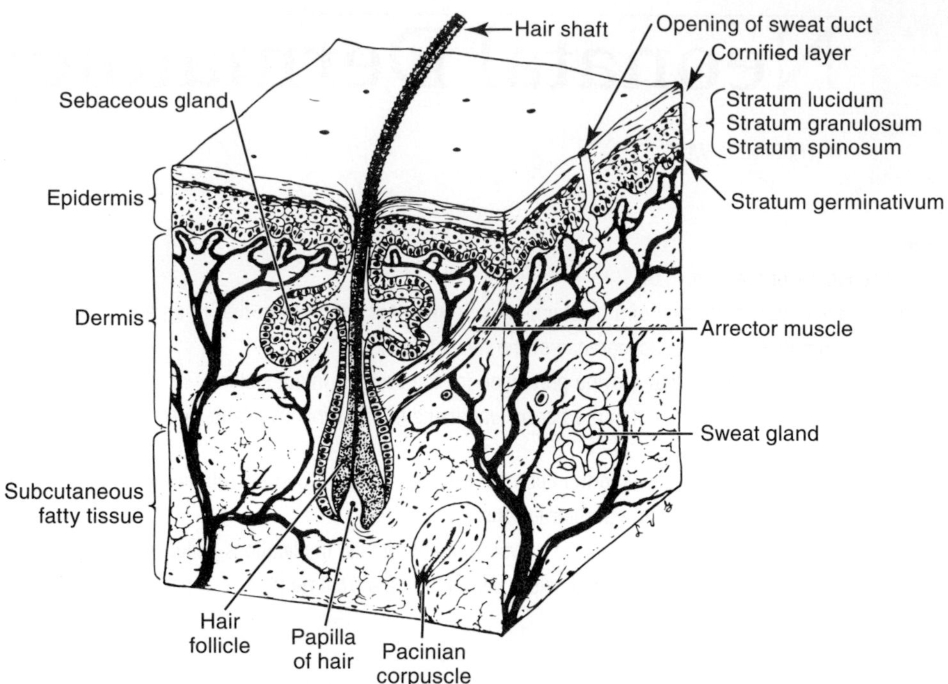


FIGURE 36-1 ■ Several layers and structures of human skin. (From Francis, C.C. and Martin, A.H.: *Introduction to human anatomy* [7th ed.]. St. Louis, 1975, Mosby.)

(1) Tightly packed, thick-walled cells, held together by intercellular lipids, provide a protective barrier against transepidermal water loss and external invasions.

(2) Process of constant sloughing and replacement of stratum corneum prevents colonization of the skin surface by bacteria and other organisms.

**b.** Chemical/bacterial.

(1) Acidic surface of skin (pH 5 to 6) provides defense against bacteria and other microorganisms (Percival et al., 2012).

(2) Production of melanin protects against damage from ultraviolet-light radiation.

**2.** Heat regulation.

**a.** Production and evaporation of sweat.

**b.** Dilation and constriction of blood vessels.

**c.** Insulation of body by subcutaneous fat.

**3.** Sense perception: heat, touch, pain, and pressure.

**C. Differences in newborn/preterm skin.**

**1.** Basic structure is same as that of the adult. The epidermis is nearly mature by 34 weeks of gestation (Dyer, 2013). Less mature neonates have less mature skin epidermis and dermis, and minimal subcutaneous fat.

**2.** Skin adaptation occurs rapidly during the first few weeks after birth. The full-term infant will achieve a stratum corneum that is structurally and functionally equivalent to the adult by approximately 2 weeks of age. The preterm infant will also experience accelerated skin maturity, although it may take as long as 4 to 8 weeks in the extremely preterm neonate (Dyer, 2013; Fluhr et al., 2011; Paller and Mancini, 2011). The acid mantle of the epidermis develops over 5 to 6 weeks, with the pH value decreasing from around 6.0 in the newborn to 5.1, which is comparable to adult levels (Fluhr et al., 2011).

**3.** The earlier the gestational age, the more thin and gelatinous is the skin, with fewer layers in the stratum corneum and a thinner dermis with fewer elastic fibers. Transepidermal water loss is inversely related to gestational age, and even at 4 weeks of age a 25-weeks-gestation infant has twice the transepidermal water loss as a term infant (Agren et al., 2006; Gilliam and Williams, 2008; Hammarlund and Sedin, 1979). Subcutaneous fat is accumulated predominantly during the third trimester.

a. Preterm babies have little fat, resulting in an inability to maintain body temperature and blood glucose level.
b. Brown fat, which is important for temperature regulation in the newborn infant, begins to differentiate during the seventh month of gestation (Loomis et al., 2008).

4. Immature skin is thinner and therefore more permeable.
   a. An infant, especially a preterm infant, quickly absorbs topically applied medications and chemicals (Blumer and Reed, 2011; Loomis et al., 2008, Paller and Mancini, 2011).
   b. Greater permeability allows for greater insensible water loss in the preterm infant.
   c. Higher surface area–body weight ratio also allows for greater absorption of chemicals and greater transepidermal water loss.
5. Fewer fibrils connect the dermis and epidermis, and they are more fragile in term and preterm skin than in the skin of an adult. The stratum corneum is thinner in the term and preterm infant. Risk of injury from tape, monitors, and handling is increased, especially in the preterm infant; this type of injury includes removal of the outermost layer of the dermis with removal of tape or electrodes (Ness et al., 2013; Sardesai et al., 2011).
6. Sweat glands are present at birth, but full adult functioning is not present until the second or third year of life. Although present in the preterm infant, sweat glands are immature and function poorly before 36 weeks of gestation (Gilliam and Williams, 2008).
   a. The newborn infant has limited ability to tolerate excessive heat.
   b. Vasodilation to increase heat loss can result in hypotension and dehydration caused by increased insensible water loss.

## CARE OF THE NEWBORN INFANT'S SKIN

A. **Term newborn infant.**
   1. Initial bath with water and a mild soap.
      a. Plain water or mild soaps with a neutral pH should be used for bathing neonates (Lavender et al., 2013).
      b. Safety of bacteriostatic soaps has not been determined. These products may be too harsh for the neonate's skin and may negatively affect normal skin colonization (Association of Women's Health, Obstetric and Neonatal Nurses [AWHONN], 2007).
      c. As soon as the body temperature is stable (>36.5° C [97.7° F]), it is advisable to bathe the healthy term infant to decrease the caregiver's risk of exposure to blood-borne pathogens. Standard Precautions, including the use of gloves, should be adhered to when handling the infant who has not been bathed after delivery and during any invasive procedure in which the caregiver may be exposed to body fluids (Dyer, 2013).
   2. Parents may prefer to give the first bath themselves.
   3. Vernix caseosa contains fats and proteins that protect the skin from the amniotic fluid and bacteria in utero, and is thought to aid in skin maturation after birth. Vernix insulates the stratum corneum and should not be removed during the initial bath (Dyer, 2013; Visscher et al., 2011).
   4. When possible, avoid puncturing the skin of babies with suspected maternal infections.
   5. Routine use of emollients is not recommended in the term infant. Creams and emollients that contain perfumes are drying and may irritate the infant's skin. Products that change the pH of the skin decrease the bacteriostatic properties. If cracking or fissures develop in the skin, a nonperfumed emollient such as white petrolatum may be used (AWHONN, 2007; Ness et al., 2013).

B. **Preterm infant.**
   1. Keep skin clean with water. Mild, nonalkaline soap may be used on soiled areas as needed; otherwise plain water is acceptable. Preterm infants should be bathed infrequently during the first 2 months of life to avoid excessive drying of the skin and to avoid overstimulation, stress, and fatigue (AWHONN, 2007).
   2. Handle infant gently and minimally to avoid trauma.
   3. Minimize use of tape and other adhesives as much as possible. Use care when removing tape to avoid stripping the epidermis (AWHONN, 2007; Sardesai et al., 2011).

a. Use of adhesive solvents is not recommended. Cotton balls soaked with warm water can be used effectively for removing tape and other adhesives.
b. Gelled adhesives and pectin-based barriers are good alternatives to tape, as removal causes less trauma to the skin (Ness et al., 2013).
c. Pectin or hydrocolloid layers applied before adhesives may protect the skin from damage when endotracheal tubes or catheters are secured (AWHONN, 2007).
d. Benzoin and other adhesive bonding agents form a strong bond between the adhesive and the epidermis, increasing the risk of stripping the epidermis when the adhesive is removed. Use of these agents with preterm infants should be avoided.

4. Increased permeability of the skin allows absorption of some medications and products such as alcohol and povidone–iodine (Pinsker et al., 2013). When these substances are used for an invasive procedure, it is recommended that they be removed completely with water as soon as possible to prevent absorption or chemical burns.
5. The skin should be disinfected before any invasive procedure. Although chlorhexidine gluconate has been shown to be more effective than other agents in reducing skin colonization, it has not been approved for use in infants less than 2 months of age. Chlorhexidine gluconate is available in single-use applicators that contain 70% alcohol but may be drying to the neonate's skin or cause burning or other injury (AWHONN, 2007; Garland et al., 2009; Stevens and Schulman, 2012).
6. Emollient creams that are free of preservatives and perfumes may be of benefit to the preterm infant as they decrease transepidermal water loss and skin breakdown when cracking, excessive dryness, or fissures are present (AWHONN, 2007; Lund and Kuller, 2007). Humidity at levels of 70% to 90% during the first week after birth reduces insensible water loss and evaporative heat loss in extremely low birth weight infants. Humidity should be gradually decreased to 50% after the first week. Transepidermal water loss in extremely low birth weight infants decreases after the first week after birth. Decreasing humidity to around 50% may improve skin barrier maturation (Agren et al., 2006).
7. Transparent adhesive dressings can be used over wounds and abrasions and to secure intravenous (IV) catheters and central lines (Lund and Kuller, 2007).

C. **Umbilical cord care.**

1. Sterile cutting of cord at delivery, rapid drying of umbilical cord, and keeping cord clean is the most effective way to prevent umbilical infections. The use of antimicrobial creams or ointments has not been shown to be more effective in preventing infection than keeping the cord clean and dry (Ness et al., 2013).
2. Some studies have suggested that chlorhexidine may be of benefit in cord care, particularly in circumstances in which infection risk is increased, although cord separation time may be lengthened (Mullany et al., 2013).
3. Bathing does not increase the rate of omphalitis or cause a delay in cord separation.
4. It is normal for the cord to appear slightly mucky, with small amounts of cloudy, mucus-like material at the junction of the cord and abdominal skin.
5. Omphalitis is characterized by serosanguineous drainage, inflammation of the surrounding tissues, and a foul odor. Poor feeding, lethargy, and fever may also be associated. Suspected omphalitis should be treated immediately with IV antibiotics.

## ASSESSMENT OF THE NEWBORN INFANT'S SKIN

A. **Factors affecting the appearance of the skin.**

1. Gestational age.
2. Postnatal age.
3. Nutritional status and hydration.
4. Racial origin.
5. Type and amount of available light.
6. Hemoglobin and bilirubin levels.
7. Environmental temperatures.
8. Oxygenation status.

**B. Definitions used to describe skin lesions (Paller and Mancini, 2011; Weston et al., 2007).**

1. Macule: a pigmented, flat spot that is visible but not palpable. Macules greater than 1 cm in diameter may be referred to as a patch.
2. Papule: a solid, elevated, palpable lesion, with distinct borders less than 1 cm in diameter.
3. Plaque: a solid, elevated, palpable lesion, with distinct borders, greater than 1 cm in size.
4. Nodule: a solid lesion, elevated with depth, up to 2 cm in size.
5. Tumor: a solid lesion, elevated with depth, greater than 2 cm in size.
6. Vesicle: an elevated lesion or blister filled with serous fluid and less than 1 cm in diameter.
7. Bulla: a fluid-filled lesion larger than 1 cm.
8. Pustule: a vesicle filled with cloudy or purulent fluid.
9. Petechiae: subepidermal hemorrhages, pinpoint in size. They do not blanch with pressure.
10. Ecchymosis: a large area of subepidermal hemorrhage.
11. Wheal: area of edema in the upper dermis, creating a palpable, slightly raised lesion.
12. Ulcer: erosion of skin with damage of the epidermis into the dermis. Will leave a scar after healing.

## COMMON SKIN LESIONS

**A. Normal variations in newborn skin.**

1. Cutis marmorata.
   a. Bluish mottling or marbling effect of the skin.
   b. Physiologic response to chilling caused by dilation of capillaries and venules.
   c. Disappears when infant is rewarmed.
   d. May be a sign of stress or overstimulation in newborn infant.
   e. Common in infants with trisomies 18 and 21.
   f. If condition persists in infants 6 months of age or older, it may be a symptom of hypothyroidism or a vascular abnormality such as cutis marmorata telangiectasia (Paller and Mancini, 2011).
2. Harlequin color change (Fig. 36-2).
   a. A difference in the amount of blood flow in the right and left sides of the body results in a sharply demarcated difference in color between one side and the other. This is most often seen in the dependent half of the body when the infant is lying on his or her side. When the infant's position is reversed, the color changes to the other side. This condition may also be seen when the infant is lying flat. It is most often visible in the trunk. It may last from a few seconds to a few minutes and changes with activity or changes in position.
   b. Caused by immaturity or temporary disturbance of the autonomic regulation of the cutaneous vessels. It is more common in preterm neonates.
3. Erythema toxicum (newborn rash) (Fig. 36-3).
   a. Small white or yellow pustules surrounded by an erythematous base (erythematous base is caused by histamine release) (Hussain et al., 2013; Lucky, 2008).
   b. Benign, found in up to 70% of newborn infants (Hussain et al., 2013).
   c. Seen in neonates and infants up to 3 months of age.
   d. Lesions come and go on various sites of face, trunk, and limbs, although they are never seen on the palms of the hands or soles of the feet.
   e. Cause unknown, but condition may be exacerbated by handling or by chafing from linen.
   f. Differential diagnosis: may resemble a staphylococcal infection. Diagnosis can be confirmed by smear of aspirated pustule showing numerous eosinophils.
   g. No treatment is necessary. Lotions or creams may exacerbate condition.
4. Milia (Fig. 36-4).
   a. Multiple yellow or pearly white papules about 1 mm in size; epidermal inclusion cysts composed of laminated, keratinous material. They occur on the brow, cheeks, and nose.
   b. Milia are observed in about 40% of term infants (Weston et al., 2007).
   c. No treatment is necessary. They resolve spontaneously during the first few weeks after birth.

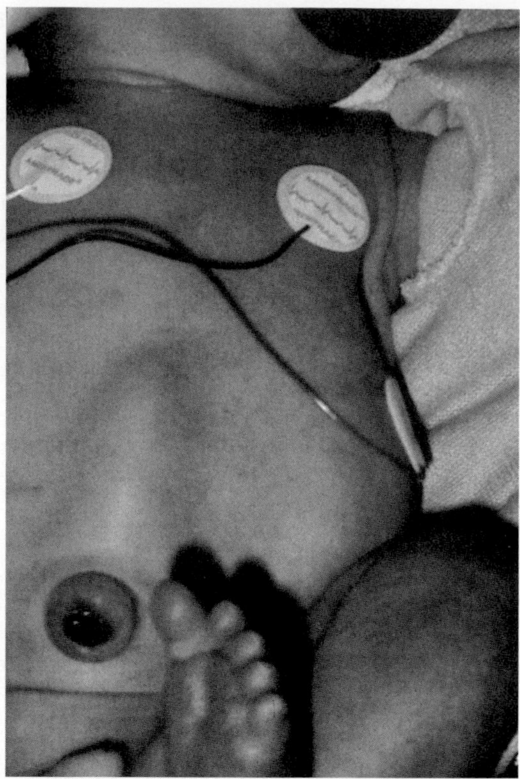

FIGURE 36-2 ■ Harlequin color change. (Courtesy Jane Deacon, RNC, M.S., NNP, The Children's Hospital, Denver, Colo.)

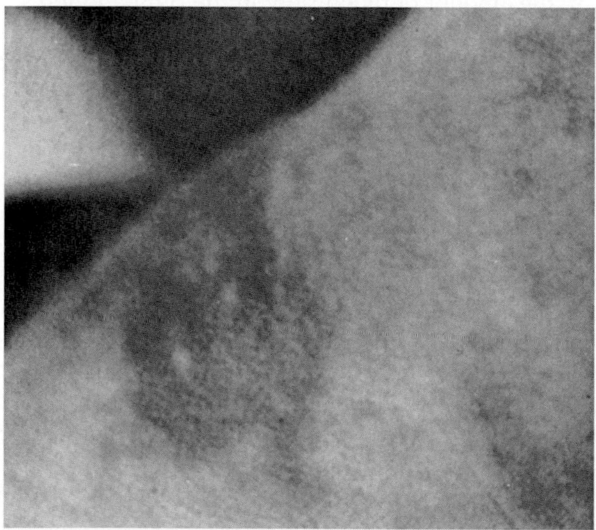

FIGURE 36-3 ■ Erythema toxicum. (Courtesy Jacinto Hernandez, M.D., The Children's Hospital, Denver, Colo.)

5. Epstein's pearls (Fig. 36-5).
   a. Oral counterpart of facial milia. They can be seen on the midline of the palate or on the alveolar ridges.
   b. Epstein's pearls occur in approximately 60% of neonates (Weston et al., 2007).
6. Sebaceous gland hyperplasia.

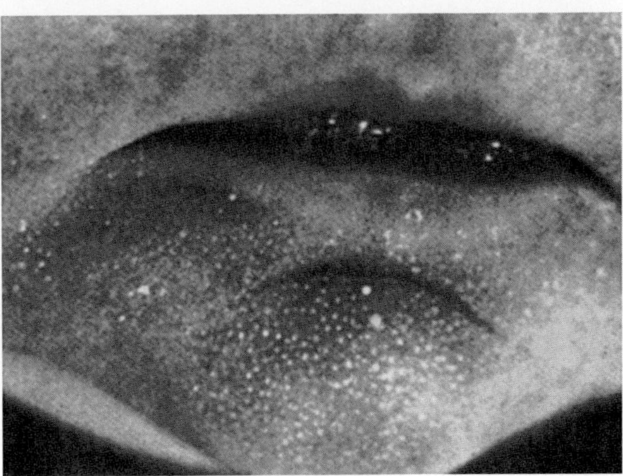

FIGURE 36-4 ■ Milia. (Courtesy Jacinto Hernandez, M.D., The Children's Hospital, Denver, Colo.)

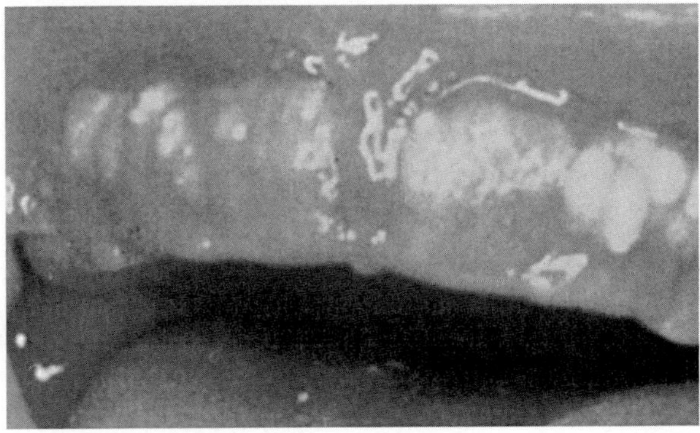

FIGURE 36-5 ■ Epstein's pearls. (Courtesy Jacinto Hernandez, M.D., The Children's Hospital, Denver, Colo.)

   a. Tiny (<0.5 mm) white or yellow papules found on the nose, cheeks, and upper lips of newborn infants.
   b. Common in term infants but rarely seen in preterm infants.
   c. Represent overactivity of the sebaceous follicles and are a manifestation of maternal androgen stimulation.
   d. They resolve without treatment within a few weeks.
7. Miliaria. Caused by occlusion of sweat ducts by keratin, resulting in retention of sweat. There are two main types of miliaria.
   a. Miliaria crystallina: clear, thin vesicles 1 to 2 mm in diameter that develop in the epidermal portion of the sweat glands. They are seen over the head, neck, and upper aspect of the trunk in newborn infants. Can be present at birth (Paller and Mancini, 2011).
   b. Miliaria rubra: commonly referred to as "prickly heat"; results from prolonged occlusion of pores, leading to release of sweat into the lower epidermis. Condition appears as pink or white papules and vesicles 2 to 4 mm in diameter, with an erythematous base. The lesions are generally found in the flexure areas, such as the neck, groin, and axillae, as well as on the face and the upper aspect of the chest.
8. Diaper dermatitis.
   a. May be caused by chafing from diapers, by prolonged contact with urine or feces, or by sensitivity to chemicals in disposable diapers or in detergent used in laundering cloth diapers.
   b. The best treatment is prevention by frequent diaper changes and by protection of the skin with a barrier product containing zinc oxide and/or petrolatum. The skin should

be cleansed with warm water after voiding or stooling. Diaper wipes that do not contain alcohol may be used (Ravanfor et al., 2012).

c. Cornstarch and baby powder should not be used. They provide a medium for growth of bacteria and yeast, and inhaled particles are irritating to the respiratory tract (AWHONN, 2007).

d. *Candida* diaper dermatitis: see 2. under E. Infectious Lesions.

**B. Lesions resulting from trauma.**

1. Forceps marks.
   a. Forceps marks are red or bruised areas seen over the cheek, scalp, or face of infants after forceps delivery.
   b. The infant should be examined for underlying tissue damage or other signs of birth trauma such as scalp abrasions, fractured clavicles, or facial palsy.
2. Subcutaneous fat necrosis.
   a. A hard, circumscribed, red or purple nodule under the dermis in the subcutaneous tissue. Nodules appear on the trunk, extremities, or face, usually during the first 2 weeks of life. They may grow larger initially and then resolve spontaneously within several weeks.
   b. Subcutaneous fat necrosis has been attributed to trauma, cold stress, shock, and asphyxia and is caused by crystallization of the subcutaneous fat cells. It has also been reported in neonates being treated with therapeutic hypothermia for hypoxic–ischemic encephalopathy (Hogeling et al., 2012).
   c. Hypercalcemia may be associated with subcutaneous fat necrosis in infants with multiple nodules. Hypocalcemia has also been reported, possibly because of the underlying cause of the nodules. Serum calcium levels should be monitored (Hogeling et al., 2012).
3. Scalp lacerations.
   a. Scalp lacerations may be caused by trauma during delivery, placement of scalp electrodes, or fetal blood pH sampling.
   b. Treatment consists of keeping the area clean and dry and assessing for infection.
4. IV extravasations.
   a. Vascular access sites in the infant should be assessed hourly to evaluate line patency and detect extravasation. The IV catheter should be removed immediately if patency is not certain or if signs of extravasation are apparent. If an infiltration of a vesicant medication has occurred, treatment should be determined before removing the catheter (AWHONN, 2007).
   b. If extravasation occurs, using a multiple-puncture technique has been reported to help avoid swelling at the site and further tissue damage (AWHONN, 2007). Using aseptic technique, make several puncture holes with a 25-gauge needle over the area of swelling and gently squeeze fluid out of the tissue, or allow the fluid to leak out on its own. Hyaluronidase injected into the tissue surrounding the site may decrease tissue damage, and phentolamine can be used as an antidote for infiltration of vasoconstrictive agents such as dopamine or norepinephrine, although evidence from randomized controlled trials is minimal (AWHONN, 2007; Gopalakrishnan et al., 2012).
   c. Application of an occlusive hydrocolloid dressing may aid in healing (AWHONN, 2007).

**C. Pigmented skin lesions.**

1. Hyperpigmented macules (Fig. 36-6).
   a. Large macules or patches, gray or blue-green, seen most commonly over the buttocks, flanks, or shoulders.
   b. Most common pigmented lesion seen at birth, occurring in 80% of African American, Asian, and Hispanic infants and only occasionally in lighter-skinned infants (Gibbs and Makkar, 2008).
   c. Hyperpigmented macules are caused by the increased presence of melanocytes dispersed in the dermis.
   d. The spots fade somewhat during the first few years after birth, particularly as surrounding skin darkens, but may persist into adulthood.
   e. It is important to document size and location to avoid question of nonaccidental trauma.
2. Congenital melanocytic nevi (pigmented nevi) (Fig. 36-7).

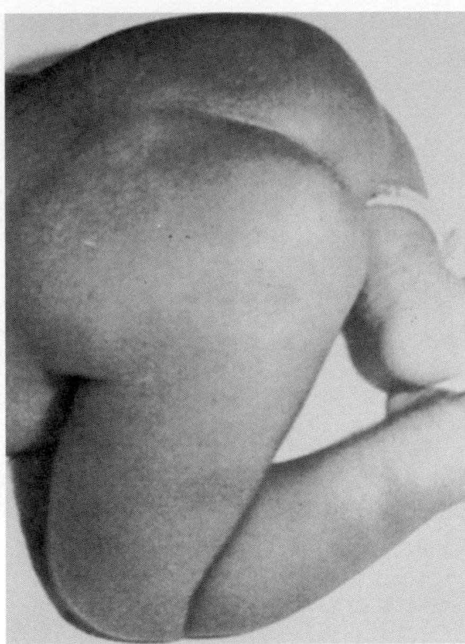

FIGURE 36-6 ■ Hyperpigmented macules (mongolian spots). (Courtesy Jacinto Hernandez, M.D., The Children's Hospital, Denver, Colo.)

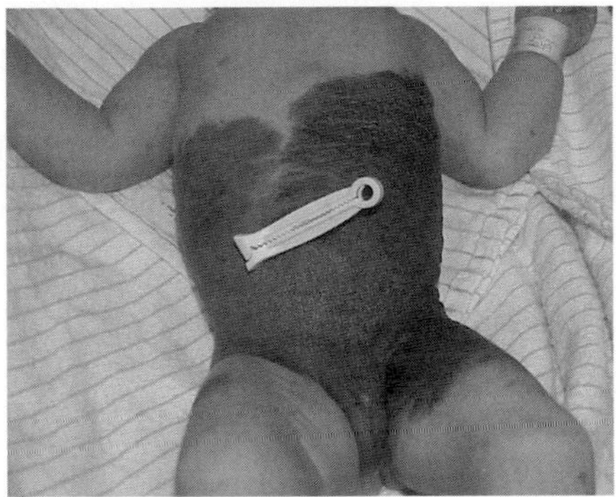

FIGURE 36-7 ■ Giant pigmented nevus. (Courtesy Catherine L. Witt, Aurora, Colo.)

a. Dark brown or black macules that may or may not be hairy. Nevi may occur anywhere on the body, with the "bathing trunk" area being the most common site.
b. Caused by collection of melanocytes under the skin.
c. Most are small, less than 2 cm, with smooth surfaces. Large nevi (>10 cm) are rare (Weston et al., 2007).
d. Pigmented nevi are generally benign. Malignant changes may occur but are rare before puberty in small nevi (Gibbs and Makkar, 2008; Paller and Mancini, 2011; Weston et al., 2007).
e. Close observation for changes in size or shape is indicated, with possible surgical excision. Large, unusually shaped nevi may be difficult to assess for changes and should be followed closely (Weston et al., 2007).
f. Pigment-specific lasers such as the Q-switched or ruby laser have been used with increasing success (Polder et al., 2011).
g. A hairy nevus present over the spine may be associated with spina bifida or meningocele (Gibbs and Makkar, 2008).
h. Pigmented nevi may also be associated with neurofibromatosis or tuberous sclerosis.

3. Transient neonatal pustular melanosis (Fig. 36-8).

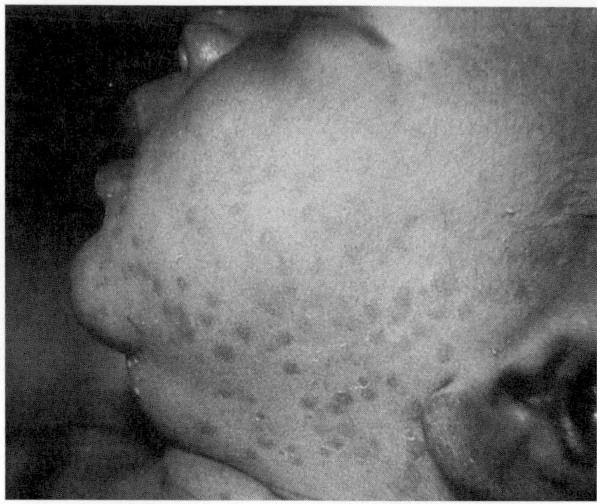

FIGURE 36-8 ■ Neonatal pustular melanosis. (Courtesy Jane Deacon, RNC, M.S., NNP, The Children's Hospital, Denver, Colo.)

   a. Superficial vesiculopustular lesions that rupture during the first 12 to 48 hours after birth, leaving small, brown, hyperpigmented macules. The macules may be surrounded by very fine white scales. They often rupture before delivery, presenting as macules.
   b. Benign; found in up to 5% of African American infants and in about 0.2% of white neonates (Paller and Mancini, 2011; Ramamurthy et al., 1976).
   c. No treatment is necessary. The macules generally fade during the first few weeks or months after birth.
   d. Aspirating the contents of the vesicles will reveal a variable number of neutrophils and few or no eosinophils.
4. Café-au-lait spots (Fig. 36-9).
   a. Tan or light brown patches with well-defined borders.
   b. When less than 3 cm in length and fewer than six in number, they are of no pathologic significance.
   c. Six or more spots may be an indication of neurofibromatosis (Gibbs and Makkar, 2008; Paller and Mancini, 2011).

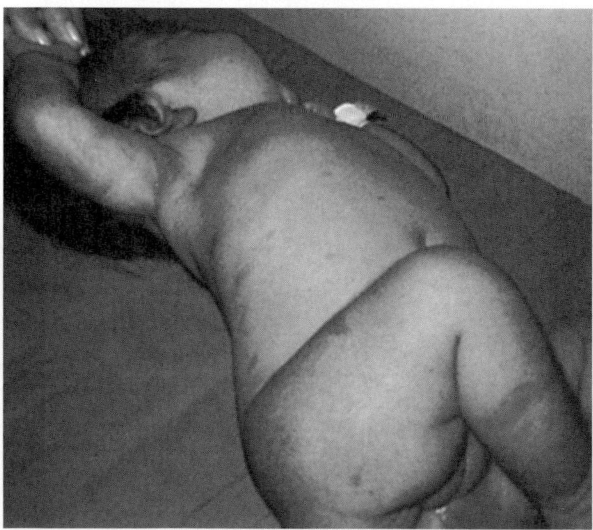

FIGURE 36-9 ■ Café-au-lait spots. (Courtesy Jacinto Hernandez, M.D., The Children's Hospital, Denver, Colo.)

(1) Neurofibromatosis is a condition in which tumors form on cutaneous nerves and along the thoracic, brachial, and lumbar nerve trunks. Cranial nerves may also be affected.

(2) It is an autosomal dominant disorder.

(3) Café-au-lait spots may be the only finding of this disease in the neonatal period.

5. Ash leaf macules.
   - **a.** White macules in the shape of an ash leaf or thumbprint; seen primarily over the trunk or buttocks.
   - **b.** Found in 90% of infants with tuberous sclerosis, although up to 5% of white infants will have hypopigmented macules (Paller and Mancini, 2011; Weston et al., 2007).
   - **c.** May be difficult to see in fair-skinned infants. Use of a Wood's (ultraviolet) lamp will aid in examination.
   - **d.** Infants with unexplained seizures should be examined for these macules.
   - **e.** May also be a normal finding or may be associated with neurofibromatosis.

**D. Vascular lesions.**

1. Nevus simplex.
   - **a.** Nevus simplex (stork bite) refers to macular pink areas of distended capillaries found on the nape of the neck, the upper eyelids, the nose, or the upper lip. They have diffuse borders, blanch with pressure, and become pinker with crying.
   - **b.** These are the most common of vascular birthmarks, seen in 30% to 50% of newborn infants (Hook, 2013; Weston et al., 2007).
   - **c.** The lesions tend to fade by the first or second year, with the exception of those on the nape of the neck, which may persist.
2. Port-wine stain.
   - **a.** A flat vascular nevus is present at birth. It is usually pink in infancy, but may be red or purple. The nevus may be small or may cover almost half of the body. It is flat, sharply delineated, and blanches minimally. Facial lesions are the most common.
   - **b.** Port-wine stains consist of mature capillaries that are dilated and congested directly below the epidermis. The cause is unknown.
   - **c.** The nevus does not grow in area or size. It will not resolve and should be considered permanent. The lesion may become darker and thicker with age.
   - **d.** The pulsed-dye laser has been successful in significantly lightening most port-wine stains. The laser works by causing intravascular coagulation (Anolik et al., 2011). Light-colored facial lesions have the best results; red or purple lesions that are thick and nodular respond less well. Most infants require several treatments.
   - **e.** Sturge–Weber syndrome (Fig. 36-10).

     (1) Port-wine stains that are confined to a pattern similar to that of the branches of the trigeminal nerve.

     (2) Their central feature is disordered proliferation of endothelial cells, particularly in the small veins. It is associated with atrophic changes in the cerebral cortex and calcium deposits in the walls of small vessels and areas of affected cortex (Weston et al., 2007).

     (3) Manifestations of the disease may include visual disturbances, headaches, focal seizures, hemiparesis, and cognitive impairments (Lo et al., 2012; Weston et al., 2007).
3. Infantile hemangioma (strawberry hemangioma) (Fig. 36-11).
   - **a.** Raised, lobulated, soft, bright red tumor located on the head, neck, trunk, or extremities. These lesions may also occur in the throat, where they can cause airway obstruction, requiring a tracheostomy in extreme cases.
   - **b.** Caused by dilated capillaries occupying the dermal and subdermal layers, in association with endothelial proliferation.
   - **c.** About 50% to 60% are present at birth, and 90% are evident by 2 months of age (Enjolras and Garzon, 2008; Leonardi-Bee et al., 2011). The lesions occur in approximately 1% to 2% of newborn infants and are more common in preterm infants (10% to 15% will have lesions), with females predominating (Haggstrom et al., 2007; Paller and Mancini, 2011). They are also more common in white infants and in twins or higher-order multiples. The lesions may also be familial (Paller and Mancini, 2011).

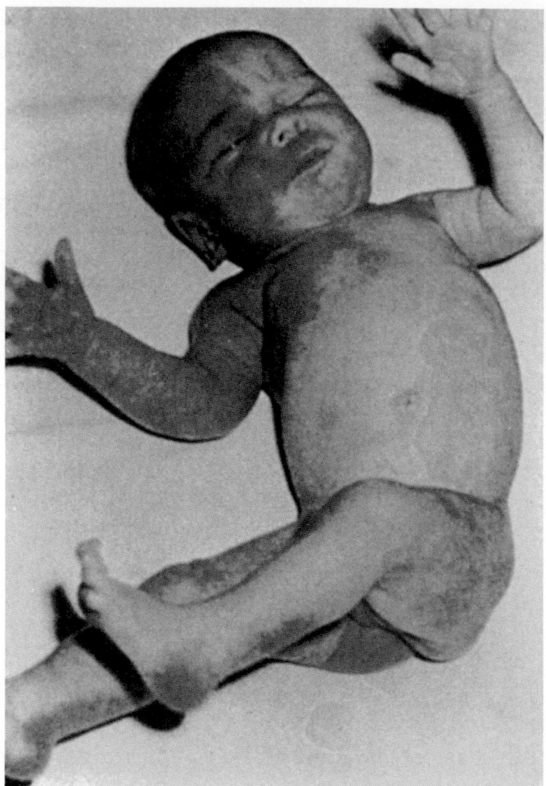

FIGURE 36-10 ■ Sturge–Weber syndrome. (Courtesy Jacinto Hernandez, M.D., The Children's Hospital, Denver, Colo.)

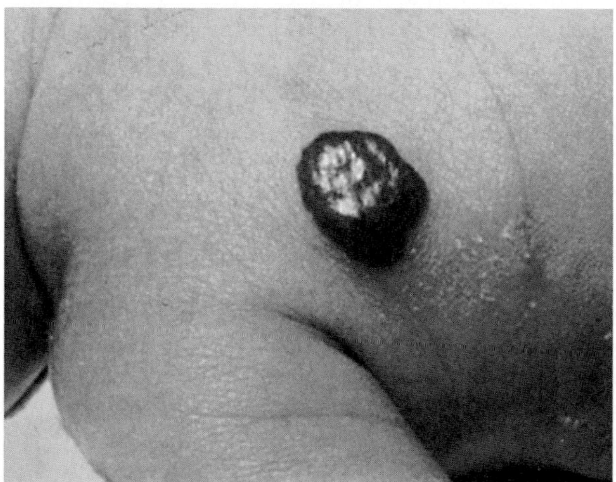

FIGURE 36-11 ■ Strawberry hemangioma. (Courtesy Jacinto Hernandez, M.D., The Children's Hospital, Denver, Colo.)

**d.** Strawberry hemangiomas will generally increase in size during the first 6 months, and then become stable in size before undergoing gradual spontaneous regression, with most leaving no trace. This may take several years. Infants will often have more than one lesion.

**e.** Treatment of choice is to allow the lesion to regress spontaneously. If the lesion is interfering with vision, is bleeding or ulcerating, or is impinging on other vital functions, treatment should be considered. There are few data on the effectiveness of various treatment options (Leonardi-Bee et al., 2011).

(1) Systemic corticosteroid therapy is the treatment of first choice for most hemangiomas (Chen et al., 2013).
(2) Flashlamp-pumped pulsed-dye laser may be effective on some lesions (Chen et al., 2013; Enjolras and Garzon, 2008).
(3) Cryosurgery may be used with small lesions, but concerns about scarring have prevented this option from becoming widespread (Enjolras and Garzon, 2008).
(4) Interferon alfa-2b may be effective in treating steroid-resistant lesions (Chen et al., 2013).

**f.** The infant should be monitored for signs of impingement on vital organs or functioning, such as stridor, poor feeding, and difficulty in swallowing, which would make treatment necessary.

**g.** The cosmetic concerns of parents require a caring, supportive approach. Pictures illustrating spontaneous regression may be helpful.

**4.** Cavernous hemangioma.

**a.** This lesion is composed of large venous channels and vascular elements lined by endothelial cells.

**b.** It involves the dermis and subcutaneous tissue and appears as a bluish red discoloration under the overlying skin.

**c.** The cavernous hemangioma has poorly defined borders and may feel cystic, like a "bag of worms," when palpated. Like the strawberry hemangioma, the cavernous hemangioma will increase in size during the first 6 to 12 months and then involute spontaneously (Enjolras and Garzon, 2008).

**d.** Treatment is not indicated unless the lesion is interfering with vital functions, including airway obstruction, in which case systemic corticosteroid treatment or interferon alfa may be helpful (Enjolras and Garzon, 2008).

**e.** Kasabach–Merritt phenomenon.
(1) Vascular anomalies resembling a hemangioma associated with sequestration of platelets and thrombocytopenia (Kelly, 2010; Lo et al., 2012).
(2) Treatment consists of systemic corticosteroid therapy. Transfusions of platelets and blood are frequently necessary (Enjolras and Garzon, 2008; Weston et al., 2007). The lesions may resolve spontaneously.
(3) Significant bleeding or impingement of vital organs may occur (Kelly, 2010).

**f.** Klippel–Trenaunay–Weber syndrome.
(1) Syndrome consists of cutaneous capillary malformations such as a port-wine stain, hypertrophy of a limb with associated vascular anomalies, and hypertrophy of underlying bone and soft tissue (Meier, 2009).
(2) No specific treatment for the disease. Severe limb hypertrophy may require orthopedic consultation, with possible amputation of the affected limb.

**E. Infectious lesions.**

**1.** Thrush.

**a.** A fungal infection of the mouth or throat, caused by *Candida albicans*.

**b.** Very common in infants.

**c.** Manifested as patches of adherent white material scattered over the tongue and mucous membranes.

**d.** Treated with an oral antifungal preparation such as nystatin (Mycostatin).

**2.** *Candida* diaper dermatitis.

**a.** Fungal infection of skin in the diaper area; may include buttocks, groin, thighs, and abdomen.

**b.** Caused by *C. albicans*.

**c.** Manifested as a moist, erythematous eruption, often with white or yellow satellite pustules.

**d.** Treatment consists of an antifungal cream or ointment preparation such as nystatin, applied to the rash several times per day. Oral antifungal treatment may be recommended in cases of persistent *Candida* dermatitis.

**3.** Systemic *Candida* infection.

**a.** Very low birth weight infants are at risk of having systemic, invasive fungal infections, with invasion of the fungus beyond the stratum corneum.

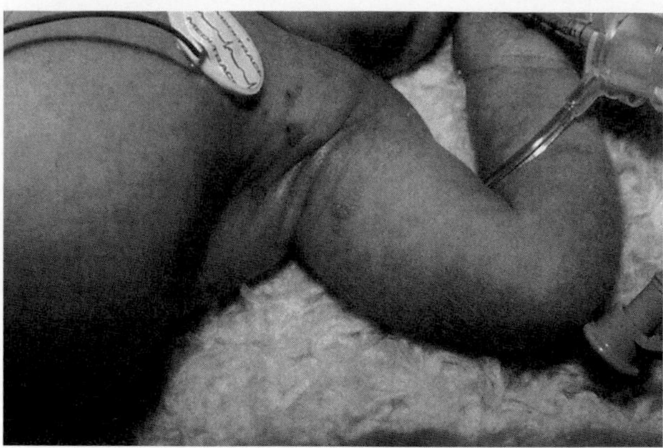

FIGURE 36-12 ■ Herpes simplex vesicles in axilla. (Courtesy Jane Deacon, RNC, M.S., NNP, The Children's Hospital, Denver, Colo.)

   **b.** Improving the barrier function of the skin by minimizing trauma and maintaining a sterile environment may help prevent onset of this infection.

**4.** Herpes.
   **a.** Neonatal herpes simplex infection is one of the most serious viral infections in the neonate.
   **b.** Rash appears as vesicular or pustular rash (Fig. 36-12).
   **c.** Seventy percent of infants with herpes will have subsequent rash but not necessarily before other signs and symptoms of illness develop. Therefore, the absence of vesicles does not eliminate the possibility of disease (Baley and Toltzis, 2011).
   **d.** Treatment with an antiviral agent such as acyclovir should begin immediately when vesicles are noted or disease is suspected. The earlier treatment is begun, the better the outcome (Baley and Toltzis, 2011; Weston et al., 2007).

**5.** Scalded skin syndrome (also known as bullous impetigo, toxic epidermal necrolysis, Ritter's disease, and nonstreptococcal scarlatina).
   **a.** An inflammatory skin disorder generally caused by the phage strain of group II *Staphylococcus aureus*. May follow an upper respiratory tract infection or otitis media.
   **b.** Manifested as a widespread, tender erythema, followed by blisters ranging from small vesicles to large bullae. Caused by the release of an endotoxin that acts on the stratum granulosum of the epidermis. The blisters, which frequently begin in the diaper area and spread to the rest of the body, rupture, leaving large, raw, scaldlike areas.
   **c.** Treatment includes isolation and aseptic handling to prevent further infection in the infected infant and the spread of bacteria to others. The infant is treated systemically with antibiotics. Many of the strains in the phage strain of group II *S. aureus* are resistant to penicillin, so methicillin or vancomycin may be required. A topical antibiotic ointment such as bacitracin may be applied locally (Smith and Sandall, 2012).

**6.** Congenital viral infection.
   **a.** Petechiae and purpuric macules erupt on the head, trunk, and extremities of affected infants. The lesions are often described as "blueberry muffin" spots and are caused by dermal erythropoiesis (Fig. 36-13).
   **b.** The lesions generally disappear in 2 to 3 weeks. Treatment is based on the underlying disorder.
   **c.** Although the lesions are most often associated with rubella, they are also seen in association with other congenital infections such as cytomegalovirus, toxoplasmosis, syphilis, and herpes.
   **d.** Affected infants may also have growth restriction, jaundice, hepatosplenomegaly, and thrombocytopenia (Baley and Toltzis, 2011).

**F. Hereditary and miscellaneous lesions.**

**1.** Epidermolysis bullosa.

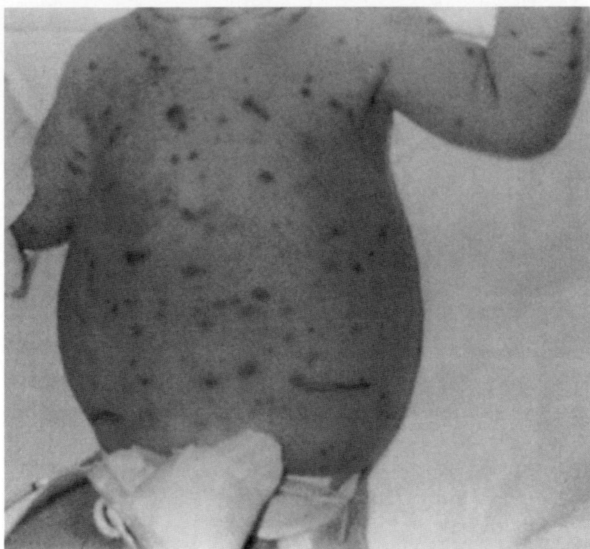

FIGURE 36-13 ■ "Blueberry muffin" rash. (From Clark, D.: *Atlas of neonatology*. Philadelphia, 2000, W.B. Saunders, p. 56.)

a. Disease characterized by the formation of vesicles and bullae over various parts of the body. Skin is extremely fragile. The underlying genetic defect may be autosomal dominant or recessive (Rimoin and Graham, 2012).
b. Vesicles may appear spontaneously or in response to minor trauma such as routine handling.
c. Lesions may appear at birth or a few weeks later.
d. Three types of vesicles may appear at birth.
   (1) Simple, nonscarring: bullae form in small numbers throughout childhood and heal without scarring. Often disappear at puberty. Prevention of trauma and infection is important.
   (2) Dystrophic, scarring: more severe form of the disease, with lesions forming scars, loss of nails, and contractures. Death may result from secondary infections.
   (3) Epidermolysis bullosa lethalis: most severe form, with large, numerous lesions, usually present at birth. Large areas of epidermis are lost, leaving red, weeping erosions. Esophageal lesions may also occur. The life span of these patients is generally short. Treatment is supportive care, minimizing trauma and infection (Rimoin and Graham, 2012; Weston et al., 2007).

2. Collodion baby.
   a. Term describes an appearance rather than a disease. These babies are born covered with a tight, shiny, transparent membrane that cracks and peels off after a few days. A few infants will have no underlying disorder, but many will have some form of ichthyosis (Weston et al., 2007) (Fig. 36-14).
   b. Treatment consists of liberal application of sterile olive or mineral oil several times a day to hydrate and lubricate the skin, careful handling, and prevention of infection.
3. Ichthyosis.
   a. Ichthyosis is a disease involving excessive scaling of the skin, caused by excessive production of stratum corneum cells or faulty shedding of the stratum corneum (Weston et al., 2007). There are four types of ichthyosis.
      (1) Ichthyosis vulgaris: an autosomal dominant disease, usually appearing after 3 months of age. This is the most common and most benign of the ichthyosis disorders, occurring in approximately 1 in 250 infants (Weston et al., 2007). It consists of fine white scales and excessively dry skin.
      (2) X-linked ichthyosis: appears at birth or during the first year of life. It occasionally occurs in a collodion baby. The disorder consists of large, thick, dark brown scales

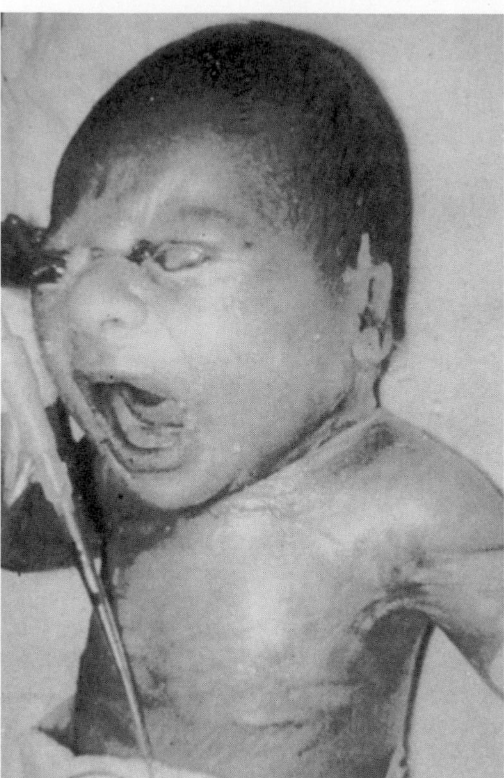

FIGURE 36-14 ■ Collodion infant. (From Solomon, L.M. and Esterly, N.B.: *Neonatal dermatology*. Philadelphia, 2001, W.B. Saunders, p. 115.)

over the entire body, with the exception of the palms and soles. It occurs in males only.

(3) Lamellar ichthyosis: an autosomal recessive trait that is manifested at birth as bright red erythema and universal desquamation. Some infants resemble collodion babies. Scales are large, flat, and coarse and may be less prominent in infancy than later in childhood. Eversion of the lips and eyelids may occur, and the palms and soles may be thickened. Hyperkeratosis may be seen on skin biopsy, although this is not diagnostic of the disorder (Weston et al., 2007).

(4) Bullous ichthyosis: autosomal dominant disorder characterized by recurrent formation of bullous lesions, erythroderma, and excessive dryness and peeling. As the child grows, the involvement generally becomes limited to small, thick, hard scales, most often found in the flexure regions. Hyperkeratosis may be seen on the palms and soles. Infection in the neonatal period with *S. aureus* is of primary concern because of the widespread skin breakdown.

b. Treatment of ichthyosis is limited to use of topical preparations to hydrate and lubricate the skin. Daily baths with a water-dispersible bath oil, with use of alpha-hydroxy acid ointments, may be helpful (Weston et al., 2007).

c. Drying soaps and detergents should be avoided.

d. Care must be taken to prevent infection of dry or cracked skin.

4. Harlequin fetus.

a. The harlequin fetus previously was considered to have a severe form of ichthyosis but may in fact have a separate rare autosomal recessive disease (Weston et al., 2007). The harlequin fetus has hard, thick, gray or yellow scales that cause severe deformities of skeletal and soft tissues.

b. The condition is untreatable, and most infants die within a few hours or days of life.

5. Cutis aplasia.

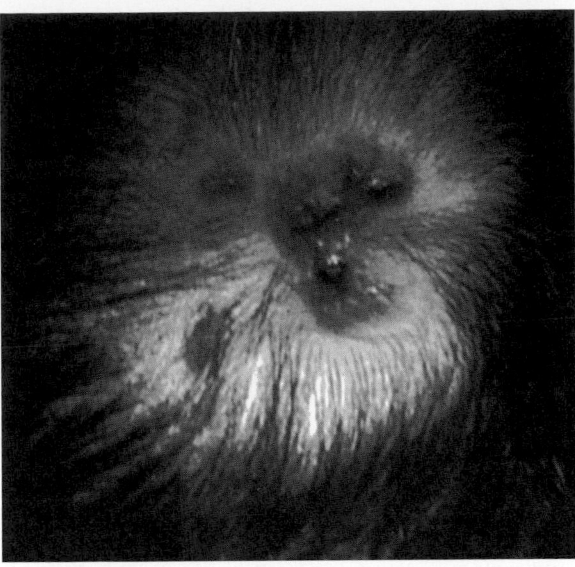

FIGURE 36-15 ■ Cutis aplasia. (Courtesy Jacinto Hernandez, M.D., The Children's Hospital, Denver, Colo.)

a. Term refers to congenital absence of skin, either as a midline defect, a posterior scalp defect, or several small or large defects involving the upper and lower extremities (Fig. 36-15).
b. Lesions heal slowly over several months, leaving a hypertrophic or atrophic scar.
c. May be associated with other defects such as cleft lip and palate, heart disease, tracheoesophageal fistula, and other midline defects. It is seen in approximately 50% of infants with trisomy 13 (Jones, 2006).

## REFERENCES


Agren, J., Sjors, G. and Sedin, G.: Ambient humidity influences the rate of skin barrier maturation in extremely premature infants. *Journal of Pediatrics*, 148(5):613–617, 2006.

Anolik, R., Newlove, T., Weiss, E.T., et al.: Investigation into optimal treatment intervals of facial port wine stains using pulsed dye laser. *Journal of the American Academy of Dermatology*, 67(5):985–990, 2011.

Association of Women's Health, Obstetric and Neonatal Nurses: *Neonatal skin care*, (2nd ed.). Washington, DC, 2007, Association of Women's Health, Obstetric and Neonatal Nurses.

Baley, J.E. and Toltzis, P.: Perinatal viral infections. In R.J. Martin, A.A. Fanaroff, and M.C. Walsh (Eds.): *Fanaroff and Martin's neonatal-perinatal medicine: Diseases of the fetus and newborn* (9th ed.). Philadelphia, 2011, Elsevier, pp. 841–886.

Blumer, J.L. and Reed, M.D.: Principles of neonatal pharmacology. In S.J. Yaffe, and J.V. Aranda (Eds.): *Neonatal and pediatric pharmacology: Therapeutic principles in practice* (3rd ed.). Philadelphia, 2011, Lippincott, Williams & Wilkins, pp. 169–181.

Chen, T.S., Eichenfield, L.F. and Friedlander, S.F.: Infantile hemangiomas: An update on pathogenesis and therapy. *Pediatrics*, 131:99–108, 2013.

Dyer, J.A.: Newborn skin care. *Seminars in Perinatology*, 37:3–7, 2013.

Enjolras, O. and Garzon, M.C.: Vascular stains, malformations, and tumors. In L.F. Eichenfield, I.J. Frieden, and N.B. Esterly (Eds.): *Neonatal dermatology* (2nd ed.). Philadelphia, 2008, Elsevier Saunders, pp. 343–374.

Fluhr, J.W., Darlenski, R., Lachmann, N., et al.: Infant epidermal skin physiology: Adaptation after birth. *British Journal of Dermatology*, 166:483–490, 2011.

Garland, J.S., Alex, C.P., Uhing, M.R., et al.: Pilot trial to compare tolerance of chlorhexidine gluconate to povidone-iodine antisepsis for central venous catheter placement in neonates. *Journal of Perinatology*, 29:808–813, 2009.

Gibbs, N.F. and Makkar, H.S.: Disorders of hyperpigmentation and melanocytes. In L.F. Eichenfield, I.J. Frieden, and N.B. Esterly (Eds.): *Neonatal dermatology* (2nd ed.). Philadelphia, 2008, Elsevier Saunders, pp. 397–421.

Gilliam, A.E. and Williams, M.L.: Skin of the premature infant. In L.F. Eichenfield, I.J. Frieden, and N.B. Esterly (Eds.): *Neonatal dermatology* (2nd ed.). Philadelphia, 2008, Elsevier Saunders, pp. 45–57.

Gopalakrishnan, P.N., Goel, N. and Banerjee, S.: Saline irrigation for the management of skin extravasation injury in neonates. *Cochrane Database of Systematic Reviews* (2):CD008404, 2012.

Haggstrom, A., Drolet, B., Baselga, E., et al.: Prospective study of infantile hemangiomas: Demographic, prenatal and perinatal characteristics. *Journal of Pediatrics*, 150(3):291–294, 2007.

Hammarlund, K. and Sedin, G.: Transepidermal water loss in newborn infants: Relation to gestational age. *Acta Paediatrica Scandinavica*, 68(6):795–801, 1979.

Hogeling, M., Meddles, K., Berk, D.R., et al.: Extensive subcutaneous fat necrosis of the newborn associated with therapeutic hypothermia. *Pediatric Dermatology*, 29:59–63, 2012.

Hook, K.P.: Cutaneous vascular anomalies in the neonatal period. *Seminars in Perinatology*, 37:40–48, 2013.

Hussain, S., Venepally, M. and Treat, J.R.: Vesicles and pustules in the neonate. *Seminars in Perinatology*, 37:8–15, 2013.

Jones, K.L.: *Smith's recognizable patterns of human malformation:* (6th ed.). Philadelphia, 2006, Elsevier Saunders pp. 18-19.

Kelly, M.: Kasabach-Merritt phenomenon. *Pediatric Clinics of North America*, 57(5):1085–1089, 2010.

Lavender, T., Bedwell, C., Roberts, S.A., et al.: Randomized controlled trial evaluating a baby wash product on skin barrier function in healthy term neonates. *JOGNN: Journal of Obstetric, Gynecologic, & Neonatal Nursing*, 42(2):203–214, 2013.

Leonardi-Bee, J., Batta, K., O'Brien, C. and Bath-Hextall, F.J.: Interventions for infantile haemangiomas (strawberry birthmarks) of the skin. *Cochrane Database of Systematic Reviews* (5)CD006545, 2011.

Lo, W., Marchuk, D.A., Ball, K.L., et al.: Updates and future horizons on the understanding, diagnosis, and treatment of Sturge–Weber syndrome brain involvement. *Developmental Medicine & Child Neurology*, 54:214–223, 2012.

Loomis, C.A., Koss, T. and Chu, D.: Fetal skin development. In L.F. Eichenfield, I.J. Frieden, and N.B. Esterly (Eds.): *Neonatal dermatology* (2nd ed.). Philadelphia, 2008, Elsevier Saunders, pp. 1–17.

Lucky, A.W.: Transient benign cutaneous lesions in the newborn. In L.F. Eichenfield, I.J. Frieden, and N.B. Esterly (Eds.): *Neonatal dermatology* (2nd ed.). Philadelphia, 2008, Elsevier Saunders, pp. 85–97.

Lund, C.H. and Kuller, J.M.: Integumentary system. In C. Kenner, and J.W. Lott (Eds.): *Comprehensive neonatal care: An interdisciplinary approach* (4th ed.). St. Louis, 2007, Elsevier Saunders, pp. 65–91.

Meier, S.: Klippel-Trenaunay syndrome. *A case study. Advances in Neonatal Care*, 9(3):120–124, 2009.

Mullany, L.C., Shah, R., Arifeen, S.E., et al.: Chlorhexidine cleansing of the umbilical cord and separation time: A cluster-randomized trial. *Pediatrics*, 131 (4):708–715, 2013.

Ness, M.J., Davis, D.M.R. and Carey, W.A.: Neonatal skin care: A concise review. *International Journal of Dermatology*, 52:14–22, 2013.

Paller, A.C. and Mancini, A.J.: *Hurwitz clinical pediatric dermatology: a textbook of skin disorders in childhood and adolescence:* (4th ed.). Philadelphia, 2011, Elsevier.

Percival, S.L., Emanuel, C., Cutting, K.F. and Williams, D.W.: Microbiology of the skin and the role of biofilms in infection. *International Wound Journal*, 9:14–32, 2012.

Pinsker, J.E., McBayne, K., Edwards, M., et al.: Transient hypothyroidism in premature infants after short term topical iodine exposure: An avoidable risk? *Pediatrics and Neonatology*, 54(2):128–131, 2013.

Polder, K.D., Landau, J.M., Vegilis-Kalner, I.J., et al.: Laser eradication of pigmented lesions: A review. *Dermatologic Surgery*, 37(5):572–595, 2011.

Ramamurthy, R.S., Reveri, M., Esterly, N.B., et al.: Transient neonatal pustular melanosis. *Journal of Pediatrics*, 88(5):831–835, 1976.

Ravanfor, P., Wallace, J. and Pace, N.: Diaper dermatitis, a review and update. *Current Opinions in Pediatrics*, 24 (4):472–479, 2012.

Rimoin, L. and Graham, J.M.: Blistering skin disorders in the neonate. *Clinical Pediatrics*, 51(7):685–688, 2012.

Sardesai, S.R., Kornacka, M.K., Walas, W. and Ramanathan, R.: Iatrogenic skin injury in the neonatal intensive care unit. *Journal of Maternal-Fetal & Neonatal Medicine*, 24(2):197–203, 2011.

Smith, J. and Sandall, M.: Staphylococcus scalded skin syndrome in the newborn: A case review. *Journal of Neonatal Nurses*, 18:201–205, 2012.

Stevens, T.P. and Schulman, J.: Evidence based approach to preventing central line-associated bloodstream infection in the NICU. *Acta Paediatrica*, 101 (Suppl. 464):11–16, 2012.

Visscher, M.O., Utturkar, R., Pickens, W.L., et al.: Neonatal skin maturation—vernix caseosa and free amino acids. *Pediatric Dermatology*, 28(2):122–132, 2011.

Weston, W.L., Lane, A.T. and Morelli, J.T.: *Color textbook of pediatric dermatology:* (4th ed.). St. Louis, 2007, Elsevier Mosby.

CHAPTER

# 37 Ophthalmologic and Auditory Disorders

DEBBIE FRASER AND WILLIAM DIEHL-JONES

**OBJECTIVES**

1. Describe the normal anatomy of the eye.
2. Identify the normal anatomy of the ear.
3. Identify the major function(s) of each structure.
4. Describe the components of a nursing assessment of the eyes and ears in the neonate.
5. Describe the nurse's role in assisting the physician with neonatal eye examinations.
6. Discuss the factors to consider in universal hearing screening of newborns.
7. For each of seven types of eye disorders in the neonatal period—traumatic injuries to the eye, conjunctivitis, nasolacrimal duct obstruction, cataracts, retinoblastoma, infections (TORCH diseases), and retinopathy of prematurity—(1) provide an overview of the pathogenesis and (2) describe commonly used treatment modalities, outlining the specific nursing care measures designed to meet the needs of neonates with these disorders.
8. Outline the most common causes of hearing loss in the newborn.
9. Outline teaching points for the family of a newborn at risk for hearing or vision problems.

An examination of the neonate's eyes and ears is an important, though often neglected, portion of a physical assessment. There is a great deal of clinically significant information that the astute nurse can glean from a thorough evaluation of these systems. Evidence of intrauterine infection, birth trauma, congenital malformations, disease, and a variety of genetic abnormalities can be detected during the course of the nurse's assessment of the neonate's eyes and ears.

This chapter provides the neonatal nurse with a review of normal anatomy of the eye and ear, together with the major function(s) of each structure; the essential components of an assessment of the newborn's eyes and ears; an overview of the most common eye disorders in the neonate; and common treatment modalities and nursing measures used in the treatment of various ocular disorders in the newborn infant. The essential elements of a universal hearing screening program for newborns are addressed, as are the most common causes of hearing loss in neonates.

## ANATOMY OF THE EYE (FIG. 37-1)

### Protective Structures

A. **Eyelids:** shade the eyes during sleep; protect from excessive light or foreign objects; spread lubricating secretions over the eyeball.
B. **Conjunctiva:** mucous membrane lining the inner aspect of the eyelids (palpebral) and onto the eyeball to the periphery of the cornea (bulbar).
C. **Lacrimal system:** manufactures and drains away tears; cleans, lubricates, and moistens the eyeball.
D. **Bony orbit or socket:** surrounds and protects the eyeball. Most important opening within the orbit is the optic foramen, through which the optic nerve, ophthalmic artery, and ophthalmic vein from each eye pass en route to the brain.

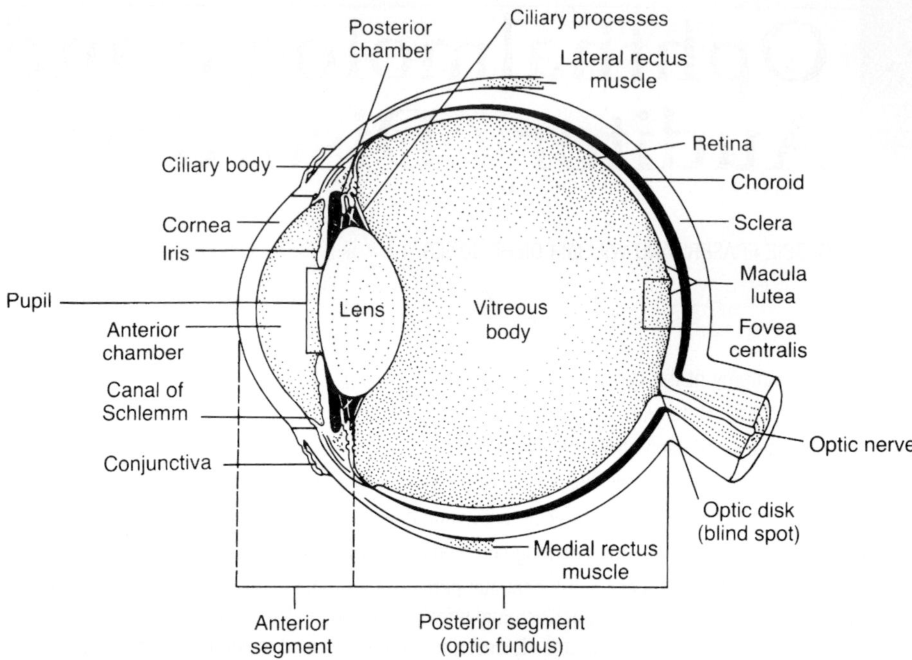


FIGURE 37-1 ■ Cross-section of eyeball. (From Boyd-Monk, H.: The structure and function of the eye and its adnexa. *Journal of Ophthalmic Nursing and Technology*, 6[5]:176-183, 1987.)

## The Eyeball

**A. Outer layer (fibrous tunic).**
   1. Cornea: transparent; reflects light rays.
   2. Sclera: the "white" of the eye; normal bluish appearance in newborn infants; gives shape to the eyeball and protects the inner parts.

**B. Middle layer (vascular tunic): the uveal tract.**
   1. Iris and pupil: a circular pigmented diaphragm with a central hole; controls the amount of light entering the eye.
   2. Ciliary body: the anterior portion of the choroid.
   3. Choroid: a vascular, pigmented membrane that lines most of the internal surface of the sclera, absorbs light rays, and nourishes the retina.

**C. Inner layer: the retina.**
   1. Extends from the ora serrata to the optic nerve.
   2. Functions in image formation.
      a. Photoreceptors: rods and cones.
      b. Bipolar cells.
      c. Ganglion cells.
   3. Optic disc: retinal blood vessels enter the eye, and optic nerve exits the eye. Blind spot in field of vision because optic disc has no photoreceptors.
   4. Optic nerve: second cranial nerve.
   5. Macula: exact center of the retina and location of sharpest vision.

**D. Anterior cavity (filled with aqueous humor).**
   1. Anterior chamber: behind the cornea, in front of the iris.
   2. Posterior chamber: behind the iris, in front of the suspensory ligament and lens.

**E. Lens:** a biconvex, transparent capsule that refracts light; the most important focusing mechanism of the eye.
   1. Lens remains cloudy until 30 to 34 weeks of gestation.

**F. Posterior cavity (filled with vitreous humor):** lies between the lens and the retina. Contributes to intraocular pressure, gives shape to the eyeball, and holds the retina in place.

### Extraocular Muscles

A. **Musculature.** Six muscles move each globe. The muscles of each eye work in conjunction with each other.
B. **Innervation.** The extraocular muscles are innervated by the oculomotor (third cranial) nerve, the abducens (sixth cranial) nerve, and the trochlear (fourth cranial) nerve.
   1. Pupillary reflex is functional by 36 weeks.
C. **Function (Blackburn, 2013; Gardner and Goldson, 2011).**
   1. At birth, newborns are able to see an object best at a distance of 8 to 10 inches with a visual acuity of 20/400 (de Alba Campomanes et al., 2012).
   2. A healthy term newborn is able to fix on an object and follow it up to 90 degrees in a horizontal arc.
   3. Newborns prefer black-and-white patterns and the human face.
   4. Color discrimination develops at 2 to 3 months of age (Graven, 2004).

## PATIENT ASSESSMENT

### History

A. **Pregnancy:** first-trimester infections (e.g., rubella), unknown rashes, fever, sexually transmitted disease, vaginal discharge, medications.
B. **Birth history:** gestational age, duration of labor, use of forceps.
C. **Family history:** incidence of ocular disorders, especially retinoblastoma; systemic diseases.

### Examination (de Alba Campomanes et al., 2012; Johnson, 2009)

The examination is performed with the baby in a quiet, alert state. To facilitate the spontaneous eye-opening, use an auditory stimulus, change the infant's position from supine to upright, or dim the lights (Johnson, 2009). Eye prophylaxis may make the examination more difficult.

A. **External assessment.**
   1. General facial configuration: should be symmetrical. Note distance between the eyes; increased width between the eyes is referred to as hypertelorism; decreased width is referred to as hypotelorism.
   2. Spontaneous eye movements: note range of motion and conjugation (the ability of the eyes to move together). Infants can track and follow objects with both eyes. Erratic or purposeless movements may be observed during the first few weeks of life. Median focal distance for the term neonate is about 8 inches (20 cm).
B. **Reaction to light or visual stimuli:** strong blink reflex to bright light or stimulation of the lids, lashes, or cornea. A somewhat unsteady gaze can be observed shortly after birth, with ability to fixate on a stimulus for 4 to 10 seconds and refixate every 1 to 1.5 seconds. Ability to maintain fixation and to follow does not occur until 5 to 6 weeks of age.
C. **Pupils:** shape should be round and reaction to light should be equal; constriction to both direct and contralateral stimulation should occur. The red reflex should be elicited bilaterally; normally appears as a homogeneous bright red-orange. Opacities or interruptions may indicate cataracts or retinoblastoma.
D. **Eyelids:** note symmetry, epicanthal folds, bruising or edema, lacerations, ptosis, and presence of lacrimal puncta.
E. **Conjunctivae:** should be pink and moist; redness or exudate is abnormal.
F. **Corneas:** may be somewhat less than transparent or slightly hazy in the first few days of life in both premature and term infants. Sclerae may be bluish in premature or small babies as a result of thinness.
G. **Irises:** should be similar in appearance; note pigmentation. A coloboma, or keyhole pupil, may be associated with congenital anomalies. Brushfield's spots are silvery gray spots scattered around the circumference of the iris—strongly associated with Down syndrome.
H. **Lenses:** should be clear and black with direct illumination. Examination of the anterior vascular capsule of the lens is a useful adjunct to determination of gestational age in preterm infants between 27 and 34 weeks.

# PATHOLOGIC CONDITIONS AND MANAGEMENT

## Birth Trauma

A. **Pathophysiology.**
   1. Direct result of duration and difficulty of delivery.
   2. Improperly applied forceps.
   3. Compression of cranial nerves.

B. **Clinical presentation.**
   1. Petechiae, ecchymoses, edema, and/or lacerations of pinna, lids, conjunctiva, or globe.
   2. Bright red patches on conjunctiva (subconjunctival hemorrhage): occurs in up to 13% of births (Isenberg, 2005).
   3. Droopy eyelids.

C. **Complications:** These injuries are generally mild and transient, often resolving spontaneously.

## Conjunctivitis

Conjunctivitis is an inflammatory reaction resulting from invasion of the conjunctivae by pathologic organisms.

## Etiology

A wide variety of infectious agents are capable of producing conjunctivitis in the newborn infant. The most common causes in North America include the following:

A. ***Neisseria gonorrhoeae*:** peripartum transmission, onset 3 to 4 days.
B. ***Chlamydia trachomatis*:** peripartum transmission, onset 5 to 7 days.
C. ***Staphylococcus aureus*:** acquired during the neonatal period, onset 5 to 14 days.
D. **Herpes simplex:** peripartum transmission, onset 6 to 14 days

## Neisseria gonorrhoeae

A. **Incidence:** One third of neonates born vaginally to infected women develop ophthalmic gonococcal infection (Embree, 2011). May be higher in areas with poor perinatal care or irregular antibiotic eye prophylaxis after birth.

B. **Onset of infection:** onset of symptoms usually between days 3 and 4 of life.

C. **Clinical presentation.**
   1. Edema of the eyelids.
   2. Purulent discharge.
   3. Redness/hyperemia of the conjunctivae.

D. **Diagnostic findings.**
   1. History.
      a. Maternal history of sexually transmitted disease.
      b. Age at onset of infection.
   2. Physical examination.
      a. Clinical signs of inflammation.
      b. Purulent discharge.
   3. Laboratory.
      a. Gram stain shows gram-negative diplococci.
      b. Culture positive for gonococci from conjunctival surface or exudate.

E. **Nursing care.**
   1. Isolate infant in accordance with infection control guidelines.
   2. Irrigate eyes with sterile normal saline solution hourly until discharge is eliminated.
   3. Promptly administer appropriate systemic therapy. Topical antimicrobial therapy is not required.
      a. Penicillin-sensitive *N. gonorrhoeae*: aqueous crystalline penicillin G, intravenous (IV) or intramuscular (IM), for 10 days (Venkatesh et al., 2011).

   b. Penicillin-resistant *N. gonorrhoeae*: ceftriaxone, 25 to 50 mg/kg (maximum 125 mg) IV or IM in a single daily dose (de Alba Campomanes et al., 2012) or cefoxitin (Venkatesh et al., 2011).
4. Parents of infected infant should be referred for evaluation and treatment.

**F. Complications.**
1. Infants with gonococcal conjunctivitis are at risk of having corneal ulceration, perforation, and subsequent visual impairment.
2. Systemic complications involving the blood, joints, or central nervous system may occur in a small number of infants.

## Chlamydia trachomatis

**A. Incidence.**
1. The most common cause of conjunctivitis in the neonatal period, especially in areas with poor perinatal care or irregular administration of erythromycin eye prophylaxis after delivery. Chlamydial eye infections occur in up to 1% of births in developed countries (Isenberg, 2005).
2. About 20% to 50% of babies born vaginally to mothers with a *C. trachomatis* infection of the cervix will develop conjunctivitis; 10% to 20% develop pneumonia (Darville, 2011).
3. Prevention of infection in the newborn infant is dependent on prenatal detection and treatment of the mother or on the use of an effective form of eye prophylaxis at birth (e.g., erythromycin ointment).

**B. Onset:** Symptoms are usually observed between 5 and 7 days of age.

**C. Clinical presentation:** Symptoms vary from mild conjunctivitis to intense edema of the lids with purulent discharge. A pseudomembrane may be present over the conjunctiva.

**D. Diagnostic findings.**
1. Identification of *Chlamydia* antigen.
2. Stains of conjunctival scrapings.
3. Culture of conjunctival scrapings.

**E. Patient management.**
1. Therapy of choice is oral erythromycin (estolate preparation), for 14 days (Darville, 2011).
2. Topical therapy alone is inadequate to eradicate the organism from the upper respiratory tract.
3. Parents of infected infants should be referred for evaluation and therapy.

**F. Complications:** Infection is spread via the nasolacrimal system to the nasopharynx, leading to *Chlamydia*-related pneumonia.

## Nasolacrimal Duct Obstruction

**A. Pathophysiology.**
1. Lacrimal apparatus consists of structures that produce tears (lacrimal glands) and structures responsible for drainage of tears (upper and lower puncta, canaliculi, lacrimal sac, and nasolacrimal duct). System functions to clean, lubricate, and moisten the eyeball.
2. Term and preterm newborn infants have the capacity to secrete tears (reflex tearing to irritants) but usually do not secrete emotional tears until 2 to 3 months of age.
3. Congenital obstruction is usually caused by an imperforate membrane at the distal end of the nasolacrimal duct.
4. Congenital nasolacrimal obstruction is the most common abnormality of the neonate's lacrimal apparatus. Incidence of this condition ranges between 5% and 10% of all newborn infants (de Alba Campomanes et al., 2012).

**B. Clinical presentation.**
1. Usually within the first few weeks of life.
2. Persistent tearing (epiphora): need to rule out congenital glaucoma.
3. Crusting or matting of the eyelashes: "sticky eye."
4. Spilling of tears over the lower lid and cheek: a "wet look" in the involved eye(s).
5. Absence of conjunctival infection.

6. Mucopurulent material refluxing from either punctum when gentle pressure is applied over the involved nasolacrimal sac.

C. **Nursing care.**
 1. Conservative management, with daily massage of the nasolacrimal sac in an attempt to rupture the membrane at the lower end of the duct.
 2. Technique consists of placing the index finger over the common canaliculus to block the exit of material through the puncta, and stroking downward firmly.
 3. Digital pressure increases hydrostatic pressure in the nasolacrimal sac, which may cause a rupture of the membranous obstruction.
 4. If a mucopurulent discharge is present, antibiotic eyedrops (sodium sulfacetamide) or ointment (erythromycin) may be required.
 5. Cleansing of eyes: eyes should be cleaned with moist compresses, with secretions mechanically removed.
 6. Duration of conservative management: conservative management is advocated for the first year of life.
 7. Resolution: the majority of nasolacrimal obstructions resolve spontaneously or with massage by 1 year of age.
 8. Surgical treatment: unresolved obstructions can be successfully treated surgically; tear duct probing is done, with the infant under general anesthesia, after the first year of life.

D. **Complications.**
 1. Acute dacryocystitis: inflamed, swollen lacrimal sac.
 2. Fistula formation.
 3. Orbital or facial cellulitis.

## Cataracts

Congenital cataracts are the main treatable cause of visual impairment in infancy. To ensure optimal visual development, congenital cataracts should be surgically removed within 6 to 8 weeks of birth (de Alba Campomanes et al., 2012).

A. **Pathophysiology.**
 1. Lens: the lens is a biconvex, transparent capsule that refracts light. It is the most important focusing mechanism of the eye.
 2. Cataract: a cataract is an opacity of any size or degree in the lens of the eye.
 3. Path of light: normally the light from an object passes directly through the lens to a focal point on the retina, producing a sharp image. Cataracts result in a degraded image or no image at all.
 4. Visual impairment: cataracts lead to varying degrees of visual impairment, from blurred vision to blindness, depending on the location and extent of the opacity. In neonates, cataracts may be transient, disappearing spontaneously within a few weeks.

B. **Etiology or precipitating factors.**
 1. Idiopathic (30%): developmental variation, not associated with other abnormalities.
 2. Genetically determined (30%): most common mode of inheritance—autosomal dominant.
 3. Congenital rubella: cataracts are present in 30% of newborn infants with congenital rubella syndrome (Plotkin et al., 2011).
 4. Other congenital infections.
  a. Toxoplasmosis.
  b. Cytomegalovirus (CMV) infection.
  c. Herpes simplex.
  d. Varicella.
 5. Metabolic disorders (e.g., galactosemia).
 6. Chromosomal abnormalities (e.g., Down syndrome, trisomy 13, Turner's syndrome).
 7. Clinical syndromes (e.g., Crouzon's disease, Pierre Robin syndrome).
 8. Prematurity.

C. **Clinical presentation.**
 1. White pupil (leukokoria).
 2. Searching nystagmus (at 1 to 2 months of age). The presence of nystagmus is a marker for poor visual prognosis.

**D. Diagnostic findings.**
1. History.
   a. Family history of ocular disease or systemic disorders.
   b. Pregnancy, especially first-trimester intrauterine infections.
2. Physical examination.
   a. Normally, when light is directed at the pupils, they appear black to the naked eye of the examiner.
   b. Examine to detect a white pupil by shining a light into each eye, with the light source held to one side.
   c. If the opacity is small, it may be identified only when the pupils are dilated and with the use of an ophthalmoscope.
   d. Consider other diseases of the eye that may produce a white pupil (e.g., retinoblastoma).

**E. Nursing care.**
1. Eye examination: assist the physician in carrying out a thorough eye examination of the newborn infant. This includes administering drops to dilate the pupils before the examination and supporting the infant's head to facilitate examination.
2. Parental education: in collaboration with the physician, assist parents in understanding the nature, possible cause, and treatment of cataracts in the newborn infant, together with the prognosis for future vision. Surgery is indicated whenever the cataract is likely to interfere with vision.
3. Explore any feelings of guilt the parents may have in relation to the cause of the cataracts; provide appropriate support.
4. Encourage parent–infant attachment: neonate may not be able to see the parents but can learn to know their voices, smell, and touch.
5. Care for the patient postoperatively.
   a. Prevent increased intraocular pressure. Keep the neonate comfortable, well fed, and free of pain to decrease crying.
   b. Administer eyedrops or ointments as ordered postoperatively.
   c. Apply clean eye patches or protective shields to protect the eye from rubbing or bumping and to prevent irritation from light.
   d. Monitor for complications of cataract surgery. These are relatively infrequent but include infection within the eye, glaucoma, and retinal detachment. Note any increased redness or haziness of the eye, increased tearing, photophobia, or cloudiness of the cornea. Increased crying, irritability, disruption in sleeping patterns, or rubbing of the eye may indicate pain.
   e. Assist the parents in understanding the essential role of optical correction devices, such as glasses or contact lenses, in their infant's vision and development.
   f. Promote appropriate visual stimulation and foster normal infant development by teaching parents about newborn visual preferences (e.g., black-and-white contrast or medium-intensity colors, the human face, geometric shapes, checkerboard designs).

**F. Complications.**
1. Varying degrees of visual impairment, leading to developmental delay.
2. Presence and/or severity of associated ocular defects, such as microphthalmos and glaucoma.

**G. Outcome.** Visual prognosis depends not only on the extent of cataracts, age at removal, surgical outcome, and rapid optical correction but also on the nature of other associated anomalies of the eye or syndromes.

## Retinoblastoma (de Alba Campomanes et al., 2012)

Retinoblastoma is the most common ocular malignancy in children, with an incidence of 1 in 15,000 to 20,000 live births.

**A. Clinical presentation.**
1. Leukokoria (54%).
2. Strabismus (19%).
3. Loss of visual acuity (4%).
4. Red eye (5%).

**B. History.**
   1. Family history of retinoblastoma.

**C. Physical examination.**
   1. Examine for presence of red reflex and to detect a white pupil.
   2. Consider congenital cataracts as an alternative cause of leukokoria.

**D. Treatment.**
   1. Enucleation.
   2. Chemotherapy.
   3. Focal destruction of the lesion.

**E. Complications.**
   1. Loss of vision in the affected eye.
   2. Survival is greater than 90% with early recognition and treatment.
   3. Long-term survival is 50% if spread outside the eye has occurred.

## Congenital Infections

The developing eyes are highly vulnerable to the damaging effects of prenatal infection (Mets and Chhabra, 2008), and ocular abnormalities may in fact be the predominant manifestation of the disease. A number of the congenitally acquired infections are associated with abnormal ocular conditions, including cataracts, chorioretinitis, corneal opacities, and glaucoma. The most common of these infections are toxoplasmosis, rubella, CMV, and herpes (see also Chapter 32).

## Congenital Rubella Syndrome

In the prevaccine era, rubella was a common childhood infection. Since the introduction of vaccinations, congenital rubella syndrome occurs infrequently. In fact, between 2001 and 2004, only 25 cases of congenital rubella syndrome were reported (Anderson and Gonik, 2011).

**A. Pathophysiology.**
   1. Timing of infection: Consequences of the transplacental infection are determined primarily by the timing of the viral insult.
   2. Infection in the first trimester of pregnancy presents the greatest hazard to organogenesis, including that of the eyes.

**B. Incidence.** Ocular abnormalities are frequently seen in congenital rubella, with "salt-and-pepper" retinopathy being the most common ocular abnormality (Plotkin et al., 2011).

**C. Clinical presentation.**
   1. Gestational age: Findings in the infant exposed to rubella in utero depend on the gestational age at which the infection occurred.
   2. Ocular manifestations.
      a. Cataracts: in approximately 30% of patients.
      b. Pigmentary retinopathy.
      c. Microphthalmos.
      d. Glaucoma.
   3. Other common manifestations include severe hearing loss, intrauterine growth restriction, hepatomegaly, thrombocytopenia, and cardiac anomalies (see also Chapter 32).

**D. Nursing care.**
   1. Virus shedding may continue for months after birth. Infants with suspected congenital rubella should be isolated from other newborn infants and from pregnant women (both in the hospital and at home after discharge).
   2. See E. Nursing Care, under Cataracts.

**E. Outcome.**
   1. Prognosis: depends on severity of symptoms and number of organ systems involved.
   2. Mortality rate: in first year of life may approach 80% when multisystem involvement occurs.
   3. Multiple disabilities: common in surviving infants.
   4. Consequences of congenital rubella: may not be evident at birth but may become apparent in subsequent months.

## Cytomegalovirus

**A. Pathophysiology.**

1. CMV can cause a perinatal viral infection.
2. Congenital illness is most severe if infection occurs early in pregnancy, the period of greatest susceptibility of the developing fetus. Congenital infections can result from either a primary or recurrent maternal infection.

**B. Etiology.**

1. Ubiquitous virus: CMV can cause infection in all age groups.
2. Route of transmission: Infection may be acquired transplacentally, during birth (via the cervix), or through breast milk. In seropositive mothers, the risk of transmission through breast milk is 30% to 59%.
3. Transfusion: An important possible cause of morbidity in premature infants is transfusion-acquired CMV. All premature infants should receive seronegative blood products.

**C. Incidence.**

1. The most common congenital viral infection, affecting 1% to 2% of all newborns in the United States (Britt, 2011).
2. In the presence of primary acute maternal infection, 30% to 40% of fetuses are affected (Anderson and Gonik, 2011).

**D. Clinical presentation.**

1. A diagnosis of congenital CMV infection can rarely be made on the basis of clinical findings alone. Only 5% to 10% of neonates infected with CMV will have symptoms at birth. When symptomatic CMV is present, disseminated disease can occur involving all major organ systems.
2. Laboratory diagnostic methods (e.g., isolation of the virus from the urine) must be used if this condition is suspected.
3. Chorioretinitis is present in 10% to 15% of infants with symptomatic CMV (Britt, 2011).
4. Other eye abnormalities include conjunctivitis, microphthalmos, strabismus, cataracts, and optic atrophy.
5. Other manifestations include intrauterine growth restriction, microcephaly, hepatosplenomegaly, jaundice, and bleeding disorders (see also Chapter 32).

**E. Nursing care.**

1. Limited research suggests some benefit from IV ganciclovir or oral valganciclovir.
2. Use of gowns and good handwashing technique are essential to prevent the spread of infection.
3. Seronegative pregnant women should not care for infants with known or suspected infection.
4. These infants require long-term follow-up.

**F. Complications.**

1. Cytomegalic inclusion disease.
2. Sensorineural hearing loss, the most important late sequela, and the most common cause of congenital hearing loss (Britt, 2011).
3. Chorioretinitis or optic atrophy.

**G. Outcomes.**

1. Mortality rate: Overall mortality rate for symptomatic congenital infection is up to 30% (Freij and Sever, 2005).
2. In 10% to 15% of infants who are free of symptoms at birth, neurologic sequelae, such as microcephaly, neurodevelopmental delay, or sensorineural deafness, may develop in the first 2 years of life.

## Toxoplasmosis (Remington et al., 2011)

**A. Pathophysiology.** Fetal damage occurs as a direct result of inflammation caused by the presence of cysts in the tissues, including the eyes.

**B. Etiology.**

1. Maternal infection by the protozoan *Toxoplasma gondii* in the first and second trimesters of pregnancy is often associated with transplacental infection of the fetus.

2. Infection is acquired through contact with the excrement of infected cats and ingestion of improperly cooked meat.

C. **Incidence.**
1. The incidence of maternal infection varies considerably according to geographic location. Estimates in the U.S. population suggest a seroconversion rate of 1 in 1000 during pregnancy (Anderson and Gonik, 2011).
2. The risk of transmission for an infection acquired during pregnancy is 20% to 50% (Anderson and Gonik, 2011).

D. **Clinical presentation.**
1. Congenital *T. gondii* may be present at birth, in the first few months of life, or with sequelae from a previously undiagnosed infection.
2. Eighty percent to 90% of infected infants are symptomatic at birth (Anderson and Gonik, 2011).
3. Chorioretinitis is the most common manifestation. Toxoplasmosis infection is the most common cause of chorioretinitis in the United States (Remington et al., 2011).
4. Other manifestations include hydrocephalus, intracranial calcifications, hepatosplenomegaly, jaundice, and bleeding disorders (see also Chapter 32).

E. **Specific nursing care.**
1. Nursing care includes pharmaceutical treatment of *Toxoplasma* infection by administering sulfadiazine and pyrimethamine. These agents will eradicate the cysts and improve outcome but may not reverse the damage already done.
2. Give supportive care to the family, with sensitivity to feelings of guilt they might have.
3. Teach parents to recognize the signs of sequelae, including visual impairment in infancy (e.g., failure to fix and focus on objects or faces).

F. **Outcome.**
1. Prognosis for infants with congenital infection is markedly improved with prompt initiation of treatment.
2. Eighty percent of treated infants with moderate to severe disease have normal psychomotor development.
3. Recurrent eye lesions develop in 10% of treated infants with mild disease and in up to 30% of treated infants with moderate or severe disease.

## Retinopathy of Prematurity

Formally referred to as retrolental fibroplasia, retinopathy of prematurity (ROP) is a vasoproliferative retinopathy that occurs primarily in low birth weight infants (Fierson, American Academy of Pediatrics Section on Ophthalmology, American Academy of Ophthalmology, American Association for Pediatric Ophthalmology and Strabismus, and American Association of Certified Orthoptists, 2013).

A. **Pathophysiology.**
1. Human retina is avascular until 16 weeks of gestation. After this time, a capillary network begins to grow, starting at the optic nerve and branching outward toward the ora serrata (edge of the retina).
2. Nasal periphery is vascularized by about 32 weeks of gestation, but the process is not complete in the more distant temporal periphery until 40 to 44 weeks. Most cases of ROP begin at 31 to 32 weeks of gestation.
3. After premature birth, this process of normal vasculogenesis may be arrested as a result of injury from some noxious agent(s) or stressor(s).
4. Vasoproliferation: This arrest of normal vasculogenesis is later followed by a phase of rapid, excessive, irregular vascular growth and shunt formation (vasoproliferation), stimulated by vascular endothelial growth factor (VEGF) and interleukin growth factor.
5. Area of new growth generally forms an abrupt ridge between the vascular and avascular retina, particularly in the temporal periphery.
6. ROP may resolve if the vasculature in the area recovers and resumes advancing normally, allowing the retina to become completely vascularized.

7. If the new vasculature proceeds to develop abnormally, these capillaries may extend into the vitreous body and/or over the surface of the retina (where they do not belong). Leakage of fluid or hemorrhage from these weak, aberrant blood vessels may occur.
8. Blood and fluid leakage into various parts of the eye can result in scar formation and traction on the retina.
9. Traction may pull the macula out of its normal position, thus affecting visual acuity. If the macula is slightly out of position, vision will be mildly affected.
10. Tractional exudative retinal detachment results in blindness.

**B. Etiology.**

1. Complex multifactorial disorder.
2. Possible risk factors (Gardner et al., 2011).
   a. Prematurity/low birth weight: most important clinical factor associated with ROP.
   b. Supplemental oxygen, hypoxia, and hyperoxia.
   c. Hyper-/hypocapnia.
   d. Growth hormone deficiency.
   e. Ventilator support.
   f. Surfactant therapy.
   g. Apnea/bradycardia.
   h. Asphyxia/acidosis/shock.
   i. Blood transfusions.
   j. Steroid exposure.
   k. Sepsis.
   l. Patent ductus arteriosus.
   m. Intraventricular hemorrhage/seizures.
   n. Nutritional deficiencies such as vitamin E and vitamin A.
   o. Hyperglycemia.
   p. Prenatal complications: maternal hypertension, diabetes, bleeding, smoking.
   q. Ethnicity—ROP is more common and more severe in white infants than in African American infants.
   r. Exposure to bright light.
   s. Elevated bilirubin and exposure to phototherapy.

**C. Incidence.**

1. Incidence of ROP appears to increase significantly as birth weight and gestational age decrease. Up to 67% of neonates weighing less than 1251 g will develop ROP; up to 37% of these infants will progress to vision-threatening disease (Hartnett and Penn, 2012).

**D. Stages of retinopathy.**

1. Standardized approach for describing ROP, developed by the International Committee for the Classification of Retinopathy of Prematurity (2005) according to five stages.
   a. Stage 1: demarcation line within the plane of the retina separating the avascular and vascular retinal regions.
   b. Stage 2: ridge or elevation at the junction of the avascular and vascularized regions of the retina.
   c. Stage 3: ridge with extraretinal fibrovascular proliferation, either
      (1) Continuous with the posterior edge of the ridge,
      (2) Posterior but disconnected from the ridge, or
      (3) Into the vitreous.
   d. Stage 4: subtotal retinal detachment.
      (1) Extrafoveate.
      (2) Involving the foveae.
   e. Stage 5: total retinal detachment.
2. Aggressive posterior ROP: significant dilation and tortuosity of posterior pole vessels, present in zone I or II.
3. "Plus" disease: an indicator of activity. Signs (in increasing order of severity) include the following:
   a. Engorgement and tortuosity of vessels of the posterior pole in two or more quadrants.
   b. Iris vessel engorgement.

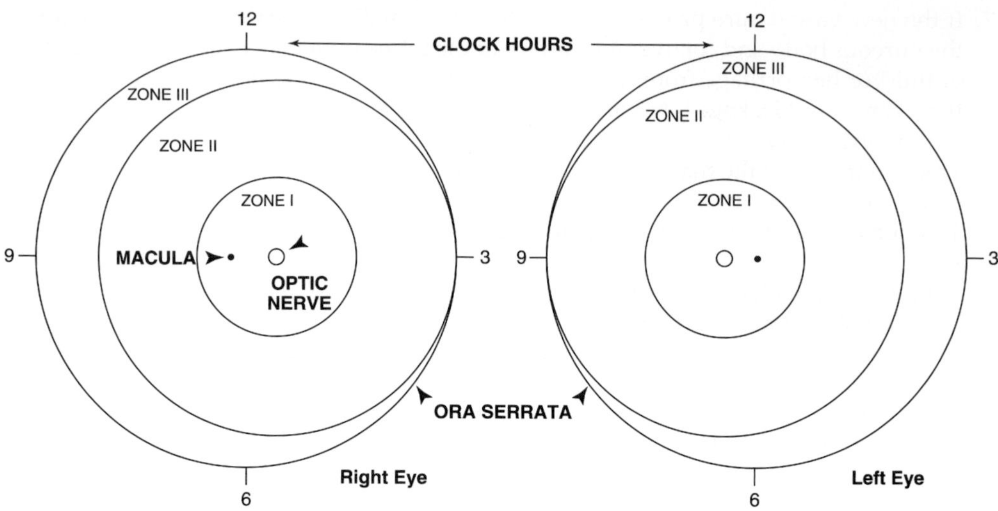


FIGURE 37-2 ■ Zones in retinopathy of prematurity. (From George, D.S.: The latest on retinopathy of prematurity. *MCN: American Journal of Maternal Child Nursing*, 13[4]:254-258, 1988.)

   c. Pupil rigidity.
   d. Vitreous haze.
4. Pre–plus disease: abnormal vessels, dilation and tortuosity in two or more quadrants not yet sufficient for a diagnosis of plus disease.
5. Zones for classification of ROP (Fig. 37-2).
   a. Zone I: extends from the optic disc to twice the disc–foveal distance—a radius of 30 degrees.
   b. Zone II: extends from the periphery of the nasal retina (ora serrata) in a circle around the anatomic equator.
   c. Zone III: anterior to zone II; present temporally, inferiorly, and superiorly but not in the nasal retina.

**E. Physical examination.**

1. Examination of the high-risk neonate: All newborn infants born at less than 30 weeks of gestation or with a birth weight of less than 1500 g, and selected high-risk infants between 1500 and 2000 g or gestational age greater than 30 weeks with an unstable clinical course, should have their eyes examined by a trained pediatric ophthalmologist when in stable clinical condition, 4 to 6 weeks after birth (approximately 31 to 33 weeks of postconceptional age) (Fierson et al., 2013). Infants born at less than 25 weeks of gestation may benefit from an ROP screen before 31 weeks to detect early aggressive ROP (Fierson et al., 2013).
2. Dilation of pupils: Infant's pupils should be dilated with a mydriatic agent before examination, to facilitate optimal evaluation. Cycloplegic mydriatic agents (e.g., cyclopentolate, tropicamide) have rapid onset of action, with peak ophthalmic effects between 20 and 60 minutes. The excess eyedrops should be wiped away promptly to avoid systemic absorption. Absorption can also be minimized by applying gentle pressure over the nasolacrimal duct for 1 minute following instillation of the eyedrops. It is necessary to protect eyes from bright light after mydriasis. Assess for symptoms of systemic absorption (e.g., tachycardia, restlessness) and notify physician immediately if symptoms are present.
3. Documentation: Location and extent of any retinopathy should be precisely documented and classified according to the guidelines developed by the International Committee for the Classification of Retinopathy of Prematurity (2005).
4. Follow-up.
   a. Infants who are found to have areas of retinal immaturity on initial examination should have repeated examinations every other week and, subsequently, every 2 to 3 weeks until vascularization has reached the ora serrata.
   b. If ROP is present during the initial examination, the infant should be examined weekly or every other week, depending on the severity of clinical findings.

F. **Prevention.**
1. Precautions while using oxygen: Although the role of oxygen in the pathogenesis of ROP is unclear, cautious and judicious administration and monitoring of oxygen remains one possible preventive measure.
   a. Continuous assessment and monitoring of the infant receiving oxygen to control arterial oxygenation. Cautious administration of oxygen while carrying out nursing procedures such as suctioning.
   b. Ongoing assessment of the oxygen delivery system, including calibration of oxygen analyzers, monitoring fractional inspired oxygen, checking/recording ventilator settings, circuit, and oxygen saturation monitors.
   c. Use of oxygen blenders to deliver precise oxygen concentrations.
   d. Lowering oxygen saturation alarm limits to 85% to 93% for neonates who weigh ≤1250 g at birth for the first week of life may decrease the incidence of threshold ROP (Sears et al., 2009). Recent research suggests that higher oxygen saturations (>94%) for infants greater than 32 weeks of gestation may decrease the progression of ROP (Chen et al., 2010).
2. Sensory stimulation: Provide a variety of forms of sensory stimulation to the infant, appropriate to level of development and behavioral cues.
3. Assessment: Assess newborn infant's ability to fix and focus.
4. Assistance: Assist the physician in carrying out a safe, minimally stressful eye examination of the newborn infant.
5. Protection against bright light: Protect the infant's eyes from bright light by shielding the incubator with a blanket and reducing the light in the nursery. The use of eye pads should be evaluated according to the principles of developmental care.
6. Parent education: Provide accurate parent education about the possibility of ROP (when parents are ready to receive information about potential non–life-threatening complications). Ensure that parents understand the importance of timely and appropriate follow-up (Fierson et al., 2013).
7. Follow-up: Unit-specific procedures for ensuring appropriate screening and follow-up should be in place and communicated to all members of the health care team, including those responsible for care after discharge.

G. **Treatment.**
1. Timing of treatment: Ablative treatment may be initiated for the following (Fierson et al., 2013):
   a. Zone I ROP: any stage with plus disease.
   b. Zone I ROP: stage 3 with no plus disease.
   c. Zone II: stage 2 or 3 with plus disease.
   d. The number of clock hours may not always be the determining factor for the strong consideration of ablative treatment.
   e. Treatment should be started within 72 hours of the finding of treatable disease to decrease the risk of retinal detachment.
2. Laser photocoagulation.
   a. Uses either an argon or diode laser to coagulate the avascular periphery of the retina.
   b. Laser surgery can be performed in the nursery with sedation and analgesia rather than general anesthesia.
   c. Is more difficult when the retina is not readily visualized (pupils cannot be dilated, presence of hemorrhage).
   d. Has fewer systemic and ocular side effects than cryotherapy and carries less risk of damage to adjacent structures (Bashour, 2013). Is less painful than cryotherapy.
   e. Complications: cataracts (Chen et al., 2011); burns to the cornea, iris, or lens; retinal, periretinal, or vitreous hemorrhage; photocoagulation of the fovea; and late-onset retinal detachment.
3. Nursing care for the infant undergoing laser photocoagulation.
   a. Preoperatively, the infant should be given nothing by mouth for 4 to 6 hours; phenylephrine with cyclopentolate (Cyclomydril) and sedation and analgesia should be given as ordered.
   b. Intraoperatively, monitor the baby and give medications as indicated.

c. After laser photocoagulation, the infant's respiratory status, oxygen saturation, and vital signs should be monitored.
d. Assess the eyes for drainage and edema.
e. Medications such as cyclopentolate and the combination dexamethasone, neomycin, and polymyxin B sulfate (Maxitrol) may be ordered to reduce postoperative complications.

4. Cryotherapy.
   a. Although the use of cryotherapy is decreasing, it continues to be used in some centers. Cryotherapy can be used in special circumstances (Isenberg, 2005).
   b. Supercooled probe is used to freeze the avascular retina, preventing vessel proliferation.
   c. Invasive procedure requires anesthesia.
   d. Complications include scarring of the retina; periorbital edema; conjunctival hematoma or laceration; elevation of intraocular pressure; retinal, periretinal, or vitreous hemorrhage; central renal artery occlusion; freezing of the optic nerve; and late-onset retinal detachment (Isenberg, 2005).
5. Anti-VEGF therapy.
   a. Still in the experimental stage, bevacizumab (Avastin) is a monoclonal antibody that inhibits angiogenesis.
   b. Avastin is administered as an intraocular injection and suppresses the development of blood vessels in the retina.
   c. A randomized controlled trial comparing Avastin to laser therapy found a greater benefit of Avastin for zone I ROP but not for ROP in zone II (Mintz-Hittner et al., for the BEAT-ROP Cooperative Group, 2011).
   d. Reported side effects of Avastin include progression to retinal detachment, persistent peripheral retinal avascularization and recurrent angiogenesis in the vitrea (Hu et al., 2012).
6. Vitreoretinal surgery results in reattachment of the retina in 30% of cases; however, following macular detachment visual prognosis is poor even if the retina is successfully reattached (Repka et al., 2011).
7. Provide emotional support and appropriate community referrals for parents whose infant will have significant visual impairment.

**H. Complications.**

1. Mydriatic eyedrops and eye examinations can produce hypertension, reflex bradycardia, and apnea as a result of drug effects and vagal stimulation.
2. Varying degrees of visual impairment (e.g., myopia) may require corrective lenses to improve visual acuity. Up to 70% of infants with ROP have some degree of myopia (Chen et al., 2011).
3. Additional complications include the following:
   a. Strabismus (20%).
   b. Glaucoma.
   c. Cataracts
   d. Amblyopia.
   e. Astigmatism (40%).
   f. Retinal detachment and blindness.

**I. Outcome.**

1. Ninety percent (or more) of cases of acute ROP resolve spontaneously, with little or no visual loss.
2. Timely treatment has been shown to decrease the risk of blinding complications of ROP by 50%. A significant number of visual impairments may result, especially in the presence of disease in zone I.

## ANATOMY OF THE EAR (FIG. 37-3)

### External Ear

**A. Auricle.**

1. Thin plate of elastic cartilage covered by skin.
2. Collects air vibrations.

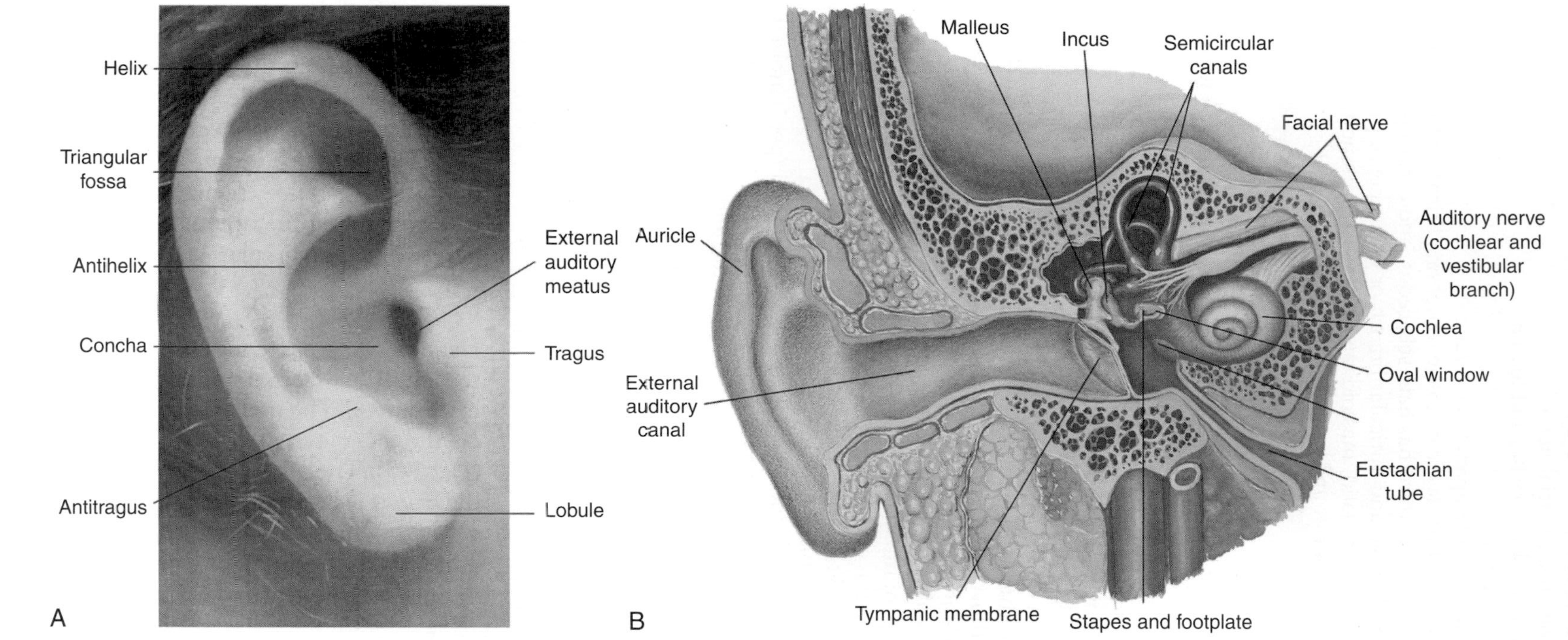


FIGURE 37-3 ■ **A,** Different parts of the auricle of the external ear. **B,** Anatomy of the ear. (From Seidel, H.M., Ball, J.W., Dains, J.E., and Benedict, G.W.: *Mosby's guide to physical examination* [6th ed.]. St. Louis, 2006, Elsevier Mosby.)

3. Possesses extrinsic and intrinsic muscle.
4. Supplied by branches of facial nerve.
5. Consists of tragus, helix, concha, and lobule.

B. **External auditory meatus.**
   1. Curved tube leading to tympanic membrane.
   2. Framework composed of elastic cartilage (outer one third) and bone (inner two thirds).
   3. Lined by skin; outer one third has hair, sebaceous, and ceruminous glands.
   4. Auriculotemporal nerve and auricular branch of vagus nerve provide sensory output.
   5. Lymph drainage is to parotid, mastoid, and cervical lymph nodes.
   6. At birth, meatus is shorter and less curved than in the adult.

## Middle Ear

A. **Slit-like air-containing cavity within petrous (bony) portion of the temporal bone.**

B. **Has roof, floor, anterior, posterior, medial, and lateral walls.**

C. **Lateral wall is the tympanic membrane.**
   1. Tympanic membrane is thin, fibrous membrane.
   2. Sound waves move tympanic membrane medially.
   3. Obliquely placed, concave laterally.
      a. Depression in concavity is called the umbo.
      b. Umbo is produced by the tip of the handle of the malleus ("hammer").

D. **Contains the auditory ossicles.**
   1. Ossicles include malleus, incus ("anvil"), and stapes ("stirrup").
   2. Malleus and incus can be recognized on otoscopic examination.
      a. Tensor tympani muscle inserts on malleus; dampens vibrations.
   3. Stapes inserts on the oval window of the semicircular canal.
      a. Stapedius muscle inserts on stapes; dampens vibrations.
   4. Movement of tympanic membrane moves ossicles.
   5. Movement of ossicles induces compression waves in fluid (perilymph) in cochlea.

E. **Communicates to the nasopharynx via the eustachian (auditory) canal.**
   1. Eustachian tube equalizes air pressure between the middle ear and the nasopharynx.

## Inner Ear

A. **Cavity in petrous portion of temporal bone, medial to middle ear.**

B. **Consists of bony labyrinth and membranous labyrinth; the latter is lodged within the former.**
   1. Membranous labyrinth filled with endolymph.
   2. Bony labyrinth consists of vestibule, semicircular canals, and cochlea.
      a. Vestibule forms base of semicircular canals.
      b. Semicircular canals (superior, posterior, and lateral) arise from vestibule; filled with perilymph.
      c. Movement of perilymph in semicircular canals induced by axial movement.
      d. Transduced by vestibular branch of cochlear nerve.
      e. Cochlea composed of two continuous chambers (scala tympani and scala vestibule) filled with perilymph and a medial chamber (cochlear duct) filled with endolymph.
      f. Sensory ("hair") cells stimulated by compression waves that cause relative movement of membranes within cochlea.

# INNERVATION

A. **Sensory afferents from cochlea and vestibule transmitted by branches of vestibulocochlear (eighth cranial) nerve.**
   1. Vestibular branch forms vestibular ganglion, which receives nerves from different regions of the vestibule.
   2. Cochlear nerve has motor and sensory branches.

B. **Motor efferents to tensor tympani and stapedius muscles.**
   1. Tensor tympani supplied by mandibular branch of trigeminal nerve.
   2. Stapedius supplied by the facial nerve.

C. **Vestibulocochlear and facial nerves enter the inner ear via the internal acoustic meatus.**

# PATIENT ASSESSMENT

## History

A. **Pregnancy:** first-trimester infections (e.g., CMV), unknown rashes, fevers, flu-like illnesses.
B. **Family history:** incidence of hearing loss, ocular disorders.
C. **History of risk factors:** see B. Etiology, under Hearing Loss.

## Examination

During all interactions, care providers should observe the neonate's response to sound. A more focused assessment is performed with the baby in a quiet, alert state.

A. **General assessment.**
   1. General facial configuration: the ears should be symmetrically positioned with the helix of the ear on or above an imaginary line drawn from the inner to the outer canthus of the eye toward the ear. Ears that fall below that line are termed low-set and are often associated with genetic syndromes and other congenital malformations.
   2. The development of the pinna correlates with the infant's gestational age. The pinna of a term infant is firm, with prompt recoil.
   3. Presence of preauricular pits or skin tags may be familial or associated with other anomalies, especially of the renal system. Pits may also communicate with the brain or inner ear and lead to infection.
   4. Poorly developed or malformed ears are associated with hearing loss and other anomalies (Johnson, 2009).
   5. Otoscopic examination of the newborn ear is not part of a routine examination. Visually inspect the auditory canal to ensure patency.
   6. As part of a complete assessment, physical features of syndromes associated with sensorineural hearing loss should be identified.

## Hearing Loss

Hearing loss in the newborn population is estimated to occur at a rate of between 1 and 2 in 1000 live births (Matthews and Robin, 2011). Low birth weight neonates demonstrate failure rates of 20% to 25% when tested at term (Volpe, 2008). Hearing loss occurs across a continuum and can be classified as mild, moderate, or severe. Some types of hearing loss, such as those caused by congenital infections, are progressive or manifest well beyond the newborn period. Ongoing monitoring is needed for those infants with risk factors but who have normal hearing at birth (Vohr, 2011; Volpe, 2008).

A. **Pathophysiology.**
   1. Conductive: dysfunction of the outer or middle ear prevents sound transmission.
   2. Sensorineural: results from damage to the sensory nerve endings in the cochlea or impairment of the auditory nerve.
   3. Mixed: a combination of conductive and sensorineural hearing loss.

B. **Etiology.**
   1. Risk factors (Vohr, 2011; Volpe, 2008).
      a. Familial.
      b. Craniofacial anomalies: especially those involving the pinna and ear canal.
      c. Hyperbilirubinemia: at levels requiring exchange transfusion.
      d. Bacterial or herpes meningitis.
      e. Low Apgar scores (<5 at 1 minute, <6 at 5 minutes).

f. Ototoxic drugs.
   (1) Gentamicin.
   (2) Vancomycin.
g. Intrauterine infections.
   (1) CMV.
   (2) Rubella.
   (3) Syphilis.
   (4) Herpes.
   (5) Toxoplasmosis.
h. Syndromes associated with hearing loss.

2. Idiopathic (up to 50% of cases).

## Hearing Screening

A. **Examination of all newborns.** The Joint Committee on Infant Hearing (2007) recommends universal hearing screening for all newborns. Prompt detection of hearing loss facilitates interventions aimed at preventing speech, language, and cognitive development impairments.

B. **Methodology.**
   1. Evoked otoacoustic emissions.
      a. Measures sound waves generated in the inner ear in response to clicks or tone bursts generated by small microphones placed in the infant's auditory canals.
      b. Advantages: results are specific to each ear; not dependent on the infant's state; short test time.
      c. Disadvantages: inaccurate in the presence of debris in the ear canal; infant must be relatively inactive during the test; does not test neural transmission of sound.
   2. Auditory brainstem response.
      a. Using three scalp electrodes, measures brain waves generated in response to mechanically generated ticks.
      b. Advantages: ear-specific results; unaffected by ear canal debris.
      c. Disadvantages: infant must be in a quiet state.

C. **Follow-up:** Hearing screening identifies infants at risk for hearing loss but is not diagnostic. Infants who fail screening tests must be referred for further testing and intervention.

---

## REFERENCES

Anderson, B.L., and Gonik, B.: Perinatal infections. In R.J. Martin, A.A. Fanaroff, and M.C. Walsh (Eds.): *Fanaroff and Martin's neonatal-perinatal medicine: Diseases of the fetus and newborn* (9th ed.). St. Louis, 2011, Elsevier Mosby, pp. 399–422.

Bashour, M.: Retinopathy of prematurity. Emedicine. 2013. Available at http://emedicine.medscape.com/article/1225022-overview. Accessed March 16, 2013.

Blackburn, S.T.: *Maternal, fetal, and neonatal physiology: A clinical perspective* (4th ed.). Philadelphia, 2013, Elsevier Saunders.

Britt, W.: Cytomegalovirus infections. In J.S. Remington, J.O. Klein, and C.B. Wilson, et al, (Eds.): *Infectious diseases of the fetus and newborn infant.* Philadelphia, 2011, Elsevier Saunders, pp. 706–755.

Chen, M.L., Guo, L., Smith, L.H., et al.: High or low oxygen saturation and severe retinopathy of prematurity: A meta-analysis. *Pediatrics,* 125(6):e1483–e1492, 2010.

Chen, J., Stahl, A., Hellstrom, A., and Smith, L.E.: Current update on retinopathy of prematurity: Screening and treatment. *Current Opinion in Pediatrics,* 23 (2):173–178, 2011.

Darville, T.: Chlamydia infections. In J.S. Remington, J.O. Klein, and C.B. Wilson, et al, (Eds.): *Infectious diseases of the fetus and newborn infant.* Philadelphia, 2011, Elsevier Saunders, pp. 600–606.

de Alba Campomanes, A.G., Binenbaum, G., and Quinn, G.E.: Disorders of the eye. In C.A. Gleason, and S.U. Devaskar (Eds.): *Avery's diseases of the newborn* (9th ed.). Philadelphia, 2012, Elsevier Saunders, pp. 1423–1440.

Embree, J.E.: Gonococcal infections. In J.S. Remington, J.O. Klein C.B. Wilson, et al, (Eds.): *Infectious diseases of the fetus and newborn infant.* Philadelphia, 2011, Elsevier Saunders, pp. 516–523.

Fierson, W.M. American Academy of Pediatrics Section on Ophthalmology, American Academy of Ophthalmology, American Association for Pediatric Ophthalmology and Strabismus, and American Association of Certified Orthoptists: Screening examination of premature infants for retinopathy of prematurity. *Pediatrics,* 131(1):189–195, 2013.

Freij, B.J., and Sever, J.L.: Viral and protozoal infections. In M.G. MacDonald, M.M.K. Seshia, and M.D. Mullet

(Eds.): *Avery's neonatology: Pathophysiology and management of the newborn* (6th ed.). Philadelphia, 2005, Lippincott, Williams & Wilkins, pp. 1274–1356.

Gardner, S.L., and Goldson, E.: The neonate and the environment: Impact on development. In S.L. Gardner, B.S. Carter, M. Enzman-Hines, and J.A. Hernandez (Eds.): *Merenstein & Gardner's handbook of neonatal intensive care* (7th ed.). St. Louis, 2011, Elsevier Mosby, pp. 270–331.

Gardner, S.L., Enzman-Hines, M., and Dickey, L.A.: Respiratory diseases. In S.L. Gardner, B.S. Carter, M. Enzman-Hines, and J.A. Hernandez (Eds.): *Merenstein & Gardner's handbook of neonatal intensive care* (7th ed.). St. Louis, 2011, Elsevier Mosby, pp. 581–677.

Graven, S.: Early neurosensory visual development of the fetus and newborn. *Clinics in Perinatology*, 31:199, 2004.

Hartnett, M.E., and Penn, J.S.: Mechanisms and management of retinopathy of prematurity. *New England Journal of Medicine*, 367(26):2515–2526, 2012.

Hu, J., Blair, M.P., Shapiro, M.J., et al.: Reactivation of retinopathy of prematurity after bevacizumab injection. *Archives of Ophthalmology*, 130(8):1000–1006, 2012.

International Committee for the Classification of Retinopathy of Prematurity: The International Classification of Retinopathy of Prematurity revisited. *Archives of Ophthalmology*, 123:991–999, 2005.

Isenberg, S.J.: Eye disorders. In M.G. MacDonald, M.M.K. Seshia, and M.D. Mullet (Eds.): *Avery's neonatology: Pathophysiology and management of the newborn* (6th ed.). Philadelphia, 2005, Lippincott, Williams & Wilkins, pp. 1469–1484.

Johnson, P.J.: Head, eyes, ears, nose, mouth and neck assessment. In E. Tappero, and M.E. Honeyfield (Eds.): *Physical assessment of the newborn* (4th ed.). Santa Rosa, CA, 2009, NICU Ink.

Joint Committee on Infant Hearing: Year 2007 Position Statement: Principles and guidelines for early hearing detection and intervention program. *Pediatrics*, 120 (4):898–921, 2007.

Matthews, A.L., and Robin, N.H.: Genetic disorders, malformations, and inborn errors of metabolism. In S.L. Garner, B.S. Carter, M. Enzman-Hines, and J.A. Hernandez (Eds.): *Merenstein & Gardner's handbook of neonatal intensive care* (7th ed.). St. Louis, 2011, Elsevier Mosby, pp. 787–811.

Mets, M.B., and Chhabra, M.S.: Eye manifestations of intrauterine infections and their impact on childhood blindness. *Survey of Ophthalmology*, 53(2):95–110, 2008.

Mintz-Hittner, H.A., Kennedy, K.A., and Chuang, A.Z.: for the BEAT-ROP Cooperative Group: Efficacy of intravitreal bevacizumab for stage 3+ retinopathy of prematurity. *New England Journal of Medicine*, 364 (7):603–615, 2011.

Plotkin, S.A., Reef, S.E., Cooper, L.Z., and Alford, C.A.: Rubella. In J.S. Remington, J.O. Klein, and C.B. Wilson et al, (Eds.): *Infectious diseases of the fetus and newborn infant* Philadelphia, 2011, Elsevier Saunders, pp. 861–898.

Remington, J., McLeod, R., Wilson, C.B., and Desmonts, G.: Toxoplasmosis. In J.S. Remington, J.O. Klein, and C.B. Wilson et al, (Eds.): *Infectious diseases of the fetus and newborn infant* Philadelphia, 2011, Elsevier Saunders, pp. 918–1041.

Repka, M.X., Tung, B., Good, W.V., et al.: Outcome of eyes developing retinal detachment during the Early Treatment for Retinopathy of Prematurity study. *Archives of Ophthalmology*, 129(9):1175–1179, 2011.

Sears, J.E., Pietz, J., Sonnie, C., et al.: A change in oxygen supplementation can decrease the incidence of retinopathy of prematurity. *Ophthalmology*, 116(3):1282, 2009.

Venkatesh, M.P., Adams, K.M., and Weisman, L.E.: Infection in the neonate. In S.L. Gardner, B.S. Carter, M. Enzman-Hines, and J.A. Hernandez (Eds.): *Merenstein & Gardner's handbook of neonatal intensive care* (7th ed.). St. Louis, 2011, Elsevier Mosby, pp. 553–580.

Vohr, B.: Hearing loss in the newborn infant. In R.J. Martin, A.A. Fanaroff, and M.C. Walsh (Eds.): *Fanaroff and Martin's neonatal-perinatal medicine: Diseases of the fetus and newborn* (9th ed.). St. Louis, 2011, Elsevier Mosby, pp. 1049–1056.

Volpe, J.J.: *Neurology of the newborn* (5th ed.). Philadelphia, 2008, Elsevier Saunders.

CHAPTER

# 38 Foundations of Neonatal Research

KAREN A. THOMAS

**OBJECTIVES**

1. Identify nurses' research competencies according to educational preparation.
2. Describe the research process and key components of research studies.
3. Identify neonatal nurses as research consumers who implement research translational strategies through clinical evidence-based practice.
4. List questions to ask when critiquing research literature.
5. Be informed about the rights of research subjects and the ethical conduct of research.

## RESEARCH AND GENERATION OF NURSING KNOWLEDGE

*Research* refers to systematic inquiry or investigation governed by scientific principles and conducted to expand knowledge and increase understanding. The research process describes a logical and orderly progression from development of a question through the conduct of a study, analysis of resultant findings, dissemination of conclusions, translation into practice, and implementation. The questions asked and the methodology that guide inquiry reflect underlying values and beliefs, worldview, or philosophy. Scientific method describes prescribed rules of logic and imposed controls, ensuring that the knowledge generated is truthful. Research generates empirical (i.e., experienced) knowledge. Although nursing, as a science-based profession, strongly subscribes to empirical research, the body of nursing knowledge is enriched by diversity in ways of knowing. Nonresearch bases for nursing knowledge—tradition, authority, trial and error, personal experience, intuition, and commonsense reasoning—have a powerful influence and are part of nursing tradition; however, nonresearch knowledge does not permit scientific predictability, nor does it provide for scientific rationale and justification for nursing actions. Within the nursing profession, research promotes health and well-being of patient populations through a variety of applications. Research improves practice by providing answers to clinical questions, evaluating the effectiveness of nursing interventions and programs of care, and expanding the body of nursing knowledge. Increasing emphasis on evidence-based practice, research-based practice, best practices, practice guidelines, and outcomes focus mandates that research occupy a central role in nursing. The American Nurses Association (ANA) research agenda addresses the value of nursing in improving safety, clinical effectiveness, and quality assurance, and promoting the health of populations (ANA, 2011).

The ANA research agenda speaks to the value and impact of nursing contributions to safety, care quality, and clinical efficiency in supporting the health of populations (ANA, 2011; LoBiondo-Wood and Haber, 2010). All nurses have a role related to research (LoBiondo-Wood and Haber, 2010). Put simply, nurses "do" and/or "use" research. While not all nurses do research, every nurse is a consumer of research. Research findings are an essential component of evidence-based practice. At the time of this writing, a search in PubMed using the terms "evidence-based practice nursing" yielded 10,719 hits. The earliest of these articles dates from the 1980s. The past three decades are marked by mounting emphasis on empirical proof as the base for nursing care as well as on the evaluation and synthesis of knowledge supporting nursing actions. There is a significant need in nursing for well-constructed systematic and integrative reviews of the literature (McGrath, 2012). Pressure for evidence-based practice is also related to cost containment and demonstrating the value of nursing care as well as cost-effectiveness of nursing interventions. Although nurses in general increasingly subscribe to the principles of evidence-based practice, nursing leadership and organizational support play an essential role in the implementation of evidence-based practice

■ TABLE 38-1
■ ■ **Processes of "Doing" and "Using" Research in Nursing**

| Research | Evidence-Based Practice |
|---|---|
| Formulate a question or hypothesis | Specify a clinical problem |
| Choose study design | Conduct literature review |
| Plan study methods and procedures | Gather evidence |
| Collect data | Critically appraise evidence |
| Analyze data and generate findings | Develop practice guideline |
| Disseminate results | Apply the practice change |
| Translate findings into practice | Evaluate patient/family outcomes and share results |

Adapted from Raines, D.A. Quality improvement, evidence-based practice, and nursing research . . . Oh my! *Neonatal Network,* 31(4):262-264, 2012; and Melnyk, B.M. and Fineout-Overholt, E.: Making the case for evidence-based practice and cultivating a spirit of inquiry. In B.M. Melnyk and E. Fineout-Overholt (Eds.): *Evidence-based practice in nursing and healthcare: A guide to best practice.* Philadelphia, 2011, Wolters Kluwer, pp. 3-24.

(Ahrens and Johnson, 2013). Neonatal clinical nurse specialists, nurse managers, and nursing administration are critical, therefore, in moving research into practice. Evidence-based practice shares elements with conducting research (Raines, 2012) and requires knowledge of the "doing" of research to evaluate existing evidence (Table 38-1).

Independently planning and conducting research requires advanced knowledge. Assuming that any nurse can do research is like assuming any nurse can insert a peripherally inserted central catheter line. Both require specific education and skill development. The conduct of research requires expertise in research design and methods as well as statistical analysis. Research is differentially emphasized in the curriculum of nursing academic programs. Table 38-2 illustrates general research competencies based on educational preparation. The American Association of Colleges of Nursing specifies research competencies as essentials in baccalaureate, master's, and advanced practice doctoral education (American Association of Colleges of Nursing, 2013) and emphasizes research and development of nursing science as the center of Ph.D. education in nursing (American Association of Colleges of Nursing, 2001).

Bridging the gap between doing and using research is the role of translational science. Though various terms are used, translational science, knowledge translation, and implementation science, in general all refer to moving science "from the bench to the bedside," including both practice and policy (Curran et al., 2011). Translation, the in-between step, is a science unto itself, with theory and methods guiding how and why knowledge is transmitted into practice. Translational science, the underpinning of evidence-based practice, examines the nature of evidence and its evaluation, synthesis of evidence, informatics, the study of knowledge-to-action gaps, factors promoting and hindering knowledge transfer, methods of knowledge transfer, and evaluation of effects (Curran et al., 2011).

Whether doing or using research, nurses assume several roles related to research ethics. Nurses independently conducting research comply with regulations governing human research subject participation. Nurses also may serve as staff on research projects conducted by others. Finally, nurses care for patients and their families who are involved in research. In all of these roles, nurses promote safety and protection of rights. In an American Association of Critical-Care Nurses draft resource document, Richmond and Ulrich (2012) outlined the ethical requirements related to the scientific value, integrity, and validity of the specific research project, benefits of the research outweighing the risks, informed consent processes, and respect for research participants. Neonatal intensive care unit (NICU) nurses face particular research ethics challenges given the vulnerable nature of infants and their parents (Franck, 2005).

## RESEARCH PROCESS AND COMPONENTS OF A RESEARCH STUDY

The nursing process and research process both represent an organized approach to critical thinking and share several similarities (Table 38-3). In essence, every patient is an "*n* of 1" research study.

■ TABLE 38-2
■ ■ **Nursing Research Education**

| Program | Educational Preparation*,†,‡,§ |
|---|---|
| ADN | Appreciate the importance of research in nursing and assist in problem identification and data collection.‡<br>Identify problems, collect data, apply research findings in care delivery.§ |
| B.S.N. | AACN B.S.N. Essential III. Translation of current evidence into practice.<br>Basic understanding of research process and translation to practice, appraise sources of information, participate in translation of evidence into practice, collaborate in collection and dissemination of evidence, understand nursing quality and safety measures.¶ |
| Master's | AACN Master's Essential IV. Translation and integration of scholarship into practice.<br>Integration and translation of multiple information sources to improve practice and subsequent outcomes for patient aggregates, ethical protections for research participants, articulate evidence base for practice, work collaboratively to improve outcomes and promote policy change through generation, dissemination, and implementation of knowledge, apply practice guidelines, rigorous examination of database evidence to guide nursing practice.¶¶ |
| DNP | AACN DNP Essential III. Clinical scholarship and analytical methods.<br>Determine best evidence for practice through critical appraisal, design and implement outcome evaluation of practice, design and conduct quality improvement processes, develop evidence-based practice guidelines, work collaboratively as a practice specialist to generate knowledge, dissemination to improve outcomes.** |
| Ph.D. | Develop the science of nursing. Research intensive, develop in-depth knowledge in substantive area, knowledge of the philosophy of science, integrative scientific perspective, generate knowledge, conduct original research, research ethics, leadership in the conduct of research, communication and dissemination of findings.† |

*AACN*, American Association of Colleges of Nursing.
*AACN Essentials: http://www.aacn.nche.edu/education-resources/essential-series
†AACN Indicators of Quality in Research-Focused Doctoral Programs in Nursing: http://www.aacn.nche.edu/publications/position/quality-indicators
‡Adapted from AACN Position Statement on Nursing Research, approved 1998, revised 2006: http://www.aacn.nche.edu/publications/position/nursing-research
§Adapted from Ayers, D.M. and Coeling, H.: Incorporating research into associate degree nursing curricula. *Journal of Nursing Education*, 44 (11), 2005, 515-518.
¶AACN BSN Essentials: http://www.aacn.nche.edu/education-resources/BaccEssentials08.pdf
¶¶AACN Masters Essentials: http://www.aacn.nche.edu/education-resources/MastersEssentials11.pdf
**DNP Essentials (advanced nursing practice): http://www.aacn.nche.edu/publications/position/DNPEssentials.pdf

■ TABLE 38-3
■ ■ **Similarities of the Research Process and the Nursing Process**

| Nursing Process | Research Process |
|---|---|
| Client assessment | Identification of problem |
| Nursing diagnosis | Questions or hypotheses |
| Plan of care | Method |
| Evaluation | Findings |
| Revision of plan | Implications and dissemination |

Adapted from Gillis, A. and Jackson, W.: *Research for nurses: Methods and interpretation*. Philadelphia, 2002, F.A. Davis.

Regardless of the topic investigated, a research study contains several key elements (Houser and Bokovoy, 2006; LoBiondo-Wood and Haber, 2010):

A. **Question:** All research derives from a purpose and begins with a problem or general question, which is refined to form specific research aims, questions, or hypotheses.
   1. The research questions or hypotheses are the focal point of a research study, driving all other aspects of the investigation, including method choices.

2. Each element of a research project fits the stated questions or hypotheses.
3. Analysis and study results direct relate to stated aims, questions, or hypotheses.

B. **Background:** Framework is derived from a review of the literature that establishes what is currently known regarding the study topic and identifies the gaps in knowledge that the study will address.
1. When a study is derived from an existing theory, the theoretical framework portrays the variables and their relationships as prescribed by the theory.
2. A conceptual framework is a description of concepts, defined for the purposes of the research, and their relationships.

C. **Method:** In some readings, the term *method* is used to define what was done to collect the data (e.g., observation, questionnaire, interview, physiologic measure); however, here *method* is defined as the entire description of how the study is conducted.
1. Design: the plan for data collection, much like a recipe or pattern. There are two general types of research design:
   a. Descriptive (sometimes divided into descriptive and exploratory).
      (1) Designs involve depicting the study sample "as is."
      (2) Provide information to help understand the variables of interest in defined sample.
   b. Experimental.
      (1) The investigator manipulates independent variables and measures the response in dependent variables.
      (2) Intervention studies are by nature experimental.
   c. The design determines the number of subject groups, the timing of data collection, and control of extraneous variables that may produce bias.
   d. These design choices contribute to scientific validity of the study and are related to how subjects are selected, the control of extraneous variables, how the independent variables are applied.
   e. Designs are described according to internal and external validity. Designs offer differing strengths and weaknesses relative to internal and external validity (Table 38-4).
      (1) Internal validity refers to lack of bias and random variation that support obtaining accurate results in the population studied.
      (2) External validity refers to the generalizability of results to a wider population.
2. Sample: represents who or what is studied.
   a. Made up of units of analysis, such as individuals, nursing units, or hospitals.
   b. Typically selected from a larger population.

**TABLE 38-4**
**Levels of Bias Control in Research Design**

| Level | Designs | Independent Variable Control* | Control Group | Outcomes Present at Enrollment |
|---|---|---|---|---|
| A | Randomized concurrent controlled trial<br>Quasi-randomized concurrent trial<br>Randomized pre–post design | Yes | Yes (concurrent) | No |
| B | Cohort concurrent study<br>Pre–post study | No | Yes (may or may not be concurrent) | No |
| C | Ex post facto study<br>Case–control study | No | Yes (may or may not be concurrent) | Yes |
| D | Descriptive | No | No | Yes or no |

Adapted from Jacob, R.F. and Carr, A.B.: Hierarchy of research design used to categorize the "strength of evidence" in answering clinical dental questions. *Journal of Prosthetic Dentistry*, 83(2):137-152, 2000.
*Independent variable or intervention controlled by investigator.

c. Specific strategies for sampling determine if results from a sample can reasonably be generalized to the larger population.
   (1) Probability sampling: Each individual in the population has an equal chance of being included in the sample. Probability sampling is not always feasible, particularly in nursing research dealing with small patient populations. In this situation, nonprobability sampling is employed.
d. Sample size is a factor in the selection of analysis strategies.

3. Variables: the attributes or properties measured in a research study.
   a. Variables are defined both conceptually and operationally.
      (1) Conceptual definition: variable is described in the abstract (e.g., hypertension).
      (2) Operational definition: defines the variable in measurable terms. For example, hypertension will be defined as a systolic blood pressure greater than 100 mm Hg in the term neonate.
   b. *Instruments* and *tools* are terms used interchangeably to indicate operational measures.
   c. The quality of measurement is critical to research. Validity and reliability describe instrument measurement characteristics.
      (1) Validity is the degree to which an instrument measures what it is purported to measure. The instrument measures truly the variable.
      (2) Reliability refers to ability of the instrument to obtain consistent results (i.e., reproducibility) over time or across administrators.
4. Setting: portrays where the study is conducted and the conditions surrounding the study.
5. Procedure: describes in stepwise fashion how the study was carried out.
6. Analysis: uses statistical or analytic techniques on the data collected to answer the research questions or compare findings with stated hypotheses.
7. Results: include a description of the study sample as well as findings from the analysis based on stated aims, questions, or hypotheses.
8. Conclusion: includes discussion of study findings, implications, limitations, and recommendations for future research. Practice recommendations are supported by the study results.

## QUANTITATIVE RESEARCH

A. **Numeric data are analyzed using a statistical approach specified as part of the planning for the research project.**
B. **Descriptive statistics include measures of central tendency (mean, median, mode) and dispersion (standard deviation, variance, range).**
C. **Inferential statistics are based on probability and allow judgments to be made about the population, and hypotheses to be tested.** In general, inferential statistics test either how things differ or how things are related.
D. **Statistical significance means that the particular finding is not likely due to chance alone.**
   1. The investigator sets an alpha or probability level that will be acceptable in interpreting results (often alpha is set at $p < 0.05$).
   2. The $p$ value is the probability associated with the test statistic calculated from the study data. If the $p$ value is less than alpha, the test is statistically significant.
   3. Statistical significance is not always consistent with clinical significance, meaning that the magnitude of the effect is not relevant or important in clinical practice.

## QUALITATIVE RESEARCH

A. **Maintains the same rigor as quantitative research.**
B. **Focus is in-depth understanding of a phenomenon, with particular emphasis on the subject's reports of personal experience, used to increase understanding of phenomena perceived by individuals, groups, and cultures (Holloway and Wheeler, 2010).**
C. **Participant observation, focus groups, and interviews are methods frequently employed in qualitative research.**

D. **The specific research approach stems from an underlying philosophical perspective.** Types of perspectives commonly used in nursing qualitative research include phenomenology, grounded theory, and ethnography (Holloway and Wheeler, 2010).
   1. Phenomenology: seeks to understand the lived experience of individuals.
   2. Grounded theory: symbolic interaction forms the basis for understanding social processes and behavior.
   3. Ethnography: describes a cultural group.

E. **The analysis is inductive and interpretive.**

F. **The process of conducting qualitative research and components of the research project are parallel with those of quantitative research.** Qualitative research entails defined specifying aims, defined approach, description of sampling and data collection procedures, analysis consistent with philosophical approach and aims, and actions to maintain rigor (validity) (Holloway and Wheeler, 2010).

## AREAS OF EXPLORATION IN NEONATAL NURSING

A. **Research supports generation of knowledge guiding evidence-based practice.**

B. **Contemporary topics in neonatal nursing research include the following:**
   1. Consequences of pain experiences in the neonate and pain management.
   2. Initiation of oral feeding in preterm infants and feeding schedules.
   3. Promotion of breastfeeding in preterm infants.
   4. Empowerment of families and family-centered care.
   5. Safe care delivery and patient safety.
   6. Cost containment.
   7. Promotion of optimal developmental outcomes.
   8. NICU nursing staff recruitment, training, and retention.
   9. NICU design and environment effects on infants and nursing staff.
   10. Ethical challenges in NICU care.
   11. Prevention of hospital-acquired infections.
   12. Care of drug-exposed neonates.
   13. Nutritional needs of high-risk infants.
   14. Innovations in care delivery structure and process.
   15. Neural protection measures such as head cooling or whole-body cooling.

## NURSES AS CONSUMERS OF RESEARCH

A. **Every nurse is a consumer of research whether or not direct participation in research activities occurs (Box 38-1).**

BOX 38-1
**RESEARCH APPLICATIONS IN PRACTICE**

Clinical practice committee
Quality improvement committee
Process improvement protocol
Policies
Procedures
Standards
Critical pathways
Protocols
Guidelines
Journal club
Product review committee

**B. Nursing activities involving consumption of research.**

1. Individually reading current research articles and attending conference research presentations to expand knowledge and support practice.
2. Conducting reviews of evidence.
3. Types of evidence review (Whittemore and Knafl, 2005).
   a. Systematic review—combine studies on specific problem or questions, the basis for evidence-based practice.
   b. Meta-analysis—statistical combining of findings from primary research studies to form aggregate results.
   c. Integrative review—address the broadest base of existing knowledge (Whittemore and Knafl, 2005).
4. Research critique and appraisal is a systematic approach to reading and assessing research articles to assess applicability of knowledge in practice and use in further research. Key questions to ask when reviewing a research article are provided in Box 38-2.

**C. Research utilization.**

1. Refers to specific application of research findings, irrespective of research method, in practice and includes critique of studies, synthesis of findings, assessing applicability to practice, development and implementation of research-based guidelines, and evaluation of practice change (Titler et al., 2001).
   a. The Iowa Model (Fig. 38-1) is an example of research-based practice that includes generation of practice-related questions and systematic assessment of research findings used to change caregiving.
   b. The Iowa Model emphasizes a variety of research sources of data and is not limited to randomized controlled trials.

BOX 38-2

**RESEARCH CRITIQUE AND APPRAISAL**

Is there a clear statement of the problem and purpose?
Are the research questions or hypotheses unambiguous and stated in measurable terms?
Does the background establish a theoretical or conceptual framework and show gaps in knowledge?
Does the background define key concepts and their measures and describe relationships among study concepts?
Is the literature review comprehensive and current?
Do the purpose, questions/hypotheses, design, method, and analysis fit together logically?
Is the design clearly described?
Are possible extraneous variables identified and controlled?
Are the sample characteristics described and sampling exclusion and inclusion criteria reported?
To whom can study results be generalized?
Is the sample size adequate to address the research questions or hypotheses?
Is loss of subjects explained?
Is the measurement of study variables described?
Are study measures valid and reliable?
Are study procedures described?
How were extraneous variables controlled?
Is the analysis described and are the statistics appropriate for addressing the questions/hypotheses?
Do the reported results address the research questions/hypotheses?
Are the findings interpreted and compared with current knowledge?
Are conclusions justifiable on the basis of the stated findings?
Are statistically significant findings also clinically significant?
Are limitations of the study presented?
Is application of findings discussed?
Are future research directions outlined?

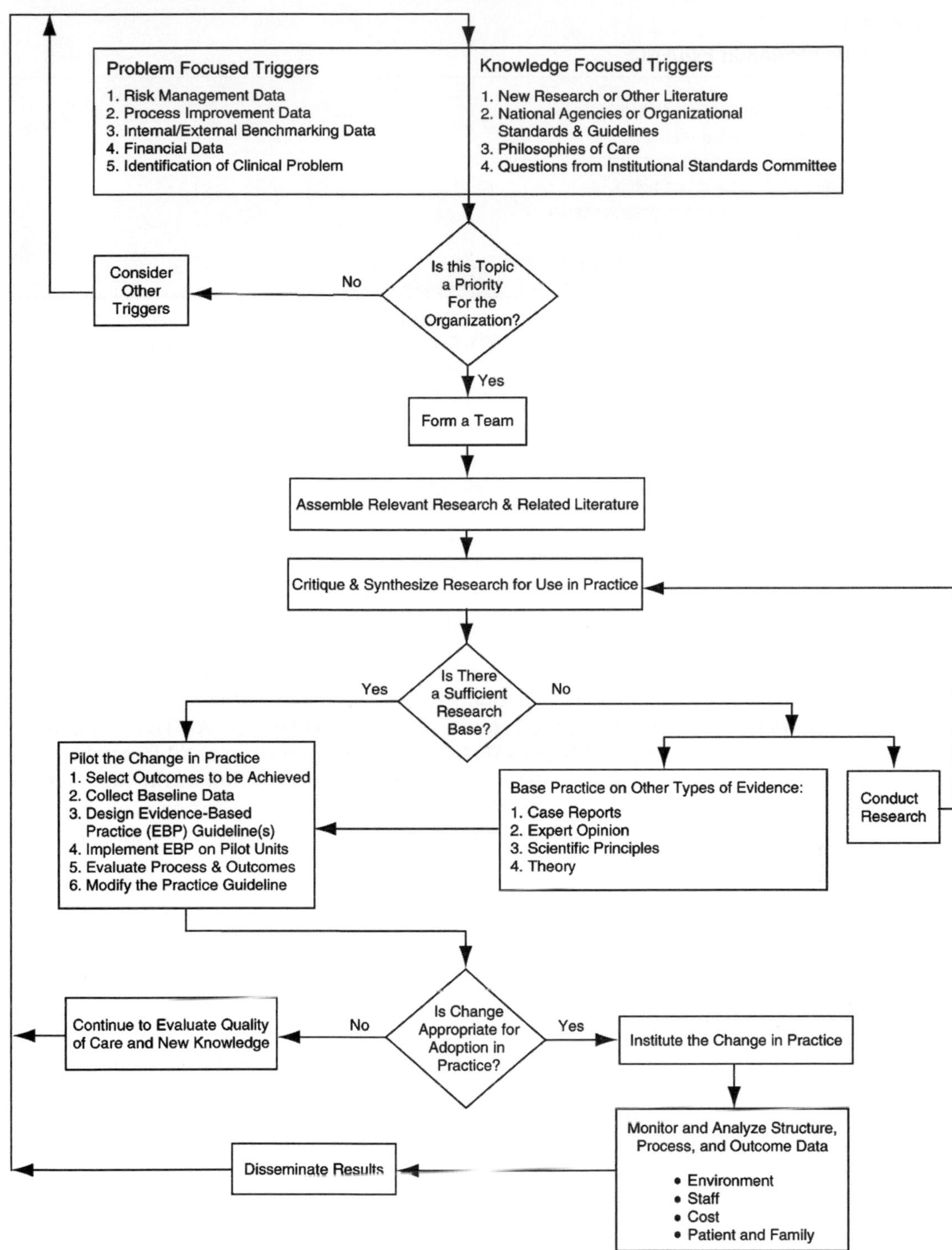


FIGURE 38-1 ■ Iowa Model of research-based practice to promote quality care. (From Titler, M.G., Steelman, V.J., Budreau, G., et al.: The Iowa Model of evidence-based practice to promote quality of care. *Critical Care Nursing Clinics of North America*, 13[4]:497-509, 2001.)

■ BOX 38-3
■ **LEVELS OF RESEARCH EVIDENCE**

Meta-analysis of randomized controlled trials
Single randomized controlled trial
Single well-designed controlled study without randomization
Single well-designed quasi-experimental study
Systematic reviews of nonexperimental research
Well-designed single nonexperimental study
Expert opinions, committee reports, consensus panels

Adapted from Agency for Health Care Policy and Research: *Clinical Practice Guideline No. 9: Management of cancer pain* (AHCPR Publication No. 94-0592). Rockville, Md., 1994, Department of Health and Human Services; and Guyatt, G., Drummond, R., Meade, M.O., and Cook, D.J.: *Users' guides to the medical literature: A manual for evidence-based clinical practice* (2nd ed.). New York, 2008, McGraw-Hill.

D. **Evidence-based practice emphasizes systemic appraisal of best evidence combined with clinical expertise and patient/family values and preferences to develop best practices (Melnyk and Fineout-Overholt, 2011).**
   1. Systematic review of data-based literature, grading studies according to level of evidence, with highest priority given to randomized controlled trials (Box 38-3).
   2. Evidence-based practice is exemplified by the Cochrane Collaboration, an organization that has established robust criteria for the systematic evaluation of research studies resulting in recommendations for practice.
   3. Evidence-based practice in general refers to established criteria for sources of knowledge and acceptable research methods (LoBiondo-Wood and Haber, 2010).

E. **The Association of Women's Health, Obstetric and Neonatal Nurses (AWHONN) and the National Association of Neonatal Nurses (NANN) have been instrumental in establishing research-based practice programs, addressing such issues as transition of the late preterm infant initiative, neonatal skin care, transition of the preterm infant to an open crib, management of neonatal hypotension, transport standards, neonatal pain assessment, and insertion of peripheral catheters (AWHONN, 2013; NANN, 2013).**

## ETHICS IN RESEARCH AND NURSES AS ADVOCATES

A. **Whether nurses are investigators conducting research or caring for patients who are research participants, careful consideration of ethics in research is essential.**

B. **It is important that nurses maintain a clear distinction between research and practice and between the roles of researcher and care provider.** Practice is aimed at caregiving to aid the well-being of an individual, whereas research involves gathering of data to generate knowledge (American Association of Critical-Care Nurses, 2013).

C. **The ethical principles guiding human research include autonomy, beneficence, and justice.**
   1. Autonomy: the ability to make an informed choice, free of coercion, regarding participation in research. The components of informed consent are provided in Box 38-4. Consent for research participation must be obtained by a member of the research team who is qualified to explain the study and answer questions. In neonatal research, parents provide consent for infant participation.
   2. Beneficence: the research benefits must outweigh the risks. Children are considered to be a vulnerable group, and federal mandates require that risks to a child must be minimal when there is no direct benefit to the child. When a research project involves more than minimal risk, the direct benefit to the child must outweigh the risk.
   3. Justice: relates to who is represented in the research sample. Groups that bear the burden for research participation should also be groups that will ultimately benefit from the results.

D. **Subject selection should be free of discrimination and represent a broad population.**

**BOX 38-4**
**ELEMENTS OF INFORMED CONSENT**

- Complete explanation of study purpose and procedures
- Duration of involvement and time commitment clearly stated
- Full disclosure of study risks
- Description of potential adverse effects and how they will be treated
- Identification of any costs that are subject's responsibility
- Accurate description of potential benefit to self and/or society
- Description of deviations from standard care
- Indication of alternatives if an intervention is to be tested
- Permission for use of medical records
- Protection of confidentiality
- Specification of possible limits to confidentiality (e.g., mandatory reporting)
- Duration of identifiable data retention
- Permission to withdraw at any time
- Permission to refuse to answer any questions
- No coercion, including assurance that refusal will not change care or other entitlements
- Opportunity to ask questions
- Consent language and literacy at the level of signatory's understanding
- Receipt of copy of consent

E. **Several documents provide guidelines for the protection of human subjects in the United States.**
   1. The Belmont Report (National Commission for the Protection of Human Subjects of Biomedical and Behavioral Research, 1979) was developed within the Department of Health, Education, and Welfare (now the Department of Health and Human Services [DHHS]).
   2. All research sponsored by any federal agencies, including the National Institute for Nursing Research (an institute under the National Institutes of Health and part of the DHHS), must comply with standards for human participation in research listed under Title 45, Code of Federal Regulations, Part 46, "Protection of Human Subjects" (Department of Health and Human Services, 2009).
   3. The Office for Human Research Protections is specifically charged with ensuring the safety and welfare of people participating in DHHS research (additional information is available at http://www.hhs.gov/ohrp/index.html).
   4. To ensure the protection of human subjects, all research should be approved by a peer review group. All research supported by federal funds requires review by an internal review board (IRB), a specific type of peer review group established according to federal regulations.
   5. Nurses conducting research should become familiar with regulations protecting human subjects. For nurses in practice, understanding of rights in research, particularly informed consent, provides a basis for advocacy and ensuring the protection of patients who are also research participants (American Association of Critical-Care Nurses, 2013). Concerns about research ethics should be raised with the local peer review group or IRB.

## REFERENCES


Agency for Health Care Policy, Research; *Clinical Practice Guideline No. 9: Management of cancer pain (AHCPR Publication No. 94-0592)*. Rockville, MD, 1994, Department of Health and Human Services.

Ahrens, S. and Johnson, C.S.: Finding the way to evidence-based practice. *Nursing Management*, 44 (5):15–19, 2013.

American Association of Colleges of Nursing: Leading initiatives. Essentials series. 2013. Retrieved April 24, 2013, from http://www.aacn.nche.edu/education-resources/essential-series.

American Association of Colleges of Nursing: *Indicators of quality in research-focused doctoral programs in nursing*, Washington, DC, 2001, American Association of Colleges of Nursing.

American Association of Critical-Care Nurses: *Ethics in critical care nursing research*. 2013. Available at http://www.aacn.org/wd/practice/content/research/

ethics-in-critical-care-nursing-research.pcms?menu=; accessed April 26, 2013.

American Nurses Association: *American Nurses Association research agenda*, Silver Springs, MD, 2011, American Nurses Association.

Association of Women's Health, Obstetric and Neonatal Nurses: *Research-based practice projects*, 2013. Available at http://www.awhonn.org/awhonn/content.do?name=03_JournalsPubsResearch/3G_ResearchBasedPracticeProjects.htm; accessed April 26, 2013.

Curran, J.A., Grimshaw, J.M., Hayden, J.A., and Campbell, B.: Knowledge translation research: The science of moving research into policy and practice. *The Journal of Continuing Education in the Health Professions*, 31(3):174–180, 2011.

Department of Health and Human Services: Code of Federal Regulations. Title 45. Public Welfare, Part 46: Protection of Human Subjects. 2009: Available at http://www.hhs.gov/ohrp/humansubjects/guidance/45cfr46.html.

Franck, L.S.: Research with newborn participants: Doing the right research and doing it right. *Journal of Perinatal & Neonatal Nursing*, 19(2):177–186, 2005.

Gillis, A. and Jackson, W.: *Research for nurses:* Methods and interpretation. Philadelphia, 2002, F.A. Davis.

Guyatt, G., Drummond, R., Meade, M.O., and Cook, D.J.: *Users' guides to the medical literature: A manual for evidence-based clinical practice* (2nd ed.). New York, 2008, McGraw-Hill.

Holloway, I. and Wheeler, S.: *Qualitative research in nursing and healthcare* (3rd ed.). Chichester, West Sussex, 2010, Wiley-Blackwell.

Houser, J. and Bokovoy, J.: *Clinical research in practice: A guide for the bedside scientist*. Sudbury, MA, 2006, Jones and Bartlett.

Jacob, R.F. and Carr, A.B.: Hierarchy of research design used to categorize the "strength of evidence" in answering clinical dental questions. *Journal of Prosthetic Dentistry*, 83(2):137–152, 2000.

LoBiondo-Wood, G. and Haber, J.: *Nursing research: Methods and critical appraisal for evidence-based practice*. Philadelphia, 2010, Elsevier Mosby.

McGrath, J.M.: Systematic and integrative reviews of the literature: How are they changing our thoughts about practice? *Journal of Perinatal & Neonatal Nursing*, 26(3):193–195, 2012.

Melnyk, B.M. and Fineout-Overholt, E.: Making the case for evidence-based practice and cultivating a spirit of inquiry. In B.M. Melnyk and E. Fineout-Overholt (Eds.): *Evidence-based practice in nursing and healthcare: A guide to best practice* Philadelphia, 2011, Wolters Kluwer, pp. 3–24.

National Association of Neonatal Nurses: NANN Research Institute agenda. 2013. Retrieved April 25, 2013, from http://www.nann.org/uploads/files/NANN_Research_Institute_Agenda.pdf.

National Commission for the Protection of Human Subjects of Biomedical and Behavioral Research: *The Belmont Report: Ethical principles and guidelines for the protection of human subjects of research*. Washington, DC, 1979, Department of Health, Education, and Welfare. Retrieved March 16, 2003, from http://ohrp.osophs.dhhs.gov/humansubjects/guidance/belmont.htm.

Raines, D.A.: Quality improvement, evidence-based practice, and nursing research . . . Oh my! *Neonatal Network*, 31(4):262–264, 2012.

Richmond, T.S. and Ulrich, C.: Ethical foundations for critical care nursing research. 2012: Retrieved from http://www.aacn.org/wd/practice/docs/research/ethical-foundations-crit-care-nursing-research.pdf.

Titler, M.G., Kleiber, C., Steelman, V.J., et al.: The Iowa Model of evidence-based practice to promote quality care. *Critical Care Nursing Clinics of North America*, 13(4):497–509, 2001.

Whittemore, R. and Knafl, K.: The integrative review: Updated methodology. *Journal of Advanced Nursing*, 52(5):546–553, 2005.

CHAPTER

# 39 Ethical Issues

TANYA SUDIA-ROBINSON

**OBJECTIVES**

1. Explore how the principles of biomedical ethics can be applied in the neonatal intensive care unit (NICU).
2. Identify alternate theoretical and case analysis approaches to examining ethical issues in the NICU.
3. Examine the nurse's role when ethical issues arise in the NICU.
4. Recognize the contribution of hospital ethics committees in exploring and resolving ethical issues in the NICU.

Ethical issues are ever present in the NICU. Each technological advance brings ethical questions to the forefront of care. How far can and should the limits of viability be extended? How can we minimize the social, emotional, and financial costs associated with NICU care? Are we providing adequate palliative care in the NICU? These are just a few of the poignant questions that warrant ongoing ethical analysis.

Nurses, nurse practitioners, physicians, and other members of the NICU health care team have professional obligations to patients. In this chapter, the emphasis is placed on the obligations and role of the nurse in collaboration with other NICU team members. For nurses and physicians, these obligations are based on the professional codes of practice and means of ethical conduct. For example, the practice of medicine evolved from the founding obligation of *Primum non nocere*, a Latin phrase meaning "First, do no harm." This has become a guiding ethical obligation for health care professionals, regardless of their practice setting.

Nurses also focus on ethical guidance as established by professional nursing organizations. For the NICU nurse, primary professional guidance is provided through the American Nurses Association (ANA) *Code of Ethics for Nurses with Interpretative Statements* (ANA, 2001); the ANA *Position Statements on Ethics and Human Rights*; and the National Association of Neonatal Nurses (NANN) *Position Statement on NICU Nurse Involvement in Ethical Decisions* (NANN, 2010). These key documents provide the foundation for ethical practice in the NICU.

## EXAMINING ETHICAL ISSUES IN THE NICU

In the NICU, ethical dilemmas arise when ethical principles and well-intended actions compete. For example, when a neonate with overwhelming sepsis and intraventricular hemorrhage begins to exhibit multisystem failure, conflict may arise regarding continuation of the most aggressive technical care measures versus deceleration of those measures to focus on more intensive palliative care. Thus, the ethical dilemma in this situation is avoiding causing harm yet doing good, ensuring that actions taken are in the best interest of this neonate at this point in time.

Among the questions that can arise are: What are best-interest actions for the neonate? Who decides what those actions should be? What happens when members of the health care team are in disagreement about the aggressiveness of treatment? What if one or both parents disagree about the best interests of the neonate? Questions such as these and the related ethical issues encountered in the NICU often arise from very complex situations that are best addressed by a team approach.

Nurses, physicians, and other members of the NICU health care team need to have a framework for understanding and resolving the ethical issues that arise in the NICU (Callister and Sudia-Robinson, 2011). Although there are many different philosophical perspectives one can use to examine ethical issues, health care professionals need to be able to directly translate those theories to bedside care. Thus this chapter's discussion of ethical approaches focuses on models from the field of applied ethics. The following sections are designed to assist the bedside caregiver to recognize and examine ethical issues as they arise in the NICU.

## PRINCIPLES OF BIOMEDICAL ETHICS

The most well-known framework for examining biomedical ethical issues was originally developed by Beauchamp and Childress in 1979. Commonly referred to as the Principle Approach or the Principles of Biomedical Ethics, this model provides the health care team with four key principles to examine: beneficence, nonmaleficence, respect for autonomy, and justice. All four principles must be taken into account when examining an ethics case (Beauchamp and Childress, 2013).

### Beneficence

The principle of beneficence focuses on the act of doing good or performing actions with the intent of benefiting another person (Beauchamp and Childress, 2013). It is an action-based principle; thus there is a requirement to act or perform actions that lead to direct benefit. In accordance with this principle, the health care team must examine their actions and overall plan of care to determine the intended direct benefit for the neonate. An important point to remember is that, as the neonate's condition changes, an ongoing consideration of beneficence should occur.

To illustrate the principle of beneficence in the NICU, consider the case of a neonate who is born extremely premature and with an extremely low birth weight. The parents are in agreement with a plan of aggressive treatment. However, at approximately 4 days of age, the neonate has a grade 4 intraventricular hemorrhage, severely distended abdomen, poor perfusion, and signs of failing organs. The plan of care that was benefiting this neonate several days ago no longer has the same effect. The care measures that have been in place are not having a direct beneficial effect and must be reexamined with the parents.

### Nonmaleficence

The principle of nonmaleficence obligates health care providers to avoid directly causing harm to a patient. Specifically, the plan of care must avoid causing intentional harm. Using the previous example of a neonate in multisystem decline, the NICU team would need to evaluate the continuing use of aggressive therapies with a neonate who is physiologically progressing through the dying process. The plan of care should not involve measures directly intended to cause the neonate's death, nor should the care plan cause harm without any direct benefit.

The key aspect of this principle resides in the intent of the health care provider's action. Ethically, health care providers cannot perform actions that are intrinsically wrong for the sole purpose of yielding a positive outcome. This is known as the principle of double effect or the rule of double effect (RDE) (Beauchamp and Childress, 2013). According to Beauchamp and Childress (2013), for an act to be considered morally justifiable under the RDE, the following four conditions must be met: (1) the actual act must be good or morally neutral, (2) the intent must be limited to the good effect, (3) the bad effect cannot serve as the means to the good effect, and (4) the good effect must outweigh the bad effect.

The RDE is best illustrated by the administration of increasing amounts of morphine in a dying patient. A nurse administers morphine with the intent of relieving the patient's pain and in the process the patient's respirations slow considerably to the point of cessation. The nurse's intent was not to cause the patient to stop breathing and die. Rather, the nurse's intent was to ease the patient's pain. Thus, upon ethical examination of this situation, the conclusion would be that this nurse did not act in a maleficent manner toward the patient.

### Respect for Autonomy

The principle of respect for autonomy emphasizes the right of an individual to make decisions for himself or herself. In health care, this principle is reflected in both the right to make decisions about a treatment plan as well as the right to refuse treatment. When an adult is the patient, the health care team seeks permission for treatment by means of informed consent. True informed consent is an actual process that involves more than obtaining a signature on a form or legal document. During the informed consent process, the patient should be provided with accurate, sufficient, and understandable information. The patient can then weigh the pros and cons of the proposed treatment options and, after adequate consideration, the patient can express an informed decision regarding his or her preferences.

In the NICU, parents serve as the legal surrogate decision makers for their neonate. NICU staff can assist parents in their decision-making role by keeping them well informed of the neonate's condition and by objectively presenting treatment options. Parents' preferences for care must be reassessed as the neonate's condition warrants, because their preferences may change in either direction. For example, parents who expressed a desire for very aggressive treatment may later decide that deceleration of care may be in the infant's best interest. Other parents may decide to continue aggressive care as planned, even though a grim prognosis is present. Regardless, in order for parents to act in their infant's best interest, they need to be kept informed of all options as well as the likely outcomes of the options.

### Justice

The principle of justice focuses on the fair distribution of the benefits, risks, and costs among members of society in relation to health care needs. In the NICU, questions of justice frequently arise. For example, two mothers are about to give birth to neonates who will require care in the NICU. The births will occur within an hour of each other. One neonate is extremely premature and will have a less than 20% chance of survival. The other neonate will have a 75% chance of survival. If the neonate with only a 20% chance of survival is born first, should he or she occupy the last available NICU bed or should that bed be reserved for the more viable neonate?

Questions of justice are difficult to resolve at the bedside. Yet pursuing these questions is an important step in achieving balance in health care. Furthermore, moving toward examining justice from a societal perspective provides an opportunity to develop and refine health policy that will assist in refining hospital policies and further translate back to the bedside.

### Utilization of the Principle Approach in the NICU

When ethical issues arise in the NICU, the principle approach can assist the health care team to organize its assessment and analysis of the situation. Examining the proposed plan of care with full consideration of benefits and burdens to the neonate can provide insight into competing goals. Fully engaging the parents in the decision-making process as early as possible will assist them in exercising their rights as surrogate decision makers for their neonate. Raising justice-related questions will help clarify how this neonate's case affects the institution and how related cases affect public policy. However, it is important to remember that all principles should be taken into account and that no one principle is inherently given precedence over the other three principles (Beauchamp and Childress, 2013).

## OTHER APPROACHES TO ETHICAL ISSUES

In addition to the principle approach to ethical issues, there are many ethical theories and case analysis models. It is beyond the scope of this chapter to adequately address all of these perspectives. However, NICU nurses should be encouraged to further explore these in clinical ethics textbooks.

### Ethical Theories

Three of the theories commonly referenced in bioethics are Kantianism, utilitarianism, and liberal individualism. Whereas these theories can assist nurses in examining ethical issues broadly, they do not provide direct guidance for resolving issues at the bedside.

### Kantianism

Kantianism, or deontology, is an obligation-based theory from the 1700s. This theory requires that individuals act with a sense of obligation, yet does not address how to act when there are conflicting obligations (Beauchamp and Childress, 2013). For example, a father may have a child who needs a kidney donation as well as his own parent who needs a kidney. The father may wish to donate, and may have an obligation to donate. Yet to whom does he owe the greatest obligation? This theory does not directly help resolve such dilemmas.

### Utilitarianism

The focus of utilitarianism is on utility, or the maximization of the goodness of an act (Beauchamp and Childress, 2013). According to this theory, the decision maker has to identify the greatest good while balancing the interests of all affected individuals. For example, the health care team may desire to provide aggressive treatment to a neonate who will require a succession of very expensive surgical procedures. The family may be unable to pay for any of the treatment. Under utilitarianism, it may be determined that providing care for this infant would not maximize utility of resource allocation for the community and thus this infant would not receive the costly extensive care that was recommended by the health care team. Although this theory provides a means of examining issues, it was developed in the late 1700s and is not easily adapted to the process of daily NICU decision making.

### Liberal Individualism

Liberal individualism addresses the rights, both positive and negative, that individuals in our society possess. A positive right requires someone to do something for another individual, such as a health care provider's duty to treat those in need of immediate care. A negative right keeps individuals from being directly harmed by others. For example, an individual requests that no experimental treatments be performed on him. Without his or her explicit consent, his right cannot be overridden.

## CASE ANALYSIS MODEL

Apart from ethical theories and principles, a model for analyzing ethical cases was developed and refined for bedside use by Jonsen et al. (2002). Their model provides four components that health care providers should examine for each case: the medical indications, patient preferences, quality of life, and contextual features.

### Medical Indications

Health care providers can begin by summarizing the neonate's diagnosis and prognosis. The treatment plan, along with the benefits and burdens, would also be discussed.

### Patient Preferences

In the NICU, the health care providers would obtain the parents' preferences for their neonate's treatment plan. It would be important to ask the parents what their goals are for the infant. In light of the current and/or proposed treatment plan, the NICU team should also ask parents how they view the benefits and burdens for their infant. It is important to elicit parental preferences as well as any other concerns the parents may have.

### Quality of Life

This component of the model provides an opportunity to examine the quality of life from the perspective of the health care team and to relate that to the stated parental preferences. This may require additional conversation with the parents to ensure correct interpretation of their values by the NICU team.

### Contextual Features

The contextual features incorporate a variety of factors, including religious beliefs and practices, financial concerns, family issues, potential conflicts of interest among the care providers or within the institution, and the legal implications of treatment options (Jonsen et al., 2002).

The case analysis model can be useful as an initial step in examining or identifying ethical issues in the NICU. It does not provide a directive for decision making, but it illuminates the issues so that further conversation and progressive steps can be taken toward resolution.

## THE NURSE'S ROLE IN ETHICAL ISSUES

The NICU nurse plays a critical role in both direct care of the neonate and support for the parents. The nurse can help prevent some ethical issues from arising by engaging the parents in both conversation and care from the time of admission throughout the neonate's hospitalization. Parents will need help understanding and coping with all of the complex dimensions and implications of their infant's NICU admission (Sudia-Robinson, 2011b). They will also need nursing support to more actively engage in the care of their neonate (Franck and Axelin, 2013; Skene et al., 2012).

### Adequate Communication With Parents

In the NICU, nurses along with other members of the health care team have an obligation to keep the parents thoroughly informed of the options for care and the associated risks and benefits (Sudia-Robinson, 2011a; Sudia-Robinson and Freeman, 2000). To adequately involve parents in the decision-making process, health care providers need to move beyond merely imparting information. Parents must have the information but also know how to interpret the information they receive. This has been described in various health care situations as the transparency model (King, 1992).

Nurses can assist in this process by incorporating the transparency model into their daily interactions with parents. Telling parents what the neonate's ventilator settings are or stating the latest blood gas results represents a nurse simply giving information to parents. The problem with this approach is that parents may or may not know how to interpret the information given to them. Information without comprehensive explanation or without the proper context is merely data and does not help parents move toward understanding. However, when a nurse explains what the ventilator settings mean for their particular neonate in relation to the course of the neonate's disease process, the nurse is actively helping parents to begin to better understand and think about the information they are given by the health care team. Nurses need to remember that sharing knowledge is different from helping with comprehension or understanding. Therefore, when nurses assist parents to understand their neonate's overall condition, nurses are preparing parents to make more informed decisions for their neonate.

Not all parents will want to be fully engaged in the decision-making process for their neonate. Sometimes parental preferences for involvement will change during the course of the neonate's hospitalization. For example, some parents may be so intimidated by the NICU initially that they may not ask many questions and may agree with whatever is presented to them. As time passes, however, they may begin to ask more questions and move toward desiring to become more involved in daily care. It is important to recognize differences in parental preferences while reassessing parental desire for involvement in daily care and decision making as the neonate's condition changes.

### Supporting the NICU Team

At times the NICU nurse may feel torn between support for the parents and support for the health care team. This can occur when the health care team advocates one plan of care and the parents disagree with the team's recommendation. For example, the NICU team may recognize that the neonate is in multiorgan system failure and that death is imminent, yet the parents continue to request that aggressive medical intervention continue. The nurse has an obligation to support the team and the parents while ensuring that the infant's best interests are being met. This is where ethical dilemmas arise, and the nurse may find it helpful to seek ethical consultation.

## CONSULTING THE HOSPITAL ETHICS COMMITTEE

When significant differences in the desired plan of care arise between the parents and NICU team, it can be beneficial to initiate an ethics consultation. In most institutions, a nurse, physician, social worker, other staff, or a parent can request an ethics consultation. The focus of the consultation should be the actual process rather than the outcome. Ethics committee members can sometimes aid in clarifying the issues and various perspectives presented. The process must be respectful of all perspectives and give full consideration of all possible options. The product of an ethics consultation will be a set of recommendations, not a mandate for a particular trajectory of care.

The ethics committee can be of assistance to the NICU in situations other than actual case consultation. Hospital ethics committees can serve as important resources about both ethically and legally permissible courses of action that can guide policy development in the NICU. Some ethics committees also prepare educational materials for families to make them aware of the process and how to access committee members (Mitchell and Truog, 2000).

## SUMMARY

Nurses are in a unique position to recognize ethical issues as they arise in the NICU. Understanding key ethical concepts and ethical principles can assist in further understanding and resolution of ethical issues. Supporting parents throughout the process by providing information in an understandable context is imperative for collaborative ethical decision making in the NICU.

## REFERENCES

American Nurses Association: *Code of ethics for nurses with interpretative statements.* Silver Springs, MD, 2001, American Nurses Association.

Beauchamp, R.L. and Childress, J.F.: *Principles of biomedical ethics* (7th ed.). New York, 2013, Oxford University Press.

Callister, L.C. and Sudia-Robinson, T.: An overview of ethics in maternal-child nursing. *MCN: American Journal of Maternal Child Nursing,* 36(3):154–159, 2011.

Franck, L.S. and Axelin, A.: Differences in parents', nurses', and physicians' view of NICU parent support. *Acta Paediatrica,* 102:590–596, 2013.

Jonsen, A.R., Siegler, M. and Winslade, W.J.: *Clinical ethics* (5th ed.). New York, 2002, McGraw-Hill.

King, N.M.: Transparency in neonatal intensive care. *Hastings Center Report,* 22(3):18–25, 1992.

Mitchell, C. and Truog, R.D.: From the files of a pediatric ethics committee. *Journal of Clinical Ethics,* 11 (2):112–120, 2000.

National Association of Neonatal Nurses. *Position Statement #3015: NICU nurse involvement in ethical decisions,* Chicago, IL, 2010, National Association of Neonatal Nurses.

Skene, C., Franck, L., Curtis, P., and Gerrish, K.: Parental involvement in neonatal comfort care. *JOGNN: Journal of Obstetric, Gynecologic, & Neonatal Nursing,* 41:786–797, 2012.

Sudia-Robinson, T.: Ethical implications of newborn screening, life-limiting conditions, and palliative care. *MCN: American Journal of Maternal Child Nursing,* 36 (3):188–196, 2011a.

Sudia-Robinson, T.: Neonatal ethical issues: Viability, advance directives, family centered care? *MCN: American Journal of Maternal Child Nursing,* 36(3):180–185, 2011b.

Sudia-Robinson, T. and Freeman, S.B.: Communication patterns and decision-making among parents and health care providers in the neonatal intensive care unit: A case study. *Heart & Lung,* 29(2):143–148, 2000.

CHAPTER

# 40 Legal Issues

M. TERESE VERKLAN

**OBJECTIVES**

1. Identify how an attorney may use the nursing process for litigation.
2. Define standards of care and guidelines for establishing the standard of care.
3. Define malpractice and the conditions that constitute malpractice.
4. Define concepts of liability and negligence.
5. Discuss the importance of documentation in the patient's record and guidelines for charting.
6. Discuss the nurse's role in informed consent.
7. Identify scope-of-practice issues in providing patient care functions.
8. Identify the risks and benefits of possessing professional liability insurance.

In the past, the specialty of obstetrics was considered the "high-risk" area for malpractice suits and loss of licensure. Today litigation is not uncommon in our own area of specialization. Neonates are seen as a "special" population that is afforded extra protection (Verklan, 2012). Thus neonatal nurses must be cognizant of the minimum standards of professional conduct that they, as health care providers, must adhere to. The purpose of this chapter is to familiarize the nurse with the concepts and ramifications of legal concerns as they pertain to the realm of neonatal intensive care nursing. Topics that will be discussed include standards of care, liability, documentation, informed consent, scope of practice, and professional liability insurance.

## NURSING PROCESS

A. **The nursing process forms the foundation for nursing education, practice, and documentation, regardless of whether the nurse graduated from a diploma, associate degree, or baccalaureate program.** Although the phrase "nursing process" is often omitted from practice standards and teaching strategies, nursing documentation should continue to be reflective of the nursing process. Failure to follow the following five steps of the nursing process is the number one cause of all patient injuries:
   1. Assessment: gathers data related to the neonate's physiologic and psychosocial status.
      a. Vital sign records, flow sheets, and nursing progress records.
      b. Body and organ-system findings (e.g., cardiopulmonary findings).
      c. Laboratory and diagnostic reports.
      d. Medical progress notes.
      e. Intake and output.
      f. Progress notes from other disciplines (e.g., respiratory, social work, pharmacy).
      g. Information from the family.
   2. Diagnosis: correctly identifies the neonate's condition using the data obtained from the assessment step, from documents on the nursing care plan, and in the progress notes.
   3. Planning: develops a plan of care that incorporates all aspects of the neonate's condition.
      a. Uses a multidisciplinary approach.
      b. Documents interventions and anticipated outcomes for the targeted diagnosis on the nursing care plan.
      c. Incorporates research-based findings into practice.
   4. Implementation: carries out the plan of care.
      a. Follows neonatologist and/or advanced practice nurse (APN) orders, provides direct care, supervises the care given by another, teaches and/or counsels the family, provides referrals for care by other disciplines.
      b. Documents all pertinent information on the neonate's medical record.

5. Evaluation: evaluates the neonate's response to the plan of care as outlined by the multidisciplinary team, noting any revisions or changes to the plan.
   a. Implementation process is not complete without evaluating the effectiveness of the intervention.
   b. Communicates patient response to treatment to members of the multidisciplinary team.
   c. Documents pertinent findings in the patient's medical record.
   d. Revises plan of care based on the patient's response and anticipated outcomes.

**B. The attorney, as well as all interested parties involved in the legal process, will use the steps of the nursing process to:**

1. Interpret the medical record.
2. Identify possible deviations from the standard of care.
3. Speak the same language as the nurse.
4. Generate questions that will be used to depose a nurse defendant.
5. Use the reports of expert witnesses who will outline how the nurse did or did not follow the nursing process.

## STANDARD OF CARE

The standard of care outlines the minimum criteria by which proficiency is defined in the clinical area. When the standard is not specifically referred to in the state nurse practice act, it becomes a guideline for practice rather than law. In the legal system, the standard of care is established by defining what a reasonable and prudent nurse would have done in the same or similar circumstances. The issue of excellence in practice or quality of care given does not pertain to the argument—what is being sought is reasonableness and prudence. A reasonable and prudent nurse is a nurse with like education, background, and experience who would behave in a corresponding manner, given a parallel set of events. The plaintiff attorney has the burden to prove that the standard(s) do exist and that the defendant nurse failed to meet the standard(s).

In addition, it is expected that the standard of care given to neonates everywhere is the same. "A neonatal nurse is a professional nurse who provides skilled nursing care for low-risk, high-risk and critically ill neonates, high-risk neonates, and their families. The neonatal nurse has specialized knowledge and develops and maintains clinical competence through standardized practice and continuing education" (Association of Women's Health, Obstetric and Neonatal Nurses [AWHONN] and National Association of Neonatal Nurses [NANN], 1997, p. 8). "Although neonatal nurses may provide basic neonatal care, they may also focus on an area of expertise, as for example, intensive or critical neonatal care, transport, lactation, grief, extracorporeal membrane oxygenation or developmental care" (American Nurses Association [ANA], 2013; AWHONN and NANN, 1997; AWHONN, 2009).

*Ewing v. Aubert* (1988) set out that a maternal–child nurse is held to the standard of care of a nurse practicing in the maternal–child specialty. Neonatal nurses, a subspecialty within maternal–child nursing, must be cognizant of what the professional practice standards are for that subspecialty:

> A nurse who practices her profession in a particular specialty owes to her patients the duty of possessing the degree of knowledge or skill ordinarily possessed by members of her profession actively practicing in such a specialty under similar circumstances. It is the nurse's duty to exercise the degree of skill ordinarily employed, under similar circumstances, by members of the nursing profession in good standing who practice their profession in the same specialty and to use reasonable care and diligence, along with his/her best judgment, in the application of his/her skill to the case (*King v. Department of Health & Hospitals*, 1999).

The quality of the nursing care provided is judged according to national standards, making obsolete the "locality rule." The locality rule permitted nurses to be judged according to the standard of care evidenced by nurses working in the same geographic area, reflecting the community's accepted practices. Recognition of national standards by professional neonatal nursing organizations and accreditation agencies is reflected in clinical policy and procedure manuals. In addition, accredited schools of nursing across the nation have similar curricula and textbooks, and nurses attend similar continuing education conferences. Thus it is expected that the professional nurse will be and remain competent and continually updated on the standards of care and practice (ANA, 2013; AWHONN, 2009).

Five basic types of evidence are used to establish the legal standard of care: (1) state and federal regulations; (2) institutional policies, procedures, and protocols; (3) testimony from expert witnesses; (4) standards of professional organizations; and (5) current professional literature.

## State and Federal Regulations

These agencies establish the standards of care and scope of practice. The national standards tend to be written in broad language to permit flexibility without compromising standards to accommodate differences within each state. The standard of practice is also defined by the state nurse practice act as mandated by each state's legislature. Here the scope of practice is delineated for each level of nursing (e.g., licensed vocational nurse, registered nurse, APN). For example, a registered nurse may not delegate the act of assessment and the formulation of a nursing diagnosis to any assistive personnel who are unqualified to perform this task (ANA, 2012). In addition, standards of nursing practice are also regulated by the state board of nursing, the department of health, The Joint Commission (TJC), and the Health Care Financing Administration, in addition to other regulatory agencies (Iyer, 2011).

## Institutional Policies, Procedures, and Protocols

The hospital's policies, procedures, and protocols also outline the standard of care. The policy establishes the purposes for performing a procedure, whereas the procedure is the guideline for how that procedure should be carried out. These guidelines must reflect the national and state standards of care, should be reviewed at least annually, and should be revised to reflect current acceptable nursing practice (TJC, 2013). In addition, these guidelines must also be (1) prepared by a qualified committee of professionals who practice in the specialty, (2) consistent with current research and practice literature, (3) archived for the length of liability, and (4) accessible to staff (Rottkamp, 2011). The policy and procedures manual should be approved by both the unit and the hospital's nursing and medical administrations.

Being unaware of the policy and procedures for the standard clinical practice at your institution is not an acceptable excuse for not being held accountable for your practice. The policy and procedures manual is often one of the first documents requested by both the plaintiff and defense attorneys because it is the best source for specific standards by which to evaluate a specific nurse's care. Because the statutes of limitations endure for 18 to 21 years and standard care practices change dramatically across the years, keeping the policy and procedures manual will also help to determine what the standard of care was at the time the neonate was hospitalized.

## Testimony From Expert Witnesses

A nurse expert is typically required to articulate what the standard of care is or was in the situation in which the nurse has deviated from the usual and customary standard of care. A nursing expert opinion requires that the person expressing that opinion possess special skill, knowledge, and experience in the neonatal area and knowledge of the standards applicable at the time of the occurrence (Zerres et al., 2011). The judge and jury have little knowledge related to neonatal physiology, pathophysiology, and the relevant neonatal nursing care. They therefore need assistance in understanding just what a reasonable and prudent nurse would have done in the given circumstances (e.g., did the nurse meet the accepted standard of care?).

Both liability and damages have to be proved in nursing malpractice cases. Thus two types of experts are usually necessary: a nurse to address the nursing standard of care and a physician to determine causation, that is, to link the breach of standard to the injuries suffered by the neonate. Professional nursing philosophies dictate that nurses be the only witnesses permitted to testify as experts outlining what the nursing standard of care is in a nursing malpractice suit. However, it is the quality of the expert's experience and education that determines the competency and credibility of the testimony (Zerres et al., 2011).

## Standards of Professional Organizations

Professional associations represent the interests of nurses. The ANA has developed standards with measurable criteria that define professional nursing practice (2010) as well as neonatal nursing (2013). Specialty organizations such as the NANN, AWHONN, American Association of Critical-Care Nurses (AACN), and National Association of Pediatric Nurse Associates and Practitioners (NAPNAP) have adapted these standards to define the standards of care and professional practice guidelines applicable to the care of neonates. For example, AWHONN publishes *Standards for Professional Nursing Practice in the Care of Women and Newborns* (2009).

## Current Professional Literature

Current texts and journal articles, although technically hearsay, aid in establishing the legal standard of care. A number of journals specific to the care of neonates focus on clinical, management, and research articles. Clinical articles are useful in helping to determine the applicable standard of care at the time of the malpractice suit, whereas nursing textbooks provide information related to the standard of care associated with nursing techniques and care (Iyer, 2011). Research articles are beginning to assume more importance in the legal arena because of the desire to document evidence-based practice. Evidence-based practice is defined as the incorporation of the current best evidence in clinical decision making. Increased use of websites such as Medline and CINAHL for research/clinical information have led to an increase in the critique of published literature by nurses. Hospitals holding Magnet status must demonstrate that nurses participate in research utilization or they will lose their designation. Despite this, the integration of research findings into clinical practice is slow, taking as long as 10 to 15 years. However, keeping theory and clinical practice on par with the literature and remaining current with regard to continuing education will assist the nurse in ensuring that his or her professional standards are synonymous with those of his or her peers.

## Further Issues: Practice Guidelines and Ethical Standards

Standards of care are often confused with practice guidelines. Standards of care are the basis for proving that the nurse had a duty to the patient and that there was a breach of that duty. Clinical practice guidelines, with reference to the standards of care, are meant to assist the health care provider in the delivery of care in specific clinical circumstances. For example, *Guidelines for Perinatal Care* outlines recommendations regarding nurse providers, nursing ratios, staffing guidelines, and outreach education for inpatient perinatal care facilities providing basic, specialty, and subspecialty care (American Academy of Pediatrics and American College of Obstetricians and Gynecologists, 2012). Critical pathways are another example of a practice guideline that is modified to reflect the neonate's clinical progress. Therefore, the difference between a standard of care and a practice guideline is that the standard always must be adhered to, whereas the guideline suggests a voluntary approach to achieve a desirable patient outcome (Iyer, 2011; NANN, 2010a).

The ethical standards of nursing practice may also be the issue in a malpractice suit:

> The Mississippi Board of Nursing charged Terry Lynn Hanson, a registered nurse, with abuse of neonatal patients. It was noted that her clinical practices included holding a baby around its neck with only one hand, carrying babies by holding them under their axillae, carrying naked babies around the NICU and washing them in the unit's sinks, and that she endangered the babies by rapidly flipping the levers on the incubators when attempting to stimulate them. The Board, finding her guilty on all charges, revoked her license. Nurse Hanson appealed to the Supreme Court of Mississippi, who held that her behavior constituted a reckless disregard of the health and safety of the neonates. The Court also ruled that she was negligent by holding babies under the axillae, permitting their bodies to dangle, removing them naked from incubators to bathe and weigh them in different areas of the NICU compromised thermoregulation and exposed them to risks of infection, and that overstimulation increased the risk of intraventricular hemorrhage (Tammelleo, 1998, p. 1).

## MALPRACTICE

The term *malpractice* means negligence on the part of the nurse, in that she or he has violated the standards of ordinary nursing practiced by nurses of similar background in the same specialty of nursing. Malpractice is professional misconduct that may be intentional or unintentional. If the individual is acting in a personal capacity, then the individual would be subject to negligence, as malpractice is limited to the omission, lack, or misuse of a professional skill.

> By undertaking professional services to the patient, a nurse represents that she/he possesses, as a duty, the degree of learning and skill ordinarily possessed by nurses of good standing practicing in the same community under similar circumstances. It is the nurse's further duty to use the care ordinarily exercised in like cases by reputable members of the profession practicing in the same or a similar locality and under similar circumstances. The nurse is to use reasonable diligence and best judgment in the exercise of her or his skills and learning in an effort to accomplish the purpose of employment. A defendant nurse must violate one of these duties before being found to have committed malpractice (Fulginiti et al., 2007, p. 1375).

It must be emphasized that the nurse need possess only the knowledge and skill possessed by the average reasonable, prudent nurse and must exercise reasonable care, skill, and judgment in carrying out her or his professional work. The nurse need not be perfect or able to predict every single difficulty or uncertainty regarding the patient. However, the nurse must act in a careful or prudent fashion in the delivery of professional care while exercising reasonable care, skill, and judgment. Occasionally an unexpected situation arises so quickly that one's actions on hindsight may not be considered to have been the perfect course of action.

A mistake in judgment is not considered malpractice:

> A mistake in judgment on the part of the nurse is not evidence of negligence. If a nurse possesses reasonable and ordinary skill and uses care ordinarily used in like or similar situations by nurses of reasonable and average skill, practicing in the community at the time in question, she/he is not guilty of negligence even though her/his judgment may be subsequently proven incorrect. (Fulginiti et al., 2007, p. 1375)

## LIABILITY

Today nurses are recognized as professionals who are responsible and accountable for the care they give to their patients. If the nurse is liable to the patient because of negligent conduct, that nurse can be held legally responsible for the harm caused to that patient (Verklan, 2012). Harm must result from the act, because without damage, no legal wrong has been committed.

> Baby R was born after a difficult labor including the presence of meconium and episodes of hypoxia. Routine orders for the admission were given despite the presence of risk factors for hypoglycemia. Over the next three hours of life, the baby's glucose values decreased from 104 mg/dL to 28 mg/dL. The nurse fed the baby, but did not notify the physician. The neonate continued to experience hypoglycemia throughout the night. The glucose level increased to normal parameters after a feeding in the morning. The physician examined the baby shortly after the feeding, noting that she was at risk for hypoglycemia. No further orders were given such as the need to begin intravenous glucose. A neonatologist was not consulted. Later that day profound hypoglycemia was evidenced by seizure activity. Nursing did not notify the physician of the seizure activity until later in the evening when the seizures became worse. The physician returned to the nursery and examined Baby R. Once the seizures were observed, the baby was transferred to another hospital. The hospital settled for $1.75 million prior to trial (Laska, 2005).

The plaintiff, the party bringing the suit, must prove the following four elements in a malpractice case:

1. The nurse had a duty to her or his patient.
2. There was a breach of that duty.
3. Harm or damages did occur to the patient.
4. Breach of that duty resulted in harm (proximal cause).

An infant, born in a depressed state, had Apgar scores of 3 and 8 at 1 and 5 minutes, respectively. Although his condition was improving, he continued to have raspy breathing that required suctioning. It was alleged that the defendants failed to provide adequate special care and observation, causing the baby to suffocate on its own secretions. The neonate was discovered in a cyanotic state two hours after birth. Resuscitative techniques restored the heartbeat in eighteen minutes. He was transferred to another hospital, declared to be brain-dead, and was removed from life support four days later. The plaintiff claimed that resuscitation was both delayed and improperly performed. The defendants argued that the baby appeared normal, that the cause of the respiratory arrest was unknown, and that inborn errors of metabolism caused the death. They also countered that failure to respond to resuscitation does not imply negligence (Du Page County [IL] Circuit Court, Case No. 94 L-318 [Laska, 1997]).

In this case the plaintiff proved that the defendant owed a duty to the neonate, in that the baby and his parents should expect the care received to be at least equal to the standard of care. However, the plaintiff was not able to prove that the defendant breached the duty (failure to respond to resuscitation does not imply negligence) or that there was proximal cause (inborn errors of metabolism may have contributed to or caused the injury). Thus, despite the neonate's death (damages), a malpractice suit cannot be won if all four elements are not present.

**A. The costs of liability when a neonate is involved are high for three reasons:**

1. The costs of health care for a damaged infant with a normal life expectancy are high.
2. The longer statute of limitations for minors may permit charges to be made years later, applicable to other medical malpractice actions.
3. There is sympathy toward the family, who may not be able to afford the needed care for the child, as opposed to the deep pockets of a corporation, who may be seen as uncaring and will not miss the money anyway.

**B. Although an individual nurse is accountable only for his or her own practice, there are three additional theories of liability that may be pursued against a facility or its management (Lewis and Krulewicz, 2011; Rottkamp, 2011):**

1. *Respondeat superior*, which, in essence, says that the employer is given the responsibility and accountability for the actions or intentions of the employee. This doctrine:
   - **a.** Holds an employer liable for the negligent acts of employees that arise in the course of the employment (i.e., employers are held responsible for the acts of those whom they have a right to supervise or control).
   - **b.** Holds the institution responsible for ensuring that the policies and procedures meet the standard of care, and that employees follow these policies.
   - **c.** Will not impose liability in most circumstances on a nursing supervisor for negligent acts of the nursing personnel he or she is supervising. This responsibility rests with the person who makes changes in the policies and procedures.
   - **d.** Obligates the nursing supervisor to ensure that the licensed and unlicensed nursing personnel under his or her supervision are able to provide patient care safely. If the supervisor does not document the personnel's deficiencies and use the chain of command, she or he can be held liable for any damages that befall a patient.
   - **e.** Holds that negligent employees are always liable for their own conduct.
2. *Corporate negligence* holds the institution's management and board of trustees liable for any breach of their duties:
   - **a.** The institution must provide a safe physical setting and monitor the quality of care provided, along with the equipment necessary for patient care.
   - **b.** An equipment standard must be implemented.
     - (1) The institution must have a management plan documenting competency validation for the proper use of medical equipment by the institution's employees (TJC, 2013).
     - (2) The institution may also name the equipment manufacturer as a third-party defendant in an attempt to shift the blame (Verklan, 2012).

Shortly after birth, Baby Wright's blood pressure decreased, necessitating a transfer to the Special Care Unit. Dr. Bloom ordered a bolus of normal saline (unconcentrated) to be given over 30 minutes. Nurse Diltz offered to prepare the bolus. The hospital stocked both the unconcentrated and the concentrated normal saline solutions in the same place. Nurse Diltz obtained a vial of the concentrated sodium chloride, that had "CONCENTRATE" and "CAUTION: MUST BE DILUTED FOR I.V. USE" in large red letters. There was also a written warning in red letters that the fluid was a 14.6% solution. Nurse Diltz did not read the physician's order nor did she note the label on the sodium chloride vial. The fluid bolus was subsequently administered to Baby Wright. After the second bolus, Baby Wright suffered severe brain damage. The Wrights sued Abbott Laboratories, the suppliers of the concentrated sodium chloride solution. Abbot never sent a warning letter to the hospital despite the Food and Drug Administration's warning to change the labeling and package inserts for the concentrated and unconcentrated normal saline products. The plaintiffs argued that Abbott had a duty to warn the hospital about the dangers of inadvertent administration of the wrong solution and that the failure to warn the hospital was the proximate cause of Baby Wright's brain injury. The court granted summary judgment for Abbott (not guilty). It also found the hospital and its staff should have been aware of the dangers of stocking the look alike products together, and therefore, Abbott Laboratories did not have a duty to warn the hospital of the risk. The Court also found that had Nurse Diltz simply read the physician's orders and the label on the vial, the concentrated solution would not have been given (*Wright v. Abbott Lab.*, 2001).

   c. The facility may be found liable for advertising a service for which it lacks the proper equipment or personnel or for failure to keep these services at the acceptable standard of care.
   d. The institution must verify the credentials of those who apply for clinical privileges (e.g., APNs) and must also query the National Practitioner Data Bank at the time clinical privileges are requested, and subsequently every 2 years, regarding those who hold practice privileges. The data bank maintains records of disciplinary action taken on licenses, hospital privileges, and payment in conjunction with malpractice suits. In addition to health care organizations, professional societies and attorneys have access to the data bank. Each APN should be familiar with the data bank and should periodically verify that the information it contains regarding her or him is accurate.
   e. Clinical competencies must also be evaluated and documented every 2 years (TJC, 2013).
3. *Apparent/ostensible authority* holds an institution liable for the acts and omissions of an independent contractor (Lewis and Krulewicz, 2011; Rottkamp, 2011).
   a. The hospital should maintain a file for each agency nurse that contains her or his nursing license, required certifications, and a current competency skills checklist.
   b. APNs working within the hospital must be aware that patients view them as hospital employees even if they are in private practice, and as such the hospital may be held liable for their acts.

**C. An area of considerable controversy in the liability arena relates to risk management and quality assurance activities (Liang and Mackey, 2011).**

1. Quality assurance, more commonly called quality management today, focuses on evaluation of the quality of patient care, continuous quality improvement, and total quality management. The department and its activities may or may not be integrated with risk management.
2. Risk management is an internal systematic process aimed at preventing injuries and accidents, and reducing financial liability for the institution. Occurrence, variance, or incident reports are reviewed to evaluate and anticipate risk associated with the provision of services.
   a. By documenting occurrences and maintaining related records, such as the organization's claims history, quality assurance and utilization review activities, and risk management and analysis, this area may have information valuable for a plaintiff's malpractice case.
   b. Many jurisdictions have provided a protective shield for quality assurance and risk management activities, which renders the materials generated and the thought processes engaged in during those activities "privileged" or otherwise nondiscoverable (defendant cannot be asked to produce the materials).
3. Risk management works closely with quality assurance as information from risk management activities may be helpful in improving the quality of patient care. TJC links these areas in that such information must be accessible to all components of the quality assessment departments (TJC, 2013).

**D. Scope of practice.** Each state has its own nurse practice act, composed of statutes passed by its legislature and defining the boundaries of nursing practice. These laws vary from state to state in their demarcation of nursing practice. In contrast to state medical practice acts, the nurse practice statutes delineate nursing responsibilities in broad, universal nomenclature that generally must be examined with reference to the pertinent local law. The crucial issue regarding the scope of practice is whether the procedure performed by the nurse is legally within or beyond the scope of a nursing license to practice (Verklan, 2012).

There are numerous areas of medical and nursing practice that overlap one another, especially in the neonatal intensive care unit (NICU). Depending on the unit and its written protocols, the same procedure may be considered within the realm of medicine when performed by a physician and within the realm of nursing when performed by a nurse. These gray areas have evolved partly in response to the nurse's increased level of educational preparation and advanced practice role and partly in response to the high-tech environment found in the NICU. Neonatal nursing is considered a specialty area of practice, and the high-risk neonatal nursing in the NICU is considered a subspecialty area of practice. Certification for both the low-risk and the high-risk neonatal nurse is available through several specialty organizations (ANA, AACN Certification Corporation, National Certification Corporation [NCC], NAPNAP).

Increasing the scope of practice, autonomy, and authority is likely to result in greater exposure to liability situations. Critical legal liability and scope-of-practice problems arise whenever the nurse assumes patient care functions of an independent nature that:

1. Have long been held to be solely within the province of physicians.
2. Are not the subject of standing orders.
3. Lack definition in the nurse practice act.
4. Are not generally recognized as legitimate nursing functions by accredited professional organizations.

The standard of care and liability for negligence may be determined by (TJC, 2013):

1. Nurse's level of training and experience.
2. Manuals and textbooks written for the specialty.
3. Actions and inactions of the nurse.
4. Protocols and instructions referred to by the nurse.
5. The accepted professional nursing practice.

The following case highlights many of these principles.

> Dr. Seal remained with Baby T, born at 0130 after a difficult labor and traumatic forceps delivery, for approximately 1 hour before the baby was taken to the nursery. He left the hospital at approximately 0300, with instructions to the nurse that the medical student was in charge, but that he was to be called if needed. Nurse Bowles was concerned about Baby T from the outset, taking vital signs every 15 minutes. She called the medical student at 0345 and 0400, both times at which she was reassured that the baby looked "fine." Nurse Bowles did not call Dr. Seal. The nurse's aide assigned to Baby T did not take vital signs as ordered, and fell asleep twice during the shift. Baby T's condition required transport to another hospital, where he was diagnosed with hypovolemic shock related to a subgaleal hematoma, likely the result of the forceps delivery. The plaintiffs brought a negligence suit against the hospital after the baby's death alleging that the hospital personnel failed to take proper action when Baby T displayed signs of distress. The jury returned a verdict against the hospital of $800,000, which was reduced to $650,000 because Dr. Seal agreed to a pretrial settlement of $150,000 (Tammelleo, 1995).

The reasonable, prudent nurse, besides being responsible to the patient, is also accountable to herself or himself and to the profession (Verklan, 2012). Both the nurse and the employer have the responsibility to determine the level of competence of the nurse who is asked to provide care outside her or his specialty area. The right of a nurse's refusal to "float" has been upheld by the Wisconsin Supreme Court (*Winkelman v. Beloit Memorial Hospital*):

> A nursery nurse, Nurse Winkelman, was asked to float to a unit that provided postoperative and geriatric care. She discussed the situation with the supervisor, indicating that she had never floated, that she was exclusively a nursery nurse, and that she was not qualified to provide the type of care being requested. It was her opinion that the floating would put the patients and her license at risk, and thus, the hospital in jeopardy. The supervisor gave her three options, (a) float; (b) find another

nurse to float; or (c) take an unexcused absence day. Nurse Winkelman left the hospital, and later received a letter informing her that the hospital took her actions to be a voluntary resignation. Although she denied that she had ever resigned, the hospital refused to reinstate her. Nurse Winkelman filed a complaint of wrongful discharge against the hospital. The case was decided in her favor, and the hospital appealed. The Supreme Court affirmed that she had identified the fundamental policy that provides for only qualified nurses to render care, and that nurses who provide care for which they are not qualified are subject to sanctions under the law (Tammelleo, 1992).

## ADVANCED PRACTICE

Coincident with evolving health care delivery systems, neonatal APNs can be found in hospitals, ambulatory care centers, and private practice. The APN is often the only health care provider in many rural areas. According to the ANA, APNs are those who have further knowledge and practice experiences that have prepared them for specialization, expansion, and advancement in the practice role (ANA, 2013).

1. Specialization: focusing on one aspect of the field of nursing.
2. Expansion: acquisition of new practice skills.
3. Advancement: encompassing both specialization and expansion and involving:
    a. New integration of theories and skills.
    b. Graduate education.

The licensing statute in each state controls advanced practice and thereby protects the use of the title of APN. All states have defined the scope of the APN by the board of nursing, with several states having the state board of nursing and the state medical board jointly oversee licensing and scope of practice for APNs. An APN is a nurse with a graduate degree in nursing who is practicing in an advanced clinical role. APNs are able to conduct comprehensive health assessments and demonstrate expert skill in the diagnosis and treatment of complex clinical issues evidenced by individuals, their families, and communities. The APN functions with a high degree of autonomy in the formulation of clinical decisions to manage acute and chronic illness and promote wellness. Education, research, management, leadership, and consultation are integrated into their clinical role. They collaborate with nurses, physicians, pharmacists, and others who influence the health care arena (ANA, 2013).

In the neonatal area, the two recognized APNs are the neonatal nurse practitioner and the clinical nurse specialist. As APN roles continue to expand, there will be further debate on what constitutes nursing functions.

**A. Neonatal nurse practitioner (ANA, 2013; AWHONN, 2009; NANN, 2010b).**

1. One of the most common APNs found in the tertiary care setting.
2. Is responsible for managing a caseload of neonatal patients with general supervision, collaboration, and consultation from a physician.
3. Exercises independent judgment in the assessment, diagnosis, and initiation of delegated medical processes and procedures by using extensive knowledge of pathophysiology, pharmacology, and physiology.
4. Is involved in education, consultation, and research.
5. Has successfully graduated from a master's program (after year 2000) with certification through the NCC.

**B. Clinical nurse specialist.**

1. Focuses on patient care, staff education, research, and consultation.
2. Responsibilities are (ANA, 2013; AWHONN, 2009; NANN, 2010b):
    a. Acting as a resource for neonatal nurses, neonatal nurse practitioners, and other care providers.
    b. Establishing and evaluating patient care standards.
    c. Assessing and identifying educational needs of the family, nursery, and community.
    d. Designing and implementing appropriate educational programs based on identified needs.
    e. Providing consultation to health care providers.
    f. Initiating research projects, participating in data collection, and instituting changes based on research findings (evidence-based practice).

By virtue of the necessary education and training required to become an APN, they are held to a higher standard than a registered nurse. Thus the standard of care expected of the APN is the degree of care expected of any reasonable and prudent APN who practices in the same specialty.

A major legal issue relates to the permissible scope of practice and how independent of physician oversight the APN may be. The nurse practice act, in reference to the APN, has been broadened to include diagnosis and treatment, areas that were exclusive to those holding medical credentials. All states have passed legislation that defines the scope of practice.

The most common areas in which APNs have incurred liability are as follows (Guido, 2013; Iyer, 2012):

1. Conduct exceeding their scope of expertise resulting in damages.
2. Conduct exceeding physician-delegated authority resulting in damages.
3. Practicing independently in a state that stipulates that APNs must have a sponsoring physician.
4. Failure to refer the patient to a physician when the APN's skills are exceeded.
   a. Is the most common cause of action.
   b. APNs must also refer the patient in a timely manner when they recognize the patient's condition requires increased medical attention.
5. Negligence in their delivery of health care.
6. Failure to adequately diagnose the patient's condition.

## DOCUMENTATION

A. **It is a professional responsibility of the nurse to document on the medical record. This will:**
   1. Facilitate care.
   2. Enhance continuity and coordination of care.
   3. Assist in the evaluation of the patient's response to treatment.
   4. Provide a legal and official record of the care provided.

B. **Thus the medical record is used by the attorney as a tool to provide evidence in legal proceedings because it also verifies that the nurse (Iyer, 2012; Iyer and Koob, 2011):**
   1. Provided the standard of care.
   2. Did so within the scope of his or her nurse practice act.
   3. Provided "routine care." Negligence could be proved if this information is absent or inappropriate. Flow sheets that list these routines, along with times, dates, patient and caregiver identification, and nursing care outcomes, are valuable in providing a means of documenting repetitious nursing activities.

C. **Although nursing notes need to be as complete as possible, the comment "If it's not documented, then it wasn't done" doesn't always hold true.** Patient care is always the number one priority. Once the emergency is past, the nurse should strive to document the events, using as much detail as possible. However, if the needs of other patients were placed on hold during a crisis, those needs must be met immediately once the crisis is past. When the medical record is incomplete, the nurse may testify as to what constitutes her or his usual practice.

D. **The most common charting systems in the NICU are (Iyer and Koob, 2011):**
   1. Flow sheets.
      a. Decrease the need to document repetitive, routine nursing functions in the narrative notes.
      b. Have column-and-row format organized according to time and/or shift.
      c. Use abbreviations, symbols, and check marks to enter information.
   2. Narrative charting.
      a. Patient care is documented by using chronologic format.
      b. Entries describe the neonate's status, interventions, evaluation of care, medical treatments and equipment (e.g., ventilator, bed, phototherapy lights) used, and the neonate's response to care.
   3. Problem-oriented charting.
      a. Problem list outlines the patient's priority problems.
      b. Updates should be entered on a regular basis as problems resolve and new ones emerge.
      c. Documentation may be directly on the care plan or in the narrative notes.

d. Specific format is followed:
   (1) S=subjective information that the patient tells the nurse.
   (2) O=objective information the nurse observes (including laboratory results).
   (3) A=assessment of the above-mentioned data, leading to a nursing diagnosis.
   (4) P=plan that the nurse will implement to address the care issue.

4. Problem, intervention, and evaluation of problems (PIE) charting: uses flow sheets, progress notes, and nursing diagnoses.
5. Charting by exception.
   a. Narrative notes are completed only when the neonate's progress and/or condition deviates from the expected or when an untoward occurrence arises.
   b. Charting system contains nursing care plans, nursing data base, flow sheets, and progress notes.
   c. Standards of practice, determined by the institution, are incorporated into the charting system to record routine, repetitive nursing interventions (e.g., observation of intravenous site, checking ventilator settings).
6. Computerized medical record.
   a. Uses a single, easily accessible site to store a detailed account of the neonate's delivery, transition, and hospital course.
   b. Accuracy in patient information is enhanced as the nurse relies less on human recall.
   c. Patient monitoring is automatically uploaded into the appropriate space (e.g., vital signs from cardiopulmonary monitoring: blood pressure, heart rate, oxygen saturation, etc.).
   d. The nurse requires training on the documentation system/computer used in order to input and retrieve patient-related data.
   e. To access the medical record, an electronic signature and password/code must be entered. This is unique for each health care provider and must never be shared.
   f. Only health care providers/staff that are caring for the patient have a legal right to access the medical record.

**E. Table 40-1 outlines the advantages and disadvantages of each charting strategy.**

**F. Guidelines for documentation (Iyer and Koob, 2011; Verklan, 2012).**

1. Sign at the end of every entry by using full name and credentials or only initials (full name and credentials noted in the appropriate space). Ensure that no vacant lines are left. An empty space may later prompt someone to fill in a "missing" piece of information.
2. Cosigning means that you have observed and/or approved the care given and that you are accepting joint responsibility (and liability) for that care. Nurses who are required by hospital policy routinely to countersign documents or information in the patient's chart should protect themselves in one of two ways:
   a. By personally verifying the information being recorded.
   b. By noting in the record that the signature is included in accordance with hospital policy and is not based on personal knowledge of the information in question.
3. Illegible, sloppy handwriting with spelling and grammatical errors will convey a negative impression of the nurse.
4. Late charting is always suspect because it is typically key information that is added. Chart the information as soon as possible, beginning with the words "late entry for [date and time]."
5. To correct a mistaken entry:
   a. Draw one line through the entry.
   b. Write "mistaken entry" above the line. (The term *error* is no longer advised because juries tend to associate it with a clinical error.)
   c. Initial or sign document and add date next to "mistaken entry."
   d. What if a nurse is instructed not to chart an error by the attending physician? Nurses who accede to the demands of a physician to cover up the true facts of an unusual clinical episode by deliberately not mentioning it in the patient's chart not only may be subject to possible loss of licensure but also, in flagrant circumstances, even subject themselves to criminal action, leading to a fine or jail sentence.
6. Avoid inappropriate comments concerning:

■ TABLE 40-1
■ ■ **Advantages and Disadvantages of Charting Systems**

| Charting Systems | Advantages | Disadvantages |
|---|---|---|
| Flow sheets | Easy to use.<br>Decrease time spent. | No note on narrative sheet.<br>Duplication of documentation on narrative sheet. |
| Narrative charting | Easy to document events as they occur in time. | Information may be disorganized and may not contain all elements of nursing process.<br>Key patient issues may vary from shift to shift and from nurse to nurse; thus it may be difficult, years later, for hospital, nurse, and/or attorney to tease out relevant information related to specific patient complaint. |
| Problem-oriented charting | Documentation is organized.<br>All disciplines use same progress notes, permitting increased collaboration and continuity of care. | Continuing same format on all patient problems becomes redundant, with same information appearing over and over.<br>Time consuming because of repetitious nature of note. |
| PIE charting | Documentation is organized.<br>Evaluation of each problem requires only the information that is specific to that particular problem, intervention, and evaluation. | Novice nurses may have difficulty where there is no traditional care plan but instead an ongoing plan of care that is documented daily. |
| Charting by exception | Complete, detailed patient information is easily accessible to the health care provider.<br>Standard of practice for documentation outlines expected normal findings. | Exceptions to the standards of practice may not be documented because nurses become accustomed to "checking off" the flow sheets. |
| Computerized medical record | Improves legibility of the record, decreasing misinterpretation and error. Correct spelling is already in the system. | The selection of phrases or words doesn't always reflect the neonate's condition as computerized records are "built" for the entire hospital. The nurse may have to input additional notes. |
| | Patient information can more easily/quickly be located, retrieved and filed. | Accidently "choosing" the wrong descriptive phrase from the dropbox may result in a misleading or inaccurate assessment. |
| | Uses a standardized and structured format for inputting data, as well as mandatory areas that require population (care plans, flow sheets, nursing assessments). | Because the nurse is charting on the same computer, he or she may inadvertently chart the assessment on a different neonate. |
| | All entries are time-stamped. Also, the time the individual accesses the medical record is time-stamped. | Privacy, security and confidentiality may be endangered. Hospital policy as well as the HIPAA provide for stern penalties, including punitive actions. |
| | Use of bar codes allows the information to be scanned immediately into the medical record. | Misinformation may be difficult to correct as the error may not be detected and the medical record can be viewed by the entire appropriate health care community. |
| | Policies and procedures may also be on the same computer for quick, easy access when needed. | |

Data from Iyer, P.W. and Koob, S.L.: Nursing documentation. In P.W. Iyer, B.J. Levin, K.C. Ashton, and V. Powell (Eds.): *Nursing malpractice: Volume I. Roots of nursing malpractice*. Tucson, AZ, 2011, Lawyers & Judges Publishing, Kindle edition.
*HIPAA*, Health Insurance Portability and Accountability Act; *PIE*, problem, intervention, and evaluation.

a. The patient's or family's personality traits or idiosyncrasies (unless such remarks are relevant to the infant's treatment).
b. Subjective views to the effect that the patient or family is a potential litigant.
c. Admissions of legal liability with respect to untoward medical or nursing events. Examples are:
(1) "The IV infiltrated because the night staff forgot to check it" (Solberg, 1986, p. 13).
(2) "Patient going into shock. Could not get Dr. Jones to come. We never can!!!" (Fox and Imbiorski, 1979).

7. Document occurrences accurately and concisely. For example, the neonate's parents (plaintiffs) may have a different view of what actually took place. In a malpractice action, the burden of proof rests with the plaintiff.

In the case of *Coleman v. Touro Infirmary of New Orleans* (1993), the plaintiff alleged that the defendants had been negligent by failing to treat an abruptio placentae before the premature delivery of the infant and that the defendants' actions or inaction had caused the child's death. There were several discrepancies between the patient's recollection of events and the medical record. The court consulted the chart and the physician, determined that the nurses' notes stated another set of events, and concluded that the plaintiff failed to prove any act or omission by the obstetrician or hospital that resulted in the wrongful death of the Coleman infant.

8. Document objectively.
a. Avoid using "appears to be" and "seems to be." These phrases are not consistent with the judgments/diagnosis made by the critical thinking nurse of today.
b. Quantify in measurable aliquots when possible. For example, "approximately 30-cc emesis" gives more information than "large emesis."
c. The patient record is not an appropriate place to refer to an incident report's having been made. What should be documented is a factual account of what transpired and what was done. Incident reports enable the hospital or agency to make necessary investigations of the situation while the patient is still hospitalized, to identify situations of increased risk, and to trend these events to determine whether they are preventable (Iyer and Koob, 2011).

9. Document promptly:
a. Any significant changes in the patient's status.
b. Nursing actions undertaken to intercede in the situation, including notifying the physician of the concern. Note the time of the phone call notifying the physician, the information relayed, any orders received, and what you did next.

The case of *Mark and Debbie Easter, etc. v. Baylor University Medical Center* (Laska, 1993) illustrates the way in which nurses can place themselves in a liability situation by ignoring the above-noted standard of conduct.

The defendant was a 29-week gestational age neonate delivered by cesarean section at the defendant hospital. His serum potassium was not measured during the first 6 days of his life, and the blood glucose level was measured once on the day of his birth. As a result, hyperkalemia and hypoglycemia were undetected until he had a severe episode of bradycardia and/or cardiac arrest, stopped breathing, and required cardiopulmonary resuscitation. He suffered permanent brain damage. A subsequent laboratory report revealed severe hyperkalemia and hypoglycemia; however, the report was not forwarded to the neonatologists for approximately 7 hours. The plaintiff brought a complaint of gross negligence for failure to properly diagnose and timely treat the hyperkalemia and hypoglycemia. The jury returned a $4,500,000 verdict.

Medical records are crucial in a court case because they provide the sequence of events, the time frame in which they occurred, and the participants in the care of the patient.

Dylan Keene was born at 0107 May 15, 1986. He was discharged from the NICU to the regular nursery at 0630 with a one-page discharge note that noted "watch for sepsis, hold antibiotics pending complete blood count [CBC] results and cultures." The medical records for the next 24 hours went missing. Dylan was diagnosed with septic shock and seizures at 0230 May 16, 1986. Testing determined he had sepsis and meningitis that resulted in profound brain damage. He was discharged from the hospital June 18, 1986. His parents brought a malpractice suit against the hospital on May 12, 1995, alleging that there was a failure to properly diagnose and treat for sepsis and meningitis. The plaintiffs requested names of health care providers involved in the treatment and care of Dylan on May 14, 15 and 16, 1986, including those involved in the decision to not give antibiotics on those dates. The hospital records for these dates could not be located. The judge applied a default sanction against the hospital as the loss of the records for which the hospital was responsible had deprived the plaintiffs of their day in court. The plaintiffs were awarded $4,108,311.66 (*Keene v. Brigham and Women's Hospital*, 755 N.E.2d 725-MA 2002 [Tammelleo, 2002]).

If a nurse is named in a suit or is called to testify with regard to what took place, sometimes many years later, the chart serves as a memory aid. Statements contained in the medical record are not, in themselves, admitted into evidence; rather, the testimony of the witness concerning the particular event, as reinforced by the medical record, becomes the direct evidence given under oath. Most cases in which the hospital records cannot be located appear to be those in which the amount of damages in question is significant and the hospital appears to be liable; seldom do "missing" records ever favor the defendant hospital (Tammelleo, 2002).

## INFORMED CONSENT

Legally, for a person to be able to give informed consent, that person must have the capability of "capacity." This usually entails that the person (1) has reached the age of majority and (2) can understand the information that is being given by the health care provider. Neonates therefore do not meet the criteria to give informed consent legally. Thus the parents typically are the surrogate decision makers for the neonate, as long as they appear to be acting in the best interests of their infant. If the parents are married (to each other), either may consent on behalf of the neonate. However, in situations involving divorce, custody battles, and teenaged and foster parenting, issues related to informed consent and patient privacy can become convoluted (Guido, 2013). A guardian *ad litum* may be appointed by the court to act in the neonate's best interests, instead of or in addition to the parent(s). To meet the legal standard of informed consent, the surrogate decision maker must receive sufficient information regarding the proposed plan of treatment, including the risks and benefits of treatment, alternative treatment strategies, and the repercussions of not consenting (Guido, 2013). The only exception to treating before obtaining informed consent is when delay of treatment could place the neonate at risk of further harm, such as in an emergency situation.

It is outside the boundaries of nursing practice to provide the patient and/or family with information regarding medical–surgical risks and benefits of treatment or to suggest alternative medical–surgical therapies. It is appropriate for the nurse to inform the physician that the family members need further clarification to enable them to come to a decision comfortably. Obtaining the informed consent is the responsibility of the physician providing the treatment. Ideally, the treating physician should also be responsible for obtaining the signatures on the appropriate form once the parent(s) have consented, because she or he is truly the only one who can ensure that the parent(s) have no further questions and fully comprehend all treatment issues.

A. **If nurses are required to obtain patient and/or family signatures on consent forms, they should limit their clarification of patient and/or family understanding to two questions:**
   1. Has your physician discussed your baby's surgery (i.e., treatment approach) with you?
   2. Are you ready to sign this consent form? This means that you consent to the procedure.
B. **It is recommended that the name of the person able to give informed consent on behalf of the neonate be recorded in the medical record or nursing care plan once identified (Guido, 2013).**
C. **What if the parents or guardian will not give consent?**
   1. If physicians heed the parents' wishes and do not treat the infant, they may be guilty of child abuse or neglect, because laws stipulate that parents must provide needed medical care. Denial of this care can constitute a form of child neglect or abuse.
   2. If physicians proceed to treat the infant, ignoring parental objections, they could be liable for battery because their touching of the infant was intentional and there was a lack of consent.
   3. Physicians may petition the court for an authorization to provide the infant with the necessary treatment (i.e., obtain a court order). The most common example of physicians' seeking court orders to intervene in treatment is that of refused consent for blood transfusions based on religious beliefs. This request is almost always granted—certainly in emergency situations.

**D. When parents refuse treatment for other reasons, the court will base its decision on several factors (Guido, 2013).**
1. The infant's overall health and development.
2. The immediacy of danger to the infant if treatment is withheld.
3. The risks and benefits of the proposed treatment.

## PROFESSIONAL LIABILITY INSURANCE

There is a growing trend to hold nurses personally liable for their acts of negligence, especially when they have assumed additional responsibility as APNs. Some believe that nurses should not carry insurance because this only provides them with "deep pockets," making them more attractive to the plaintiff. Others insist that being well insured will serve as good protection. How much insurance is enough? Is the insurance coverage provided by the employer enough, or should nurses also invest in a personal policy for additional protection? These questions need to be answered by the individual nurse after examination of her or his practice.

**A. Principal benefits afforded by an individual malpractice policy (Guido, 2013).**
1. Insurer's agreement to defend all malpractice claims filed against the nurse. Also generally included are claims alleging assault, battery, invasion of privacy, and defamation of character and claims that the nurse/APN practiced outside the scope of his or her license.
2. Insurer's agreement to pay the amount that the nurse is legally liable to pay the plaintiff, up to the limits of the policy.
3. Coverage of all costs associated with an appeal of an adverse verdict.
4. Coverage for instructional and supervisory activities, as well as off-duty and non–hospital-related nursing activities, such as volunteer work.

**B. Reasons to obtain malpractice insurance (Guido, 2013).**
1. The hospital may have liability insurance policies that limit coverage and cover employees only when they work as hospital employees. No institutional policy covers a nurse for any acts or omissions that occur outside the normal work environment.
2. Hospital's policy is designed to meet its needs, and may not be able to protect the nurse's best interests.
3. If the hospital decides that what you did was not covered under its policy, it will not defend you. In fact, the hospital may actually assume an adversarial position to demonstrate that you are the legally responsible party. The institution may bring an indemnity claim against the nurse for monetary contributions if the nurse's actions or failure to act resulted in the patient's original injury. You will now have to defend yourself on your own.
4. Hospital policies do not have supplementary payments for the nurse's additional expenses related to investigating the claim or loss of work while defending the claim. The nurse will have to pay for his or her own out-of-pocket expenses.
5. You will be protected if the hospital is not insured.

The case of *Wake County Hospital System v. National Casualty Co.* (1992) involved alleged nursing malpractice of a neonatal nurse. The hospital had a self-insured retention, or a deductible, of up to $750,000 per person/event before its commercial insurance coverage became effective. The defendant nurse's policy was deemed to be excess coverage over other valid and collectible insurance. The U.S. District Court ruled that self-insurance by a hospital is not really insurance in the legal sense. It also ruled that the nurse's insurer had to pay the full amount awarded in the case. This case is a good illustration of a nurse's needing her or his own malpractice coverage.

6. When an insurance carrier makes payment to a plaintiff on the basis of malpractice, the insurer is legally entitled to sue the nurse to obtain reimbursement for the amount paid.
7. Cost of a policy for staff nurses is low; however, the insurance for the APN may cost several hundred dollars a year.

**C. Most health care providers do carry their own professional liability insurance. There are two types of insurance policies (Guido, 2013).**
1. Claims-made policy: covers damages only when the damages occurred during the policy period (when the policy was in effect) and only if the claim is reported to the insurance company during the policy period or the extending reporting endorsement (tail). This is typical of policies held by institutions.

2. Occurrence-basis policy: covers damages occurring during the period covered by the policy, even if the claim is made after the policy period has ended. This is typical of policies held by individuals.
   a. Preferable for neonatal nurses because the lawsuit may not be filed until an extended period after the infant is discharged from the hospital.

D. **There are differences in coverage between an institutional and an individual liability policy (Guido, 2013).**
   1. Institutional liability policy.
      a. Employer purchased and provided as typical "claims-made" coverage.
      b. Institution is the primary insured party, holding fullest rights and responsibilities.
      c. Policy covers specific professional activities in the work environment.
      d. Institution may be able to sue the nurse for all or part of the money paid in settlement, judgment, and legal fees.
      e. Insurance company employs the attorney; the individual nurse may not have a right to select counsel.
      f. Individual nurse has no right to refuse or authorize settlement.
   2. Individual liability policy.
      a. Commercially purchased insurance that typically has an "occurrence" coverage.
      b. Individual nurse is the primary insured party.
      c. Policy covers specific professional activities of the insured at any time and place.

E. **All nurses can practice preventive legal maintenance by avoiding 18 legal pitfalls (Guido, 2013; Monarch, 2002):**
   1. Neglecting to make safety a high priority.
   2. Failing to spot and report possible violence. For example, the number of kidnapping occurrences has increased in recent years. Nurses play a role in the security plan by wearing photographic identification badges, enforcing visiting policies, and, along with risk management, developing a preventive program to anticipate neonatal kidnapping.
   3. Not following institutional policies and standards of care.
   4. Responding unwisely in a short-staffing or floating situation. Courts have generally upheld the validity of the hospital's floating policy; thus a nurse's refusal to accept the assignment may place the nurse in jeopardy. It is suggested that the prudent course is to accept the assignment after clearly informing the nurse manager or charge nurse concerning your limitations and concerns.
   5. Neglecting to use due care in physical procedures, such as the dispensing of medications.
   6. Not checking equipment.
   7. Assuming that others are responsible for your duties.
   8. Assuming responsibility for informed consent.
   9. Wrongfully disclosing confidential information.
   10. Making reckless accusations.
   11. Failing to act like a professional.
   12. Confusing licensure issues with malpractice.
   13. Failing to communicate.
   14. Failing to monitor and assess.
   15. Failing to listen to information provided by family and friends, and to patient's or parent's requests for assistance.
   16. Neglecting to follow principles of risk management.
   17. Not following documentation principles.
   18. Confusing legal and ethical questions.

## REFERENCES


American Academy of Pediatrics and the American College of Obstetricians and Gynecologists: *Guidelines for perinatal care* (7th ed.). Elk Grove Village, IL, 2012, American Academy of Pediatrics.

American Nurses Association: *Neonatal nursing: Scope and standards of practice* (2nd ed.). Washington, DC, 2013, American Nurses Association.

American Nurses Association: *ANA's principles for delegation by registered nurses to unlicensed assistive personnel.* Washington, DC, 2012, American Nurses Association.

American Nurses Association: *Nursing: Scope and standards of practice* (2nd ed.). Washington, DC, 2010, American Nurses Association.

Association of Women's Health, Obstetric and Neonatal Nurses: *Standards for professional nursing practice in the care of women and newborns* (7th ed.). Washington, DC, 2009, Association of Women's Health, Obstetric and Neonatal Nurses.

Association of Women's Health, Obstetric and Neonatal Nurses and National Association of Neonatal Nurses: *Neonatal nursing: Orientation and development for retired and advanced practice nurses in basic and intermediate care settings.* Washington, DC, 1997, Association of Women's Health, Obstetric and Neonatal Nurses.

*Coleman v. Touro Infirmary of New Orleans*, 506 So. 2d 571-LA, 1993.

*Ewing v. Aubert*, 532 S. 2d 876 (Lo. App. 1988).

Fox, L. and Imbiorski, W.: *The record that defends its friends*. Chicago, 1979, Care Communications.

Fulginiti, K.F., Davis, S.L., Chalierl, H.G., and Neggers, W.: Trial techniques. In P.W. Iyer (Ed.): *Nursing malpractice* (3rd ed.). Tucson, AZ, 2007, Lawyers & Judges Publishing1343–1384.

Guido, G.W.: *Legal and ethical issues in nursing:* (5th ed.). Upper Saddle River, NJ, 2013, Prentice Hall, pp. 44-46.

Iyer, P.W.: Foundations of nursing practice. In P.W. Iyer, B.J. Levin, K.C. Ashton, and V. Powell (Eds.): *Nursing malpractice: Volume I. Roots of nursing malpractice* (4th ed.). Tucson, AZ, 2011, Lawyers & Judges Publishing, Kindle edition.

Iyer, P.W. The roots of patient injury. In P.W. Iyer, B.J. Levin, K.C. Ashton, and V. Powell (Eds.): *Nursing malpractice* Volume II. *Foundations of nursing practice claims* (4th ed.). Tucson, AZ, 2012, Lawyers & Judges Publishing, Kindle edition.

Iyer, P.W., and Koob, S.L.: Nursing documentation. In P.W. Iyer, B.J. Levin, K.C. Ashton, and V. Powell (Eds.): *Nursing malpractice: Roots of nursing malpractice. Volume I.* Tucson, AZ, 2011, Lawyers & Judges Publishing, Kindle edition.

The Joint Commission: *2013 Hospital accreditation standards.* Oakbrook Terrace, IL, 2013, The Joint Commission.

*Keene v. Brigham and Women's Hospital*, 755 N.E.2d 725-MA, 2002.

*King v. Department of Health & Hospitals*, 728 So. 2d 1027, 1030 (La. Ct. App.), writ denied, 741 So. 2d 656 (La. 1999).

Laska, L. (Ed.): Failure to treat newborn's hypoglycemia. *Medical Malpractice Verdicts, Settlements & Experts*, 4: 26, 2005.

Laska, L. (Ed.): Newborn suffers cyanosis soon after birth due to lack of suctioning: Brain damage leads to death—defense verdict. *Medical Malpractice Verdicts, Settlements & Experts*, 1: 25–26, 1997.

Laska, L. (Ed.): Failure to timely diagnose and treat hyperkalemia and hypoglycemia in premature infant: Brain damage—$4.5 million Texas verdict. *Medical Malpractice Verdicts, Settlements & Experts* 9:1, 1993.

Lewis, T., and Krulewicz, E.D.: The intersection of nursing and employment law. In P.W. Iyer, B.J. Levin, K.C. Ashton, and V. Powell (Eds.): *Nursing malpractice: Volume I. Roots of nursing malpractice* (4th ed.). Tucson, AZ, 2011, Lawyers & Judges Publishing, Kindle edition.

Liang, B.A. and Mackey, T.: Moving from traditional law and medicine to promote safety and effective risk management. In P.W. Iyer, B.J. Levin, K.C. Ashton, and V. Powell (Eds.): *Nursing malpractice; Volume I. Roots of nursing malpractice* (4th ed.). Tucson, AZ, 2011, Lawyers & Judges Publishing, Kindle edition.

Monarch, K.: The nurse as a civil litigation defendant. In K. Monarch (Ed.): *Nursing and the law: Trends and issues.* Washington, DC, 2002, American Nurses Association53–94.

National Association of Neonatal Nurses: *Neonatal nursing transport standards: Guideline for practice:* (3rd ed.). Chicago, IL, 2010a, National Association of Neonatal Nurses.

National Association of Neonatal Nurses: *Requirements for advanced neonatal nursing practice in neonatal intensive care units:* (3rd ed.). Chicago, IL, 2010b, National Association of Neonatal Nurses.

Rottkamp, J.: Inside the healthcare environment. In P.W. Iyer, B.J. Levin, K.C. Ashton, and V. Powell (Eds.): *Nursing malpractice Volume I. Roots of nursing malpractice* (4th ed.). Tucson, AZ, 2011, Lawyers & Judges Publishing, Kindle edition.

Solberg, D.: Legal implications of patient charting. *Nursing Business News*, 13, 1986.

Tammelleo, A.D.: "Lost" hospital records lead to default and 4 million-dollar award. *Nursing Law's Regan Report*, 43(5):2, 2002.

Tammelleo, A.D.: Neonatal nurse's reprehensible conduct results in revocation. *Regan Report on Nursing Law*, 38(9):4, 1998.

Tammelleo, A.D.: Nurses fail to "go over doctor's head": Death results. *Regan Report on Nursing Law*, 36(4):4, 1995.

Tammelleo, A.D.: Court upholds nurse's refusal to float. *Regan Report on Nursing Law*, 33(2):2, 1992.

Verklan, M.T.: Neonatal nursing malpractice issues. In P.W. Iyer, B.J. Levin, K.C. Ashton, and V. Powell (Eds.): *Nursing malpractice: Volume II. Foundations of nursing practice claims* (4th ed.). Tucson, AZ, 2012, Lawyers & Judges Publishing, Kindle edition.

*Wake County Hospital System v. National Casualty Co.*, 804 F. Supp. 768 (N.C. 1992).

*Wright v. Abbott Lab. Inc.*, No. 99-333 I (10th Circ. Aug. 6, 2001).

Zerres, M., Iyer, P., and Banes, C.: Working with nursing expert witnesses. In P.W. Iyer, B.J. Levin, K.C. Ashton, and V. Powell (Eds.): *Nursing malpractice: Volume I. Roots of nursing malpractice* (4th ed.). Tucson, AZ, 2011, Lawyers & Judges Publishing, Kindle edition.

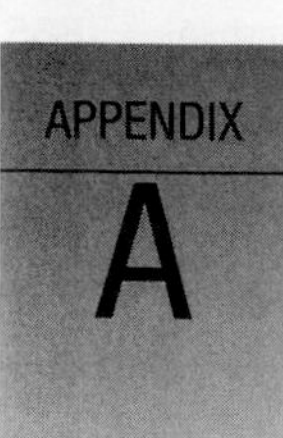

APPENDIX A

# Newborn Metric Conversion Tables

## TABLE A-1
### Temperature Conversion: Fahrenheit (F) to Centigrade (C)

| °F | °C | °F | °C | °F | °C | °F | °C |
|---|---|---|---|---|---|---|---|
| 95.0 | 35.0 | 98.0 | 36.7 | 101.0 | 38.3 | 104.0 | 40.0 |
| 95.2 | 35.1 | 98.2 | 36.8 | 101.2 | 38.4 | 104.2 | 40.1 |
| 95.4 | 35.2 | 98.4 | 36.9 | 101.4 | 38.6 | 104.4 | 40.2 |
| 95.6 | 35.3 | 98.6 | 37.0 | 101.6 | 38.7 | 104.6 | 40.3 |
| 95.8 | 35.4 | 98.8 | 37.1 | 101.8 | 38.8 | 104.8 | 40.4 |
| 96.0 | 35.6 | 99.0 | 37.2 | 102.0 | 38.9 | 105.0 | 40.6 |
| 96.2 | 35.7 | 99.2 | 37.3 | 102.2 | 39.0 | 105.2 | 40.7 |
| 96.4 | 35.8 | 99.4 | 37.4 | 102.4 | 39.1 | 105.4 | 40.8 |
| 96.6 | 35.9 | 99.6 | 37.6 | 102.6 | 39.2 | 105.6 | 40.9 |
| 96.8 | 36.0 | 99.8 | 37.7 | 102.8 | 39.3 | 105.8 | 41.0 |
| 97.0 | 36.1 | 100.0 | 37.8 | 103.0 | 39.4 | 106.0 | 41.1 |
| 97.2 | 36.2 | 100.2 | 37.9 | 103.2 | 39.6 | 106.2 | 41.2 |
| 97.4 | 36.3 | 100.4 | 38.0 | 103.4 | 39.7 | 106.4 | 41.3 |
| 97.6 | 36.4 | 100.6 | 38.1 | 103.6 | 39.8 | 106.6 | 41.4 |
| 97.8 | 36.6 | 100.8 | 38.2 | 103.8 | 39.9 | 106.8 | 41.6 |

Note: °C = (°F − 32) $\infty$5/9. Centigrade temperature equivalents are rounded to one decimal place by adding 0.1 when second decimal place is 5 or greater. The metric system replaces the term "centigrade" with "Celsius" (the inventor of the scale).

■ TABLE A-2
## ■ ■ Length Conversion: Inches to Centimeters

**1-inch increments.** Example: to obtain centimeters equivalent to 22 inches, read "20" on top scale, "2" on side scale; equivalent is 55.9 cm.

| Inches | 0 | 10 | 20 | 30 | 40 |
|---|---|---|---|---|---|
| **0** | 0 | 25.4 | 50.8 | 76.2 | 101.6 |
| **1** | 2.5 | 27.9 | 53.3 | 78.7 | 104.1 |
| **2** | 5.1 | 30.5 | 55.9 | 81.3 | 106.7 |
| **3** | 7.6 | 33.0 | 58.4 | 83.8 | 109.2 |
| **4** | 10.2 | 35.6 | 61.0 | 86.4 | 111.8 |
| **5** | 12.7 | 38.1 | 63.5 | 88.9 | 114.3 |
| **6** | 15.2 | 40.6 | 66.0 | 91.4 | 116.8 |
| **7** | 17.8 | 43.2 | 68.6 | 94.0 | 119.4 |
| **8** | 20.3 | 45.7 | 71.1 | 96.5 | 121.9 |
| **9** | 22.9 | 48.3 | 73.7 | 99.1 | 124.5 |

**One-quarter (¼) inch increments.** Example: to obtain centimeters equivalent to 14¾ inches, read "14" on top scale and "¾" on side scale; equivalent is 37.5 cm.

**10 TO 15 INCHES**

| | 10 | 11 | 12 | 13 | 14 | 15 |
|---|---|---|---|---|---|---|
| 0 | 25.4 | 27.9 | 30.5 | 33.0 | 35.6 | 38.1 |
| ¼ | 26.0 | 28.6 | 31.1 | 33.7 | 36.2 | 38.7 |
| ½ | 26.7 | 29.2 | 31.8 | 34.3 | 36.8 | 39.4 |
| ¾ | 27.3 | 29.8 | 32.4 | 34.9 | 37.5 | 40.0 |

**16 TO 21 INCHES**

| | 16 | 17 | 18 | 19 | 20 | 21 |
|---|---|---|---|---|---|---|
| 0 | 40.6 | 43.2 | 45.7 | 48.3 | 50.8 | 53.3 |
| ¼ | 41.3 | 43.8 | 46.4 | 48.9 | 51.4 | 54.0 |
| ½ | 41.9 | 44.5 | 47.0 | 49.5 | 52.1 | 54.6 |
| ¾ | 42.5 | 45.1 | 47.6 | 50.2 | 52.7 | 55.2 |

Note: 1 inch = 2.540 cm. Centimeter equivalents are rounded one decimal place by adding 0.1 when the second decimal place is 5 or greater; for example, 33.48 becomes 33.5.

■ TABLE A-3

## ■ ■ Weight (Mass) Conversion: Pounds and Ounces to Grams

**Example:** To obtain grams equivalent to 6 pounds, 8 ounces, read "6" on top scale, "8" on side scale; equivalent is 2948 g.

| | Pounds | | | | | | | | | | | | | | |
|---|---|---|---|---|---|---|---|---|---|---|---|---|---|---|---|
| **Ounces** | **0** | **1** | **2** | **3** | **4** | **5** | **6** | **7** | **8** | **9** | **10** | **11** | **12** | **13** | **14** |
| 0 | 0 | 454 | 907 | 1361 | 1814 | 2268 | 2722 | 3175 | 3629 | 4082 | 4536 | 4990 | 5443 | 5897 | 6350 |
| **1** | 28 | 482 | 936 | 1389 | 1843 | 2296 | 2750 | 3203 | 3657 | 4111 | 4564 | 5018 | 5471 | 5925 | 6379 |
| **2** | 57 | 510 | 964 | 1417 | 1871 | 2325 | 2778 | 3232 | 3685 | 4139 | 4593 | 5046 | 5500 | 5953 | 6407 |
| **3** | 85 | 539 | 992 | 1446 | 1899 | 2353 | 2807 | 3260 | 3714 | 4167 | 4621 | 5075 | 5528 | 5982 | 6435 |
| **4** | 113 | 567 | 1021 | 1474 | 1928 | 2381 | 2835 | 3289 | 3742 | 4196 | 4649 | 5103 | 5557 | 6010 | 6464 |
| **5** | 142 | 595 | 1049 | 1503 | 1956 | 2410 | 2863 | 3317 | 3770 | 4224 | 4678 | 5131 | 5585 | 6038 | 6492 |
| **6** | 170 | 624 | 1077 | 1531 | 1984 | 2438 | 2892 | 3345 | 3799 | 4252 | 4706 | 5160 | 5613 | 6067 | 6520 |
| **7** | 198 | 652 | 1106 | 1559 | 2013 | 2466 | 2920 | 3374 | 3827 | 4281 | 4734 | 5188 | 5642 | 6095 | 6549 |
| **8** | 227 | 680 | 1134 | 1588 | 2041 | 2495 | 2948 | 3402 | 3856 | 4309 | 4763 | 5216 | 5670 | 6123 | 6577 |
| **9** | 255 | 709 | 1162 | 1616 | 2070 | 2523 | 2977 | 3430 | 3884 | 4337 | 4791 | 5245 | 5698 | 6152 | 6605 |
| **10** | 283 | 737 | 1191 | 1644 | 2098 | 2551 | 3005 | 3459 | 3912 | 4366 | 4819 | 5273 | 5727 | 6180 | 6634 |
| **11** | 312 | 765 | 1219 | 1673 | 2126 | 2580 | 3033 | 3487 | 3941 | 4394 | 4848 | 5301 | 5755 | 6209 | 6662 |
| **12** | 340 | 794 | 1247 | 1701 | 2155 | 2608 | 3062 | 3515 | 3969 | 4423 | 4876 | 5330 | 5783 | 6237 | 6690 |
| **13** | 369 | 822 | 1276 | 1729 | 2183 | 2637 | 3090 | 3544 | 3997 | 4451 | 4904 | 5358 | 5812 | 6265 | 6719 |
| **14** | 397 | 850 | 1304 | 1758 | 2211 | 2665 | 3118 | 3572 | 4026 | 4479 | 4933 | 5386 | 5840 | 6294 | 6747 |
| **15** | 425 | 879 | 1332 | 1786 | 2240 | 2693 | 3147 | 3600 | 4054 | 4508 | 4961 | 5415 | 5868 | 6322 | 6776 |

Note: 1 pound = 453.59237 g; 1 ounce = 28.349523 g; 1000 g = 1 kg. Gram equivalents have been rounded to whole numbers by adding 1 when the first decimal place is 5 or greater.

# Index

Note: Page numbers followed by *f* indicate figures, *t* indicates tables, and *b* indicates boxes.

**M**

## V